AMBULATORY SURGERY

and the Basics of Emergency Surgical Care

AMBULATORY SURGERY
and the Basics of Emergency Surgical Care

Second Edition

Edited by

Mark W. Wolcott, M.D.
Assistant Chief Medical Director for Clinical Affairs
Veterans Administration Central Office;
Clinical Professor of Surgery
George Washington School of Medicine
Washington, DC

38 contributors

J. B. LIPPINCOTT COMPANY
Philadelphia
London Mexico City New York St. Louis
São Paulo Sydney

Acquisitions Editor: Lisette Bralow
Sponsoring Editor: Sanford J. Robinson
Manuscript Editor: Lee Henderson
Indexer: Betty Herr Hallinger
Design Coordinator: Caren Erlichman
Production Manager: Carol A. Florence
Compositor: Bi-Comp, Inc.
Printer/Binder: Maple Press Company, Inc.

2nd Edition

6 5 4 3 2 1

Library of Congress Cataloging-in-Publication Data

Ambulatory surgery and the basics of emergency
surgical care.

Includes bibliographies and index.
1. Surgery, Outpatient. 2. Surgical emergencies.
I. Wolcott, Mark W. [DNLM: 1. Ambulatory Surgery.
2. Emergencies. WO 192 A497]
RD110.A48 1988 617'.024 87-3401
ISBN 0-397-50805-0

The authors and publisher have exerted every effort to ensure that drug selection and dosage set forth in this text are in accord with current recommendations and practice at the time of publication. However, in view of ongoing research, changes in government regulations, and the constant flow of information relating to drug therapy and drug reactions, the reader is urged to check the package insert for each drug for any change in indications and dosage and for added warnings and precautions. This is particularly important when the recommended agent is a new or infrequently employed drug.

Contributors

Kenneth N. Buchi, M.D.
Assistant Professor of Medicine
Division of Gastroenterology
Consulting Physician
Gastroenterology Section
University of Utah School of Medicine
Salt Lake City, Utah

Terry Clemmer, M.D.
Director of Critical Care Medicine
Latter-Day Saints Hospital;
Associate Professor of Medicine
University of Utah School of Medicine
Salt Lake City, Utah

Benjamin L. Crue, Jr., M.D.
Emeritus Clinical Professor of Neurological Surgery
University of Southern California School of Medicine
Los Angeles, California;
Medical Director
Durango Pain Rehabilitation Center
LaPlata Community Hospital
Durango, Colorado

Douglas S. Dahl, M.D.
Associate Clinical Professor of Urology
University of Utah School of Medicine
Salt Lake City, Utah

John A. Dixon, M.D.
Professor of Surgery
Director, Laser Institute
University of Utah School of Medicine;
Attending Surgeon
Veterans Administration Medical Center
Salt Lake City, Utah

Nancy Futrell, M.D.
Special Fellow in Cerebrovascular Disease
University of Miami School of Medicine
Miami, Florida

Andrew A. Gage, M.D.
Professor of Surgery
School of Medicine
State University of New York at Buffalo;
Deputy Director
Roswell Park Memorial Institute
Buffalo, New York

William A. Gay, Jr., M.D.
Professor and Chairman
Department of Surgery
University of Utah School of Medicine
Salt Lake City, Utah

Linda S. Georges, M.D.
Assistant Professor (Clinical)
Medical Director, Ambulatory Surgery Unit
University of Utah Medical Center
Salt Lake City, Utah

James E. Goodnight, Jr., M.D., Ph.D.
Associate Professor
Chief, Division of Surgical Oncology
Department of Surgery
University of California–Davis School of Medicine
Davis, California

M. Peter Heilbrun, M.D.
Professor of Neurosurgery
Chairman, Division of Neurosurgery
Consultant, Veterans Administration Medical Center
Salt Lake City, Utah

Aaron A. Hofmann, M.D.
Associate Professor
Orthopaedic Surgery
University of Utah School of Medicine
Salt Lake City, Utah

Bruce A. Houtchens, M.D.
Associate Professor of Surgery
Attending Surgeon
Trauma Service and Surgical Critical Care Unit
The University of Texas Health Science Center at Houston
Houston, Texas

J. Preston Hughes, M.D.
Clinical Instructor
Department of Surgery
University of Utah School of Medicine
Salt Lake City, Utah

Gary R. Hunter, M.D., B.S.
Assistant Professor of Surgery
Division of Plastic Surgery
University of Utah School of Medicine
Salt Lake City, Utah

Dale G. Johnson, M.D.
Professor of Surgery
Professor of Pediatrics
University of Utah School of Medicine;
Head, Division of Pediatric Surgery
Chairman, Department of Surgery
Primary Children's Medical Center
Salt Lake City, Utah

Leland P. Johnson, M.D.
Associate Professor of Surgery
Division of Otolaryngology–Head and Neck Surgery
University of Utah School of Medicine
Salt Lake City, Utah

S. V. Karwande, M.D.
Assistant Professor of Surgery
University of Utah School of Medicine;
Chief of Cardiothoracic Surgery
Veterans Administration Medical Center
Salt Lake City, Utah

Peter F. Lawrence, M.D.
Associate Professor of Surgery
Chief of Vascular Surgery
University of Utah School of Medicine;
Chief of Surgery
Veterans Administration Hospital
Salt Lake City, Utah

Ronald J. Mann, M.D.
Professor of Orthopaedic Surgery
Department of Surgery
University of Utah School of Medicine;
Chief of Orthopaedic Surgery
Veterans Administration Medical Center
Salt Lake City, Utah

James B. Manning, M.D.
Chief Resident
Orthopaedic Surgury
University of Utah School of Medicine
Salt Lake City, Utah

Michael E. Matlak, M.D.
Associate Professor of Surgery
Associate Professor of Pediatrics
University of Utah School of Medicine;
Staff Pediatric Surgeon
Division of Pediatric Surgery
Primary Children's Medical Center
Salt Lake City, Utah

J. M. McGreevy, M.D.
Associate Professor of Surgery
University of Utah School of Medicine
Salt Lake City, Utah

Richard G. Middleton, M.D.
Professor of Surgery
Chairman, Division of Urology
University of Utah School of Medicine
Salt Lake City, Utah

Clark A. Millikan, M.D.
Professor of Neurology
University of Utah School of Medicine
Salt Lake City, Utah

Alan P. Newman, M.D.
Assistant Professor of Surgery, Orthopaedics
Adjunct Assistant Professor of Bioengineering
University of Utah School of Medicine;
Staff Surgeon
Veterans Administration Medical Center
Salt Lake City, Utah

James L. Parkin, M.D., M.S.
Professor of Surgery
Chairman, Division of Otolaryngology–Head and Neck Surgery
University of Utah School of Medicine
Salt Lake City, Utah

Raymond W. Postlethwait, M.D.
Professor of Surgery Emeritus
Former Chief of Surgery
Duke University
Durham, North Carolina

Preston N. Richards, M.D., B.S.
Resident, Department of Surgery
University of Utah School of Medicine
Salt Lake City, Utah

Layton F. Rikkers, M.D.
Professor and Chairman
Department of Surgery
University of Nebraska Medical Center
Omaha, Nebraska

Andrew C. Ruoff III, M.D.
Clinical Professor of Surgery
Uniformed Services University of the Health Sciences;
Orthopaedic Surgeon
Veterans Administration Hospital
Salt Lake City, Utah

Clifford C. Snyder, M.D., B.S.
Professor of Surgery
Chairman Emeritus, Division of Plastic Surgery
Consultant, University of Utah School of Medicine
Salt Lake City, Utah

Hunter R. Stokes, M.D.
Professor (Clinical)
University of South Carolina
Charleston, South Carolina

Jon S. Thompson, M.D.
Associate Professor
Department of Surgery
University of Nebraska Medical Center;
Chief of Surgery
Veterans Administration Medical Center
Omaha, Nebraska

Glenn D. Warden, M.D.
Shrine Professor of Surgery
University of Cincinnati College of Medicine;
Chief of Staff
Shriners Burn Institute
Cincinnati Unit;
Director, Burn Special Care Unit
University of Cincinnati Hospital
Cincinnati, Ohio

James C. Warenski, M.D.
Professor, Department of Obstetrics and Gynecology
University of Utah School of Medicine
Salt Lake City, Utah

Mark W. Wolcott, M.D.
Assistant Chief Medical Director for Clinical Affairs
Veterans Administration Central Office;
Clinical Professor of Surgery
George Washington School of Medicine
Washington, DC

K. C. Wong, M.D., Ph.D.
Professor of Anesthesiology and Pharmacology
Chairman, Department of Anesthesiology
University of Utah Medical Center
Salt Lake City, Utah

Preface

The second edition of *Ambulatory Surgery and the Basics of Emergency Surgical Care* is the seventh edition of *Ferguson's Surgery of the Ambulatory Patient* and is being published 46 years after publication of the first edition by L. K. Ferguson, M.D., in 1942. His experience over a period of 10 to 12 years as Chief of Ambulatory Surgery at the University of Pennsylvania thoroughly convinced him of the value of ambulatory surgery and led him to publish the first edition, which was in fact the first textbook devoted exclusively to this area. It has been well received over the intervening years and has been widely used in emergency rooms, military dispensaries, and private offices.

Over these years, tremendous advances have been made. Antibiotics have come onto the scene, new forms of anesthesia have developed, and whole new specialty areas of surgery have emerged. Moreover, the entire medical care arena is evolving and continues to evolve rapidly, precipitated by the enormous cost of medical care, which in recent years has led to concerted efforts toward cost control. Among these efforts has been the rediscovery of ambulatory surgery.

Several new chapters have been added to this volume, including one on arthroscopy, and there has been a major expansion of the chapter on ophthalmology. The addition to the previous edition of a chapter on emergency surgical care (Chap. 23) was well received; that chapter has been updated significantly, indicating the volatility of that special area. The chapter on the unconscious patient links well with the chapter on emergency surgical care, as does the chapter on outpatient management of acute and chronic pain. The other chapters have been revised to reflect the current practice and understanding in these special areas. Most importantly, the basics of sound surgical care have remained unchanged and unchanging.

Mark W. Wolcott, M.D.

Contents

1 Ambulatory Surgery—Part of the Revolution in Medicine

MARK W. WOLCOTT

American medicine has changed enormously in the past 200 years, and this change has accelerated in the last 30 years. A brief review of these changes and their cause and effect will enable one to understand the current status of medicine and what its future may be.

Medicine is a power that has grown from a weak profession of minor economic significance to a huge system of hospitals, clinics, health plans, and insurance companies employing a vast labor force. Although the history of modern medicine is an epic of scientific progress, it is also a story of the assumption of power and authority. The medical profession has had a very pervasive claim to authority because of its close bonds with science and direct and intimate contact with patients. This is quite different from, let us say, the profession of law. Sickness promotes reliance on medical judgment, and this has provided physicians with other social privileges, economic power, and political influence. Today all of these are in considerable jeopardy.

Physicians have not always been held in high esteem. In ancient Rome physicians were slaves, freed men, or foreigners and were considered unimportant. In the England of the 17th and 18th centuries, physicians ranked only slightly above surgeons or apothecaries. They were not gentry, and they struggled for the patronage of the rich.

In the America of the mid-18th to mid-19th centuries a few doctors tried to establish medicine as a profession, but most failed because of schisms in their own ranks and the public's strong democratic bent to grant privileges to the physician reluctantly and to assert the right of individuals to treat themselves. The quality of medicine was poor and practitioners were concerned primarily with money and with undercutting their colleagues. Between 1850 and 1930 the medical profession finally began to become an "authority" and achieve its place in society. Most of this success can be attributed to markedly increased cohesiveness among doctors. Physicians were learning about the physiology of the body, cause of diseases, x-rays, aseptic techniques, and anesthesia. The Flexner Report in 1911 was a further manifestation of physicians' recognition of the need to improve education and, not coincidentally, to limit the numbers of doctors and to continue an ongoing effort to suppress other health care disciplines and cults (a suppression that continues today). Reform of medical education really started, however, in the 1870s, when the universities began to evolve into true institutions of learning and research. Leadership came from such notables as Eliot of Harvard and Gilman of Johns Hopkins, and enough money to support reform was donated by wealthy men who were concerned about the miserable state of the universities and about the need to upgrade the curriculum and quality of teachers.

From the 1930s to the 1970s American medicine was in its heyday: Increasing dollars from third-party payers and the availability of government Medicare and Medicaid in 1965 resulted in increased consumer expectations and demand for more and more medical care. The medical professional came to believe that private, voluntary institutions were better equipped to organize and provide those services than other organizations. Unfortunately, such institutions were often wrongly motivated and were unqualified to provide the requested services. The increased funding for research and for the support of education and hospital construction resulted in the awe-inspiring deluge of scientific and technological breakthroughs of the 1950s, 1960s, and 1970s.

In 1970 our mandate to provide medical care regardless of the cost ran out. Instead of a limitlessly expanding future, medical professionals suddenly encountered the economic facts of life: Enormous increases in costs were apparent, but improvements in health care were not.

A revolution in American health care was under way during the past 30 years. It included:

The field of science. The pace of ever more sophisticated diagnostic and therapeutic breakthroughs blurred the line between life and death and held the promise of remarkable cures available at "unacceptable" cost.

Demography. The aging of America raised the specter of a rapidly expanding population that today requires a third of our medical care dollars. Opening Pandora's box of medical discoveries has led inexorably to decisions, with ethical and legal implications, of who gets what and how much.

Multiple factors have contributed to the health care revolution. Third-party reimbursement beginning after World War II removed the reality of health care costs, as did Medicare–Medicaid, the government's third-party payer, beginning in 1965. Enormous advances in technology and medical knowledge raised the physician to preeminence and power with control of more than 70% of health care expenses. Increased consumer interest in and demand for health care has stressed the physician–patient relationship.

Prospective payment DRGs (diagnosis related groupings) have dramatically increased the competitiveness in medicine (without sacrificing quality, it is hoped). Health maintenance organizations (HMOs) and PPOs are putting even more pressure on the individual physician.

Ambulatory surgery is part of the revolution taking place in health care delivery. Many factors have conspired to bring about these enormous changes that have occurred since the mid-1970s. American medicine is being wrenched by multiple events, the most persuasive being the enormous cost of health care delivery. Health care currently accounts for 10.5% of the gross national product (GNP), exceeding $400 billion in 1986, and employs one of every 20 persons in the work force—some 8 million people.

Ambulatory surgery is the oldest form of surgery. Initially, surgery was performed in the home, in the office, or in makeshift facilities without anesthesia. In 1840, as pointed out by Thomas,[4] the discovery of anesthesia resulted in hospitals becoming the primary site for performing major and minor surgery.

Ambulatory surgery in the hospital is not new; it was performed as early as the early 1900s, documented by Nicoll,[3] who reported performing over 7000 operations on ambulatory patients. Its rate of growth in the past 15 years is astounding. Today over 20 million procedures are done annually on an ambulatory basis. According to the American Hospital Association's *Annual Survey of Hospitals*, 28% of all surgery performed in the United States in 1984 was ambulatory. Thirty percent of all ambulatory surgeries are performed in hospitals with less than 400 beds; approximately 25% to 27% are performed in hospitals with more than 400 beds. Free-standing and office surgeries account for the rest. This enormous increase largely resulted from the effort to avoid the costs of hospitalization, nor can the contribution of improved short-acting anesthetics be ignored. The hospital industry has responded well with the development of better and more efficient physical plants to care for the ambulatory surgery load. Eighteen to 40% of all surgery can probably be done safely on an ambulatory basis.

Ambulatory surgery may be provided in several different settings:

The Physician's Office or Clinic. The advantages of surgery in the physician's office or clinic are low cost, efficient use of the surgeon's time, and rapid service to the patient. The disadvantages include potential absence of quality control, lack of facilities for care of emergent situations, and limits on sophistication of procedures that can be performed. The significant increase in the number of procedures done in the physician's office or clinic is partially due to several policies instituted by Blue Cross–Blue Shield[1] that have begun to make this arena attractive to the doctor for carefully selected cases.

The Hospital-Based Facility. The hospital-based facility can consist of an administrative, physically separate facility connected by bridge or tunnel to the parent hospital or unused beds in the main hospital. In both situations many of the hospital's ancillary facilities are used. The patient comes into the hospital in the morning and leaves in the late afternoon, which provides the availability of many people and ancillary services, thus maximizing use of such facilities as laboratory, radiology, and operating rooms. It also provides a safety factor in case of untoward results. The disadvantage of a hospital-based facility is a hospital's own inertia generated by the routines of inpatient care. Separating the ambulatory unit administratively from the regular hospital hierarchy seems imperative if some of these problems are to be overcome.

The Free-Standing Ambulatory Surgery Unit. The free-standing unit can provide a convenient, well-controlled, cost-effective, and pleasant experience, but it cannot provide in-depth emergency care. In a community that is already overbedded, it may hurt some hospitals seriously and actually lead to increased overall cost to the public because of the less efficient occupancy rate in the hospitals.

The Emergency Room. The hospital emergency room is mentioned only to condemn its use for ambulatory surgery. It adds confusion to an often tense situation, staff are overtaxed, and the patient is educated to a less than desirable mode of obtaining surgical care.

It is important to note that no single type of ambulatory surgery unit satisfies the questions of cost effectiveness, consumer satisfaction, and quality of care. Studies have addressed this question and continue to do so. According to Grossman[2] it would seem that:

> If the "need" for additional ambulatory surgery capacity is shown, free-standing facilities are preferable. However, if the surgical capacity in a community is excessive, hospital-based ambulatory surgery programs are preferable, and the incremental unit costs incurred could be minimal and the savings to the community could be greater than constructing a free-standing facility. Furthermore, if a hospital can justify only one ambulatory-surgery operating room, it probably should not pursue a program of "in-hospital based" ambulatory surgery let alone a free-standing unit.

It is projected that ambulatory surgery centers will increase from 330 in 1985 to 832 by 1990 and that 80% of all hospitals will have ambulatory surgery capability.

The range of procedures is quite wide. The procedures performed at the SurgiCenter in Phoenix, Arizona, are fairly characteristic (see list). Some centers include diagnostic bronchoscopy, esophagoscopy, and esophageal dilatation. The medical staff decides what is to be done, but the decision obviously is influenced by many factors, including patient safety, available time, and available personnel. One can note from this list that the ambulatory surgery performed at the Phoenix SurgiCenter consists of 33% gynecology, 31% ENT, 19% orthopaedics or plastic surgery, and 16% general surgery. These also are average figures from other services. Maurene Fedeson, M.D., of Henry Ford Hospital identified 700 procedures that are done at that hospital and believes that as much as 60% of all surgeries can be done on an ambulatory basis.

(*Text continues on p 6.*)

PROCEDURES CARRIED OUT IN AMBULATORY SURGICAL CENTER, PHOENIX, ARIZONA

Ear, Nose, Throat

adenoidectomy and myringotomy
antral puncture
antral window
arch bars, removal
branchial arch appendages, excision
Caldwell–Luc operation
closed reduction (nose or zygoma)
ethmoidectomy
foreign body removal (ear)
inclusion cyst, excision
inferior turbinate resection
laryngoscopy
laryngoscopy with operative procedure
lip, wedge resection
mouth biopsy
myringoplasty or tympanoplasty
myringotomy with or without tubes
nasal polypectomy
otoscopy
otoscopy (with removal of foreign body)
palate biopsy
polyethylene tubes, removal
preauricular cyst excision
septal reconstruction, SMR septoplasty
stapedectomy
tongue biopsy
tonsillar tag excision
tonsillectomy, with or without adenoidectomy
tympanoplasty

Eye

canthus excision
cataract
chalazion, removal
conjunctiva, repair

(*continued*)

cryocoagulation
cyst excision
ectropion, repair
entropion, repair
enucleation
eye examination
eye muscle operation, recession or resection
  unilateral
  bilateral
eyebrow, dermoid cyst, excision
eyelid, wedge resection
lacrimal duct, probing lacrimal duct, reconstruction
photocoagulation
pterygium, removal

General Surgery

abscess, incision and drainage
anal tag, excision
Baker's cyst, excision
breast implant, removal
  single
  double
breast mass, excision
bronchoscopy
  with operative procedure
cervical node biopsy
colostomy, revision
cyst, excision
epigastric herniorrhaphy
esophagoscopy
  with operative procedure
fistulectomy
foreign body removal
  without x-ray
  with x-ray
frenulectomy, tongue
gynecomastia, excision
hemangioma, removal
hemorrhoidectomy
hydrocelectomy
hyperhidrosis axillas, bilateral, excision
inguinal herniorrhaphy
  infant, unilateral
  infant, bilateral
  adult, unilateral
  adult, bilateral
lacerations, repair
  under 1 hr
  over 1 hr
lipoma, excision
lysis of abdominal adhesions
mass, excision
melanoma, excision
muscle biopsy
orchiectomy
orchiopexy
pilonidal cyst, excision
rectal biopsy
rectal dilation
rectal polypectomy
sigmoidoscopy
  with operative procedure
skin graft
skin lesion, excision
stitch granuloma, removal
suture removal
  superficial
  deep
thyroglossal duct cyst, excision
torticollis, repair
umbilical herniorrhaphy
  with bilateral inguinal herniorrhaphy
umbilical sinus, excision
varicose vein ligation with or without stripping
  under five
  five or more, unilateral
  five or more, bilateral
ventral hernia
vermilionectomy
  upper or lower lip
  both lips
lacerations
  under 1 hr
  over 1 hr

Gynecologic

adhesions of clitoris, release
Bartholin cystectomy
cervical amputation, Sturmdorf
cervical conization
cervical dilation
cervical polypectomy
colpotomy
condylomata acuminata, removal or fulguration
cryolaparoscopy
cryotherapy
  with biopsy and/or dilatation and curettage
culdocentesis
culdoscopy
dilatation and curettage
  with conization
  with culoposcopy
  with hysteroscopy
  with laparoscopy
  with laparoscopy and conization
episiotomy
examination under anesthesia
hymenotomy
hysterosalpinography
hysteroscopy
IUD, removal
labial lesion, excision
laparoscopy
  bilateral tubal coagulation
MacDonald's procedure
pelvic endoscopy
perineoplasty
perineorrhaphy
phlebography

rectovaginal fistula repair
transvaginal ligation of tubes
tubal insufflation
vaginal cyst, cautery
vaginal stenoses, release
vaginal tumor, excision
vaginal web, excision
vaginoplasty
vulvar biopsy

Neurosurgical

carpal tunnel decompression
intercostal neurectomy
Morton's neuroma
neuroma
temporal artery, resection
ulnar nerve transfer

Orthopaedic

Aristospan injection
Arthrodesis
  phalanges
  other joints
arthroplasty
  phalanges
  other joints
arthroscopy
arthrotomy, meniscectomy
bone biopsy
bone graft
bone reconstruction
bunionectomy
  unilateral
  bilateral
bursectomy
capsulectomy
carpal tunnel decompression
carpal tunnel ligament release
cast change with roentgenography
corn, removal
debridement
exostosis, excision
fasciectomy
  finger
  palm
fingernail, removal
foreign body excision
  with x-ray
fracture, closed reduction
  with roentgenography
  without roentgenography
fracture, open reduction
  with roentgenography
  without roentgenography
fusion
ganglionectomy
hammertoes, correction of
  bilateral
hand fasciectomy for arthritis
hand surgery, reconstructive
hardware, removal
joints, manipulation
  with roentgenography
ligament repair
mass excision with scar revision
metatarsal head, excision
  unilateral
  bilateral
Morton's neuroma
nerve repair
  finger
  other
neurolysis
  finger
  other
neuroma, removal
  finger
olecranon bursa, excision
osteotomy
phalangectomy
plantar wart, excision
sequestrectomy
skin graft, 45 min
synovectomy
tarsorrhaphy
tendon release (tenotomy)
tendon repair
tendon sheath, release
tenosynovectomy
toenail, removal
trigger finger, release
ulnar nerve transfer
xanthoma, excision
Z-plasty
Zygomatic arch

Plastic Surgery

basal cell cancer, excision
blepharoplasty, upper or lower bilateral
  combined
breast capsule, rupture
breast hematoma, bilateral, evacuation
breast implant, exchange unilateral
capsulotomy
  unilateral
  bilateral
chemical peel
chin augmentation
dermabrasion
  partial
  full
face lift, partial (2 hr)
facial wire, removal
flap revision
lesion excision with graft
lipectomy
mammoplasty, augmentation, unilateral
mammoplasty, reconstruction
  unilateral
  bilateral
mastopexy

(*continued*)

otoplasty
  unilateral
  bilateral
rhinoplasty
rhytidectomy
  with blepharoplasty
scar revision
skin graft

Urologic

bladder tumor, transurethral resection
circumcision
  pediatric
  adult
cystoscopy
hydrocelectomy
litholapaxy
meatotomy
orchiectomy
perineal needle biopsy
prostate biopsy
testicular biopsy
testicular prosthesis insertion
urethral dilation
vasectomy
vasovasotomy

Blocks

caudal
celiac (splanchnic)
intercostal
lumbar sympathetic
roentgenography with block
stellate
visit with treatment

Special Cases

cryotherapy, alone
impacted wisdom teeth, removal
  two or less
  more than two
multiple teeth extractions, 1 hr
operative dentistry, 3 hr
periodontal surgery, 4 hr

(Used with the kind permission of R. C. Williams, Executive Director, SurgiCenter, Phoenix, Arizona.)

Health care costs now represent over 10% of the GNP, nearly $400 billion in 1985. What then are our options to curtail these escalating costs? Never have all communities (perhaps never has any community) satisfied all the needs of the consumer. The idea of rationing health care is not new. However, with increasing costs, greater knowledge, more sophisticated machinery, and ever-increasing inflation, remedial efforts must be made.

As physicians we can do several things. First of all, we must recognize that at least 60% to 70% of the health care dollar is under our control. Judicious ordering of tests and prescribing practices can reduce health care costs significantly. Most of the practicing physicians today have been trained within the last 30 years. Those years have seen perhaps the greatest explosion in development of knowledge, laboratory tests, and high technology that has ever occurred. Yet in few medical schools today is a meaningful effort being made to teach young physicians the economic facts of life. Recent studies have shown an abysmal lack of knowledge among physicians of what it costs for tests, procedures, and the like. Therefore great effort needs to be made to educate physicians, especially those now in training. Even the older ones might be taught some new approaches.

Ambulatory surgery is a part of all this since it has been shown that a given procedure done in a well-run ambulatory surgical unit can cost one-third to one-half less than in a hospital. Therefore we must educate physicians to this fact.

Another important factor is educating the patient that ambulatory surgery is not only less expensive but in most cases as good as in-hospital surgery and that it has the added benefit of permitting recovery in the patient's own home. Such education will occur slowly by word of mouth from satisfied patient to patient. It can be spread more rapidly by enthusiastic support from physicians and nurses and, of course, the media.

Ambulatory surgery is going to continue to grow for all the reasons stated, but its acceptance by the patient will be the most important factor in the speed with which it grows.

REFERENCES

1. Blue Cross Blue Shield of North Carolina: Blue Shield Bulletin, 1982
2. Grossman RM: Is ambulatory surgery less expensive? Hospitals 3:112, 1979
3. Nicoll JH: The surgery of infancy. Br Med J 2:753–754, 1909
4. Thomas FT: Office Surgery for Family Physicians, p 3. Woburn, MA, Butterworth, 1981

2 Planning and Management of a Surgical Ambulatory Care Operation

MARK W. WOLCOTT

The purpose of this chapter is to give a brief overview of some aspects of planning an ambulatory surgical unit; a description of how one might be organized, staffed, and equipped; and a few observations regarding management, including quality assurance. It will in no way attempt to cover these subjects in depth, as there are many very adequate writings on this subject.

PLANNING

Before plans for an ambulatory surgical unit are implemented, community needs must be carefully considered. If there is pressure for hospital beds for short-term patients, then construction of a free-standing unit or addition of an ambulatory surgical unit to the present hospital should be considered. If there is overbedding then conversion of some of those hospital beds to the 1-day surgery concept, long-term care, or nursing home care should be carefully considered.

It is important to assess the growth rate of the community to be served. If the community is stationary or shrinking, the need for more hospital beds of any kind must be questioned.

Weltman has said that "establishing an ambulatory short-stay surgical center is justifiable only when it can be shown that the center will bring an overall decrease in the total cost of health care to the community itself." If a community has too many hospital beds, adding an ambulatory care unit, either free-standing or as part of an existing hospital, will further reduce the bed occupancy and increase the cost per patient in the in-hospital setting. This is true because a reduction of, for example, 10% in bed utilization cannot be matched by a 10% reduction in costs, many of which are fixed.

What is the planning procedure after a decision has been made that an ambulatory surgical unit is needed, based on the community hospital-bed situation, the number of functioning ambulatory surgical units, and the growth rate and potential of the community?

The first consideration is the attitude of the surgical staff toward an ambulatory unit. Unless they are in accord, the unit probably will have a very difficult time. One of the first things then will be to establish a broad-based working committee of surgeons and administrators to consider the type of facility (free-standing or hospital based), size, and complexity.

The impact of an increase in office ambulatory care should be considered. Insurance companies are experimenting with incentives for physicians to perform some procedures in their office.

It must be recognized that a hospital that loses some bed occupancy by developing an ambulatory surgery unit in the long run may so improve the utilization of its beds and operating rooms that there will be a significant increase in admissions from the physicians who found trouble gaining patient admission or adequate operating time.

Kraft suggested several other ways of persuading surgeons to use ambulatory surgery, including a longer wait for inpatient elective surgery; holding a spare operating room available for only ambulatory surgery up until 2 weeks before the scheduled operating date;

TABLE 2-1. An Evaluation of the Factors That Tend to Differentiate Ambulatory Hospital Surgery From Independently Operated Free-Standing Short-Stay Surgical Facilities

CRITERIA	IN-HOSPITAL SHORT-STAY SURGERY VS.	INDEPENDENTLY OPERATED FREE-STANDING AMBULATORY CARE SURGERY FACILITY
Cost to patient	Probably higher, because of present hospital pricing structure, but the cost could be lower because of the potentially more efficient use of capital by hospitals	Usually lower
Cost to community	Probably lower, only if sufficient in-hospital surgical facilities existed in a given area	Probably higher if it duplicates hospital surgical facilities that are not highly utilized
Quality of care	Tendency toward being higher, but not in all cases	May be very good, but peer review and other safeguards must be part and parcel of it
Access to care		
If hospital facilities are at total capacity in the local area	Restrictive	Would increase access by providing for much-needed additional facilities (depending on how carefully placed they were)
If hospital facilities are not at total capacity	Then access is not aided by duplicating services	No increase in access
If patients lack ability to pay	The nonprofit community hospital tends to render care based more on need of care than on ability to pay; hence access to care is increased in those instances	Depends on individual situation
Continuity of care	Tendency toward increase	A decrease, but this is not the purpose of come-and-go surgery
Comprehensiveness of care	Tendency toward increase	A decrease, but this is not the purpose of come-and-go surgery
Patient satisfaction	Reduced; hospital admission policies are often bureaucratic and inefficient, but this could certainly be improved; other areas besides admission policies must be evaluated, however	Tendency toward increase, especially if admission procedures are highly streamlined and efficient
Fragmentation of health care delivery system	Tendency toward low fragmentation	In first-rate facility, such as Phoenix SurgiCenter, there may be consolidation because better division of labor may be provided
Dynamics of responsiveness to changing community	Free-standing advocates claim that hospitals are too bureaucratic to be highly responsive; however, many hospitals may respond well because of their great community contact and broad range of services	Possibly greater, depending on how well they are managed

(Courtesy of Thomas R. O'Donovan, Ph.D.)

filling the midweek operating room bulge with ambulatory surgery; and bringing in overnight-stay patients for ambulatory surgery Friday to leave on Saturday, which would utilize one day of the weekend slump.

The Washington, D.C., Professional Standards Review Organization (PSRO), with full concurrence of the Medical Society of the District of Columbia, has mandated that it will grant Medicare–Medicaid reimbursement for 51 selected surgical procedures only if they are done on an outpatient basis. There are some contingent situations in which these procedures may be done in hospital, such as medical conditions that may prolong postoperative observation; an unrelated procedure that requires hospitalization being done simultaneously; lack of proper supervision at home for postoperative care; another surgical procedure following the first; and technical difficulties, documented by admission or operative note. This is now a generally accepted policy with many insurance companies.

There are two main types of ambulatory care units: free-standing and hospital based. The emergency room is not an appropriate site for ambulatory surgery, and the physician's office can handle at best only the most trivial ambulatory surgical cases. The argument over which type of unit is best is still not settled. O'Donovan has listed nine criteria that may be helpful in decision making (Table 2-1). These express the differences and advantages very well and should enhance decision making. Office-based ambulatory surgery is being advocated by some. This is a return to the 1930s, when many surgeons did a fair amount of minor surgery in their offices.

DESIGN OF SPACE AND EQUIPMENT

The primary effort should be to design into an ambulatory surgical care unit a synthesis of the physical and practical aspects of a unit. Both a free-standing and a hospital-based unit should have a warm and inviting atmosphere. Certainly one of the pluses of 1-day surgery is its partial replacement of the severe atmosphere of the acute-care hospital. However, within this much more inviting milieu must be housed all the equipment and support facilities required to provide care as good as that in the hospital.

The actual design depends on many factors—projected workload, facilities in the community, sophistication of the medical community, and space available if it is to be an

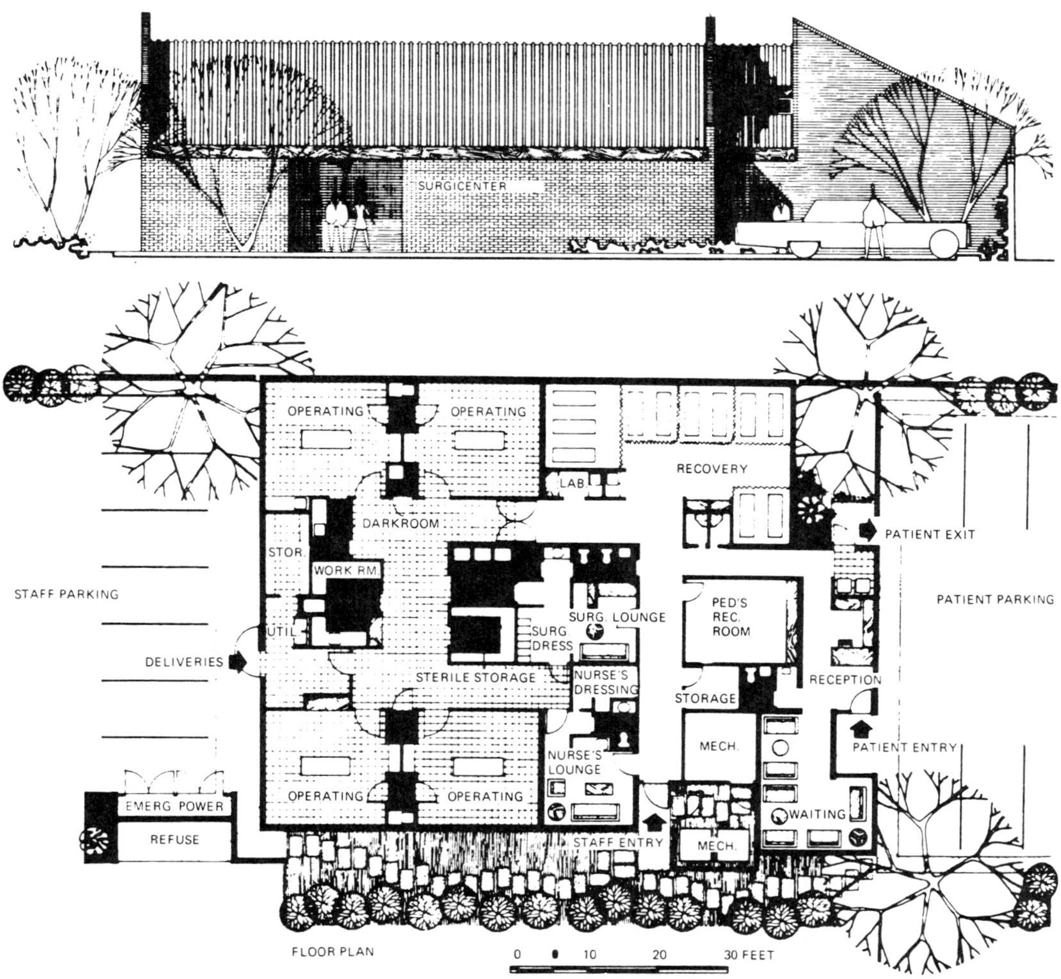

Figure 2-1. The SurgiCenter in Phoenix is an example of a free-standing ambulatory surgery unit.

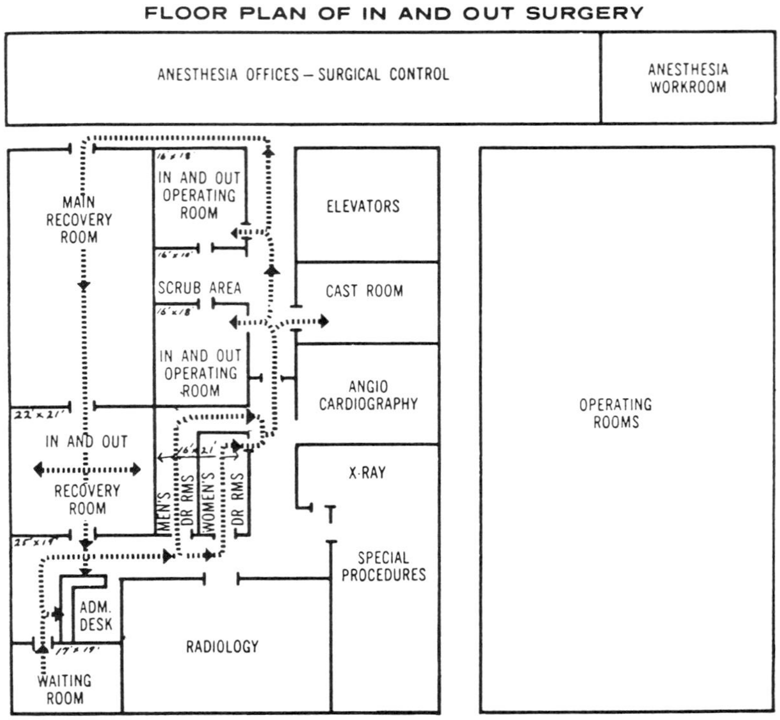

Figure 2-2. The ambulatory surgery unit of the George Washington University Hospital, Washington, DC, is an example of an in-hospital surgical facility. (Levy ML, Coakley CS: South Med J 61:995, 1968

in-hospital facility. Architects who have the expertise to design a functional and tasteful unit should be sought. This chapter will not attempt to discuss this matter. Figures 2-1 and 2-2 show floor plans of a free-standing unit and an in-hospital unit. In some situations motel-like accommodations serve best (e.g., in areas where large distances are involved in getting to a medical care unit). Recently, the number of "ambulatory health hospitals" designed primarily for the patient not yet ready to go home has increased significantly. These facilities mainly accommodate hospitalized patients but could serve ambulatory surgical patients who either do not have an adequate support person at home or live far away. They also could provide a place for family members to stay.

The design teams, in addition to the architect, should include a chief administrator for the project, a representative of the hospital staff, a building committee representative, a member of the biomedical engineering department, and a nursing representative. Special consultants in areas such as laboratory, physical therapy, and radiology should be used as necessary on an ad hoc basis.

Of course, equipment is different in the free-standing and in-hospital units, because the in-hospital unit relies much more heavily on the hospital's support services—radiology, laboratory, central supply, and the like. The in-hospital unit also depends on the volume of work expected and the number of operating rooms. The staff must decide whether certain types of procedures, such as bronchoscopy, esophagoscopy, colonoscopy, thoracoscopy, and cystoscopy, will be done in the ambulatory surgery unit. There are arguments pro and con, so this must be a combined medical and administrative staff decision.

OPERATION OF THE AMBULATORY SURGERY UNIT

BASIC CRITERIA

The ambulatory surgery unit must be based on the premise that, for the types of operation proposed and for most patients, it will offer less expensive care of a quality as good as that in the hospital, and, it is hoped, in a friendlier environment. The accomplishment of such aims depends on the cooperation and good will of all involved, from the orderlies, nurses, and support personnel to the surgical and administrative staff. Leadership by a strong, dedicated individual is of the highest importance. The importance of attitude and conduct of personnel cannot be too strongly stressed. This ambience in most ambulatory surgical units has been central to the growth of ambulatory surgery.

OPERATING POLICIES

Operating policies are the guidelines for day-to-day operation of the unit and include such things as block scheduling by a specialty, length of procedures permitted, types of procedures permitted, criteria for staff privileges, admission policies, use of simplified admissions, treatment and discharge forms, and development of a clear and distinct organizational plan. All of these policies must be in writing and accepted by the majority before the unit opens.

A well-designed, simple but complete chart for recording the process of care from initial contact to the assessment of problems to the intraoperative and postoperative period and finally to follow-up after discharge is a necessity. A number of these charts are available and care should be taken to select a good one.

STAFFING PATTERN

With the appearance of many new paramedical personnel, such as physician assistants, patient ombusdmen, medical technicians, and the upgrading of nurses to nurse practitioners and nursing specialists, has come a blurring of the lines of authority and mission. Add to this the increased involvement of social workers and it becomes obvious that we must have a multidisciplinary approach to health care delivery. Nowhere is this more true than in the ambulatory care setting. The mix that is appropriate for one setting may be inappropriate for another. To a fairly large degree, the type of personalities available helps determine this mix. The administrator, with advice and consent from his people—surgeon, anesthetist, nurse—must sit down and decide this mix. Visiting operational units is of vital importance to this team prior to decision making in order to see variations and to decide what approach is most appropriate.

ANCILLARY SERVICES

The in-hospital unit needs to have a clear understanding with the ancillary services (laboratory, radiology, central service, physiotherapy, and so on) and have guidelines well worked out in advance. The free-standing unit must decide how much of such service it will have to provide and how much can be obtained elsewhere. The free-standing unit must provide a basic minimum of ancillary services, such as some diagnostic radiology and basic laboratory procedure capabilities. Additionally, the unit needs to be self-supportive concerning central service of supplies and equipment.

FISCAL AND MARKETING

Who will be the third-party payer? What will be the status and level of Medicare and Medicaid payments? How will financing be handled for the indigent? The answers to these questions will vary with the local community, but such questions must be considered in advance.

Marketing may have connotations similar to those of the "money changers in the temple," but it is a very important function, for ambulatory surgery is still "selling a product" to many physicians and the consumer. The day may come when government, convinced of its long-term cost effectiveness, may mandate that certain procedures be done in an ambulatory setting. Marketing today is important, and a person (or persons) knowledgeable in this area should be engaged, if only as a consultant. If the product is good, it will sell.

QUALITY ASSURANCE

The need for strong quality assurance procedures has been a concern of many considering ambulatory surgery as a method of health care delivery. Concern arises because of the short length of stay, the abbreviated medical records, and the potential problems in follow-up.

Perhaps the most important measure to assure quality care and avoidance of complications is care in the selection of patients. Not every patient is a candidate for ambulatory surgery, even though the planned procedure is considered normally to be an accepted procedure for ambulatory care. One must start from this premise and after a careful history and physical examination and discussion with the patient and family decide on the desirability of choosing the ambulatory route.

Quality assurance is the same in the ambulatory setting as it is in the hospital. It consists of checking the licenses of each health care provider who is from a profession that requires licensure. It requires delineation of privileges initially and a periodic review to increase or maintain current privileges. Policy and procedure must be established according to the Joint Commission from American Hospital (JCAH) and must consist of long-range plans, current objectives, determined schedules, and identification of areas to be monitored on a continuing basis. Identification and resolution of problems may surface spontaneously, but continuous review of risk areas is necessary (e.g., deaths, infections, cardiac arrests, accidents, need for admission to the hospital following surgery, and atypical anesthesia). Chart review to monitor completeness and continuity of care, justification for surgery, and appropriateness of the surgery performed is a key element of quality assurance. Once a problem has been identified, precise evidence that appropriate and corrective action was initiated must be well documented.

BIBLIOGRAPHY

General

Bartlett MK, Batlit GE, Rockett AM et al: The role of surgery on ambulatory patients in one teaching hospital. Arch Surg 114:319–329, 1979

Cughani A, Meyers D: Who needs ambulatory surgery? Hospitals 49:15–54, 1975

Davis JE: Ambulatory surgery care: Basic concept and review of 1,000 patients. Surgery 73:843–845, 1973

Delany HM: A surgeon's view of a community health center. Surgery 73:486–489, 1973

Egdahl RH: Editorial: Ambulatory health-care delivery and the surgeon. Surgery 73:637–638, 1973

Griner PF: Innovations in ambulatory care and teaching: A house staff group practice. J Med Educ 49:607–608, 1974

Grossman RM: Is ambulatory surgery less expensive? Hospitals 53:112, 1979

O'Donovan TR: Ambulatory Surgery Centers: Development and Management. Germantown, MD, Aspen Systems Corporation, 1976

Rogers DE: The American health care scene. N Engl J Med 288:1377–1383, 1973

Ryan GB: Can free standing surgical centers and hospitals coexist? Mod Med p 22, May, 1975

Planning

Kraft O: Quoted in Same Day Surgery 3:55–56, 1979

O'Donovan TR: Criteria for in hospital stay vs free standing care. Mich Hosp June:12, 1973

O'Donovan, TR: Hospital ambulatory surgery in the 1980's. Hospital and Health Services Administration 1 Special II 1981

Patterson JF, Bechtoldt AA, Levin KJ: Ambulatory surgery in a university setting. JAMA 235:266–268, 1976

Phillips DF: Ambulatory care has come of age. Hospitals 50:53–58, 1976

Wegmiller DC, Platow CN: Looking backward, planning forward. Hospitals 49:57–59, 1975

Weltman AJ: Maybe you can't afford a short stay surgical center. HFM 11:32–37, Oct, 1976

Design and Organization

Arneill BP: Guidelines for design of facilities. Hospitals 49:85–86, 1975

Burgun JA: Construction consideration for ambulatory care facilities. Hospitals 50:79–84, 1976

Grubbs J, Bobrow ML: Centralized ambulatory care unit convenient and efficient. Hospitals 50:127–133, 1979

Redmond JM: Ambulatory care: Current problems center around organization and management. Hospitals 52:58–61, 1978

Marketing and Fiscal

Berarducci AA: Toward economic self sufficiency. Hospitals 49:63–65, 1976

Berkowitz EN, Flexner WA: The marketing audit: A tool for health service organizations. Germantown, MD, Aspen Systems, 1978

Ireland RG: Using marketing strategies to put hospitals on target. Hospitals 51:54–58, 1977

Redmond JM: Apply effective fiscal techniques to improve ambulatory care. Hospitals 50:93–95, 1976

Quality Assurance

Ambulatory Health Care Standards Manual of Joint Commission on Accreditation of Hospitals, 1986

Gonnella J: Towards an effective system of ambulatory health care evaluation. QRB 3:7, 1977

Kingsley J, Bradley D, Leary J: Quality assurance: Guidelines/workbook for surgery, office and clinic. Mid Columbia Surgical Associates, P.L. The Dalles, OR, 1984

3 Anesthesia for Ambulatory Surgery

LINDA S. GEORGES AND K. C. WONG

Health care cost containment remains a national priority, and ambulatory surgery is a major development as an outgrowth of this concern. Well-organized hospital-based and free-standing ambulatory surgery programs are becoming common throughout the United States and Great Britain.

The advantages of ambulatory surgery are obvious. There is less disruption of family life, particularly with pediatric patients; reduced exposure to hospital infections; and, of course, reduced cost. However, there are several disadvantages to ambulatory surgery. There is less available time for the development of rapport between the patient and medical personnel, which increases the risk of developing efficient but impersonal care, and the time required to evaluate the patient is reduced. In a well-run unit, however, these disadvantages can be minimized, and the standard of patient care can be of high quality.

Ambulatory surgical facilities in the United States are organized in several ways: There are office-based facilities, where surgeons perform superficial procedures; hospital-affiliated programs; and free-standing centers. Hospital-affiliated units, which are the most common facility, are of three types: satellite facilities, located some distance from the hospital; separated units, located within the hospital but with totally separate patient care facilities; and totally integrated units, which utilize the same operating suite for both ambulatory patients and inpatients. Free-standing ambulatory centers are independently operated but usually have an agreement with one or more nearby hospitals for the transfer of occasional patients who need hospitalization. The standards of care should be the same in each type of facility and should be of the same high quality as those provided for inpatients.

Surgical techniques are identical to inpatient techniques; however, anesthesia and recovery room procedures, although following some basic principles, are far from identical. If traditional inpatient techniques are used, more patients would be admitted for delayed recovery from anesthesia or would have longer outpatient surgery stays. With the development of new short-acting anesthetic and analgesic agents, anesthesiologists caring for outpatients play a crucial role in the success of an ambulatory surgical facility. The goals of anesthesia for ambulatory patients are to provide adequate anesthesia and analgesia, to provide an acceptable surgical field, to maintain homeostasis in the anesthetized patient, and to help speed the recovery and safe discharge of the patient.

PREOPERATIVE PREPARATION

PATIENT SELECTION

Proper selection of patient and surgical procedure and preoperative preparation are the keys to successful ambulatory surgery. For a number of years only patients who met the American Society of Anesthesiologists' Class I and II criteria were considered candidates for ambulatory surgery. These patients were healthy or had mild to moderate systemic disturbances (e.g., mild diabetes, hypertension, and moderate obesity) that were well controlled.

More recently, Class III patients, those with more severe systemic disturbances—such as insulin-dependent diabetes, coronary artery disease with angina pectoris or previous myocardial infarction, or moderate degrees of pulmonary insufficiency—are being considered as possible candidates for ambulatory surgery.

Class IV patients, who have severe, already life-threatening disorders, may be candidates for surgery on an ambulatory basis when admission to the hospital may put the patient at risk for acquiring hospital-borne infections. An example would be the immunosuppressed patient who requires some vascular access or diagnostic procedure.

Special consideration must also be given to patients at the extremes of age. Neonates, particularly ex-prematures, may be at increased risk for problems such as postoperative apnea, temperature instability, and hypoglycemia. Geriatric patients may have multiple systemic disorders, as well as the physiologic consequences of aging, thus making them more sensitive to the effects of narcotics, sedatives, and other drugs.

Patients in each of these categories may receive excellent outpatient surgical care, if they are properly prepared preoperatively and if their anesthetic management is suited to their particular needs.

PROCEDURE SELECTION

Selection of surgical procedures plays an important role in the success of an ambulatory surgical facility. Procedures performed must include only those that result in minimal bleeding and metabolic derangements. There should be no major intervention in the cranial vault or in the abdominal or thoracic cavities. The procedure should be of moderate to short duration, cause minimal or no postoperative complications, and not require a prolonged recovery phase. Poor candidates include patients who may develop severe nausea and vomiting, patients whose pain cannot be controlled by oral analgesics, and those who strongly desire to be admitted to the hospital.

PHYSICIAN SELECTION

The surgeon who performs ambulatory procedures must have sufficient skill to perform the procedures safely and in reasonable time. He or she can be very valuable in the preoperative assessment and preparation of the patients.

The anesthesiologist has the unique opportunity to provide safe, high-quality anesthetic care in a cost-effective manner. He or she interacts with alert patients and their families and thus participates in the patients' total care. Finally, the anesthesiologist serves as a consultant to evaluate possible candidates for ambulatory surgery.

Medical consultants, either a patient's own physician or a consultant called on to evaluate a complicated patient preoperatively, can provide a valuable service. Merely giving "clearance" for surgery is rarely helpful. Providing specific information about a patient's medical history, as well as arranging postoperative consultations, will allow for safer, more comprehensive perioperative care. Notes concerning a patient's medical problems, evaluation of how successfully these problems are controlled, management suggestions, and a list of medications that the patient is presently taking facilitate successful ambulatory surgery.

PREOPERATIVE SCREENING AND EVALUATION

All ambulatory surgical programs must have some mechanism whereby patients can be screened properly and evaluated prior to the day of surgery. Currently, about half the existing programs use telephone screening procedures, with a complete history and physical examination done when the patient arrives in the center on the day of surgery. Any problems that arise during the screening process are brought to the attention of the anesthesiologist in charge of the unit and to the attending surgeon. Likewise, any laboratory data that prove to be abnormal are brought to the physician's attention, so that he or she can take the appropriate action. Consultations with appropriate specialists can also be obtained at this time.

Other centers require that patients visit the ambulatory surgery department prior to the day of their scheduled surgery for an interview with the anesthesiologist and nursing personnel. Patients then become familiar with the facilities and are introduced to the perioperative routine. Although orientation procedures may vary considerably, the important goal for all programs is that patients are screened and appropriately recommended and that patients are adequately prepared for the surgical experience.

Screening laboratory tests at most centers include a complete blood count and urinalysis.

Other studies, including electrolytes, blood sugar, liver function tests, arterial blood gases, chest x-ray, and electrocardiogram, are ordered at the discretion of the anesthesiologist and/or surgeon, as the patient's condition indicates.

Natof has published two reviews concerning the complication rate in ambulatory surgery patients with preexisting medical problems compared with that of "healthy" patients and finds the rate of complications to be essentially the same. He stresses, however, that all ambulatory patients were optimally prepared and carefully managed perioperatively.[1–2]

PREOPERATIVE INSTRUCTIONS

Precise verbal and written preoperative instructions are always valuable to patients who are anxious about their scheduled surgery and who may not remember conversations with their surgeons, anesthesiologists, or ambulatory surgery nurses. Specific fasting instructions, for example, must be given to diabetics and the parents of pediatric patients. Likewise, medication instructions should be clearly detailed for patients with complicated conditions. Patients should also be reminded to notify the center or their surgeon if their physical status has changed. Examples include a child who develops a runny nose or an older patient who experiences the new onset of chest pain.

Equally important for the patient's total care are specific postoperative instructions. It is wise to review these in the preoperative period, allowing the patient and family to ask questions. Safe transportation home following surgery and adequate home care for the subsequent 24 hours are essential and should be emphasized strongly. The responsibility of the physicians and the ambulatory center does not end when the patient leaves the facility! Safe transportation and home care must be assured before the procedure is undertaken.

PREOPERATIVE MEDICATIONS

Most anesthesiologists feel that pharmacologic premedication prior to ambulatory surgery is unnecessary if the patient has been prepared psychologically. They argue that the preoperative medications slow the recovery and delay discharge. Although such medications have been used effectively, the trend is to avoid pharmacologic agents unless specifically indicated.

Anticholinergic drugs are so named because they compete with acetylcholine at various effector organ sites. Atropine, an alkaloid of the belladonna plant, in the usual dose of 0.01 mg/kg to 0.02 mg/kg (max, 0.6 mg) parenterally, exerts its primary action at the postganglionic parasympathetic receptor, producing tachycardia and antisialorrhea. Some anesthesiologists administer glycopyrrolate 0.005 mg/kg to 0.01 mg/kg (max, 0.2 mg), a quaternary ammonium compound, to provide a prolonged antisecretory effect with less tachycardia and central nervous system excitement.

Because the inhalation anesthetics used at this time cause infrequent problems with excessive secretions, anticholinergics are not indicated for routine premedication of the ambulatory patient. They may be useful to decrease secretions in endoscopy procedures, and in small infants anticholinergics may reduce secretions as well as prevent dangerous bradycardia.

Antacids and Cimetidine

Ong has demonstrated that ambulatory surgery patients may be at greater risk for aspiration of gastric contents than inpatients, because they come to surgery with larger volumes of acidic gastric contents.[3] Another study showed that 60% of ambulatory patients had gastric volumes greater than 25 ml and pH less than 2.5.[4] Thus anesthesiologists have sought ways to minimize this risk.

Antacid therapy aims at increasing the gastric pH, so that aspiration of gastric material is less damaging to the lungs. A soluble, nonparticulate antacid such as sodium citrate (30 ml) is preferred. It decreases gastric acidity but does not decrease gastric volume.

Cimetidine, an H_2-receptor histamine antagonist, also may be used to decrease the risk of aspiration in ambulatory surgical patients. In one study 300 mg given orally 1 to 4 hours preoperatively increased gastric pH to above 2.5 in 84% of treated patients, and the gastric volume was less than 20 ml in 88% of patients.[5]

Metoclopramide is a gastroprokinetic drug that has no effect on gastric acidity yet increases lower esophageal sphincter tone and facilitates gastric emptying. Although it has been found to have little antiemetic effect alone, the combination of metoclopramide (10 mg) with cimetidine (300 mg) given orally 2 hours prior to induction of anesthesia has been shown by Rao to reduce gastric volume and increase pH in laparoscopy patients.[6] The combination of metoclopramide and sodium citrate may also be useful.[7]

Until more conclusive data are available, each surgical center should determine the need for antacids or cimetidine for each patient on an individual basis.

Narcotics

The primary indication for narcotics is relief of pain. The use of narcotics for premedication can produce side-effects such as respiratory depression, rigidity, nausea, and postural hypotension. Fentanyl is a synthetic narcotic with 100 times the potency of morphine but with a duration of action of 30 to 45 minutes from a single injection of 100 μg. Conner has shown fentanyl alone to be a poor preoperative sedative drug, as 100 μg produced a minimal decrease in anxiety and an increase in sedation in fewer than half the patients studied.[8] Long-acting narcotics such as meperidine and morphine are not desirable for ambulatory surgery patients, unless the patients are to be admitted postoperatively.

Barbiturates

The short-acting barbiturates pentobarbital and secobarbital have been used widely as premedicants in inpatients. They are good hypnotics and lack the side-effects of nausea and vomiting. Their long duration of action, however, makes them poor choices as premedicants in the outpatient setting.

Nonbarbiturate Sedatives

Phenothiazines. Phenothiazines are potent antiemetic drugs because of their inhibition of the chemoreceptor trigger zone as well as their anticholinergic activity. However, postural hypotension resulting from central depression of vasomotor reflexes, peripheral adrenergic blockade, and direct vasodilation are potential problems. Also troublesome are the possible extrapyramidal effects and long duration of action.

Phenothiazines are of little use in ambulatory surgery.

Benzodiazepines. The benzodiazepines allay anxiety by depressing the limbic system and the amygdalae, where fear, anxiety, and aggression are generated. There is little soporific effect if given orally. Diazepam has been used widely in the past as a premedicant, as it possesses good sedative and amnestic properties at the dose of 5 mg to 10 mg orally or parenterally. Peak drug levels occur at 60 to 90 minutes following oral administration, with drowsiness persisting up to 120 minutes. Larger doses, up to 20 mg, result in a more rapid peak blood level, but drowsiness may persist for up to 4 hours. Intramuscular injection of diazepam results in poorly predictable absorption and blood levels. Additionally, parenteral diazepam is quite painful.

When injected intravenously, diazepam can cause depression of the respiratory and cardiovascular systems. These effects are additive in the presence of narcotics. One is reminded that patients vary in their clinical response to the drug and that it should be administered in small increments and titrated to effect. The recommended dose for ambulatory patients is 0.05 mg/kg to 0.15 mg/kg.

The redistribution half-life of diazepam is 2.5 hours. However, recurrence of drowsiness and increase in plasma concentration occur at 6 to 8 hours, probably because of enterohepatic recycling. This effect is more pronounced if fatty foods are ingested 3 hours after diazepam is administered. The elimination half-life is 1.5 days resulting from primarily hepatic metabolism and clearance.

Oral absorption of diazepam is slow; therefore administration of an oral dose of diazepam immediately prior to transport of a patient to the operating suite has little or no sedative effect preoperatively and often slows the patient's recovery due to prolonged sedation. To have the proper effect, the oral dose must be given at least 1 hour prior to surgery.

When diazepam is administered intravenously, it is desirable to flush the injection site with intravenous fluid because diazepam is very irritating to tissues. It is insoluble in water and is formulated in organic solvents, including propylene glycol and ethyl alcohol, resulting in frequent phlebitis.

Midazolam, a new water-soluble benzodiazepine, is useful both as a premedicant and as an induction drug. It is twice as potent as diazepam. A dose of 5 mg administered intravenously produces sedation and axiolysis in 1 to 2 minutes, and marked sedation persists for approximately one-half hour. Anterograde amnesia is present in over 90% of patients in 2 minutes and persists for 20 to 40 minutes. Recovery of motor performance occurs at approximately 30 minutes, and subjects are fully awake at 70 minutes. Plasma half-life is 60 to 90 minutes, without apparent enterohepatic recycling and recurrence of drowsiness. Phlebitis is rare.

Doses of 1 mg to 2 mg midazolam intravenously given immediately prior to transporting the patient into the operating room have proved very effective in producing sedation and amnesia for short procedures.

Butyrophenones. Droperidol is the most commonly used butyrophenone. Patients given this drug exhibit marked tranquilization with easy arousability. However, significant drug levels of metabolite are present in the plasma for 8 to 12 hours. Tests for coordination and attention remain abnormal at 10 hours postinjection. Some patients who receive droperidol experience restlessness, anxiety, and agitation. Low doses, less than 1.25 mg, appear to produce minimal problems. In general, the long action of droperidol makes it an unsuitable premedicant for ambulatory surgical patients. Droperidol can potentiate the analgesic as well as the respiratory depressant effects of opiates.

ANESTHESIA TECHNIQUES

Anesthesia techniques vary according to the procedure, the surgeon, the patient, the anesthesiologist, and the surgery center's past experiences. The technique itself is not as important as the drugs and dosages employed.

Each surgical center must provide the same standards of care for delivery of anesthesia, monitoring, and resuscitation as those provided for inpatients.

Minimal monitoring should include a precordial or esophageal stethoscope, blood pressure cuff, continuous electrocardiograph display, temperature probe, and measure of inspired oxygen concentration. Pulse oximetry may soon be the standard of care in all operating suites, as it has proved valuable not only in general anesthetic cases, but in local and regional anesthesia as well.

LOCAL AND REGIONAL ANESTHESIA

Local Anesthetic Agents

Local anesthetics produce their effect by interfering with the initial step in the excitation-conduction process in nervous tissue by decreasing the rate and degree of depolarization without altering the resting potential, threshold potential, or repolarization phase. When the degree of depolarization fails to reach threshold potential, a propagated action fails to develop and nerve conduction is blocked. The receptor site for local anesthetic agents is believed to reside in the nerve membrane. However, the specific receptor location varies according to the type of local anesthetic agent employed.

Local anesthetic agents are classified according to their chemical structure. The two major groups are those containing either an ester or an amide link between their aromatic portion and the intermediate chain. The aminoesters include cocaine, procaine, tetracaine, and chloroprocaine. The aminoamides include lidocaine, mepivacaine, prilocaine, bupivacaine, and etidocaine. The basic differences between the ester and amide compounds reside in the manner in which they are metabolized and in their allergic potential.

The ester agents are hydrolyzed in the plasma by pseudocholinesterase, whereas the amide agents undergo enzymatic degradation in the liver. Para-aminobenzoic acid, one of the metabolites formed from the hydrolysis of esterlike compounds, is capable of inducing allergic reactions in a small percentage of the population. The amide drugs are not metabolized to para-aminobenzoic acid, and reports of allergic phenomena are rare.

On the basis of differences in anesthetic potency and duration of action, it is possible to classify the clinically useful injectable local anesthetic compounds into three categories:

Group I—agents of low anesthetic potency and short duration of action (procaine and chloroprocaine).

Group II—agents of intermediate anesthetic potency and intermediate duration of action (lidocaine, mepivacaine, prilocaine).

Group III—agents of high anesthetic potency and long duration of action (tetracaine, bupivacaine, etidocaine). These agents are rarely used for ambulatory anesthesia.

Local Infiltration Anesthesia

Infiltration anesthesia involves administration of a local anesthetic agent into an extravascular space in or around the operative site and diffusion to the nerve endings, where excitation is inhibited. Onset of action is almost immediate for all agents following intradermal or subcutaneous administration. The concentration and volume of local anesthetic required for adequate infiltration anesthesia depend on the extent of the area to be anesthetized and the expected duration of the surgical procedure. Epinephrine may be added to prolong the effect of infiltration anesthesia. It should be used in concentrations no higher than 1:200,000, and its use is contraindicated in nerve blocks of the hands, feet, and digits, when blood supply to the area may already be compromised by the presence of peripheral vascular disease.

The most commonly used drugs for infiltration anesthesia include 1% to 2% procaine, 0.5% to 1% lidocaine, 2% chloroprocaine, 0.5% to 1% mepivacaine, and 1% prilocaine. Refer to Table 3-1 for a summary of recommended dosages and durations.[9] The surgeon and scrub nurse must be meticulous in accounting for the total amount of local anesthetic administered in order to avoid overdose.

The infiltration is generally done by the surgeon with or without monitored anesthesia care ("stand-by"). Complex or extremely anxious patients are better managed with an anesthesiologist monitoring the patient's vital signs and administering supplementary drugs. In the event that intraoperative problems demand general anesthesia, the anesthesiologist is already present and is not called to treat a patient with whom he is unfamiliar.

Premedication for local anesthesia patients may be useful in allaying anxiety and reducing the pain of injection. If given orally, the medication must have adequate time to take effect before the procedure. A preferable route is to titrate the drug in small doses to the desired effect to avoid oversedation, thus resulting in prolonged postoperative recovery.

The ultra-short-acting barbiturates in subanesthetic doses are well suited for producing temporary obtundation of consciousness during a painful local anesthetic injection, such as retrobulbar block. Thiopental (25 mg to 50 mg) or methohexital (10 mg to 20 mg) given intravenously may be very useful for this purpose. Caution must be exercised in the care of all patients, particularly the elderly, who must be monitored closely for signs of respiratory and cardiovascular depression.

Field Block Anesthesia

Field block is accomplished by injecting a wall of anesthetic solution across the path of the nerves supplying an operative field (Fig. 3-1). In the majority of cases the layer of soft tissue in which the nerves are situated is injected. The anesthesia produced by a field block is generally of longer duration than that obtained from local infiltration. Another advantage of field block is the absence of edema and distortion of the anatomic landmarks along the line of incision.

Intravenous Regional Anesthesia

Intravenous regional anesthesia involves the intravenous administration of local anes-

TABLE 3-1. Infiltration Anesthesia for Ambulatory Surgery

AGENT	CONCENTRATION (%)	PLAIN SOLUTIONS Max. Adult Dose (mg)	Max. Dose (mg/kg)	Duration (min)	EPINEPHRINE-CONTAINING SOLUTIONS Max. Adult Dose (mg)	Max. Dose (mg/kg)	Duration (min)
SHORT DURATION							
Procaine Chloroprocaine	1–2	800	11	15–30	1000	14	30–90
MODERATE DURATION							
Lidocaine	0.5–1	300	4	30–60	500	7	120–360
Mepivacaine	0.5–1	300	4	45–90	500	7	120–360
Prilocaine	0.5–1	600	7	30–90	Not available		

(Philip BK, Covino BG: Local and regional anesthesia. In Wetchler BV [ed]: Anesthesia for Ambulatory Surgery. Philadelphia, JB Lippincott, 1985)

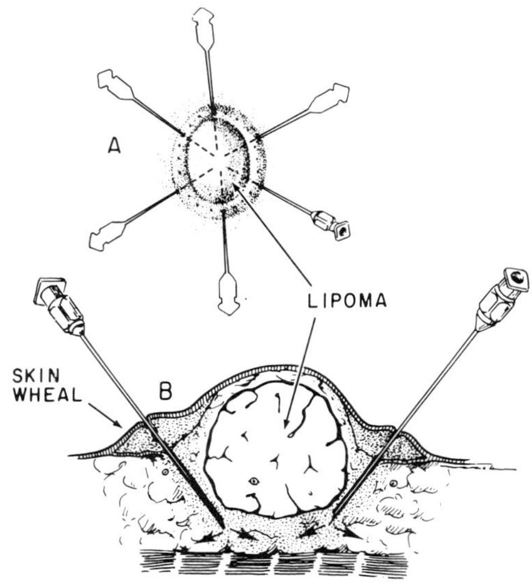

Figure 3-1. Field block for superficial surgery. (*A*) Intradermal wheals are raised to circumscribe a lipoma, followed by (*B*) subcutaneous infiltration to surround the surgical specimen.

thetic into a tourniqueted limb. Calibration of an occlusive double pneumatic tourniquet is of great importance, in order to prevent leakage of the local anesthetic solution, loss of anesthesia, and possible systemic toxicity. Exsanguination of the limb should be accomplished by elevation and wrapping, distal to proximal, with an Esmarch bandage. One can also accomplish exsanguination by elevating the limb for 5 minutes. Prior to exsanguination, an intravenous catheter should be inserted in a distal vein.

After exsanguination has been accomplished, the proximal tourniquet cuff should be inflated to 100 mm Hg above systolic blood pressure. Local anesthetic is then injected into the intravenous catheter when the bandage is removed. Commonly, 40 ml of 0.5% lidocaine has been found to give satisfactory analgesia for the upper extremity, but volumes as large as 75 ml to 100 ml of dilute anesthetic solution, 0.25% to 0.35% lidocaine, may be required for the lower extremity. Children have been successfully treated with intravenous regional anesthesia using 3 mg/kg to 5 mg/kg of 0.25% to 0.5% lidocaine.

The proximal cuff should remain inflated for 15 to 20 minutes to allow for adequate tissue binding of the anesthetic drug. The distal tourniquet is then inflated, followed by deflation of the proximal cuff. At the conclusion of the surgery intermittent tourniquet release is advocated in 10- to 15-second intervals, in order to decrease peak concentrations of local anesthetic in the systemic circulation.

Minor Nerve Blocks

Minor nerve blocks are defined as procedures involving single nerve entities, such as the ulnar or radial nerves at the wrist and the anterior or posterior tibial nerves at the ankle. These can be quite useful for superficial procedures of the extremities.

See Table 3-2 for dosages and durations.

Major Nerve Blocks

Major nerve blocks consist of those procedures in which two or more distinct nerves or a nerve plexus are blocked. For example, a brachial plexus block at the axilla is commonly used for operations of the hand, forearm, and distal part of the arm. A flooding technique is used for brachial plexus block that involves the use of larger volumes of local anesthetic (up to 40 ml) injected within the brachial plexus sheath (Fig. 3-2).

TABLE 3-2. Minor Nerve Blocks for Ambulatory Surgery

		PLAIN SOLUTIONS			EPINEPHRINE-CONTAINING SOLUTIONS
AGENT	USUAL CONCENTRATION (%)	Usual Adult Volume (ml)	Usual Adult Dose (mg)	Average Duration (min)	Average Duration (min)
Procaine Chloroprocaine	2%	5–20	100–400	15–30	30–60
Lidocaine Mepivacaine Prilocaine	1%	5–20	50–200	60–120	120–180

(Philip BK, Covino BG: Local and regional anesthesia. In Wetchler BV [ed]: Anesthesia for Ambulatory Surgery. Philadelphia, JB Lippincott, 1985)

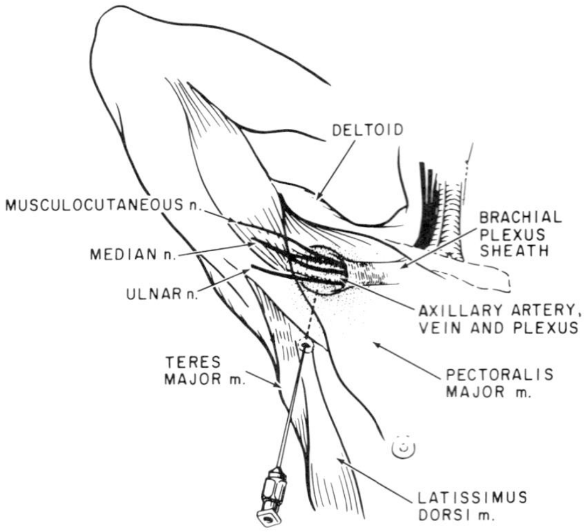

Figure 3-2. Brachial plexus block by axillary approach. Pulsation of the axillary artery provides the target for insertion of needle. Paresthesia of the arm or hand indicates the needle is in the brachial plexus sheath and near the nerves. The entire volume of local anesthetic solution is injected with frequent attempts at aspiration. If blood is aspirated, the needle is carefully advanced or withdrawn to clear the intravascular position; then the injection is continued. Frank pain in the arm or hand during injection indicates neuronal irritation, and the needle is immediately repositioned. *Dotted area* depicts expansion of axillary plexus sheath with injection of local anesthetic.

While aspirating frequently, 30 ml to 40 ml of local anesthetic is injected. A small-gauge needle minimizes hematoma. Anesthesia using this procedure is generally achieved within 30 to 45 minutes of injection and persists for 2 to 3 hours.

In general, the agents of moderate duration, such as lidocaine and mepivacaine, produce anesthesia for 2 to 4 hours, whereas short-acting agents such as chloroprocaine provide 1 to 2 hours of anesthesia. Epinephrine (1 : 200,000) prolongs the duration of most local anesthetics and may be used when indicated.

Other approaches, such as the interscalene, supraclavicular, and infraclavicular, may produce somewhat more intense blocks of peripheral brachial plexus nerve distribution, but they also increase the risk of complications such as pneumothorax and subarachnoid injection.

See Table 3-3 for drugs and dosages.

Central Neural Blockade

Epidural Anesthesia. Lumbar epidural anesthesia is useful for surgical procedures involving the lower abdomen, pelvis, perineum, and lower extremities. Caudal anesthesia may be appropriate for procedures in the pelvic and perineal areas. Lumbar epidural anesthesia requires the use of 10 ml to 20 ml of local anesthetic solution to obtain the desired effect, in contrast to the 20 ml to 30 ml needed for caudal anesthesia. Drugs commonly used include 1.5% to 2% lidocaine or mepivacaine, 2% prilocaine, and 2% to 3% chloroprocaine.

For epidural or caudal block in children, the dose can be calculated using the formula 0.1 ml per year, per segment blocked (±0.2 ml), using 1% lidocaine, 1% mepivacaine, or 0.25% bupivacaine, up to age 12. For caudal block it is often easier to use 0.5 ml/kg, as this amount consistently provides spread to L2 to L3, and sometimes to T10 to T11.[10]

Patient position has been demonstrated to influence the spread of an epidural block, as more anesthetic agent is required to obtain the desired level in a patient who is in a sitting position than in a patient who is in the supine position. Additionally, dose requirements are directly proportional to patient height. Although controversial, doses may be propor-

TABLE 3-3. Major Nerve Blocks for Ambulatory Surgery

		PLAIN SOLUTIONS				EPINEPHRINE-CONTAINING SOLUTIONS			
AGENT	USUAL CONCENTRATION (%)	Usual Adult Volume (ml)	Max. Adult Dose (mg)	Usual Onset (min)	Usual Duration (min)	Usual Adult Volume	Max. Adult Dose	Usual Onset	Usual Duration
Chloroprocaine	2–3	25–40	800	10–20	30–50	30–60	1000	10–20	60–120
Lidocaine	1–1.5	20–30	300	10–20	60–90	30–50	500	10–20	120–140
Mepivacaine	1–1.5	20–30	300	10–20	60–120	30–50	500	10–20	180–300
Prilocaine	1–2	30–50	600	10–20	60–120		Not available		

(Philip BK, Covino BG: Local and regional anesthesia. In Wetchler BV [ed]: Anesthesia for Ambulatory Surgery. Philadelphia, JB Lippincott, 1985)

TABLE 3-4. Epidural Blockade for Ambulatory Surgery

		PLAIN SOLUTIONS				EPINEPHRINE-CONTAINING SOLUTIONS			
AGENT	USUAL CONCENTRATION (%)	Usual Adult Volume (ml)	Total Adult Dose (mg)	Usual Onset (min)	Usual Duration (min)	Usual Adult Volume	Max. Adult Dose	Usual Onset	Usual Duration
Chloroprocaine	3	15–25	150–750	5–15	30–60	15–30	150–900	5–15	30–90
Lidocaine	1–2	15–30	150–300	5–15	60–90	15–30	150–500	5–15	60–180
Mepivacaine	1–2	15–30	150–300	5–15	60–120	15–30	150–500	5–15	60–180
Prilocaine	1–3	15–30	150–600	5–15	60–120	Not available			

(Philip BK, Covino BG: Local and regional anesthesia. In Wetchler BV [ed]: Anesthesia for Ambulatory Surgery. Philadelphia, JB Lippincott, 1985)

tional to patient age up to 18 years, then inversely proportional to age after 18 years.

Lidocaine, mepivacaine, and prilocaine are commonly used for surgical procedures of 1 to 2 hours, whereas chloroprocaine is often employed for procedures for 1 hour or less. Epinephrine (1 : 200,000) may be added to prolong the block but is rarely appropriate for ambulatory surgery (Table 3-4).

Autonomic blockade occurs with the onset of epidural anesthesia and may cause significant changes in blood pressure, heart rate, and cardiac output. This blockade usually occurs slowly, but profound alterations may occur in some patients. The higher the block, the greater the number of sympathetic fibers that are affected, leading to a reduction in vascular tone and a decrease in blood pressure. Blocks below T5 are seldom associated with profound hypotension, whereas blocks affecting T1 through T5 may result in hypotension and profound bradycardia. These patients are extremely sensitive to any postural changes. Cardiovascular depression is also more profound in the hypovolemic patient. Normal vasoconstrictive responses are blocked and marked cardiovascular collapse may occur. Adequate intravascular volume is essential before the block is administered.

Patients who have had lumbar epidural or caudal anesthesia for ambulatory surgery may begin to ambulate with assistance when clinical examination reveals resolution of sympathetic and motor blockade. Risks of the procedure include dural puncture, with subsequent development of spinal headache, neurologic sequelae, systemic local anesthetic toxicity, and allergic reaction. In the hands of a skilled anesthesiologist, however, these complications are rare.

Spinal Anesthesia (Subarachnoid Block; Fig. 3-3). Spinal anesthesia is a subject of great controversy in ambulatory surgery. Most centers discourage its use due to concern about prolonged sympathetic blockade and increased numbers of hospital admissions. On the other hand, a few centers use this technique frequently and find it quite satisfactory.

Performance of subarachnoid block involves entering the subarachnoid space under sterile conditions with a small-gauge spinal needle (25-gauge or 26-gauge) and depositing a small amount of local anesthetic solution in

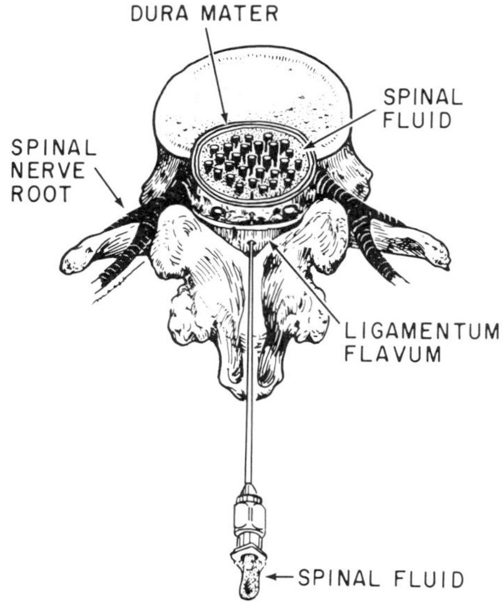

Figure 3-3. Subarachnoid (spinal) block. The needle is positioned in a midline approach. Distinct resistance is felt as it penetrates the tough ligamentum flavum. The arachnoid membrane is closely adherent to the dura mater, and penetration of both membranes is felt as a single pop.

TABLE 3-5. Spinal Anesthetic Agents for Ambulatory Surgery

AGENT	USUAL CONCENTRATION (%)	USUAL ADULT VOLUME (ml)	TOTAL ADULT DOSE (mg)	BARICITY	GLUCOSE CONCENTRATION (%)	USUAL ANESTHETIC DURATION (min)
Lidocaine	5	1–2	50–100	Hyperbaric	7.5	45–60
Tetracaine	0.25–1	1–4	5–20	Hyperbaric	5	75–150
	0.1–0.3			Hypobaric		
	0.5			Isobaric		
Dibucaine	0.25	1–2	2.5–5	Hyperbaric	5	75–180
	0.5	1–2	5–10	Isobaric		
	0.06	5–20	3–12	Hypobaric		
Bupivacaine	0.5	3–4	15–20	Isobaric		75–150
	0.75	2–3	15–22.5	Hyperbaric	8	75–150

(Philip BK, Covino BG: Local and regional anesthesia. In Wetcher BV [ed]: Anesthesia for Ambulatory Surgery. Philadelphia, JB Lippincott, 1985)

the spinal fluid. The effect of the block is influenced by patient position, volume of the subarachnoid space, and dosage of the drug used. Venocaval compression in the pregnant patient and decreased spinal fluid volume in the elderly make these patients more prone to higher block levels than predicted.

Lidocaine is the drug of choice for subarachnoid block in the ambulatory patient. Tetracaine may be appropriate if the surgery is scheduled early in the day and there is sufficient time for full recovery before the patient is discharged. Epinephrine (0.2 mg to 0.3 mg) may produce a 50% prolongation of the spinal anesthesia. Phenylephrine (1 mg to 5 mg) added to the local anesthetic solution is an alternative way to extend the length of anesthesia. See Table 3-5 for recommended dosages.

Spinal anesthesia, like epidural anesthesia, is associated with hypotension secondary to sympathetic blockade. This effect may be profound, particularly in the hypovolemic patient. Its treatment includes the administration of fluids, slight Trendelenburg position, and use of a vasopressor such as ephedrine, in doses of 5 mg to 10 mg intravenously.

TABLE 3-6. Spinal Anesthetic Agents for Pediatric Ambulatory Surgery

AGENT	CONCENTRATION (%)	DOSE (mg/kg)
Lidocaine	5	2 (under 3 yr) 1 (3–10 yr)
Tetracaine	1	0.2
Dibucaine	0.5	0.2

(Philip BK, Covino BG: Local and regional anesthesia. In Wetchler BV [ed]: Anesthesia for Ambulatory Surgery. Philadelphia, JB Lippincott, 1985)

Spinal anesthesia has been used for pediatric ambulatory patients (Table 3-6). The increased dose for lidocaine anesthesia in infants is due to a higher volume of cerebrospinal fluid relative to body weight.

The complications of subarachnoid block are the same as those described for epidural block and include headache, neurologic sequelae, systemic local anesthetic reactions, and allergic reactions. The incidence of headache after subarachnoid block is reported to be 1.5% if a 25-gauge or 26-gauge spinal needle is used.[11]

Criteria for ambulation after subarachnoid block include return of perianal sensation (S4 to S5), plantar flexion of the foot, and proprioception of the great toe. Discharge criteria should include demonstrated normal strength, proprioception, and ability to urinate. Specific instructions as to activity at home should be given on discharge. The patient should be told to rest in bed for 24 hours. He may prop himself up on pillows and sit up to eat. He may go to the bathroom with assistance, but all lifting and Valsalva's maneuvers should be avoided. If any complications, such as headache, stiff neck, or fever, develop that do not respond to acetaminophen, the patient should call the anesthesiologist or surgery center immediately.

GENERAL ANESTHESIA

General anesthesia is the technique used most frequently in all ambulatory surgery centers. The techniques and combinations of drugs are as variable as the number of anesthesiologists using them. The key to successful ambulatory anesthesia is choosing the appropriate short-acting drugs and administering them in the proper doses in a timely manner.

Induction

The preferable method of induction is chosen contingent on the age and general condition of the patient. Young children may be quite apprehensive and thus better managed with an inhalation or rectal induction, whereas most adults prefer intravenous induction. Sometimes the primary planned technique may not be feasible, therefore an alternate plan should be available.

Rectal Induction. The rectal administration of an ultra-short-acting barbiturate such as methohexital has proved very useful in small children. The 10% solution (100 mg/ml) is administered to the child through a well-lubricated catheter in a dose of 20 mg/kg to 30 mg/kg. The onset of sleep occurs in 7 to 8 minutes. The advantages of this technique are that the child can be anesthetized in the parents' arms and then carried into the operating room, where a peaceful inhalation induction can be performed or intravenous line inserted as needed. Care must be taken to keep the airway patent as the child falls asleep, and the anesthesiologist must remain at the child's bedside until he is transported to the operating room. The disadvantage of this technique is the added time required to administer the drug. This problem can be eliminated if it can be performed in an induction area by a team approach.

Intramuscular Induction. Intramuscular injections are painful and for that reason are not commonly used for induction of anesthesia. However, with a struggling child or retarded patient, where intravenous access is difficult, IM injection may be most appropriate. An injection of ketamine 2 mg/kg to 4 mg/kg plus atropine 0.02 mg/kg provides adequate conditions for successful mask induction or intravenous line placement in 3 to 5 minutes. Atropine is added to avoid the copious secretions that accompany the administration of ketamine and make the airway management difficult. When patients are administered low-dose ketamine as an induction agent, the incidence of nightmares and unpleasant emergence phenomena is significantly reduced.[12]

Methohexital (6 mg/kg) administered as a 5% solution is another choice for intramuscular induction. It is reported to produce sleep in 6 minutes. An advantage of both of these agents is that they allow the child to go to sleep in the parent's arms, relieving both the patient's and parent's anxiety.

Inhalation Induction and Potent Inhalation Agents. Inhalation induction is the most commonly used technique to anesthetize children. The child is allowed to breathe the anesthetic gases through a mask that has been scented with a fruit-flavored oil of the child's choice. The child can be distracted with puppets or stories or by an attempt to blow up the anesthesia rebreathing bag while he becomes anesthetized. In the hands of a skilled anesthesiologist, this technique works well for most children.

NITROUS OXIDE. Nitrous oxide in oxygen is the most commonly used carrier gas used in anesthesia. It is used in combination with potent inhalation agents and/or narcotics for the induction and maintenance of anesthesia. It is almost odorless, which makes it ideal for the induction of inhalation anesthesia. It is used in concentrations of 70% or less and reduces the required amount of concurrently administered inhalation agents (MAC).

HALOTHANE. Halothane represents the first of a new generation of inhalation anesthetics introduced into clinical practice in the 1950s. Induction of anesthesia is achieved in 3 to 5 minutes with inspired concentrations of 1% to 4% in combination with oxygen and nitrous oxide. Although it is well tolerated by the respiratory tract, rapid increases of inspired halothane concentration can irritate the respiratory mucosa and produce breath holding or coughing. Maintenance of anesthesia requires a concentration of 1% to 2%.

Halothane is a potent cardiovascular depressant, decreasing arterial blood pressure, myocardial contractility, and heart rate. These effects are dose dependent and are especially profound in the young, fasting infant. Halothane renders the heart more sensitive to catecholamines; thus local infiltration with epinephrine for hemostasis should be monitored carefully. The total dose administered should not exceed 2 μg/kg to 3 μg/kg over an hour.

Recovery after brief halothane anesthesia is usually rapid and smooth. After prolonged administration, however, emergence may be delayed. The incidence of nausea and vomiting is rare. Repeated halothane anesthetics are avoided in adults because of the possibility of sensitization resulting in postoperative "halothane hepatitis." This does not appear to be a problem with the preadolescent child.

ENFLURANE. Enflurane was introduced into general use in 1972. It is a stable, nonflammable liquid that produces rapid induction of anesthesia and rapid emergence. Enflurane is about half as potent as halothane; therefore 2% to 3% is required for maintenance of anesthesia. This concentration requirement is reduced with the addition of nitrous oxide to the inspired gas mixture. In clinical practice, inhalation induction with enflurane is associated with an increased incidence of coughing and breath holding, compared with induction with halothane. Although emergence may be slightly more rapid, recovery room stay and time until discharge for the two agents are comparable.

Cardiac rhythm tends to be stable, and there is less sensitivity to catecholamines during enflurane anesthesia compared with halothane anesthesia. Vasodilation and hypotension are common. A peculiar side-effect of enflurane is that about 2% of patients exhibit signs of hyperactive skeletal muscle movement with abnormal EEG seizure patterns, which are more prevalent during hyperventilation and hypocarbia.

Enflurane is metabolized by the liver by defluorination to produce free fluoride ion, which is a potential renal toxic agent. Thus a relative contraindication to the use of enflurane is the existence of renal failure and decreased urinary output in a patient.

ISOFLURANE. Isoflurane, an ether anesthetic, was introduced into clinical practice in 1983. Its low blood : gas solubility coefficient suggests that induction and recovery from anesthesia should be rapid. Its pungent smell and tendency to irritate the respiratory mucosa, however, have limited its usefulness in inhalation inductions. The coughing, breath holding, and laryngospasm can be reduced somewhat by having the patient breathe 60% to 70% nitrous oxide for 2 minutes and by increasing the inspired concentration of increments of 0.25%. Postoperative recovery is rapid, even after cases of longer duration. Only 0.2% of the drug is metabolized in the body, and repeated exposure does not present problems. Isoflurane has proved to be a very valuable drug in ambulatory anesthesia and is used primarily for maintenance of anesthesia following intravenous induction.

Intravenous Inductions. ULTRA-SHORT-ACTING BARBITURATES. Sodium thiopental is a sulfurated barbiturate used clinically as a 2.5% solution. Standard induction doses of 3 mg/kg to 4 mg/kg produce sleep immediately. Recovery is rapid (10 to 15 minutes) because of redistribution of the drug from the vessel-rich group (brain, heart, etc.), to muscle, and then to fat. Rapid induction is aided by the fact that the drug is very lipid soluble and 50% ionized at physiologic pH (pKs = 7.4).

Small doses of thiopental are commonly used for a sedative effect. Its short duration of action is useful in many clinical situations. If repeated doses of thiopental are administered, eventually the tissue depots become saturated and the equilibrium of the drug between blood and tissue favors the blood, resulting in prolonged sedation. Generally, when cumulative doses exceed 10 mg/kg, prolonged sedation is expected.

Thiopental produces dose-dependent cardiac depression. Because systemic vascular resistance is usually reflexly increased, blood pressure is generally maintained. This may not be the case in the physiologically compromised patient, such as one who is hypovolemic. For this reason most anesthesiologists use a "test dose" of thiopental (50 mg) to evaluate the patient's cardiovascular response prior to giving the entire induction dose. Thiopental is also a respiratory depressant, and equipment to support ventilation must be available whenever the drug is administered.

Extravascular injection of thiopental can result in tissue necrosis because of the solution's alkalinity (pH 11). Elimination of the drug is via metabolism by the liver at a rate of 10% of the amount of drug in the body per hour.

Methohexital is an oxybarbiturate, used as a 1% solution. Standard induction doses of 0.75 mg/kg to 2.2 mg/kg produce rapid loss of consciousness. Its redistribution half-life is similar to that of thiopental, but its elimination by the liver is faster, resulting in a more rapid return of psychomotor function. Significant side-effects occur with administration of methohexital, and these include cough, hiccough, and involuntary muscle movements. These effects can be minimized by the administration of fentanyl (1 μg/kg) as a preoperative medication.

MIDAZOLAM. Midazolam may be used as an induction drug. Dose requirements range from 0.1 mg/kg to 0.4 mg/kg, resulting in loss of lash reflex and unresponsiveness to command. Dose requirements may be decreased by increasing the speed of injection, suggesting that acute tolerance may be developed if the drug is administered very slowly. Dose requirement also may be reduced by premedication with narcotics such as fentanyl or sufentanil. Older and less fit patients require less drug for induction.

Emergence from intravenous midazolam induction is 1.5 to 2.5 times longer than that from induction with thiopental.

Addition of potent opiates to the technique tends to prolong the recovery. Amnesia with midazolam is excellent.[13]

ETOMIDATE. Etomidate is a short-acting hypnotic, used in induction doses of 0.2 mg/kg to 0.4 mg/kg. Both induction and awakening time are on the order of 4 to 10 minutes. It has minimal cardiovascular and respiratory side-effects. It does, however, cause pain on injection in 50% of patients, and 55% experience nausea and vomiting. Myoclonic movements occur in 70% of patients.[14] These side-effects can be reduced by using fentanyl (100 μg) 3 minutes prior to induction. Etomidate has limited usefulness in ambulatory anesthesia.

KETAMINE. Ketamine is a phencyclidine derivative that induces a state of disinterest and detachment from the environment termed *dissociative anesthesia*. It is effective for the induction and maintenance of anesthesia, characterized by cataplexy, catatonia, amnesia, and analgesia. Airway and respiration are usually well maintained, but obstruction is not uncommon with slight overdose.

Intravenous injection of 2 mg/kg produces unconsciousness in 60 to 90 seconds and lasts 15 to 30 minutes. Repeated small doses or continuous infusion may be used to maintain anesthesia in combination with nitrous oxide and oxygen. Hyperactive oropharyngeal reflexes and salivation are common. Preoperative anticholinergic premedication is essential to prevent excessive oral secretions. Stimulation of oropharyngeal structures should be minimized, because laryngospasm is common.

Ketamine stimulates the cardiovascular system, resulting in increases in heart rate and blood pressure of 20% to 25%. These qualities make it useful for management of hypovolemic patients, but undesirable for hypertensive patients or those with increased intracranial pressure.

The use of ketamine is associated with postanesthetic confusion, disorientation, bad dreams, hallucinations, and restlessness. The incidence of the unwanted effects can be minimized by the administration of benzodiazepines prior to the ketamine. The use of ketamine has found limited acceptance in ambulatory anesthesia because of prolonged emergence.

Maintenance of Anesthesia

Anesthesia is usually maintained with a combination of nitrous oxide, oxygen, and a potent inhalation agent, and/or intravenous agents such as short-acting narcotics and muscle relaxants. The technique used depends primarily on the individual patient, procedure, and the anesthesiologist's personal preference. The goal is to administer adequate anesthesia for the procedure and to allow the patient to return rapidly to his preoperative state of well-being. The potent inhalation agents halothane, enflurane, and isoflurane have been discussed in the section on induction of anesthesia. The following section reviews intravenous agents, including narcotics and muscle relaxants.

Intravenous Anesthetics. Intravenous techniques for the maintenance of anesthesia include bolus administration and infusions of barbiturates, narcotics, and ketamine. Emergence from anesthesia depends on the rate of administration and total dose of the drugs. The requirement that the patient recover rapidly from anesthesia in the ambulatory setting has somewhat limited the range of appropriate agents. Intravenous anesthetics are more controllable if given by continuous infusion. Compared with bolus administration, the "peaks and valleys" are minimized, and less total drug is used.

FENTANYL. Fentanyl is a potent synthetic narcotic. After intravenous administration, its effects are noted within 2 minutes and last 45 to 60 minutes. Termination of its effect is due to redistribution into blood and peripheral tissues. Distribution half-life is 13.4 minutes, and elimination half-life is 219 minutes. These rapid kinetics illustrate why fentanyl is the most widely used narcotic supplement in ambulatory surgery.

Fentanyl causes marked respiratory depression accompanied by decreases in PaO_2 and pH and an increase in $PaCO_2$. Respiratory depression occurs first at 30 to 60 minutes and again at a later time, which is variable. This is due to hepatobiliary secretion of fentanyl and its subsequent reabsorption from the small intestine or to redistribution of unchanged fentanyl back into the bloodstream.

Continuous infusion of fentanyl has been useful for ambulatory patients. After a loading dose of 100 μg, fentanyl is administered as a 2 μg/ml infusion at a rate of 0.1 μg/kg/min. This technique has been shown to result in a 45% decrease in the total dose of fentanyl administered compared with bolus administration.[16]

ALFENTANIL. Alfentanil is a new fentanyl analog with one-quarter the potency and one-third the duration of action of fentanyl. The pharmacokinetics of alfentanil include a rapid redistribution half-life (11.6 minutes) and an elimination half-life of 94 minutes. Termination of effect is primarily dependent on hepatic metabolism rather than redistribution, and prolongation of action after large or repeated doses should not occur. Recovery after ambulatory procedures has consistently been rapid if appropriate doses are used.

The pharmacokinetics of alfentanil suggest that it may be most effectively administered by continuous administration. Patients are given a loading dose of 250 μg to 500 μg of alfentanil, followed by an infusion of 40 μg/minute to 70 μg/minute of a 10 μg/ml solution.

NARCOTIC AGONIST–ANTAGONISTS. The narcotic agonist–antagonists butorphanol and nalbuphine have potential use in ambulatory surgery. Butorphanol is five times as potent as morphine, and nalbuphine is equipotent. Neither drug causes significant respiratory depression, and the onset of action is rapid and pleasant. Unfortunately, duration of action is long, similar to morphine; thus acceptance for ambulatory procedures has been limited.

KETAMINE. Ketamine has been used as a continuous infusion of 50 μg/kg/min after a 50-mg loading dose. A concentration of 1 mg/ml is generally used. Emergence reactions in adult patients are unpredictable; thus the use of ketamine for ambulatory patients is uncommon.

Muscle Relaxants. **SUCCINYLCHOLINE.** Succinylcholine is most frequently used to facilitate endotracheal intubation. Skeletal muscle relaxation is achieved through persistent depolarization of the muscle end-plate, which is then unable to respond to further stimulation. Structurally, succinylcholine is two acetylcholine molecules joined together, and hydrolysis by plasma pseudocholinesterase constitutes the primary metabolic pathway for terminating the neuromuscular blocking action of succinylcholine.

The usual intravenous dose of 1 mg/kg produces immediate blockade of diaphragmatic movement for 7 to 10 minutes. Succinylcholine may be used in divided doses or as a continuous intravenous drip to provide muscle relaxation for short surgical procedures. However, two potential problems arise from such practices: (1) repeated doses of succinylcholine can produce bradycardia and other cardiac arrhythmias, especially in children, and (2) cumulative doses exceeding 4 mg/kg may change the mechanism of the initial depolarizing blockade (phase 1) to a blockade not characterized by depolarization (phase 2). The mechanism of phase 2 block is not clear. Prolonged neuromuscular blockade following succinylcholine administration demands respiratory support until the patient regains muscle strength.

Prolonged succinylcholine blockade can also be the result of abnormal pseudocholinesterase, which is a heterozygous genetic problem that occurs in 1 out of 4000 patients. In addition, succinylcholine should not be administered to patients with burns, multiple trauma, or spinal cord injuries, because of the possible development of dangerous hyperkalemia.

The muscle pain experienced by patients following the administration of succinylcholine is cause for concern. It appears to be less in inpatients than in outpatients, who are awake and active sooner. The incidence may be as high as 66% and is most frequently reported in the neck and shoulder muscles.[17] There is no correlation between the intensity of fasciculations produced by succinylcholine and the severity of the postoperative myalgias. Pretreatment with a variety of drugs, including diazepam, d-tubocurarine, pancuronium, and a "self-taming" dose of succinylcholine, has been used in an attempt to decrease the incidence of myalgias. However, the incidence reported was never below 8%.[18] When these aches and pains related to anesthesia outlast the pain of surgery, they are a great source of consternation for the patient and the anesthesiologist.

Malignant hyperthermia is a potentially fatal syndrome consisting of muscle rigidity, severe combined metabolic and respiratory acidosis, and a fulminating rise in temperature. Body rigidity and a tightening of the jaws, instead of muscle relaxation, following the administration of succinylcholine may be an early sign of the syndrome. Halothane is also known to trigger the malignant hyperthermia response. Patients should be questioned about any family history of abnormal responses to anesthesia and about the existence of any neuromuscular disease that would put the patient at increased risk for malignant hyperthermia syndrome.

INTERMEDIATE-ACTING NONDEPOLARIZING RELAXANTS. Prior to 1984 the available nondepolarizing muscle relaxants, d-tubocurarine, pancuronium, metocurine, and gallamine, found limited usefulness in ambulatory surgery because of their long duration of action. The introduction of two intermediate-acting nondepolarizing muscle relaxants, atracurium and vecuronium, has offered anesthesiologists more flexibility in their choice of muscle relaxants for ambulatory patients.

Both drugs are relatively devoid of cardiovascular side-effects in their clinical dose range. Atracurium produces minimal histamine release, whereas vecuronium produces none. The drugs differ in their mode of degradation in the body. Vecuronium undergoes hepatic excretion, whereas atracurium's primary mode of elimination is through Hofmann degradation, a spontaneous breakdown at normal body temperature and pH.

Atracurium and vecuronium both provide acceptable alternatives to succinylcholine for intubation when speed is not critical. The minimal acceptable intubating dose for atracurium is 0.25 mg/kg, with doses up to 0.5 mg/kg providing good to excellent conditions. However, histamine-related side-effects increase with larger dosages. A pretreatment or "primary dose" of atracurium (0.075 mg/kg) followed by 0.3 mg/kg provides adequate intubating conditions in 2 minutes.

Vecuronium is also a safe and predictable relaxant. Used in doses of 0.1 mg/kg to 0.15 mg/kg, it provides adequate intubating conditions in about 3 minutes. This time can be shortened and the dose can be decreased by "priming" the patient with 15% of the intubating dose (0.015 mg/kg). The priming dose should be given 5 to 7 minutes before the intubating dose of 0.05 mg/kg. Another advantage of this technique is a more rapid return to baseline of the muscle twitch measurement, thus requiring less reversal of the action of the muscle relaxant by an anticholinesterase.

REVERSAL OF MUSCLE RELAXATION. It is imperative that muscle strength be adequate at the end of the procedure. If this cannot be achieved by appropriately timed dosages of muscle relaxants, chemical reversal of relaxant effect must be ensured. Reversal can be accomplished with administration of quaternary ammonium compounds that facilitate cholinergic transmission. Their actions are secondary to both anticholinesterase and direct cholinomimetic effects. An anticholinergic drug, atropine or glycopyrrolate, is administered with the facilitatory drug to minimize the muscarinic side-effects such as bradycardia and excessive salivation.

Clinically used facilitatory drugs differ in their time of onset and duration. Edrophonium (0.5 mg/kg to 1 mg/kg) has the fastest onset of action but has weaker muscarinic activity than neostigmine. Pyridostigmine has the slowest onset of activity, requiring 10 to 15 minutes to achieve adequate reversal. The dosage is 0.2 mg/kg to 0.4 mg/kg. Neostigmine (0.05 mg/kg to 0.07 mg/kg) is intermediate in its onset of action. All three drugs are cleared from the plasma at comparable rates (neostigmine, 80 minutes; pyridostigmine, 112 minutes; edrophonium, 110 minutes).

THE RECOVERY PERIOD

In no area of anesthesia is the recovery period of greater importance than in ambulatory surgery. Not only should the anesthesia be tailored to the needs of the ambulatory patient, but the nursing and medication techniques used in the primary and secondary recovery periods should encourage early return to the patient's preoperative state of well-being. The wellness of the patient should be emphasized, and he or she should be urged to return to modified normal activities as soon as appropriate.

OBJECTIVE EVALUATION OF THE RECOVERING PATIENT

Because of the need to evaluate patients who are recovering from anesthesia and surgery in an objective and consistent manner, many systems have been developed. The one most commonly used for inpatient surgery is that developed by Aldrete.[19] This list provides an easily scored evaluation performed on the patient at timed intervals during the course of his stay in the postanesthesia recovery unit. It includes evaluation of activity, respiration, circulation, consciousness, and color. Scores range from 0 to 2 for each category, and a patient must achieve a total score of 10 to be allowed to progress to secondary recovery.

A two-phase recovery system is common in ambulatory surgery centers. Primary recovery is the area in which the patient is first cared for upon returning from the operating room. Once the patient is alert and all vital signs are stable, he or she can be transferred to secondary recovery, where further recovery may take place in a relaxed atmosphere in the presence of a family member or friend. Many centers use reclining chairs in this phase to encourage a feeling of recuperation and well-being. The patient is urged to ambulate with assistance, take liquid nourishment when appropriate, and void.

Secondary recovery must be equipped to handle any patient emergencies that might arise, and a physician must be readily available at all times to evaluate recovering patients.

An anesthesiologist must discharge the patient from secondary recovery in most centers. When objective criteria have been met, the clinical judgment of the physician examining the patient becomes the single most important factor in determining the patient's home readiness. The patient is then discharged in the care of a responsible adult for transportation home and care for the next 24 hours. Prior to discharge, written instructions for postambulatory surgical care from the surgeon and anesthesiologist are reviewed with the patient and the home care provider.

CRITERIA FOR DISCHARGE HOME

1. Stable vital signs for at least one-half hour.
2. No new signs or symptoms postoperatively that may threaten a safe recovery.
3. Cessation of oozing or bleeding if bleeding was a feature of the operation.
4. No nausea or vomiting for one-half hour or evidence that nausea is decreasing.
5. Good circulation in, and return of sensation to, the operated extremity when a tourniquet has been used.
6. No evidence of swelling or impaired circulation in an extremity when a cast has been applied.
7. Voided clear urine following cystoscopy.
8. The ability to recognize time and place.
9. Little or no dizziness after changing clothes and sitting for 10 minutes.
10. Control of postoperative pain by oral analgesics.

(Phoenix SurgiCenter criteria)

MEDICATION OF THE RECOVERING PATIENT

Medication in the postoperative period must be administered in a manner different from that with inpatients if rapid recovery and discharge are to be achieved. In primary recovery, judicious use of a short-acting narcotic such as fentanyl in a 1-μg/kg to 2-μg/kg dose is usually effective. In the secondary recovery area, oral analgesics are encouraged. Long-acting narcotics such as morphine and demerol are discouraged, as they will prolong the recovery period.

COMPLICATIONS AND REASONS FOR ADMISSION

The most commonly encountered problems in the postoperative period in ambulatory surgery are nausea and vomiting, pain, drowsiness, and dizziness. Other more serious problems include bleeding, hypotension, postintubation croup, arrhythmias, perforated viscus, and other surgical misadventures. If these cannot be managed appropriately prior to discharge, the patient should be transferred to an inpatient facility.

SUMMARY

In summary, the goal of anesthesia for the ambulatory patient is to provide satisfactory anesthesia for the patient, optimal operating conditions for the surgeon, and a rapid return of the patient to his or her preoperative state. Although the manner in which these desirable conditions are achieved varies, all health care personnel involved with the patient must emphasize the patient's wellness and encourage a speedy recovery.

REFERENCES

1. Natof HE: Complications associated with ambulatory surgery. JAMA 244:1116, 1980
2. Natof HE: Ambulatory surgery: Patients with pre-existing medical problems. IMJ 166:101, 1984

3. Ong BY, Palahniuk RJ, Cumming M: Gastric volume and pH in outpatients. Can Anaesth Soc J 25:36, 1978
4. Manchikanti L, Merrero TC: Effect of cimetidine and metoclopromide on gastric contents in outpatients. Anesthesiol Rev 10:9, 1983
5. Manchikanti L, Rousch JR: Effect of preanesthetic glycopyrrolate and cimetidine on gastric fluid pH and volume in outpatients. Anesth Analg 63:40, 1984
6. Rao TLK, Madharareddy S, Chinthagada M et al: Metoclopramide and cimetidine to reduce gastric fluid pH and volume. Anesth Analg 63:1014, 1984
7. Manchikanti L, Grow JB, Colliver et al: Bicitra (sodium citrate) and metoclopramide in outpatient anesthesia for prophylaxis against aspiration pneumonitis. Anesthesiology 63:378, 1985
8. Conner JT, Herr G, Katz RL et al: Droperidol, fentanyl, and morphine for I.V. surgical premedication. Br J Anesth 50:463, 1978
9. Philip BK, Covino BG: Local and regional anesthesia. In Wetchler BV (ed): Anesthesia for Ambulatory Surgery. Philadelphia, JB Lippincott, 1985
10. Schulte-Steinburg O: Neural blockade for pediatric surgery. In Cousins MJ, Bridenbuagh PO (ed): Neural Blockade in Clinical Anesthesia and Management of Pain. Philadelphia, JB Lippincott, 1980
11. Burke RK: Spinal anesthesia for laparoscopy: A review of 1063 cases. J Reprod Med 21:59, 1978
12. Krantz EM: Low-dose intramuscular ketamine and hyaluronidase for induction of anesthesia in non-premedicated children. S Afr Med J 58:161, 1980
13. Reeve JG, Fragen RJ, Vinik HR, Greenblatt DJ: Midazolam: Pharmacology and uses. Anesthesiology 62:310, 1985
14. Giese JL, Stanley TH, Pace NL et al: Fentanyl pretreatment reduces side effects associated with etomidate anesthetic induction. Anesthesiology 59:A 320, 1983
15. White PF, Way WL, Trevor AJ: Ketamine—Its pharmacology and therapeutic uses. Anesthesiology 56:119, 1982
16. White PF: Use of continuous infusion versus intermittent bolus administration of fentanyl or ketamine during outpatient anesthesia. Anesthesiology 59:294, 1983
17. Churchill-Davidson HC: Suxamethonium (succinylcholine) chloride and muscle pains. Br Med J 74:209, 1954
18. Perry J, Wetchler BV: Outpatient anesthesia: The effects of diazepam pretreatment of succinylcholine on fasciculation or postoperative myalgia. AANA 52:48, 1984
19. Aldrete JA, Kroulik D: A postanesthetic recovery score. Anesth Analg 49:924, 1970
20. Philip BK: Supplemental medication for ambulatory procedures under regional anesthesia. Anesth Analg 64:1117, 1985
21. Wetchler BV (ed): Anesthesia for Ambulatory Surgery. Philadelphia, JB Lippincott, 1985

4 Soft-Tissue Injuries and Foreign Bodies

MARK W. WOLCOTT

SOFT-TISSUE INJURIES

Soft-tissue injuries range from abrasions to severe lacerations, puncture wounds, burns, and frostbite. Foreign bodies may be of many types and may be simple or complex.

The more severe soft-tissue injuries involving vascular structures or nerve injuries are discussed in Chapter 20.

Accurate evaluation of a soft-tissue injury is important, since only minor lacerations, contusions, or abrasions should be cared for on an ambulatory basis. Foreign bodies should also be evaluated carefully before a decision is made to attempt removal on an ambulatory basis.

CLOSED WOUNDS

Contusions

Contusions, or bruises, result from injury to the capillaries and other tissues by a blow or fall that does not break the skin. They are painful and rapidly (minutes to hours) become discolored because of capillary bleeding into the tissues.

Hematoma

A hematoma, which is a discreet collection of blood, may develop if bleeding is sufficient to disrupt the cleavage planes of the traumatized tissue or if the bleeding is in continuity with a preexisting bursa or fascial plane.

Myositis Ossificans

Occasionally, especially after repeated trauma to the thigh muscles, as in football or basketball, an indurated "tumor" may develop. Roentgenograms reveal diffuse amorphous cloudiness, and calcification occurs in the mass.

Management

Contusions. Cold compresses or an ice pack should be applied within the first hour or two of injury. After 12 to 24 hours, heat may hasten reabsorption of the blood, but if it is used too early it can add to the amount of hemorrhage and fluid extravasation.

Hematomas. If a fluctuant hematoma is present, aspiration with a large-bore, 16- to 18-gauge needle and a 20-ml syringe may reduce pain and hasten healing. Great care must be taken not to infect the hematoma. The skin is carefully prepared with antiseptic solutions such as iodine, sterile gloves are used, and the aspiration site is covered with a sterile bandage.

Occasionally, because of the large size of the hematoma or because clotting has occurred, incision and drainage under local or general anesthesia are required. In this case, packing and drainage are important. The hematoma must be opened widely, all clots removed, and the wound packed open. Daily redressing is necessary until the wound is clean, normally 4 to 7 days. If the hematoma becomes secondarily infected, it must be drained by means of an adequate incision that permits complete evacuation of the infected clot and packing of the space. Subsequently, repeated removal and replacement of the packing are necessary until the wound is clean and heals from the bottom out.

Myositis Ossificans. Occasionally a biopsy is necessary to exclude a bone tumor. Rest, minimum activity, and avoidance of further trauma usually result in slow resolution of the mass and even disappearance of the calcification over a period of months.

OPEN WOUNDS

Principles of Wound Care

Healing of wounds has a high biologic priority, and once the mechanism has started it is almost impossible to stop. The role of the surgeon in wound management is to provide an environment in which optimum healing can take place, the primary objective being to restore continuity in the least possible time with a minimum of deformity and loss of function.

Puncture Wounds

Puncture wounds are caused by nails, knives, gunshot, glass, or other relatively sharp objects. A puncture wound that has penetrated a body cavity or injured vital structures such as blood vessels and nerves must be cared for in the hospital, where close observation is possible.

A danger of puncture wounds is clostridial tetanus or other infection, because of the essentially closed nature of the wound or deep embedment of foreign material, allowing anaerobic growth of bacteria.

Management. The edges of the wound are carefully debrided by simple excision of a few millimeters of skin around the opening; the wound is irrigated with a syringe and needle and left open under a sterile dressing. Tetanus toxoid should be given. Foreign bodies should be removed in most cases. (See section on "Foreign Bodies" later in this chapter.)

Both exit and entry tracks of superficial gunshot wounds should be debrided and left open. The track does not need to be explored unless suspected of being contaminated with clothing or some other foreign material.

Lacerations

In management of a traumatic open wound the surgeon has a number of options available: primary closure, delayed primary closure, and open treatment.

Selection of the technique to be used in a specific case and the decision on using ancillary measures must be based on a thorough knowledge of the repair mechanism. A careful history should be obtained, with particular attention being paid to the time of the injury and the causative agent. Close inquiry should be made into those systemic factors that may influence healing. Careful inspection of the wound itself is absolutely necessary. The most important factor in this decision is the physician's estimate of the risk of infection—a judgment based on the preceding information. Repeated reevaluation during the course of healing may dictate a change in method.

Primary Closure. In the technique of primary closure the tissues of the wound are carefully approximated after thorough cleansing and debridement of foreign material and devitalized tissue. Most surgical incisions are managed in this fashion, and the technique can be applied to many clean accidental wounds in which the risk of infection is considered small. Closure may be by suture or Steri-Strips. Primary healing produces minimal scarring and deformity and the least functional impairment. Because of the dangers of infection in a closed space, primary closure should not be considered when there is more than minimal risk of infection. A drain should not be placed in the subcutaneous tissue of a clean wound. Careful attention to hemostasis should make drainage unnecessary; placement of such a drain to provide a route for pus to escape if infection occurs later indicates poor judgment in the choice of management technique. Paradoxically, such a drain may allow bacteria to enter and infect a wound. If the risk of infection is considered great enough to suggest use of a drain, primary closure should not be employed.

Delayed Primary Closure. Delayed primary closure is applicable to many dirty wounds. It may be used with excellent results when the degree of contamination or the delay between injury and treatment is such that the risk of infection appears high. It is the standard method of the military for most battlefield injuries. In this technique the wound is debrided and irrigated as in primary repair, but instead of being closed immediately it is carefully packed open and a sterile dressing is applied.

The wound is inspected daily, using strict precautions against infection. If by the third or fourth day there is no evidence of infection and the entire wound appears healthy without any necrosis or debris, closure is accomplished by tying previously placed sutures, preferably of wire or a monofilament synthetic. Since closure is accomplished prior to the proliferative phase of healing, no delay in healing is measurable, and repair progresses in the same fashion and with the same benefits as outlined earlier. If, however, infection or necrotic debris is evident, the technique of delayed primary closure should be abandoned and open treatment, as described later, should be employed.

Open Treatment. Open treatment is the method of choice in infected or grossly contaminated wounds and in wounds in which the presence of devitalized tissue is known or suspected. It should also be used in wounds that have been closed primarily but have later become infected. The technique is essentially that of open-wound management, and the mechanism of healing is by wound contraction, granulation tissue formation, and epithelialization. Although ultimate results in terms of function and deformity may be quite good, considerable delay in healing and formation of excess scar tissue can be anticipated with this method.

Avulsion Injuries

In avulsion injuries a segment of skin or skin and subcutaneous tissue is torn from its bed, but it is sometimes still attached by a more or less large pedicle. Often it contains foreign material and requires very careful debridement and irrigation prior to closure.

Management. (Management is essentially the same as that for lacerations.)

1. If the edges are viable, simply suturing the skin back to its original position suffices.
2. It is usually not wise to trim thinned-out edges and use as a split graft.
3. Large U-shaped avulsion flaps usually cannot be sutured back successfully. Several buried interrupted sutures, working from the base outward, starting at the base of the pedicle and drawing together subcutaneous tissue and the flap, help prevent contracture.
4. With large avulsions in which there is tissue loss a split-thickness graft of moderate thickness can be used to fill in the noncovered space.
5. Advancement of rotational or bilobed flaps should be utilized rarely, if ever, and then only in a hospitalized patient.

Placement of a simple pressure dressing over a petrolatum-gauze dressing completes the procedure.

Anesthesia. Adequate anesthesia can be obtained by infiltration of procaine, lidocaine, or another suitable anesthetic into the wound margins. The same agents can be used to obtain a field block of the area or a regional nerve block. A regional block is of considerable value in management of traumatic wounds, particularly of the upper extremity and face, because of the danger of spreading contamination from the wound to the surrounding tissue is eliminated. Experience and skill in its use are required, however, and sufficient time must be allowed for the block to become fully effective. General sedation and administration of analgesics may be indicated in certain patients, but general anesthesia is seldom necessary.

ADJUNCTIVE MEASURES IN WOUND MANAGEMENT

Dressings, Bandages, and Splints

Sound wound management in an ambulatory patient includes proper use of dressings, bandages, and splints. A plain dry dressing of sterile gauze held in place by adhesive tape is suitable for most simple wounds treated by primary closure. The main purpose of such a dressing is to protect the wound, and therefore it must be fastened securely so that it is not displaced before the patient's next visit to the physician. In addition, the dressing absorbs any oozing from the wound and serves to splint the area to some degree. A nonadherent layer of Telfa gauze or petrolatum gauze should be used next to the wound in abrasions and fresh skin grafts. A bulky dressing should then be applied to absorb exudate. Fine mesh gauze is used next to exposed tissue in preparation for delayed primary closure, with an overlying protective and absorptive bulky dressing.

Wet dressings are used primarily in the management of open wounds, particularly if inflammation is present (see Chapter 8). To be maximally effective they must be changed at least four times a day. Most patients and their families can be instructed to use the proper aseptic technique for ambulatory management. Sterile saline (2 teaspoonfuls of table salt in 1 quart of water boiled for 15 minutes and allowed to cool) is the simplest and safest solution. Dakin's solution is useful when debridement of patchy areas of necrotic tissue is necessary, but the solution should be diluted and the skin edges protected with Vaseline gauze if any irritation occurs. For maximum debridement effect, dressings should be applied wet and removed without remoistening. If debridement is not necessary, remoistening prior to a dressing change usually prevents additional trauma to the wound and unnecessary discomfort to the patient.

Bandages of gauze, cloth, or elastic material may be used for additional fixation of dressings, partial immobilization, or compression. Splints of plaster, wood, metal, or other rigid material may be used for further immobilization. This is particularly indicated when a wound is located in proximity to a joint and would be subject to excessive motion. Slings and crutches are valuable protective devices for wounds of the upper and lower extremities, respectively.

Heat

The use of heat is a valuable adjunct in the management of inflammation. A well-insulated and well-padded electric heating pad is excellent for this purpose. Local application of heat increases local blood flow, local metabolic activity, and phagocytosis, aiding the body defense mechanisms and repair process. Caution must be observed to avoid excessive heat, particularly in the aged and the very young. Application of heat is contraindicated in areas of circulatory impairment.

Elevation

Elevation of an injured part, usually an extremity, is effective in limiting the edema associated with trauma or inflammation: Circulation is improved and healing aided. It is of particular importance in injuries involving the lower extremity and increases in value with the extent of the injury; with the patient recumbent the extremity is raised above the level of the heart and supported with pillows.

Antibiotics

Routine prophylactic use of antibiotics in patients with clean wounds is to be condemned except where a prosthetic foreign body has been implanted. Use in situations in which body defense mechanisms are impaired, however, is certainly justified. Prophylactic antibiotic treatment of dirty wounds is still controversial, but clinical experience and experimental evidence tend to support it in many injuries of this type. Administration of antibiotics does not, however, substitute for strict adherence to proper wound care. An infected wound surrounded with cellulitis is a clear indication for systemic antibiotic therapy. Cultures should always be obtained prior to institution of antibiotic treatment. Broad-spectrum drugs should be used at least until culture results are obtained.

Enzyme Treatment

There is no evidence that oral or intramuscular administration of various enzymes has any beneficial effect on wound healing; therefore it cannot be recommended.

Topical use of proteolytic enzymes to aid in the debridement of necrotic debris in open wounds is also controversial. It has been our experience that careful surgical debridement and proper dressing techniques are at least as effective as proteolytic enzymes in aiding natural mechanisms, and enzyme therapy neither offers additional benefit nor substitutes for good surgical management.

FOREIGN BODIES

GENERAL CONSIDERATIONS

Foreign bodies in soft tissues present many problems in the treatment of ambulatory patients.

The first is infection in the primary wound. Almost all wounds due to foreign bodies have the potential for infection, and because of the small wound of entrance, tetanus bacilli and the common pyogenic organisms must be considered likely invaders. Tetanus prophylaxis should be routine, therefore, in the primary management of soft-tissue foreign bodies.

The second problem is whether to remove the foreign body. When it has entered the tissues recently, it is easily located and accessible. In such instances removal is usually attempted. If, however, no symptoms are produced and removal would entail an operation that might do more harm than the presence of the foreign body in the tissues, it may be better to let it remain. This is a matter of careful judgment, and the patient must be informed. Many foreign bodies, especially metallic ones, may become encysted by scar tissue and give no symptoms whatever. At any time, however, as a result of trauma or latent infection, the encysted body may become painful and demand treatment. The patient must be told if a foreign body is not going to be removed. It is good to remember that a foreign body may migrate and later lead to serious problems such as nerve injury, injury to tendons, and so on. For these reasons, and often the peace of mind of the patient, most foreign bodies should be removed.

When the decision is made to remove a foreign body, the foreign body must be located in the tissues. This may not be difficult if the object can be palpated or if it is relatively large and the wound of entrance is plainly visible. When the foreign body is small and located deep in fat or muscle, removal is difficult, particularly when it cannot be definitely localized in the tissues with reference to some point on the skin surface. This is especially true of small sharp-pointed objects such as needles or parts of needles, which may move in the tissues as a result of pressure or the movement of tendons and muscle.

In localizing a foreign body in the soft tissues by roentgenography, a point on the skin is selected that can be identified later. The wound of entrance, if visible, is usually the point chosen, since it is identified easily at the time of operation. If the wound of entrance has already healed, however, some other point on the skin may be selected and marked with silver nitrate in the region in which the foreign body appears to be located. This makes a black stain that lasts for several days. The head half of a pin is placed on the skin with a small piece of adhesive, the head being located at the site of the wound of entrance or on the silver nitrate dot. The part is then immobilized with a split. Wooden splints are best because they are radiolucent. Roentgen films are then exposed in the anteroposterior and lateral positions, and the location of the foreign body in relation to the wound of entrance may be determined definitely, its distance from the skin surface may be seen, and its direction in the tissues may be ascertained. The splint should be left in place until the time of operation. This is very important because if movement of the part is permitted, the foreign body may move to a different place in the tissues and the orientation value of the roentgenograms may be lost. Thus after a roentgenogram has been obtained of a foreign body in the foot the patient should not be permitted to walk before the operation. Computed tomography is an extremely valuable new tool for localizing foreign bodies, especially wood, which has a density close to tissue and is often not identified by routine x-ray, tomography, or ultrasound. In the current highly litigious society the nearly routine use of x-rays when a foreign body may be present is wise.

There are several important aids to operative removal of a foreign body. First, the field should be absolutely bloodless. When the foreign body is in an extremity, hemostasis is best obtained by using a tourniquet. Use of an Esmarch bandage prior to application of the tourniquet further assures a bloodless field. When tourniquets cannot be used, administration of a local anesthetic plus epinephrine aids visualization very materially by keeping the field dry. The tension produced by retraction of the tissues also helps to prevent the slight ooze that may come from the capillaries or the veins.

Second, although general anesthesia is usually not necessary in the removal of foreign bodies, adequate local anesthesia is imperative. Block anesthesia is often preferred to local infiltration anesthesia because tissue edema is not associated with it. On the other hand, if the foreign body is superficial, local infiltration anesthesia can be used without difficulty.

Third, localization of the foreign body as described earlier using fixed points, good radiography or CT scans, splints (of wood) when radiologic localization is necessary can be essential so that no movement occurs from the time between x-ray and surgery.

Fourth, the intraoperative use of portable imaging devices at times can be most helpful.

Finally, selection of the proper incision is important. The incision must be made so as to permit adequate exposure and easy removal of the foreign body. Also, the underlying tissues must be considered so that the wound will not be made where it will damage important structures. When possible, the wound is made to cross the axis of the foreign body transversely. This is especially helpful in locating foreign bodies deep in fatty or muscular tissue. If the wound of entrance can be located it frequently is possible to enlarge it, with the direction taken by the foreign body being known from the roentgen film. In many cases of recent entrance of a foreign body, an area of blood stain can be traced to the site of the body in the tissue. The operative procedure is discussed in greater detail in discussion of the various types of foreign bodies encountered.

TYPES OF FOREIGN BODIES

Wood Splinters

Wood splinters are very common foreign bodies in soft tissues. They are found in any part of the body, but most frequently in the hands, feet, and buttocks. Most often, the foreign body is a piece of floor or other board that has been exposed to all sorts of bacterial contamination. Toothpicks are also common. Therefore the potential of such wounds becoming infected is high, and the danger of tetanus is especially great. As a rule, the wound of entrance is so large and the pain so marked that the patient seeks treatment immediately. Roentgenography is usually not employed to locate the splinter because wood is not radiopaque unless it has been painted (Fig. 4-1). Computed tomography is often quite helpful and has been shown to be superior to xeroradiography or sonography. Conservative treatment in this type of case is most dangerous. If the foreign body can be removed easily and early and the entire wound excised, the wound can be sutured primarily, and healing with primary union can be expected. If an attempt is made to incise the skin conservatively at the wound of entrance and to pull out the splinter, there is considerable danger that bits of splinter will be left in the wound, with resulting certainty of prolonged infection. Adequate incision is therefore desirable.

When a splinter is superficial and lies more or less parallel to the skin surface, it is wise to infiltrate the area around the wound of entrance and along the course of the foreign body with procaine solution. The entire wound of entrance is excised, and after the skin is divided over the line of the splinter, good retraction is obtained to permit exposure of the entire foreign body in the tissues. Every part of the bed of the splinter should be visible, and the fatty tissues in which it lies should be completely excised. If this comparatively radical procedure is carried out early, the wound may be irrigated with saline and closed primarily with a good prospect that primary healing will occur. In this treatment, of course, tetanus toxoid and/or tetanus immune

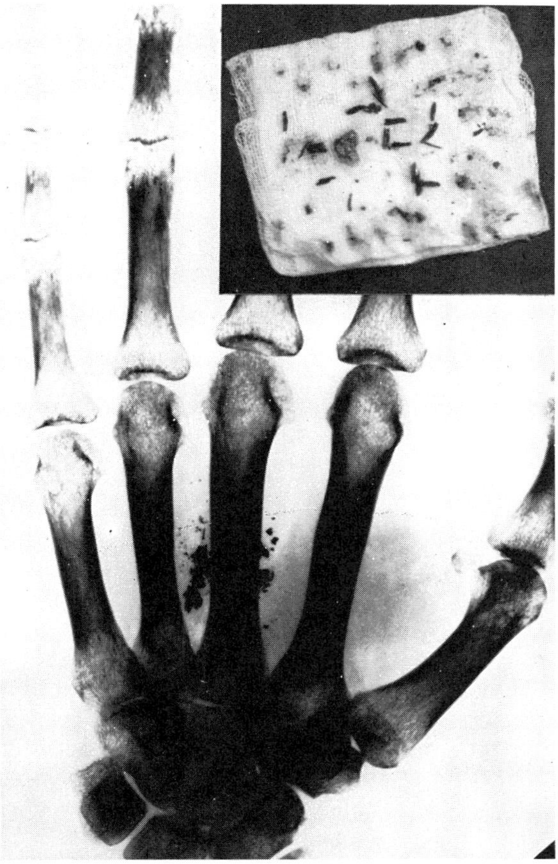

Figure 4-1. Painted wood produces a roentgen shadow. The removed splinters are shown on the gauze sponge.

globulin (human) must be administered as a prophylactic measure. (See Chapter 9 for tetanus prophylaxis.)

Splinters under the fingernail are treated by excision of that portion of the nail that overlies the splinter. This usually can be performed without anesthesia; the scalpel area of nail over the splinter is excised (Fig. 4-2). By this method the entire splinter may be removed and an anaerobic wound converted into an aerobic one. A simple finger dressing is all that is necessary until the wound is healed.

Rees reported an ingenious method for removal of foreign bodies such as needles, thorns, and splinters that break off under the dermis at nearly a right angle to the surface of the skin. Such objects are often difficult to remove because the incision may pass on one side or the other of the foreign body, and it is difficult to determine on which side it lies.

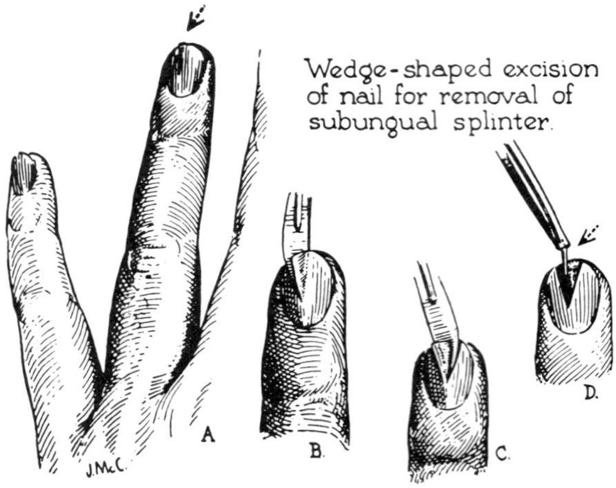

Figure 4-2. Excision of a portion of the nail for removal of a subungual splinter.

Rees suggested that the incision be made only through the skin and that the skin then be undercut on all sides for a distance of about 0.25 inch. In this way the fatty tissue in which the foreign body lies is not disturbed, and by exertion of pressure on the sides of the wound the fat may be extruded into the wound, bearing the foreign body with it (Fig. 4-3). Excision of the fat containing the foreign body is advised rather than simple removal of the object. When the foreign body projects at the skin surface, Rees makes an elliptical incision centered on the entrance wound. Removal of the elliptical piece of skin in the center then shows the exact location of the foreign body, which may be removed as described earlier (Fig. 4-4). In such exploration for foreign material he advised that local anesthesia be produced not by infiltration but by means of a field block around the area in which the foreign body is believed to lie. In this way the thickening of the tissues by edema is avoided.

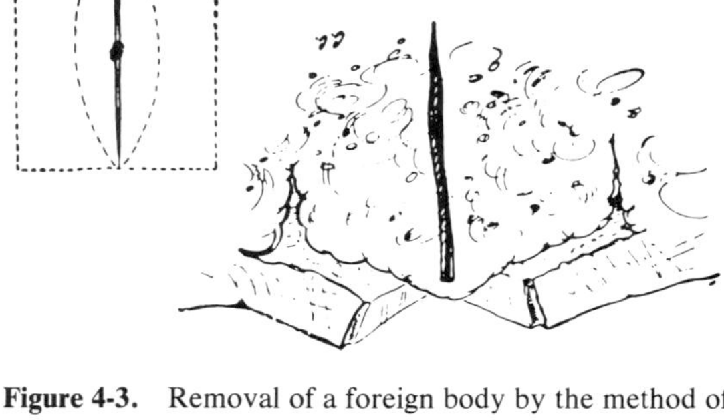

Figure 4-3. Removal of a foreign body by the method of Rees (see text for description).

Steel Splinters

Steel splinters are frequently seen in those who have been hammering on chisels or other metal objects. These splinters may enter the tissues at any point, and because of their small size are often unnoticed by the patient, except for a slight sting at the time of wounding. Later some bleeding may be observed, which calls the patient's attention to the tiny wound. When such a history is obtained, one can be almost certain that a small foreign body is embedded in the tissues, and a roentgen film will demonstrate it. A metal splinter entering the tissues in this way may be embedded very deeply and is especially difficult to find. Furthermore, the heat that is generated by the pounding may render it sterile. The question then is whether it is advisable to remove it. Occasionally, when a splinter lies deep, it may be better surgical judgment to leave it. On the other hand, if the splinter lies superficially under the skin and removal is easy, an operation for its extraction should be performed. A lesion due to this type of foreign body should be examined to ascertain if there is injury to important structures; (e.g., severed tendons or nerves). Frequently, although the skin opening is relatively minor, rather serious difficulty may be produced in the deeper tissues.

Cinders, Coal, and Stone

Cinders, bits of coal, stone, and similar materials are foreign bodies commonly found in the tissues in accidental wounds, especially in children. Often their presence is not recognized at the time the primary wound is treated; as a result they lie embedded in the tissues for

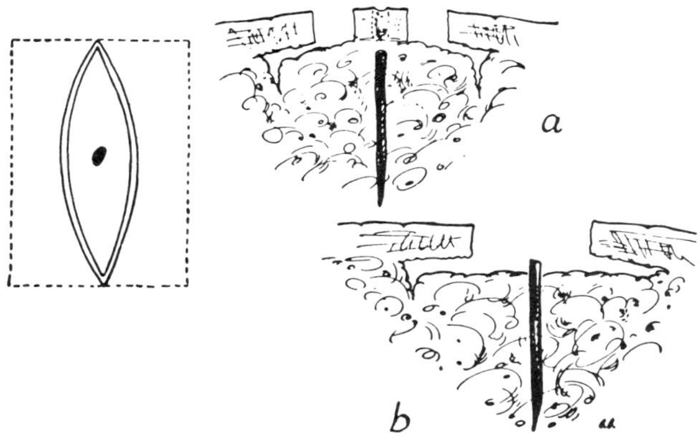

Figure 4-4. Removal of a contaminated foreign body by the method of Rees (see text for description).

a considerable time. As a rule they are not embedded very deeply, but because they carry with them considerable amounts of infective material, they almost always cause local infections. Although the primary wound apparently has been treated adequately, the embedded foreign body produces a chronic draining sinus. This is so common that we have come to suspect that any traumatic wound that continues to drain septic material has a foreign body in it. Investigation of such a wound with a needle or other searching object frequently locates the embedded object. When the wound is incised and the foreign material is removed, healing takes place rapidly.

Clothing

Bits of clothing frequently occur as foreign bodies. They have the same potential for causing infection as other foreign materials. The possibility that clothing has become embedded in the tissues is often overlooked. Cloth is not radiopaque; hence roentgenograms do not reveal its presence. Puncture wounds through sneakers, for example, can carry a minute piece of rubber into the depths of the wound and are not seen on x-ray. A search should be made for such foreign bodies.

Sutures

With a surgical wound that becomes infected and where there is a small draining area, the possibility that a suture is acting as a foreign body must be kept in mind. Silk sutures are the worst offenders; next are large catgut knots. Search for possible sutures may be facilitated by use of a small crochet hook, sterilized and inserted into the wound. It is often possible to catch the offending suture with the hook and draw it out of the wound. Healing then takes place.

Glass

Broken glass is a common foreign body. It is seen most frequently in the hands and fingers, the result of breaking a glass object in the hands. In automobile accidents glass from the shattered windshield may be found anywhere in the body, frequently in the forehead and face. It is also often found in the feet. Diagnostic difficulty arises frequently because the patient does not know whether the glass has simply cut him or has remained embedded in the tissues. Palpation of the wound frequently gives no indication. A roentgenogram is usually worthwhile when embedded glass is suspected. Many types of glass show on the roentgen film, especially glass from a windshield. Unless the glass can be seen, palpated, or demonstrated on the roentgen film, it is usually wise to treat the wound primarily as a laceration. After healing has occurred, glass makes itself evident by the pain produced by pressure on it. An incision can then be made over the painful spot and the glass removed. In an operation for removal of bits of glass from the tissues, absolute hemostasis is necessary because glass is seen with a great deal of difficulty even under the best conditions.

Fish Bones

Fish bones are radiopaque and therefore can be demonstrated on a roentgen film. They are usually not deeply embedded in the tissues and are almost invariably in the hands or fingers. Removal is usually easy because they can be well localized. Instead of suturing the wound it is wise to leave it open and to treat it as a primary infection.

Needles

A needle or parts of needles of various sorts are common foreign bodies in the hands and feet. These are among the most difficult foreign bodies to localize because they are small and, in the feet at least, are frequently embedded in the fatty adipose tissue. Accurate localization is the secret to their removal. They are best located through an incision designed to cross transversely the long axis of the object. Most needles after they have been in the tissue for a time become oxidized and black and therefore are seen fairly easily if the field is bloodless. If the incision is made along the line of entrance of the needle, it has been found that frequently a dark-stained area of hemorrhage can be followed.

I have rarely found it necessary to use a fluoroscope to locate a needle in the hands or feet, where they are most commonly embedded. A needle occasionally embedded in other parts of the body, however, is removed with a great deal of difficulty, and a fluoroscope is a considerable aid.

Occasionally a hypodermic needle breaks off in the subcutaneous tissues. The danger from this type of foreign body is not great because most needles of this type are sterile. Nevertheless, removal is usually attempted if it can be done easily. Diabetics who administer their own insulin often break a needle in the thigh. Removal is very difficult unless it can be well localized in the soft tissues. It may be wiser to leave it in place rather than to attempt excision.

Bullets

Various types of bullets are often embedded in the tissues. When they are of a very large caliber, in most cases the foreign body has penetrated so deeply and has caused so much damage that the patient should be admitted to the hospital for care. On the other hand, small shot (BB or bird shot) may be embedded only superficially in the tissues and the patient may be ambulant. These foreign bodies are radiopaque, and their localization by roentgen examination is therefore comparatively easy. Recently the development of aluminum-jacketed ammunition has made localization of the bullet more difficult, since such bullets are only faintly radiopaque and can be missed. In many cases the heat generated by the firing of the gun and passage of the bullet through the air renders such foreign bodies relatively sterile; thus when they are inaccessible, removal may be delayed until it is determined whether it is going to cause any trouble.

Fishhooks

Fishhooks are occasionally embedded in the soft tissues, usually in the fingers. Because of the barb, removal is difficult, but this may be accomplished by pushing the point through the remaining portion of the soft tissues, cutting off the barbed portion of the hook with pliers, and then withdrawing the hook in the direction from which it entered. The wound can be treated with hot moist dressings until the danger from infection is past. If the hook is small, another technique is to tie a suture around the curve of the hook and then, while constant traction is maintained on the fish line still attached to the eye of the hook, jerk the newly placed suture upward, which causes the hook to pop out. A little anesthetic is placed around the barb first, of course.

BIBLIOGRAPHY

Anderson MA, Newmeyer WL, Kilgore ES: Diagnosis and treatment of retained foreign bodies in the hand. Am J Surg 144:63, 1986

Bauer RA: Computed tomography: Localization of wooden foreign bodies in childrens' extremities. Arch Surg 118:1064, 1983

Bernard CW, Herrman JB, Woodward SC, Pulaski EJ: Healing of incisions closed with surgical adhesive tape. Am J Surg 107:591, 1964

Bernardino ME et al: The extremity soft tissue lesion: A comparative study of ultrasound, computed tomography and xeroradiography. Diagn Radiol 139:53–59, 1986

Boswick JA: Wound care. Postgrad Med 55:171–177, 1974

Connolly WB, Hunt TK, Zederfeldt B, Cafferata HT, Dunphy JE: Clinical comparison of surgical wounds closed by suture and adhesive tapes. Am J Surg 117:318–322, 1969

Conradi S: New aluminum-jacketed ammunition. Am J Forensic Med Pathol 3:153, 1982

Craig EV: Delayed laceration of ulnar nerve following hand trauma. JAMA 253:1014, 1985

Emerson EB: Fishhooks. NY State Med 2414–2416, 1966

Howells CHL, Young HB: A study of completely undressed surgical wounds. Br J Surg 53:436–439, 1969

Hudspeth AS: Elimination of wound infection by delayed primary closure. South Med J 66:934–936, 1973

Kuhns LR et al: An *in-vitro* comparison of computed tomography, exroradiography and radiography in the detection of soft-tissue foreign bodies. Radiography 132:218–219, 1979

Lawrence RR: Infection and healing in superficial wounds. Calif Med 100:100, 328, 1964

Lehr HB, Fitts WT: The management of avulsion injuries of soft tissues. J Trauma 9:261–273, 1969

Nichols RL: Use of prophylactic antibiotics in surgical practice. Am J Med 70:686–692, 1981

5 Burns and Frostbite

GLENN D. WARDEN

BURNS

Burns are the destructive changes occurring in tissue due to excessive heat, chemicals, ultraviolet radiation, and other agents. Small burns, generally treated on an outpatient basis, constitute approximately 95% of all burns treated in the United States. These burns are generally superficial and rarely exceed 8% to 10% of the body surface area and rarely require hospitalization.

Although survival is usually not an issue and most minor burns ultimately heal regardless of therapy, undertreatment and, more commonly, overtreatment may result in infection or delay in healing with discomfort and prolonged morbidity. The goals of outpatient burn management include wound healing, patient comfort, and rapid rehabilitation.

SEVERITY OF BURN INJURY

In ambulatory patients, one must treat only relatively minor burns. The more serious aspects of burns—shock, hypermetabolism, and other serious disturbances—cannot be well cared for in all ambulatory patients. The seriousness of thermal injury can be defined by the following factors: (1) extent, (2) depth, (3) location, (4) age, (5) general health, and (6) cause. The extent of the injury is related to the total area of burn. Estimation of the total surface area burned is necessary for immediate fluid replacement and for determining the severity of thermal injury. Even in minor burns an accurate estimation of the surface area is mandatory. The rule of nines is an accurate means of estimating body surface in individuals more than nine years of age; however, the Lund and Browder chart should be available in every emergency room and should be used in children under 10 years of age to correct for the greater surface area of the head and the lesser surface area of the lower extremities (Fig. 5-1).

Burns have classically been divided into first, second, and third degrees, according to depth. In first-degree burns, tissue destruction is superficial, involving only the epidermis. There is local pain and erythema without blister formation, and systemic response is mild to absent. First-degree burns require no treatment except large burns of infants or the elderly; however, various antiseptic and anesthetic ointments have been recommended and used for years. Oily ointments that exclude air from the burned area may give considerable relief. Incorporation of an anesthetic agent into the ointment, however, is not recommended, for it can be toxic if large areas are treated. First-degree burns usually result from contact with hot fluids or from exposure to sun lamps, sunlight, or an ultraviolet lamp. Occasionally they are secondary to flash burns due to an explosion.

Second-degree burns are now divided into superficial partial-thickness injury and deep partial-thickness injury. Superficial partial-thickness burns involve only the epidermis and dermis. The wounds appear red and are moist. There is blister formation, and the tactile and pain sensors are intact. Superficial partial-thickness burns are extremely painful since the pain sensors are intact. Superficial partial-thickness burns heal in 14 to 21 days with minimal scarring. They are generally caused by flash, scalds, or brief contact with hot objects. Deep partial-thickness burns involve the entire epidermis and dermis, leaving only the skin appendages, the hair follicles, and the sebaceous glands intact. In contrast to superficial partial-thickness burn, these injuries have a mottled appearance with larger areas of waxy-white injury. The surface is dry and anesthetic. Clinically it is difficult to distinguish deep partial-thickness from full-thickness injury; however, a deep partial-thickness

BURN ESTIMATE AND DIAGRAM
Age vs. Area

Area	Birth 1 yr.	1-4 yr.	5-9 yr.	10-14 yr.	15 yr.	Adult	2°	3°	Total	Donor Areas
Head	19	17	13	11	9	7				
Neck	2	2	2	2	2	2				
Ant. Trunk	13	13	13	13	13	13				
Post. Trunk	13	13	13	13	13	13				
R. Buttock	2½	2½	2½	2½	2½	2½				
L. Buttock	2½	2½	2½	2½	2½	2½				
Genitalia	1	1	1	1	1	1				
R. U. Arm	4	4	4	4	4	4				
L. U. Arm	4	4	4	4	4	4				
R. L. Arm	3	3	3	3	3	3				
L. L. Arm	3	3	3	3	3	3				
R. Hand	2½	2½	2½	2½	2½	2½				
L. Hand	2½	2½	2½	2½	2½	2½				
R. Thigh	5½	6½	8	8½	9	9½				
L. Thigh	5½	6½	8	8½	9	9½				
R. Leg	5	5	5½	6	6½	7				
L. Leg	5	5	5½	6	6½	7				
R. Foot	3½	3½	3½	3½	3½	3½				
L. Foot	3½	3½	3½	3½	3½	3½				
						TOTAL				

Cause of Burn ____________________

Date of Burn ____________

Time of Burn ____________

Age ____________

Sex ____________

Weight ____________

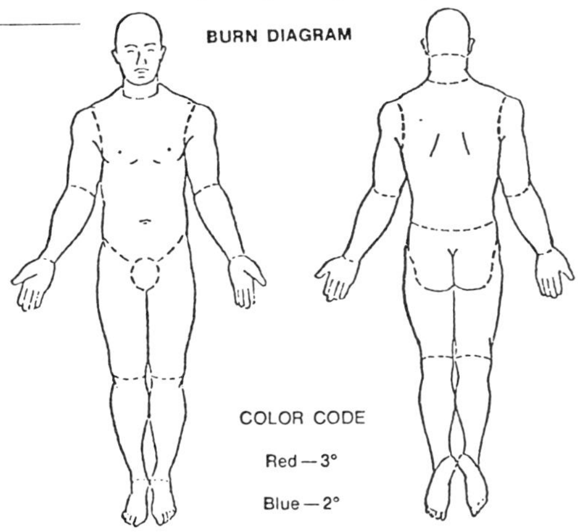

Figure 5-1. Chart for estimating body surface burn.

burn will heal spontaneously in about 4 to 6 weeks. The deep partial-thickness burn, however, heals with unstable epithelium, late hypertrophic scarring, and marked contracture formation. The current treatment for this injury dictates excision and skin grafting.

Third-degree or full-thickness burns involve the epidermis, dermis, and underlying subcutaneous tissue. The wounds appear white, cherry red, or black and may or may not contain deep blisters. Frequently thrombosed veins are visible. The elasticity of the dermis is destroyed, giving the wound a dry, hard, leathery appearance. Marked edema and decreased elasticity may necessitate removal of eschar from circumferential deep partial-thickness injuries and full-thickness burns. Ironically, full-thickness burns are painless and are completely anesthetic. Full-thickness burns require skin grafting if larger than 2.5 cm or if in an area of potential cosmetic deformity. A full-thickness injury is generally caused by flame, high-intensity flash, chemicals, electricity, or prolonged contact with the source of heat.

The location of the burn is extremely important in regard to severity, with the critical areas being the eyes, ears, face, hands, feet, and perineum. Other factors that influence severity include age, associated major trauma, inhalation injury, or health status.

The cause of the burn is also important, for a small burn may be associated with severe inhalation injury or, if the wound was second-

TABLE 5-1. Modified ABA Injury Severity Grading System

	DEPTH			COMPLICATIONS	
	Second Degree				
MAGNITUDE OF BURN INJURY	Adult (% BSA)	Children (% BSA)	Third Degree (% BSA)	Special Location	Poor Risk, Trauma, Fx
Major	>25	>20	10 or >	+	+
Moderate	15–25	10–20	<10	−	−
Minor	<15	<10	< 2	−	−
	< 5	< 5	< 1	+	−

(Edlich RF et al: Modification of American Burn Association Injury Severity Grading System. JACEP 7:226, 1978)

ary to electrical injury, the entrance and exit sites may be extremely small. There may be underlying muscle necrosis.

A modification of the American Burn Association injury severity grading system (Table 5-1) defines the group of thermally injured patients who may be treated as outpatients. A second-degree burn that involves less than 15% of the total body surface in an adult and less than 10% in a child may be treated on an outpatient basis. Third-degree burns covering less than 2% of the body, and excluding those involving critical areas—namely, the eyes, ears, face, hands, feet, and perineum—can also be treated outside the hospital. Burns due to electricity, smoke injury, and inhalation, and burns complicated by other major trauma should be treated in a burn center. Poor-risk burn patients should be hospitalized. Individuals with burns involving critical areas but covering less than 5% of the total body surface and those with third-degree burns covering less than 1% may be treated as outpatients.

TREATMENT AT THE SCENE OF THE ACCIDENT

At the scene of the accident, after elimination of the heat source, areas with minor burns should be placed in tepid water rather than ice water. The burn area should be wrapped in a clean towel and the victim taken to an emergency facility. The potential benefits of cooling burn wounds are controversial. It has been suggested that such beneficial effects, if they do exist, last only for the first two or three minutes following thermal injuries, and the application of ice water following this initial period may result in prolonged edema and impairment of healing and may convert a partial-thickness injury to full-thickness injury.

Chemical burns should be irrigated with copious amounts of water. Tar burns should be cooled with water, but the tar should not be removed at the scene of the accident.

Initial Medical Management

A protocol for immediate wound care in the emergency room or outpatient facility is mandatory for efficiency in treating thermal injury that is often characterized by panic, confusion, and a multiplicity of approaches. An accurate history of the burn should include when and where the accident occurred and the burning agent (e.g., flame, hot liquid, electricity). The history should also elicit any possibility of smoke inhalation injury. Evaluation for possible associated injuries, depending on the circumstances of the accident, is also important. Pertinent past medical history, including drug allergies, medication history, and history of systemic illnesses, should also be obtained at this time.

Tetanus prophylaxis is the same for minor burns as for any other injury. A tetanus toxoid booster is given for any patient who has not received one for 10 years or who cannot recall the date of last immunization. Patients not previously immunized should receive 250 units of tetanus human immune globulin and the first of a series of active immunization with tetanus toxoid.

Burn wounds may be soaked in tepid water or covered with saline-soaked sponges, which decrease the pain until the physician can evaluate the patient. However, it must be stressed that ice water should not be used. The wounds should be washed with mild soap and warm water, excessive debris trimmed, and hair shaved within margins of at least 1 inch around the burn wound.

The removal of tar and asphalt is best accomplished with the use of Medisol (Orange-Sol, Inc., Chandler, AZ), a citrus and petroleum distillate with hydrocarbon structure that consists of 70% petroleum distillate (base oil),

25% to 27% limonene (orange oil), 2% to 3% lanolin, and 1% surfactant (dioctyl sodium sulfosuccinate). This product has proved to be the most efficient in removing tar without damaging the underlying burn wound. Mineral oil and petroleum ointments, such as bacitracin and Neosporin (Burroughs-Wellcome, Research Triangle Park, NC), may also be used to remove tar. The tar should not be peeled off because of potential damage to the hair and skin incorporated in the tar.

Chemical burns should be irrigated with water for 20 minutes, if this was not done previously at the scene. A neutralizing agent should not be applied, as the neutralizing reaction is always exothermic (heat producing) and can result in a more severe injury.

Debridement of blisters is controversial. Blisters may be managed in three ways: (1) the blister may be left intact and the underlying wound allowed to heal in the blister fluid environment; (2) the blister fluid can be evaluated and the overlying skin allowed to cover the underlying wound; or (3) the blister may be debrided. The technique that is used depends not only on the location and size of the blister, but also on the social status of the patient. If there is a question of reliability of a patient or of the potential infection of the wound, it is generally more practical and safer to debride the blister.

After the wound is cleansed and debrided, the extent and depth of injury and areas involved are estimated. If the burn is minor, the patient can be treated as an outpatient. If there is any question regarding the social feasibility of outpatient management, it is safer to admit the patient to the hospital for 24 to 48 hours, after which outpatient management can be accomplished if everything is favorable.

Follow-up Wound Care

Wound care and follow-up of minor thermal injury remain controversial. Probably no wound in surgery has more "voodoo" associated with its management than the treatment of the minor burn wound. Both public and medical personnel have a marked fear of burn injury. The problems associated with major thermal injury are frequently extrapolated erroneously to the minor burn wound. Minor burn injury is not associated with immunosuppression, hypermetabolism, or increased susceptibility to infection. A useful philosophy of care is that minor burn injuries are very similar to abrasions and should be treated as such. Basic principles include keeping the wound clean and in a moist environment while the wound heals. Powerful topical chemotherapeutic agents, such as mafenide acetate (Sulfamylon, Winthrop-Breon Laboratories, New York, NY), silver sulfadiazine (Silvadene, Marion Laboratories, Kansas City, MO), or providone-iodine (Betadine, Purdue Frederick Company, Norwalk, CT) should not be applied to minor burn wounds, since they have been shown to delay wound healing. They were introduced to prevent burn wound sepsis in major thermal injuries. In addition, systemic antibiotics are rarely indicated in small burns and may predispose the wound to later opportunistic infection with bacteria, fungi, or viruses.

The follow-up care should include (1) washing the wound with bland soap and water in a bathtub or shower; (2) patting the wound dry with a clean towel; (3) applying a bland ointment, such as bacitracin, and a nonstick porous gauze, such as Adaptic (Johnson & Johnson, New Brunswick, NJ), then wrapping the wound lightly with gauze rolls (Kerlex, Kendall, Boston, MA). This regimen is performed twice daily (see "Guidelines for Burn Management in the Emergency Room").

Initially, follow-up may be performed daily if there is some question regarding the extent or depth of the wound or the reliability of the patient or his family. However, generally with education, the patient is followed at weekly intervals in the burn clinic.

As in major thermal injury, the patient with a minor burn is instructed in a vigorous program of range-of-motion exercises. Prolonged edema is a deterrent to wound healing and may be minimized with adequate physical therapy. Rehabilitation time may also be decreased with an active exercise program.

If the wounds are deep partial- or full-thickness burns, the patient may still be treated as an outpatient until primary excision and grafting can be performed. In children, the thickness of the epidermis and dermis is decreased, and thus the depth of injury is difficult to determine. If there is any question regarding depth of injury, the wounds are treated conservatively for 10 to 14 days before performance of excision and grafting.

In order to obtain satisfactory results, the burn wound should be totally epithelialized in 2 to 3 weeks. In general, a prediction of wound

GUIDELINES FOR BURN MANAGEMENT IN THE EMERGENCY ROOM

Classification

1. Burns less than 15% in adults; 10% in children.
2. No serious involvement of critical areas.
3. No respiratory injury.

Scene of Accident

1. Place under tepid water.
2. Wrap in clean towel and proceed to emergency facility.

Emergency Room

1. Soak in tepid water.
2. Cleanse wound with bland soap and water.
3. Shave hair in areas of, and adjacent to burns.
4. Debride or evacuate all blisters and remove dead tissue.
5. Wound Care. Apply bland ointment (Bacitracin, Mycitracin, Neosporin, Vaseline, etc.) and wrap with Kerlex.

Follow-up Care

1. Twice daily wash with bland soap and water, apply bland ointment, and wrap with Kerlex.
2. Return to clinic, office or physical therapy every four to five days.
3. Encourage vigorous range of motion exercises.

healing can be made by 14 days postinjury. If the wounds are not healing within this time period, then primary excision and grafting should be performed. Waiting for eschar separation and formation of granulation tissue delays wound closure, prolongs wound healing, and results in increased scarring and prolonged rehabilitation time.

A superficial partial-thickness injury should be followed until epithelial coverage has been obtained and then examined at 6 weeks for evidence of hypertrophic scarring. If hypertrophic scarring occurs, compression dressings should be fitted and worn until the wound becomes quiescent, which usually requires 12 to 18 months. A problem in a healed burn is the formation of very thin water blisters, which occur as a result of minor trauma. These blisters, which rarely exceed 1 cm, occur 2 to 6 weeks following wound closure and leave small open areas that heal without incidence in 3 to 5 days if they are kept clean with bland soap (e.g., Ivory) and water and are covered with a bland ointment (e.g., bacitracin). Recently healed partial-thickness burn wounds become very dry. A mild lanolin cream (e.g., Nivea, Beiersdorf, Norwalk, CT) or lotion (e.g., Nivea; Vaseline Intensive Care, Chesebrough Ponds, Inc., Greenwich, CT) should be used until the natural skin lubrication mechanisms return, which is usually 6 to 8 weeks.

The patient should also be instructed to avoid sun exposure during time of wound maturation, as the wound may become hyperpigmented, which is frequently permanent. The use of a sun block (sun protection factor 15) is recommended for healed areas that must be exposed to direct sunlight.

Pruritus is a common complaint in maturing burn wounds, and when it is severe it is extremely difficult to treat. The antipruritics diphenhydramine hydrochloride (Benadryl, Parke-Davis, Morris Plains, NJ) and hydroxyzine (Vistaril, Pfizer Laboratories, New York, NY; Atarax, Roerig, New York, NY) have proved beneficial. Using a moisturizing cream is also beneficial for itching.

Alternative Methods of Wound Management

There are multiple methods for managing outpatient burn wounds. Some advocate bulky dressings for as long as 10 to 14 days. Although a bulky dressing prevents pain, there is a potential hazard of bacterial overgrowth in the warm, moist dressing. In addition, range-of-motion exercising cannot be performed, which prolongs edema and rehabilitation. Topical chemotherapeutic agents, such as silver sulfadiazine, are frequently used in the management of minor burn injury. If this form of management is used, it is important to remember that silver sulfadiazine is inactivated by tissue secretions and must be changed at least twice a day. In addition, a pseudomembrane forms over the partial-thickness injury, which is frequently painful and difficult to remove.

The use of prosthetic skin substitutes in the treatment of partial-thickness outpatient burns has recently become popular. Two substitutes useful on partial-thickness injury are Biobrane (Winthrop-Breon Laboratories, New York, NY) and Op-Site (Acme United Corporation, Bridgeport, CT). Biobrane can be used effectively in partial-thickness burns. Physicians who use this product report that it is well tolerated, is capable of compressing underlying fluid collection, and can transmit any bacterial activity to its membrane. It has been used successfully in outpatient management and may be left on until epithelialization occurs. Op-

Site is a synthetic barrier and has also been used on partial-thickness wounds. It requires some expertise as fluid collections beneath the barrier frequently occur. The problem of accurate diagnosis of depth of injury is a drawback with both of these prosthetic skin substitutes. If the wound is a medium to deep partial-thickness injury, then an eschar does form, necessitating frequent dressing changes.

Biologic dressings, including allograft, xenograft, and amnion, have been used in the past to treat outpatient burns. The cost of cadaveric allograft is prohibitive. Xenografts should not be used on superficial partial-thickness injury because of the incorporation of xenograft tissue into the healing donor sites, which occurs in as many as 35% of the patients so treated.

Management of Critical Areas

Face. Superficial burns of the face should be treated by exposure. The face is washed twice daily with a mild soap and water, and a thin layer of a bland ointment (e.g., bacitracin) is applied to the open wounds to prevent drying.

Ears. Superficial burns of the ear should be treated with a bland ointment. Deeper injuries must be treated with topical chemotherapy and the avoidance of excessive pressure to avoid chondritis.

Eyes. Suspected corneal burns should be stained with fluorescein for confirmation of diagnoses. Superficial corneal burns not asymptomatic by 48 hours and all more serious injuries should be evaluated by an ophthalmologist.

Hands. Hands with superficial burns should be elevated for 24 to 48 hours to minimize swelling. Circumferential hand burns may require hospitalization for observation of adequate circulation. Range-of-motion exercises should begin as soon as possible after injury. Instructions for the exercise program should be part of the initial management protocol.

Feet. Although burns of the feet are painful, the patient should walk and do range-of-motion exercises. Crutches should not be allowed. To prevent edema, burned feet should be elevated when the patient is not walking or exercising. An elastic bandage should be applied over the wound dressing when ambulating or sitting; however, this should be removed at night when the feet are elevated.

Perineum. Perineal burns frequently require hospitalization for 24 to 48 hours for observation of urinary obstruction secondary to edema. Minor perineal burns may be treated with a bland ointment, but extensive superficial perineal burns, as seen in pediatric bathtub scald injuries, are best treated with topical chemotherapy (Silvadene) utilizing a diaper as the wound dressing.

Complications

Most complications in small burn injuries result from overtreatment, either too vigorous dressing changes that pull off newly formed epithelium or the use of a variety of topical and systemic antibiotics that may result in secondary infection or formation of a pseudomembrane that may require debridement. What is necessary aggressive therapy in larger burns is overtreatment of small burns. In small burns systemic antibiotics are rarely indicated and topical agents are generally not necessary. Local infection may occur or healing may be delayed as a result of overtreatment.

FROSTBITE

Cold injury is a form of trauma resulting from exposure to cold. Perhaps no other injury has been managed in so many ways with so little regard for the essential pathophysiology. Management of cold injury has been in dispute for many years. Therapy has often been based on folklore rather than controlled experimentation. Apparently logical thinking and seemingly reasonable analysis have often led to conclusions that controlled experimentation has since proved erroneous.

CLASSIFICATION

Cold injuries can be classified into two major categories: (1) frostbite and (2) nonfreezing cold injury. The term *frostbite* should be applied only to those injuries in which the tissue water has actually been converted to ice. Conditions such as chilblain (pernio), trenchfoot, and immersion foot are cold injuries in which the tissue has not been frozen. Nevertheless, the pathophysiology of these lesions is like that of frostbite.

PATHOPHYSIOLOGY

For tissue to freeze, the heat lost from the exposed part must exceed the heat gained by the part. The temperature of the tissue will fall as long as heat loss exceeds gain. When tissue temperatures drop below about −6°C, freezing begins, although occasionally supercooling, that is, cooling below the freezing point without solidification or crystallization, is possible. The wind velocity at the time of exposure to cold and the humidity are important factors in regard to the temperature that will initiate the freezing process.

The pathophysiology of both freezing and nonfreezing injuries is a direct consequence of dysfunction of microcirculation. This dysfunction is initiated by vasospasm, but development of tissue damage parallels neither distribution of vasoconstriction nor the cooling gradient; rather, it corresponds closely to the extent of secondary erythrostasis. The tissue necrosis following frostbite has been attributed to the mechanical effects of ice crystals, cellular dehydration, and microvascular occlusion. When tissues are frozen rapidly, crystals of ice form within both the cells and the extracellular spaces. However, practically all clinical freezing injuries occur by a slower process in which ice crystal formation is exclusively an extracellular process. Water from within the cell is "sucked out" through the cellular membrane to be incorporated into the developing crystals, thus dehydrating the cell and leading to cellular collapse. Spicules of ice, many times the size of the adjacent cells, compress and distort the cell wall.

In spite of this frightening microscopic picture, mechanical distortion of tissue does not appear to be lethal, at least over a short period. During thawing the cells regain their water and become histologically indistinguishable from normal cells. Although the mechanical action of extracellular ice crystals is almost never responsible for clinical tissue injury, the cellular dehydration that accompanies ice crystal formation can be lethal.

CLINICAL SIGNS AND SYMPTOMS

Cold injury can be classified according to degree of severity: first degree, hyperemia without blistering; second degree, hyperemia with vesicle formation; third degree, necrosis of the skin and subcutaneous tissue (Fig. 5-2); fourth degree, deep necrosis and loss of the part. The extent of tissue loss in cases of frostbite depends on (1) the length of time the tissue was frozen, (2) the temperature of the tissue while frozen, and (3) the temperature during thawing.

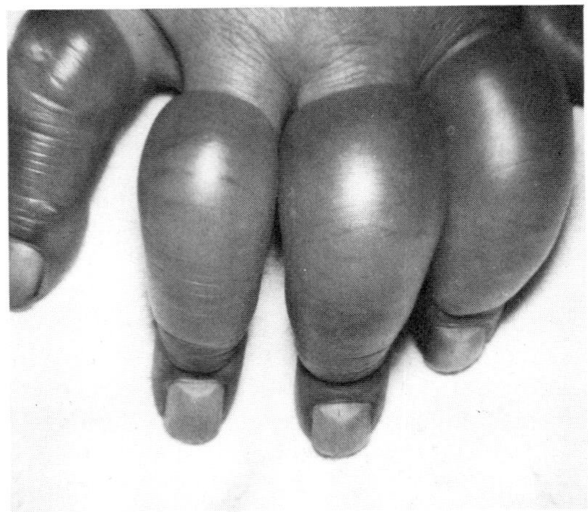

Figure 5-2. Vesicle formation on the fingers early after frostbite.

The history given by the patient is usually quite characteristic after exposure to cold: the victim notices, in the hands, feet, ears, or nose, at first a sticking, burning sensation and then definite numbness or anesthesia. The part of the body involved becomes waxy white. The numbness should be a warning that further exposure to cold is dangerous. If the patient goes into a warm room, the ischemic area becomes intensely red and edematous and is associated with an itching and tingling sensation. Chilblain may develop. This consists of nodules surrounded by a reddened area of hyperemia or of cyanotic flat swelling in the area exposed. Chilblain causes symptoms long after the exposure to cold is over.

Trenchfoot and immersion foot are the result of long exposure to wet cold at temperatures above freezing. Immersion foot occurs several days to weeks after submersion in cold or cool water. Trenchfoot develops more rapidly, usually after one to several days of exposure to dampness at temperatures at or near the freezing point. Both injuries are associated with dependency and immobility. Both lead to paresthesias, hypersensitivity to cold, muscle weakness or atrophy, and, in severe cases, superficial gangrene.

Pernio, or chilblain, is characterized by

small superficial ulcers that appear on the exposed area of the body, particularly the legs, after exposure to dry, cold air. The lesions tend to appear during the winter and disappear during the warmer months. Massive tissue loss is not seen.

As in the case of frostbite, the mechanism leading to gangrene in nonfreezing cold injuries seems to involve microcirculatory impairment, progressive stasis of erythrocytes in the capillaries, and venules appearing 2 to 3 days after the cold exposure.

TREATMENT

Merymen expressed the realistic though pessimistic view of the treatment of cold injury: "These injuries, unlike many medical problems, are not in progress, they have already happened, and tissue may be irrevocably dead, although some is not. The goal is primarily to prevent the subsequent and unnecessary loss of the latter, much as in the management of any traumatic injury."* Thus tissue cells can be affected by freezing in three different ways: (1) a certain number of cells are killed, (2) a certain number remain unaffected, and (3) a large number are injured. They may recover and survive under the right circumstances. It is the third group to which therapy must be directed. Essential principles of therapy include (1) the avoidance of further mechanical or thermal injury and (2) the prevention of bacterial contamination. This approach is entirely analogous to that used in the treatment of major burns, including the removal of eschar, fasciotomy, topical chemotherapy (e.g., silver sulfadiazine), daily hydrotherapy, and debridement of devitalized tissue with removal of blisters (see "Management of Cold Injury").

Optimal salvage of tissue requires restraint on the part of the surgeon, who must avoid the temptation to amputate until complete demarcation has occurred. This may occur as early as 4 or 5 days, but in the usual case, 5 to 6 weeks are required.

Although the preceding precepts are practically indisputable and are the essence of frostbite therapy, other measures, predicated on the preservation of marginally viable tissue, have evoked dispute; however, they may offer some promise.

One great advance has been demonstrated both experimentally and clinically: Rapid thawing of frozen tissue improves the degree of tissue survival considerably. This demonstration makes untenable the previously held position that rapid warming should not be used in management of frostbite because it produces greater pain and edema than slow warming. Rapid warming of a frozen part is accomplished by immersion of the part in a water bath heated to 42°C. The rapid inflow of heat into the frozen tissue quickly raises the temperature of the tissue to the freezing point, prevents a long delay between euthermic conversion of ice into water, and assures rapid reestablishment of blood flow. Because of the conductivity and high thermal capacity of water, even deep tissues are rapidly returned to a near-normal temperature.

All of the other methods that have been suggested for improving blood supply remain controversial. These methods include sympathectomy or sympathetic block, which may be of value. However, since this requires an anesthetic and an operation on a patient who may otherwise be injured, it should be performed only when there is a high degree of suspicion that the injuries are third or fourth degree. Most surgeons, including me, prefer to reserve sympathectomy for the late complications of frostbite. Low-molecular-weight dextran may also be of benefit, but if it is not given within 1 or 2 hours after the thawing process, it is of little value. Vasodilators, anticoagulants, antihistamines, steroids, and hyperbaric oxygen appear to be of little benefit.

MANAGEMENT OF COLD INJURY

Emergency Treatment

Rapid thawing at 42°C
Debridement of nonviable tissue
Apply topical agent (Silvadene, Sulfamylon).
Low-molecular weight dextran
Fasciotomies if indicated

Wound Management Principles

Prevention of infection
- Daily debridement
- Topical chemotherapeutic agent (e.g., Silvadene)

Optimal salvage of tissue
- Restraint until demarcation occurs

* Quoted in Strandness, DE, Summer DS: Cold injury. In Hemodynamics for Surgeons, p 594. New York, Grune & Stratton, 1975.

In conclusion, the best results in the management of cold injury are achieved first of all by avoiding additional mechanical, thermal, or infectious trauma and by delaying operative intervention until the tissues are well demarcated.

BIBLIOGRAPHY

Burns

American Burn Association Injury Severity Grading System, 1976

Artz CP, Moncrief JA, Pruitt BA Jr (eds): Burns: A Team Approach. Philadelphia, WB Saunders, 1979

Bruck HM: The management of small burns. In Artz CP, Moncrief JA, Pruitt BA Jr (eds): Burns: A Team Approach, pp 165–168. Philadelphia, WB Saunders, 1979

Demling RH, Mazess RB, Wolbert W: The effect of immediate and delayed cold immersion on burn edema formation and resorption. J Trauma 19:56, 1979

Edlich RF et al: Modification of American Burn Association Injury Severity Grading System. JACEP 7:226, 1978

James JH, Watson ACH: The use of Op-Site, a vapour permeable dressing, on skin graft donor sites. Br J Plast Surg 64:107, 1975

Lund CC, Browder NC: The estimate of areas of burns. Surg Gynecol Obstet 79:352, 1944

MacMillan BG: Present status of bioadherent materials, barrier dressings, and biosynthetics as skin substitutes. In Wise DL (ed): Burn Wound Coverings, Vol. 1, pp 115–136. Boca Raton, FL, CRC Press, Inc., 1984

Nance FC, Lewis VC, Hires JC et al: Aggressive outpatient care of burns. J Trauma 12:144, 1972

O'Neil JA: Burns—office evaluation and management. Primary Care 3:531, 1976

Salisbury RE, Wilmore DW, Silverstein P et al: Biological dressing for skin graft donor sites. Arch Surg 106:705, 1973

Stratta RJ, Saffle JR, Kravitz M, Warden GD: The management of tar and asphalt injuries. Am J Surg 146:766, 1984

Tavis MJ, Thornton JW, Bartlett RH, Roth JC, Woodroof EA: A new composite skin prosthesis. Burns 7:123, 1981

Frostbite

Bouwman DL, Morrison S, Lucas CE, Ledgerwood AM: Early sympathectomy for frostbite—is it of value? J Trauma 20:744–749, 1980

Carpenter HM, Hurley LA, Hardenberg E, Williams RB: Vascular injury due to cold. Arch Pathol 92:153, 1971

Kulka JP: Cold injury to the skin. Arch Environ Health 11:484, 1964

Lazarus HM, Hutto BS: Electric burns and frostbite: patterns of vascular injury. J Trauma 22:581–585, 1982

Mundth ED, Lung DM, Brown RB: Treatment of experimental frostbite with low molecular weight dextran. J Trauma 4:246, 1964

Porter JM, Wesche DH, Rosch J, Baur GM: Intraarterial sympathetic blockade in the treatment of clinical frostbite. Am J Surg 132:627, 1976

Strandness DE, Summer DS: Cold injury. In Hemodynamics for Surgeons, pp 582–619. New York, Grune & Stratton, 1975

6 Management of Infections and Wounds

GLENN D. WARDEN

Infection is a complicated process involving invasion of a body by pathogenic microorganisms and reaction of the body tissues to the organisms and their toxins. Infections treated in the outpatient department should be restricted to those that do not represent a serious risk of fatality or long-term morbidity. In borderline situations it is always wiser to hospitalize a patient for the first few days of treatment than to risk progression of the infection in the event that outpatient treatment is inadequate. Treatment should take into consideration the cause of the infection, the organism involved, the general health of the patient, the location and extent of the infection, and the social environment of the patient.

A surgical infection is an infection that requires surgical treatment and has developed before or as a complication of surgical treatment. Almost all infections encountered in ambulatory surgical patients are of two varieties: infections resulting from accidental or surgical wounds or infections from nontraumatic origins for which surgical therapy must be considered. In addition, most infections treated in an ambulatory patient are superficial, involving skin or mucous membranes and adjacent tissues.

DIAGNOSIS

The classic signs and symptoms of infection are redness, swelling, heat, and pain. Redness of the skin is due to hyperemia and is seen only in infections of the skin itself; it may not be seen in infections involving the deeper subcutaneous tissues. Swelling always accompanies infection. Heat results from hyperemia and may be detected in the absence of redness. The most universal sign of infection is pain. Associated with pain is tenderness over the infected area. Another local sign of infection is loss of function, which is brought about by reflex and voluntary immobilization.

Depending on the type and extent of the infection, systemic symptoms of varying degree may arise as a result of infection. They include malaise, anorexia, and fever. Leukocytosis also accompanies acute infection; however, in most superficial surgical infections the total leukocyte count is slightly or only moderately elevated. A massive pyogenic abscess may occur without leukocytosis, fever, or tenderness.

Laboratory diagnosis of infection should include examination of any exudate obtained from the infected area. Culture and sensitivity determinations under both aerobic and anaerobic conditions are essential. In certain circumstances, such as chronic granulomatous infection, biopsy may be performed. The surgeon must initiate treatment immediately on the basis of clinical judgment, although he will often make appropriate changes after he receives the laboratory report.

LOCAL CARE OF INFECTION

The basic surgical principles are the same in all types of infection; however, the local treatment of an infection must vary with the type and situation of the infection. Treatment of a "closed" infection such as a furuncle or cellulitis differs from that of an "open" infection such as an infected wound. The three nonspecific principles of local infection are application of heat, elevation, and immobilization.

APPLICATION OF HEAT

Heat in any form when applied to the body surface causes an increased rate of blood flow due to vasodilatation. This results in a rise in capillary pressure associated with an increased rate of transfer of fluid from the blood to the tissues, accelerated metabolic activity, and increased phagocytosis. Excessive local temperatures are prevented by distribution of heat throughout the body by increased blood flow. Since the advent of antibiotics, which are employed routinely in the management of infection, application of heat, particularly in the form of hot soaks or hypertonic solutions, has largely given away to dry heat treatment. The electric heating pad is probably the most effective method of applying heat for long periods. Care must be taken that the pad does not become wet, since a short circuit and burning may occur. To avoid producing a troublesome burn, extreme care must be exercised, particularly in very young children, in old people, in patients who are debilitated, and in those suffering from chronic disease such as atherosclerosis or other form of impaired peripheral circulation.

ELEVATION

Elevation as a nonspecific treatment for infection is easy when the infection is in the extremities. For elevation to be effective the infected area should be above the level of the heart; the marked swelling associated with the infection may be decreased and venous and lymphatic drainage aided by making sure the part is not dependent. In addition, elevation affords relief of pain and spasm.

IMMOBILIZATION

For the superficial infections treated in ambulatory patients, immobilization of the part is required to attain physiologic rest. The extremities are best immobilized by the use of splints, bandages, slings, and adhesive strappings. In addition, immobilization affords protection of the inflammatory lesion from external trauma. Ironically, the most common type of trauma is the pinching and squeezing of open infections by the patient or by the energetic surgeon. There is no better way to break down the protective wall of induration and produce an extension of the inflammatory process. It is mentioned only to be condemned. Other trauma, such as bumping or striking an area of infection, has the same result, which is why it is necessary to protect the area with a dressing, splints, or both.

SURGICAL TREATMENT

The immediate decisions that must be made by the surgeon caring for infection in an ambulatory patient include: (1) Is the infection fluctuant and therefore suitable for drainage? (2) If drainage is needed, can it be accomplished in the outpatient department or is hospitalization required? (3) Are antibiotics required? The nature of the lesion and the character of its response to treatment determine whether surgical intervention is needed.

The extraordinary efficacy of antibiotic therapy in such lesions as cellulitis and lymphadenitis is evidenced by the rapid control and resolution of the infection. Surgical intervention in these infections is necessary only when treatment was late in a case in which localized abscess or gangrene occurred. As a general rule, drainage is required in all fluctuant staphylococcal lesions to limit further breakdown of infected tissues, to reduce tension in the area of inflammation, to relieve pain, to provide for ingress of blood-borne antibiotics and phagocytes, and to allow wound healing. The philosophy concerning removal of sutures, reopening of infected incisional wounds, and removal of foreign bodies, infected necrotic tissue, and sequestra is important for the same reasons. Although effective chemotherapy has resulted in marked reduction in the number of cases in which extensive drainage is required for resolution, incision and drainage are still indicated when (1) the infection has localized and fluctuation is evident, (2) there is no likelihood of spontaneous rupture with adequate drainage, and (3) there is no danger of extension of the infection as the result of the surgical trauma.

INCISION AND DRAINAGE

Fluctuation points to the presence of fluid within an abscess cavity and is an indication for incision and drainage. Experience is the best guide to the presence of fluctuation and the indication for drainage. If doubt exists as to fluctuation, diagnostic needle aspiration should be performed before incision. Compression of a suspected abscess with two fingers will sometimes reveal fluctuation. In certain closed locations, such as the breast, perirectal area, and distal space of the finger, incision must be accomplished before fluctuation is apparent if extensive necrosis is to be avoided.

Incision should not be performed in cellulitis since this opens tissue planes for more extensive spread of the infection. If identification of the organism is desired, needle aspiration of the area for culture is permissible, although it is not usually rewarding.

Although specific details depend somewhat on the nature and localization of the infection, certain general principles of incision and drainage should be followed. Strict aseptic techniques should be used to prevent spread of the patient's infection to others and to prevent new and possibly more virulent organisms from spreading to the patient. This includes careful skin preparation and use of sterile drapes, instruments, gloves, mask, and the like. Local infiltration with lidocaine (Xylocaine) is satisfactory, but care must be taken not to spread infection to the surrounding tissue. Local intradermal infiltration of the proposed line of incision is safe in this regard. Regional area blocks are ideal and applicable in many circumstances. The surgical incision should be precise, in the direction of natural skin lines, and only as long as necessary to provide adequate drainage. The contents of the abscess cavity should be evacuated and a specimen removed for culture and determination of antibiotic sensitivity. The cavity should be carefully explored to detect and open any undrained pockets of pus.

PACKING AND IRRIGATION

Initially the wound should be cleaned mechanically of liquid, pus, and necrotic tissue. The surrounding area should be kept free of pus and crusts and should be protected from excoriation due to irritating discharges.

Following incision and drainage of a closed fluctuant wound it should be packed loosely with cotton gauze $\frac{1}{8}$ in. to 1 in. wide, which is removed in 24 hours. It should be "packed tightly" only in cases of marked bleeding. A packed abscess should have all of the initial packing material removed within 24 hours, and a loose wick should then be inserted. Iodoform gauze may be used initially as a local antiseptic; however, its prolonged use may exert damage to the surrounding healing tissues. The usual management following incision and drainage consists of packing the wound with iodoform gauze for 24 hours followed by removal of the packing and beginning a treatment regimen of irrigation of the wound with either saline or 2% hydrogen peroxide solution. Following irrigation the wound is packed lightly with plain gauze moistened with saline. This routine is performed twice daily. Treatment of an infected traumatic wound or after reopening an infected incisional wound differs somewhat from the program outlined earlier. The wound itself should be cleaned and mechanically debrided. Following irrigation of the wound with saline or 2% hydrogen peroxide, the surface of the wound is covered with a layer of saline-moistened fine-mesh gauze over which compression dressings are applied. Absorbent dressings permit early and rapid removal of liquefied wound secretions and thus promote continued flow of serum, lymph, and leukocytes into the wound. These dressings should be bulky enough to prevent soaking through. Dressings are generally changed twice daily. In addition, the beneficial effects upon healing of heat, moisture, elevation, and mobilization are added to the treatment regimen.

ANCILLARY MEASURES

The role of topical antiseptics, or antibiotics, and other chemotherapeutic agents in the management of open infected wounds is still highly controversial. If our concept of the body's method of handling infections is correct, then there is no place for topical application of antiseptics or antibiotics in the treatment of infected wounds unless it can be shown that they enhance the action of the natural process. It is clear that antiseptics are ineffective against organisms immediately beneath the surface of the wound. Furthermore, the destructive action of most antiseptics is exerted against all cells with which they come in contact, whether tissue cells or bacteria. The result is lessening of local tissue viability and retardation of healing. There is therefore no rational basis for the use of these agents in the treatment of open infected wounds.

In recent years, however, topically applied chemotherapeutic agents have been developed that have a definite antibacterial effect without appreciable toxicity for tissues. Silver sulfadiazine, aqueous silver nitrate (0.5% solution), and mafenide (Sulfamylon) are three such agents that have revolutionized the treatment of major thermal injuries; their use in smaller burns has been questioned, however. The effectiveness of these agents in management of open infected wounds, other than burns, has not been established. Nitrofurazone (Furacin) has also been used for topical application to infected wounds, but hypersensitivity and superinfection with resistant organisms have been problems. Povidone-iodine (Betadine) and other organic iodine preparations have also been used for this purpose. Numerous topical antibiotic preparations have been developed, but because of the risk of sensitization it has generally been considered unwise to use, for topical application, antibiotics that are normally employed systemically. Most topical antibiotic preparations therefore contain antibiotics that are rarely used systemically. These include neomycin, bacitracin, and polymyxin. Even when used in combination, these agents are not effective against all bacteria. Consequent to their use, overgrowth of resistant organisms may occur. Local hypersensitivity has also been observed.

It appears, therefore, that despite wide usage, there is little rationale for the use of topical antibiotics and antiseptics in routine ambulatory surgical infections. Personal experience indicates that these often expensive preparations offer little advantage over simple moist saline dressings. At the present state of our knowledge, it appears rational to avoid using these topical agents except in the management of major thermal injuries, unless their use is clearly indicated because of delayed wound healing, as evidenced by high concentrations of surface bacteria. Cultures of both bacteria and fungi at the time of initiating treatment can provide help in selecting the appropriate topical agent.

The use of porcine xenograft and cadaveric homograft may also be helpful in the management of infected wounds. Although not warranted in routine infected wounds, they may be beneficial in the management of indolent skin ulcers that remain chronically infected despite correction of the underlying cause such as postphlebitic stasis or intensive topical therapy.

SYSTEMIC TREATMENT OF INFECTION

Although antibiotic therapy has revolutionized the treatment of infections, due consideration must be given to various supportive measures designed to maximize host resistance. The adjunctive use of antibiotics in the treatment of infection is dependent on adequate blood supply and is most effective against acute infections such as cellulitis, septicemia, and peritonitis. Antibiotics have slight access to abscesses and penetrate by slow diffusion, if at all. In these situations, they should be used in conjunction with incision and drainage. Antibiotics are the primary treatment for acute spreading infections and should result in clinical improvement in 24 to 48 hours. Change to a more effective antibiotic should be based on culture and sensitivity reports.

The two basic requirements for effective antibiotic therapy of an infection are: (1) The antibiotic must be capable of inhibiting the growth of the agent or agents causing the infection. This requires identification of the infecting bacterium and selection of antibiotic against the organism. (2) A therapeutically effective concentration of antibiotic must reach the infected tissue for a long enough time to permit antimicrobial activity if the compound is to be effective. This requires knowledge of the dosage of the antibiotic that gives antimicrobial concentration in the blood, and it requires a blood supply capable of delivering the antibiotic in the blood to the infected tissues. The general indications for systemic antibiotic therapy are lesions associated with a wide area of cellulitis, lymphangitis, and lymphadenitis; systemic symptoms such as fever, chills, or malaise; or depressed host resistance due to other illnesses. In addition, multiple simultaneous lesions and lesions of the face, neck, and hands should be treated with systemic antibiotics.

SELECTION OF ANTIBIOTIC THERAPY

In most cases of infection seen in an outpatient clinic or in an ambulatory setting, a physician is called upon to make an empirical selection of an antibiotic without laboratory investigation of the bacteria or without specificity tests. As a general rule he should be able to distinguish the types of inflammation produced by streptococcus (spreading cellulitis, lymphangitis, lymphadenitis) from those produced by staphylococcus (boil, carbuncle, paronychia). This should give the physician sufficient information to make a primary selection of an antibiotic because most infective inflammations seen in an ambulatory setting are produced by one of these two organisms. If the infection responds to the chemotherapeutic agent selected, culture and specificity tests are not needed. It is known, however, that many species of staphylococci have developed resistance to antibiotics, especially to penicillin. In such cases cultures and specificity tests are important, and laboratory help is necessary to obtain the information required for antibiotic selection. The empirical choice in antibiotic therapy for staphylococcal infection depends on whether the patient developed the infection in the hospital or outside the hospital and, to a certain degree, whether he did or did not receive antibiotic therapy within a 3-month period prior to onset of the present illness. If the patient has not been hospitalized and has not received penicillin before or in recent months, the chances are excellent that the staphylococcus causing the infection is susceptible to penicillin. For hospital-acquired infections, culture and sensitivity tests become more important because of the varying pattern of resistance found in these infections. Penicillinase-resistant penicillins or the cephalosporins are frequently effective alternative drugs.

Prophylactic antibiotics in the management of traumatic wounds are useful only if antibiotics are administered in the early, preinvasive phase before bacteria have become established in the wound. Despite ample experimental evidence to support this concept, there is no clinical evidence that antibiotic prophylaxis has any influence on the course of soft-tissue wounds that have been adequately and promptly debrided and cleansed. Prophylactic antibiotic therapy is reserved for extensive musculoskeletal injuries, compound fractures, and penetrating injuries of the abdomen, mouth, esophagus, central nervous system, and eye. The choice of agent or agents is dependent on the bacterial flora expected to be encountered.

Regardless of the indication, the dosage of antibiotic selected should be adequate to produce the desired antibacterial effect on the blood and extracellular fluids. The duration of therapy should be sufficient to permit the natural defense mechanism of the body to eradicate the inhibited organisms in the lesion. Unnecessary prolonged therapy is unwise and may be harmful. After 72 hours, antibiotic therapy should be reviewed, reevaluated, and changed if indicated.

Antibiotics and chemotherapeutic agents currently used in surgical practice are listed in Table 6-1. The selection of antibiotic and dosage for a specific infection depends on clinical judgment, bacterial sensitivity tests, and awareness of the toxicity of the drug.

SPECIFIC SURGICAL INFECTIONS

FOLLICULITIS, FURUNCLES, AND CARBUNCLES

Stages of Infection

Folliculitis, furuncles, and carbuncles are the names applied to local staphylococcal infections of the skin and subcutaneous tissues. Each begins as an infection of a hair follicle or sebaceous gland and progresses to produce a small area of induration with central necrosis known as a pimple or a pustule. By further extension, the infection involves the underlying subcutaneous tissues, and a single area of central necrosis surrounded by a well-formed area of redness and induration is formed; this is called a furuncle or a boil. In areas in which there are dense fibrous septa extending from the skin to the underlying fascia, as in the back of the neck, the infection may extend from one area of subcutaneous tissue to another without effective walling-off of the process, thus attaining considerable size. This lesion is known as a carbuncle. It may be noted, therefore, that these lesions must be looked on as progressive stages of the same process, and the variations in progress may be considered, in part, to be indicative of the patient's general and local "resistance" to the staphylococcal infection and of the architecture of the infected tissues.

Predisposing Factors

In many instances the recognition and the appropriate management of predisposing factors may be as important as the administration of specific measures. Therefore it is essential

TABLE 6-1. Choice of Antibiotics for Organisms Found in Surgical Infections

MICROORGANISM	FIRST CHOICE	ALTERNATE AGENT
GRAM-POSITIVE COCCI		
Diplococcus pneumoniae	Penicillin G	Erythromycin; a cephalosporin; chloramphenicol; vancomycin
Staphylococcus aureus		
Non–penicillinase-producing	Penicillin G	A cephalosporin; erythromycin; vancomycin; clindamycin
Penicillinase-producing	Nafcillin or other penicillinase-resistant penicillins	A cephalosporin; gentamicin; erythromycin; clindamycin; vancomycin
Peptostreptococcus	Penicillin G	Erythromycin; clindamycin; a tetracycline
Streptococcus faecalis	Penicillin G (with streptomycin or kanamycin for endocarditis or septicemia)	Vancomycin or erythromycin with or without streptomycin, kanamycin, or gentamicin
Streptococcus pyogenes groups A, B, C, and G	Penicillin G	Erythromycin; a cephalosporin; clindamycin
Streptococcus viridans	Penicillin G with or without streptomycin	Erythromycin with or without streptomycin, vancomycin, or a cephalosporin
GRAM-NEGATIVE COCCI		
Neisseria gonorrhoeae	Penicillin G	Ampicillin; amoxicillin; spectinomycin; erythromycin; a tetracycline
Neisseria meningitidis	Penicillin G	Chloramphenicol; a sulfonamide
GRAM-POSITIVE BACILLI		
Clostridium tetani	Penicillin G	A cephalosporin; a tetracycline; erythromycin
Clostridium welchii (*Bacillus perfringens*) (gas gangrene)	Penicillin G	A tetracycline; a cephalosporin
Corynebacterium diphtheriae	Penicillin G	Erythromycin
GRAM-NEGATIVE BACILLI		
Bacteroides fragilis	Chloramphenicol or clindamycin	A tetracycline or erythromycin or carbenicillin or penicillin or metronidazole
Bacteroides melaninogenicus or *oralis*	Penicillin	Erythromycin; clindamycin
Enterobacter (*Aerobacter*) species	Gentamicin or tobramycin	Carbenicillin; kanamycin; chloramphenicol; tetracycline
Escherichia coli	Gentamicin, tobramycin	Ampicillin; carbenicillin; kanamycin, a tetracycline; a cephalosporin; chloramphenicol
Hemophilus influenzae	Ampicillin	Chloramphenicol; a tetracycline
Klebsiella pneumoniae	Gentamicin or tobramycin	A cephalosporin; kanamycin; chloramphenicol
Proteus mirabilis	Ampicillin	Gentamicin; tobramycin; ticarcillin; a cephalosporin; kanamycin
Proteus (other species)	Gentamicin or tobramycin	Ticarcillin; chloramphenicol; a tetracycline and streptomycin; cephalosporin
Providencia species	Amikacin	Gentamicin; kanamycin, tobramycin; carbenicillin; ticarcillin
Pseudomonas aeruginosa	Gentamicin or tobramycin	Amikacin; carbenicillin, ticarcillin; piperacillin
Salmonella species	Ampicillin	Chloramphenicol
Serratia species	Gentamicin or tobramycin	Kanamycin; amikacin; chloramphenicol; carbenicillin or ticarcillin
Shigella species	Ampicillin	A tetracycline; oral kanamycin

to keep in mind the following recognizable local and systemic factors that determine the degree of "resistance" of the skin to pyogenic infection: (1) trauma of any form, which includes exposure to irritants, deodorants, and defatting agents; (2) poor hygiene; (3) local causes of pruritus, such as insect bites and pediculosis capitis; (4) excessive sweating, especially of intertriginous sites, hands, and feet; (5) climatic factors; (6) diabetes; and (7) blood dyscrasias. To treat these infections effectively it is essential for the physician to recognize and correct these predisposing factors whenever they are present.

Location and Description

These lesions may occur on any part of the body, but the most frequent sites are the face, back of the neck, the axillae, the groin, the buttocks, the arms, and the proximal phalanges of the fingers.

The earliest lesion is characterized by a small reddened firm mound of induration, which is itchy and tender and in a few days shows a central yellow point. This furuncle, or pimple, may extend no farther, and the process may subside with the discharge of a drop or two of pus or may simply "dry up." Frequently, however, there is deeper extension, with gradual enlargement of the area of inflammatory induration. Pain, which is a common manifestation, is present and increases with motion. In this case the area of inflammation has extended beyond the skin into the subcutaneous tissues, and, in the untreated lesion, the protective wall of inflammatory induration usually takes from 4 to 6 days to become well formed. By this time the central necrotic core, with serosanguineous pus, is prominent, and drainage of pus and necrotic material may occur spontaneously or after surgical incision. As soon as drainage is established, tension is relieved, pain decreases, and the process subsides when the necrotic material has all been evacuated.

In the carbuncular type of infection, most often seen on the back of the neck or on the dorsum of the hand, the walling-off process does not seem to keep pace with the tendency of the infection to spread in the poorly resistant fat lobules lying between the fibrous tissue septa beneath the skin. As a result the encircling inflammatory wall of induration is frequently wide, and pointing takes place at the multiple sites in the skin over the underlying necrosis. Elevation of the temperature and "toxemia" due to absorption from the area of infection usually are present.

The prognosis depends on the clinical type of infection, the site of involvement, the predisposing factors, the duration of infection, and the nature of the causative organisms. Superficial pustular folliculitis and furuncles tend to have a more or less self-limited course and to clear up readily with various types of therapy. A dominant etiologic factor may be underlying dermatitis, in which case proper treatment of the dermatitis may result in a permanent cure of the furunculosis. Through the process of autoinoculation, staphylococci may be carried from a lesion and infect other parts of the body. Unless suitable precautions are taken, the microorganisms are conveyed by fingers or handkerchief to other parts of the body, such as the nose, the eyes, and the external ear, where they are liable to persist. Recurrent infection in the axilla, a warm, moist hairy area with apocrine glands, is readily understandable. All physicians recognize that furuncles and carbuncles in the center of the face may give off small emboli and give rise to cavernous sinus thrombosis, septicemia, or metastatic infection some distance from the original infection. It is also well known that staphylococcal infections in the newborn and in children may lead to serious sequelae, such as osteomyelitis. Appropriate antibiotic therapy has significantly reduced the mortality and morbidity from these serious complications of cutaneous infections.

In general, cutaneous pyogenic infections of brief duration are more amenable to therapy than are those that are chronic. The causative organism also influences the prognosis. If the offending *Staphylococcus aureus* is sensitive to the antibiotic selected, institution of adequate effective local therapy as quickly as possible after the infection becomes apparent is likely to result in its prompt resolution.

Treatment

The treatment of established local staphylococcal infections still rests chiefly on the surgical principles of rest, elevation, and heat and drainage when pus has formed. Scrupulous cleanliness is the first principle of management. For smaller furuncles and carbuncles, effective treatment further consists of protecting and immobilizing the area with a dry gauze dressing over an application of bacitracin (Mycitracin) or other antibiotic ointment at the site of pointing. The area around the furuncle or boil is shaved, and after the necrotic bleb has been removed with a needle or forceps a small dot of ointment is placed at the point of the lesion. In many cases the infection may be aborted by this treatment; in others the use of 95% phenol, cautiously applied with a toothpick swab to enlarge a small sinus or to open an abscess that is pointing near the surface, is still good practice. After 2 or 3 days the area of central necrosis may be lifted out with a sterile forceps or mosquito hemostat. This treatment is continued until all the central slough has liquefied and drained away.

In some boils, when movement of a part prevents effective walling off of the process and when there is associated cellulitis of the adjacent tissues, as, for instance, in furuncles on the dorsum of the proximal phalanx of the finger, the application of splints and dry heat is beneficial.

Penicillin is administered parenterally or one of the other antistaphylococcal antibiotics is given to hasten localization of the infection process. Under this regimen the cellulitis surrounding the lesion will subside in 36 to 48 hours, and, with localization of the process, there will be a discharge of the central necrotic area followed by rapid healing. Incision in such cases is not performed until localization has taken place, and usually by this time spontaneous drainage begins. It may be necessary to incise this drainage site slightly.

The use of penicillin and other antibiotics has revolutionized the treatment of this condition. When antibiotics are administered early and in sufficient dosage, they aid the body defenses in bringing under control the general and local manifestations within 48 to 72 hours, and they have so modified the subsequent course that both mortality and morbidity are reduced significantly.

Since the invasive qualities of this lesion now are so effectively controlled by antibiotics, radical excision has become obsolete. Instead, limited surgical intervention is recommended when indicated; this consists of incision and drainage of abscesses when they occur during therapy, and excision of tissue hopelessly devitalized by suppuration and necrosis. Penicillin or one of the newer synthetic penicillinase-resistant drugs is administered in adequate doses, either intramuscularly or orally. Patients with extensive carbuncles and systemic manifestations are usually best treated in a hospital until localization and adequate drainage have been obtained.

In some cases, furuncles are recurrent. Usually this is due to one or more of the predisposing factors previously listed, although in some instances the most exhaustive studies do not reveal any apparent cause. The most thorough attention to skin hygiene and to the nutrition and general health of the patient is important. Trauma, such as that due to the pulling of hairs from the nares, the wearing of chafing, dirty clothes, or the rubbing or fingering of the lesions, should be avoided. The possibility of underlying allergic dermatitis should be borne in mind, and, if it is present, it should be treated suitably. Sugar metabolism should be investigated and controlled if abnormal. Restriction of carbohydrates, even in the absence of demonstrable elevation of the blood sugar level, may be beneficial. It is difficult to evaluate the utility of toxoids and vaccines. All of these preventive measures are not uniformly successful, but in some cases they seem to be effective in checking recurrence.

It is now recognized that in chronic furunculosis of the upper respiratory tract, the anterior nares, even though apparently healthy, are often colonized with *Staphylococcus aureus*. Occasionally, instead of the nose, the eye, the ear, the axilla, or some other region is the reservoir from which infection persists in the neighborhood of a lesion until it is completely healed.

LYMPHANGITIS

Etiology and Symptoms

Acute lymphangitis is an infection that extends along the lymphatic vessels. It frequently originates from a superficial wound, which may be small, such as a pinprick, and spreads proximally through the lymph channels to the lymph nodes. A hemolytic streptococcus is the most common causal organism. Lymphangitis of the upper extremity often arises from a hand infection resulting from a puncture wound by a needle, pin, or wire; from a blister; or from an infected incised wound. Lymphangitis of the lower extremity may arise from an infected blister, callus, or toenail; from an interdigital fungus infection; or from the numerous scratches or bites on the legs of children.

Most patients suffering from lymphangitis have had one of the foregoing wounds of entry for the microorganisms, but an occasional patient may not remember having sustained such a wound. The limb is swollen and painful, but the initial edema does not pit on pressure as in thrombophlebitis. It is tender to palpation, particularly along the course of the affected lymphatics, which may be recognized by their giving rise to red streaks that run up the extremity. These red streaks are tender to palpation, as are the regional lymph nodes.

The general condition of the patient may be one of malaise or of prostration. There may be a chill if the infection is severe, and the temperature and the pulse rate are both elevated. As in any infection, the severity varies according to the virulence of the organism, the degree of contamination and inoculation, and the resistance of the patient. The onset of symptoms and the systemic reaction are more fulminating in the severe infection, and the local signs develop more rapidly in those cases. Injudicious incision or other trauma, neglect, or continued functional use of the part favors rapid spread, complications such as septicemia, and even death. There is little tendency for abscesses to form. When local breakdown of tissue does occur, it is characterized either by gangrene of the overlying skin or the development of thin, watery pus.

Treatment

Much of the fear of lymphangitis has been dispelled by early proper treatment with antibiotic drugs. Their extraordinary efficacy in combating these infections has been proved beyond question. Thus the treatment of acute lymphangitis consists primarily in the control of its invasive characteristics by antibiotic therapy, rest, and heat and secondarily in incision and drainage of collections of pus and necrotic tissue should they present themselves. Penicillin is the drug of choice in hemolytic streptococcal lymphangitis. One of the other broad-spectrum antibiotics may be employed if allergy or resistance to penicillin exists. With therapy, usually the lymphangitis subsides in 24 to 48 hours, but treatment should be continued for 2 or 3 days after the inflammatory process has disappeared. Of equal importance in treatment are rest, heat, and elevation of the infected part, and it is usually advisable, even in the less severe cases, to confine the patient to bed during the acute phase of the infection. In mild cases, enforced bed rest may seem to be drastic treatment from the patient's viewpoint, but a safe and a rapid recovery is thereby ensured. Application of heat may be instituted for the comfort of the patient, although this is no longer as essential to resolution of the infection as it was in the prechemotherapy era. When the infection is in the leg, arm, or hand, the immobilization accomplished by elevating the part on several pillows is sufficient. After control of the invasive characteristics of the infection by penicillin or one of the other chemotherapeutic agents, drainage of the local lesion may be instituted in the event that pus or necrotic tissue has formed, which is rare.

CELLULITIS

Etiology

Cellulitis is a diffuse inflammation of the tissues caused by pyogenic bacteria. It differs from lymphangitis in that it is not limited to the lymphatic vessels. As does lymphangitis, cellulitis arises from an infected wound, which is usually superficial, and the offending organism is again most often a hemolytic streptococcus, although a staphylococcus or mixed flora may be involved. The portal of entry may be an obvious open laceration, ulcer, callus, or blister, or it may be a small puncture wound or abrasion. The spread of infection is usually less rapid than in acute lymphangitis, and the systemic reaction is not as severe. Cellulitis may initiate lymphangitis if it is not promptly treated.

Diagnosis

Increased heat of the affected part, diffuse redness, slight pain and tenderness, and soft edema of the skin and subcutaneous tissues are characteristic of cellulitis. Care must be taken to differentiate between primary cellulitis and the indurated skin over a deep abscess that has become localized and is pointing toward the surface. Timed incision and drainage are indicated in the latter case, whereas conservative therapy is advisable in cellulitis.

Treatment

Rest, elevation of the part of the extremity that is involved, and application of heat constitute the essential local therapeutic measures in the treatment of cellulitis. Penicillin usually produces rapid control of the infection and resolution of the inflammatory process. Not uncommonly, however, the infection becomes localized, and a discrete abscess forms. When induration has diminished and the abscess has become fluctuant and well walled off, incision and drainage facilitate recovery. If there is no clinical response after 48 hours of penicillin and supportive therapy, penicillin-resistant organisms should be suspected as the cause of the infection, and change to another antibiotic may be advisable.

ERYSIPELAS

Symptoms

Erysipelas is an acute infectious disease of the skin or, more rarely, of the mucous membranes, due to infection of the superficial lymphatics, particularly in the corium, by a hemolytic streptococcus. It often originates in a wound. For some reason, erysipelas is rarely seen today. It occurs most frequently in individuals past midlife, and tends to recur unless there is prompt, adequate, specific therapy. The infection seems to have seasonal variation, appearing most often during the fall and the spring. It is characterized by an abrupt onset of systemic symptoms, usually with a chill, headache, severe malaise, and fever. The local lesion, which occurs about the face or the forehead in the majority of cases, is distinctive. The skin becomes hot, red, and indurated and has a well-defined, palpably raised, and sharply demarcated margin. The burning local pain and redness that occur may precede the systemic reaction, although the skin lesion usually does not appear until 6 to 12 hours after the onset of the symptoms. The redness and the induration spread by direct continuity from the periphery, often quite rapidly, and vesicles or even large blebs may form in the area of earlier involvement as the lesion progresses.

Treatment

Treatment of erysipelas usually cannot be carried out in an ambulatory patient, although patients with mild cases without marked systemic symptoms may not require hospitalization. A brief discussion of the present-day therapy of this disease is especially indicated, as erysipelas in its milder forms or earlier stages may be seen first in the physician's office or in the outpatient clinic, and abortive treatment may be given.

Antistreptococcal chemotherapy is the most important single measure in the management of erysipelas, and it has made older forms of treatment obsolete. Penicillin is considered to be the treatment of choice. It is given intramuscularly or intravenously in doses of 600,000 to 1,000,000 units once or twice daily, and it is continued until the patient has been afebrile for at least 3 days. Supportive measures, including generous administration of fluids, are essential for the comfort and the safety of the patient. Recurrence, which is controlled by additional treatment, is seldom as severe as the original attack; lymphatic damage is often responsible for persistent swelling, especially in the extremities.

Prophylaxis

Disinfection of the hands of attending physicians and nurses and scrupulous care of contaminated instruments are essential. Although strict isolation is not necessary, these patients should not be cared for by those who must simultaneously attend obstetric or surgical patients.

ACUTE LYMPHADENITIS

Etiology

Lymphadenitis is an inflammatory process of the lymph nodes that is almost invariably due to lymph-borne infections, although occasionally it may result from blood-borne infections or direct trauma. Although any organism capable of producing infection in tissues may produce lymphadenitis, streptococci and staphylococci are most frequently responsible. The infection is usually secondary, but it may be primary or it may be superimposed on a primary disease of lymphatic tissue. Single nodes or groups of nodes may be affected, or involvement may be widespread, depending on the nature of the etiologic agent.

Diagnosis

A regional lymph node or a chain of enlarged nodes often provides a clue to the diagnosis. Thus acute inflammation of the neck may follow oral sepsis, scalp sepsis, superficial wounds of the head, or infections of the tonsils or respiratory tract. Chronic infectious cervical adenitis may be due to delayed resolution of acute cervical adenitis, or it may be due to tuberculosis, syphilis, anthrax, actinomycosis, or other infection.

In the upper extremity the antecubital and the epitrochlear glands may be involved early in infections involving the ulnar side of the hand. In infections of the radial side of the hand the axillary glands are first to be involved. Infections of the middle finger may drain into either the antecubital or the axillary glands, but in some instances they drain directly into the supraclavicular glands.

Enlarged inguinal nodes occur in sepsis of the lower extremity, for example, in interdigital infection, infected varicose ulcers, and cellulitis or infection in the rectal or the genital area.

Ulcerating lymph nodes, regardless of their location, suggest tuberculosis, tularemia, anthrax, actinomycosis, specific venereal disease, or malignant disease. Differentiation between infection and malignant disease is necessary.

Course

The course of the inflammatory process within the lymph nodes may vary greatly, depending particularly upon the virulence of the invading organism, the nature of the primary infection, and the resistance of the patient. Lymphadenitis appears in the neck, the axilla, or the groin at the height of the primary infection. There is often no evidence of intervening lymphatic involvement. The lymph nodes become tender, hard, and enlarged. In the majority of cases, bacterial lymphadenitis will quickly subside when the primary infection has been adequately controlled. In some cases the primary area of infection may have healed, so that retreatment of the primary lesion is not helpful. In some instances, necrosis and abscess formation result. The infection may extend beyond the lymph nodes and involve adjacent tissues, thus spreading cellulitis.

Treatment

The treatment of lymphadenitis must be directed primarily toward the original portal of infection. This holds true whether the lymphadenitis is of a fulminating, suppurative type or of a low-grade, smoldering type. The management of the primary lesion will, of course, depend entirely upon its nature.

Rest is important during the acute stages. In severe infections, rest in bed with elevation of the affected part, if the primary lesion involves an extremity, is advocated. Immobilization with dressings, splints, or even plaster affords a means of complete rest for an affected extremity in an ambulatory patient. Heat applications are indicated, as they are for any acute inflammation. Antibiotics, usually penicillin given intramuscularly or intravenously in dosage of 500,000 to 1,000,000 units daily, are indicated; in the early stages the infection may be aborted, and in the later stages, even if fluctuation is present and incision is indicated, antibiotics hasten healing.

When suppuration occurs, as evidenced usually by fluctuation of the node, incision and drainage are necessary. If done too early, however, this tends to spread the infection. It is best to delay incision until the induration has practically disappeared and a localized abscess has formed. In the neck it is frequently difficult to demonstrate fluctuation in the enlarged deep nodes. However, lymphadenitis that persists as an enlarged, hard swelling for 10 days or more after an acute infection has subsided usually is found to be the seat of a suppurative necrotic process, and incision is indicated.

In incising lymphadenitis, it is best to make a small incision over the most prominent part of the mass and then to enter the suppurative process with a closed blunt hemostat. When pus is found the hemostat is removed with the blades open, thus enlarging the wound. The wound is then explored with a curved hemostat or a probe, and the incision is enlarged in the direction of the longest diameter of the abscess, the edges of the wound being held open with rake retractors or Allis forceps. When the abscess is completely open the lips of the wound are filled loosely with gauze, which is to be removed in 24 hours; otherwise it may prevent drainage. In suppurative lymphadenitis of the neck the same method of opening the abscess is used, but frequently it is inadvisable to enlarge the opening to the full extent of the abscess because of important structures that must be protected against trauma. Following incision and drainage the wound is managed as described earlier with packing and irrigation.

Penicillin is usually the drug of choice in pyogenic infections, with erythromycin and the cephalosporins as alternatives. Streptomycin is specific therapy for tuberculosis and tularemia; chlortetracycline or oxytetracycline may be used with benefit in actinomycosis.

TETANUS

Tetanus is an acute disease caused by the action on nerve tissue of a diffusible exotoxin produced by *Clostridium tetani*. The portal of entry may be located in any part of the body, but most often tetanus occurs in wounds of the feet, calf, thigh, buttock, or axilla. The patient gives a history of a wound of entry for infection, and usually there is no physical evidence of such a wound. Nail punctures, splinter injuries, burns, and traumatic wounds are common portals. Superficial suppuration under a gauze dressing or a crust provides sufficiently anaerobic conditions for the tetanus bacillus. The incubation period varies from 4 days to 3 weeks, depending somewhat on the character, extent, and location of the wound.

Surgical Prophylaxis

The surgical prevention of tetanus is based on the fact that *C. tetani* is a strict anaerobe, which means that its spores can germinate and give rise to actively growing, toxin-producing bacilli only in an environment free from oxygen. It follows that all open wounds due to violence must be carefully debrided, all necrotic tissues and foreign bodies being removed with as little trauma as possible. If the tissues in the wound following debridement have an adequate blood supply, then all parts of the wound may be considered to be sufficiently oxygenated, and tetanus spores, even if they are present, do not find conditions suitable for germination. Conversely, if debridement has not been adequate, if the wound contains foreign bodies, blood clot, and areas of necrotic tissue, or if the blood supply is precarious, then conditions readily become suitable for germination of spores and production of toxin. Puncture wounds, particularly if contaminated, may require incision and drainage.

Immunoprophylaxis

The Committee on Trauma of the American College of Surgeons recommends the following guidelines in management of the tetanus-prone wound:

I. General Principles:

- A. For each patient the attending physician must determine the adequate prophylaxis against tetanus.
- B. Meticulous surgical care, including removal of all devitalized tissue and foreign bodies, should be provided immediately for all wounds regardless of the active immunization status of the patient. Such care is an essential part of the prophylaxis against tetanus.
- C. Each patient with a wound should receive adsorbed tetanus toxoid intramuscularly at the time of the injury, as an initial immunization, unless he has received a booster or has completed his initial immunization series within the past 12 months. As the antigen concentration varies in different products, specific information on the volume of a single dose is provided on the label of the package.
- D. Need for passive immunization with homologous (human) tetanus immune globulin must be considered in relation to the characteristics of the wound, the conditions under which it was incurred, and the previous active immunization status of the patient.
- E. Every wounded patient should be given a written record of the immunization provided, and instructed to carry the record at all times and, if indicated, to complete active immunization. For precise tetanus prophylaxis, an accurate and immediately available history regarding previous active immunization against tetanus is required.
- F. Basic immunization with adsorbed toxoid requires three injections. A booster of adsorbed toxoid is indicated 10 years after the third injection or 10 years after an intervening wound booster.

II. Specific measures for patients with wounds

- A. For previously immunized individuals
  1. When the patient has been immunized within the past 10 years
     - a. For non–tetanus-prone wounds, no booster dose of toxoid is indicated.
     - b. For tetanus-prone wounds and if more than five years has elapsed since the last dose, give 0.5 ml adsorbed toxoid. If excessive prior toxoid injections have been given, this booster may be omitted.
  2. When the patient has had two or

more prior injections of toxoid and received the last dose *more than 10 years previously,* give 0.5 ml adsorbed toxoid for both tetanus-prone and non–tetanus-prone wounds. Passive immunization is not considered necessary.

B. When the patient has received only one or no prior injection of toxoid, or the immunization history is unknown:
   1. For non–tetanus-prone wounds: Give 0.5 ml adsorbed toxoid.
   2. For tetanus-prone wounds:
      a. Give 0.5 ml adsorbed toxoid.
      b. Give 250 units (or more) of human T.A.T.
      c. Consider providing antibiotics, although the effectiveness of antibiotics for prophylaxis of tetanus remains unproved.

HUMAN BITES

Definition

Human bites are traumatic wounds inoculated with the organisms found in the mouth. The most common site for the lesion is over the metacarpophalangeal joint on the dorsum of the hand, when the clenched fist of one combatant strikes the teeth of his opponent (Fig. 6-1). Sometimes the injury is intentional. Bites acquired by attendants caring for psychiatric patients and by policemen bringing in prisoners are not uncommon. Finally, the injury may occur as a result of accidental puncture by utensils (forks) or instruments (dental) contaminated with human saliva. The aerobic and the anaerobic cocci, fusiform bacilli, and spirochetes present in the mouth are thus transferred to a broken area of the skin, into which may also enter any or all of the bacteria present on the skin when the wound was incurred. Anaerobic streptococci seem to be the most important of these microorganisms, although, because all act in synergism with each other, none can be ignored. The spread of infection is by way of the tissue planes contaminated by the injury. The lesions include soft-tissue necrosis, cellulitis, abscess formation, tenosynovitis, thenar and palmar space infections, and dorsal subcutaneous and subaponeurotic space infections.

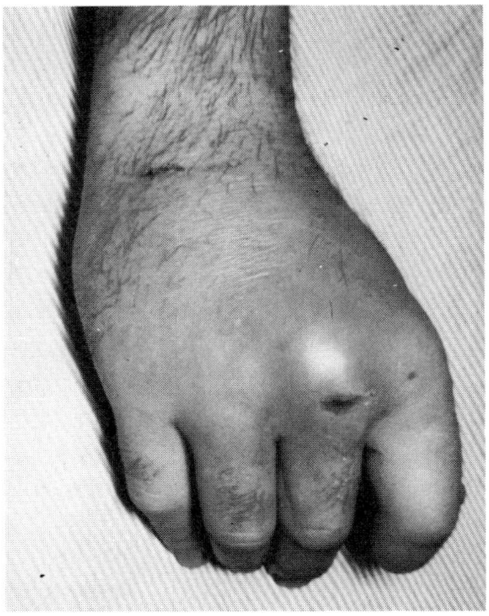

Figure 6-1. Cellulitis around human bite over metacarpophalangeal joint.

Prophylaxis

These are potentially dangerous injuries, especially when they are ignored or treated incorrectly. The general lack of comprehension of the pathologic process, combined with outright mismanagement, accounts for a major portion of the poor results that follow them. In the preantibiotic era, mutilating surgery and amputation of digits, or even of an extremity, were sometimes performed, and an occasional fatality occurred.

Ideal prophylaxis in human bites of the hand begins with cleansing the part for at least 10 minutes with an antibacterial soap and water. Sterile technique is used, and the depths of the wound receive special attention. Only after careful and thorough cleansing are the depth, the extent, and the characteristics of the injury determined. Needless to say this entire process must be performed with good anesthesia of the affected part and gentle handling of the tissues. Debridement is carried out if gross devitalized tissue is present. It is never advisable to attempt primary closure of these wounds, and tightly packed gauze in the wound is avoided. The hand is splinted in the position of function, whether or not surgery is indicated. In any event, penicillin therapy is begun as soon as the patient is seen, and all surgery is performed under its protection. Although no cases of tetanus have been reported from human bites, tetanus immune globulin or toxoid is given.

Treatment

If, as often happens, the victim is not seen until the infection is established, the affected part resembles ordinary cellulitis, with or without lymphangitis and constitutional symptoms, and is very painful, especially on movement. There is a slight to moderate discharge, which frequently has a foul odor. The infection spreads progressively with time.

In the treatment of the infected human-bite wound, the main reliance is on chemotherapy based on culture and sensitivity of the organism. The part is cleansed and swathed in dressings, and, if it is the hand, it is splinted in the position of function and kept elevated. Incision and drainage are resorted to after localization has occurred. Necrotic tissue, if it is not extruded spontaneously, is meticulously debrided. Physical therapy and repair of severed tendons are delayed until after the infection has resolved and the wound has healed.

ANIMAL BITES

Treatment

Bites inflicted by dogs, cats, and other domestic animals, although usually limited to minor abrasions, may result in lacerated or penetrating wounds that are usually badly contused. Such wounds demand the careful, immediate care given any potentially infected contused wound. In addition, the possible transmission of rabies, a specific infectious disease of mammals, always must be considered in the treatment of animal bites.

The first step in the treatment of a bite wound is careful cleansing of the wound and the surrounding skin area. Good anesthesia, with either an adequate local or regional block or general anesthesia, is essential. All badly traumatized and nonviable tissue should be debrided. Primary suture of the wound usually is not advisable. If the animal concerned is rabid, has suggestive symptoms, or cannot be identified, it is recommended that the wound be treated as if rabies might result.

RABIES

Rabies, or hydrophobia, is encephalitis due to a neurotropic virus acquired from the saliva of a rabid animal, usually as a result of a bite. It is usually fatal. Although rabies is now well under control in regions in which public health service programs are in operation, sporadic outbreaks do occur from time to time. Dogs are most commonly responsible for transmitting the virus to man, although other mammals may do so on occasion. Bats are an important reservoir in the Western Hemisphere. Although most human cases occur during hot weather, the disease affects lower animals in all seasons.

Prophylactic Treatment

Prevention and control of rabies entail the impounding of stray ownerless dogs and the restraint of other dogs by their owners. In most communities mass immunization of the canine population is required on an annual basis. The principal threat in the United States now comes from skunks, bats, foxes, and raccoons.

In dealing with bites from animals suspected of having rabies all factors of the case should be considered in deciding if antirabies vaccine should be administered. If the animal responsible is known to have rabies or cannot be examined, immediate immunization is indicated. Otherwise a veterinarian should observe the dog for 14 days. If the dog was infective at the time of the bite, it will die during this period, and immunization of the patient must then be started. However, since rabies due to bites about the face and neck tends to have a shorter incubation period, it may be advisable in such cases to begin immunization at once and to continue it until a full course of vaccine is given. The incubation period varies from 10 days to 12 months and depends largely on the amount of virus introduced and the severity of the laceration.

Rabies Antiserum

For the most serious types of exposure, passive immunization with rabies antiserum is available. Because of the possibility of a very serious type of reaction to the equine serum, a careful history of allergy and of possible sensitization to serum by previous injections should be obtained and tests for sensitivity should be carried out. (As a precaution against a severe anaphylactic reaction it is good to have at hand a syringe containing 1 ml of 1:1000 epinephrine for immediate use.) The dose of antiserum given is 40 units/kg, and half of it should be given locally into the wound. To be maximally effective, passive immunization with antiserum should be instituted within 24 hours after the bite of a rabid animal. Existing laboratory and human studies support the view that the rabies virus remains at the wound site for probably about 3 days, during which time it is subject to the action of the injected antiserum. After that time it is believed to become fixed in the nervous tissue itself, where it cannot be neutralized by rabies antibody.

A hyperimmune rabies immune globulin obtained from human volunteers, HRIG, has been licensed. This product will eliminate serum sickness from passive immunization; however, because of limited supply, it should be reserved for persons who have a history of allergy to equine products, whose skin test of the equine product is positive, or who are pregnant. The recommended dose of HRIG is 20 I.U./kg. Up to 50% of the antiserum should be used to infiltrate the wound, and the rest should be administered intramuscularly.

All bites inflicted by possibly rabid animals should be treated by copious flushing with 20% soap in water, benzalkonium chloride 1%, or ethanol 43% to 70%. Whiskey of 86 proof or greater can be used in emergencies. The decision whether to immunize or not should be based on the local incidence of rabies, the type of animal inflicting the bite, and the circumstances surrounding the incident.

If the biting animal is a domestic one, such as a dog or cat, its behavior during and after the attack is most important. Healthy animals that appear to have been provoked into biting should merely be observed, without treatment of the victim. Animals with signs suggestive of rabies should be sacrificed and their brains examined for rabies infection. Treatment should be started at once and stopped if the laboratory report is negative.

Bites of sylvatic animals, when unprovoked, must be considered contaminated by rabies virus unless the biting animal can be captured and shown to be free of rabies. Rodent bites, such as those inflicted on slum children by rats or on middle-class children by pet hamsters, ordinarily need no antirabies treatment. However, strains of rabies virus developed for vaccination of dogs, when given to other species, may not be sufficiently attenuated. Rabies can thereby be provoked in the pet rodent, resulting in a hazard for human contacts.

Antiserum should be used locally and parenterally, in addition to vaccine, whenever exposure to rabies has been proved or is highly likely, based on the fact that in the clinical situation it is impossible to estimate the amount of virus introduced into the wound. In infection of guinea pigs with small doses of rabies virus, vaccine alone sufficed for protection, but when moderate doses were given, antiserum was necessary in addition to vaccine. The combination of antiserum and vaccine provides an immediate rise in the level of antibody, which should result in maximal neutralization of the virus while it is still susceptible to the action of antibody. A single dose of antiserum (40 units/kg) followed by vaccine results in immediately detectable circulating antibody, which persists through the period of 10 to 14 days before a response to vaccine takes place. This therapy is a double-edged sword, however, because even one dose of antiserum may slightly suppress the response to vaccine unless the latter is given in adequate antigenic mass.

Antirabies Vaccine

Duck embryo inactivated vaccine is the only currently licensed vaccine available in the United States. The vaccine must be given daily for at least 14 days. Some authorities recommend 21 daily injections when the vaccine is used with hyperimmune serum. The inoculations cannot be given over a shorter period or in a larger volume less frequently; daily stimulus is necessary. In order to insure that antiserum does not suppress the active antibody response, booster doses of vaccine must be administered 10 days and 20 days after the last injection of the initial series.

BIBLIOGRAPHY

General Principles: Surgical Infections

Alexander JW: Emerging concepts in the control of surgical infections. Surgery 75:934, 1974

American College of Surgeons Committee on Control of Infection in Surgical Patients, 2nd ed. Philadelphia, JB Lippincott, 1984

Meleney FL: Clinical Aspects and Treatment of Surgical Infections. Philadelphia, WB Saunders, 1949

Pulaski EJ: Common Bacterial Infections: Pathophysiology and Clinical Management. Philadelphia, WB Saunders, 1964

Antibiotic Therapy

Crofton J: Some principles in the chemotherapy of bacterial infections. Br Med J 2:137, 1969

Kagan BM (ed): Antimicrobial Therapy, 3rd ed. Philadelphia, WB Saunders, 1980

Pratt WB: Fundamentals of Chemotherapy. New York, Oxford University Press, 1973

Smith H: Antibiotics in Clinical Practice, 3rd ed. Baltimore, University Park Press, 1977

Treatment of Local Infections

Altemeier WA, Giuseffi J: Treatment of surgical infections in the ambulatory patient. Surg Clin North Am (Nation Wide Number), p 1259, 1951

Blumer JL, O'Brian CA, Lemon E, Capretta TM: Skin and soft tissue infections: Pharmacologic approaches. Pediatr Infec Dis 4:336–341, 1985

Koch SL: Boils and carbuncles. Surg Gynecol Obstet 117:231, 1963

Pulaski EJ: Treatment of soft tissue infections. Antibiot Med Clin Ther 4:657, 1957

Tetanus

Altemeier WA, Hummel RP: Treatment of tetanus. Surgery 60:495, 1966

American College of Emergency Physicians: Tetanus immunization recommendations for persons seven years of age and older. Ann Emerg Med 15:1111–1112, 1986

American College of Surgeons Committee on Trauma: A guide to prophylaxis against tetanus in wound management. Bull Am Coll Surg, 1982

Center for Disease Control, Department of Health and Human Services: Diphtheria, tetanus and pertussis: Guidelines for vaccine prophylaxis and other preventive measures. Ann Intern Med 103:896–905, 1985

Human and Animal Bites

Callahan M: Dog bite wounds. JAMA 244:2327–2328, 1980

Dreyfuss UY, Singer M: Human bites of the hand: A study of one hundred six patients. J Hand Surg 10:884–889, 1980

Edlich RF, Spengler MD, Rodeheaver GT: Mammalian bites. Compr Ther 9:41–47, 1983

Kerr R: Human bite infections of the hand. Orthopedics 9:761, 763–765, 1986

Rabies

Corey C, Hottwick M: Treatment of persons exposed to rabies. JAMA 232:272, 1975

Gross EM, Bearman JE: Post-exposure rabies prophylaxis: Establishing effectiveness of abbreviated treatments. Vaccine 3:283, 1985

Marwick C: Changes recommended in use of human diploid cell rabies vaccine. JAMA 254:13–14, 1985

Ubol S, Phanuphak P: An effective economical intradermal regimen of human diploid cell rabies vaccination for post-exposure treatment. Clin Exp Immunol 63:491–497, 1986

7 Sutures and Suturing

RAYMOND W. POSTLETHWAIT

The choice of material for a surgical suture or ligature is, within reasonable limits, less important than the technique employed. The suture must be properly placed and securely tied with appropriate tension to fulfill its purpose. Although any of several types of sutures may be satisfactory in a specific situation, one may be more advantageous than another, and some knowledge of the characteristics of a suture will influence proper selection. The composition of the material, strength, knot efficiency, tissue response, and other factors are important.

A number of these factors must be considered for an ideal suture (see "Characteristics of Ideal Surgical Suture"). Some of these are obviously mutually exclusive but help form a basis for suture selection. The variety of sutures, discussed below, that are now available indicates the developments in this field in the past few years.

HISTORY

The original use of sutures and ligatures is obscure, but ancient Greek and Egyptian medical writings describe such materials as linen, cotton, leather, animal tendon, catgut, and metal wire. Rhoads and his associates reviewed in detail the use of catgut.[18] In 1816, Philip Syng Physick published the results of his experiments and receives credit for the general use of catgut. Lister in 1868 described the first of his many experiments with catgut. Macewen in 1881 first recommended chromicizing catgut to increase the strength. Over the years numerous studies of absorption and changes in strength in implanted catgut were reported, notably those of Howes and of Jenkins and their associates.[4–6] The work of Meleney and Chatfield eventually assured sterility of the catgut.[8]

Halsted, after observing the use of silk by Kocher, utilized this material for years before his definitive description of the silk technique in 1913.[3] Whipple in 1933, as well as others, confirmed the superiority of silk in clean wounds. Meade and Ochsner in 1940 described their experimental and clinical results with cotton[7]; Babcock in 1947 recorded his extensive experience with stainless-steel wire.[1]

Nichols and Diak in 1940 first compared nylon with other suture material and concluded that the synthetic suture is satisfactory for clinical use.[9] Since then a number of synthetic sutures, described later, have been offered by suture manufacturers and have been used extensively.

CHARACTERISTICS OF IDEAL SURGICAL SUTURE

- May be used in any operation
- Handles comfortably
- Adequate tensile strength
- Tissue reaction minimal
- Not conducive to infection
- Knots securely
- Does not fray
- No shrinkage or excessive extension
- Nonelectrolytic, noncapillary, nonallergenic, noncarcinogenic
- Sterilized without alteration
- Absorbed after purpose served
- Inexpensive

ABSORBABLE SUTURES

CATGUT

Catgut in either plain or chromicized form is initially uniform in finish and strength. It handles well, knots securely when properly tied, and, because it is absorbed, may be indicated when a wound may be contaminated. The disadvantages are the erratic behavior in loss of strength, absorption, and tissue reaction.

In situations such as fascial closure, the rate of loss of breaking strength is unpredictable.

Implantation studies in animals show that breaking strength may be retained near the initial level for 2 to 3 weeks in some, whereas in others, a decided loss of strength occurs during this period. Absorption is equally erratic; remnants of the catgut may persist for months.

Early after implantation in tissues, catgut acts as any other monofilament suture (the tissue reaction to all sutures for 5 to 7 days is secondary to the trauma of passage of the needle and insertion of the suture). The perisutural tissue reaction occurs when absorption of the catgut begins (Fig. 7-1). A mononuclear cell infiltrate first develops about the suture, then about the fragments of suture as absorption progresses. Polymorphonuclear leukocytes are seldom an important component, although occasionally eosinophils may be. After absorption is complete a collection of mononuclear cells with foamy brownish cytoplasm remains for a variable period.

SYNTHETIC ABSORBABLE SUTURE

Two types of absorbable sutures are available: polyglycolic acid, a homopolymer of glycolic acid, and polyglactin, a copolymer made from lactide and glycolide. They are made by melt extrusion under controlled temperature and pressure, both are multifilament, and their characteristics are so similar that they may be considered together. Both feel slightly rough but handle well and knot securely.

Their initial tensile strength is greater than that of silk or catgut but less than that of Dacron. After implantation in tissue the loss of strength is predictably linear to a zero point in about 21 to 25 days. The absorption is equally predictable, beginning in the fourth week and being complete in the fourth month.

The tissue reaction is unique. After the initial reaction has subsided, perisutural cellular reaction of any type rarely develops (Fig. 7-1).

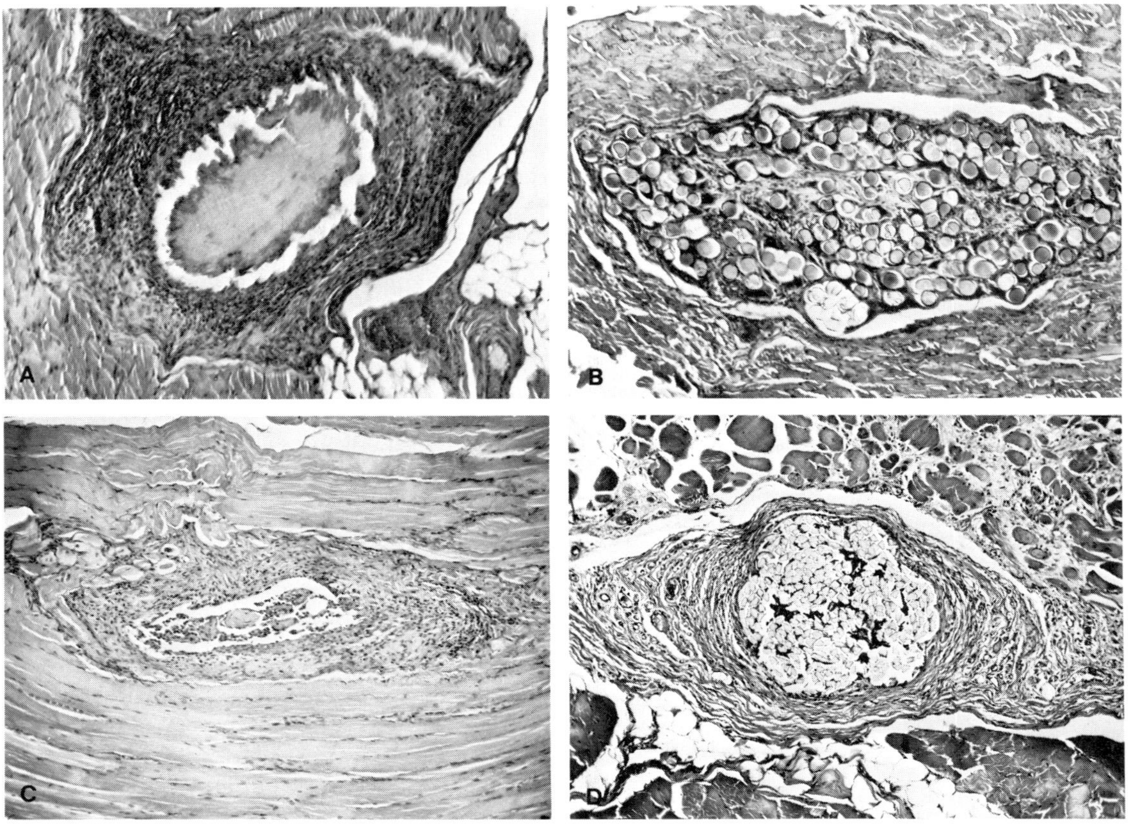

Figure 7-1. (*A*) An intense cellular reaction develops as catgut is absorbed. (*B*) Synthetic absorbable suture shows cellular invasion about the fibers but no reaction around the suture. (*C*) Site of wire suture with fibrous tissue cuff and minimal reaction. (*D*) Compact silk suture with modest cellular response.

The interstices of the suture are invaded by mononuclear cells, with some lymphocytes and occasionally giant cells. As absorption takes place the suture fibers become smaller, although not uniformly, and then disappear. The cells that have invaded gradually decrease in number at the same time.

In addition to the two materials described previously, more recently a third synthetic absorbable suture has become available. This is a polymer, polydioxanone (PDS), which is monofilament and uniquely flexible. Young's modulus is about a fourth that of polyglycolic acid or polyglactin; the initial tensile strength exceeds that of polypropylene and nylon. Absorption is by hydrolysis with minimal tissue reaction, beginning about the 90th day and being complete in 180 days. Most important, the implantation studies of Ray and colleagues[17] show the loss of breaking strength to be almost linear to zero in 8 to 10 weeks. After 4 weeks, 71% of the initial strength of size 2-0 remained and 46% of size 6-0.

From the clinical standpoint the advantages of the synthetic absorbable sutures over catgut are apparent: adequate initial tensile strength, a predictable rate of loss of strength and of absorption, and minimal tissue reaction. Although catgut may be indicated in specific situations the synthetic absorbable sutures should generally replace catgut.

NONABSORBABLE SUTURES

SILK

Silk is generally considered the standard nonabsorbable suture, more from tradition than from fact, as silk may be absorbed. In some patients, however, silk will persist unchanged (microscopically) for at least 20 years. Silk is a protein with a core of fibroin analogous to horn, hair, and similar dermal products, according to Meade and Ochsner.[7] It is a dyed, waxed, multifilament suture with an initial tensile strength greater than cotton but less than the synthetic nonabsorbable materials. The wide usage of silk is at least in part due to the surgeons trained by Halsted and their subsequent generations of trainees. Silk handles most comfortably, because of its pliability, and knots satisfactorily.

The strength of silk is dependable to the range of 6 to 8 weeks. After this, wide variation is found. In animal implantation studies extending through 5 years, an occasional strand of silk was found that had retained appreciable strength. Absorption is equally variable, as noted earlier.

Histologically, three patterns of reaction to silk are found. Usually the silk remains as a compact bundle surrounded by a connective tissue zone of variable thickness. Within this and nearest the suture, two or more layers of mononuclear cells, mainly histiocytes, persist for years (Fig. 7-1D). In the second pattern the interstices are invaded by fibroblasts, histiocytes, and lymphocytes. Giant cells may be present. Least often, and usually about a knot, a granulomatous reaction is seen with or without fragmentation of the silk.

To define precisely the current indications for silk as sutures and ligatures is not feasible. The synthetic materials, both absorbable and nonabsorbable, have replaced silk in many operations.

COTTON

For use as sutures and ligatures, the properties of silk and cotton are so similar that detailed description is unnecessary. The handling, knot stability, changes in strength, and tissue reaction do not differ greatly. One decided advantage of cotton is that it is the most inexpensive of the sutures.

WIRE

Stainless-steel wire has a high tensile strength that is not altered by implantation in tissue. The surface allows smooth gliding through tissue, and the knot holds firmly. Wire is stiff and the ends sharp, which causes problems in its use until the surgeon becomes accustomed to it. Multifilament wire is more easily handled. Wire used for such purposes as abdominal closure may be seen to have broken in x-ray films made later. If the cut ends of the wire are not turned in they may erode to or through the skin in a thin patient. A major advantage of wire, other than strength, is that it does not tend to support infection.

The tissue reaction to wire is modest, the area about the wire showing a variable concentration of mononuclear cells and a small amount of fibrous tissue (Fig. 7-1). Monofilament wire may have a slight tendency to cut into enclosed tissues.

After technical proficiency has been attained in using wire, it provides a versatile suture for a number of uses.

NYLON

Nylon is a polyamide that had most extensive use as a monofilament but in recent years has become available in a multifilament form that handles much like silk. The monofilament is somewhat stiff, and a secure knot can be obtained only with multiple loops. The initial tensile strength is excellent and in tissues decreases slowly over a period of years.

In our animal implantation studies,[13–16] monofilament nylon has most consistently stimulated the least tissue reaction of any material examined. The usual finding is a narrow, nearly acellular type of fibrous tissue (Fig. 7-2). The multifilament suture is prone to incite more reaction, similar to Dacron, as noted later.

Nylon is another suture material with a wide range of applications. Extremely fine nylon is used in microsurgery. Small-caliber nylon as a continuous suture provides precise skin closure. Heavy nylon may be useful for difficult abdominal closure.

DACRON

Dacron has gained extensive application because of sustained strength, low tissue reactivity, and good handling properties. It is a multi-

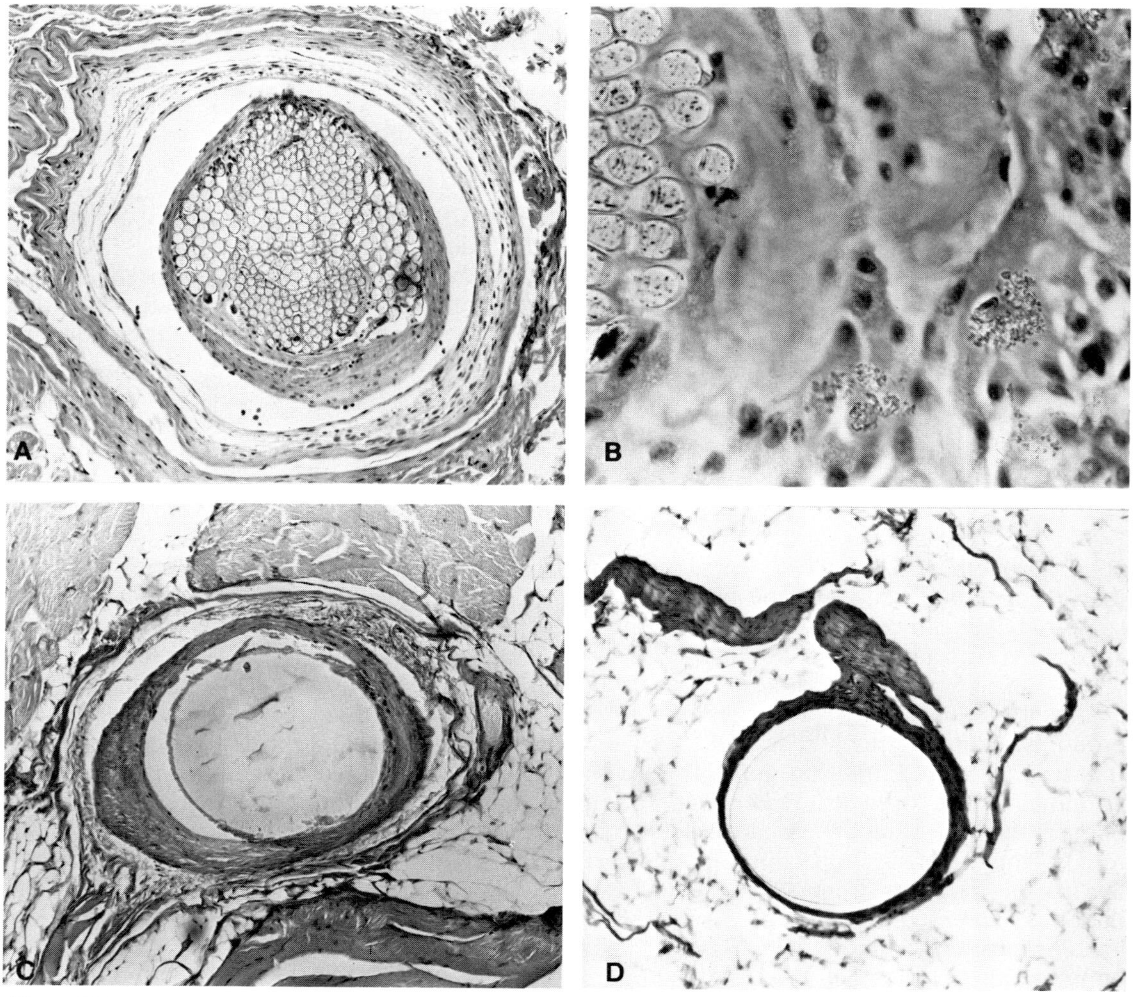

Figure 7-2. (*A*) Dacron suture stimulates little cellular reaction. (*B*) Teflon shed from coated Dacron suture is seen as granular appearing material. Cellular reaction to both nylon (*C*) and polypropylene (*D*) sutures is essentially absent.

filament suture and may be obtained uncoated or coated with such materials as Teflon, silicone, or polybutylate. The coated sutures hold a knot less well than the uncoated and require additional loops in the knot, the number varying with the specific suture. The initial tensile strength is high and is maintained in tissues.

Dacron stimulates a very moderate tissue reaction, much less than silk or cotton but more than nylon (Fig. 7-2). The fibers tend to remain compact, surrounded by a connective tissue zone invariably containing a number of mononuclear cells near the suture. Occasionally fibrous tissue invades the interstices of the suture. The Teflon-coated sutures, for an unknown time extending from months to years, appear to shed the Teflon into the adjacent tissues. These fragments in turn stimulate a secondary mononuclear cell reaction (Fig. 7-2). After the Teflon has disappeared the reaction is similar to that of uncoated Dacron. We have not investigated the other two coatings, but from previous experiments with silicone-treated silk, we would not anticipate the reaction to differ from that of uncoated Dacron.

Dacron, either uncoated or coated, is useful in essentially any application in which silk has been employed, in addition to some operations in which silk is now known to be contraindicated, namely, synthetic grafting to vessel anastomoses. Teflon shed from the suture should cause no problems except in the most delicate operations such as nerve or tendon suture.

POLYPROPYLENE

A polyolefin, polypropylene is provided as a monofilament suture of excellent, maintained strength with a major advantage of sliding through tissues very easily. As a monofilament synthetic material with a memory, and relatively low coefficient of friction, knot security is obtainable only with multiple loops.

The very minor tissue reaction stimulated by polypropylene is the same as that by nylon (Fig. 7-2). Infrequently, however, fibrillation of the polypropylene occurs, and each fragment then causes a reaction about it.

The most extensive use of polypropylene sutures has been in cardiac and vascular operations; in minor surgery its application has been more limited.

HEALING OF SKIN

Since an important component of minor surgery relates to healing of the skin, a brief discussion seems appropriate. The following is based mainly on the excellent studies of Ordman and Gillman.[10–12] Their investigations were carried out on pigs, whose skin closely resembles that of humans. They emphasized that a healing cutaneous wound is not a thin line but a vertically placed block of new tissue extending down into the subcutaneous fat for the entire depth of the incision.

Blood and serum rapidly form a linear scab over the wound after closure, and the epithelium grows beneath this. Within a few hours of injury, epithelium on either side of the incision thickens and begins to migrate across the deficit as two long sheets. The gap is bridged in 24 to 48 hours. The new epithelium then thickens, and some downward growth extends into the dermal breach. The epithelium then acquires some of the structural features of the uninjured epidermis, and about the fifth day, keratin forms with resultant loosening of the overlying scab.

In the dermis, vertically oriented strands of fibrin enmesh erythrocytes and white cells, mainly polymorphonuclear. Phagocytosis begins about the second day, and the cellular exudate changes to a primarily mononuclear one. Fibroblasts, also vertically oriented, are present about the fourth day with the first appearance of collagen 24 hours later. After the seventh day, the collagen lies across the incision to interdigitate with adjacent normal tissue or nearby transected preexisting collagen bundles. After the 21st day the cellular and vascular elements decrease gradually, and the scar usually widens, even with sutures in place. The collagen then thickens and forms bundles, and the junction between old and new tissue becomes more difficult to define.

Depending on the body area involved, a variable number of skin appendages are divided. Throughout the incision, epithelial growth may occur from each divided end of, for example, a hair follicle. The epithelial aggregation may be solid or cystic but is absorbed after several weeks.

The major emphasis of Ordman and Gillman was the advantage of microporous adhesive tape over sutures for skin closure, and for this reason, they provided detailed descriptions of the reaction about the suture as it traverses the skin. Briefly, the suture stimulates an inflammatory reaction along its track. A granulomatous, then fibrous, tissue response develops. In addition, from each point of penetration of the skin, epidermis grows along the suture, first on the convex side but eventually as a tube surrounding the suture. Keratin is formed between the fifth and tenth day, and even in the absence of infection the inflammatory response is manifested grossly by a reddish halo about the points of entry and exit of the suture. After the suture is removed the reaction subsides and the epithelium is eventually absorbed.

METHODS OF SUTURING

The variety of incisional, excisional, and traumatic wounds, as well as the various tissues that may be involved in minor surgery, make a detailed description of all applicable suture techniques too extensive to be discussed here. Therefore, assuming that the deeper structures have been approximated appropriately, emphasis will be given to skin closure.

Suture closure of the skin is usually interrupted or continuous, simple or mattress in type (Fig. 7-3). Other methods have been described, but these generally are most satisfactory. The beginner is well advised to learn first the proper use of the interrupted mattress suture. The spacing and amount of tissue within the suture loop are dependent to a degree on the site being closed. However, an effort is made to encompass the same amount of tissue on each side of the wound, as well as to maintain the same angle of insertion and egress. A straight or curved cutting needle with material such as nylon or silk swedged on is used. The first insertion is sufficiently deep to approximate the skin and relieve any tension; the return insertion is in the most superficial layer of the epidermis, encompassing only enough tissue to allow approximation.

As the knot is formed the tension applied to the suture loop must be precise: Excessive tension results in cutting of the suture and increased tissue necrosis, whereas insufficient tension does not appose the wound surface. The same principle applies when a continuous suture is used. The surgeon should keep in mind that some swelling of the tissues occurs after closure, which increases the possibility

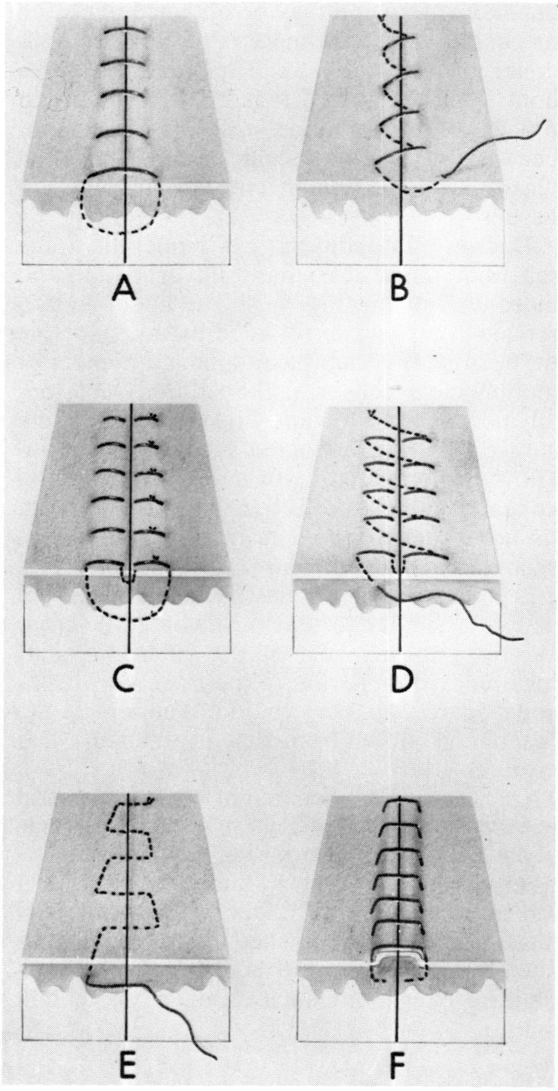

Figure 7-3. Methods of skin closure: (*A*) interrupted simple suture, (*B*) continuous simple suture, (*C*) interrupted mattress suture, (*D*) continuous mattress suture, (*E*) subcuticular closure, (*F*) staples.

of the skin suture cutting into the epidermis and leaving the characteristic ladder pattern.

Although the surgeon and patient hope for a minimal scar in any situation, in some areas, such as the face, this is more important than in others. Accordingly, tension is relieved by subcutaneous sutures with the knots deep, and the skin is approximated with very fine suture material, meticulously placed and tied.

A continuous subcuticular suture provides good apposition while avoiding the necessity for suture removal and the possibility of suture scars. Although the use of nonabsorbable material, usually as a pullout suture, has been described, a fine synthetic absorbable suture is preferable. The knots can be buried, and the suture linearly placed in the inner aspect of the dermis to provide good apposition of the epidermis with slight eversion.

The time for removal of skin sutures depends on a number of factors, one being the tensile strength of the skin. Through the fourth day the tensile strength is slight as it is dependent on the adherence of the fibrin in the dermis and the strength of the epithelial bridge. The tensile strength increases rapidly from the fifth through the fifteenth day, then increases more slowly. Theoretically, sutures would be removed about this time, but their prolonged presence in tissue has adverse effects. Granulation and epithelialization of the suture track, noted earlier, will develop; the presence of a foreign body increases the chances of infection; the puncture wounds of entry and exit are more likely to cause a visible scar. As a general rule, therefore, sutures should be removed between the sixth and tenth day, as recommended by Ordman and Gillman. Exceptions are obvious. For example, in the face half the sutures may be removed the second or third day (reinforcing if necessary with tape) and the remainder on the fourth or fifth day. In areas under tension such as those on the back or extremities, sutures may be left in for 10 to 14 days.

OTHER METHODS OF CLOSURE

The tissue adhesives (cyanoacrylates) have not fulfilled the early hopes for use except in a few specific locations and have little role in wound closure. Skin clips, which have long been available, have not been very satisfactory, but recently skin staplers have been developed. To increase rigidity the staple wire is larger than the usual wire suture. The staple is in the form of a wide inverted U, and as the staple is inserted the cross arm is bent, directing the legs of the staple into the skin. This elevates the enclosed skin and approximates the edges. A special instrument is needed for removal of the staples. The skin stapler provides rapid, satisfactory closure in many situations.

Microporous surgical adhesive tape has not attained wide popularity, in spite of the strong recommendations of investigators such as Ordman and Gillman. Grabb and Smith have noted the advantages and disadvantages of tape.[2] Tape saves time in application and removal, causes no skin reaction, avoids suture puncture scars, can be applied without an anesthetic, and can be left in place for long periods beneath dressings or casts. The disadvantages are the lack of eversion of skin edges, failure to adhere to wet skin, and the possibility of its coming off during bathing and of its premature removal by children or uncooperative patients.

REFERENCES

1. Babcock WW: Metallic sutures and ligatures. Surg Clin North Am 27:1435, 1947
2. Grabb WC, Smith JW: Plastic Surgery. Boston, Little, Brown & Co, 1973
3. Halsted WS: Ligature and suture material. Employment of fine silk in preference to catgut and the advantages of transfixion of tissues and vessels in control hemorrhage. JAMA 60:1119, 1913
4. Howes EL: Factors determining the loss of strength of catgut when embedded in tissue. JAMA 90:530, 1928
5. Howes EL, Harvey SC: The strength of the healing wound in relation to the holding strength of the catgut suture. N Engl J Med 200:1285, 1929
6. Jenkins HP, Hrdina LS, Owens FM, Jr, Swisher FM: Absorption of surgical gut (catgut). III. Duration in the tissues after loss of tensile strength. Arch Surg 45:74, 1942
7. Meade WH, Ochsner A: The relative value of catgut, silk, linen and cotton as suture materials. Surgery 7:485, 1940
8. Meleney FL, Chatfield M: The sterility of catgut in relation to hospital infections with an effective test for the sterility of catgut. Surg Gynecol Obstet 42:430, 1931
9. Nichols HM, Diack AW: An experimental study of nylon as a suture material. West J Surg 48:42, 1940
10. Ordman LJ, Gillman T: Studies in the healing of cutaneous wounds. I. The healing of incisions through the skin of pigs. Arch Surg 93:857, 1966
11. Ordman LJ, Gillman T: Studies in the healing of cutaneous wounds. II. The healing of epidermal, appendageal, and dermal injuries inflicted by suture needles and by the suture material in the skin of pigs. Arch Surg 93:883, 1966

12. Ordman LJ, Gillman T: Studies in the healing of cutaneous wounds. III. A critical comparison in the pig of the healing of surgical incisions closed with sutures or adhesive tape based on tensile strength and clinical and histological criteria. Arch Surg 93:911, 1966
13. Postlethwait RW, Dillon ML, Reeves JW: Experimental study of silk suture. Arch Surg 84:698, 1962
14. Postlethwait RW: Long-term comparative study of nonabsorbable sutures. Ann Surg 171:892, 1970
15. Postlethwait RW: Polyglycolic acid surgical suture. Arch Surg 101:489, 1970
16. Postlethwait RW, Willigan DA, Ulin AW: Human tissue reaction to sutures. Ann Surg 181:144, 1975
17. Ray JA, Doddi N, Regula D, Williams JA, Melveger A: Polydioxanone (PDS), a novel monofilament synthetic absorbable suture. Surg Gynecol Obstet 153:497, 1981
18. Rhoads JE, Hottenstein HF, Hudson IF: Decline in strength of catgut after exposure to living tissues. Arch Surg 34:377, 1937
19. Whipple AO: The use of silk in the repair of clean wounds. Ann Surg 98:662, 1933
20. Whipple AO: The choice and use of ligature and suture material in the repair of clean wounds. Int Abstr Surg 69:109, 1939

8 Dressings

MARK W. WOLCOTT

Dressings are used for protection, pressure, immobilization, absorption, debridement, comfort, and appearance. The requirements of dressings and bandages for ambulatory patients are somewhat more exacting than those for patients in hospitals or at home and in bed. They must stay absolutely in place until the time for replacement, and they should permit, as far as possible, the patient to resume or continue his normal activities with the least amount of inconvenience. There has been recent evidence that surgical wound infection in undressed wounds is less than in the dressed. However, this is not likely to apply to an ambulatory patient subjected to many other sources of contamination.

FUNCTIONS

PROTECTION

The applied dressing should protect the wound from further trauma and from both endogenous and exogenous sources of contamination from bacteria. It should therefore be of adequate bulk and well applied so that it does not slip from its position. It is well to consider application of either petrolatum gauze or Telfa to the wound before the dressing is applied to prevent further trauma to the wound when the dressing is removed.

PRESSURE

A well-applied dressing can apply a modest amount of pressure that prevents oozing from wound edges and can help to prevent edema of the transudate that accumulates in traumatized tissue. A correct amount of pressure can therefore prevent some fluid accumulation and bleeding and potential development of a hematoma. Prevention of both of these reduces the chances of infection in a hematoma and the amount of scar formation and may prevent wound dehiscence. One must be careful not to apply a dressing too tightly, creating a tourniquet effect; therefore the dressing should be applied from distal to proximal. It is well also to increase the bulk of the dressing over the wound as convexity increases the amount of pressure that the circular dressing applies. One must always keep in mind the danger of pressure on nerves or impairment of arterial and venous flow. Therefore after the application of a pressure dressing, one should check carefully for any neurologic signs or color changes as a result of compression of arterial or venous supply. The patient should be instructed to report immediately any numbness, temperature, or color change to the physician.

ABSORPTION

A dressing should act as a passageway and storage for drainage of blood serum as it accumulates in the wound. A dressing should therefore be hydrophilic, encouraging the movement of water from the wound to the absorbent layers. If much drainage is expected, a bulky dressing should be applied, which further protects the wound from trauma.

IMMOBILIZATION

A well-applied dressing tends, to a modest degree, to prevent motion of the affected part. This promotes wound healing, minimizes the amount of discomfort, and prevents bleeding.

DEBRIDEMENT

In some situations, especially in burns and other types of scraped wounds, the dressing can act by a combination of capillary action and maceration of the foreign and necrotic material so that when the dressing is removed, there is a cleansing debriding action. The material used for this debridement should be free of lint to minimize contamination of the wound. The original dressing applied at the time of operation should provide sufficient absorbent material to take care of the wound secretion for at least 24 to 48 hours and should be applied well enough to remain in place for that period.

Occasionally, packing is placed in an infected wound following an incision. A plain gauze dressing or commercial type of gauze dressing containing a film of cotton should be applied over the wound. Pressure is applied by placing one or two strips of adhesive tape across the dressing and on the skin and applying a firm bandage, often with a Kerlex type of gauze dressing.

REDRESSING OF WOUNDS

The time for redressing depends on the type of wound, or more exactly, the amount of secretion from it.

DRESSING OF CLEAN WOUNDS

With a clean wound, unless pain, swelling, or other evidence of infection appears, redressing is not necessary until it is time to remove the sutures—anywhere from 3 to 7 days. Every patient with a clean wound, therefore, is instructed to return in 3 days or sooner if the lesion does not become increasingly uncomfortable. At the third day visit the dressing is inspected. If it is not soiled and there is no discomfort in the region of the wound, the patient is asked to return between the fifth and seventh day for removal of the sutures. When there is some soiling of the superficial parts of the dressing, the gauze on the top may be changed, with care being taken not to disturb the layers underneath, where there is usually a brownish hard stain of dried blood that acts as an excellent splint for the wound.

When the patient complains of discomfort in the area of the wound and, on inspection, some edema of the tissues is noted, the dressing is removed and the wound inspected. This situation is usually found in cases in which there has been considerable dissection in the subcutaneous fatty tissues and low-grade localized cellulitis has resulted. In such cases it is rarely necessary to open the wound, although removal of one or two sutures to relieve tension may be helpful. Experience has shown that this type of wound reaction subsides in 24 to 48 hours if 70% alcohol is applied to the dressing; the patient is instructed to apply this three or four times a day and to keep the injured area elevated. Cleansing with soap and water is often desirable. No ointments should be used because they tend to macerate the tissues.

At the patient's second visit, between the fifth and the seventh day after operation, the sutures are removed. If the integrity of the wound might be affected by movement of the part, splints are included as part of the dressing for a week or so after removal of the sutures. In other cases, adhesive strips may be applied across the wound at right angles to its long axis. These provide continued support at the wound edges and may be left in place for a week or 10 days if desired. They are especially valuable for wounds of the shoulder and back, where the skin is quite thick and motion tends to pull the wound edges apart.

DRESSING OF INFECTED WOUNDS

The patient with an infected lesion should be asked to return for redressing on the second day after operation. As a rule, it is unwise to change the dressing on the day following operation, because this usually causes renewed bleeding, and the secretions are usually not excessive enough to demand a change of dressing.

On the second day after operation the superficial dressings are removed and the wound is inspected to be sure the packing or the drain is still in place. The surgeon then decides the type of dressing to be applied, and it must be applied before the instruments and the dressing tray become soiled. He should be provided with sufficient cotton balls soaked in hydrogen peroxide to wash away the dried secretions on the edge of the wound and to use as sponges in removing purulent secretions from the wound itself. A few alcohol sponges or organic iodine solution is useful for a final cleansing of the skin around the wound. If packing is to be replaced, sterile instruments should be reserved for removing packing from its sterile container and for cutting it without contaminating the remainder. Unless the packing in the wound seems to be acting as a plug and preventing drainage of the wound secretions, it is usually wise to leave it in place or to remove it only partly at the time of this dressing because a sufficient amount of inflammatory induration has not developed in the walls of the wound to keep its lips from falling together. It should be mentioned that when gauze packing is adherent to the edges of the wound, considerable pain is produced by pulling it away at this second-day dressing, whereas this gauze usually is removed easily without pain at later renewals of the dressing.

After this initial dressing the interval between future dressings depends to a great extent on the amount of secretion. If it is profuse, daily dressings are necessary, whereas if the breakdown of sloughing tissue is slow, dressings may be maintained for 2 or 3 days. Usually at the second dressing all packing is removed from the wound, and by this time, if an adequate incision has been made, an opening of sufficient size remains. Unless the infected area is deep there is no necessity for reinserting packing or other drainage material. The inflammatory induration in the walls of the wound does not permit its closure until all the purulent material has been discharged. When the wound is exposed, an effort should be made to remove all the liquid necrotic material and as much of the loosened necrotic tissue as possible.

Two methods are of particular value for removal of liquid material, irrigation and mopping of the wound with a sponge. The easier and less painful method is irrigation of the wound with warm sterile saline solution. A glass syringe with a rubber bulb or a disposable sterile plastic bulb syringe has been found to be most useful; either type can be handled with one hand, and the force of the stream can be regulated so that the solution may be forced with good pressure into the deeper recesses of the wound cavity. This method of cleaning the wound is of particular value when the wound is deep and when there is considerable sloughing of fascia and connective tissue. Hanging a bottle of sterile saline and connecting an intravenous tube to it provides copious gentle irrigation. Large bottles of solutions for irrigation are now available commercially containing up to 2 liters apiece. In surface infections the liquid secretion and the slough may be removed by mopping the wound surface gently with a cotton sponge moistened with saline or hydrogen peroxide. Once the wound and the surrounding tissues have been cleaned of purulent material, areas of sloughing tissue that has not yet liquefied may be seen. Often these areas may be loosened gently by applying slight tension with forceps, or they may be cut away carefully with scissors from the surviving tissue adjacent to them. If the sloughs are not loose it is better to leave them alone until the next dressing rather than to run the risk of causing the patient pain and of causing bleeding.

When the wound and the surrounding tissues have been cleared of purulent secretions, it is often well to bathe the skin around the wound with 70% alcohol on a cotton sponge or with an organic iodine solution. This may prevent infection of the hair follicles in the adjacent skin and furunculosis, which frequently occur. When the secretion is profuse, the surrounding skin may become excoriated. This is treated by applying a small amount of zinc oxide ointment after the skin has been thoroughly cleaned with 70% alcohol. Packing with povidone-iodine (Betadine) soaked gauze may be helpful in cleaning deeper wounds.

Dressings are changed daily or every other day as long as there is much drainage from the wound. Moistening the dressing prevents crusting and permits the escape of the wound secretions. Applying petrolatum gauze or Telfa after the first several dressing changes helps prevent sticking once the need for absorptive material is no longer as great. It should be borne in mind, however, that the best results are obtained and maceration of the skin is avoided by permitting the dressing to dry at frequent intervals, so that after the fourth or fifth day the dressings need be moistened only once or twice a day.

As soon as all the slough has disappeared and the wound has become covered with a base of granulation tissue, an effort may be made to hasten the closure of the wound by pulling its lips together with adhesive straps. Generally this is necessary only in cases in which there has been considerable skin slough, as for instance, following incision and drainage of a carbuncle. In a few such cases, epithelialization may be hastened by the application of pinch skin grafts. These can be obtained with use of local anesthesia in the office and placed on the granulating bed.

HOT WET DRESSINGS

In the treatment of inflammatory lesions, hot moist dressings are applied both before and after incision. A wet dressing must be able to be kept warm for a considerable period and must allow drying to take place. In addition, because the patient is ambulatory, some provision must be made to protect clothing; waxed paper, Saran Wrap, or cellophane is most useful. Special attention must be paid to the security of the dressing. In almost all hot moist dressings of the extremities a splint or some other form of immobilization is employed to keep the part at rest. The inflammatory lesion is overlaid with several gauze compresses. These are applied dry and are so placed and built up over the wound as to provide a large dressing of gauze fully 0.5 inch thick at its center, which spreads for a considerable distance on all sides of the infected wound.

To keep the moisture and heat from escaping, a protection of one or two layers of crumpled waxed paper, cellophane, or Saran Wrap is then applied over the compress. A disposable plastic trash-can liner makes an excellent outer cover (Fig. 8-1). In some cases a plastic tube or a rubber catheter, through which solutions may be added, is placed between the gauze layers and is brought out to the surface above the protective covering. The whole is then securely wrapped with a gauze bandage. Finally, the securing strips of adhesive are applied in circles so that the end of each strip lies on adhesive. When the dressing is applied to the hand or forearm, a sling is provided.

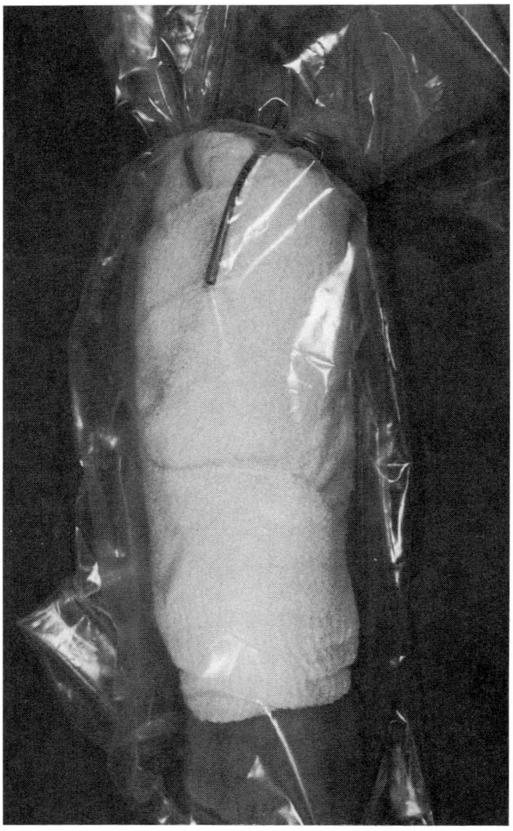

Figure 8-1. Hot wet dressing technique for extremities.

The patient is then instructed to moisten the gauze compress with a designated solution. This is best done with a small rubber ear syringe, the nozzle of which is inserted at one end of the bandage while the part is so held that the solution will moisten the gauze compress by gravity and by capillary attraction. When a plastic tube is used, the solution may be introduced through it. This directs the solution on to the gauze compresses, and as a rule, a smaller amount of solution may be used because there is no doubt about its getting to the right place. Dressings do not need to be moistened more often than three or four times a day.

When hot wet dressings are to be applied to large areas, for instance, in treatment of lymphangitis of the arm, and when there is no open wound, it is often possible to use nonsterile materials such as absorbent cotton or surgical lint. The arm is flexed at a right angle, and the entire arm, from hand to shoulder, is covered with the cotton or lint and then with crumpled waxed paper or Saran Wrap, which in turn is held in place by bandages such as Kerlex gauze or a proper-sized tubular elastic net bandage. In such cases, openings may be left in the waxed paper and marked on the surface of the bandage; through these the patient later may moisten the dressing at intervals.

DRESSINGS FOR INDIVIDUAL PARTS

FINGER AND TOE

For dressings of the fingertip, as, for instance, following incision and drainage of an infection of the distal closed space, the 3-inch gauze compress is cut as shown in Fig. 8-2. The loose ends are then folded over the fingertip, and the dressing is completed with circular turns of a bandage about the gauze and recurrent turns over the tip of the finger; the latter are finally held in place by additional circular

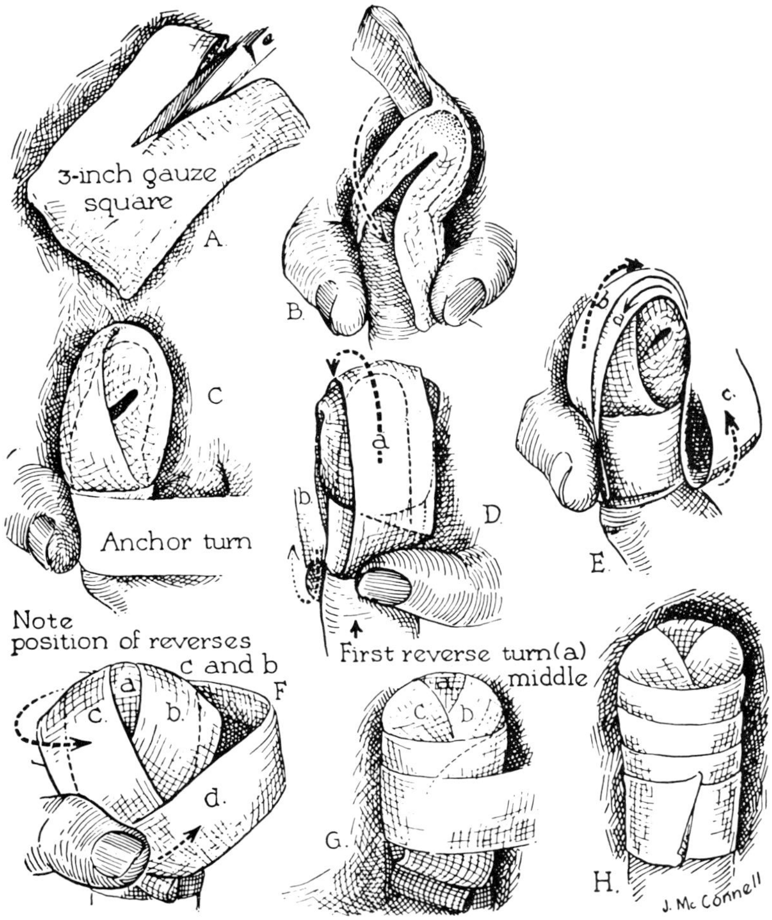

Figure 8-2. Dressing for the finger.

turns. The bandage is then anchored with a longitudinal adhesive strip held in place by circular anchoring strips. In many cases it is advisable to apply a hairpin or opened paper clip as a splint for extra protection (Fig. 8-3).

In lesions at the base of the finger, for instance, a furuncle of the proximal phalanx, there is frequently considerable associated cellulitis and edema over the dorsum of the hand. In these cases it is good to apply a splint that includes the adjacent finger. The splint that has been found to be most useful is the swabstick-adhesive splint (Fig. 8-4). This is applied with two or three circular turns of adhesive, which include the sterile gauze over the lesion. More gauze is then applied as indicated, and the whole is held in place by a 1-inch bandage about the palm and the proximal fingers. Circular turns of 0.5-inch adhesive anchor the dressing.

Dressings for the toe are applied in the same manner as for the finger.

HAND

Dressings for the palm and the dorsum of the hand are best applied with 2-inch bandage and must be anchored by figure-of-eight turns around the hand and wrist (Fig. 8-5). The new, but somewhat expensive, loose-weave bandages are extremely useful for bandaging irregularly shaped regions of the body. When a splint is used with this dressing, it should be long enough to include the entire length of the fingers and to extend upward beyond the midforearm. Padding should be provided in the palm to allow the fingers to lie comfortably in partial flexion.

FOREARM

Dressings for the forearm are held in place with 2-inch gauze bandage applied in spiral and spiral-reverse turns. The bandage should be anchored by diagonal strips of 0.5-inch ad-

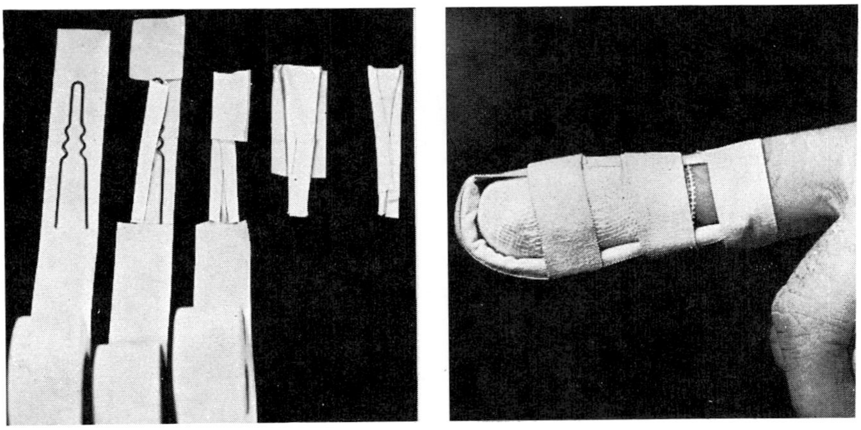

Figure 8-3. (*Left*) Hairpin splint. This splint is readily available and useful in immobilizing fingers. It is small, compact, and molds easily to the part. (*Right*) Hairpin splint applied to the finger. The splint is molded to fit over the finger dressing, covering the palmar surface of the finger and the fingertip. It is held in place with a longitudinal strip of adhesive, which begins and ends on the skin and is anchored by three circular turns of adhesive applied in such a way that the ends lie on adhesive. In this way the dressing may be soaked without fear of its coming loose. (Ferguson LK: Pa Med J 40:909, 1937)

A B C

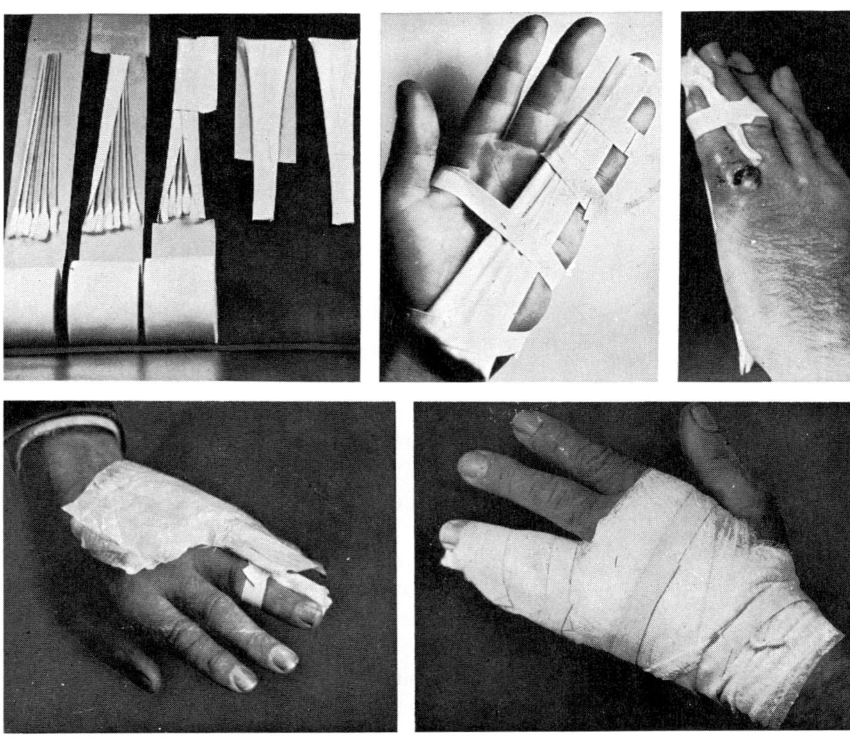

D E

Figure 8-4. Methods of applying hot moist dressings for a furuncle of the dorsal surface of the proximal phalanx. The swab-stick splint (*A*) is made and is applied to the hand with adhesive (*B*). The fingers are separated with gauze (*C*); sterile gauze dressings are applied and overlaid with waxed paper (*D*), and the entire dressing then is enclosed in gauze bandage held in place with adhesive circles (*E*). (Ferguson LK: Pa Med J 49:909, 1937)

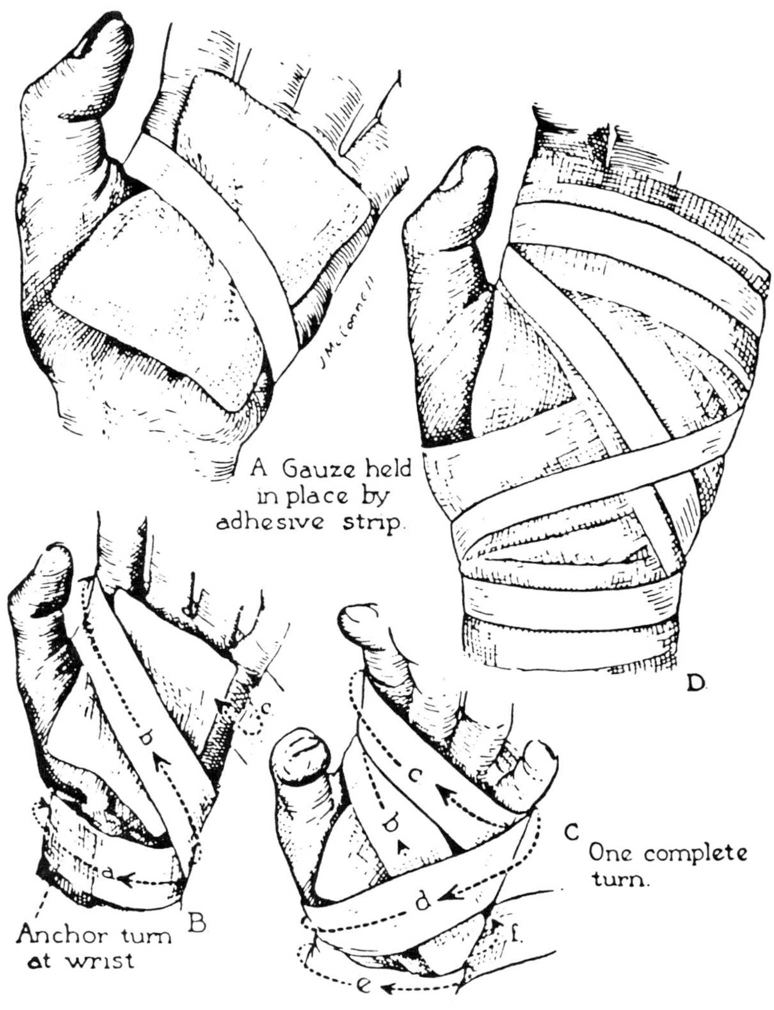

Figure 8-5. Application of a hand dressing.

hesive applied to the skin above and below the bandage; these in turn are fixed by circular turns of 0.5-inch adhesive (Fig. 8-6). Again Kerlex or a similar loose-weave bandage is advisable.

ELBOW

For dressings at the elbow, large gauze compresses are used, usually 4 × 8 inches. With the elbow flexed at a right angle, these are anchored by a circular turn or two of 2-inch bandage on the forearm side. The bandage is then applied in figure-of-eight turns, one loop above and one below the elbow, until the area is covered. Longitudinal anchoring strips of 0.5-inch adhesive are applied to the skin above and below the bandage, and circular turns are used to hold these in place (Fig. 8-7).

UPPER ARM

Dressings for the upper arm are applied in the same way as they are to the forearm, except that in this area reverse turns are less often necessary, since the upper arm is more uniform in size.

AXILLA

Dressings are most often applied to the axilla for superficial infections or abscesses. After a sufficient gauze has been used to cover the wound, one large piece of gauze should be spread out to cover the entire underlying dressing and to extend for a distance of about 3 or 4 inches downward along the lateral chest wall and for the same distance along the inner side of the upper arm. A strip of 1-inch adhesive is then placed across the middle of the

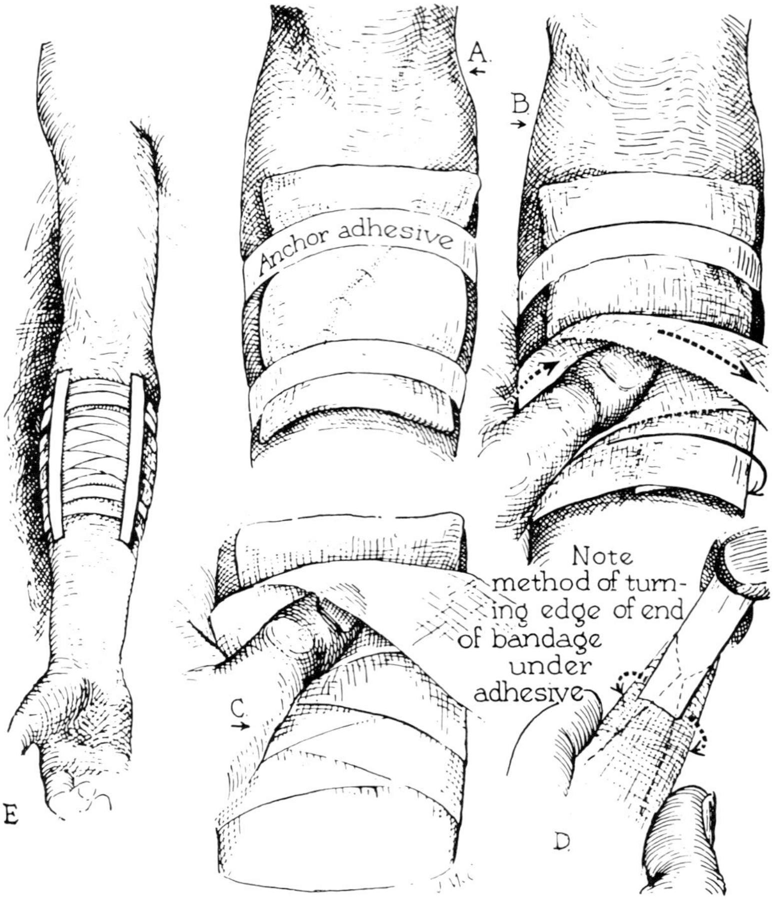

Figure 8-6. Application of a forearm bandage dressing.

gauze in the uppermost part of the axilla; the adhesive should be long enough so that the cut ends reach over the top of the shoulder (Fig. 8-8). The arm is then placed down against the side of the chest wall, and the adhesive is attached to the skin in front and back, one end overlying the other over the acromion. The arm then is raised, and a second strip of adhesive is applied over the gauze and fixed front and back over the chest wall. A third strip is applied in the same manner over the gauze and around the upper arm. Large-sized tubular net bandages that include the chest and the arm can be useful.

SHOULDER

The spica bandage is used occasionally for the application of dressings to the top of the shoulder and the upper chest. It is applied in what amounts to figure-of-eight turns, beginning in the axilla of the normal side and coming up across the anterior portion of the chest and the shoulder and around the arm from behind forward. Sometimes a circular turn is made around the arm in the first lap of bandage, and then the roll is carried across the back to its original starting place in the sound axilla. These turns are repeated, crossing each other higher and higher on the shoulder, each succeeding turn overlapping about half of the previous one, until sufficient turns have been applied to cover the desired area. A 3-inch gauze bandage or Kerlex gauze is best for this purpose. The spica is fixed with 1-inch adhesive strips (Fig. 8-9). Here again the elastic net dressing of proper size can hold dressings in place quite well.

NECK

Dressings are most often applied to the neck for furuncles or carbuncles at the back of the neck or for abscesses of the cervical glands in

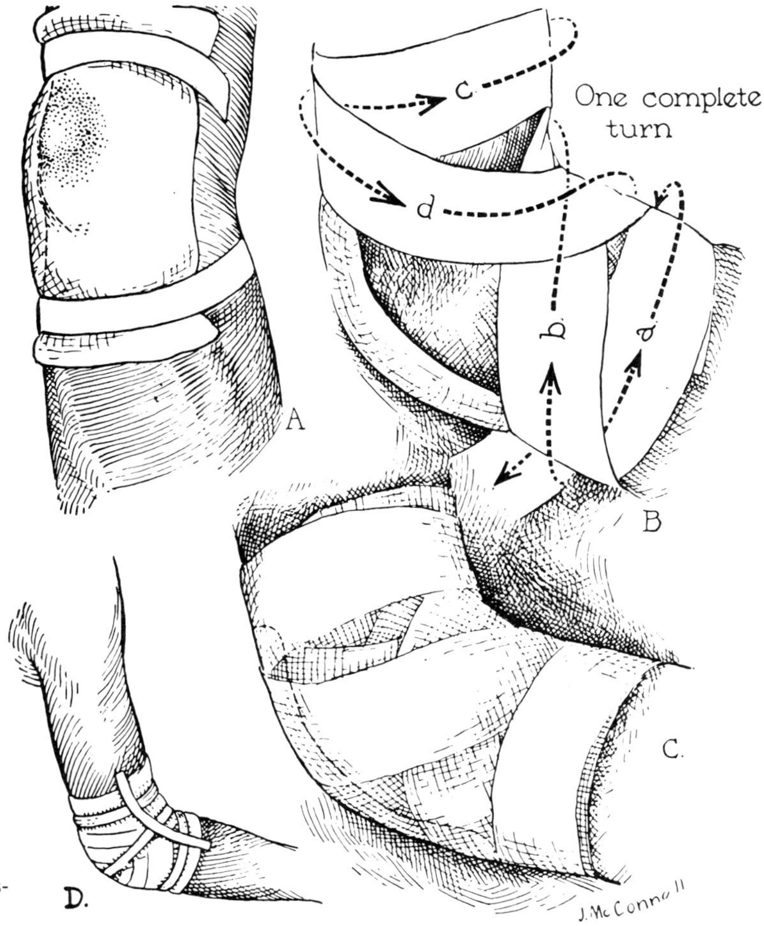

Figure 8-7. Application of a dressing and bandage at the elbow.

the anterior area of the neck. After application of a sufficient number of gauze compresses, the dressing is held in place by circular turns of 2-inch gauze bandage; Kerlex gauze is extremely helpful. This dressing cannot be applied well with the patient lying down. Therefore when it is to be applied immediately after operation, it is best to hold the dressing in place until the patient has recovered sufficiently from the anesthetic and can sit up. The dressing is usually wider at the site of the lesion than it is at other portions of the circumference of the neck, and the bandage should be so applied at this area as to cover completely and to hold in the top and the bottom of the gauze compresses. The bandage is anchored in place by 0.5-inch adhesive strips. Experience has shown that it is more secure if the adhesive strips are applied first at the site of the lesion, at the top and bottom of the bandage, and in such a manner as to form an ellipse. The ends are then covered by a circular strip of adhesive applied over the middle of the bandage (Fig. 8-10). After such a dressing has been applied it should be inspected carefully to make sure that it is not so tight as to compress the veins of the neck, with resulting hemostasis of the face and head. Occasionally it is necessary to snip the bandage a little in several places to relieve this compression.

LOWER FACE AND JAW

As a rule, ordinary dressings of the face and the jaw may be applied with gauze and adhesive, or a spray adhesive may be applied. In some instances, however, and especially following trauma or operation, a dressing must be held in place with bandage for compression or for application of hot wet dressings. In these cases loose-knit roller dressing is ideal (Fig. 8-11).

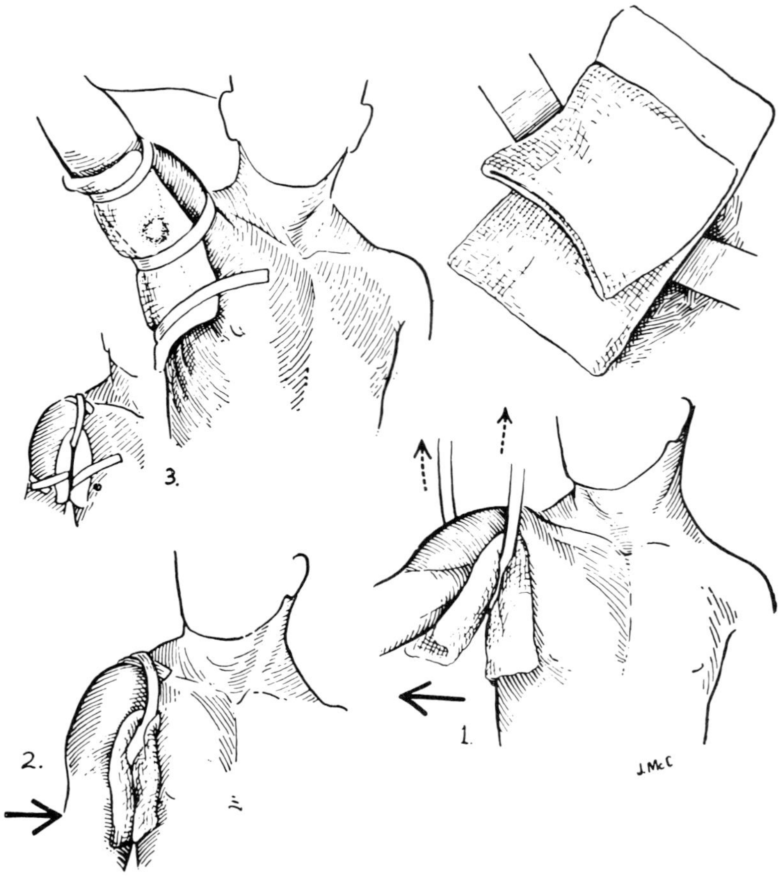

Figure 8-8. Application of a dressing to the axilla using adhesive.

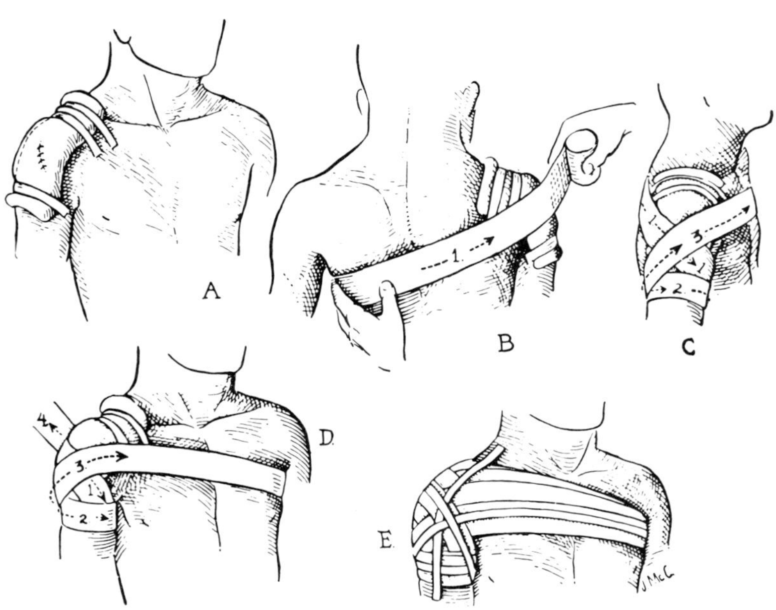

Figure 8-9. Application of a spica bandage over a dressing on the shoulder.

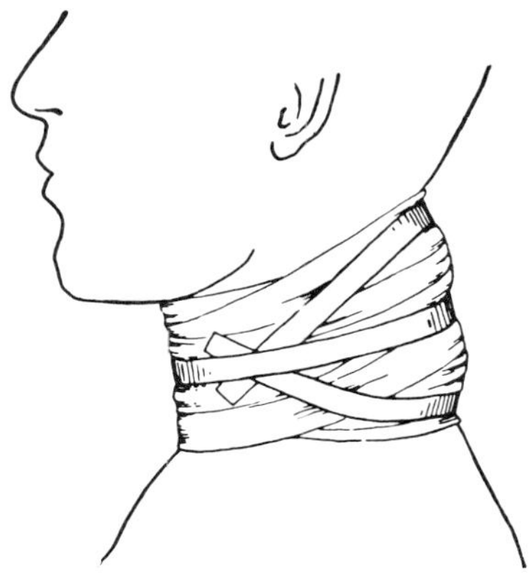

Figure 8-10. Neck dressing. Note method of applying adhesive strips.

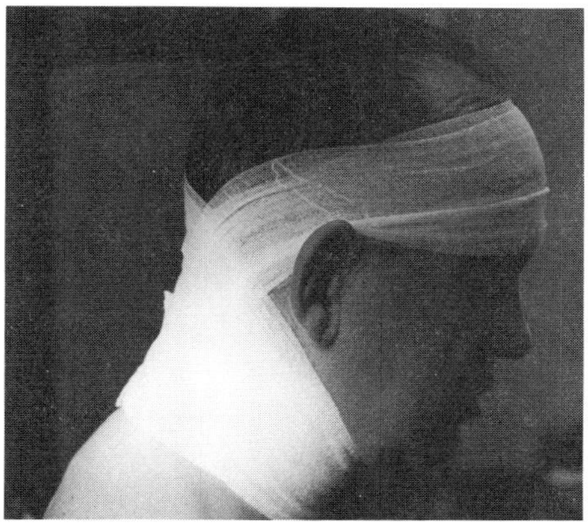

Figure 8-12. A figure-of-eight bandage for neck and back of the head and forehead.

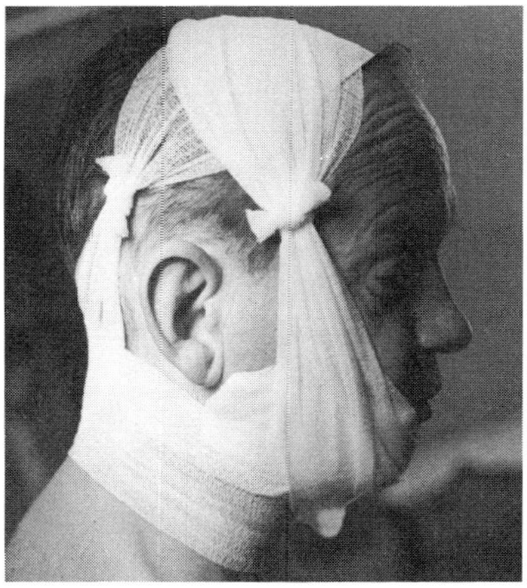

Figure 8-11. Barton type of bandage for lesions of the jaw. Note method of tightening bandage with ties of gauze.

BACK OF THE NECK AND HEAD

The dressings of the back of the neck and the lower scalp are held in place best by figure-of-eight turns around the head and the neck. The bandage is started at the back of the neck and carried forward around the head and above the ears to its starting place, thence around the neck and back again to its beginning. Several such turns are applied to cover the compress. The bandage is strengthened by a figure-of-eight turn of 0.5-inch adhesive applied over it (Fig. 8-12).

SCALP

Most traumatic or operative wounds of the scalp may be treated by application of a spray adhesive dressing. When the ooze has been controlled by digital or palmar pressure, the wound is sprayed with the adhesive. A small amount of fluff cotton is then applied over the wound while the adhesive is still moist, and the cotton is moistened with additional spray. This dries rapidly, and as a rule, no other dressing needs to be applied. Occasionally there is a slight ooze, which may be absorbed by application of a small amount of gauze over the wound for a short time.

When there is considerable secretion from an infected wound, or hemorrhage demanding pressure, a skullcap dressing is most satisfactory. Gauze compresses are placed over the lesions, and the entire skull is then covered by two of the 4 × 8-inch gauze compresses, which have been unfolded so as to make a double layer of gauze about 8 × 8 inches. These pieces of gauze are held tightly over the scalp by an assistant while the surgeon applies two or three circular turns of 3-inch or 4-inch looseweave gauze bandage snugly around the scalp below the occiput and well down over the forehead (Fig. 8-13). When the gauze has thus been anchored, it is pulled down snugly in all directions so as to provide pressure over the gauze compress and the lesion. The edges of the gauze are then turned upward and are included in additional circles of bandage, some turns of which extend well down behind the occiput and high on the forehead, while others extend low on the forehead and high on the occiput. Then 0.5-inch strips of adhesive are applied over the gauze across the head from in front backward and from side to side. Finally, two anchoring circles of 0.5-inch ad-

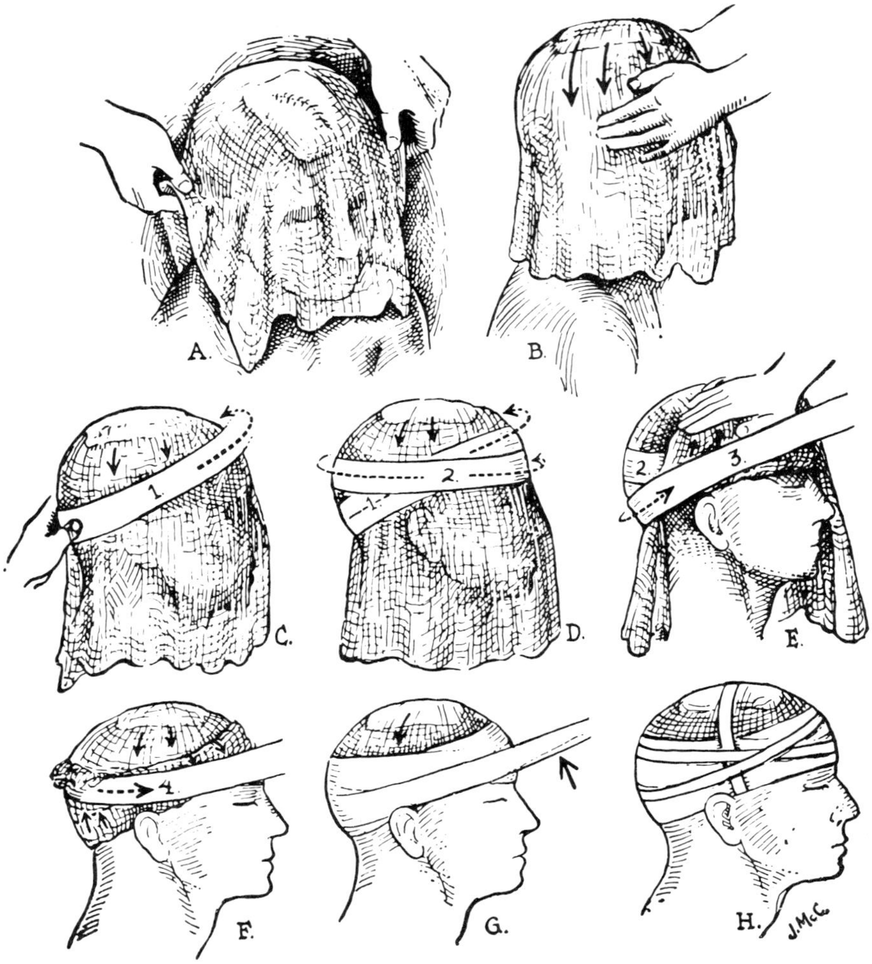

Figure 8-13. Preparation of a Frazier head dressing for lesions of the scalp.

hesive are applied, the first extending well down behind the occiput and high over the forehead and the second passing across the forehead at the lowermost part of the bandage and high up on the occiput. This dressing will be found to give excellent compression and will remain securely in place for 5 or 6 days if necessary.

BREAST

Dressings for the breast are applied most often for inflammatory lesions, either before or after incision. Gauze compresses are placed over the lesion and are held in place with transverse circles of the bandage so placed that they lie above and below the breast. As a rule, those turns lying above the involved breast are pulled downward so that they lie below the opposite breast, and those that are applied below the involved breast cross the chest in an upward direction to lie above the normal breast. In effect, the bandage is a cross-bandage of the breast. Circular strips of adhesive and occasionally longitudinal ones are applied (Fig. 8-14). This bandage must be applied with the patient in the sitting or standing position. A dressing can also be held in place by a brassiere.

GROIN

A spica bandage of the groin is usually applied to provide pressure or to hold compresses in place. Here a loose-weave roller gauze such as Kerlex or Kling is great help. It

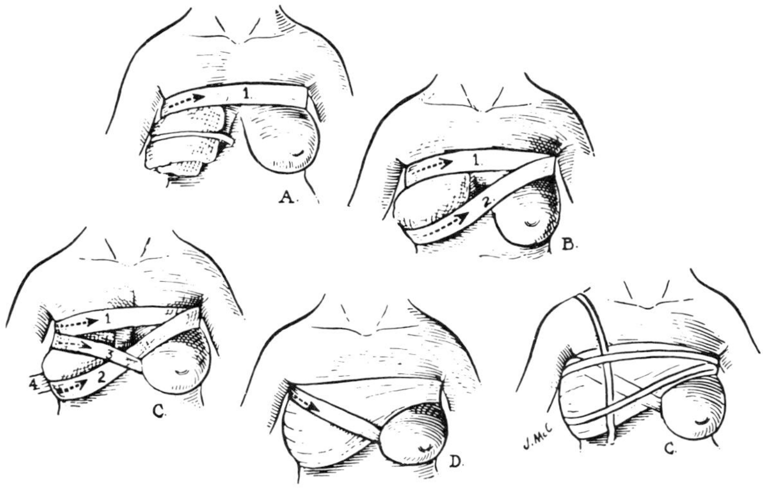

Figure 8-14. Application of a bandage to the breast.

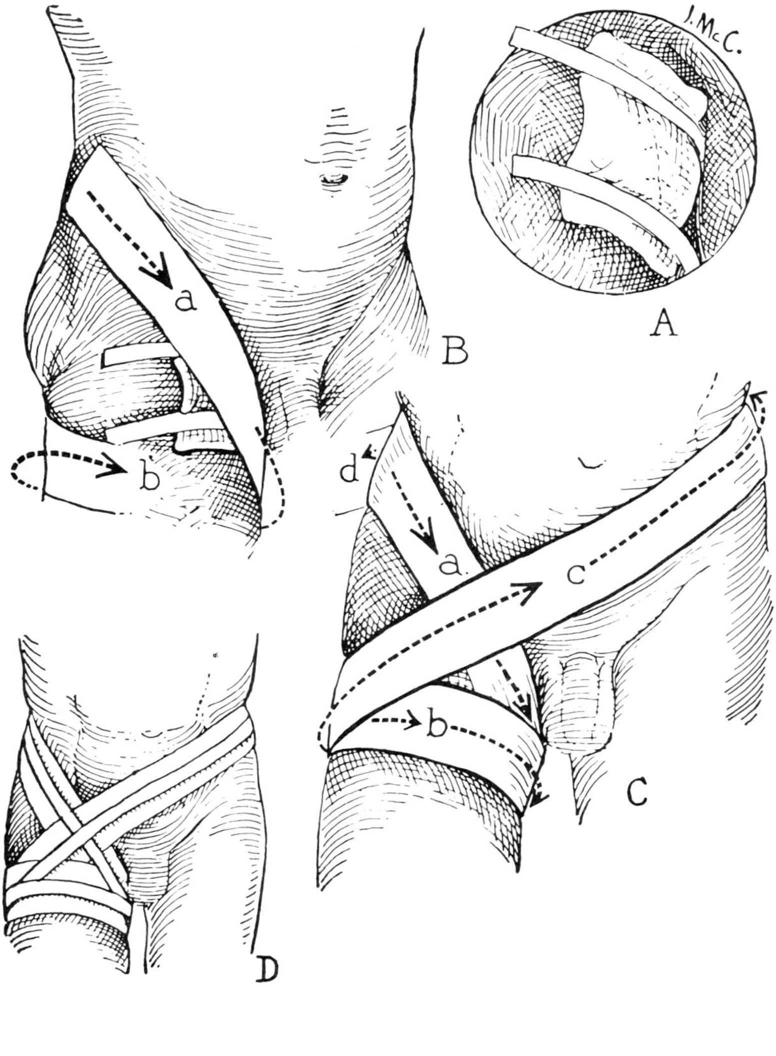

Figure 8-15. Application of a dressing to the groin.

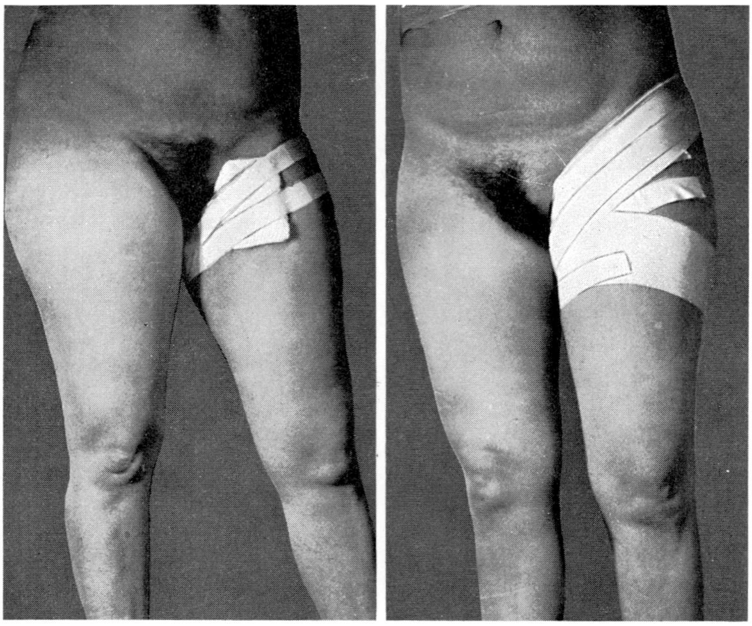

Figure 8-16. Application of a dressing to the groin using elastic adhesive. This gives firm compression and does not necessitate a bandage round the abdomen; therefore it is more convenient and is especially serviceable after ligation of varicose saphenous veins.

is begun with a circular turn around the upper thigh and is best applied with the patient standing and holding the legs spread slightly apart. After the first circular or anchoring turn, the bandage is carried upward across the groin and the lower abdomen. A circular turn is then made around the low back and downward across the groin to the thigh. This constitutes one turn of the bandage; several such turns are applied, and the bandage is anchored with a similar turn of 0.5-inch or 1-inch adhesive (Fig. 8-15).

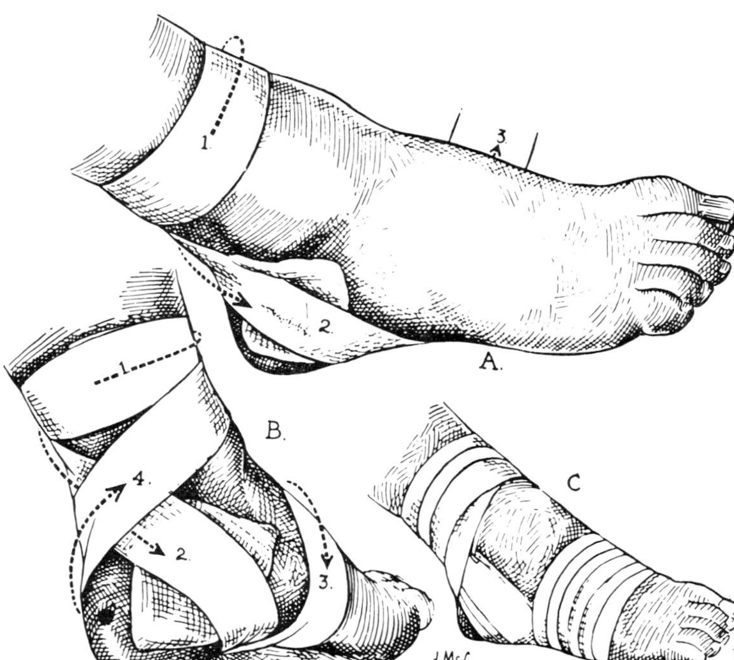

Figure 8-17. Application of a dressing to the heel.

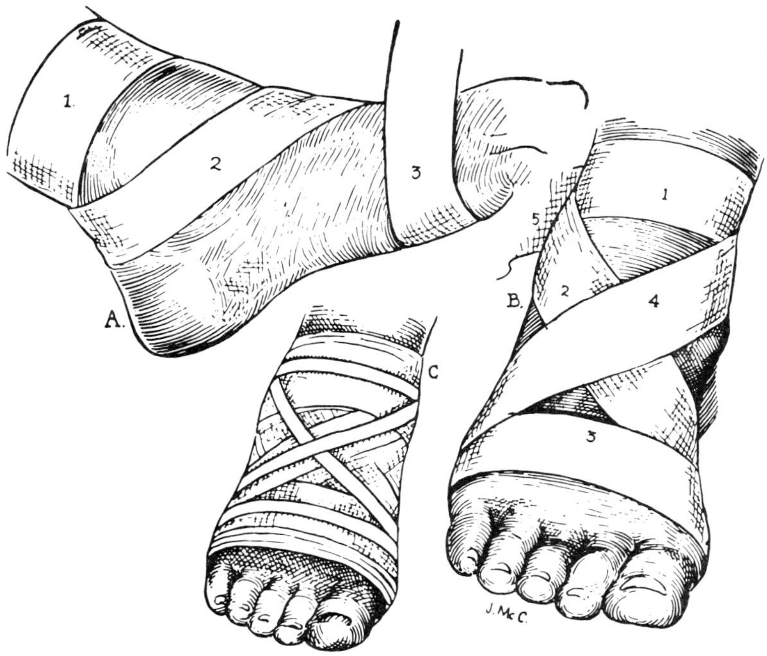

Figure 8-18. Application of a dressing to the foot.

If elastic adhesive is used, a groin dressing is more easily applied: After the compress has been fixed with one or two strips of adhesive, the elastic adhesive is started below and lateral to the anterior spine of the iliac crest and is carried down parallel to and below Poupart's ligament and around the thigh to finish the original turn. The ends of the bandage are fixed with strips of 1-inch adhesive to prevent rolling (Fig. 8-16).

THIGH AND LEG

When dressings are to be applied to the thigh and the leg, it is usually wise to fix the compresses in place with one or two transverse strips of 1-inch adhesive. The bandage is applied in spiral and then spiral-reverse turns until the compress is covered sufficiently. Two longitudinal strips of adhesive fix the bandage to the skin above and below, and the whole is held in place by two or three fixation circles of 0.5-inch or 1-inch adhesive. When the lesion is anterior, in placing the adhesive circles on a conical part the adhesive should be stretched and applied to the back of the part first. The cut ends are then brought around the part. To lie flat they must ascend slightly. Dressings are applied to the opposite side of the part in a similar manner. For the thigh 3-inch bandage is best, and for the leg 2-inch is best.

ANKLE AND FOOT

Bandages for the ankle and the foot are most conveniently applied in figure-of-eight turns around the foot and ankle; 2-inch bandage is usually used, with fixation by 0.5-inch adhesive (Figs. 8-17 and 8-18). A splint may be

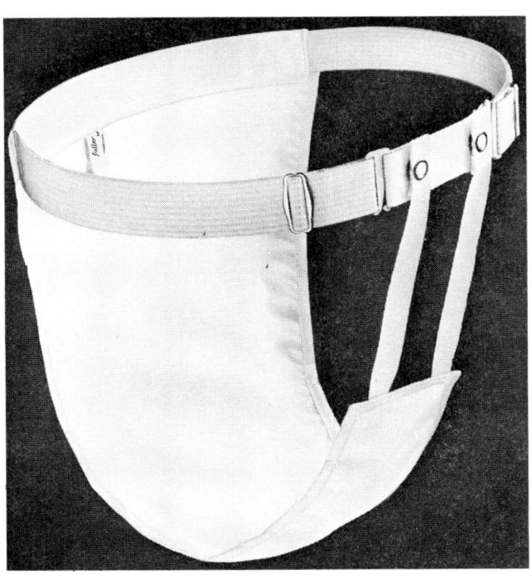

Figure 8-19. The Fuller shield is a protective pouch designed to hold anal, perianal, and sacral dressings in place without binding and without adhesive. It may be used in male or female patients. (Courtesy of Fuller Laboratories, a subsidiary of Parke-Davis)

desirable if there is likely to be much movement of the injured area.

PERINEUM

It is difficult to hold perineal dressings in place with adhesive. The best is composed of one sterile gauze pad over the wound, held in place by an ordinary sanitary pad (Kotex). The elastic sanitary belt that may be applied with a snap is the most convenient type.

Also available is a protective dressing designed especially to hold anal, perianal, and sacral dressings in place without the use of adhesive tape. It is rubberized to prevent soiling and is held in place by an adhesive, adjustable waistband (Fig. 8-19).

BIBLIOGRAPHY

Ajao OG: Surgical wound infection: A comparison between dressed and undressed wounds. J Trop Med Hyg 80:51–52, 1978

Jackson IT: A method to keep dressings moist prior to delayed skin grafting. Plast Reconstr Surg 56:347–348, 1975

Noe JM, Kalish S: The mechanism of capillarity in surgical dressings. Surg Gynecol Obstet 143:1–3, 1976

Westaby S, Everett WG: Wound irrigation device. Lancet 2:503, 1978

Wood RAB, Williams RHP, Hughes LE: Foam elastomer dressing in the management of open granulating wounds: Experience with 250 patients. Br J Surg 64:554–557, 1977

Zide B, Pardoe R: The many uses of polyurethane foam. Am J Surg 132:424–426, 1976

9 Bites and Stings—Vertebrates and Invertebrates

CLIFFORD C. SNYDER AND GARY R. HUNTER

When the first human appeared on this earth, he encountered a barrage of poisonous insects and venomous animals, and being without protective garb, he was vulnerable. With a little imagination one may conceive the frustrations that primitive man encountered combatting venomous attacks for which he had no defense. Through the ages therapeutic approaches have not differed a great deal. The ancient papyri of Edwin Smith (1800 B.C.) and Ebers (1500 B.C.) reveal that advice for dealing with attacks from snakes, scorpions, and spiders was not much different then from what it is today. The Egyptian physician-priests used incisions and drainage of the fang punctures, various soothing balms, wound irrigations, bandages, and elevation of the injured part. Celsus (ca. A.D. 50) suggested "opening the bitten arm and place a piece of chicken fat into the bite site." Galen (A.D. 131–201) recommended excision of the bitten area, wound suction, cautery, and astringents—"with excellent results." Paul of Aegina (A.D. 625–690) described his treatment of mad dog bites and attacks from snakes, bees, and lizards, as "sucking the wound of its poison, cupping the wound, and follow with dressings of hot wine, vinegar, and onions." Ambrose Paré (1510–1590) wrote of incision, excision, and suction of the venom from the bite wound. Fontana (1720–1805), an Italian biologist, performed over 6000 experiments using 4000 animals and 3000 snakes and concluded that, depending on the bite severity, the therapies should include retrieval of the venom by "incision or excision and suction, cauterizing with alkalies and acids, wound care with herbs and oils, and lastly amputation when necessary to save a life." Henry Sewall, in 1887, with pigeons as subjects, achieved immunity against rattlesnake venom; and this was affirmed by Calmette and Frazer in 1895.

The medical history of human inflictions by bugs and beasts continues to be dictated and dispersed (10,000 publications yearly), and though our knowledge of venoms and their sequelae is improving, much is left to be achieved, for over 100,000 human victims worldwide continue to succumb from envenomations yearly.

SNAKEBITES

Rarely is a medical problem encountered that causes more speculation and professional disagreement than the therapy for snakebite. The poisonous snakes of medical significance native to the United States are rattlesnakes, cottonmouth moccasins, copperhead moccasins, and coral snakes. The first three belong to the family Crotalidae, which is represented by 210 species and subspecies. They have a heat-sensitive organ called a pit below and in front of each eye, hence the name *pit vipers*. Coral snakes do not have this pit and are members of the Elapidae family, which is represented by 87 species and subspecies. The largest of the domestic serpentine venomers is the *Crotalus adamanteus* (eastern diamondback rattlesnake). The *C. adamanteus, C. atrox* (western diamondback rattler), and *C. scutulatus* (Mohave rattlesnake) are responsible for most of the critical bites in the United States. These are followed, in *numerical* sequence of serious envenomation, by the *Agkistrodon piscivorus* (cottonmouth water moccasin), the genera *Micrurus* and *Micruroides* (coral snakes), and the *Agkistrodon mokeson* (copperhead moccasin).

Throughout the world, deaths due to snakebite are more frequent than most doctors realize. Recent indications, as determined by an attentive review of the literature and correspondence with physicians abroad, are that

TABLE 9-1. Snakebite Age Groups (30-Year Study)

AGE GROUP	NO. OF SNAKEBITES
Adults	118
Adolescents	191
Children	279
TOTAL	588

ENVIRONMENT OF BITE

Theater stage	Hunting preserve
Serpentarium	Home yard
Research lab	Forest
Golf course	Swamp
Auto camper	Desert
Fraternity house	Garage
Living room	Bedroom

the total human death rate is more likely to be around 75,000. This does not include an untold number of bites that are never treated or reported. The authors have been consulted and have treated 588 human snakebites. Children have been by far the most numerous victims (Table 9-1). The bite sites on the human torso mostly involve the leg (knee to ankle), because children are bitten more, and people tend to walk in occult foliage (Table 9-2). The environment in which the victim is bitten is very interesting (see "Environment of Bite"). In our series of human beings struck by snakes, most inflictions took place in such rural regions as woods, swamps, and deserts. Two bites were purposeful, both being attempts at homocide. The first incident involved an Eastern diamondback rattler that was placed by a husband in a sleeping bag in an auto camper to kill his wife, and although she was bitten twice on the lower extremity she survived. A similar episode occurred when a mistress attempted to slay her lover by hiding a Mohave rattler between the sheets in a warm bed. A bite on the dorsum of the hand terminated with a loss of soft tissues and a portion of the middle finger. One other bizarre snake infliction may be mentioned. It took place in a fraternity house while a student was being hazed. The initiate was prompted to kiss a nonpoisonous snake, which, apparently perplexed and harassed, bit the student's extended tongue. The resultant megaloglossia nearly necessitated a tracheotomy, but the edematous tongue responded to frozen desserts, and resumed its normal size.

TABLE 9-2. Body Sites

SITE	NO. OF SNAKEBITES
Foot	89
Leg	279
Thigh	13
Arm	21
Forearm	5
Hand	88
Head	89
Torso	4
TOTAL	588*

* 2 Deaths

A poisonous snake is endowed with a pair of specialized glands, relatively comparable to the salivary glands of humans but variable in that the serpent's glands comprise in addition a venomous excreting portion. The principal salivary duct empties its contents into the hollow fang on the anterior surface at its base. This injecting apparatus is a specially constructed, canalized tooth that serves to expel the toxin (Fig. 9-1).

Protein fractionation of poisonous venom discloses a diversity of active principles, the names and descriptions of which depend on the interpretations of individual investigators who sometimes are not in agreement. Regardless, it is the consensus that Elapidae venom contains potent neurotoxins and respiratory toxins but only mild hemolytic and cytolytic enzymes. These factors account for the extreme systemic reaction yet rather mild local reaction, observed in Elapidae (cobra and coral) envenomation. In comparison, Crotalidae venom is moderately neurotoxic but, because of its powerful hemolysins, cytolysins, and coagulant factors, produces severe proteolysis, necrosis, and slough of tissue at the bite site. Venom from the Viperidae simulates many of the actions of Crotalidae poisoning (Fig. 9-2).

An early correct diagnosis of envenomation is important because immediate therapeutic procedures can be life-saving (see "Human Reactions to Snake Envenomation"). In contradistinction, vigorous therapy with horse-serum antivenom for misdiagnosed poisonous serpent bites may terminate in misfortune. If possible, the venomer should be retrieved and taken to an authority on herpetology for identification. The presence of fang marks in the skin is diagnostic of venomation. There may

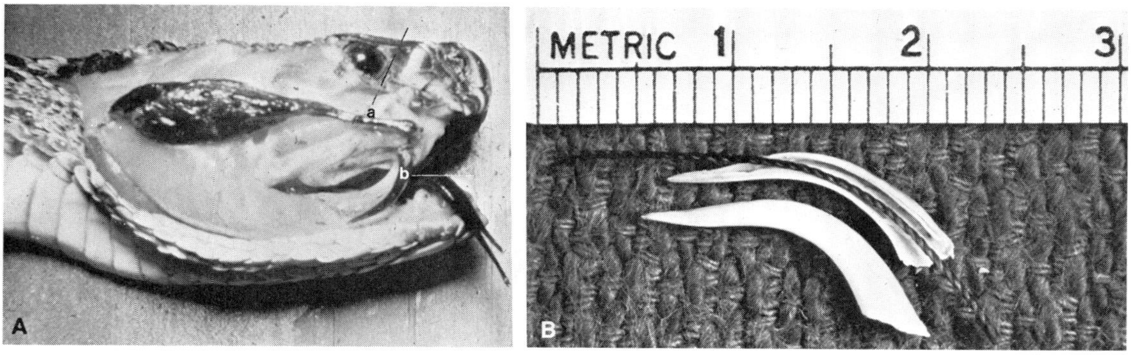

Figure 9-1. (*A*) The venom gland is a salivary organ enveloped in muscular and fibrous connective tissue. On contraction of the masseter muscle, the venom is compressed through the main duct (*a*) and propelled out the canalized or grooved fang (*b*). (*B*) Fangs are specialized teeth, some solid, some grooved, and others canalized as in this rattlesnake specimen. They simulate hypodermic needles with the distal orifice not precisely at the tip. Some have an outer plate, a diploe, and an inner plate to reduce the chance of fracture.

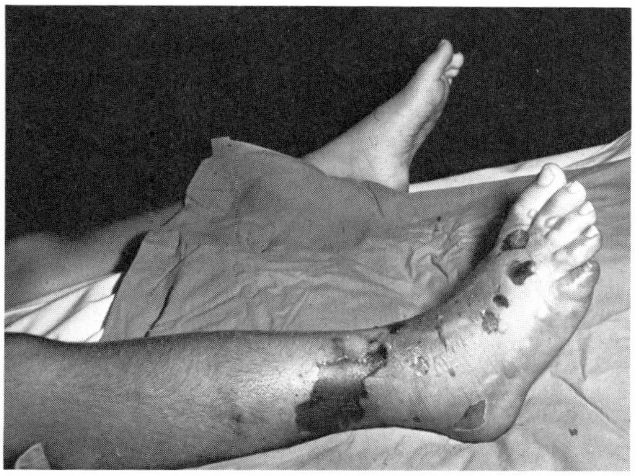

Figure 9-2. Necrosis and slough, due to Viperidae venom, in the area of the bite. Crotalidae and Viperidae venoms consist of powerful hemolysins, cytolysins, and coagulants that are responsible for these as well as for vascular clotting and proteolysis.

HUMAN REACTIONS TO SNAKE ENVENOMATION

Cardinal Findings

Fang marks (1–6)
Immediate pain
Rapid swelling

Ancillary Findings

Hemorrhagic transudate
Petechiae
Bullae
Paresthesias
Cyanosis
Necrosis
Tissue slough

be only one fang mark, or there may be two, three, four, or even more. We have observed six marks (Fig. 9-3) in a victim. Pain is the most common finding in Crotalidae and Viperidae bites, the average onset occurring within 10 minutes. The discomfort may be only slight, or it may be moderate or severe. Local erythema becomes evident and is incessant. Edema usually appears in a few minutes and is definitely progressive (Fig. 9-4). The bites of Elapidae (cobra and coral snakes) usually are painless and initially without swelling; edema usually starts immediately or may be delayed an hour or so after the bite and reaches a plateau in 24 to 48 hours; other signs are eyelid ptosis, hemoptysis, and incoagulable blood. The victim may worsen and exhibit symptoms of shock (weakness, syncope, hypotension), become nauseated, vomit, exhibit urinary and fecal incontinence, begin to twitch, and not respond to external stimuli. If the patient becomes moribund, the pupils dilate, respiration is difficult, the pulse is hardly palpable, and unconsciousness follows. Following snakebite without venomation, none of these symptoms occurs routinely or in this sequence. Reid reported a most important observation: It is incorrect to assume that snakebites are fatal and to assume that snakebites that do not produce symptoms of poisoning are always inflicted by nonpoisonous snakes; 53% of the victims of "lethal" viper, cobra, and sea-snake bites escape with mild or no poisoning, and more than half of the bites inflicted by poisonous serpents do not produce serious envenomation. He says in summary

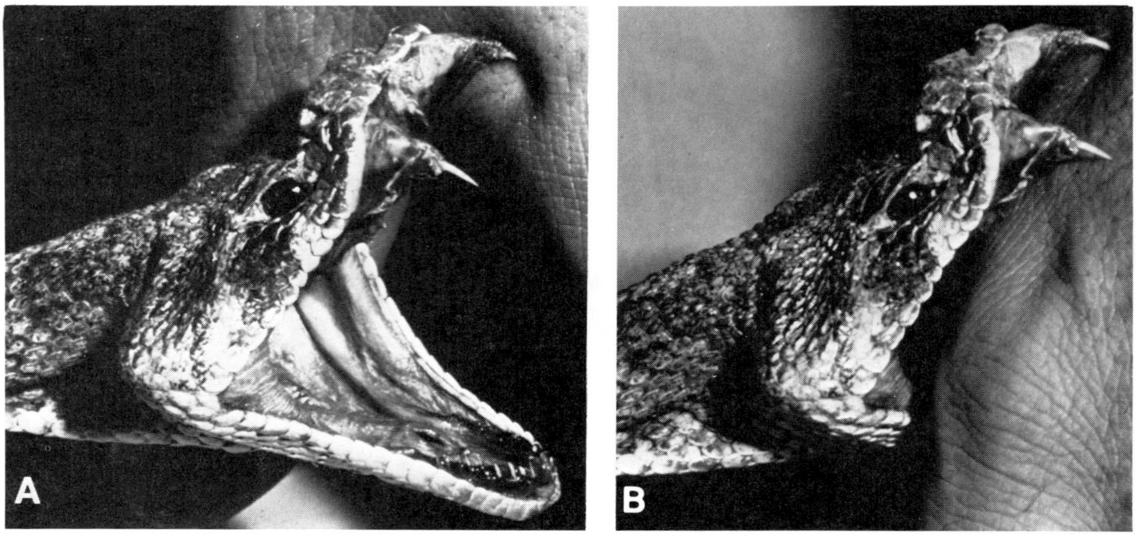

Figure 9-3. Puncture wounds (fang marks) are pathognomonic of envenomation. They may be numerous or merely one, as depicted in this glancing strike of a rattlesnake (*A*). Two puncture wounds due to a direct strike (*B*) are in contrast to the near-miss of one fang mark.

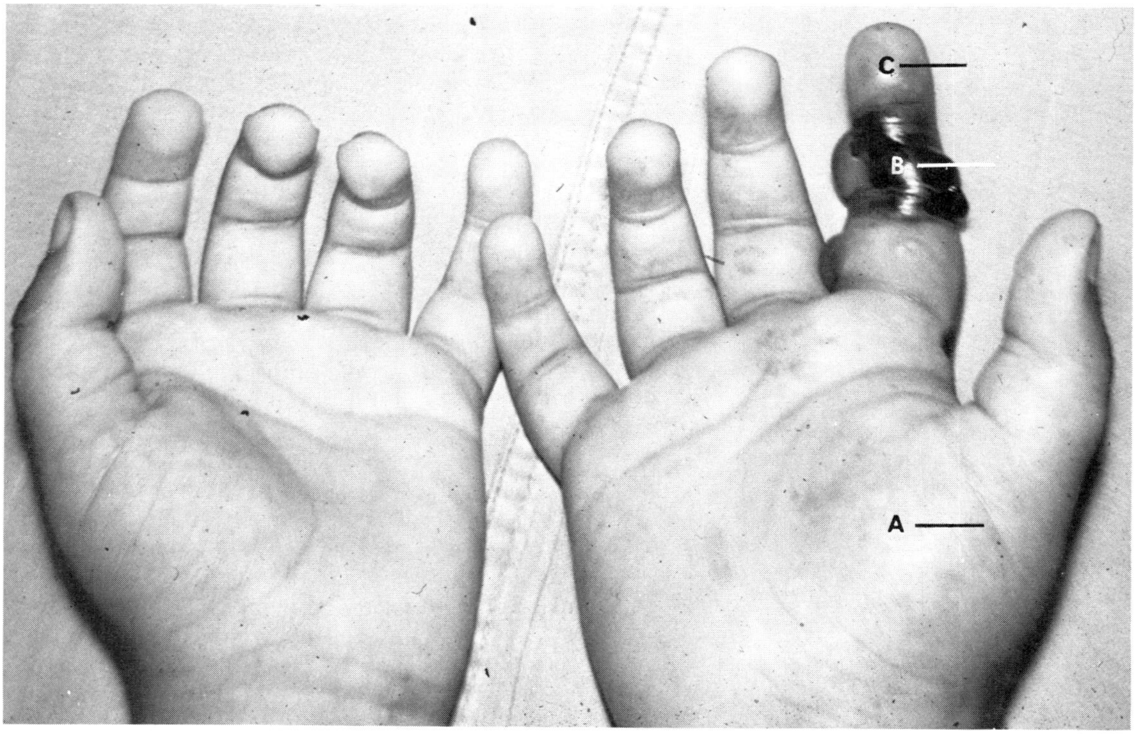

Figure 9-4. Among the early findings of snake envenomation are swelling (*A*), hemorrhagic transudate (*B*), and cyanosis (*C*).

that snakes bite human beings strictly as a defense mechanism, that little venom is injected, and that poisonous snakebite is therefore not synonymous with snakebite poisoning.

Because the effects of snakebite differ in severity, their treatment should be varied according to their classification:

Mild: scratch marks, no pain, minimal swelling
Moderate: fang marks, pain, local swelling, no systemic symptoms
Severe: fang marks; immediate, excruciating wound pain; progressive swelling, cyanosis, bullae, and systemic symptoms

For mild envenomation the wound should be cleansed with soap and water or alcohol and dressed if necessary. Incisions and antivenin are not indicated. For moderate envenomation the fang marks should be incised and antivenin given. Severe snakebite should be treated vigorously by application of a tourniquet, excision of the fang mark area, administration of antivenin, and hospitalization of the patient (Fig. 9-5).

Treatment for venomous snakebite consists of (1) immediate (first-aid) treatment in the field and (2) hospital therapy. Snake-infested areas, occult foliage, old logs, caves, and dens should be avoided. A vehicle should be kept near for emergencies, and one should carry a snakebite kit (and know how to use it) (Fig. 9-6) containing a flat tourniquet (25¢), two alcohol-prep sponges (10¢), a disposable scalpel in sterile foil (20¢), polyvalent antivenin (about $35), 100-mg vial of hydrocortisone sodium succinate (Solu-Cortef) (75¢), a sterile disposable syringe and needle (8¢), a packet of polymyxin B (Neosporin) ointment, sterile sponges, and a 100-ml vial of normal saline solution with tubing (90¢).

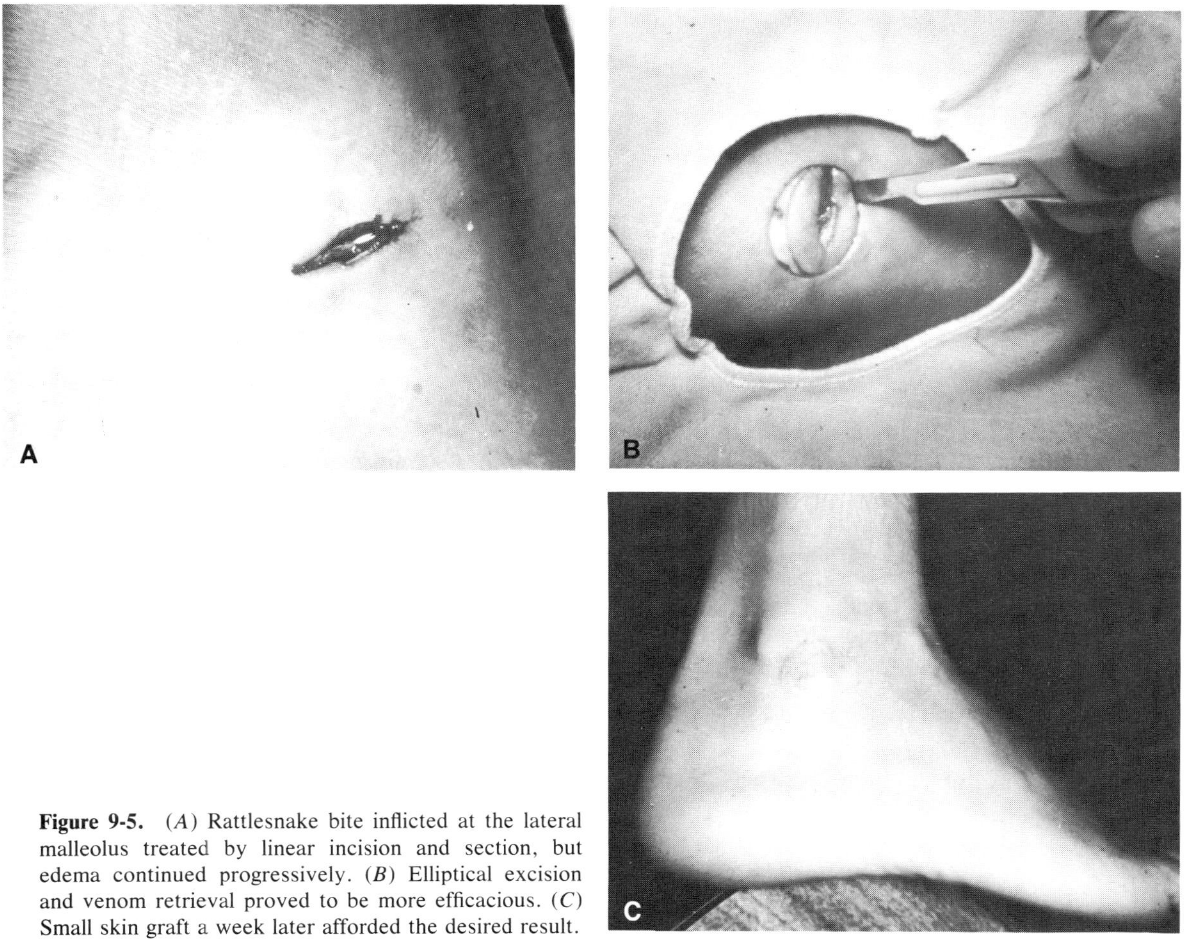

Figure 9-5. (*A*) Rattlesnake bite inflicted at the lateral malleolus treated by linear incision and section, but edema continued progressively. (*B*) Elliptical excision and venom retrieval proved to be more efficacious. (*C*) Small skin graft a week later afforded the desired result.

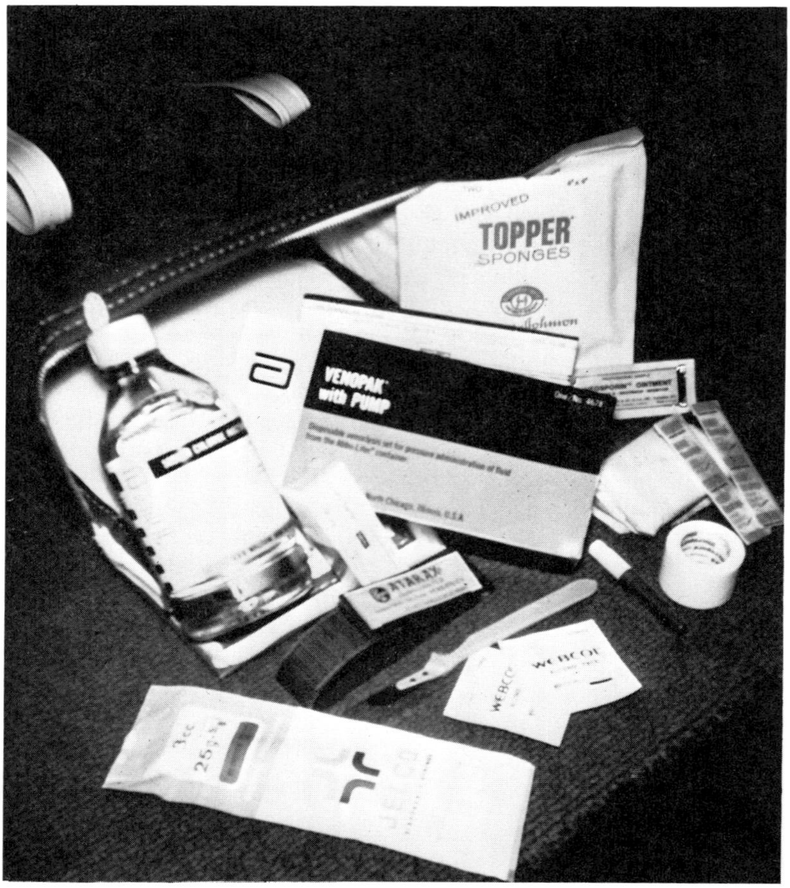

Figure 9-6. Snakebite kit (see text for contents).

IMMEDIATE FIELD TREATMENT

Incarcerate the antigen, using a flat tourniquet applied between the bite and the heart; this should be tight enough to impede the superficial venous and lymphatic return but not so tight as to obstruct the arterial supply or produce ischemia (Fig. 9-7). The tourniquet should admit a finger beneath it easily and should not be removed and reapplied at short intervals because this perpetuates the spread of the venom. Every effort should be made to avoid elevation of blood pressure by activity or acceleration of circulation with stimulants or drugs. The affected bite area should be kept at heart level, without elevation or dependency. The victim should be taken to the nearest physician or hospital as soon as feasible. The snake, if slain, should be retrieved for identification.

Retrieve the antigen, after cleansing the wound with the alcohol sponges, by making only one linear incision (not cruciate incisions) through the fang mark(s) with the disposable scalpel. The incision is extended 0.25 inch beyond the punctures, avoiding vital structures such as nerves, tendons, and large vessels. Cruciate incisions are condemned, as they macerate, necrotize, and harbor anaerobes. Digitally express or mechanically suction the wound for 5 to 10 minutes but avoid trauma to the soft tissues. Oral suction is not advocated, as it introduces bacteria into the wound.

Neutralize the antigen, using polyvalent antivenin. It is disadvantageous to inject the antivenin into the snakebite area, which is edematous and inhibits absorption of the antivenin. When the antivenin is given in this way or intramuscularly, it is also difficult to retrieve it or to treat the victim if he is allergic to the antivenin. It is permissible for a lay person to inject the antivenin intramuscularly to achieve faster absorption. (Intravenous and intraarterial administration are discussed later.) Never

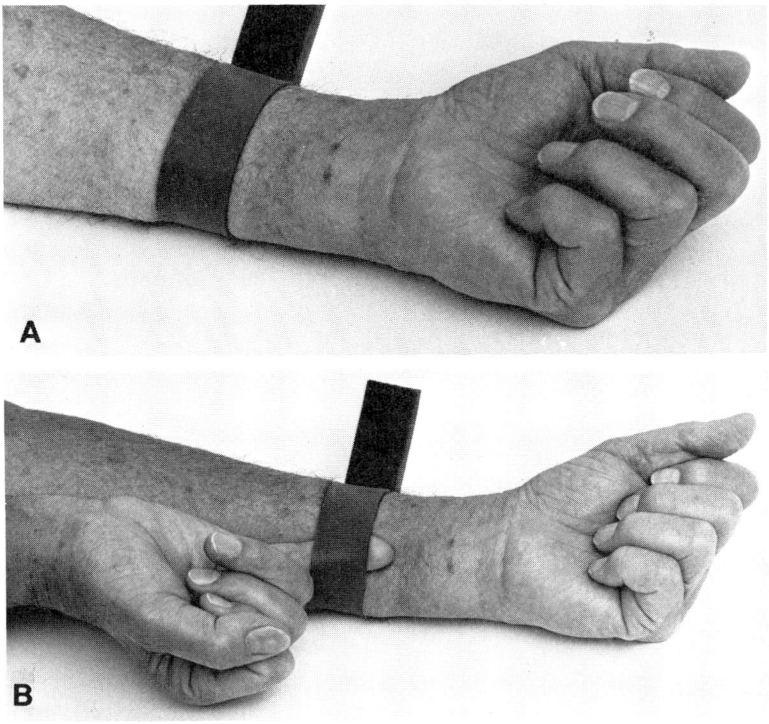

Figure 9-7. To incarcerate the venom and excise the snakebite site for retrieval of the poison, a flat elastic tourniquet, comparable to a wristwatch band, is applied between the bite and the heart (*A*). It would easily admit a finger under it (*B*).

inject antivenin into the base of a digit because this may obliterate the vessels by causing pressure or spasm and may result in loss of the digit. Because the antivenin is a horse-serum product, allergy precautions listed in the packet flyer should be followed.

HOSPITAL TREATMENT

The physician or the nurse should immediately become acquainted with the traumatic incident by recording a *rapid history and physical examination*. Patients with allergic manifestations should be treated cautiously.

With the tourniquet still in position, the *fang marks should be excised,* with the excision extending 0.5 inch beyond each fang mark and down to the vital structures beneath the skin.

If the victim is not allergic to horse serum, one vial of polyvalent antivenin should be administered intravenously or intraarterially to effect rapid neutralization of the venom. The antivenin is diluted by adding it to 100 ml isotonic saline to which has been added 100 mg hydrocortisone sodium succinate; it is given over a 20-minute period. The intraarterial antivenin route reaches and neutralizes the venomous antigen faster. If the patient is known to be allergic or if the skin test is positive, host desensitization is required, and the dosage of antivenin must be tempered to the severity of the snakebite. The initial dose, given subcutaneously, may be 0.1 ml of 1 : 10, 1 : 100, or 1 : 1000 dilution of the antiserum, and subsequent doses should be doubled and given every 15 min until 1 ml of undiluted antiserum is accepted by the host without reaction. The rest of the material is then administered slowly watching for any undue reactions.

Hypersensitivity reactions range from local urticaria and erythema to severe anaphylaxis with bronchocongestion and vascular collapse. Immediate therapy includes administration of epinephrine, corticosteroids, and antihistamines. It has been proved that some antihistamines act synergistically with snake venom, and these drugs are therefore contraindicated in snakebite therapy. The tourniquet should be removed if the extremity is ischemic or cyanotic; otherwise tourniquets are left in position for 2 hours if necessary but must be loosened in relation to the ensuing edema. Children, because they have less blood volume, and thus the venom concentration is greater, need more antivenin than do adults. If more than one vial of antivenin is necessary, it should be administered without hesitation. In 15 canines and 84 humans only one vial of antivenin per patient given intraarterially was necessary to neutralize *C. adamanteus, C. atrox,* or *A. piscivorus* antigen successfully.

Cooling a bitten area is beneficial when it is used to decrease metabolic processes in the area of the bite. Frostbite induced by extensive ice application and superimposed upon a snakebite modifies a serious condition into a critical one. Cooling the inflammatory process with mild hypothermia is beneficial, but freezing it is detrimental because of local tissue damage and the increased escape of venom into the soft tissues when the ice is removed.

A steroid may be of value as an antigen inhibitor or an antiinflammatory agent and to counteract allergic manifestations of the horse-serum antivenin. Several clinicians and investigators have concluded that ACTH, cortisone, hydrocortisone, and procaine neither effect absolute recovery nor present tissue damage and inflammation. We use 1 ml to 5 ml (depending on the victim's age and condition) of 0.5% lidocaine in 1000 ml of normal saline. The intravenous administration should be slow. Alcoholic beverages are contraindicated because they accelerate circulation and camouflage important symptoms when respiratory depression is present.

When their use is indicated, tetanus antitoxin or booster, antibiotics, analgesics, oxygen, transfusion, calcium, tracheostomy, fascial incisions, and hemodialysis are all helpful. All victims of venomous snakebite should be observed closely for 72 hours following the bite.

HYMENOPTERA

The order Hymenoptera includes bees, wasps, hornets, ants, and other insects of which the venomers are the females. The venom is expelled by an ovipositor that has the dual purpose of injecting poison and depositing eggs. Some ovipositors are smooth and others are barbed; the former type may sting repeatedly, whereas the latter hooks into the victim and tears from the insect, causing its death. The lancet deposited in the recipient adds antigens to the bee venom. Responses in the unfortunate prey may range from only a slight histamine wheal to dramatic, fatal anaphylactic shock. The interval between the envenomation and death is usually rapid—less than an hour. Drop for drop the venom of a bee is just as dangerous as that of a rattlesnake. The findings vary and include pain at the site of the sting, swelling, erythema, fever, arthralgia, pruritus, and urticaria. If allergic systemic symptoms ensue, the venom's hemolytic and neurotoxic effects appear, with development of petechial hemorrhages, malaise, weakness, nausea, vomiting, abdominal cramps, dyspnea, vascular collapse, and death.

Treatment of severe hymenopterous envenomation must be prompt. If indicated, establish an open airway, start oxygen and artificial resuscitation, and prepare an intravenous infusion of diphenhydramine (Benadryl) 3 mg/kg of body weight, followed by 10 ml of 10% calcium lactate or gluconate solution. Immediate but slow injection of 0.5 ml to 1.0 ml of 1 : 1000 epinephrine into the vein may be lifesaving. Other antihistamine or corticoid therapy is also of benefit. Cold packs and local applications of antihistamine ointments are adjunctive measures to relieve pain and soft-tissue irritation. Emergency kits for treating allergic reactions to insect stings should contain a tourniquet to be used for extremity bites, a no. 11 scalpel blade to remove the stinger, a disposable syringe for injection of epinephrine, and antihistamines. For desensitization and prophylaxis, there is a commercial polyvalent hymenopteran antigen available from Center Laboratories, Port Washington, New York. Instructions are included in the package, but a physician should instruct the patient on its use.

SPIDERS

All spiders are venomous, but the majority transmit so little venom that their bites are inconsequential. There are two groups of poisonous spiders in the United States, *Latrodectus* (widow spiders) and *Loxosceles* (brown spiders), which merit medical attention. Black widow spiders are found in all the states, and bites have been reported from most of them. There are three species of *Latrodectus* in America: *geometricus, mactans,* and *curariensis*. Spiders propagate the poison from their venom glands via a pair of appendages near the mouth.

Black widow spider envenomation of humans usually occurs at chance intrusion into the spider's domain. The venom is a most potent biologic toxin that is histolytic to cell membranes and degranulates nerve cell terminals, resulting in the release of neurotransmitters. There have been thousands of clinical cases and many deaths have been reported, but these represent only a fraction of the true number, because many cases have been misdiagnosed and many patients never reported for treatment.

Unless the patient actually felt the sting or saw the spider inflict the bite, a history is wanting. Minute red fang marks on the skin may be the only finding, yet the bite may be severe, one in which the major symptoms are severe pain, cramps, and muscle spasms that eventually affect the whole body. There is usually leukocytosis, and many times there is hematuria. About 4% of widow bites end in death. Misdiagnoses include acute appendicitis, cholecystitis, ruptured peptic ulcer, coronary thrombosis, lobar pneumonia, and tetanus.

Immediate treatment consists of cold compresses to reduce local pain, 10 ml of a 10% solution of calcium gluconate intravenously every 4 hours, diazepam 10 mg intravenously or orally if the patient is not nauseated, and methocarbamol 10 ml intravenously. We advocate prompt local excision of the bite site, which relieves the pain and sequelae. There is a specific antivenin available; 2.5 ml is given intravenously.

A most popular spider to receive current medical attention is the *Loxosceles reclusa* (brown recluse spider) (Fig. 9-8). This drab fellow is found along the Mississippi River and many of the states in the South. A cache of over 50 recluse spiders were recently found in a Salt Lake City home basement. The brown recluse spider has emerged as a potent venomous creature. Loxoscelism is no longer an infrequent medical problem. The average *L. reclusa* has long legs and measures about 12 mm long and 6 mm wide and is light tan to deep brown in color. It sports a dark brown violin-shaped insignia on its dorsal cephalothorax, hence its nickname *fiddler spider*. Another distinguishing characteristic of the fiddler spider is the six eyes positioned on the cephalic end in a semicircle. It prefers the indoors but also lives in outhouses, woodpiles, and under leaves.

The physician should use caution when making the definitive diagnosis of brown recluse spider bite. Unless the victim actually senses the bite, catches the spider scurrying away, or has expert confirmation of the species, the diagnosis is only presumptive by signs and symptoms that later develop. There is no diagnostic laboratory test for loxoscelism. Lymphocytes of a previously envenomated patient undergo blast formation when exposed to *Loxosceles* venom. Henderson demonstrated that these lymphocytes incorporate thymidine into a nucleoprotein, and this test has potential for confirming the diagnosis. Although no symptoms may be initially apparent, in a few hours at the envenomation site a small bluish hemorrhagic blister with a

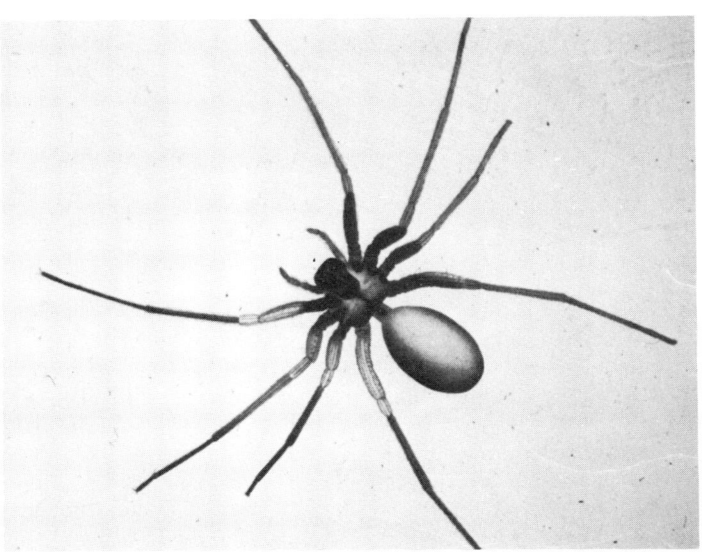

Figure 9-8. The brown recluse spider is also known as the fiddler because of the dark guitar- or violin-shaped insignia on its back.

blanched ischemic periphery appears and is surrounded by an erythematous halo. If seen early this "red, white, and blue" configuration is typical of *Loxosceles* poisoning. Later the central area becomes necrotic, sloughs, and forms an ulceration (Fig. 9-9). In addition to the cutaneous lesions, generalized findings may include headache, fever, chills, nausea, vomiting, skin rash, and arthralgia. Thrombocytopenia, hemolytic anemia, and pulmonary embolism have been responsible for deaths.

The management of loxoscelism is controversial. If the victim is seen early following the brown recluse bite, corticosteroids are effective, but they must be given in adequate doses. Solu-Medral should immediately be given I.V. in 125-mg doses at 12, 24, 36, and 48 hours. This should inhibit necrosis and eliminate systemic sequelae. Dapsone is an effective agent used to treat skin disease in which polymorphonuclear leukocytes play a prominent role. In experimental loxoscelism, agents that deplete or inhibit PMN leukocyte functions ameliorate the venom's effects. Thus the judicious use of dapsone in low doses, 50 mg to 100 mg per day, is found to be helpful in eliminating necrotic skin ulcers produced by the brown recluse spider bite. This may be the most effective specific therapy to date available aside from the specific antivenins, which are only available in South America. Reese has been experimenting with an antivenin on animals that shows promise. Excision of the lesion and immediate closure has proved to be effective in the subacute stage. Local application of silver-impregnated porcine xenograft helps prevent spreading infections.

Antibiotics are indicated to avoid secondary infection.
Analgesics are used for pain.
Tetanus prophylaxis as indicated.

Loxoscelism due to brown recluse spider venom is exhibited by anorexia, apathy, and dehydration during the first 8 hours after the bite. The bite site becomes erythematous and then forms a blister surrounded by a halo of ischemia. In a week or so the central area becomes depressed and necrotic (Fig. 9-9). The necrosis spreads and forms an ulceration. Systemic reactions consist of chills, fever, nausea, vomiting, arthralgia, and a petechial eruption within 24 hours of envenomation. A diagnosis of loxoscelism is only presumptive if the venomer has not actually been seen. Patients have been protected against brown recluse spider venom with methylprednisolone. We use total excision and primary closure of the site and recommend this in human cases. Early skin grafts to the excised ulcer site take poorly.

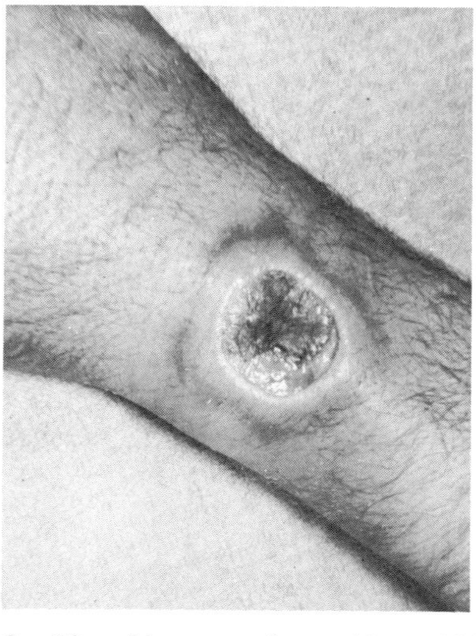

Figure 9-9. Bite of brown recluse spider exhibiting an ulcer with an elevated periphery and an umbilicated center, which are typical.

SCORPIONS

All scorpions are venomous, but instead of biting they inject their venom via a tail stinger. Some produce a local reaction, whereas others produce a systemic effect. Stings of scorpions found in Arizona and the southwest are potentially lethal (Fig. 9-10). In Arizona twice as many deaths are due to scorpion venom as to venom from all other animals. Scorpion venom seems to increase circulating cathecholamines, which cause myocardial damage and cardiac failure. The lethal species of scorpions found in these areas are *Centruroides sculpturatus* and *C. gertschi*.

Usually there is little or no edema or discoloration at the injection site. The victim experiences a sharp instant pain, and within minutes the area becomes numb. Itching of the nose and mouth is common, followed by tongue sluggishness and speech impairment. Copious salivation and difficulty in opening the mouth become apparent. Soon the patient becomes

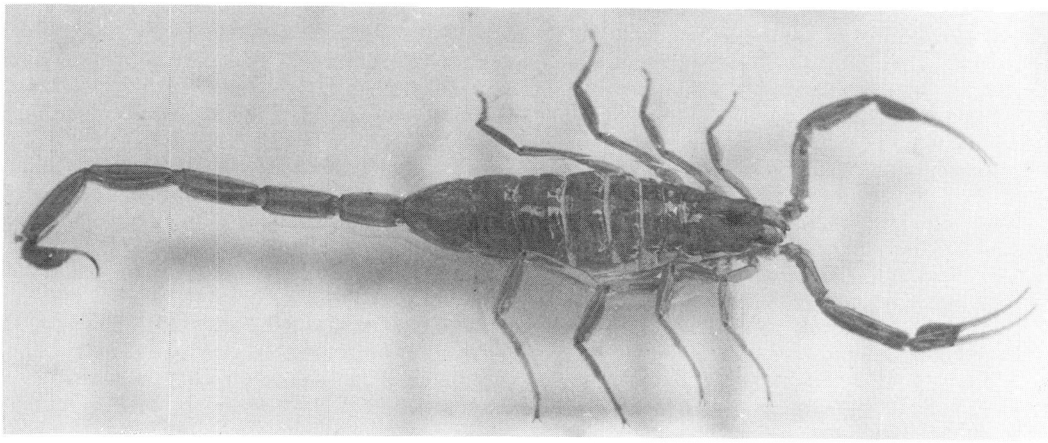

Figure 9-10. Scorpions do not bite but inject their venom through a tail stinger.

restless, exhibiting muscular twitching and spasms. If treatment is wanting, nausea, vomiting, incontinence, convulsions, and death ensue.

To relieve the local pain, betamethasone valerate (Valisone) ointment 0.1% or betamethasone dipropionate (Diprosone) ointment 0.05% is applied to the infliction and 2 ml lidocaine (Xylocaine) 2% with epinephrine 1 : 100,000 is injected into the affected area. Intravenous administration of 10 ml of 10% calcium gluconate (repeated as necessary), of 0.6 mg atropine sulfate, and of 100 mg pentobarbital (Nembutal) inhibits the general manifestations. Morphine and demerol are contraindicated and may convert a sublethal envenomation into a lethal one. Antivenin is available to Arizona physicians.

BIBLIOGRAPHY

Andrews CE: Venomous Snakebite Committee Annual Report. J Fla Med Assoc 55:308, 1968

Arbesman CE: The allergic response to stinging insects. IV. Cross-reactions between bee, wasp, and yellow jacket. J Allergy 36:147, 1965

Berger RS: Management of brown recluse spider bite. JAMA 251:889, 1984

Bogen E: The treatment of spider bite poisoning. In Buckley EE, Porges N (eds): Venoms, pub 44, p 101. Washington, American Association for the Advancement of Science, 1956

Davidson T: Inside the world of the honey bee. National Geographic 154:188, 1959

Dillaha CJ, Jansen GT, Honeycutt WH, Carlson RH: North American loxoscelism—necrotic bite of the brown recluse spider. JAMA 188:33, 1964

Ditmars RL: The Reptiles of North America, p 119. Garden City, NY, Doubleday, 1951

Ellis ER, Smith RT: Systemic anaphylaxis after rattlesnake bite. JAMA 193:151, 1965

Ersek RA et al: Treatment of spider bites with silver-impregnated porcine xenografts. Texas Med 81:32, 1985

Fardon DW, Wingo CW, Robinson DW, Masters FW: Treatment of brown spider bite. Plast Reconstr Surg 40:483, 1968

Frazier CA: Insect sting reactions in children. Ann Allergy 23:37, 1965

Garfan SR, et al: Rattlesnake bites and surgical decompression. Toxicon 22:177, 1984

Glass TG: More on snakebites. Texas Med 78:13, 1982

Glass TG: Treatment of rattlesnake bites. JAMA 247:461, 1982

Grazier DB, Carler FH: Use of the artificial kidney in snakebite. Calif Med 97:177, 1962

Gueson M: Catecholamines and myocardial damage in scorpion sting. Am Heart J 75:715, 1968

Holmes MM: Scorpion bites. Br Med J 2:353, 1957

Horen WP: Arachnidism in the United States. JAMA 185:839, 1963

Jensen H, Westphal U: Chemical structure and interrelationship of toad poisons. In Buckley EE, Porges N (eds): Venoms, pub 44, p 75. Washington, American Association for the Advancement of Science, 1956

Kennedy CB: Insect stings and bites; diagnosis, treatment, and prevention. Postgrad Med 37:193, 1965

King LE, Reilly SR: Dapsone treatment of a brown recluse bite. JAMA 250:648, 1983

Levi HW: The number of species of black widow spiders Theridiidae Latrodectus. Science 127:1055, 1958

Lockhart WE: Treatment of snakebite. JAMA 193:36, 1965

McCollough NC, Gennaro JF: Evaluation of venomous snakebite in the southern United States from parallel clinical and laboratory investigations; Development of treatment. J Fla Med Assoc 49:959, 1963

Mead R: The Medical Works of Richard Mead, p 35. Edinburgh, Donaldson and Elliot Co., 1747

O'Connor R, Erickson R: Hymenoptera antigens: An immunological comparison of venoms, venom sac extracts, and whole-insect extracts. Ann Allergy 23:151, 1965

Parrish HM, Scatterday JE: A survey of poisonous snakebites among domestic animals in Florida. Vet Med 52:135, 1957

Rauber A: Black widow spider bites. J Toxicol Clin Toxicol 21:473, 1984

Rees R, et al: Management of the brown recluse spider bite. Plast Reconstr Surg 68:768, 1981

Reid HA: Symptomatology, pathology, and treatment of land snake bite in India and Southeast Asia. In Bucherl W et al (eds): Venomous Animals and Their Venoms, p 611. New York, Academic Press, 1968

Shaffer JH: Stinging insects—a threat to life. JAMA 177:473, 1961

Snyder CC: AAHA Scientific Presentations 61:65, 1963

Snyder CC, Hunter GR, Browne EZ Jr: Malevolent inflictions: Bites and Stings. In Shires GT (ed): Care of the Trauma Patient, p 176. New York, McGraw-Hill, 1979

Snyder CC, Knowles RP: Snakebite! Consultant, July–Aug, 1963. Pathogenesis and treatment of poisonous snakebites. J Am Vet Med Assoc 15:1635, 1967

Snyder CC, et al: A definitive study of snakebite. J Fla State Med Assoc 55:330, 1968

Snyder CC, Knowles RP, Pickens JE, Emerson JL: Snakebite poisoning. In Catcott EJ (ed): Canine Medicine, p 253. Wheaton, IL, American Veterinary Publishers, 1968

Snyder CC: Bites and stings. In American College of Surgeons: Early Care of the Injured Patient, Chap 7, p 73. Philadelphia, WB Saunders, 1972

Stahnke HL: Hypothermia and scorpion venomation. Southwest Med 44:285, 1965

Stark DR, et al: Emergency treatment of snake venom poisoning. Curr Concepts Trauma Care 9:16, 1986

10 Tumors

JAMES E. GOODNIGHT

Establishing the correct diagnosis is fundamental to management of accessible tumors in ambulatory patients. Many times it is possible to identify a lesion as clearly benign from its external characteristics, but unless this certainty exists, biopsy is mandatory. Initial mismanagement of a malignant tumor can lead to tragic results, for example, electrodesiccation of a malignant melanoma without biopsy or dismissal of a soft-tissue sarcoma on physical examination as a lipoma or organizing hematoma.

This chapter will cover the ambulatory care of tumors of the skin and soft tissues, masses in the neck, and biopsy techniques. A more detailed discussion of cancer management can be obtained in texts by DeVita and colleagues (1985), Haskell (1985), and Holland and Frei (1982).

BIOPSY METHODS

GENERAL CONSIDERATIONS

Combined with initial examination of the patient, biopsy is the major feature of ambulatory surgical management of tumors. Since malignant neoplasms are often treated by multiple physicians, there must be careful recording of the measurements, location, and characteristics of a lesion plus good records regarding the biopsy and histologic diagnosis. Subsequent treatment decisions depend heavily on this information.

The decision to perform a biopsy in the outpatient setting versus the operating room requires good judgment. Most lesions discussed in this chapter can be managed in a well-equipped biopsy suite. The requirements are good lighting plus adequate instruments and assistance to obtain good visualization and hemostasis, particularly for masses in the neck or deep subcutaneous lesions. Some malignant soft-tissue tumors are highly vascular, and hemorrhage from biopsy can be significant. An additional consideration is the pain tolerance of the patient. The patient must have confidence that pain can be controlled. However, concentrated anesthetics are not required for most biopsies. A very adequate drug is 1% lidocaine without epinephrine. Epinephrine should be particularly avoided in diabetic patients and in the hands or feet. Always ask the patient about allergies to local anesthetics. Although they are rare, one must be prepared to treat severe allergic reactions to these agents.

Meticulous sterile technique must be used, including careful preparation of the skin, adequate draping to isolate the field thoroughly, and properly sterilized equipment. The operator should wear mask and gloves and, frequently, a sterile gown to help protect the field from contamination. Again it is emphasized that a properly equipped biopsy suite and adequate assistance are essential to performing efficient and safe outpatient surgery.

TECHNIQUES

EXCISIONAL BIOPSY

Complete excision of the lesion is preferred when primary closure of the skin can be obtained; it is the procedure of choice for diagnosis as well as therapy for most skin lesions and benign soft-tissue tumors. There are two considerations in placement of incision for excisional biopsy. The first is cosmesis, and if possible the incision line should be placed parallel to the tension lines of the skin (Fig. 10-1). The second consideration that may supersede cosmesis is the possibility of further surgery for the lesion in question. Should the lesion be malignant and require radical resection, the biopsy incision must be removed to help prevent local recurrence of tumor.

In excisional biopsy all the lesion is re-

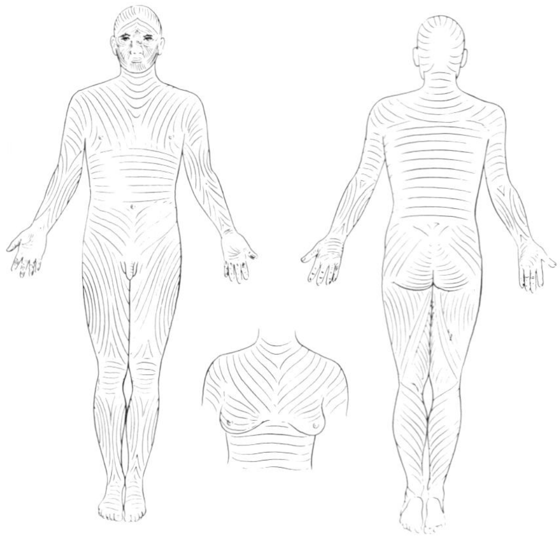

Figure 10-1. Tension lines of the skin. Scars oriented parallel to these lines undergo less spreading.

moved plus a margin of normal skin and a cuff of normal tissue on the undersurface and sides of the lesion (Fig. 10-2). For skin tumors a full thickness of skin is excised with the lesion so that it can be evaluated completely by the pathologist. This maneuver is essential for biopsy of nevi. If the lesion is suspected to be malignant, clean instruments should be obtained for skin closure. To obtain closure without tension the skin may be undermined with sharp scissors or a scalpel. In cosmetically vulnerable areas the skin should be approximated with subcuticular sutures (see Chap. 7). Instruct the patient regarding signs of infection and care of the wound, including cleanliness and limitation of motion and trauma. Sutures are generally removed as early as is consistent with good healing. This is approximately 4 days for the face and neck, 7 days for the upper extremity and the trunk, and 10 days for the lower extremity and back. Application of Steri-Strips to wounds after suture removal helps prevent late wound separation.

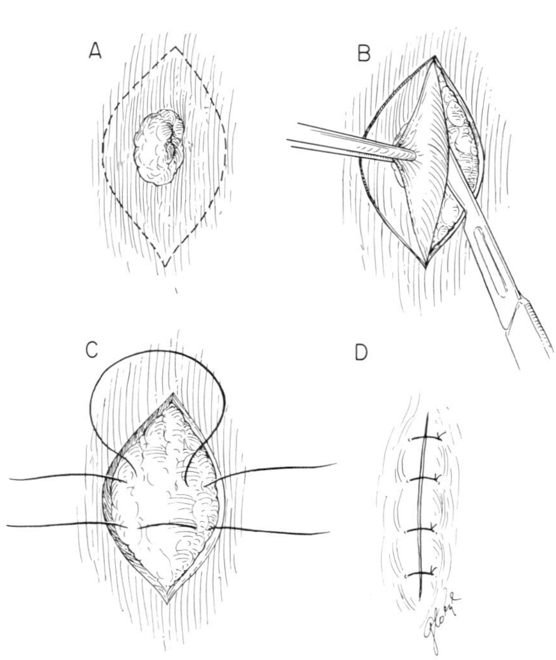

Figure 10-2. Excisional biopsy of skin lesion.

INCISIONAL BIOPSY

For initial evaluation of large tumors of the skin or soft tissues incisional biopsy is excellent in that it allows the work-up of the patient and the plans for further therapy to proceed on the basis of a firm diagnosis. Patients with benign lesions may be spared extensive unnecessary studies. The value of the information gained outweighs the risk of spreading tumor cells. Most oncologists now believe that malignant tumors shed cells early in their course and that the development of metastatic disease is the result of a struggle between the biologic aggressiveness of the particular neoplasm and host resistance factors (DeVita, 1977). It has been shown that circulating tumor cells present at the time of extirpation of a malignant neoplasm do not preclude ultimate cure of the patient (Roberts et al., 1967).

The same considerations for placement of incision previously outlined hold for incisional biopsy (Fig. 10-3). For lesions in the neck the biopsy site must be placed so that it can be removed by subsequent radical neck dissection. For biopsy on the extremity the incision should be placed longitudinally so that it can be removed if the lesion proves to be malignant. Select a representative area of the neoplasm for biopsy. It is frequently helpful to send a portion of the specimen for frozen-section diagnosis to make sure that viable tumor has been obtained. Otherwise, a report from permanent sections may show fibrous capsule containing no tumor. If a strong clinical suspicion of malignancy exists, a normal result (i.e., no malignant lesion seen) from incisional biopsy requires additional sampling of the lesion.

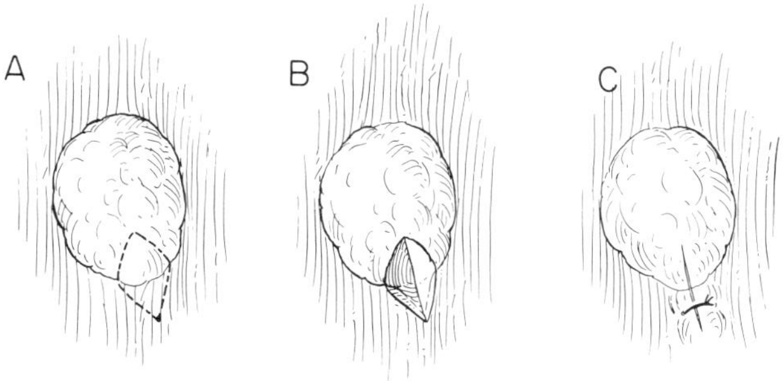

Figure 10-3. Incisional biopsy of skin lesion.

PUNCH BIOPSY

A punch, a circular cutting device, is a simple, neat means for performing either excisional or incisional biopsy of skin growths, depending on the size of the particular lesion. The punch should be well sharpened and a full thickness of skin should be removed. A scalpel or scissors is usually necessary for undercutting the specimen to remove it (Fig. 10-4). Several portions of a large lesion may be sampled with the punch. The same proviso holds for normal results of punch biopsy. Closure of the punch biopsy site with a single suture promotes rapid healing.

NEEDLE BIOPSY

Various needle devices are available for obtaining small cores of tissue for histologic examination. The Vim–Silverman needle has been used for many years, but excellent disposable needles are now available. Because of its simplicity and ease of use, this technique is valuable for evaluating tumors that can be reached easily with a needle. Care must be exercised to place the needle directly in the tissue in question. The hands must be steadied so that there is complete control of the needle at all times. Virtually all needle biopsies are done with a device whereby the entire unit is advanced into the lesion, then an inner cutting needle is advanced, followed by advancement of the outer sleeve to remove the core of tissue. The entire assembly is then withdrawn (Fig. 10-5). Since the risk of sampling error exists, a normal result from the biopsy (i.e., no malignant lesion seen) cannot be accepted as the definitive diagnosis.

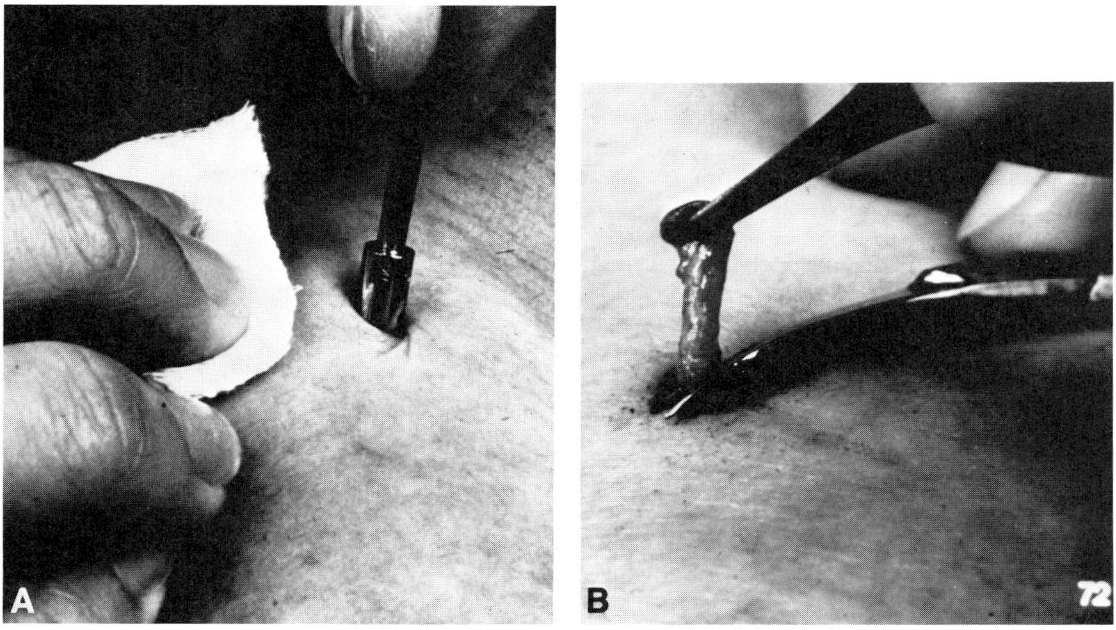

Figure 10-4. Punch biopsy. (*A*) Insertion of punch with circular motion. (*B*) Excision of specimen.

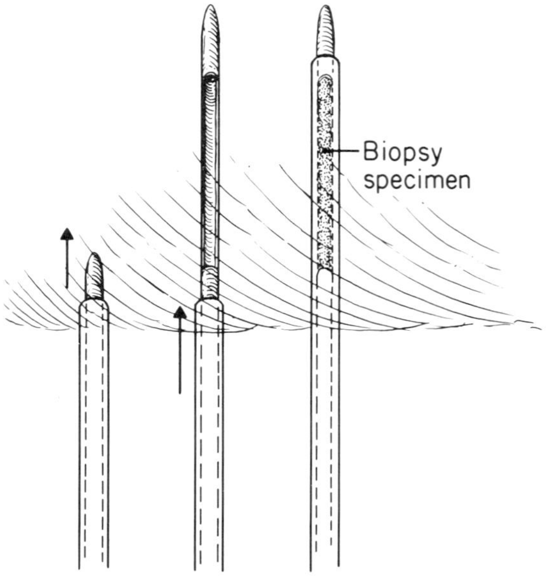

Figure 10-5. Needle biopsy (see text for explanation).

FINE NEEDLE ASPIRATION BIOPSY (FNA)

Aspirating a few cells into a conventional hypodermic needle passed percutaneously into a tumor for cytologic diagnosis has been used for over 50 years. However, this approach has become much more sophisticated in the last decade. Appropriately trained pathologists can make accurate histologic diagnosis by examination of individual cells. Morbidity and discomfort for the patient are minimal.

The biopsy specimen is obtained by first cleansing and anesthetizing the skin overlying the tumor. A 22-gauge hypodermic needle attached to a well-fitted syringe (3 ml to 10 ml) is advanced into the lesion. The plunger is pulled back to create a vacuum in the barrel of the syringe. The needle is gently moved in several directions within the tumor to obtain a representative sample of tissue. Before withdrawing the needle from the tumor, pressure on the plunger is released to eliminate the vacuum. Otherwise the biopsy specimen may be lost if aspirated into the barrel of the syringe. The unit is withdrawn from the lesion and the needle removed from the syringe. Air is drawn into the syringe and the needle is replaced. Material in the needle is expelled onto a glass slide and a thin smear is prepared. The smear should be fixed immediately in alcohol or with commercially available spray fixative as used for Papanicolaou smears. The slide is delivered to the cytopathologist for staining and examination. Smears that do not contain cellular material are unsatisfactory.

In the hands of an experienced cytopathologist, results from this type of biopsy are excellent. If the biopsy result agrees with the clinical impression and the surgeon and pathologist have developed impeccable communication relative to the biopsy technique, the diagnosis can be established by this method. However, the surgeon must be cognizant of sampling errors, unsatisfactory specimens, the experience of the surgeon and the pathologist in FNA, and variance of the biopsy results from clinical impressions. False-positive diagnoses are infrequent (0.3% or less), but including unsatisfactory specimens, sampling errors, and false-negative results, overall sensitivity for detecting malignancy by FNA is between 80% and 85%. Nevertheless, FNA is very helpful in evaluating breast masses, thyroid masses, and other superficial subcutaneous lesions.

FLUID ASPIRATION

Fluids, such as ascites or pleural effusion, aspirated from a large body cavity should be submitted for cytologic examination. The fluid can be centrifuged and the pellet fixed as a cell block for histologic examination. This technique has not been helpful in evaluating fluid from breast cysts, however.

PRESERVATION OF SPECIMEN

Most lesions are preserved in 10% formalin. However, lymph nodes should be delivered promptly to the pathologist in a fresh state (kept moist with saline). Breast cancers require evaluation for hormone receptors that by standard techniques cannot be assayed in formalin-fixed tissue. A portion of the specimen should be frozen (−70°C) to be available for determination of these hormone receptors if the breast biopsy specimen proves to be carcinoma.

Proper labeling of the specimen is imperative, as is reliable transport to the pathologist. This is the responsibility of the surgeon and requires close attention if this responsibility is delegated. Loss of the specimen is a disaster.

TUMORS OF THE SKIN

CYSTS

Sebaceous Cysts

Sebaceous cysts arise from blockage of the duct of sebaceous glands located in hair follicles. Sebaceous material continues to be secreted, and the gland slowly enlarges to form a cystic structure. These cysts are a common benign skin problem and are most often seen on the scalp, back of the neck, or upper back. They are characteristically discrete, firm masses that are readily visible and palpable in the skin.

Sebaceous cysts are excised primarily for cosmetic reasons, although occasionally they may be painful. It is necessary to remove the cyst wall completely with careful sharp dissection to prevent recurrence of the lesion (Fig. 10-6). Sebaceous cysts may become infected and require incision and drainage. After the infection is controlled, complete excision should be performed.

Epidermal Inclusion Cysts

Epidermal inclusion cysts occur secondary to a penetrating injury in which epidermis is carried into the deeper layers of the skin. Overgrowth of epidermal elements and secre-

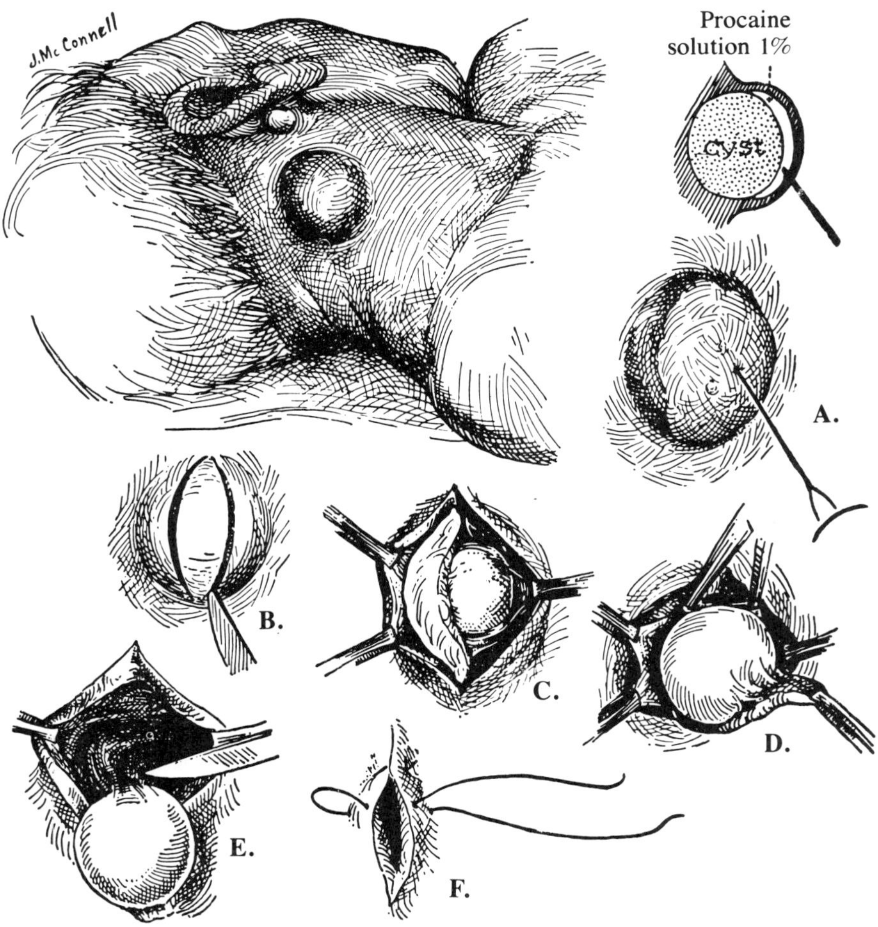

Figure 10-6. Excision of sebaceous cyst of the neck. (*A*) It is frequently possible to inject local anesthetic between the cyst capsule and the surrounding tissues so that dissection may be partly performed. (*B*) When the cyst is so large that the skin is stretched over it, an ellipse of skin may be excised with the cyst. (*C*) If the lips of the wound are kept on tension by finger pressure or by grasping the edges of the wound with Allis forceps, the dissection may be partly accomplished without manipulation. (*D,E*) The tissues under the cyst are dissected. (*F*) The wound is closed with careful approximation of skin edges.

tion of sebaceous material result in a cystic mass. They are most often found on the palmar surfaces of the hands or fingers or on the soles of the feet. These cysts are completely benign and are usually removed because they become painful. They are treated by excisional biopsy.

Dermoid Cysts

Dermoid cysts are congenital in origin. They are found most frequently in children in the periorbital area but may also be palpated in subcutaneous locations on the scalp, nose, abdomen, and sacral region (Fig. 10-7). They generally cause no difficulty but are frequently excised to differentiate them from other lesions or for cosmetic reasons. Treatment is excisional biopsy.

KERATOSIS

Senile (Actinic) Keratosis

Senile keratosis is a hypertrophy of the epidermis that appears early as small, red, scaly lesions in sun-exposed areas of aging skin, usually associated with a small telangiectasis, and later as a hyperkeratotic growth. It can degenerate to carcinoma and represents a premalignant lesion. Treatment is by excisional biopsy with careful histologic examination for malignant cells. Patients with these lesions should protect their skin from sunlight.

Seborrheic Keratosis

Seborrheic keratosis also represents overgrowth of the epidermis appearing with aging but usually earlier than senile keratosis. It presents as circumscribed, raised, black or brown skin nodules with an oily appearance to the surface that are seen primarily in sun-exposed areas (Fig. 10-8). They are removed for cosmetic reasons, although a very rare case of degeneration to basal cell carcinoma has been observed. Treatment is excisional biopsy.

Cutaneous Horn

A cutaneous horn is a raised, hard, keratin structure that has become cornified. Cutaneous horns arise from senile keratoses (Fig. 10-9). They represent tissue that should be shed but is not. Cutaneous horns should be removed by simple excision and examined histo-

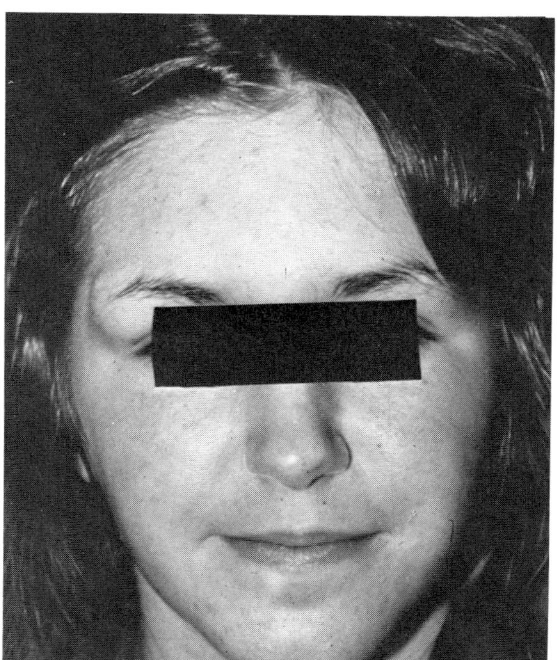

Figure 10-7. Dermoid cyst in right periorbital region.

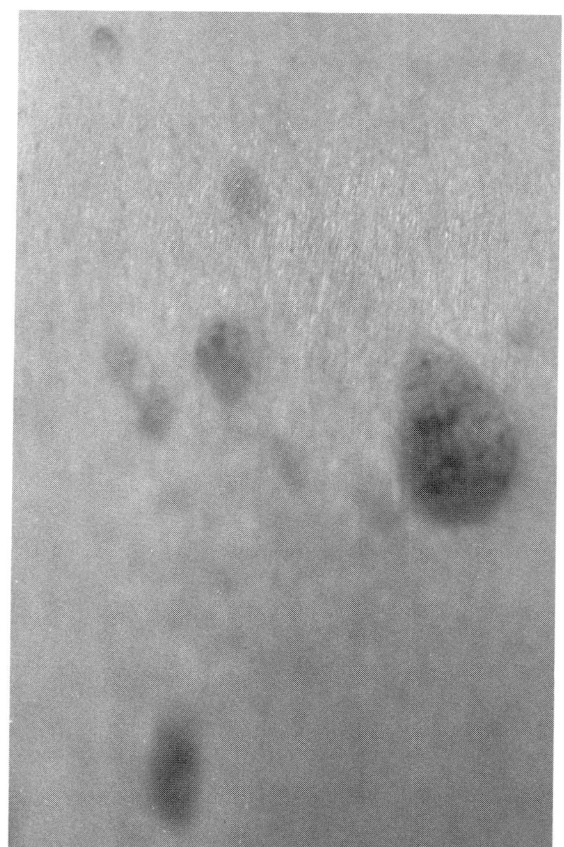

Figure 10-8. Seborrheic keratosis.

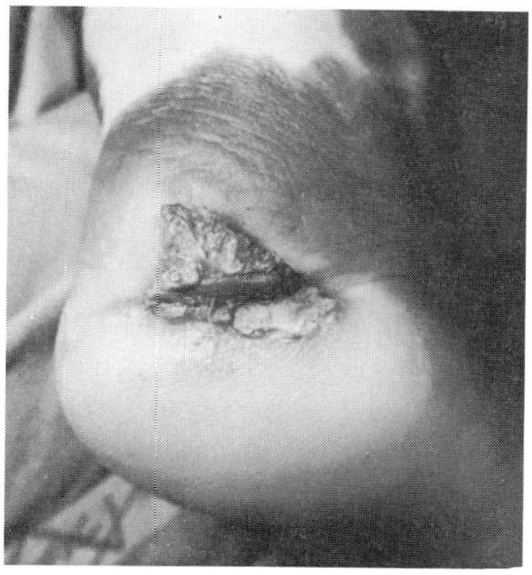

Figure 10-9. Cutaneous horn on heel.

logically because they may degenerate to carcinoma.

WARTS (VERRUCA VULGARIS)

Warts are viral infections of the skin that may present in a variety of patterns of epidermal overgrowth. They are readily recognized as sessile, pedunculated, or more commonly vegetating growth (Fig. 10-10). They most often appear on the hand but may be widespread and are found in the anogenital region as well (venereal warts). In the moist anogenital area they may produce exuberant growth. The presence of extensive anogenital warts should alert the clinician to possible HTLV-III infection. A disabling wart can appear on the plantar surface of the foot (plantar wart). Because of their infectious etiology, warts are contagious and autoinoculable. They come in crops but are a self-limited disease. However, the cosmetic deformity may be very disturbing while they last, and some warts are very refractory to treatment. In treating warts it must be remembered that they are self-limited and that the growth involves only the epidermis. The cure must not be worse than the disease by producing scarring from treatment. Warts respond very well to electrodesiccation with gentle curettage. However, this form of therapy should be avoided for plantar warts because a painful scar may result. Electrodesiccation requires local anesthesia. The needle is inserted into the wart several times, with a very mild current being used. The dehydrated wart is then removed with a sharp curette, taking care to remove the "core." Then the base is very mildly and superficially desiccated, leaving a dry scab.

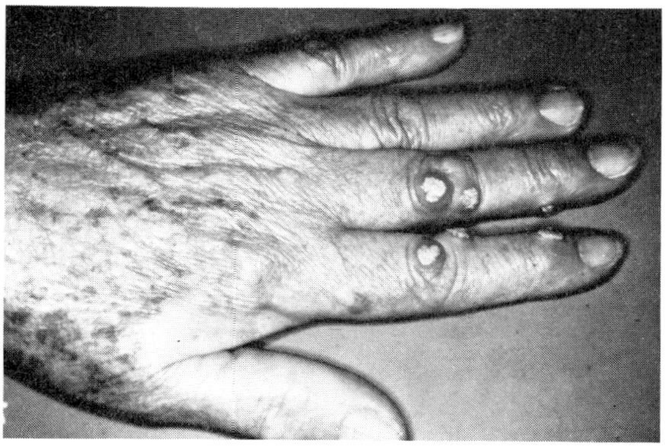

An alternative therapy that is particularly useful for venereal warts and plantar warts is the application of podophyllin. A 20% concentration of podophyllin in tincture of benzoin (which prevents spread of the solution) is applied to the warts once a week. It usually requires three to four applications. Plantar warts may be trimmed, but very carefully and gently, and this form of therapy should be avoided in diabetics. Freezing of the lesions with liquid nitrogen or with a cryotherapy probe is also effective. Radiation therapy can be used for warts, but the indications are very restricted and limited to disabling, refractory lesions. Radiotherapy is absolutely contraindicated if there is scarring or vascular compromise in the vicinity of the wart.

PAPILLOMAS

Papillomas are pedunculated growths of fibrous tissue on a stalk covered by skin. They occur primarily in the axilla or on the back or neck. They are completely benign and removed only for cosmetic reasons. They may be excised or the stalk may be ligated with thread, resulting in infarction of the lesion, which spontaneously drops off.

VASCULAR TUMORS

Intradermal Capillary Hemangiomas (Nevus Flammeus; Port-Wine Stain)

Hemangiomas are vascular malformations rather than true neoplasms. Intradermal capillary hemangiomas are made up of multiple dilated abnormal capillaries residing in the dermis and subdermal region. They appear at birth, and although they may undergo some involution during growth to adulthood, they usually do not go away. Unfortunately, they occur commonly on the face and are often large but are not raised above the level of the skin (Fig. 10-11). There is no danger of significant hemorrhage from these lesions.

Small capillary hemangiomas may be excised for cosmetic reasons. Resection of large lesions requires extensive skin grafting for resurfacing. Although gratifying results can be obtained, scarring and recurrence of the hemangioma at the graft margin complicate this approach. A satisfactory form of therapy is to cover the lesion with appropriately matched paste makeup. Patients, including children, can become surprisingly adept at applying this covering. However, men usually do not accept this treatment. Attempts at sclerosis of capillary hemangiomas with various escharotics may result in a white, atrophic scar, and the procedure is not recommended.

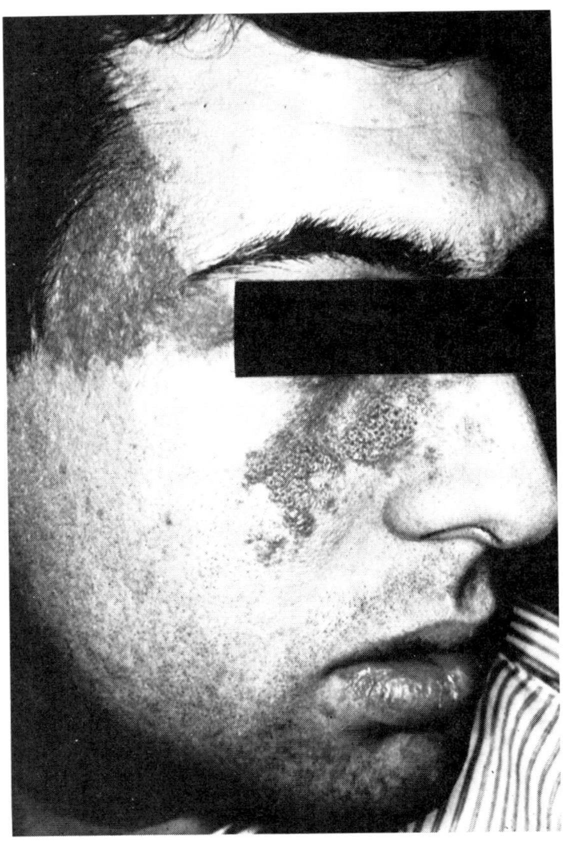

Figure 10-11. Capillary hemangioma (nevus flammeus).

Immature or Juvenile Hemangiomas (Strawberry Marks; Strawberry Capillary Hemangioma)

Immature or juvenile hemangiomas are obvious at birth and consist of a large mass of small arterioles and venules. Strawberry hemangiomas have a striking bulging appearance that is made worse by the infant's crying. They may enlarge steadily for a time after birth, but fortunately almost all these lesions involute in the period between 1 and 4 years of age (Fig. 10-12). The most important aspect of therapy is to try to keep the epidermis intact over the hemangioma to prevent scarring. Because of the high rate of involution, it is best to try to avoid treatment of this lesion. Some authorities do advocate early excision of small lesions. Escharotics result in scarring. Hemorrhage from these lesions can be significant but is of the capillary type and can be controlled easily with pressure on the lesion.

To demonstrate to concerned parents that immature hemangiomas will involute, it is wise to keep photographic records of other children. Photographs are also helpful for parents to follow the progress of involution in their own child.

Cavernous Hemangiomas

Cavernous hemangiomas are mature lesions made up of well-developed dilated vessels, arteriovenous fistulas, and shunts, and they may contain a large amount of connective tissue. They appear at birth and do not involute. The cosmetic and functional problems from cavernous hemangiomas may be significant, and they may bleed heavily when traumatized (Fig. 10-13). Disseminated intravascular clotting can result from platelet trapping within these lesions. Cavernous hemangiomas often involve deep structures as well as external surfaces. Examples are cavernous hemangiomas in the trigeminal distribution where the facial lesion is associated with deep lesions in the brain (Sturge–Weber syndrome).

Cavernous hemangiomas should be protected from trauma to prevent ulceration and infection. Smaller lesions may be excised for cosmetic deformity or for repeated trauma, but surgical resection is a major undertaking for large lesions. Cavernous hemangiomas often undergo rapid growth during the first year of life. Prednisone, administered in 20-mg to 40-mg doses daily or every other day for 30 to 90 days during this growth period, causes the

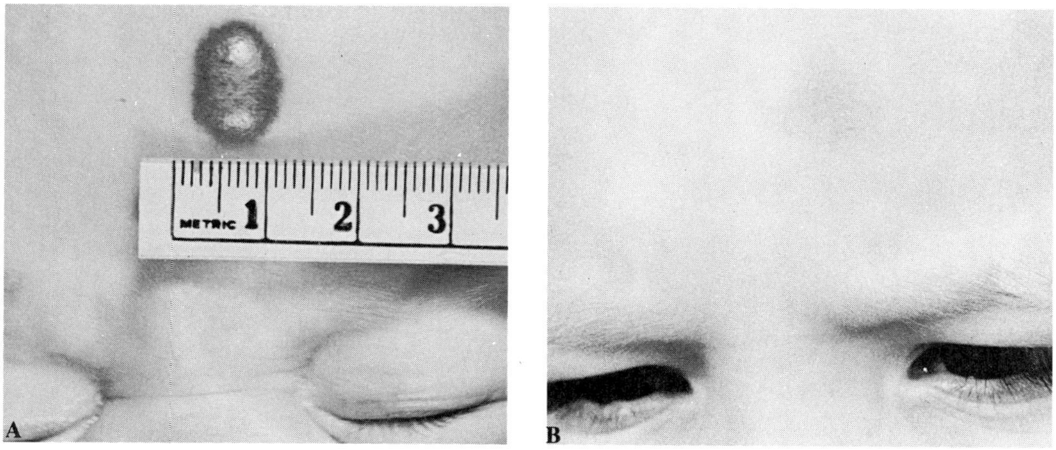

Figure 10-12. Immature hemangioma (strawberry hemangioma) (*A*) at birth and (*B*) at 3 years of age. The lesion was not treated. (Margileth AM, Museles M: Current concepts and management of congenital cutaneous hemangiomas. Pediatrics 36:410, 1965)

majority of these lesions to regress significantly. Although involution is rarely complete, this reduction in size lessens cosmetic deformity and makes subsequent surgical approaches easier.

Injection of sclerosing solutions such as 5% sodium morrhuate may be beneficial, but this approach is hazardous and may result in scarring and additional cosmetic deformity. A needle is introduced into the vascular space and the location is confirmed by withdrawing blood. The amount of sclerosing agent injected varies from a few drops to about 2.5 ml. Manual compression is maintained until a rubber-sponge-compression bandage has been applied over the area. Cavernous hemangiomas also respond to radiation therapy, but this can cause serious scarring and ulceration and probably should be avoided.

Pyogenic Granulomas

A pyogenic granuloma is an overgrowth of normal capillaries apparently in response to an injury. It appears as a bright red, nodular growth, which, when traumatized, bleeds easily and profusely (Fig. 10-14). Coloration may vary from red to blue-black. Pyogenic granulomas are found primarily on the hands, fingers, lips, and face. Treatment is excisional biopsy. Alternatively, pyogenic granulomas can be eliminated by repeated applications of silver nitrate as a sclerosing agent.

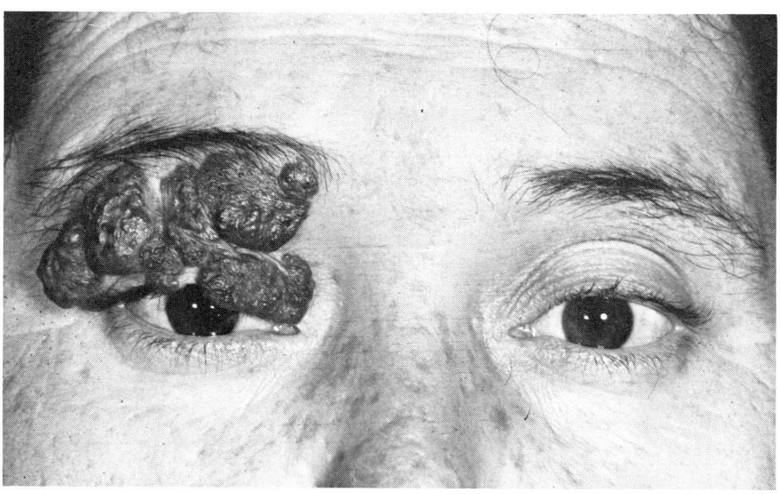

Figure 10-13. Cavernous hemangioma of right eyelid.

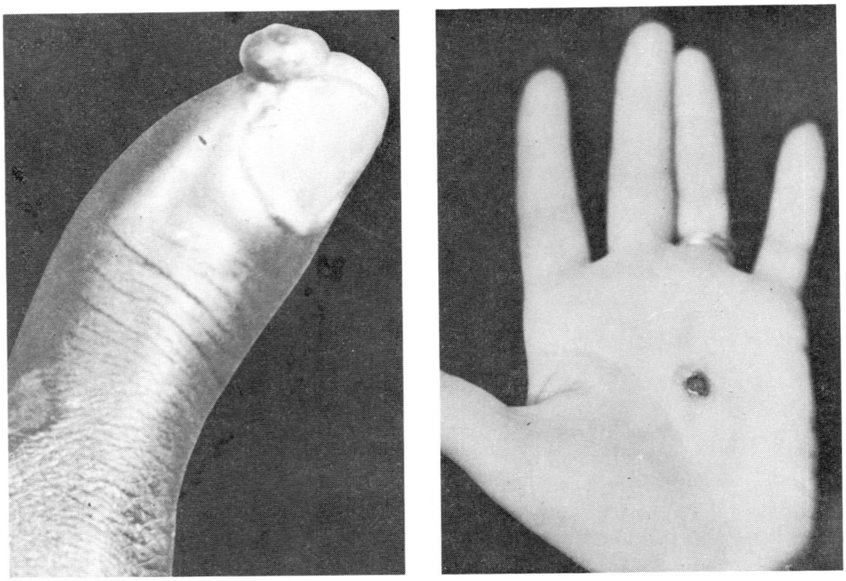

Figure 10-14. Two cases of pyogenic granuloma.

Glomus Tumors

Glomus tumors are an outgrowth of the glomus organ, which is a neurovascular bundle consisting of small arteriovenous shunts involved in temperature control of an extremity. A glomus tumor is also known as glomangioma and angiomyoneuroma. Hemangiopericytomas are the malignant counterpart of glomus tumors. The vascular endothelium is surrounded by "glomus cells," and the lesions are well supplied with sympathetic nerve fibers. Glomus tumors appear as small red or blue or reddish-blue nodules, most often on the finger where they may be subungual. They are also found over the coccyx, joints, and scapula. Their most striking feature is that they can be quite painful, either spontaneously or with pressure. The primary reasons for removal are control of pain and differentiation from malignant lesions. Complete excision is necessary to prevent recurrence. These lesions are radioresistant, and radiation therapy is not indicated.

Histiocytomas

Histiocytomas are small, hard nodules lying just under the skin and attached to it. A histiocytoma is also known as dermatofibroma. The color of the nodule varies from pink or red to yellow, dark brown, or black (Fig. 10-15). They are usually asymptomatic but can be painful over a pressure point. Histiocytomas consist of fibroblasts and histiocytes. Pigmentation results from hemosiderin deposition in the histiocytes. Histiocytomas are benign, but excision may be required because of their location or cosmetic change or to confirm the diagnosis when the pigmentation suggests melanoma. Treatment is simple excisional biopsy.

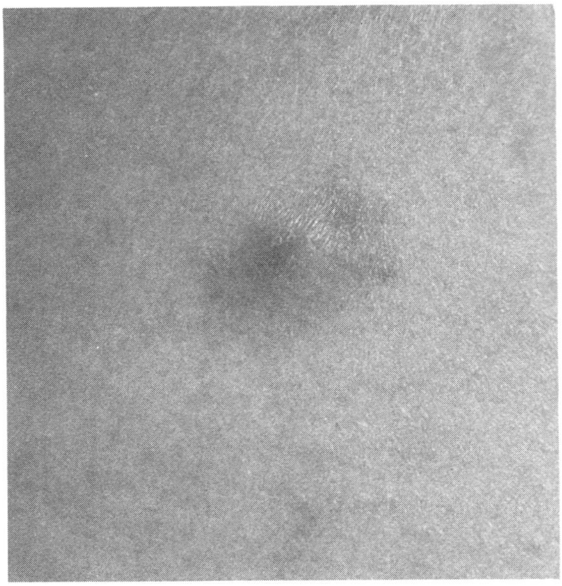

Figure 10-15. Histiocytoma.

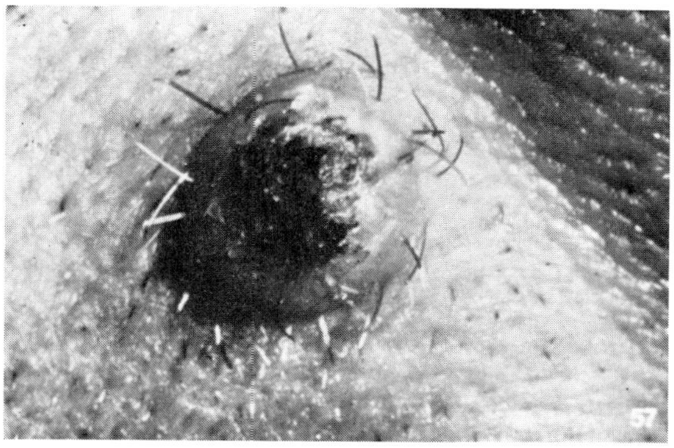

Figure 10-16. Keratoacanthoma. Note keratin plug in center of nodule.

Keratoacanthomas

Keratoacanthomas are rapidly growing, nodular lesions that appear on the skin surface in sun-exposed areas. These epithelial lesions appear as a slightly reddish nodule with a depressed center containing a keratin plug (Fig. 10-16). Because of their rapid growth and appearance they are difficult to distinguish from squamous cell carcinoma. This difficulty is true also for microscopic examination. Their natural history is spontaneous resolution after a few months. Nevertheless, because of the difficulty in distinguishing them from squamous cell carcinoma, they should be removed by excisional biopsy and examined histologically. Although considered a benign lesion, a few keratoacanthomas (less than 5%) progress to squamous cell carcinoma.

Keloids

Keloids are unsightly, bulging, tumorlike collections of fibrous tissue resulting from excess formation of collagen in healing skin wounds (Fig. 10-17). Histologically, they are composed of large bundles of collagen in a highly disorganized array. The etiology of keloids is unclear, but they can result from very slight skin trauma such as insect bites, acne, or piercing of the ears for cosmetic reasons. Their chief offense is cosmetic deformity, but large keloids can interfere with function and movement. Black people have a much greater incidence of keloid formation. These lesions are notorious for reforming after excision.

Preventive measures help reduce keloid formation. These include orientation of wounds parallel to tension lines (see Fig. 10-1), avoiding tension in wound closure, and reducing inflammation by limiting the amount of buried suture.

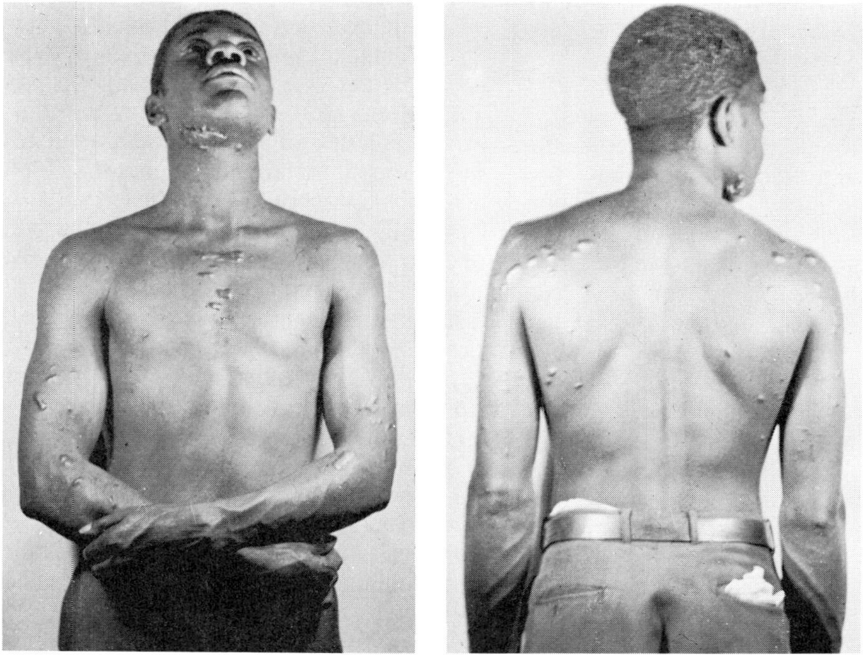

Figure 10-17. Multiple keloids. Every slight injury to the skin in this patient resulted in a keloid.

Keloids in formation (first few months) respond to steroid injection, pressure application, or radiation therapy. Triamcinolone, up to 120 mg to 150 mg (diluted up to 10 ml by mixing with 2% lidocaine), can be injected directly into a wound at closure or into the newly forming scar. Injection should attempt to distribute the drug uniformly throughout the lesion. This dose should not be repeated more often than monthly, and the dose should be reduced accordingly for children. Continuous pressure applied to a newly forming scar with a custom-fitted elastic stocking or compression bandage for a period of at least 9 months reduces keloid formation. This procedure is applicable to large wounds such as burn scars. Radiation therapy administered to developing keloids in relatively low doses is effective treatment, but there is legitimate concern over the use of radiation for benign conditions in young people.

Mature keloids (present for many months) respond to direct injection of steroids. The dose of triamcinolone is as indicated previously and is repeated at monthly intervals for up to 10 to 12 months. The patient must be observed carefully for steroid side-effects, and lower doses must be used in children. Overtreatment is possible, resulting in an atrophic, depressed scar. Some lesions require excision with careful closure, followed by application of pressure, steroid treatment, or both.

Pigmented Nevi and Malignant Melanoma

Everyone has a few nevi (moles), but for some individuals these skin neoplasms number in the hundreds. Benign nevi are of no consequence other than cosmetic, but differentiating them for malignant melanoma assumes a major significance in the ambulatory surgical clinic. Except for lung cancer in women, malignant melanoma has the fastest rate of increase in incidence of any cancer seen in the Western world. Approximately 26,000 new cases of malignant melanoma appeared in the United States in 1986, which is more than double the number of cases seen a decade ago. This increase in frequency of malignant melanoma, plus its potential lethality, gives added importance to early recognition of this lesion, which can be difficult.

Nevi are collections of melanocytes that migrate to the junction of the epidermis and dermis and then gradually mature into intradermal nodular growths. Nevi are classified as junctional, compound, or intradermal. Junctional nevi are composed of melanocytes located at the junction of the dermis and epidermis. This lesion is evolving and immature and is more likely to degenerate to malignant melanoma. Compound nevi contain both junctional and intradermal elements. Compound nevi are still maturing and are at risk for becoming melanoma. Intradermal nevi are mature lesions and have a relatively low propensity to become malignant melanoma. Intradermal nevi assume a variety of shapes from a sessile structure to markedly pedunculated or globular. They are usually uniform in color and soft to the touch. In contrast, junctional nevi are flat lesions and are more irregular in shape and color. Guidelines for determining which nevi to biopsy will be discussed later. However, any nevus that is removed for any reason should be treated by excisional biopsy and histologic examination by a competent pathologist. Nevi should never be removed by electrodesiccation.

Malignant melanoma appears much more commonly in white-skinned persons, particularly in sun-exposed areas. However, malignant melanoma is found on the palms and soles of black people and occasionally on mucous membranes throughout the gastrointestinal tract. People with sandy brown hair and diffuse freckling with multiple small pigmented nevi seem to have a greater propensity for development of malignant melanoma. This cancer is extremely rare in prepubertal children. However, rapid evolution of nevi whose growth and appearance are suggestive of malignant melanoma can occur in children. These lesions should be biopsied, but they are usually identified as juvenile melanomas that have a very favorable prognosis.

Recognition of the classic jet-black malignant melanoma with bleeding, ulceration, or satellite nodules is straightforward. However, there are a disturbing variety of presentations of malignant melanoma. Any new nevus that is growing steadily usually raises suspicions, but malignant melanoma can arise in pigmented areas that have been present for a lifetime, including birthmarks. The onset of malignancy may be heralded by relatively little change in the birthmark. An excellent article with color illustrations of malignant melanoma by Mihm and colleagues in the New England Journal of Medicine in 1973 is well worth review. They thought the most significant finding was irregularity of color, with blue or black shades being most important but with red or white spots also significant. The more variegated the color, the greater the risk of melanoma. The second most important finding was irregularity in the border of the lesion. Superficial spreading melanomas tend to have a large notch at their edge. The third finding of importance was surface irregularity, which can be best appreciated by shining a light from the side of the melanoma. Any nevus that has these features should definitely have biopsy (Fig. 10-18).

Nevi or pigmented lesions that are growing, changing, or regressing or that are pruritic, ulcerated, or bleeding should undergo excisional biopsy. Nevi that are frequently traumatized should be excised. Lesions with a pigmented halo or a halo of depigmentation should be removed. Junctional nevi appear on the palms of the hands, the genitalia, and the sole of the foot as well as mucous membranes; in general they should be removed. However, care should be exercised in removing nevi from the sole of the foot, since a painful scar can result. If a patient questions the appearance of a nevus, it should be carefully examined, since there is usually some reason for the patient to take notice of it. Choosing the lesions for biopsy can be difficult and anxiety-provoking for the physician and patient. Unfortunately, it is not possible to remove all moles effectively from a patient.

A major prognostic determinant in malignant melanoma is the depth of skin invasion of the primary lesion. Primary malignant melanomas are microstaged on the basis of the depth of skin invasion either by the levels of Clark and associates (1969) or, more important, by actual measurement in millimeters (Breslow, 1970). This information is essential for treatment planning. Shave biopsies preclude accurate microstaging and should be avoided. Biopsy of nevi should include removal of a full thickness of skin.

Incisional biopsy of large pigmented lesions is acceptable. An alternative means of evaluating these large lesions is multiple punch biopsies. However, if a nevus is clinically suspicious and biopsy has not included the whole lesion, one must be reluctant to accept a benign diagnosis based on limited sampling. Malignant melanoma can exist in only a portion of a pigmented lesion.

The definitive treatment of malignant melanoma, which is the radical wide excision of the primary site and in some cases regional lymph node dissection, has been reviewed by Siegler and Fetter (1977), Eilber and co-workers (1979), Balch and Milton (1985), Gumport and

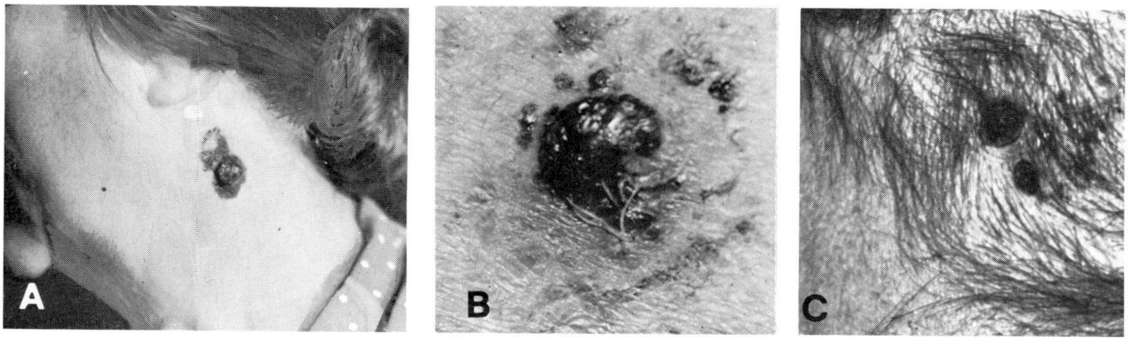

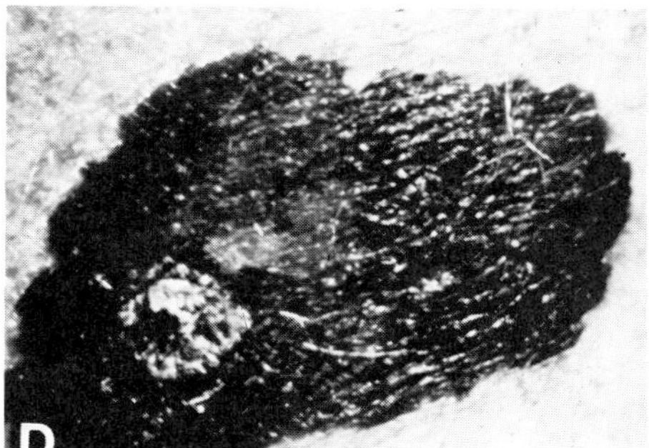

Figure 10-18. Malignant melanoma: (*A*) malignant melanoma arising in a preexisting nevus; (*B*) nodular malignant melanoma; (*C*) malignant melanoma on scalp; (*D*) superficial spreading malignant melanoma. Note multiple colors, notched border, and irregular surface.

Harris (1985), and Mastrangelo, Baker, and Katz (1985). Lesions that should be referred for definitive treatment are those with a frank diagnosis of malignant melanoma and lesions that any well-trained pathologist considers malignant melanoma even if other consultants disagree. A diagnosis that causes consternation is atypical melanocytic hyperplasia. This lesion has cellular features of malignant melanoma but is limited to the epidermis and shows no invasion (Clark and associates level I malignant melanoma). Atypical melanocytic hyperplasias should also be treated by reexcision to obtain a 1-cm margin of uninvolved skin around the lesion.

A variation of malignant melanoma, called Hutchinson's melanotic freckle or lentigo maligna, appears in exposed areas of skin in elderly patients. This lesion is tan or dark brown, grows slowly, and is seen most often on the face. Lentigo maligna becomes invasive at later stages and is described then as lentigo maligna melanoma. It is thought that approximately 30% of these lesions become invasive. Lentigo maligna should be excised, which, because of size and location of the lesion, is usually a formal operative procedure.

MALIGNANT SKIN TUMORS

BASAL CELL CARCINOMA

Skin cancers are the most frequent neoplasms afflicting mankind. There are approximately 500,000 new cases of skin cancer in the United States each year. Basal cell carcinoma is the most common skin cancer. It appears later in life and occurs predominantly on the face, neck, and dorsum of the hands. Usually there is no prior lesion visible. The neoplasm arises in the basal layer of the skin. It is a low-grade cancer that grows slowly and may take 2 to 3 years to reach 1 cm in size. It very rarely metastasizes (approximately 0.1% of lesions).

Basal cell carcinoma is characteristically a round lesion with rolled borders and an ulcerated necrotic center (Fig. 10-19). It may begin as a nodular, slightly scaly lesion before developing the classic appearance. The lesion spreads outward and downward and can invade deeply. It can present as a rodent ulcer in which most of the growth is downward into adjacent tissue.

The principles of treatment of basal cell carcinoma are (1) complete eradication of the lesion, (2) determination that all the margins are free of invasion, (3) obtaining good functional and cosmetic results. In general, 0.5-cm margin should be taken in every direction, including the undersurface. Larger basal cell carcinomas may require incisional biopsy for diagnosis, then definitive resection. Radiation therapy is relatively effective for basal cell carcinomas and is an acceptable alternative. However, the lesion must be followed very carefully to determine the adequacy of treatment.

An alternative form of treatment of basal cell carcinomas is local immunotherapy, which is the intralesional injection or topical application of agents to induce delayed cutaneous hypersensitivity responses in the immediate vicinity of accessible tumors. Klein (1968) demonstrated that patients sensitized to dinitrochlorobenzene (DNCB) showed regres-

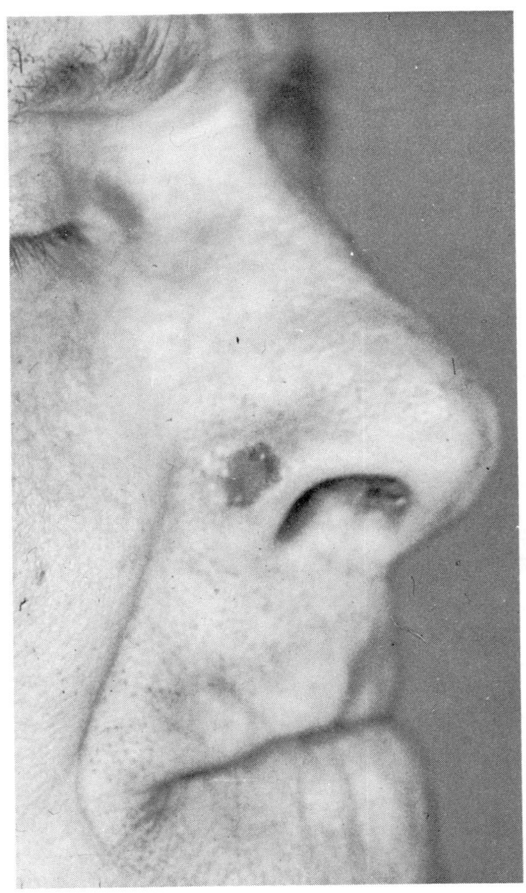

Figure 10-19. Basal cell carcinoma.

sion of superficial basal cell or squamous cell carcinomas when this agent was topically applied to the lesions. The mechanism underlying tumor destruction following this treatment is not known. Toxicity of local immunotherapy is minimal, and normal skin is relatively unaffected.

Local immunotherapy with DNCB is obtained by first sensitizing the patient to the agent. This is done with 2000 μg in 0.1 ml acetone applied to the skin with a 2-cm polyethylene ring, allowed to evaporate, and covered with a bandage. After 2 weeks, patch testing is performed on normal skin with concentrations of 10^{-1} g to 10^{-6} g DNCB/100 g cream base to determine the lowest concentration producing erythema and induration. This concentration is applied daily to the tumor and covered. Treatment should continue through necrosis of the lesion. Healing then may be allowed, but the lesion should be followed very carefully to make sure that it has been eradicated.

Therapeutic benefit can be improved by adding a second sensitizing agent, topical 5-fluorouracil (5-FU). Topical 5-FU as a 5% solution or cream is applied daily to the lesion for several weeks. There is initial erythema followed by blistering, then erosion and necrosis of the lesion, and finally epithelialization. Williams and Klein (1970) reported that topical 5-FU produced resolution of 56% of nodular basal cell carcinomas.

Local immunotherapy is beneficial for multiple superficial lesions that are not readily amenable to surgical excision. For single or large basal cell carcinomas, surgical excision is the treatment of choice.

SQUAMOUS CELL CARCINOMA

Squamous cell carcinoma arises from the epidermis. It consists of nodular growths of squamous epithelial cells with keratin formation seen as a whorled "pearl" formation on histologic examination. The lesion also commonly appears as a nonhealing skin ulceration (Fig. 10-20). It is somewhat less common than basal cell carcinoma, but the epidemiology is similar. Sun exposure is implicated as an etiologic stimulus as in basal cell carcinoma. These cancers also appear in areas of chronic trauma such as burn scars (Marjolin's ulcer), in areas of radiation dermatitis, and after arsenic exposure. For all of these lesions there is a long latent period between the trauma and the appearance of the neoplasm.

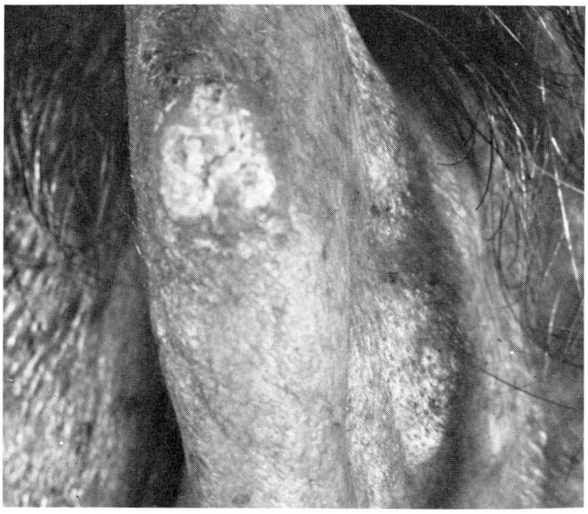

Figure 10-20. Squamous cell carcinoma on the helix of the ear (lateral surface).

Squamous cell carcinoma is most commonly seen on the vermilion border of the lip, on the paranasal fold, or at the edge of the axillary fold. It may arise in a prior skin lesion, particularly senile (actinic) keratosis. Squamous cell carcinoma grows much more rapidly than basal cell carcinoma. It can and does metastasize, although the frequency of this finding is somewhat disputed. It has been suggested that lesions of the hand are more likely to metastasize than lesions of the face. The physician must be alert to enlarged regional lymph nodes. The treatment is similar to that of basal cell carcinoma, in that complete surgical excision is recommended. Prompt diagnosis and eradication are important to prevent the erosion of surrounding tissue and metastases. These lesions are less radiosensitive than basal cell carcinomas so that surgery is generally the preferred treatment. For multiple superficial squamous cell carcinomas, local immunotherapy is an acceptable alternative treatment.

KAPOSI'S SARCOMA

Prior to the onset of the acquired immune deficiency syndrome (AIDS) epidemic, Kaposi's sarcoma was a rare tumor in the United States. Since 1980 the incidence in San Francisco has increased 30-fold. Approximately one third of all AIDS patients die of Kaposi's

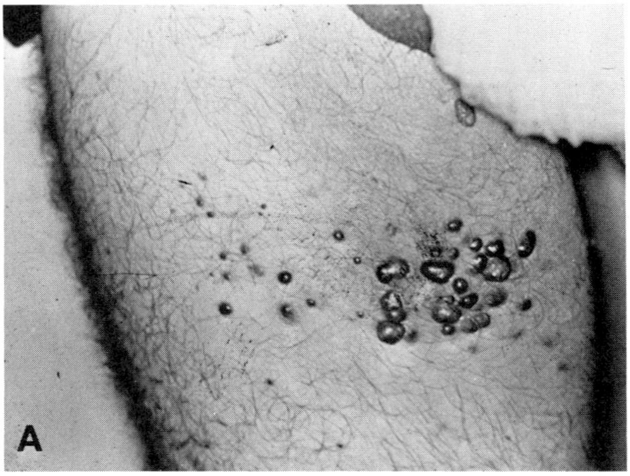

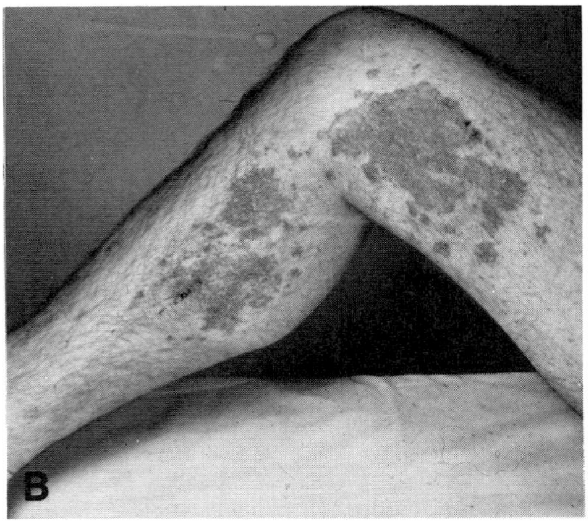

Figure 10-21. Kaposi's sarcoma: (*A*) nodules, (*B*) plaque lesions.

sarcoma. The tumor arises in the skin presumably from endothelial cells and presents as raised nodules and plaques that are red or bluish but that vary from pink to purple (Fig. 10-21). Macular lesions are seen, and in AIDS patients the disease may present as lymphadenopathy. In AIDS patients the disease rapidly disseminates to gastrointestinal organs, lungs, and other viscera. It may make its appearance as a multifocal systemic disease. In this current form Kaposi's sarcoma most resembles the form seen in young adult Africans in Zaire, where the disease presents on the extremities and is locally aggressive. Previously in the United States and Europe, Kaposi's sarcoma was seen only rarely and primarily in adult men of Mediterranean extraction. The disease in this population follows a very indolent course and is frequently associated with lymphorecticular malignancy.

The main consideration for the ambulatory surgery clinic is recognition of the lesion and biopsy plus the awareness of its close association with AIDS. Treatment is primarily chemotherapy and radiation therapy.

MYCOSIS FUNGOIDES

Mycosis fungoides is a rare T-cell lymphoma that manifests itself in the skin. It begins as eczematous dermatitis and progresses to plaques that coalesce to form very large lesions. Nodular growth develops and then spreads to the viscera. It is an insidiously progressive disease lasting many years. Mycosis fungoides present as large bluish-red raised plaques that are usually quite pruritic (Fig. 10-22). Again the main consideration in the ambulatory patient is recognition and biopsy of the disease. Treatment is topical nitrogen mustard for extensive skin disease or radiation therapy or chemotherapy for systemic disease. The diagnosis should be considered in older patients who present with eczematous dermatitis or a large, red, scaly eruption that is resistant to steroid therapy.

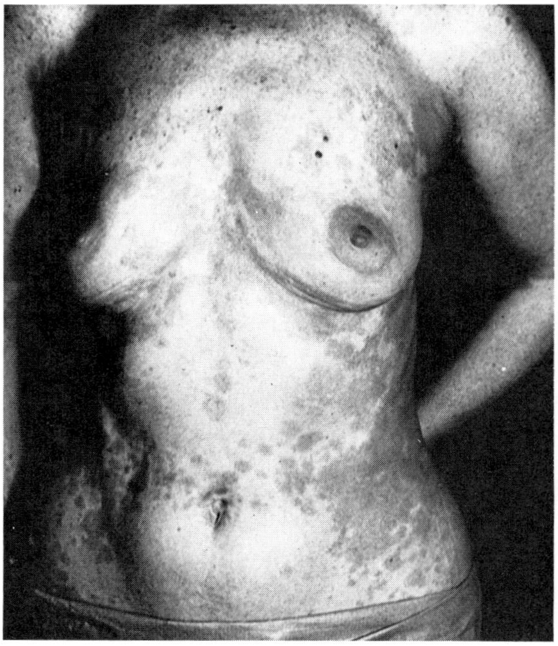

Figure 10-22. Mycosis fungoides.

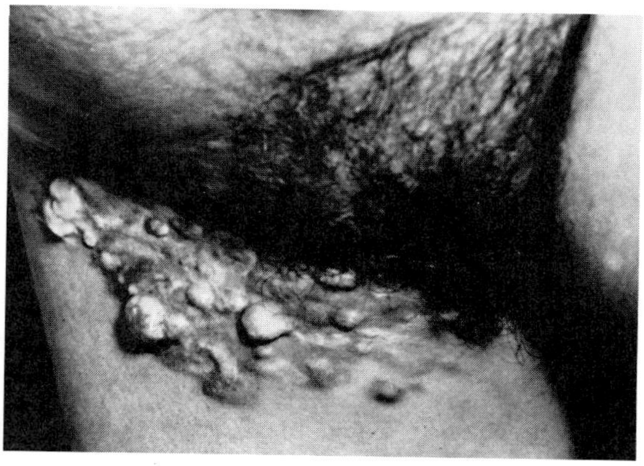

Figure 10-23. Dermatofibrosarcoma protuberans in groin.

DERMATOFIBROSARCOMA PROTUBERANS

Dermatofibrosarcoma protuberans is a sarcomatous tumor resembling a keloid and is made up of fibrous tissue. Many fibroblasts are seen on histologic examination. In the first stage it appears as plaques in the skin. These coalesce to form progressively larger lesions. The growth finally becomes tumorous, with its most striking feature being its protuberant nature (Fig. 10-23). In the initial stage the growth is very slow, but in the tumorous phase the growth can be quite rapid. The protuberant tumors are characteristically dark red, violet, or purple. This skin is sometimes ulcerated with tumor fungating through the ulcerations. This is a tumor that involves primarily the skin but rarely spreads through the subcutaneous tissue to fascia. Only very rare cases of metastases from dermatofibrosarcoma protuberans have been reported. Treatment is wide local excision with a 3-cm to 5-cm margin plus dissection deep to the fascia. Wide excision is necessary to prevent local recurrence, which is a common problem with this disease. Radiation is not an alternative treatment, as these lesions are radioresistant.

SOFT-TISSUE TUMORS

Most soft-tissue masses are benign and unfortunately produce a complacency among physicians and patients. A history of trauma prior to development of a soft-tissue mass can be very misleading. These lesions are frequently diagnosed as organized hematomas, despite persistence and gradual enlargement of the mass. Soft-tissue sarcomas are rarely painful. In evaluating soft-tissue masses, consideration should always be given to the possibility of malignancy. Simple removal or "shelling out" a presumably benign mass that on histologic examination proves to be a sarcoma creates a problem. The margins of the tumor have been obscured and subsequent resection is more difficult and more uncertain. If there is any question about a malignancy in a mass that is greater than 3 cm in diameter, the mass should undergo incisional biopsy as a first step. If it proves to be malignant, definitive therapy can be performed.

BENIGN TUMORS

Lipoma

Lipomas are very common benign lesions consisting of fat tissue contained within a capsule. They usually arise in the subcutaneous space and are quite soft and mobile (Fig. 10-24). Occasionally, these lesions are subfascial, giving them a consistency more like that of a malignant tumor. Lipomas can occur anywhere on the body but are seen most often on the back. Lipomas themselves need to be removed only for cosmetic reasons, but if the clinical diagnosis is in question, the mass should be removed for histologic diagnosis. Excisional biopsy is the treatment of choice. Lipomas may have multiple lobules that usually can be delivered easily with careful dissection. If a large cavity is created by removal of the lesion, the space should be obliterated with sutures or drained with a plastic catheter attached to a closed-drainage suction system. Excised lipomas always should be submitted for histologic examination because they occasionally contain liposarcoma.

Neurofibromas

Neurofibromas are usually freely movable, soft, pedunculated tumors. They may occur as isolated neoplasms or as multiple lesions in von Recklinghausen's disease. In this disease neurofibromas are associated with pigmented *café au lait* spots on the trunk. The lesions in the skin are primarily of fibroblastic origin but usually contain small nerve trunks. These lesions occasionally undergo sarcomatous degeneration. Lesions suspected of malignant transformation because of enlargement or a hard, fixed feeling should be removed for diagnosis. There are also neurofibromas that inter-

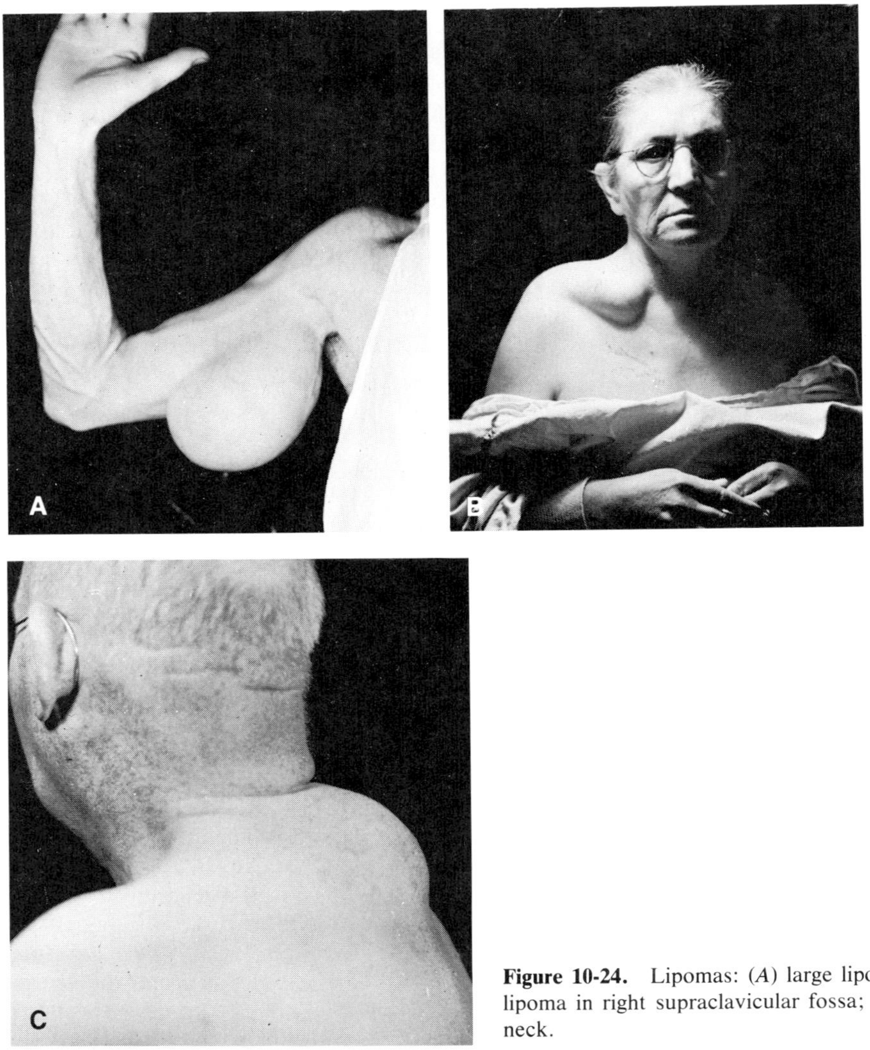

Figure 10-24. Lipomas: (*A*) large lipoma of upper arm; (*B*) lipoma in right supraclavicular fossa; (*C*) lipoma of back of neck.

fere with function and should be excised. Unfortunately, all lesions in von Recklinghausen's disease cannot be removed, since new crops of lesions appear continually throughout the patient's life.

MALIGNANT TUMORS

Sarcomas

Sarcomas are malignant neoplasms of mesenchymal origin and thus may appear in any part of the body. They generally present as painless swellings that often become quite large (Fig. 10-25). There is frequently a delay in diagnosis because the tumors are relatively rare, they are usually painless, and the mass is

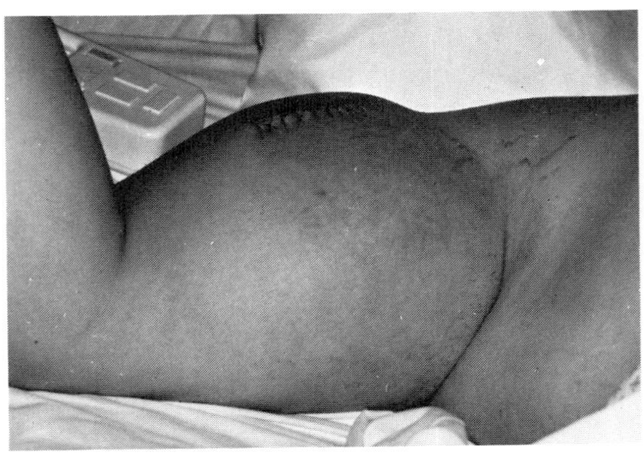

Figure 10-25. Large rhabdomyosarcoma in right biceps muscle. Note incisional biopsy. Swelling of the arm was initially attributed to trauma.

attributed to some other cause. Physical examination is not particularly helpful in distinguishing sarcomas from benign masses. The initial step in management is to obtain a histologic diagnosis. This is best accomplished by open incisional biopsy (unless the mass is very small, <2.5 cm, in which case excisional biopsy of the lesion is acceptable). Needle biopsy may be used, but the small amount of tissue obtained is usually not satisfactory for thorough characterization of the tumor by the pathologist. Histologic classification of these lesions is often difficult.

Definitive treatment of sarcomas is complex and frequently involves multimethod therapy that is beyond the scope of ambulatory management. It is essential that soft-tissue sarcomas be handled properly, since recurrence following inadequate primary therapy carries a much worse prognosis. Soft-tissue sarcomas require extensive resection of the tumor, including wide removal of skin and subcutaneous tissue, origin to insertion resection of involved muscles, and removal of other tissues involved. Amputation may be required to resect the primary tumor adequately. However, investigations have shown that combination therapy, including appropriate anticancer drugs, radiation therapy, and careful surgical dissection, provides adequate control of the primary tumor while allowing the limb to be spared (Morton et al., 1976). The prognosis of soft-tissue sarcomas is related primarily to the histologic grade of malignancy of the tumor (Russell et al., 1977). Higher-grade tumors have a very great propensity to metastasize to the lungs.

Lymphadenopathy

Persistently enlarged lymph nodes should have biopsy, particularly if they are associated with unexplained fever and chills or diffuse lymphadenopathy. Considerations are lymphoma, leukemia, metastatic carcinoma, or acquired immune deficiency disease (AIDS). In the case of lymph nodes in the head and neck region, biopsy should be undertaken only after a thorough search for a primary carcinoma in the head and neck region. In dealing with diffuse lymphadenopathy, the neck and supraclavicular areas are most likely to yield a positive diagnosis. Placement of biopsy incisions should always be with consideration that removal of the incision may be necessary in subsequent radical dissection. Lymph node biopsies can be done very well in the outpatient suite, but a thorough knowledge of the anatomy of the particular nodal region is essential, especially in the neck. The node must be located carefully by palpation prior to making the skin incision, since lymph nodes can be very difficult to find in the subcutaneous tissue, particularly in the axilla. The entire node should be removed and submitted to the pathologist in a fresh state for immediate examination.

MASS IN THE NECK

In the ambulatory surgical patient with a mass in the neck, management is directed toward making a diagnosis. In adults 42% of masses appearing in the lateral area of the neck are malignant; 80% of these malignant tumors are metastatic carcinoma from other sites; 85% of the metastatic lesions are from a primary head and neck carcinoma; the other 15% arise from neoplasms below the clavicle, usually lung, colon, kidney, or gastric carcinoma. Palpable lymph nodes may appear as part of a diffuse process such as lymphoma, leukemia, or AIDS. Benign lymphadenopathy may occur in response to head and neck infections, upper respiratory infections, or allergies. Besides benign lymphadenopathy, other nonmalignant lesions in the neck are cystic hygromas, hemangiomas, lipomas, salivary gland tumors, or neuogenic tumors.

The history and initial examination of masses in the neck are very important. It should be determined whether the mass is localized or is related to a systemic process. The length of time present, the growth characteristics of the mass, and associated complaints such as dysphagia, hoarseness, or a nonhealing ulcer in the mouth are very important. Patients with oropharyngeal carcinoma invariably have a history of smoking and heavy alcohol intake. Rapid growth is suggestive of carcinoma, as in hardness or fixation to other tissues on palpation. Benign lesions tend to be soft and mobile.

Evaluation of the mass should include a thorough head and neck examination with inspection of the skin; palpation for other masses, particularly in the floor of the mouth or tongue; and examination of the mucous membranes about the tongue, floor of the mouth, buccal mucosa, and the pharynx. The examination should include indirect laryngoscopy and visualization of the posterior nasopharynx. Biopsy should be done of any mucosal abnormality. Since lung neoplasms can metastasize to the neck, careful evaluation of the chest is essential. If no primary tumor can be found, it is reasonable to proceed to biopsy of the mass. This procedure should be performed as described for lymph node biopsy. If the lesion is large, incisional biopsy or fine needle aspiration is acceptable.

If on biopsy the neck mass is shown to be metastatic carcinoma and no primary lesion is found, the patient should have triple endoscopy, including direct laryngoscopy with careful examination of the piriform sinus and the base of the tongue as well as the larynx. Bronchoscopy and esophagoscopy should be performed. Random biopsies of the base of the tongue and piriform sinus are indicated if no other lesions are seen. Consideration should be given to obtaining laryngograms, esophagograms, sinus x-rays, and computed tomography scans of the head and neck. See "Sites of Metastases in the Neck as a Guide to the Primary Tumor" for the most common sites of primary tumors metastasizing to particular regions in the neck. Definitive treatment depends on results of the biopsies and associated findings. For therapy of head and neck cancer the reader should review tests by Lore (1973) or Batsakis (1979).

Isolated masses that appear posterior to or overlying the angle of the mandible are very likely to be parotid tumors. These tumors should not have needle biopsy where a core of tissue is obtained (see Needle Biopsy and Fig. 10-14). This procedure increases the likelihood of local recurrence. Biopsy of masses in this area is best performed in the operating room by a surgeon who is capable of performing superficial parotidectomy. However, fine needle aspiration biopsy is acceptable.

Midline masses presenting low in the neck are usually thyroid lesions. If a thyroid nodule is palpated, a thyroid scan should be obtained to determine whether the nodule is functional. If the nodule shows as a hot or functioning lesion, the chance of malignancy is low. Cold nodules are more likely to be malignant. Ultrasound studies can distinguish whether the mass is solid or cystic. Cystic lesions are very unlikely to be carcinoma. Tests of thyroid function should be obtained. Needle biopsy of thyroid masses is considered acceptable and accurate, as is fine needle aspiration biopsy.

In regard to tissue damage or hemorrhage, the technique is safe, and implantation of the needle track with cancer cells does not appear to be a significant problem. However, distribution of disease in the thyroid, particularly neoplasia, is not uniform, so that adequacy of the biopsy specimen is a limitation. Thyroiditis is readily diagnosed by needle biopsy and a positive diagnosis of cancer is reliable. However, there may be difficulty in distinguishing adenoma from well-differentiated cancer, so that a diagnosis of follicular adenoma from needle biopsy, as, for example, in a solitary cold nodule, cannot be accepted. Needle biopsy results must be considered in the context of other findings.

In children, neck masses are usually enlarged lymph nodes, but persistent swellings

SITES OF METASTASES IN THE NECK AS A GUIDE TO THE PRIMARY TUMOR

- Submental area
  - Lip
  - Anterior floor of mouth
  - Buccal walls
- Submaxillary (level I)
  - Floor of mouth
  - Tongue, anterior
  - Submaxillary glands
- Carotid bulb (level II)
  - Soft palate
  - Tonsil and pharyngeal wall
  - Nasopharynx
  - Parotid gland
  - Scalp
  - Base of tongue
  - Piriform sinus
  - Larynx
- Midjugular (level III)
  - Piriform sinus
  - Larynx
  - Thyroid
- Lower jugular (level IV)
  - Larynx
  - Piriform sinus
  - Thyroid
  - Lung
  - Cervical esophagus
- Posterior cervical triangle (level V)
  - Thyroid
  - Scalp
  - Breast
  - Nasopharynx

should have biopsy. Common neck masses in children (also diagnosed in adults) are branchial cleft cysts, thyroglossal duct cysts, and cystic hygromas. Branchial cleft cysts appear early in life and often present with a sinus tract, lateral in the neck, that connects with the oropharynx. Treatment is complete excision. Thyroglossal duct cysts present in the midline of the neck and are a remnant of the thyroglossal duct running from the thyroid gland to the base of the tongue. These cysts plus the duct are excised. Cystic hygromas are a form of lymphangioma. Most cystic hygromas present in the neck posterior to the sternocleidomastoid. There are no distinct borders between the lesion and normal tissue. Complete removal of cystic hygromas usually requires multiple partial excisions. Branchial cleft cysts, thyroglossal duct cysts, and cystic hygromas are best treated in the operating room.

BIBLIOGRAPHY

Cancer Management

DeVita VT, Hellman S, Rosenberg SA (eds): Cancer: Principles and Practices of Oncology, 2nd ed. Philadelphia, JB Lippincott, 1985

Haskell CM: Cancer Treatment. Philadelphia, WB Saunders, 1985

Holland JF, Frei E: Cancer Medicine. Philadelphia, Lea and Febiger, 1982

Biopsy

Barrows GH, Anderson TJ, Lamb JL, Dixon JM: Fine needle aspiration of breast cancer. Cancer 58:1493–1498, 1986

Christopherson WM: Cytologic detection and diagnosis of cancer. Cancer 51:1201–1208, 1983

Coulson WF: Surgical Pathology. Philadelphia, JB Lippincott, 1978

DeVita VT: Adjuvant therapy—an overview. In Salmon SE, Jones SE (eds): Adjuvant Therapy of Cancer, pp 613–641. Amsterdam, North Holland Press, 1977

Roberts SS, Hangesh JW, McGrath RG, Valaitis J, McGraw EA, Cole WH: Prognostic significance of cancer cells in circulating blood: A ten year evaluation. Am J Surg 113:757, 1967

Cysts and Benign Tumors of Skin

Brown SH, Neerhout RC, Fonkalsrud EW: Prednisone therapy in management of large hemangiomas in infants and children. Surgery 71:168, 1972

Edgerton MT: The treatment of hemangiomas: With special reference to the role of steroid therapy. Ann Surg 183:517–532, 1976

Ketchum LD: Hypertrophic scars and keloids. Clin Plast Surg 4:301–310, 1977

Margileth AM, Museles M: Current concepts in diagnosis and management of congenital cutaneous hemangiomas. Pediatrics 36:410, 1965

Moschella SL, Hurley HJ: Dermatology. Philadelphia, WB Saunders, 1985

Strahan J, Bailie HWC: Glomus tumor: A review of 15 clinical cases. Br J Surg 59:91, 1972

Zarem HA, Edgerton MT: Induced resolution of cavernous hemangiomas following prednisone therapy. J Plast Reconstr Surg 39:76–83, 1967

Pigmented Nevi and Malignant Melanomas

Balch CM, Milton GW: Cutaneous Melanoma. Philadelphia, JB Lippincott, 1985

Breslow A: Thickness, cross-sectional areas and depth of invasion in the prognosis of cutaneous melanoma. Ann Surg 172:902, 1970

Clark WH, From L, Bernardino EA, Mihm MC: The histogenesis and biologic behavior of primary human malignant melanomas of the skin. Cancer Res 29:705, 1969

Eilber FR, Holmes EC, Morton DL: Malignant melanoma. In Grabb WC, Smith JW (eds): Plastic Surgery—A Concise Guide to Clinical Practice, pp 511–517. Boston, Little, Brown & Co, 1979

Gumport SL, Harris MN: Melanoma of the skin. In Andrade R, Gumport SL, Popkin GL, Rees TD (eds): Cancer of the Skin: Biopsy, Diagnosis, Management, pp 950–973. Philadelphia, WB Saunders, 1985

Mastrangelo MJ, Baker AR, Katz HR: Cutaneous melanoma. In DeVita VT, Hellman SG, Rosenberg SA (eds): Cancer: Principles and Practice of Oncology, 2nd ed, pp 1371–1422. Philadelphia, JB Lippincott, 1985

Mihm MC, Fitzpatrick TB, Lane Brown MM, Raker JW, Malt RA, Kaiser JS: Early detection of primary cutaneous malignant melanoma: A color atlas. N Engl J Med 289:989–996, 1973

Siegler HF, Fetter BF: Current management of melanoma. Ann Surg 186:1–12, 1977

Malignant Skin Tumors

Andrade R, Gumport SL, Popkin GL, Rees TD: Cancer of the Skin: Biopsy, Diagnoses, Management. Philadelphia, WB Saunders, 1983

Blattner WA, Harvey RN: Cancer in the immunosuppressed host. In DeVita VT, Hellman S, Rosenberg SA (eds): Cancer: Principles and Practice of Oncology, 2nd ed, pp 1999–2006. Philadelphia, JB Lippincott, 1985

Cotran RS: Metastasizing basal cell carcinomas. Cancer 14:1036, 1961

DeVita VT, Jaffe ES, Hellman S: Cutaneous T-cell lymphomas. In DeVita VT, Hellman S, Rosenberg SA (eds): Cancer: Principles and Practice of Oncology, 2nd ed, pp 1670–1691. Philadelphia, JB Lippincott, 1985

Gelman EP, Broder S: Kaposi's sarcoma in the setting of the AIDS pandemic. In Broder S (ed): AIDS: Modern Concepts and Therapeutic Challenges, pp 219–232. New York, Marcel Dekker, 1987

Klein E: Tumors of the skin—immunotherapy of cutaneous and mucosal neoplasms. NY State J Med 68:900–911, 1968

Levis WR, Kraemer KH, Klinger WG, Peck GL, Terry WD: Topical immunotherapy of basal cell carcinomas with dinitrochlorobenzene. Cancer Res 33:3036–3042, 1973

Soft-Tissue Tumors

Brasfield RD, Das Gupta TK: Von Recklinghausen's disease: A clinicopathological study. Ann Surg 175:186, 1972

Eilber FR, Morton DL: Soft tissue sarcomas. In Nora PF (ed): Operative Surgery: Principles and Techniques, 2nd ed. Philadelphia, Lea & Febiger, 1979

Morton DL, Eilber FR, Townsend CM, Grant T, Mirra J, Weisenburger TH: Limb salvage from a multidisciplinary treatment of approach for skeletal and soft tissue sarcomas of the extremity. Ann Surg 184:268–278, 1976

Rosenberg SA, Suit HD, Baker LH: Sarcomas of soft tissue. In DeVita VT, Hellman S, Rosenberg SA (eds): Cancer: Principles and Practice of Oncology, 2nd ed, pp 1243–1291. Philadelphia, JB Lippincott, 1985.

Russell WO, Cohen J, Enziger F, Hajdu SI, Heise H, Martin RG, Meissner W, Miller WT, Schmitz RL, Suit HD: A clinical and pathological staging system for soft tissue sarcomas. Cancer 40:1562–1570, 1977

Mass in the Neck

Batasakis J: Tumors of the Head and Neck, 2nd ed. Baltimore, Williams & Wilkins, 1979

Conley J: The "lump in the neck" and radical neck dissection. In Nealon TF (ed): Management of the Patient with Cancer, pp 239–246. Philadelphia, WB Saunders, 1976

Lore JM Jr.: An Atlas of Head and Neck Surgery. Philadelphia, WB Saunders, 1973

Wang C, Vickery AL, Maloof F: Needle biopsy of the thyroid. Surg Gynecol Obstet 143:365–368, 1976

11 Cryosurgery

ANDREW A. GAGE

Cryosurgery is a method of producing tissue necrosis by freezing in situ. It is an excellent method for the destruction of diverse lesions, and the feasibility of use with local anesthesia makes the technique suitable for ambulatory surgery. Cryosurgery is most useful for lesions in those areas of the body that are easily accessible to treatment, either by unaided visualization or by endoscopy. In certain circumstances the advantages of cryosurgery exceed those of surgical excision, electrocoagulation, and other methods of local tissue destruction. Its special suitability for high-surgical-risk patients, including the blood coagulopathies, is noteworthy. Though useful for selected clinical problems difficult to manage by other methods of treatment, the cryosurgical techniques are more often used for the treatment of common relatively minor conditions or lesions. This chapter emphasizes applications for patients whose disease may be treated under local anesthesia in the office or outpatient clinic.

CRYOSURGICAL APPARATUS

Development of the several types of cryosurgical instruments using various cryogenic agents has been in response to the differing needs of physicians in various specialities. The surgeon has a choice of apparatus varying from the simple hand-held devices suitable for skin lesions to the sophisticated automated apparatus required for neurologic surgery. The cryogenic agents, gases in the normal state, commonly used with the apparatus are nitrogen, carbon dioxide, Freon, and nitrous oxide, all of which are nonexplosive. Liquid nitrogen is readily obtainable, easy to handle, and nontoxic and has a boiling point of about −196°C at atmospheric pressure. Its low temperature makes extensive freezing possible and makes it the most suitable of the cryogenic agents for destruction of large volumes of tissue. The other cryogens have wide usefulness when lesser degrees of freezing will suffice. With solidified carbon dioxide the lowest attainable temperature is −78.5°C. Freon-22 has a boiling point of −40.8°C but can achieve about −70°C. Liquid nitrous oxide has a temperature of −89.5°C. Nitrous oxide and liquid nitrogen are the dominant freezing agents in cryosurgery.

Nitrous oxide, easily available in the familiar E cylinders, has attractive features for cryosurgery. Its characteristics permit construction of mobile lightweight apparatus with rapid response time in the freezing and thawing cycles in comparison to some apparatus using liquid nitrogen. Nitrous oxide is commonly used in probe systems, which are cooled by the Joule–Thomson principle (expansion of a compressed gas passed through a small orifice). The probes are thin, lightweight, and suitable for endoscopic use (Fig. 11-1). All have a mechanism for heating the probe for quick release from the tissue.

Liquid nitrogen apparatus cools by a change in phase (liquid to gas) of the cryogen. The types of apparatus range widely in expense and sophistication (Fig. 11-2). Most types can be used either as closed systems, so that the liquid nitrogen is not released on the tissue, or as open systems, which spray liquid nitrogen onto the lesion. In closed systems, freezing is done with probes that are applied to the tissue. Liquid nitrogen circulates through the probe tip, conductance of heat from the tissues causes change of phase, and the gas is vented in a convenient way. Automated units have controls on the console to make possible accurate control of the temperature of the probe tip, and after termination of freezing, a heater in the probe near its tip speeds its release from the tissues. Quick release from the tissue makes this type of unit more suitable for freezing via endoscopy than is the apparatus with-

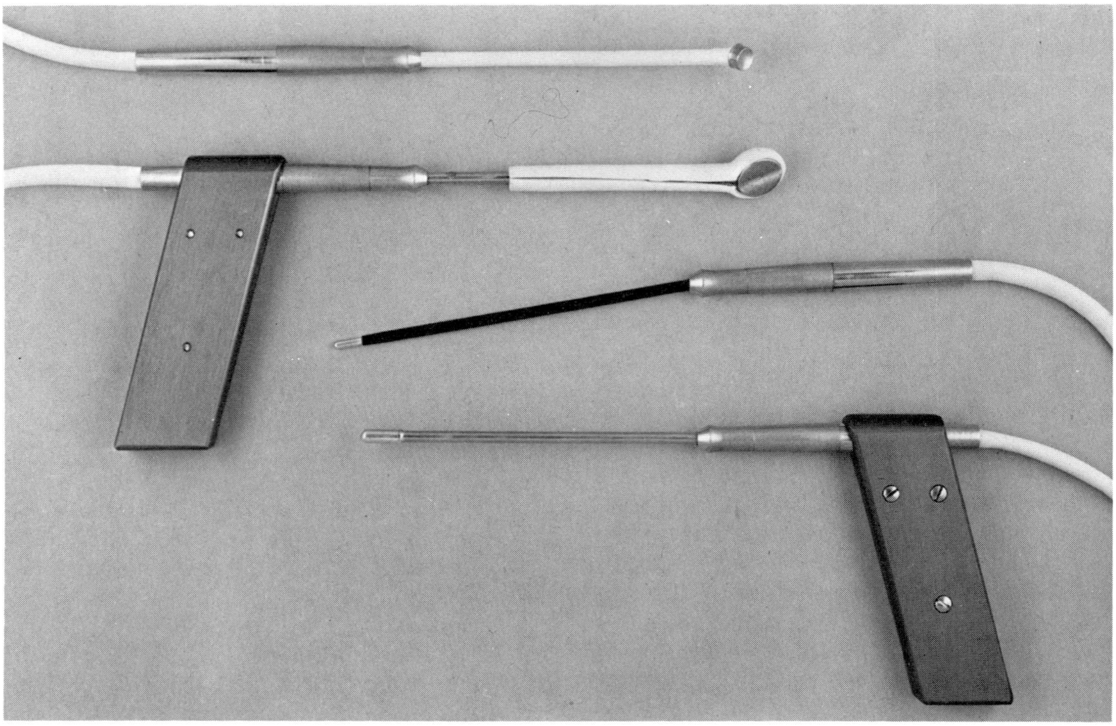

Figure 11-1. Cryosurgical probes, cooled by nitrous oxide. The top one may be used for proctologic work. The second from the top may be used for tonsillectomy. The lower probes have general usefulness and are suitable for endoscopic uses. Various other probes (not shown) are available for specialty uses.

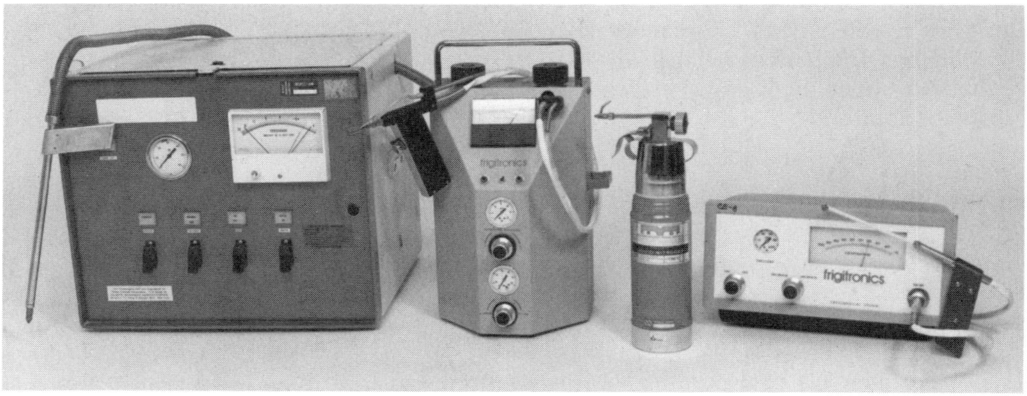

Figure 11-2. Four models of cryosurgical apparatus. On the right is a nitrous oxide unit. The E cylinder containing nitrous oxide is not shown. A probe suitable for intraoral or hemorrhoidal freezing is attached.

The other three are liquid nitrogen units. The smallest is a hand-held apparatus, weighing about 1 kg when empty, which is basically of vacuum bottle construction with limited cryogen storage capacity. It is commonly used as a spray device but may be fitted with probes.

Next to the hand-held unit is a large portable apparatus with a flexible feed line leading to a lightweight handle constructed to accept spray or probe devices, so it may be used with a variety of spray nozzles, spray cones, or closed-end probes.

On the left is automated apparatus that almost always is used with probe techniques. The feed lines are vacuum insulated. The temperature of the probe can be precisely controlled down to −180°C. A heater in the probe tip speeds release from the tissue at the conclusion of freezing. The large probe shown with the apparatus is used for general cancer cryosurgery. The apparatus, used with thinner probe, is suitable for freezing tissue via endoscopy.

out a heater. Except in neurologic surgery, control of probe temperature is not necessary; for most applications, the probe is always used at the coldest temperature. On the other hand, the heater is advantageous in many clinical applications.

The choice of equipment depends on the nature of the lesion being treated. Inflammatory lesions can be treated satisfactorily with nitrous oxide apparatus. Small benign tumors or epithelial dysplasia may be treated with nitrous oxide also. However, invasive cancer of any degree, large benign tumors, or large masses of tissue in general require the greater freezing capability of liquid nitrogen units.

TECHNIQUE

In general, the basic objective of cryosurgery is to freeze tissue in situ, without excision, thus avoiding hemorrhage. The devitalized tissue is slowly absorbed or sloughs. Healing of the wound follows. Careful application of technique is essential to be sure that the desired result is obtained.

Since the goal of cryosurgery is the production of a predictable volume of tissue necrosis, it is important to use techniques that will achieve maximal lethal effect. The important points in technique may be summarized as follows: (1) use a cryogen suitable for the lesion; (2) maintain good tissue–cryogen contact; (3) use equipment as cold as possible; (4) freeze as quickly as possible; (5) thaw slowly and unassisted; (6) overlap frozen areas (if the lesion is too large to be frozen from a single site); (7) repeat freezing after thawing; (8) include a margin of normal tissue.

Special features of technique necessarily vary in different parts of the body and with different types of lesions. The treatment of malignant tumors must be more aggressive than the treatment of benign disease. On the other hand, inflammatory disease requires only single freezing–thawing cycles. Treatment also varies according to the apparatus chosen and possibly with the adjunctive use of other methods of treatment.

The two basic techniques are (1) freezing in closed systems with probes so that the cryogen does not directly contact the tissue and (2) freezing in open systems by direct application of the cryogen as with a spray (Fig. 11-3).

FREEZING WITH CRYOPROBES

For freezing in a closed system a cryoprobe is chosen that is suitable for the size and location of the lesion. The end of the probe (at a temperature above freezing) is pressed firmly on the lesion. If contact is poor, as might be the case if the abnormal tissue is dry, is irregular, or overlies bone, a small amount of water-soluble hospital lubricating jelly is placed on the tissue to improve contact with the probe. Soft bulky tumors may be penetrated by the cryoprobe to obtain greater contact with the tissue and to produce more extensive freezing. Usually, however, surface-contact freezing is preferable because no wound is produced, the chance of bleeding is lessened, the tissue planes are not disrupted, and the chance of dissemination of tumor cells is minimized.

When freezing begins the probe becomes fixed to the tissue and cannot be moved. Removal of heat from the tissues largely depends on the temperature of the cryoprobe, the area and quality of contact between the cryoprobe and the tissue, and the duration of freezing. The probe is always used as cold as possible because a large probe–tissue temperature gradient is a prime factor in achieving a rapid cooling rate and producing extensive freezing. The larger the gradient, the more rapid the enlargement of the frozen area. Seemingly identical cooling conditions may yield variation in tissue freezing unless careful attention is given to heat exchange. Good contact between the probe and the tissue is critical. When freezing begins, the probe must be held motionless, because even slight movement of the probe can cause fracture in the bond between the tissue and the probe and interfere with heat exchange, the result being deficient freezing.

The extent of freezing is judged by inspection and palpation as the frozen tissues turn white and hard (Fig. 11-4). Freezing is allowed to continue until the frozen area encompasses the entire lesion and a reasonable amount of surrounding normal tissue. During probe contact the rate of expansion of the frozen area slows as equilibrium is established between heat brought to the area by the circulation and heat loss to the cryoprobe. Most small lesions (1 cm to 2 cm) can be frozen adequately in 1 to 3 minutes. Larger lesions may require longer tissue cooling time. Usually after 7 to 8 minutes, freezing no longer progresses, so the

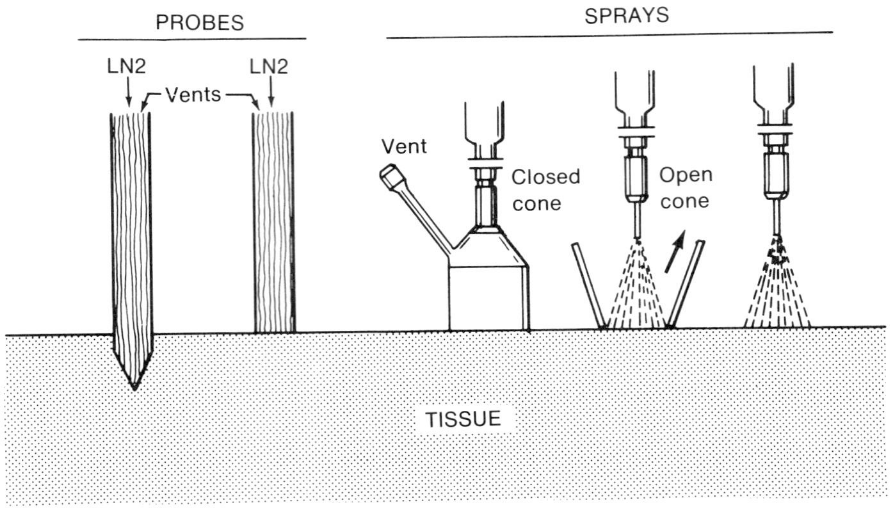

Figure 11-3. Diagrammatic representation of differences and similarities in the several probe and spray techniques in liquid nitrogen apparatus. The two probes shown on the left are closed systems in which the cryogen does not come into direct contact with the tissues. In the closed systems the liquid nitrogen, after change of phase, is vented as a gas somewhere along the return line, usually in the console of the apparatus. Surface freezing techniques (by pressing a probe against the tissue) are commonly used. However, the pointed probe may be inserted into the tissue to achieve deeper freezing. This penetration of the tissue causes a wound, which may cause problems with bleeding or infection.

In the open systems, the three devices on the right, the liquid nitrogen is sprayed directly on the tissues. The open spray technique is effective in treating wide areas with irregular outline, but care must be taken to avoid dispersion of the spray in unwanted areas. In the cone techniques the dispersion of the spray is limited. The effect of confining the spray is to produce an open probe. With the cones the heat exchange surface is on the skin and the venting of the gas is at the side or top of the device.

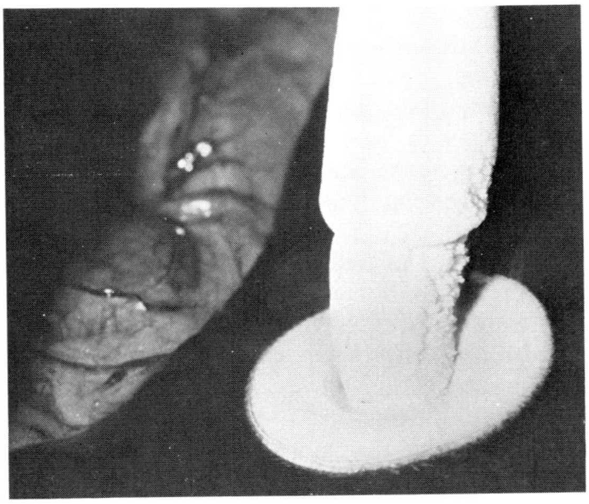

Figure 11-4. Canine liver being frozen with a large probe cooled with liquid nitrogen to −160°C. The white frosted area is the frozen tissue after 3 minutes of contact. The depth is about the same as the spread of frost from the side of the probe. With proper technique the area of necrosis will correspond closely to the visibly frozen area.

probe is thawed for removal. Lesions too large to be frozen in a single application of the probe are treated by immediate successive applications overlapping the frozen zones. When repetitive freezing is required, as is always true for treatment of tumors, the tissue is allowed to thaw, and in a few minutes, when the frosted appearance has passed, the entire area is frozen again. Successive applications to the same site slightly widen the frozen area but increase depth of freezing only little. Treatment is completed when the volume of tissue frozen and refrozen is equivalent to that excised in conservative local excision.

The duration of freezing time on each application varies and cannot be prescribed beforehand because of the many variable factors involved in treatment. Before clinical use the physicians should have some knowledge of the freezing capability of each probe by trials with test materials, such as gelatin or meat, in order to determine the size of the frozen area resulting in any chosen duration of the freezing cycle. With surface contact freezing, the shape of the frozen area is roughly hemispheric, the depth of the freezing being about the same as the lateral spread of the freezing from the side of the probe. Heat sources, such as the proximity of major blood vessels, and the shape of the probe modify the volume and shape of the frozen area (Fig. 11-5).

LIQUID NITROGEN USED AS A SPRAY

Liquid nitrogen is used as a spray far more commonly than other cryogens. In this technique a spray of liquid nitrogen, produced by flow through small apertures in nozzles or needles at the end of a feedline, is directed on the lesion and causes freezing. When a cryogen is used as a spray, it is being used at its coldest possible temperature, and it can be moved about so that freezing is extensive and wide rather than deep. If the spray is directed only at a small area, then deep freezing may be achieved as well. The disadvantage of the spray is that as the tissue freezes, vaporization is slowed and liquid nitrogen may run off the frozen tissue and produce tissue injury where it is not wanted. Therefore the spray is more difficult to control than the closed system. Runoff may be prevented and at the same time freezing may be limited to a small area by using open cylinders and cones to confine the spray. Another disadvantage is gas insufflation of tissues, which can be avoided if care is taken not to use excessive spray pressure on open wounds.

Whether to use liquid nitrogen as a spray or in a cryoprobe depends on the lesion and its location. Probes offer the advantage of more accurate control of freezing, and their use therefore results in a more predictable area of necrosis. Tissue compression by the probe increases the depth of freezing. Probe techniques are especially well chosen for the oral cavity or pharynx and are absolutely necessary to freezing through endoscopes. Probes can be used on any skin lesion and can be used to penetrate tumors for freezing. In general, freezing with probes has a wider range of usefulness than does the use of spray devices. The use of liquid nitrogen as spray is best for accessible lesions, such as those in the skin, hence its popularity with dermatologists. Spray techniques are well suited to the treatment of irregular surfaces and are best used to produce superficial freezing, which may be over wide areas. Sometimes the spray technique is well suited to the extensive freezing required for bulky external cancers, perhaps in combination with partial removal by electrocoagulation.

USE OF THERMOCOUPLES

Many cryosurgical procedures, especially those for inflammatory disease, are performed using only observation and palpation to determine the progress of treatment and judge its adequacy. Physicians with considerable experience in cryosurgery can achieve satisfactory results without the use of monitoring techniques to guide therapy, even in the treatment of cancer. Nevertheless, clinical judgment is subject to error, especially since the temperature of frozen tissue cannot be determined by its appearance, and depth of freezing is some-

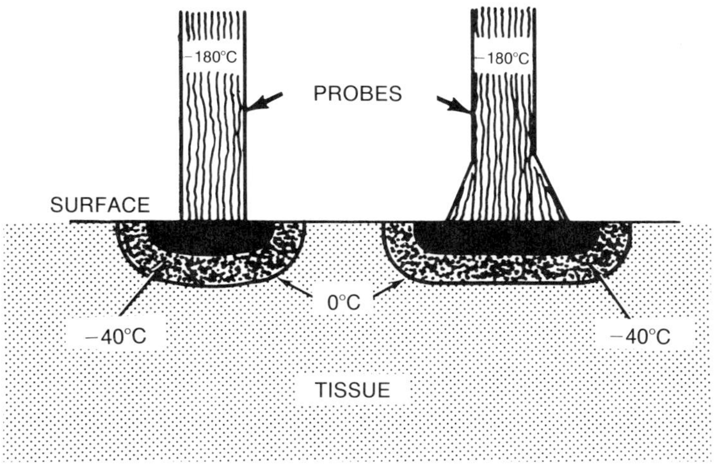

Figure 11-5. The volume and shape of the frozen area can be modified by using probe freezing surfaces of different shapes. A broader area of contact, as shown on the right, produces a wider area of freezing, but with little or no change in depth. Change in probe shape may be achieved easily by adding a metal adapter to the end of the probe. In each frozen zone, the −40°C isotherm is shown to delineate its approximate location. The location of this isotherm varies slightly with the rate of cooling the tissue. Rapid cooling moves the isotherm slightly more toward the periphery.

times difficult to evaluate. The best way to supplement clinical judgment is the use of thermocouples to measure tissue temperature during the cryosurgical procedure. The use of thermocouples to monitor cryosurgery always requires a longer freezing time than the use of clinical judgment alone. Their use is more important early in experience with cryosurgery. Later, after becoming familiar with the technique, many physicians omit their use, especially in the treatment of inflammatory disease or of small skin lesions.

In the treatment of cancer, the use of thermocouples to measure tissue temperature is of prime importance because it is important to know that destructive temperatures are produced in the tissues. In the freezing–thawing cycles tissue destruction is a multifaceted process involving the freezing rate, the tissue temperature, the duration of freezing, the thawing rate, and repetition of the freezing–thawing cycle. Separation of the relative destructive effects of these components is difficult, but the easiest to control and measure is the coldest temperature attained in the tissue during the cryosurgical treatment.

Thermocouples (copper constantan) are used to assess the progress of treatment by determining the tissue temperature during freezing. They are inserted at the periphery of the lesion to monitor tissue temperature changes that are read off the dial of a pyrometer or written on a recorder. This provides evidence that lethal temperatures are reached. They also offer protection against undesired destruction of normal tissue at the periphery of the lesion. A thermocouple measures the temperature only where it is located. The physician must use the evidence from one or more thermocouples to help visualize a thermal profile throughout the entire frozen area (Fig. 11-6).

Extreme gradients in temperature develop in the frozen area during cryosurgical treatment. The tissues adjacent to the probe cool rapidly, but the rate of freezing decreases with increasing distance from the probe. The coldest temperatures and the most extensive freezing damage occur close to the site of the probe–tissue contact. Remote from the probe, freezing is slower, tissue temperatures are higher, and the probability of cell survival increases. The temperature at the border of the frozen zone is about 0°C, and here cell survival is possible.

The important temperature measurements are at the periphery of the lesion. Extensive tissue damage occurs at −30°C produced in single short freezing–thawing cycles, which are often satisfactory for inflammatory or nonneoplastic disease but they are not sufficient for malignant disease. Repetitive freezing substantially increases the extent of destruction. Small skin cancers are cured by freezing to −25°C to −30°C in repetitive freezing cycles. However, more aggressive cancers require temperatures at least as cold as −50°C in all the tumor area. In cancer therapy it is best to produce temperatures of −40°C in the apparently normal tissue adjacent to the tumor. This provides a margin of safety. It is difficult to freeze too much in the treatment of cancer.

OTHER MONITORING TECHNIQUES

Other techniques of monitoring the freezing process have had clinical trial in recent years. None have achieved wide usefulness. These include:

- The measurement of electrical impedance or resistance in tissue
- The measurement of heat lost from the tissue by a heat flowmeter
- Ultrasound
- Computerized tomography
- Thermography

Impedance–resistance measurements are based on electrical changes in the tissue during freezing. Unfrozen tissue is a conductor of electricity because of the electrolyte content of the tissue fluid. During freezing the formation of ice crystals in tissue and removal of water from the tissue result in decreased electrical conductivity. When practically all the extracellular water is crystallized, electrical impedance or resistance rises to the high levels. This change is interpreted as being associated with death. The technique requires the insertion of needle electrodes in or about the diseased tissue and the measurement of the impedance or resistance changes to the passage of a small electric current (10 Å or less) between the electrodes. A rise in impedance to the megohm level signals complete crystallization of water and tissue death. At this time, devices to measure tissue impedance–resistance during cryosurgical procedures are still in clinical investigation status. The devices

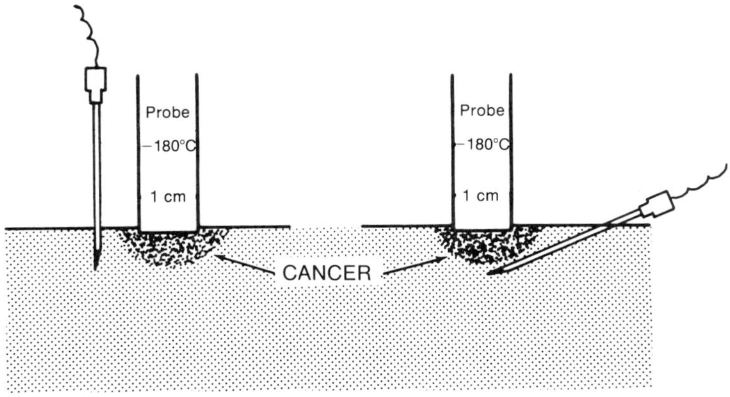

Figure 11-6. Typical sites of thermocouple insertion. Two useful methods of thermocouple insertion are shown. Either yields satisfactory results when performed by an experienced practitioner. On the right is shown a thermocouple inserted at an angle from the side of the lesion through normal tissue. The thermocouple tip rests directly beneath the tumor at a depth of 5 mm. This thermocouple confirms the temperature at the depth of the tissue in the center of the lesion. It probably is the most common method of thermocouple usage in skin cancer.

On the left is shown an alternative method of thermocouple usage. The thermocouple is inserted at the border of the tumor, 5 mm from the border and 3 mm deep. With this technique the temperature registered at this thermocouple is interpreted as being the same temperature at the depth of the tissue beneath the tumor. This method assumes that the depth of freezing is approximately the same as the lateral spread of freezing from the probe. The advantage of this technique is that the thermocouple remains outside of the frozen area until the advancing ice front incorporates it. This technique is relatively free of the error of conduction, which occurs with improper thermocouple usage. More than one thermocouple may be used and the two depicted techniques may be used jointly.

may prove especially useful in the determination of depth of freezing.

The remaining techniques have limited clinical usefulness. The heat flowmeter uses a differential thermocouple and measures total heat exchange into a probe. Ultrasound shows the frozen area as a hyperechoic border in front of a region of low reflectivity. Computerized tomography can be used because water, which is the major component of most biologic tissues, changes density on freezing and can be visualized to show the tissue lesion due to freezing. Thermography defines the isotherms in a frozen area. These techniques have only research application at this time.

EFFECT OF FREEZING ON TISSUE

Freezing kills cells. The lethal effects are due to cellular changes such as crystallization of water, toxic concentration of electrolytes within the cells, and irreversible damage to cell membranes. Cell injury is enhanced by the effect of freezing on the circulation. After freezing and thawing, the treated area becomes congested, and circulation through small vessels stagnates in less than 30 minutes. Loss of circulation deprives all cells of any possibility of survival.

The cryogenic lesion is characterized by a sharply circumscribed area of necrosis (Fig. 11-7). Although tissue death has occurred, a few days must pass before the extent of necrosis is evident. In the skin an eschar forms. In the oral cavity and the rectum, necrotic tissue appears more quickly, and an eschar does not form; instead the tissue sloughs. The time required for slough of necrotic tissue depends in part on its composition. Tissues rich in collagen, such as skin, resist structural change, and complete separation of necrotic tissue re-

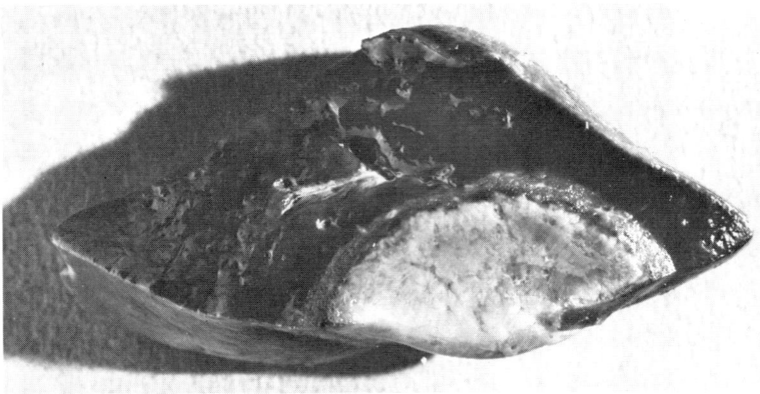

Figure 11-7. Canine liver frozen 10 days previously shows the typical cryogenic lesion. There is a sharply circumscribed, roughly hemispheric necrotic area. The necrotic tissue will slough or be absorbed.

quires many days. On the other hand, cellular tissue sloughs quickly.

Cells vary in their sensitivity to freezing. Melanocytes, skin glands, muscle, and osteocytes die with minor freezing injury. Nerves regenerate readily if their continuity was not interrupted. Small blood vessels become occluded as a result of endothelial damage and thrombosis. Major blood vessels resist freezing injury. The major change in arteries is hyperplasia of the intima of the blood vessel, which in small vessels leads to occlusion but in larger vessels only narrows the lumen until final healing occurs.

Healing of the cryogenic wound has often been judged favorable, that is, healing occurs with minimal scarring. In the skin the preservation of collagen structure during freezing and thawing is partially responsible for the minimal scarring evident after complete healing. In experiments contraction is less in wounds produced by freezing than in wounds produced by burning. Nevertheless, if the full thickness of the skin is lost, some scarring is inevitable.

Bone devitalized in situ by freezing is slowly resorbed and simultaneously replaced by new bone, a process of repair that requires many months. In the meantime the devitalized bone continues to maintain form and function during the healing stage. This favorable response permits extensive freezing of the mandible and the maxilla in the treatment of oral tumors and permits extensive freezing of rodent ulcers and other cancers overlying bone, invading its foramina, or eroding its structure.

DISEASES OF THE SKIN

The wide use of cryosurgery in dermatologic practice attests to its value in diseases of the skin, including cancers. A large number of benign lesions of the skin are suitable for cryosurgery. Verrucous and keratotic lesions, keloids, tattoos, hemangiomas, and a variety of benign tumors and inflammatory lesions of the skin are successfully treated. Freezing with nitrous oxide is satisfactory only for minor nonneoplastic lesions because the cryogen is not effective at a depth of more than 3 mm. The same is true of liquid nitrogen applied intermittently with a cotton swab. Deeper freezing requires use of apparatus cooled by liquid nitrogen. For nonneoplastic lesions, usually no anesthesia is necessary and no thermocouples are used. Treatment is given in a single cycle so that tissue destruction is no more than necessary. It is best to be conservative in nonneoplastic disease; treatment can be repeated if necessary.

SKIN CANCER

Skin cancers are satisfactorily treated by surgical excision, curettage, electrocoagulation, and radiotherapy as well as other special techniques. Cryosurgery successfully competes with these alternate methods of treatment. Almost all skin cancers are suitable for treatment by freezing (Fig. 11-8). The histologic type of the cancer is not important because there is no meaningful difference in sensitivity of squamous cell and basal cell carcinoma to freezing injury. Melanomas are also easily destroyed by freezing, but primary melanomas are best treated by excision, which offers histologic evidence of the adequacy of treatment.

Cryosurgery should be preferentially considered for certain skin cancers. These are the following: (1) multiple skin cancers; (2) cancer arising in irradiated skin; (3) cancer located over bone, so that periosteal lymphatics may

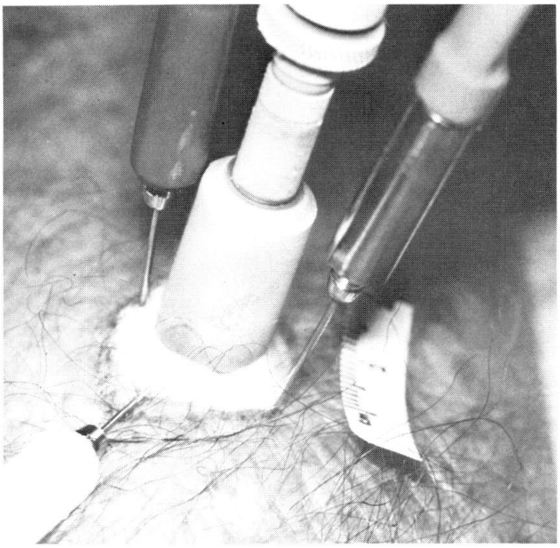

Figure 11-8. Small skin cancer (squamous cell carcinoma) on forearm is being frozen with liquid nitrogen apparatus. Visible is a skin marking 5 mm outside of the edge of the tumor. Two thermocouples are shown in this marking on opposite sides of the cancer. Freezing will be continued until these thermocouples register −40°C. The third thermocouple is placed between the probe and the tissue and is not essential to the technique; it is useful for detecting lack of progress of freezing at the earliest possible time.

be invaded or the underlying bone may be eroded; (4) cancer located about the ear, the eye, or the nose; (5) large cancers in areas difficult to excise and close primarily; and (6) cancer that persists after radiotherapy or excision.

Multiple small skin cancers are ideal for cryosurgery because many lesions can be treated at the same visit more quickly than by excision. Cancers arising in irradiated skin often are not large but are located in areas about the face, where tissue loss is costly from a cosmetic viewpoint. Freezing permits conservative treatment, with minimal tissue sacrifice in achieving cure (Fig. 11-9). If treatment is inadequate the first time, it can be repeated as often as necessary to eliminate the tumor. This is also true of cancers located about the ear, eye, or nose.

More difficult problems in treatment are presented by infiltrating carcinomas that have resisted other forms of treatment and that involve deep structures about the nose, eye, or ear. Such patients may be given palliative treatment on an ambulatory basis, but attempts at cure require hospitalization for general anesthesia. Some cancers that persist after surgical excision or radiotherapy that involve areas about the face, or neglected extensive cancers of the external ear, may be successfully treated by cryosurgery. Facial nerve paralysis commonly occurs after freezing of lesions in the ear canal, but function usually returns in several months if nerve continuity has not been interrupted. This surprisingly rapid return of function is an indication that cryosurgery may be the best method of treatment in certain situations in which there is risk of undesired major neurologic damage from conventional surgical excision.

In general, the cryosurgical method for the treatment of large tumors is to freeze as much

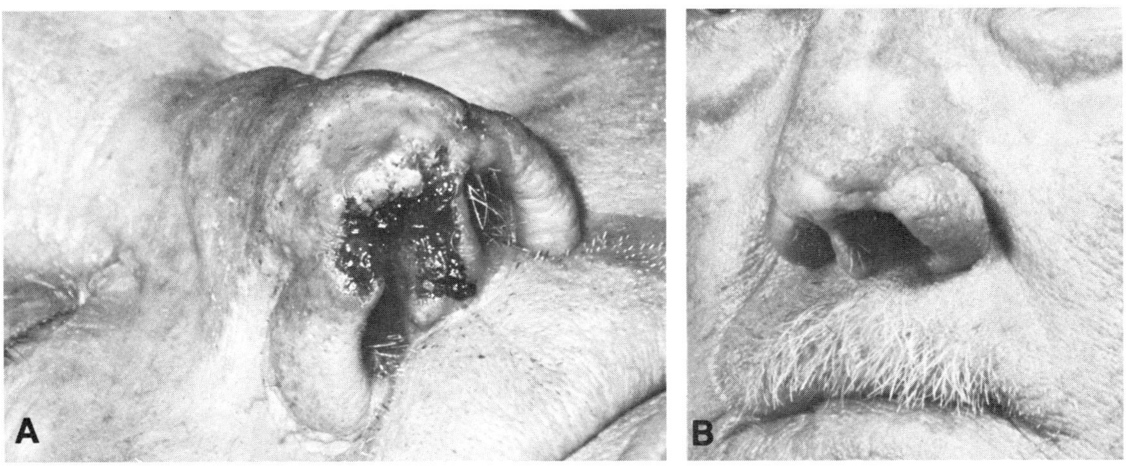

Figure 11-9. (*A*) Squamous cell carcinoma of the ala nasi and nasal septum occurring in skin severely damaged by radiotherapy for skin disease many years earlier. Scars of previous excision of skin cancers are seen. (*B*) A year after cryosurgery the cosmetic effect of treatment is excellent. There is no evidence of disease.

as possible, wait for the necrotic tissue to slough, then obtain biopsy of suspicious areas of the wound to guide repetition of cryosurgery. The wound should be left open to permit detection of persistent cancer at the earliest possible moment. Sometimes it is advantageous to partially excise or remove the bulk of tumor before freezing in order to expedite the treatment, but this debulking sometimes negates the advantages of cryosurgery from the point of view of ambulatory surgery.

Cryosurgery is also useful for palliation in advanced primary or metastatic cancer of the skin, especially bulky protuberant carcinomas, anywhere on the body. Tumor size is easily reduced. Discomfort or pain is relieved, and hemorrhage is prevented. However, only in unusual circumstances can these benefits be provided on an ambulatory basis. The palliation is not lasting because invasion continues and symptoms recur, and life probably is not prolonged. Repetition of treatment every few months is needed to control growth. Extreme care is necessary in treatment of ulcerating tumors of the neck. After freezing of cervical carcinoma involving the carotid artery, the risk of disastrous hemorrhage during the period of sloughing is considerable.

Postoperative care depends in part on the extent of freezing and the site of the disease. After thawing, the frozen skin becomes progressively reddened with congestion, and edematous. After freezing areas of the face, especially about the eyes, extensive edema (perhaps closing the eyelids) may occur on the first day, even though the skin cancer was small. This soon relents, but to avoid alarm, the patient should be informed of this possibility before the procedure. In most areas little discomfort is experienced. In a few patients headaches accompany freezing in the region of the forehead or in other areas, and pain may be more than minimal and require drugs for relief. Longer-lasting neurologic discomfort is unusual.

Initially, a dry gauze dressing is placed on the wound. When the eschar forms, a dressing is not necessary. When the eschar separates, a dressing, perhaps with an antibiotic ointment, is used to collect secretions. Healing is delayed by the need for the necrotic tissue to separate spontaneously. This depends on the amount of necrotic tissue. As an example, however, a skin cancer 2 inches in diameter, treated cryosurgically, requires about 3 weeks to heal. The final cosmetic result is good. Some changes in pigmentation are usual. With minor freezing of skin, temporary hyperpigmentation may occur. With extensive freezing, complete return of pigmentation may not occur. Therefore the techniques must be used with the knowledge that the cosmetic effect may not be favorable in brown- or black-skinned individuals.

DISEASES OF THE ORAL CAVITY

Benign and malignant tumors and precancerous conditions of the oral cavity are well suited to cryosurgery. The nature and the amount of disease determine the suitability for ambulatory treatment. Inflammatory or dysplastic disease or small tumors that can be treated with use of local anesthesia can be managed on an outpatient basis. Large lesions, requiring use of general anesthesia to provide operative exposure and extensive freezing, are usually not suitable for ambulatory therapy. The special advantages to use of cryosurgery in oral diseases: (1) the oral cavity is easily accessible to treatment; (2) often local anesthesia can be used, so operative risk is reduced; (3) the effect of treatment is readily observed in the postoperative period; (4) repetition of treatment, if necessary, is easy; (5) cryosurgery offers the outstanding advantage of permitting local treatment without sacrifice of bone of the oral cavity. Hemangiomas and mixed tumors of the oral cavity are among those that respond quickly. Tumors that overlie bone are especially suited to freezing, and the probability of cure is excellent.

BENIGN TUMORS

Benign tumors of the oral cavity are usually ideal for cryosurgery. Local or topical anesthesia is adequate for treatment of most lesions. Most often a cryoprobe is used because it offers better control of freezing than does the liquid nitrogen spray. The treatment must include the entire tumor area and an area of surrounding normal tissue. It is best to control treatment by use of thermocouples so that a temperature of $-40°C$ is achieved in the normal tissue at the periphery of the tumor. Repeated treatment after thawing is necessary. Treatment should be conservative so that normal tissue is not unnecessarily destroyed.

Treatment can always be repeated later if the first one was not adequate. In comparison with cancer, a margin of safety is present with benign tumors.

DYSPLASIA AND OTHER MUCOSAL LESIONS

Various mucosal diseases, some of which are included in the general descriptive terms *leukoplakia* and *erythroplasia,* are easily treated by cryosurgery. The nature of the disease must be established by preliminary biopsy. Papillary epithelial hyperplasia, hyperkeratosis, dysplastic epithelium, and carcinoma in situ are examples of mucosal diseases that are well suited to cryosurgery.

Since the disease is superficial, either nitrous oxide or liquid nitrogen apparatus is satisfactory, and either a probe or liquid nitrogen spray may be used. Small lesions, especially in the posterior part of the oral cavity, are best treated with a probe. The spray of liquid nitrogen is best chosen for extensive lesions in the anterior part of the oral cavity. Treatment need be given only to a depth of about 3 mm.

Treatment is usually given in the clinic; local anesthesia is utilized. Normal tissues of the oral cavity must be protected from unwanted freezing. A thermocouple is inserted submucosally beneath the area to be frozen, and treatment is given until the tissue temperature reaches −40°C, which usually requires 1 to 2 minutes (Fig. 11-10). The tissue is allowed to thaw spontaneously and then refrozen immediately. During freezing, high-volume vacuum suction is necessary to clear clouds of frozen water vapor that obscure vision, especially when a liquid nitrogen is used.

After the operation, postoperative edema is ordinarily not troublesome. Only mild analgesic drugs are needed. The patient is able to eat a soft diet, and healing is rapid. A clean granulating wound develops in around 10 days and heals with minimal scarring in about 3 weeks. The patient is cautioned against the use of alcohol, tobacco, and other irritants. Prolonged follow-up is necessary for dysplastic disease because new areas of mucosal involvement often develop months later if the original etiologic factors have not been corrected. The in-

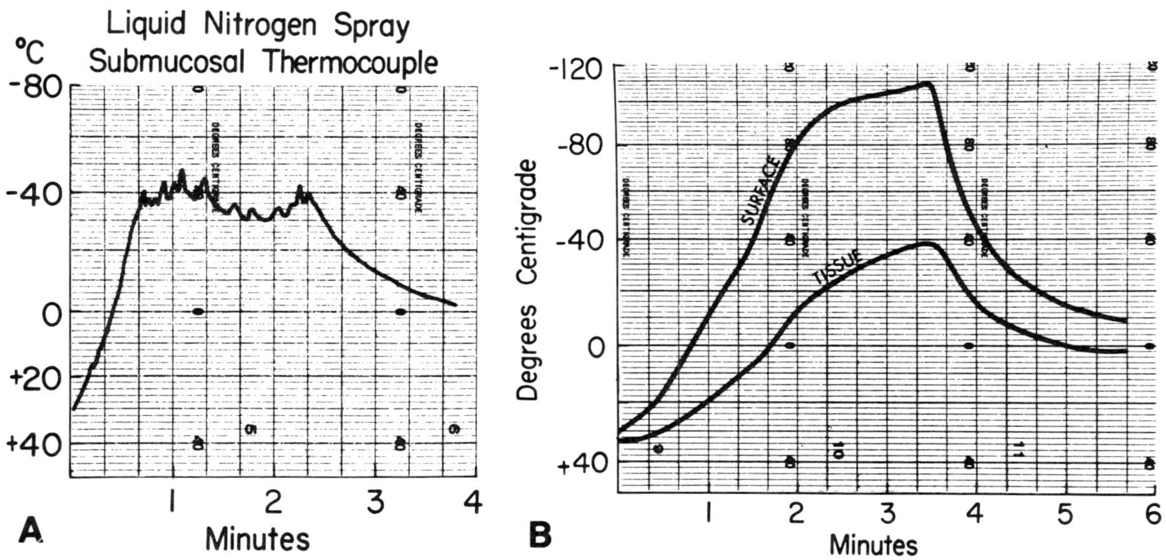

Figure 11-10. (*A*) Record of temperature from a submucosal thermocouple during treatment of carcinoma in situ of the buccal mucosa with liquid nitrogen spray. Treatment was continued until the submucosal temperature reached −40°C; then the tissue was allowed to warm. The weaving of the temperature record is due to movement of the spray over the tissues. After thawing of the tissue the freezing–thawing cycle was repeated. The entire treatment requires about 15 minutes. (*B*) For comparison, this is a record of temperatures during probe treatment of a small squamous cell cancer of the buccal mucosa. The surface temperature was recorded from a thermocouple placed between the probe and tumor. Although the probe temperature reached −160°C, it can be seen that the actual contact temperature reached only −109°C. The tissue temperature was recorded from a thermocouple placed in normal tissue lateral to the tumor. Freezing was continued until this thermocouple showed −40°C. After thawing of the tissue the freezing–thawing cycle was repeated.

cidence of persistent or new disease is about 10%.

ORAL CANCER

The usual treatment of oral cancer is surgical excision or radiotherapy. These commonly accepted methods of treatment are associated with a number of problems related to the effects of treatment or to failure of treatment to cure. Loss of form and function of the mouth and jaws after radical surgery is associated with disabilities that should not be minimized, and radiotherapy is associated with disagreeable sequelae in relation to radionecrosis of bone. Some individuals have problems related to untreated neglected cancer. Some patients with apparently curable oral cancer are not candidates for surgical excision because of the operative risks imposed by associated disease, and others refuse surgical treatment. These considerations mean that cryosurgery may be used for widely different reasons in oral cancer.

Primary Treatment of Oral Cancer

Some patients with small oral cancers may be treated by cryosurgical techniques under local anesthesia. This departure from standard methods of treatment requires careful selection of patients in order not to compromise the chance of cure through faulty judgment of the extent of the disease. Selection of patients for cryosurgery is based on the following criteria: (1) if the cancer is on or adjacent to bone so that excision would require removal of a portion of the mandible or palate; (2) if the patient has extensive cardiopulmonary disease so that the risk of extensive operation is prohibitive. Either one of these reasons is sufficient to consider a patient for cryosurgery. In addition, cryosurgery may be offered to patients who refuse suggested radical excision or radiotherapy or who are not suitable for such treatment for a variety of reasons (e.g., because of a blood dyscrasia such as coagulopathy).

Small cancers of the oral cavity (T1, N0) can be treated successfully by cryosurgical techniques, and as a method of local management, the results compare favorably with alternate methods of conservative management. Larger cancers of the tongue and the floor of the mouth are not as suitable for cryosurgery because the limits of the tumor are more difficult to define, and invasion by way of the lymphatics may be early. On the other hand, small- to moderate-sized cancers of the anterior portion of the floor of the mouth are acceptable for treatment because the extreme disability caused by resection of the anterior part of the mandible encourages acceptance of the risk of cryosurgery. Cryosurgery is particularly well suited for tumors overlying the palate or mandible because the underlying bone limits the depth the cancer can penetrate and enhances the chance of cure (Fig. 11-11). Conservation of the bony structure of the oral cavity is the outstanding reason cryosurgery deserves a place in the surgical management of oral cancer. In selected cases a survival rate comparable to that afforded by surgical excision can be achieved at less cost to the patient in terms of operative mortality and postoperative functional disability.

Cryosurgery is more likely to cure small tumors than large ones, but that is also true of any other treatment method. Advanced cancers of the oral cavity, especially those of the floor of the mouth, the base of the tongue, and the pharynx, are probably not curable by cryosurgery, and the technique should not be used for extensive cancer unless necessitated by the general condition of the patient.

Patient care following intraoral freezing for the cure of small cancer is ordinarily simple. Most problems are related to the edema, which begins to form after thawing and increases to a maximum within a day, interfering with deglutition to some extent, according to the amount of swelling in the area that has been frozen. Oral secretions are copious. The tongue after freezing becomes remarkably edematous, but obstruction to deglutition or danger to the airway should not be a problem in the type of patient chosen for ambulatory cryosurgery. Postoperative pain is usually minimal, and only analgesics are required for the discomfort caused by swelling of the tissues in the oral cavity. Since some fever and leukocytosis appear, a broad-spectrum antibiotic is given for several days after treatment.

Over several days the previously frozen tissue becomes necrotic, and a mass of malodorous tissue develops in the oral cavity. The use of a pleasant-tasting mouthwash is helpful during this period. The partially necrotic, liquefying tissue sloughs in small pieces over a 3-week period, until the wound has a clean granulating base. Then, in patients with tumors, the wound is examined closely and a

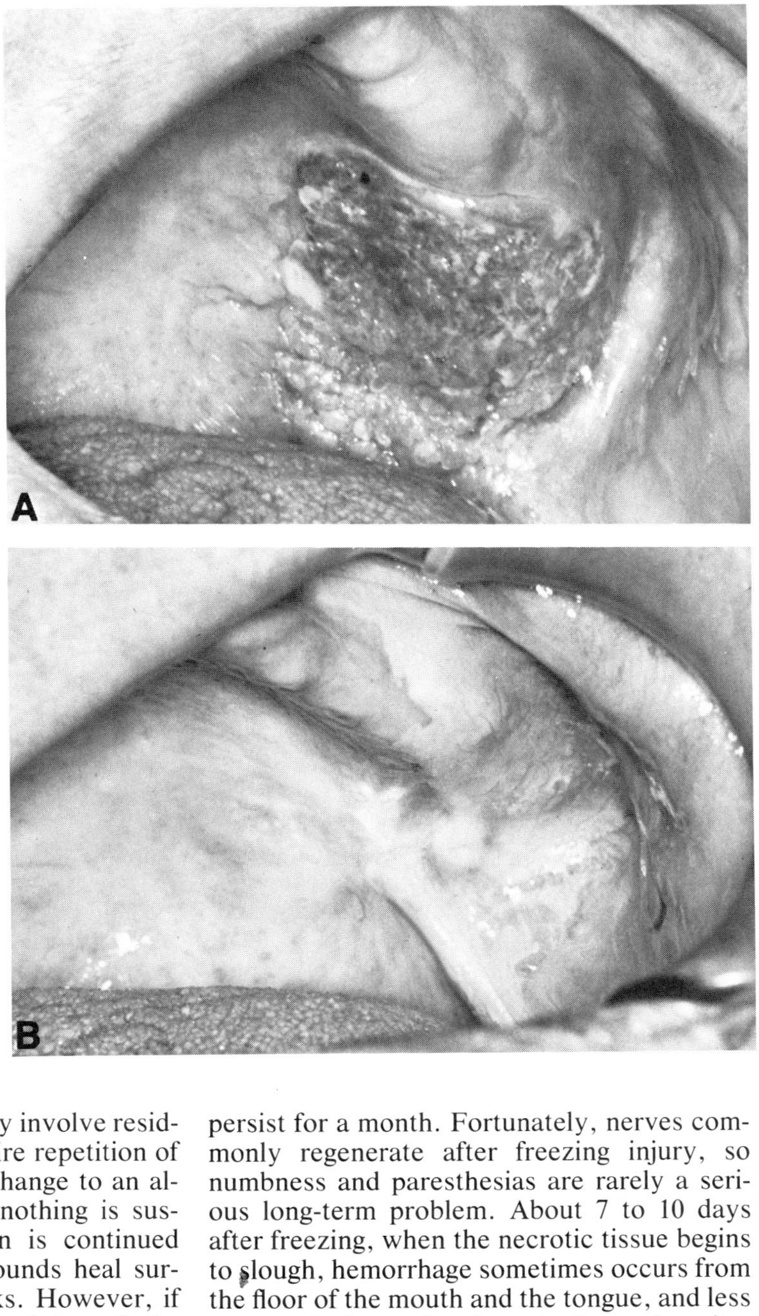

Figure 11-11. (*A*) Squamous cell carcinoma of the upper alveolar ridge and adjacent palate. There is no cervical adenopathy. Because the underlying bone limits the penetration of the tumor, the tumor is ideal for cryosurgery. (*B*) A year after treatment there is some fibrosis of the treated tissues. The tumor did not recur.

biopsy is done of areas that may involve residual disease, which would require repetition of cryosurgery or a decision to change to an alternate treatment method. If nothing is suspicious of tumor, observation is continued during the healing period. Wounds heal surprisingly well in about 4 weeks. However, if the bone is exposed by slough of the soft tissue, then healing is prolonged, and soft tissue may not completely cover the exposed bone for many months.

After freezing therapy for oral tumors, the potential delayed complications are paresthesias, trismus, hemorrhage, and sequestration of bone. Paresthesias usually subside within a few days, but occasionally sensory loss over the lip and chin and part of the tongue may persist for a month. Fortunately, nerves commonly regenerate after freezing injury, so numbness and paresthesias are rarely a serious long-term problem. About 7 to 10 days after freezing, when the necrotic tissue begins to slough, hemorrhage sometimes occurs from the floor of the mouth and the tongue, and less commonly from elsewhere in the oral cavity. Bleeding is controlled by suture-ligature or by electrocoagulation. Trismus is a serious postoperative problem. It occurs after the freezing of tumors in the retromolar area and apparently is due to edema and, later, to fibrosis of the pterygoid muscles. Exercise of the jaw during the postoperative period is a partial solution to this problem. Devitalization of bone occurs during the freezing of tumors overlying the mandible or the palate, but only minor sequestration has occurred even though bone repair may require as long as 2 or 3 years, depending on the volume of bone frozen. The effect of freezing on bone is less deleterious than that of radiotherapy.

Palliation of Advanced Oral Cancer

Neglected oral cancer causes pain and bleeding and interferes with mastication and deglutition. Few such patients are suitable for treatment on an ambulatory basis. Lesions in the posterior portion of the oral cavity are not suitable for freezing in a clinic because edema is a potential threat to the airway. In such patients tracheostomy is often done at the time of freezing in order to avoid any difficulty in the postoperative period. In bulky tumors the goal of treatment is principally to reduce their size. The palliative results of cryosurgery for large bulky tumors are often disappointing because the presence of large volume of necrotic tissue in the oral cavity is often difficult for aged or debilitated patients to tolerate. Therefore, except for relief of pain, radiotherapy is probably preferable to cryosurgery for large cancers. Painful lesions are especially suitable for treatment by freezing. Relief of pain is occasionally immediate and complete, but more often it is partial.

During the first days after freezing of large, bulky tumors, nourishment by nasogastric tube or parenteral route is needed. However, rapid reduction in tumor size usually permits ingestion of food within a few days. The tumor regrows, of course, so ordinarily treatment must be repeated in 3 or 4 months; sometimes it can be given on an ambulatory basis.

In some patients the disease persists after radiotherapy or excision, but often further surgery is not possible and more radiotherapy is considered inadvisable. Cryosurgery is an excellent alternative method of therapy and affords a chance of cure as well as relief of pain. The occasional long-term survival of such patients is an indication of the usefulness of cryosurgery as a method of salvage when disease persists after other methods of treatment.

DISEASES OF THE NOSE AND THROAT

Cryosurgery is useful in a wide variety of diseases of the nose and throat, including mucosal dysplasia, rhinitis, chronic tonsillitis, nasal polyps, and tumors. Ability to see these areas is not as good as that with the skin or oral cavity, so special probes and techniques are necessary. Ordinarily, spray techniques cannot be used in these locations. Thermocouples generally are not used. The procedure usually can be performed in the outpatient clinic with use of local or topical anesthesia, and it is necessary only to keep the patient under observation for several hours until the effect of premedication has worn off. A cooperative patient is essential.

HYPERTROPHIC RHINITIS

Chronic nasal airway obstruction due to hypertrophy of the nasal turbinates often associated with excessive nasal drainage may be treated successfully by cryosurgery and use of topical anesthesia with cocaine. Freezing of the turbinates is followed by slough of the hypertrophic tissue, which improves the nasal airway and decreases the secretions. Selection of patients is facilitated by choosing those whose symptoms are relieved by inferior turbinate shrinkage achieved with a spray of 0.25% phenylephrine hydrochloride. With freezing, the surgeon attempts to achieve an equivalent decrease in the size of the swollen tissue.

Liquid nitrogen or nitrous oxide apparatus may be used. The larger the volume of turbinate tissue, the more advisable the use of the liquid nitrogen apparatus. On the other hand, although nitrous oxide apparatus has less freezing capability, the quickness of control of freezing and thawing is better. With either apparatus, properly designed probes are needed so that insertion into the nasal passage is easy and accurate placement of the probe on the swollen turbinate is possible. Treatment should be conservative so that normal tissue is not unnecessarily frozen and the middle meatus, which contains the ostia of several paranasal sinuses, should be avoided. The duration of freezing of each turbinate is about 60 to 90 seconds (using nitrous oxide) and refreezing should not be necessary. The turbinates in each side of the nasal passage are treated alternately in order to allow thawing of previously frozen tissue.

Postoperative care features oral analgesics, oral decongestants, and an antibiotic. Some of the necrotic tissue may be removed in clinic visits as healing occurs over a 2- to 3-week period. The final result is a reduction in the amount of turbinate tissue and a normal appearance of the mucosa.

CHRONIC TONSILLITIS

Cryosurgery is not widely used for tonsillectomy. Too often it fails to remove all the tonsillar tissue, and the tonsillar remnants may cause persistent symptoms. In addition, the adenoids are rather inaccessible. However, especially in adults, cryosurgery may be chosen to prevent recurrent attacks of acute tonsillitis. It may be preferred in adult patients who have blood dyscrasias or who are at high surgical risk. Cryosurgery may be performed with little or no operative blood loss and low risk of postoperative bleeding.

Nitrous oxide or liquid nitrogen apparatus can be used. Generally speaking, the freezing capacity of the nitrous oxide apparatus is insufficient to destroy the entire tonsil, so the liquid nitrogen apparatus is preferred. Effort must be made to freeze all tonsillar tissue, which means that the probe must be applied to upper and lower portions of each tonsil, and two freeze–thaw cycles must be used. Destruction often is not as complete as removal with surgical excision. The tonsillar remnants may be removed by repeated freezing at a later date. Careful attention to technique may avoid this problem.

GYNECOLOGIC DISEASES

In recent years cryosurgical treatment has become common in gynecologic practice. A wide variety of inflammatory and neoplastic diseases of the vulva, vagina, and cervix are treated. Tissue diagnosis is important; advances in colposcopy have added to diagnostic acumen. Cryosurgical treatment is performed in the physician's office or in the outpatient clinic without need for anesthesia. Nitrous oxide or liquid nitrogen apparatus may be used, but the former is preferred for inflammatory disease.

CHRONIC CERVICITIS

Benign cervical lesions, such as chronic cervicitis, endocervical polyps, dysplastic disease, and condylomata acuminata may be treated by cryosurgery. Its principal use is in chronic cervicitis. The extent of the disease must be evaluated carefully and the possibility of invasive carcinoma excluded. Treatment should be given within 2 weeks of the last menstrual period.

Probes for cervical freezing have special shapes that are designed to fit within the cervical canal for a short distance for effective contact with the diseased tissue. Treatment can be conservative; it is necessary to freeze only about 3 mm beyond the edge of the diseased area. Only a single freezing–thawing cycle is used. To cover the entire area, repeated applications may be necessary in some instances. In unusual cases, to achieve a greater degree of tissue necrosis and deeper penetration, freezing is repeated immediately after thawing.

Immediately after treatment, some patients have headaches, dizziness, and flushing. This is a vasomotor reaction and soon disappears. In the postoperative period, mild, intermittent cramps, which may be treated with aspirin or similar analgesics, may be present. Usually a clear watery vaginal discharge develops and lasts about 10 to 14 days, gradually lessening as healing progresses. Slight bleeding may occur during the slough of necrotic tissue, but severe hemorrhage is unlikely. Because of the possibility of cervical bleeding due to trauma, abstinence from sexual intercourse for about 3 weeks is advised. Healing occurs in about 8 to 10 weeks.

CARCINOMA OF THE CERVIX

Cryosurgery is effective treatment for dysplastic disease or carcinoma in situ. It is not used for primary treatment of invasive cervical cancer, the presence of which must be excluded by cell smears and biopsy in the patients selected. The technique of treatment should be more aggressive than that for inflammatory disease, so liquid nitrogen apparatus should be used. The results of therapy are excellent, but persistent disease will be seen later in about 9% of patients. Hence careful follow-up at intervals after treatment is important.

Cryosurgical techniques are seldom used for the treatment of invasive malignant disease of the cervix. Cryosurgery has been used in some potentially curable patients who were not candidates for conventional therapy. In such patients excellent results have been achieved at times, but too few patients have been treated to permit evaluation of its ability to cure cancer in this site. More commonly, cryosurgery has been used to achieve palliation of symptoms, especially control of tumor growth and amelioration of pain due to cervical cancer when other methods of treatment have failed. Generally speaking, substantial freezing of tissue is required to produce palliative benefits. Commonly, hospitalization for a few days is necessary to achieve more than control of tumor bulk.

DISEASES OF THE VULVA

Vulvar condylomata acuminata, treated by a variety of therapeutic methods with imperfect results, may be treated by cryosurgery as well. Only local anesthesia is needed, and the lesions may be treated in one visit to the clinic. Good visual control of the freezing process is possible, and freezing should include about 2 mm of normal tissue beyond the lesion. In cases of condylomata acuminata with extensive involvement of the vulva, it is prudent to stage the freezing over several visits in order to avoid excessive vulvar edema.

Benign tumors and small cutaneous malignant tumors are treated effectively by freezing. The techniques are the same as those used for diseases of the skin, including cutaneous cancer, described earlier in this chapter.

Extensive cancers of the vulva have been treated by cryosurgery also. Such cases are few, but occasionally excellent results in difficult problems in therapy have been reported. Hospitalization is generally required for large cancers, but continued control of tumor bulk to maintain palliative benefits may be provided on an outpatient basis.

PILONIDAL DISEASE

In the treatment of pilonidal disease in recent years, emphasis has changed from eradication by wide excision to more conservative management. This change has resulted from increasing acceptance of the idea that pilonidal disease is a foreign-body reaction, because of hairs penetrating the skin, later complicated by infection. Most pilonidal disease may be managed by opening the infected tract, removing the foreign material and embedded hairs, and treating the wound in such a way as to promote proper healing. A conservative technique, combining incision and curettage with cryosurgery, is satisfactory for office or clinic use and permits the patient's early return to work. The addition of cryosurgery to the curettage improves the chances of cure by acting as a debriding maneuver and perhaps by retarding healing for a short period.

The diverse forms of pilonidal disease may be treated with cryosurgery. A common form is a simple infected sinus. After local anesthesia is produced by infiltration with 1% lidocaine (Xylocaine) a small quantity of methylene blue–hydrogen peroxide solution instilled through a small catheter into the sinus opening to stain the diseased tissue and to aid in identification of sinus extensions. Then the sinus is opened in the midline with a scalpel to expose the extent of the disease. Hair and granulation tissue are removed by gentle curettage, which should cause little bleeding. The entire open wound is then frozen with a spray of liquid nitrogen to a depth of about 5 mm (Fig. 11-12). Care must be taken to avoid runoff of liquid nitrogen down the gluteal cleft to the perineal region. Only a single freezing cycle is used. The depth of freezing is judged by manipulation of the wound because the hard frozen tissue is easily palpable and movable as a mass. There is seldom reason to freeze as deep as the sacrococcygeal fascia. After thawing, since no tissue is excised, bleeding from the wound is ordinarily minimal. The wound is loosely packed with iodoform gauze and a dressing is applied.

Multiple sinus tracts are treated in a similar manner but with modifications to suit the more complicated state. In pilonidal abscess in which there is no external opening, an incision is made sufficiently long to empty the abscess and expose its interior to a spray of liquid nitrogen. This combined technique substantially increases the chance of cure by incision and drainage, and it is quite likely that subsequent operation will not be needed.

Postoperative care stresses wound management and patient education. The packing is removed on the day following the procedure, and sitz baths are taken twice daily at home. The patient is seen weekly in the clinic for careful attention to the course of the wound healing. Periodic shaving of the area around the wound is necessary to control hair growth. The instructions given to the patient early in the illness are repeated on clinic visits.

Necrosis is obvious in the wound in about 48 hours after treatment. The slough separates

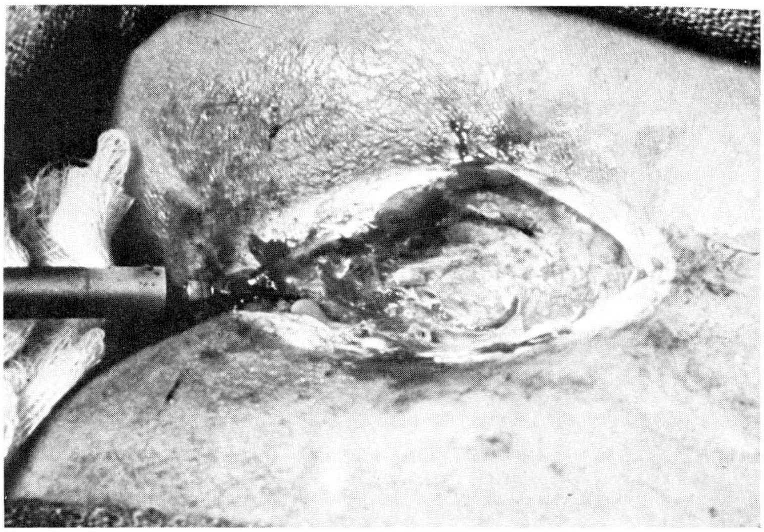

Figure 11-12. Pilonidal disease is treated by opening the diseased area in the midline and connecting the sinus openings. The wound then gapes. The granulation tissue is removed by curettage. Then the entire area is frozen with a spray of liquid nitrogen to a depth of about 5 mm, as shown in this photograph.

in about 2 weeks to leave a clean granulating wound, which then slowly heals in another 4 weeks. The slow healing time of the wound and the close attention to wound care are the important factors in the success of this technique. The recurrence rate with this technique is about 10%, which compares favorably with the more aggressive surgical methods.

DISEASES OF THE ANUS AND RECTUM

Cryosurgery is of prime usefulness in anal and rectal diseases. In general, any local lesion that can be excised or treated by electrocoagulation can also be treated by freezing in situ. At times cryocoagulation is preferable because little anesthesia is required and no bleeding is caused. In the anal region there is little difficulty determining the extent of disease, but in the rectum adequacy of visualization of the lesion may be a problem. Good treatment can be given in the anus and lower rectum through a large-diameter proctoscope, but vision through a sigmoidoscope is poor when a large-diameter cryoprobe must be used in its lumen.

Cryosurgery has been used to treat a variety of proctologic disorders, ranging from minor conditions as anal fissures and hemorrhoids to large incurable cancers. The minor conditions are easily treated in the office or clinic. Anal fissures respond well to conservative freezing. Occasionally in the treatment of an apparently minor anal condition, the biopsy made during cryosurgery reveals an unsuspected anal carcinoma. In such instances, even though the entire lesion was encompassed in the cryosurgical treatment, it is prudent to give radiotherapy to the site. Anal papillomas can be cured easily. Condylomata acuminata are difficult to treat successfully because the disease is often so extensive and often extends into the anal canal. In most cases, podophyllin therapy or electrocoagulation, as described elsewhere in this text, is a better choice. When cryosurgery is used, careful follow-up observation is required for lesions missed or inadequately frozen on the first occasion. In freezing, care must be taken to encompass the entire lesion and to include about 2 mm of normal skin.

HEMORRHOIDS

A wide variety of techniques are available for the treatment of hemorrhoids and most are used with success. Generally the trend has been toward conservative treatment, such as injection sclerotherapy in the office, and surgical hemorrhoidectomy has been reserved for severe hemorrhoids. Cryosurgical techniques have also been used successfully in recent years, perhaps more so in other countries than in the United States. The method has advantages in terms of ease of treatment, low cost, and suitability for office use that merits wider use. Conflicting opinions of the value of cryosurgery in the treatment of hemorrhoids can be found, but the results of cryohemorrhoidectomy are excellent if care is taken to use the technique properly for appropriate patients.

Cryohemorrhoidectomy is a practical, conservative method of treating any type of hemorrhoidal tissues, from irritating external skin tags to large edematous prolapsing hemorrhoids in patients at high surgical risk. However, it is best used for hemorrhoidal disease above the dentate line because drainage and offensive odors are minimized when the necrotic tissue remains internal and pain is substantially lessened. When there is combined disease, it is better to use cryosurgery only for the component above the dentate line and manage the external disease by another therapeutic method to avoid the problems of the external necrotic tissue and attendant discomfort. For external hemorrhoids, excisional techniques are preferable.

It is important to explain the procedure carefully to the patient so that swelling of tissue, drainage, and malodor are anticipated. Commonly, injection of a local anesthetic drug is used, but local freezing of internal hemorrhoids is tolerable without anesthesia. After positioning the patient and exposing the hemorrhoids, the freezing is done. Either liquid nitrogen or nitrous oxide apparatus may be used. In unusual patients with very large hemorrhoids, the greater freezing capability of liquid nitrogen may be necessary, but generally nitrous oxide, which is more convenient to use through an anoscope, is sufficient.

Several techniques are practiced:

1. In the most commonly used method, the freezing surface of the probe is applied to the hemorrhoid and becomes adherent as the freezing begins. A slight rocking motion of the shaft of the probe rolls additional hemorrhoidal tissue onto the freezing surface. When the tissue is broadly adherent, the probe is used as a retractor to lift the hemorrhoidal tissue away from the underlying sphincter. To avoid stricture, freezing of the entire circumference of the anal canal should be avoided. Whatever technique is used, care must be taken to avoid freezing the anal sphincter. (Some physicians place a thermocouple in this region but it should not be necessary.) Treatment is complete when the entire hemorrhoid is frozen. When sufficient tissue has been frozen, the probe is allowed to warm and is removed. Then the other hemorrhoids are treated in the same way. In some advanced disease, it may be desirable to treat the remaining hemorrhoids on subsequent clinic visits.

2. A clamp is applied to the base of the hemorrhoid and the probe is applied to the tissue within the clamp. Freezing is allowed to extend to include the entire hemorrhoidal area. It is not repeated.

3. Rubber-band ligature of the hemorrhoid has been combined effectively with freezing in situ. Placed just before freezing, the rubber bands occlude the circulation and encourage thrombosis and necrosis. If used below the dentate line, freezing should extend beyond the rubber ligature to reduce postoperative pain.

In the days after freezing, a serous discharge may be copious while the hemorrhoid undergoes necrosis. Gradually the necrotic tissue separates to leave a clean granulating wound in about 5 to 10 days. Mucosa grows over the wound to complete healing, which is somewhat delayed, as is true with all cryosurgical procedures, because the necrotic tissue must be eliminated before wound healing can occur. Healing is generally complete in 3 weeks.

Postoperative care is important, as with any operation in the anal region. Generally, there is little pain after freezing. Sitz baths and, occasionally, the use of lidocaine (Xylocaine) ointment ease postoperative discomfort. Many patients can return to work in a day. A few have postoperative urinary retention and require catheterization, especially if hypertrophic prostatic disease is present. Bleeding is seen occasionally. External skin tags sometimes occur and infrequently require excision under local anesthesia.

VILLOUS ADENOMA

Benign polypoid tumors of the rectum respond extremely well to freezing because their lack of dense fibrous tissue facilitates quick sloughing. Freezing is probably not the best treatment for adenomatous polyps because the commonly used snare-and-fulguration technique affords a specimen for histologic examination. However, cryocoagulation may be used instead of fulguration to destroy any residual cells that may be in the base. Freezing will perform this task better than electrocoagulation, but it does not control bleeding as well.

Villous tumors of the rectum, with their superficial and exophytic growth pattern, are nearly ideal for cryocoagulation. Freezing is easily accomplished, and the tumor sloughs readily after freezing. In comparison with electrocoagulation, often used for this tumor, freezing affords the advantages of careful control of the treatment process and avoidance of hemorrhage. Either technique has the shortcoming that biopsy shows only the nature of the tissue removed, and malignant degeneration may exist elsewhere in the specimen. This risk must be assumed when any treatment method short of total excision is used. After treatment the patient is examined periodically, and treatment is repeated as often as needed to eliminate the disease. Extensive lesions commonly require repetition of treatment.

RECTAL CANCER

In carefully selected patients, who are at high surgical risk for conventional surgical therapy, cryosurgery may be considered as a reasonable alternative, even for cure. If cure is the consideration, the criteria for selection are the same as those for electrocoagulation; that is, the neoplasm should be within reach of the examining finger, should be predominantly exophytic, and should be on the lateral or posterior wall of the rectum. Lesions higher in the rectum are too difficult to treat because of inadequate visualization. Lesions on the anterior wall of the rectum are unsatisfactory for cryosurgery because of the risk of fistula formation with the urethra or vagina. Ulcerative lesions usually have invaded to a sufficient extent to preclude cure.

Cryosurgery may be used for palliative benefit in more advanced disease. The object is simply to control the growth of the tumor by cryosurgical destruction every several months. The lower in the rectum, the better the accuracy of treatment. Lesions higher in the colon, which must be visualized through a sigmoidoscope, are difficult to freeze accurately, and risk of perforation by subsequent necrosis is considerable.

COMPARISON WITH OTHER METHODS OF TREATMENT

The advantages of cryosurgery are simplicity of use, little need for anesthesia, lack of hemorrhage, few complications in the postoperative period, and favorable healing. These advantages are most evident when cryosurgery is used to treat an accessible lesion, avoiding the excision of tissue. The devitalized tissue is allowed to become necrotic and slough. This method of use is the basis for the suitability of the technique for the high-surgical-risk patient, including those with a blood coagulopathy. Most patients have little discomfort after surgery because of the desensitizing effect of cold on sensory nerves. Nerve function, lost as a consequence of freezing, commonly returns after several months. Wound healing is surprisingly good but is delayed by the need to await necrosis and sloughing of the devitalized tissues. Healing is remarkably favorable, and extensive scarring is rare. Conservation of tissue, especially bone, is possible. The lethal effect of freezing extends into the bone and destroys any tumor cells that may be present, and the devitalized matrix remains as a structural basis for later repair. Bone repair may require a year longer for completion.

The principal disadvantages of cryosurgery are that the entire specimen is not available for tissue examination and healing is slower than that with excision and closure. The lack of a specimen is a condition shared by other methods of treatment, such as electrocoagulation and radiotherapy. Slow healing is not entirely disadvantageous, since the interval provides time to observe the open wound for persistent disease and the slow healing commonly provides a favorable end result.

The limitations of the technique are related to evaluation of the depth of freezing and to the difficulty in freezing large volumes of tissue. The extent of surface freezing is easy to evaluate but depth of freezing cannot be judged by vision. Palpation of the frozen mass provides a good idea of how much tissue is frozen, but still confirmation of depth depends on the use of monitoring techniques. Evaluation of the extent of freezing is especially difficult when treatment is given by means of endoscopy. The other limitation is the difficulty in freezing large volumes of tissue even though liquid nitrogen is used as the cryogenic agent. Depth of freezing beyond 2 cm to 3 cm is difficult to achieve. Multiple applications of the probe, insertion of the probe into bulky tumors, and repetition of freezing at a later date are methods of compensating for the difficulties of freezing sufficient tissue. Partial removal of the tissue, either by excision or by electrocoagulation, in order to expose the base of the lesion to the effect of freezing, is another effective technique of achieving depth, but this negates some of the advantages of cryosurgery and often removes it from the feasibility of performing the procedure on an outpatient basis.

Cryosurgery has some similarity to Moh's technique of treatment. Whether done by fixation or by fresh tissue technique, serial excision and immediate histologic monitoring by the Moh's technique has yielded outstanding results, even in some advanced cancers that are difficult problems in management. Cryosurgery may be used in a similar manner, monitoring the course of treatment by interval biopsies and repeating treatment as necessary in order to eradicate the disease. Cryosurgical techniques are faster in producing and are capable of destroying a larger amount of tissue at the initial treatment.

Cryosurgery must also be compared with laser therapy. Cryosurgical apparatus is less expensive and has fewer safety considerations. Experience with lasers is small but increasing rapidly as the techniques evolve. Although laser therapy requires expensive apparatus, it appears reasonable to expect that laser destruction will become competitive with other methods of therapy. The advantages of laser therapy closely resemble those of cryosurgery from the standpoint of healing, the speed of treatment of multiple lesions, and usefulness in certain anatomic sites. Like cryosurgery, the limitation of laser therapy is the difficulty in determining the depth of tumor invasion into the underlying tissue.

Radiation therapy is of wide general usefulness in the treatment of cancer and has advantages in certain difficult areas around the eyelids, nose, and ears. The results of radiotherapy indicate that it is an excellent alternate choice in many patients with cancers. Nevertheless, cryosurgery can achieve the same results in a shorter period of time. Cryosurgery has a substantial advantage in lesions overlying bone or when the tumor involves bone.

In comparison with the many other tools used by the surgeon, cryosurgical apparatus is simple to use and its techniques are learned easily. As with any other techniques that surgeons use to treat disease or to correct pathologic states, the key to success in therapy is in the selection of patients and in the proper use of the technique.

BIBLIOGRAPHY

General

Ablin R: Handbook of Cryosurgery. New York, Marcel Dekker, 1980

Bald W, Fraser, J: Cryogenic surgery. Rep Prog Physics 45:1381–1434, 1982

Gage A: Cryosurgery for cancer. Compr Ther 10(1):61–69, 1984

Gage A, Augustinowicz S, Montes M, Caruana S, Whalen D: Tissue impedance and temperature measurements in relation to necrosis in experimental cryosurgery. Cryobiology 22:282–288, 1985

Gage A, Caruana AJ, Garamy G: A comparison of instrument methods of monitoring freezing in cryosurgery. J Dermatol Surg Oncol 9:209–214, 1983

Gage A, Guest K, Montes M, Caruana S, Whalen D: Effect of varying freezing and thawing rates in experimental cryosurgery. Cryobiology 22:175–182, 1985

Mazur P: Freezing of living cells: Mechanisms and implications. Am J Physiol 247:C125–C142, 1984

Tanaka S: Immunologic aspects of cryosurgery in general surgery. Cryobiology 19:247–262, 1982

Torre D: Depth dose in cryosurgery. J Dermatol Surg Oncol 9:219–225, 1983

Skin Disease

Gage A: Cryosurgery for skin disease: Variants in technique. In E Epstein (ed): Controversies in Dermatology, pp. 151–162. Philadelphia, WB Saunders, 1984

Gage A: Deep cryosurgery. In E Epstein (ed): Skin Surgery, 5th ed, pp 857–877. Springfield, IL, Charles C Thomas, 1982

Shepherd J, Dawber R: The response of keloid scars to cryosurgery. Plast Reconstr Surg 70:677–681, 1982

Torre D: Cryosurgical treatment of epitheliomas using the cone-spray technique. J Dermatol Surg Oncol 3:432–436, 1977

Zacarian S: Cryosurgery for Skin Cancer and Cutaneous Disorders. St. Louis, CV Mosby, 1985

Diseases of Oral Cavity

Bradley P: Cryosurgery of the Maxillofacial Region. Boca Raton, FL, CRC Press, 1986

Gage A: Five-year survival following cryosurgery for oral cancer. Arch Surg 111:990–994, 1976

Gongloff R, Gage A: Cryosurgical treatment of oral lesions: Report of cases. J Am Dent Assoc 106:47–51, 1983

Diseases of Nose and Throat

Bumsted, R: Cryotherapy for chronic vasomotor rhinitis: Technique and patient selection for improved results. Laryngoscope 94:539–544, 1984

Principato J: Chronic vasomotor rhinitis: Cryogenic and other surgical modes of treatment. Laryngoscope 89:619–638, 1979

Scoppa J: Vasomotor rhinitis: A review and management by intranasal cryotherapy. Med J Aust 143:448–450, 1985

Gynecologic Disease

Bryson S, Lenehan P, Lickrish G: The treatment of grade 3 cervical intraepithelial neoplasia with cryotherapy: an 11-year experience. Am J Obstet Gynecol 151:201–206, 1985

Crisp W: Cryosurgical treatment of neoplasia of the uterine cervix. Obstet Gynecol 39:495–499, 1972

Kirwan P, Smith I, Naftalin N: A study of cryosurgery and the CO_2 laser in treatment of carcinoma *in situ* (CIN III) of the uterine cervix. Gynecol Oncol 22:195–200, 1985

Wallach RC: Cryosurgery of advanced vulvar carcinoma. Obstet Gynecol 47:454, 1976

Pilonidal Disease

Gage A: Cryosurgery for pilonidal disease. Am J Surg 133:249–254, 1977

Diseases of the Anus and Rectum

Desmond J, O'Callaghan M, Matheson T, Hall R: Inpatient treatment of prolapsing piles: Cryosurgery versus Milligan–Morgan haemorrhoidectomy. Br J Surg 69:157–159, 1982

Oh C: One thousand cryohemorrhoidectomies. Dis Colon Rectum 24:613–616, 1981

Traynor O, Carter A: Cryotherapy for advanced haemorrhoids: a prospective evaluation with 2-year follow-up. Br J Surg 71:287–289, 1984

12 Outpatient Management of Acute and Chronic Pain

BENJAMIN L. CRUE, JR.

Pain is probably the most common complaint that brings a patient to a physician's office or the hospital emergency room. It must be remembered that pain is usually a symptom and not a diagnosis. Many aspects of the treatment of pain have been discussed in earlier chapters, in which pain was only one aspect of the specific disease or traumatic entity under discussion in regard to diagnosis, treatment, and disposition. In this chapter I would like to focus primarily on the complaint of pain itself, although it will be difficult not to be repetitious on occasion.

DEFINITION, DIAGNOSIS, AND CLASSIFICATION

Pain defies adequate satisfactory definition, as Lewis pointed out in 1942. (He then wrote a book about the subject anyway.[22]) Sternbach, however, gave a very detailed definition of pain in 1968, but it fails to satisfy all aspects of the problem. He wrote, "Pain is an abstract concept which refers to (1) a personal, private sensation of hurt; (2) a harmful stimulus which signals current or impending tissue damage; (3) a pattern of responses which operate to protect the organism from harm. These responses can be described in terms which reflect certain concepts, i.e., in neurological, physiological, behavioral, and affective 'languages'."[31] Merskey and Spear emphasize a much simpler definition of pain: "An unpleasant experience which we primarily associate with tissue damage, or describe in terms of tissue damage, or both."[25] I prefer a very pragmatic but useful definition of pain: "Pain is anything the patient says it is." This definition adequately covers the subjective individual nature of the patient's pain experience, but it does leave the physician open to possible exploitation by the relatively infrequent malingerer or the sociopath.

In addition to the problem of defining pain is the still unresolved problem of classifying pain syndromes, which has been approached in many ways. Disregarding for the present any consideration of etiology, pain mechanism, severity of pain, verbalization of suffering by the patient, patient's behavioral response, or the anatomic location and extent of the pain, it is still possible to come up with a useful, although understandably limited, classification based only on the temporal duration of the pain (see "Temporal Classification of Pain Complaints"). This can then be modified further in many ways [e.g., whether the pain is due to cancer or is benign (nonmalignant)].

Whatever the original cause, there is usually a *peripheral* etiology. Then evaluation of possible central neurophysiologic and concurrent psychologic mechanisms that potentiate and continue the pain across time must be evaluated in each patient.

TEMPORAL CLASSIFICATION OF PAIN COMPLAINTS

1. *Acute pain* (up to a few days). Mild or severe; cause known or unknown.
2. *Subacute pain* (few days to a few months). Though no longer an emergency, in most ways treat like acute.
3. *Recurrent acute pain*. Examples: arthritis (either rheumatoid or osteoarthritis), migraine, primary trigeminal neuralgia. The underlying pathology may be chronic.
4. *Ongoing pain*. Due to uncontrolled *malignant* neoplastic disease.
5. *Chronic–benign pain*. Nonneoplastic; seemingly adequate coping by the patient (usually over 6 months). No nociceptive input believed involved.
6. *Chronic intractable benign pain syndrome* (CIBPS). Chronic pain; poor patient coping

Fortunately, in both the physician's office and the emergency room, the most common pain complaint is *acute* pain, which often accompanies tissue damage or disease with inflammation. The characteristics of acute pain often serve as the central clue in helping to establish a correct diagnosis. Treatment of the acute pain is then usually accomplished in the classical sense by treating the underlying cause and thus alleviating the pain. Modern medicine also offers most patients good relief from pain when the underlying etiologic agent cannot be promptly treated, as in pain from uncontrolled malignant disease or from tissue damage in which treatment and the reparative processes of the body take time (e.g., obvious fracture in an extremity). Here the proper use of peripherally acting analgesics and short-term use of centrally acting narcotics usually gives adequate, if not excellent, relief of suffering.

The diagnosis, classification, and proper treatment of patients with the various chronic pain syndromes (to be discussed later) try the patience of the physician, both in office practice and in the emergency room, especially in the evening hours or on weekends, and in seemingly ever-increasing numbers. Although the clinician interested in the phenomenon of pain must have some understanding of the underlying structure and physiology involved in both acute and chronic pain, he is referred elsewhere for perusal of the history, neuroanatomy, neurophysiology, neurochemistry, neuropharmacology, and even the psychology and psychiatry of pain.[1–7,9–12,15–16,20,29–33] In very recent years, with much interest in the neuropharmacology of acute pain and with a definite clinical correlation to the use of analgesics peripherally and narcotics centrally, a knowledge of prostaglandin metabolism peripherally and of the endorphin or enkephalin systems within the brainstem is also a prerequisite for understanding some aspects of analgesic and narcotic medications. Space precludes discussing this further here.[21]

ACUTE VERSUS CHRONIC PAIN

Before presenting some of the differences between acute and chronic pain it is very important that the reader keep in mind in each instance the *difference* between the *etiology* of pain and the subsequent neurophysiologic *mechanism* underlying the complaint of pain. Most pain, regardless of its duration, starts with an organic peripheral tissue injury or inflammation. Although it is true that there are pain syndromes in which the underlying etiologic factor is still unknown, the overwhelming number of patients with pain have a known initiating event that starts the syndrome. This then often culminates in the complaint of pain, for which the patient seeks relief. In *acute* pain with known trauma or disease as the cause, the neurophysiologic mechanism of the pain is relatively well understood, with afferent input by the peripheral nervous system to the central nervous system referred to as "nociceptive input." The problem is that each individual patient, with his own idiosyncratic central nervous system, then takes that nociceptive input and modulates it and demonstrates pain behavior (or verbalizes the complaint of pain) to the physician, often in unique ways. This leads the interested neurophysiologist reluctantly to the realization that even acute pain is not a pure primary sensation, but from a clinical standpoint, pain is really a perception.

Treatment, even in acute pain, often requires simultaneous attention to the peripheral etiologic factor and the psychological dysfunction reflected in the obvious anxiety on the part of the acutely suffering patient. Therefore the central mechanisms underlying how the patient deals with acute pain are important to evaluate and understand before adequate treatment can be instituted. With this in mind the physician must undertake therapy without being fixed entirely on the originating peripheral cause of the pain complaint itself. For example, with *acute recurrent* or *subacute* pain after an injury that occurred a few days to a week or more before, one often has to spend considerable time trying to ascertain just why the patient waited until this particular time to seek medical care. There may be tissue-level complications making the pain suddenly more severe, or litigation may now be pending, or there may be conflict or abuse in the home.

When the complaint is constant, *chronic* pain, the physician is not dealing with the same basic problem. There is not just a difference in time or even in magnitude when compared with the original acute pain problem. Acute pain functions as a useful, albeit unwanted, alarm system, warning against tissue injury. This quality of the nervous system is apparently inherited not only by humans but by most members of the animal kingdom. This is clearly observable in laboratory animals' and man's adversive behavior when subjected to nociceptive stimulation. However, chronic pain in the human often becomes almost a "thing in itself" and no longer serves a useful warning purpose. Unfortunately, since we still lack adequate knowledge of the neurophysiology of the human central nervous system, we often resort to psychological terminology. This is true in relation both to human sensation and perception and to the more obvious response to pain (human pain behavior), as we attempt to talk about these still imperfectly understood underlying neurophysiologic pain mechanisms. This attempt by the clinician to use psychological terms to attempt to explain neurophysiologic mechanisms often leads to much confusion. However, this is only a specific example (related to pain) of the dilemma that medicine and psychiatry have always faced.

TWO MODELS FOR THE NEUROPHYSIOLOGY OF CHRONIC PAIN

Basically, practitioners divide into two camps when it comes to the neurophysiology of chronic pain, the *peripheralists* and the *centralists*. The *peripheralists* believe that chronic pain is merely a continuation of an acute pain process that has lasted for an unusual time (usually accepted to be about 6 months). For some reason in chronic pain it is presumed that the underlying nociceptive input from an abnormal peripheral factor has been continued in some manner and to some degree because

- The tissue injury has "not healed properly."
- The abnormality has "not been fixed properly" by the surgeon in previous attempts at reconstruction or improvement.
- There are abnormal pain impulses (nociceptive input) coming from the abnormal damaged area, referred to as "the scar" (conveniently forgetting that all patients with former injury have scar but that in most patients the pain "decays" and "turns off").

Most patients consider their chronic pain introspectively in this manner, essentially a peripheralist position. They approach the physician in the emergency room or private office with this acute pain organic medical model, wanting and expecting to be "fixed." Trying to treat patients with chronic pain definitively with this acute model in mind does not work very often. Treating the original area of injury, blocking the peripheral sensory nerves from the area by anesthesiologic nerve blocks, cutting or burning appropriate sensory pathways within the spinal cord or brain neurosurgically, or using pharmacologic analgesics and narcotic agents over a long period has proved, over many years, largely unsuccessful in patients with chronic pain.

In contrast to its success in treating most acute pain, the medical profession has continually had to ask why its treatment of chronic pain syndromes is so often unsuccessful. Experienced physicians have come to realize that, regardless of whether one uses a neurophysiologic or psychologic model to conceptualize the underlying mechanism, patients with chronic pain seem to have more or different central nervous system aspects involved in their complaint of pain. The peripheralists consider this central mechanism to be a psychological type of potentiation and prolongation of continued peripheral nociceptive input, and they refer to "functional overlay."

Chronic pain appears to become a thing in itself and no longer serves a useful purpose. Instead it seems to reflect underlying mechanisms within the idiosyncratic brain and spinal cord of the individual patient. Thus there is a second way to view the mechanism of continued chronic pain, even with known original acute pain from peripheral organic tissue damage, that of the *centralist*.[5,13,17] The centralist holds that although the original nociceptive input may have started the sequential chain of events, as the pain becomes more chronic and more central (in both the psychologic and neurophysiologic sense) a point is reached in many patients at which there is no longer any evidence or reason to assume there is continued peripheral nociceptive input from the original tissue damage that initiated the pain. Therefore continued nociceptive input is no longer related to the continuation of the pain syndrome of such patients. This is a possibility, even though subsequent input (often nonnociceptive, such as proprioceptive input from weight bearing or from movement of a limb or pressure on the scar in a previously injured area) may increase the patient's subjectively felt pain. It is believed that subsequent input can potentiate the pain centrally but that the underlying pain (which in most chronic pain syndromes often becomes constant) is probably now neurophysiologically entirely central in its generation. Thus in any attempt to block peripheral nerves in chronic pain, probably the only chance of temporary success lies in a placebo response. In many circumstances and in many patients the placebo effect may be far greater than the usually assigned one-third that has been recognized as the average. If, because of a hyperactive neurophysiologic central mechanism, chronic pain continues, it is extremely difficult to study experimentally and even to discuss. Once again I fall back on psychologic terminology and state that the individual patient's continued pain probably represents a learned response to an "unconscious need" to continue the hurt. Although I believe this view of chronic pain is as close to fact for most chronic patients as I can presently formulate, it is admittedly not acceptable to the patient himself, or to most physicians. Medical training stresses the acute pain organic medical model, wherein pain is conceptualized as resulting from present and continuing nociceptive input from damaged tissue. However, these two contending conceptualizations point out the fact that, regardless of which hypothetical model of chronic pain is believed to be nearer the truth, the treatment of chronic pain largely involves working with the patient's central mechanisms. Whether this is by a placebo response (maximizing suggestion), by sedation (tranquilization), or, as many patients hope, by reeducation [using visual or verbal language (or symbolic inputs) to reprogram the central computer (often referred to as psychotherapy)], it means that the physician treating the patient with chronic pain must function in a supportive role, more as a psychiatrist than as an emergency room surgeon.

Discussion of these conceptualizations is warranted because many patients demonstrate both continuing acute nociceptive input and central factors in their complaint of chronic pain. Only a small percentage of patients seen in anyone's medical practice develops the chronic benign intractable pain syndrome that is entirely central.

It is difficult to respond with a centralist orientation to a patient with chronic pain who is actively seeking help. This is largely because such a patient most often appears to join forces with and respond positively to an activist physician trained with a peripheralist orientation. The latter's position is reinforced if he interacts only briefly with such a patient (i.e., in the emergency room situation). If a physician also treats patients with a chronic pain syndrome over time, many patients continue to respond to periodic changes in combinations of invasive procedures (i.e., nerve blocks) and analgesic medications. It often seems that the continuation of this type of patient–physician relationship maintains an ebb and flow within a given status quo under these circumstances as long as the physician's tolerance level to patient demands and manipulations is not exceeded. Thus, over the short term, one often can discern no differences in results between a peripheralist and centralist approach to the treatment of patients with chronic pain. Both approaches usually include placebos, sedatives, tranquilizers, or listening and counseling. Some physicians even include nerve block procedures as a placebo or a break in the "vicious cycle of pain." In this regard it is also important to remember the extremely effective placebo effect of surgical procedures.

Let us now consider the six groups in the time classification listed under "Temporal Classification of Pain Complaints." However, this needs to be done in the context of whether the physician is treating outpatients in a hospital emergency room or in private office practice. The treatment of a patient complaining of pain may vary according to the treatment location (see Fig. 12-1). Since this chapter discusses only ambulatory outpatient treatment, no attempt will be made to explain in depth any of the treatments for pain performed in a hospital on an inpatient basis. Furthermore, although ambulatory surgery in hospital-based or free-standing "surgicenters" has increased dramatically in recent years (usually because of cost savings[27]), the treatment of acute pain remains largely based in the ER (or cause for hospital admittance). Chronic pain in general *never* requires surgical intervention. Causalgia requiring sympathectomy, trigeminal neuralgia requiring operative intervention when anticonvulsants fail, and pain from cancer with indications for surgical pain-relieving procedures are all *not* chronic pain syndromes. These surgeries (except for percutaneous

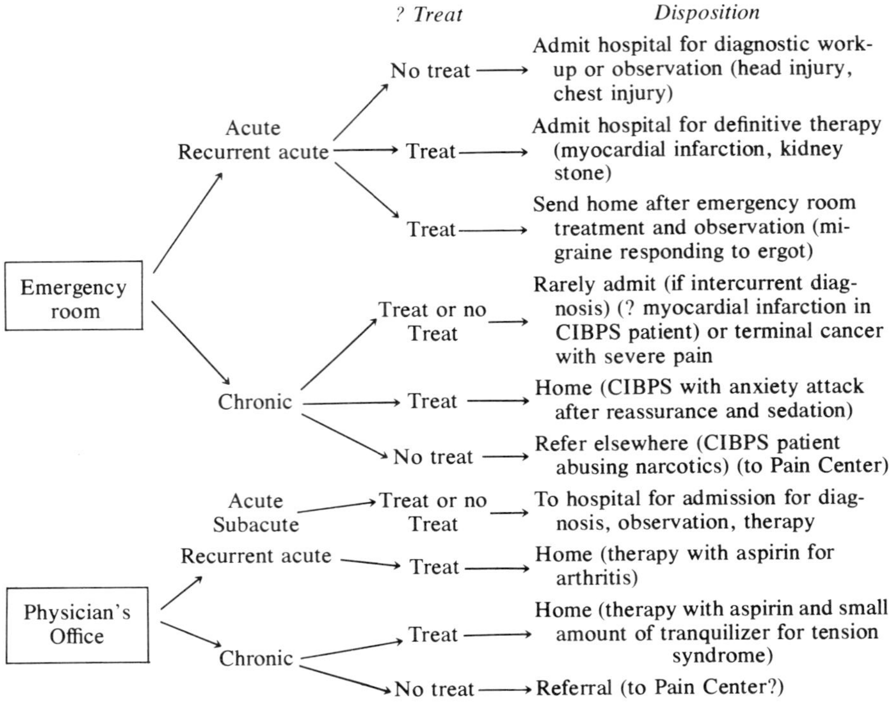

Figure 12-1. Treatment logistics: Outpatient, inpatient, or home.

chordotomy, for example) usually still require hospital admission. We are thus discussing here disposition in the ER versus the physician's private office. In each instance a decision has to be made about whether to treat the pain and, if it is to be treated, whether to do so on an outpatient or inpatient basis.

If treatment is not undertaken by the physician (either in his office or in an emergency room), disposition of the case must be made. Fortunately, in most circumstances it remains possible for an individual physician (in a nonemergency situation) to decline to accept any patient for treatment. This is especially important in patients with a chronic pain syndrome. However, there are many situations in which, particularly with a patient in severe pain, the physician is under considerable pressure to instigate treatment. If treatment is to be continued by someone else, some type of referral must be made, either back to the patient's regular physician (who may have been unavailable) or to someone else (either within the community or within the hospital if admission is indicated). Simple as this may sound, it is often extremely difficult with patients whose pain is due to an undetermined cause or whose interactional behaviors are demanding or manipulative without signs of specific acute illness. This is made more difficult when there is a history of chronic pain with many unsuccessful treatment attempts with many previous physicians and when a clearly diagnosable chronic intractable benign pain syndrome is present. Few physicians are willing to accept, or skillful enough to treat, such a patient with chronic pain. Therefore referral to a comprehensive pain center, which by definition means that it accepts patients with chronic pain syndromes,[8,17,19] should be considered.

Besides the individual qualifications and desires of the physician seeing a patient with a complaint of pain, either in private practice or in the emergency room, there are often overriding local ground rules that may limit his choices. For example, some physicians working in emergency rooms are limited to truly emergency situations or at most one or two follow-up visits. Other physicians may have the concurrence of their parent institution to utilize the emergency room as an intake for their own medical practice and can accept patients to whom they intend to continue giving necessary ambulatory care. Some emergency room physicians also continue to follow the patient after hospital admission.

SYNDROMES BY DURATION OF PAIN

ACUTE PAIN

It must be stated at the outset that there is often no relation between the severity of the patient's complaint of pain, even acute pain, and the significance of the underlying etiologic tissue disorder.[23] It is true that both the severity and the type of pain are often clues to diagnosis (e.g., sudden severe pain over the costovertebral angle in a male with known tendency for gout certainly fits a diagnosis of renal calculus). But even awesomely severe pain is not an immediate threat to the life of the individual, although, understandably, the patient may demand prompt medication for pain relief. However, there often does appear to be some correlation between the severity of the pain in myocardial infarction and the extent of the damage to the heart muscle, but this correlation is far from absolute, because many life-threatening and extensive myocardial infarcts occur in individuals who report only minor pain.

After recent trauma some generalizations about acute pain may be useful. For example, although it may sound cynical, after many years of observing patients in the emergency room (after they have been involved in an automobile or motorcycle accident and complain that they cannot move their lower extremities) in whom a fracture of the lumbar or thoracic spine with paraplegia is suspected, it is almost always valid to assume that the severity of the injury is inversely proportional to the loudness of the complaint of pain. One might expect pain with severe tissue damage (e.g., where the spine is injured and the legs organically paralyzed), with all the implications of future disability and a life of paraplegia that this carries. However, it is rare to see patients under these circumstances (even with no other injuries) complain too loudly of pain or even display much obvious fear or anxiety. In contrast, a patient with a more minor fall who is brought in complaining of inability to move his legs often complains loudly of severe pain and exhibits severe anxiety. Often, of course, in the latter situation, the reflexes are maintained; it further helps in diagnosis when the roentgenograms show no fracture and the patient, in spite of anxiety, can be distracted easily. Such a patient may show inappropriate smiling or laughter and aid in establishing the diagnosis of a conversion reaction, astasia-abasia. The same is generally true of many severe fractures in which, for a varying time, there is often little immediate pain. Obviously, this can in no way relate to patients with severe head injury and often a concomitant decrease in mental awareness.

It must always be remembered that in acute pain, even with obvious peripheral etiologic damage, as the patient is under observation for an increasing time, analgesics may not continue to bring sufficient pain relief. The inevitable fear may increase the anxiety to the point that treatment of the pain is not simply a matter of analgesics or narcotics but one of reassurance and short-term use of sedation or tranquilization. Valium on occasion works far better than more Demerol.

The underlying diagnosis in patients with acute pain often dictates the treatment of the pain. For example, a patient with moderate to severe chest pain who is believed to have a myocardial infarct requires prompt supportive measures and further diagnostic work-up as well as prompt judicious use of narcotics to relieve the pain. However, sometimes therapy to control the pain totally may not be indicated. For example, in severe chest injury where pain is acute, it is often not in the patient's best interest to give narcotics until the thoracic surgeon has had a chance to evaluate the status of the patient, because they may cause some respiratory depression. This may confuse the diagnosis and complicate the subsequent treatment. Often it takes considerable expertise and patience on the part of the emergency room physician to convince both the patient and his family that postponing pain relief is in the patient's best interest. This has to be done skillfully to prevent increasing anxiety and even frank hostility.

In general, however, physicians tend to undertreat acute pain. This is true not only in physician's offices and emergency rooms but also in intensive care units and in postoperative recovery rooms.[11] Unfortunately, it is also true in treatment of pain due to terminal cancer. In general, narcotics are often underutilized and ordered by the physician either in suboptimal doses or on an as-needed basis, with too much time between doses (which may be compounded further by the nurse's timidity in administering narcotics because she has been educated about their unwarranted side-effects and the possibility of addiction). This problem stands in stark contrast to the overutilization of medicines such as narcotics in chronic benign pain syndromes.

Although little research substantiates the clinical impression, in severe acute pain the body's chemistry is often such that the expected deleterious reactions from narcotics are seldom seen or are not major problems. However, the phenomenon of additive narcotic effect must be guarded against when narcotics have been repeated while the patient was in shock and must be looked for as treatment corrects the hypovolemia.

Narcotics are seldom needed for pain resulting from head injury and must be used sparingly when a patient has painful traumas in addition to a significant blow to the head. Narcotics may confuse subsequent clinical observation after head trauma. This is due largely to two factors: (1) Increasing lethargy may signal a normal reaction to morphine, for example, or it may be a clue to an enlarging intracranial hematoma. (2) Subsequent vomiting may represent an idiosyncratic drug reaction, or it may be a sign of increasing intracranial pressure.

SUBACUTE PAIN

The discussion of treatment of subacute pain can be brief. In general, if the patient comes to a physician a few days to a few months after the pain has started, there is an increasing likelihood that the diagnosis will be obscure. There is also a relatively good chance that the severity of the pain will be moderate, because more severe pain usually brings the patient to the emergency room or the physician's office much sooner. Although subacute pain is not often a true emergency, treatment is usually similar to that for acute pain. However, certain treatment rules of thumb can be applied with some correlation to subsequent results. For example, acute pain after soft-tissue injury is often treated by cold (i.e., the application of ice), whereas subacute pain from a soft-tissue injury of a few days' duration is more apt to respond to heat.

Again it must be emphasized that one should find out why the patient delayed in coming to the physician, unless the patient clearly describes a pain that started with much less severity and gradually (and perhaps intermittently) increased in severity or duration, ultimately becoming unbearable (often at 2:00 A.M., as sensory input from distractions around the patient decrease to a minimum and anxiety and lonesomeness take over). For example, the guilt, shame, and fear that often follow rage may be noted, along with some delay in seeking medical help, in the syndrome of the battered child or abused wife, and must also be kept in mind. Fearfulness about an impending serious illness often results in a temporary denial of pain.

RECURRENT ACUTE PAIN

Many pain syndromes labeled as chronic are in reality recurrent acute pain, although this state may have been present over many years. Often these are pain syndromes in which the underlying etiology is not known. Typical examples are migraine headaches or tic douloureux (primary trigeminal neuralgia). The treatment of recurrent acute pain is often directed, as in acute pain, to the underlying peripheral causative condition when it is known. For example, rheumatoid arthritis with recurrent flare-ups, increasing pain, and stiffness, redness, warmth, and swelling of the joints is not so much a matter of treating pain as of treating the underlying organic condition. At times the treatment of both can be combined, that is, by the use of aspirin, which apparently acts on both the inflammation of arthritis and the pain, rather than by the use of corticosteroids. Recurrent acute pain also often occurs in osteoarthritis. Often pain is a symptom secondary to degenerative arthritis of the cervical or lumbar spine in which any unusual or prolonged extra activity may again result in increased pain. Although recognition of the chronic underlying osteoarthritic condition is necessary and may lead to the proper diagnosis, it is treated in general like any acute or subacute pain syndrome. But it must be remembered that as some patients have recurrent acute pain (e.g., from underlying chronic osteoarthritis), over time they are also apt to develop central psychological mechanisms that can lead them to abuse drugs, to become manipulative and demanding, or to have a reactive depression. These patients have then developed a secondary or superimposed true chronic intractable benign pain syndrome also.

ONGOING PAIN DUE TO UNCONTROLLED MALIGNANT NEOPLASM

Although ongoing pain resulting from uncontrolled malignant neoplasm is most often treated in the hospital or by the physician in the patient's home (or in more recent years in so-called convalescent homes, which are more apt to be houses for terminal care, very few of which adhere to the hospice concepts), it is also being seen more often in the older population in the physician's office and especially in hospital emergency rooms. There can be little doubt that patients with underlying pain due to cancer (when treatment by surgery, radiation, chemotherapy, or immunotherapy has failed to halt the spread of the disease or to bring relief from the pain syndrome) do require compassionate, skillful, understanding management.

Often the cancer patient's pain is undertreated. When the cancer is truly preterminal there is no humane reason to undermedicate. The possibility of creating drug dependence or addiction ought not to be a consideration, as has been so well pointed out by McCaffery.[24] However, some patients approaching death do become anxious or depressed. If their lives are prolonged by such medical agents as chemotherapy, they may indeed also develop central chronic pain mechanisms that are secondary psychological mechanisms. They may occasionally abuse, or at least misuse, not only narcotics and analgesics, but especially tranquilizers such as diazepam (Valium). But this is relatively rare and is a short-range problem because of the primary disease. Furthermore, the truly terminally ill cancer patient with pain is not often ambulatory; most of these patients are confined to bed or at least to home if there is significant severe pain.

From a physiologic standpoint, advancing cancer pain is rarely a chronic, constant pain; it is more apt to be classifiable as a recurrent acute pain. There is known disease peripherally, which is increasing as the tumor invades and in fact becomes a series of new peripheral tissue insults. This is in accord with our assumptions regarding underlying advancement of tumor (often involving invasion of the perineurium of the peripheral nerves or plexi). Often the cancer patient has periods of relief from acute pain. Moreover, his pain frequently can be well controlled by both intermittent mild tranquilization for the anxiety and antidepressants for the depression, along with analgesics. When oral narcotics finally become necessary, I prefer oxycodone (Percodan or Percocet-5). Most patients can be taken almost to death's door before they need to be switched to methadone.[18] Parenteral narcotics are usually used only for the last few days and are often not used at all. If they are needed to control pain, then the question of intravenous setups and prolongation of needless suffering becomes an individual philosophical, ethical, and legal question that cannot be discussed here. At times neurosurgical procedures for relief are indicated.[6,9,26,34] From a physiologic standpoint, cancer pain can be considered as being due to continuing nociceptive input, with the central mechanisms and psychologic potentiation usually being a secondary but increasingly important factor and the fear of impending death compounding the situation in many patients.

CHRONIC BENIGN (NONNEOPLASTIC) PAIN WITH WHICH THE PATIENT APPEARS TO BE ADEQUATELY COPING

Pain is often intermittent. It may be due to some originally known underlying chronic condition (such as arthritis), but may last so long, or become so common a complaint, that the patient must be considered to have chronic pain. However, the important thing is that the patient adapts adequately most of the time. Frequently, he may still be working or, if older and retired, may still be spending many hours outside of his home enjoying life. In fact, there are many uncounted chronic pain patients in this category who never seek medical care. This group may help to account for the large amount of analgesics sold without prescription over drugstore counters. We have no true epidemiologic information concerning this type of chronic pain. These are the patients who usually do not require referral to pain centers and only occasionally come to the physician's office for help. They are very rarely seen in emergency rooms, perhaps in the small hours of the night or on weekends, when their own physician may be out of town. In many ways these patients can also be treated as having acute pain problems, but several factors must be kept in mind. Since many such patients do have a history of underlying chronic conditions that have led to their present complaint of pain, if possible they should not be given narcotics, because there is a potential for future drug abuse. Furthermore, a thorough evaluation must be done in each case to see that the underlying condition is receiving adequate medical treatment and has been diagnosed accurately in the past. Furthermore, with this patient more often than in any other, the rule that we as physicians should always look first for a single cause as the etiologic agent underlying patients' complaints is probably insufficient. For example, many patients have been coping well with chronic underlying osteoarthritis and some recurrent acute pain. When new pain comes along, it is often self-diagnosed as an exacerbation of the underlying condition. In fact, it may well be due to an unsuspected second cause and may require entirely different treatment. Therefore when a patient with a known chronic pain syndrome reappears with exacerbation of pain, time has to be taken, if the consulted physician is going to be responsible for that patient's treatment, to ascertain that this is indeed a pain problem related to the previous chronic condition and not a new intercurrent problem. This should be the case even in a busy physician's practice or in an emergency room.

CHRONIC INTRACTABLE BENIGN PAIN SYNDROME

The chronic intractable benign pain syndrome, although it may involve only a small percentage of the patients with pain seen in any physician's office or in the emergency room, represents a disproportionately large problem with regard to diagnosis, patient care, and disposition. The patient with this syndrome is often at the end stage of an evolving process that began with a previous acute injury and that has long since healed, but for some reason the patient's central nervous system has been unable to "turn off" the pain. This very rarely, if ever, represents any continued nociceptive input (in the acute pain model) from an improperly healed injury or from the subsequent scarring process. The central internuncial connections may be physiologically hypersensitized by deafferentation from the area that was injured (where there may now be a lack of normal sensory input). However, from a practical standpoint the patient with a chronic intractable benign pain syndrome who is unable to cope usually demonstrates a tremendous "potentiation from above" in the form of psychologic need to continue with his pain syndrome.[28] This is usually entirely at an unconscious level. Consequently, from a moral as well as a medical aspect this patient has pain, just as he states that he has. At times, if there is much of a conversion reaction (hysterical component), it seems almost unbelievable to the medical observer that the patient can be unaware of this potentiation mechanism, which often appears to others to be so superficial. Although it certainly behooves every physician to be cautious of being lied to by a malingerer or sociopath, most patients with chronic pain who go so far as to seek treatment, if they are not frank drug addicts, have totally unconscious mechanisms that continue their pain syndrome.

As time passes and the patient's pain becomes more and more constant, the chronic pain syndrome may take over his entire existence and become the center of his life. He then fails to cope, loses his job, may spend more and more time in bed, often antagonizes his spouse or significant other, and becomes an abuser of drugs—including alcohol, tranquilizers, or narcotics—until he often becomes a totally demanding, highly manipulative patient who is unwanted and unloved by most members of society, including the physicians he seeks out, still hoping to be cured. It would be wonderful to be able to give some easy or even satisfactory way to treat such patients on an ambulatory basis. Frankly, it has been my experience that this is impossible. It is also nice to theorize that with the proper previous management of acute, subacute, or recurrent acute pain problems in the physician's office or emergency rooms and with the concurrent help of the patient, his family, and other support structures in society, it might be possible to prevent the formation of what appears to be an ever-increasing number of patients with a chronic benign pain syndrome. However, we do not at present have adequate evidence to support this possibility. Instead it appears that many of our laws and workmen's compensation remuneration practices may have evolved in such a way that, along with our court systems for personal injury, they really intensify the chronic pain problem.[2,3]

At the present time chronic pain is one of the most catastrophic problems in American society and is a medical problem that has been neglected by many in both our medical profession and our health care delivery system.[3,14] The cost of medical care, pharmaceuticals, hospitalization, lost wages, disability awards, ongoing medical retirement payments, and litigation awards in the 50 states each year now totals between $80 and $90 billion. Most such patients are not treatable in a physician's office or in an emergency room and should be referred to pain centers that specialize in such individuals.[5,12] Whether this can be accomplished in a significant percentage of patients when secondary gain is involved (such as litigation or workmen's compensation proceedings that have not been settled) is still a matter for study. However, the local doctor can still assist in pain rehabilitation in the following ways:

If the patient with a noncancer chronic pain problem seeks medical help before pain center rehabilitation, the physician should be careful not to contribute to another case of drug dependence or abuse, especially with narcotics; the patient should be referred to a pain center.

If after rehabilitation attempts in a pain center have been concluded the patient returns to the care of his local physician, a cooperative effort should be undertaken jointly between the physicians at the pain center and the patient's treating physician.

The second point is easy to write about but extremely difficult for the individual physician. For example, often a young surgeon managing a hospital emergency room at night is confronted by a patient who comes in complaining loudly of intractable pain for which he insists he must have his Valium prescription renewed and a Demerol injection on the spot. All that can usually be accomplished under these circumstances is to withhold narcotics, counsel the patient (and it is hoped his more understanding and accepting family), and refer the patient back to either the treating physician or the pain center. Chronic pain of this type is a multifaceted, idiosyncratic, continuing problem for which there is no easy solution.

REFERENCES

1. Aronoff GM (ed): Evaluation and Treatment of Chronic Pain. Baltimore, Urban & Schwarzenberg, 1984
2. Aronoff GM (ed): Pain Centers in the USA—A Revolution in Health Care. New York, Raven Press (in press)
3. Brena S: Chronic Pain—America's Hidden Epidemic. New York, Atheneum/SMI, 1978
4. Brena SF, Chapman SL: Management of Patients With Chronic Pain. New York, Spectrum, 1983
5. Brena SF, Crue BL, Stieg RL: Comments on the classification of chronic pain: Its clinical significance. Bull Clin Neurosci 49:67, 1984
6. Crue, BL (ed): Pain and Suffering—Selected Aspects. Springfield, IL, Charles C Thomas, 1970
7. Crue, BL (ed): Pain—Research and Treatment. New York, Academic Press, 1975
8. Crue BL, Pinsky JJ, Agnew DC et al: What is a pain center? Bull Los Angeles Neurol Soc 41:160, 1976
9. Crue BL (ed): Chronic Pain—Further Observations. New York, Spectrum, 1979
10. Crue BL: A physiological view of the psychology of pain. Bull Los Angeles Neurol Soc 44:1, 1979
11. Crue BL: Severe chronic postoperative pain. JAMA 246:164, 1981
12. Crue BL, Pinsky JJ: Chronic pain syndrome—Four aspects of the problem. New Approaches to Treatment of Chronic Pain Research #36, Monograph Sem., National Institute of Drug Abuse, May 1981
13. Crue BL: The centralist concept of chronic pain. Semin Neurol 3:331, 1983
14. Crue BL, Chronic pain and narcotic therapy. JAMA 249:292, 1983
15. Crue BL, Pinsky JJ: An approach to chronic pain of nonmalignant origin. Postgrad Med J 60:30, 1984
16. Crue BL: Foreword. In Aronoff GM (ed): Evaluation and Treatment of Chronic Pain. Baltimore, Urban & Schwarzenberg, 1984
17. Crue BL: Multidisciplinary pain treatment programs—Current status. J Clin Pain 1:31, 1985
18. Crue BL: Treatment of patients with pain due to cancer. In Gross SC, Garb S (eds): Cancer Treatment and Research in Humanistic Perspective. New York, Springer-Verlag, 1985
19. Ghia JN (ed): Organization of Pain Clinics and Function of Personnel, Boston, Martinus Nerhaus (in press)
20. Hill GJ: Excruciating pain. In Hill GH II (ed): Outpatient Surgery. Philadelphia, WB Saunders, 1973
21. Kruger L, Liebeskind JC (eds): Neural Mecha-

nisms of Pain: Advances in Pain Research and Therapy, Vol. 6. New York, Raven Press, 1984
22. Lewis T: Pain. New York, Macmillan, 1942
23. Lim KS: Pharmacologic viewpoint of pain and analgesia. In Way EL (ed): New Concepts in Pain and Its Clinical Management. Philadelphia, FA Davis, 1967
24. McCaffery M: Nursing Management of the Patient With Pain. Philadelphia, JB Lippincott, 1972
25. Merskey H, Spear FG: Pain: Psychological and Psychiatric Aspects. London, Bailliere, Tindall, Cassell, 1967
26. Nashold B, Crue BL: Stereotaxic mesencephalic trigeminal tractotomy. In Youman (ed): Neurosurgery, 2nd ed. Philadelphia, WB Saunders, 1982
27. Nordberg M: Ambulatory surgery—The suture of the future? Options for Physicians in Transition 1:8, 1986
28. Pinsky JJ: Chronic, intractable, benign pain: A syndrome and its treatment with intensive short-term group psychotherapy. J Human Stress 4:17, 1978
29. Pinsky JJ, Crue BL: Intensive group psychotherapy. In Wall PD, Melzack R (eds): Textbook of Pain. New York, Churchill Livingstone, 1984
30. Smith WL, Merskey H, Gross SG: Pain—Meaning and Management. New York, Spectrum, 1980
31. Sternbach RA: Pain: A Psychophysiological Analysis. New York, Academic Press, 1968
32. Sternbach, RA: Pain Patients—Traits and Treatment. New York, Academic Press, 1974
33. Sternbach RA (ed): The Psychology of Pain. New York, Raven Press, 1978
34. White, JC, Sweet WH: Pain and the Neurosurgeon: A Forty-Year Experience. Springfield, IL, Charles C Thomas, 1969

13 Ambulatory Pediatric Surgery

DALE G. JOHNSON AND MICHAEL E. MATLAK

The general approach to the pediatric patient requiring ambulatory surgery differs significantly from that for the adult. The child's fears and anxieties may mask or exaggerate physical findings. Rapport is often difficult or impossible to establish, especially when parental apprehension is detected by the child. The general appearance of the child should be carefully observed while a careful history is obtained from a responsible adult or parent. As a child witnesses the communication between his parents and the physician he usually senses that the physician is deeply interested in his overall welfare. Most children appreciate simple but honest explanations regarding the physical examination and the required therapy. The child should be forewarned of painful procedures and simply told that it is acceptable to cry but unacceptable to move during these maneuvers. It is surprising how often children will follow these simple commands.

Children between 18 months and 3 years of age may not be willing to cooperate during a surgical procedure or an uncomfortable examination. Proper restraint of such a child with a folded sheet or a restraining board is invaluable (Figs. 13-1 and 13-2). The psychological trauma is quickly forgotten, especially when the surgical result is satisfactory.

At our institution pediatric anesthesiologists are always available to assist us when appropriate with ambulatory surgical procedures. During a recent 4-year interval, more than 16,000 children who were low-risk candidates underwent a general anesthesia without a serious complication. Whenever possible, then, our bias is to perform most outpatient procedures in the operating room, but we recognize that this policy is not practical in every situation.

FOREIGN BODIES

Infants and children put small objects of all descriptions into a variety of body cavities, and not infrequently these objects are either aspirated or ingested. The population at risk includes children between 9 months and 3 years of age and the mentally handicapped child. Foreign body aspiration or ingestion is a major cause of accidental death in childhood.

FOREIGN BODIES OF THE AIRWAY

Most foreign objects that reach the airway are either coughed out or passed through the glottis into the trachea. Sometimes aspirated material becomes lodged in the glottic region, however, resulting in an immediate threat to life. Objects most commonly reported to cause suffocation include hot dogs, nuts, grapes, round candy, chunks of apple, marbles, pacifiers, rattles, balls, and other material. Children with a laryngeal foreign body generally present with either partial or complete airway obstruction. Both groups require expeditious therapy to prevent asphyxiation.

Children with partial airway obstruction may have compromised but adequate air exchange. The child is able to breathe, cough effectively, and make sounds. Hoarseness and stridor are usually present. Encourage the youngster to breathe slowly and remain calm. A cooperative patient may be instructed to take a deep breath and cough vigorously to expel the object. Methods that induce an artificial cough are potentially dangerous unless the obstruction becomes complete. Any maneuvers that will agitate the child should be avoided. Supplemental oxygen is usually helpful. Most authorities prefer to prepare these children quickly for the operating room,

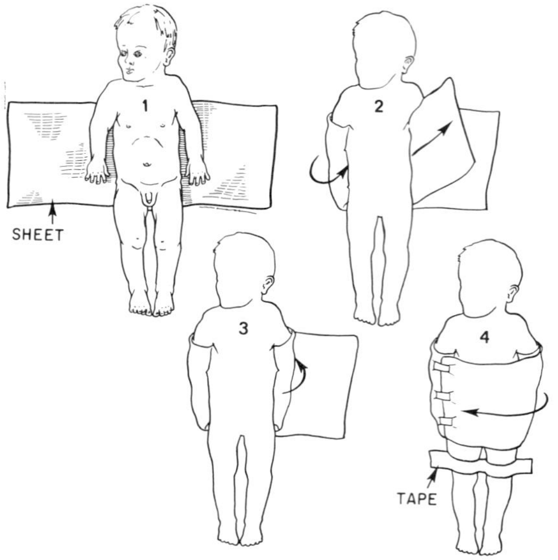

Figure 13-1. To restrain a child for a surgical procedure the child is placed on a heavy folded sheet, which is then passed around the arms and torso as shown sequentially. Two-inch tape across the torso and above the knees helps ensure proper restraint.

where direct laryngoscopy and tracheoscopy are performed. If time permits, radiographs of the neck may be helpful in determining the exact nature and location of the foreign body. A successful outcome requires expert management by the anesthesiologist and endoscopist.

A child with complete or nearly complete airway obstruction has inadequate ventilation. If a cough is present, it is ineffective. Stridor may still be present, but usually the child is unable to make sounds. Cyanosis indicates the immediate need for treatment. The guidelines for the first aid of the choking child were recently revised. The abdominal thrust—the Heimlich maneuver—is now recommended as the exclusive method of treating foreign body airway obstruction for children older than 1 year. Six to ten abdominal thrusts are applied until the foreign body is expelled. In infants, a series of back blows and chest thrusts is recommended. The Heimlich maneuver is not advised during infancy because of the potential for injury to the abdominal organs. In the hospital setting alternative therapy includes direct laryngoscopy or a cricothyroidotomy. Fortunately, the annual number of deaths due to choking has fallen from 600 to 170 over the past decade.

The majority of foreign bodies in the upper airway pass through the trachea into one of the bronchi or bronchial segments. The typical situation involves a child who starts choking and coughing with a mouthful of peanuts. The child may have a violent coughing spasm and some cyanosis and then appear to recover. The parents often ignore this situation for a few days until persistence of coughing or a rattle in the chest promotes medical consultation. A single chest film taken at this time is often normal, and a common error is to discharge the patient without bronchoscopy. Sequential inspiration and expiration films or chest fluoroscopy will usually show some air trapping in the expiration film on the side of

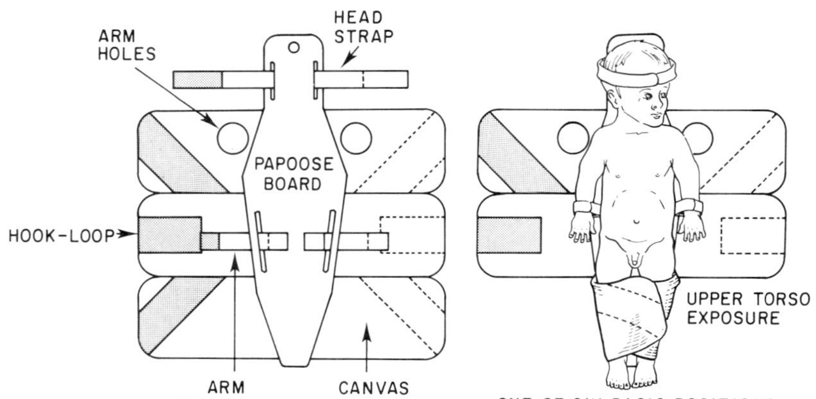

Figure 13-2. Many types of restraint boards are available. For a "papoose board" the canvas flaps are covered with Velcro, thus allowing easy application and removal. The boards are quite versatile and offer many advantages over restraint with a folded sheet.

the foreign body (Fig. 13-3). Most foreign bodies aspirated into the airway are not radiopaque. If the foreign object has been present in the airway for some time and has produced total occlusion of a bronchial segment, the roentgenogram will show atelectasis and a shift of the mediastinum toward the foreign body, rather than air trapping and a shift away from the foreign body, as is the case with partial obstruction. If the foreign body is small and moves around within the airway, the inspiration–expiration films and even chest fluoroscopy may be normal. It is most important to remember that a clear history of aspiration, signified by a choking episode, and subsequent persistence of any respiratory symptoms mandates endoscopic evaluation of the airway. It is not at all uncommon at endoscopy to find peanut fragments in the airway of a child with normal radiographic evaluation.

Although aspirated peanuts are the most common airway foreign body in our society, children aspirate a variety of other objects. Accidental inspiration of a pea from a peashooter is not uncommon, and we have removed rocks, dried potato, beans that have been in the lung sufficiently long to develop a sprout, chalk, glass beads, ball-point-pen tops, pins, needles, Christmas tree ornaments, carrots, seeds, and a long list of strange objects infants and children explore with their mouth. Occasionally, small objects such as a carrot fragment or a foreign body that does not swell and cause a lot of reaction in the airway can be expelled by chest physiotherapy if this is instituted promptly. The method is uncertain, and only an exceptional child successfully expels the foreign body. Furthermore, there is the danger of dislodging the object into the subglottic region, where it can obstruct the airway completely.

Endoscopic evaluation of all bronchial segments and subsegments is the safest procedure to avoid a retained foreign body and subsequent lung infection and destruction. The history of initial aspiration and the persistence of symptoms are the most important factors in deciding on bronchoscopy in the child. The presence of atelectasis or air trapping on a roentgenogram makes endoscopy mandatory.

Newer endoscopic equipment provides a magnified view with sharp resolution of the deep bronchial segmental anatomy, and diagnostic evaluation and foreign-body extraction can be done with safety and precision. Following endoscopy, short-term observation in the hospital is advised to watch for respiratory distress secondary to edema of the airway.

FOREIGN BODIES IN THE NOSE AND EARS

Foreign bodies in the nose and ears are also common in small children. Crayons, chalk, beans, dried peas, and buttons seem to be favorite objects to hide in these locations.

Foreign bodies of the ear typically present with pain and persistent purulent drainage from one ear despite antibiotic therapy. Prior to instrumentation, mild sedation or topical anesthesia may be useful in decreasing pain. If the child cannot cooperate, evaluation under anesthesia is safer than risking a perforated eardrum. The foreign object is easily seen unless obscured by pus. Suctioning is done gently to avoid bleeding or deeper impaction. Small alligator forceps, a cerumen curette, or

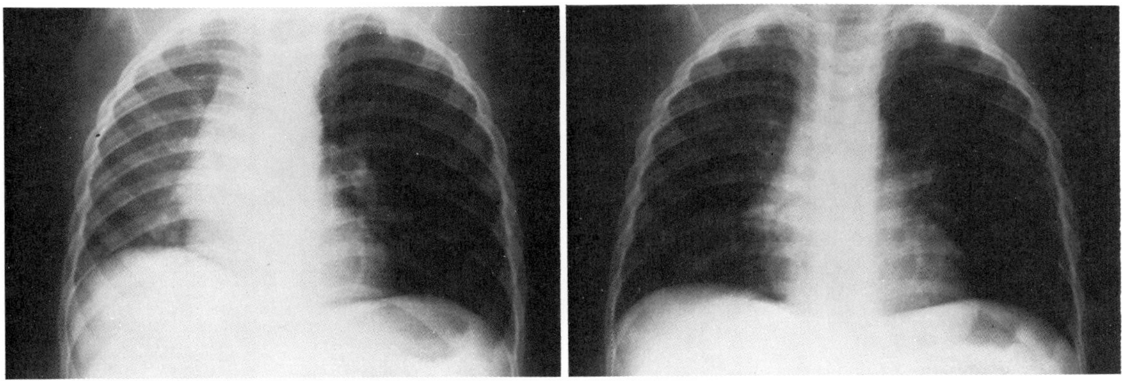

Figure 13-3. The left main stem bronchus is partially obstructed by a fragment of a peanut. The expiratory film on the left demonstrates air trapping and a shift of the mediastinum away from the foreign body.

angled hooks can be used for removal. Irrigation with warm water may deliver the object, but this should not be done with a history of a perforated tympanic membrane or if blood is present in the ear canal. Live insects should be killed before removal by filling the ear canal for several minutes with mineral oil, alcohol, or lidocaine.

Nasal foreign bodies present with persistent, foul-smelling, unilateral nasal discharge. Topical anesthetics (lidocaine or cocaine) permit a more complete evaluation and safer removal. The foreign object is usually located beneath the middle turbinate, where it can be grasped with a forceps, hooked with a curved probe, or extracted with a small balloon-tipped catheter. The object should not be pushed into the posterior nasopharynx because removal is more difficult and there is danger of aspiration. The child is placed on antibiotics and carefully followed to make certain that sinusitis does not develop.

FOREIGN BODIES IN THE GASTROINTESTINAL TRACT

The majority of ingested foreign bodies pass uneventfully through the digestive tract. The most dangerous site for lodgement is the esophagus. The child is in constant danger of aspiration, asphyxiation, and perforation until the object is removed. A foreign body in the esophagus should be suspected when a child has been known to choke, gag, or cough while having something in his mouth. An asymptomatic interval is not unusual, and this does not necessarily imply that the object has been coughed out or passed into the stomach. Symptoms of esophageal obstruction include dysphagia, a change in eating habits, excessive salivation, regurgitation of food, substernal pain, a panicky suffocating sensation, or respiratory symptoms due to impingement of a large esophageal foreign body on the larynx or trachea. On occasion the first symptom is acute asphyxia with death or shock from erosion of the object through a major blood vessel.

Radiographic examination should include several projections of the neck and chest. These films may reveal the exact location and nature of the foreign body, the presence or absence of complications, and the presence of more than one foreign body. Radiopaque objects such as coins, safety pins, and pens are easily demonstrated, but a contrast medium may be necessary to identify semiopaque ob-

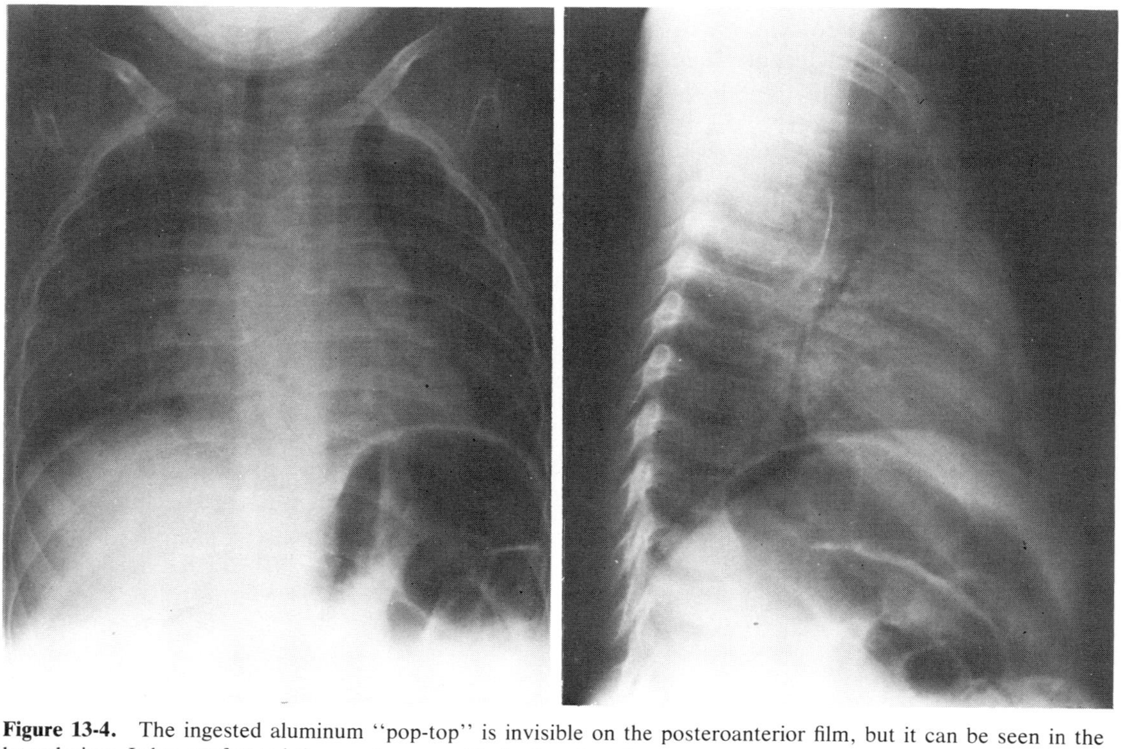

Figure 13-4. The ingested aluminum "pop-top" is invisible on the posteroanterior film, but it can be seen in the lateral view. It has perforated the esophagus and lodged against the aorta.

jects such as glass or bones or nonopaque objects.

Coins are the most common ingested foreign body in children. They become lodged in the cervical esophagus, and they rarely cause complications unless they are undetected or do not move for several weeks. Pork and chicken bones and other pointed foreign bodies such as safety pins and needles must be removed promptly to prevent perforation. Fish bones usually lodge in the pharynx or hypopharynx, and they can usually be removed with the help of topical anesthesia, a tongue blade, and hemostat. Parents should be cautioned that placement of an aluminum "pop top" into a soda can produces a dangerous situation. The presence of an aluminum pop top is easily overlooked unless a lateral roentgenogram of the chest is obtained (Fig. 13-4). Pop tops have been reported to obstruct, lacerate, or perforate the esophagus, resulting in traumatic tracheoesophageal fistulas, mediastinal abscess, or massive gastrointestinal hemorrhage from erosion of a major vessel. Fortunately, the incidence of this type of foreign body ingestion has decreased dramatically with the introduction of new safety tabs.

All foreign bodies in the esophagus must be removed. Watchful waiting is not indicated unless the child has had a completely normal roentgenographic examination.

Blunt, smooth, round, soft opaque, or nonopaque foreign bodies can be removed with a balloon-tipped catheter by an experienced radiologist (Fig. 13-5). Extraction by this method is safe, is inexpensive, and avoids general anesthesia and hospitalization. Pointed or sharp objects should never be removed by this technique, and one must be certain that a bone fragment is not present if the object is a piece of meat.

A rigid open esophagoscope is usually employed for endoscopic removal of esophageal foreign bodies. General anesthesia is required in children, and this may be particularly hazardous because of the danger of aspiration. The complications of retained esophageal foreign bodies include asphyxia, perforation with abscess formation, bleeding, hemopericardium and cardiac tamponade, endocarditis, tracheoesophageal fistula, esophageal obstruction and ulceration, and pulmonary disease.

Once in the stomach, the vast majority of ingested foreign bodies pass through the gastrointestinal tract without causing harm. Only rarely will a foreign body below the diaphragm result in perforation, obstruction, or bleeding. The usual treatment is watchful waiting, regular diet, and avoidance of cathartics. Most objects successfully navigate the gut in 3 or 4 days, but some require 3 to 4 weeks.

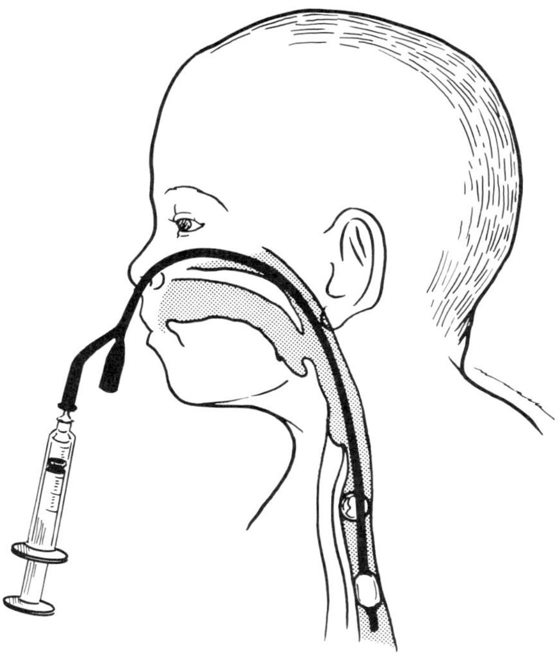

Figure 13-5. Removal of many esophageal foreign bodies can be done with a balloon-tipped catheter. First, the secretions above the object are aspirated. Then a balloon-tipped catheter is passed through the nose and beyond the foreign body. The balloon is filled with barium, and under fluoroscopic control the object is gently disimpacted, withdrawn, and coughed out.

Endoscopic removal from the stomach is suggested for long or sharp foreign bodies such as large open safety pins, brooches, nails, or bobby pins that are unlikely to negotiate the entire gut in a small child (Figure 13-6). As a general rule, an object 2 inches or longer in length in a 2-year-old will not pass through the intestine without significant risk of perforation. If endoscopic removal is unsuccessful or if the object has entered the small intestine, hospitalization is required and daily radiographs are performed. Exploratory laparotomy is indicated if complications develop, the object fails to change position daily, a toxic substance has been ingested, or a foreign body is too large or long to pass spontaneously.

A very worrisome ingested foreign body is a small alkaline battery. Leakage of highly caus-

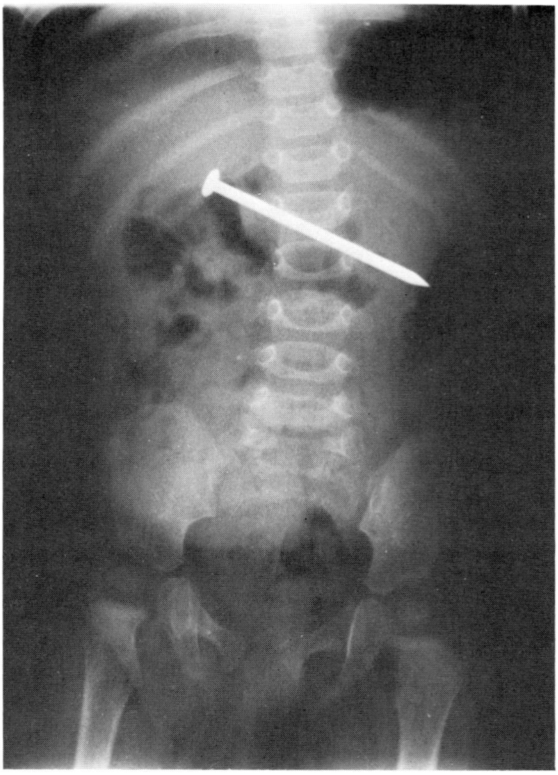

Figure 13-6. A long, sharp foreign body such as this nail in the stomach should be removed endoscopically.

tic lye may produce liquefaction necrosis and perforation. Fatalities have resulted from esophageal perforation. Batteries in the esophagus or stomach should be removed immediately. When the battery is in the stomach, a magnet attached to a catheter can be used to advance the object back into the esophagus. Balloon-tipped catheter extraction is then employed to complete the removal avoiding anesthesia and hospitalization. If these maneuvers fail, endoscopic removal is indicated.

VAGINAL FOREIGN BODIES

For some little girls the vagina is a favorite hiding place for small objects. The presence of a foreign body is often manifested by a foul discharge or odor from the vagina. Occasionally the foreign object can be detected by transrectal examination of the vagina, but often the foreign material is soft enough to elude detection by the finger in the rectum. Blind instrumentation of the vagina in a small child is traumatic and difficult without anesthesia. Light anesthesia for examination of the vagina with an infant cystoscope or nasal speculum is the most satisfactory way to determine the presence of a vaginal foreign body.

INGUINAL HERNIA

INCIDENCE

Excepting circumcision and tonsillectomy, repair of inguinal hernia is the most frequent operation performed on infants and children. The peak clinical appearance is in the first year of life, and more infants appear with hernias in the first 6 months than in the second. Inguinal hernias are eight to ten times more common in males than in females. Bilateral hernias are more commonly found in premature infants, in females, when the symptomatic hernia is on the left side, and in any child under 1 year of age.

EXAMINATION IN THE ABSENCE OF A GROIN MASS

The diagnosis of inguinal hernia must be made on direct evidence when a mass in the groin is not present. Male children are most easily examined for hernia in the supine position (Fig. 13-7), and the spermatic cord should be placed on tension by downward traction on the ipsilateral testicle. This is key to the examination. Otherwise it is possible for a casual examiner to confuse a coiled spermatic cord or a retracted or undescended testicle for a hernia. With the cord on tension, an attempt should be made to assess the size of the spermatic cord both in relation to the cord on the opposite side and in relation to the size of a normal cord for the child's age. The examiner's perception of normal, of course, is dependent on his own experience. If one spermatic cord is obviously much larger than the other, or much larger than one would expect for a normal child of the same age, it is presumed the cord "thickening" is due to a hernia sac on the anteromedial aspect of the normal cord structures.

The "silk glove sign," a slippery, silky sensation elicited when the cord is rolled under the examining finger, has been recommended for hernia diagnosis and is alleged to indicate the presence of two peritoneal surfaces sliding against each other in a hernia sac. This sign is not reliable, and the slippery sensation with

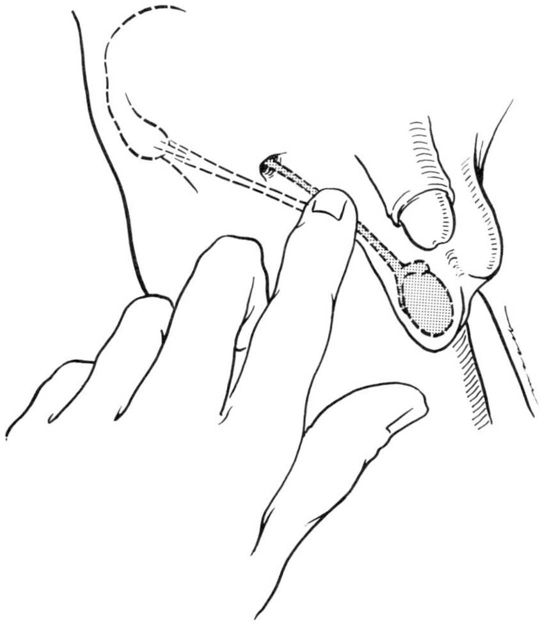

Figure 13-7. The spermatic cord can be rolled beneath the index finger just over the pubic tubercle while the testis is placed on traction to maintain tension. The presence of a hernia sac on the anteromedial aspect of the cord will give a sensation of increased cord volume.

cord palpation may be elicited with many normal children. Unequal or abnormal cord volume is a much more reliable presumptive sign of hernia, but even with this sign the diagnosis is only probable and not certain. If the examiner feels a tiny squirt of fluid pass into the peritoneal cavity as he palpates the cord at the internal ring, he has diagnosed a patent processus vaginalis but not necessarily a clinical hernia. The presence of bowel, omentum, ovary, or even uterus in a hernia sac establishes the diagnosis with certainty.

Small females with no mass in the groin are much more difficult to examine and to evaluate for the presence of hernia. Unlike the situation in males, the examiner may often find it useful to press gently on the female infant's abdomen to force fluid, bowel, or ovary through the internal ring. For the older child who can stand erect, it is helpful to stand behind her while exerting abdominal pressure downward. Simultaneous palpation of the inguinal canals is used to detect any change resulting from this abdominal pressure. If fluid or abdominal viscera are palpated in the inguinal canal, the diagnosis of hernia, of course, is confirmed.

EVALUATION OF A GROIN MASS

A "lump" that suddenly appears in the groin of a child should be evaluated on an emergency basis. Incarceration of bowel in a hernia is more common in small infants than in older children, and persistent incarceration not only jeopardizes the viability of the bowel but may also cause thrombosis of the adjacent testicular vessels and subsequent infarction of the testis. Infarction of an ovary incarcerated in a hernia is uncommon because the vascular pedicle of the ovary is small in relation to the internal inguinal ring that has allowed passage of the larger ovary. It is possible to develop secondary incarceration of bowel following incarceration of an ovary. In this case the ovarian pedicle can be compressed by the bowel and result in ovarian infarction.

Every groin mass should be examined with regard to position medial or lateral to the spermatic cord and contiguous or separate from the internal inguinal ring. The following anatomic aphorisms will solve the diagnostic dilemma for most groin masses:

A mass clearly lateral or inferior to the spermatic cord placed on tension cannot be an indirect hernia (Fig. 13-8). If it is lateral to the femoral vessels and inferior to the inguinal ligament it is almost certainly an enlarged inguinal lymph node. Any attempt at reduction will be unsuccessful and painful. Femoral hernia must be considered if the mass originates below the inguinal ligament and is medial to or overlying the femoral artery. Femoral hernias are rare in children, but they do exist. If the mass is below the inguinal ligament and medial to the femoral artery and has appeared suddenly, a gentle attempt at reduction should be made. If reduction cannot be accomplished and if femoral hernia is still a likely possibility, exploration must be undertaken.

A mass clearly anteromedial and attached to the cord on tension is related to the processus vaginalis of the peritoneum. If normal cord (without associated medial thickening) can be palpated between the mass lying anteromedial to the cord and the inguinal ring the mass is not a bowel-containing hernia—it is almost certainly a hydrocele of the cord as demonstrated in Figure 13-9. In the majority of cases these lesions are tense, freely movable with the cord, irreducible, and purely elective from the standpoint of surgical correction.

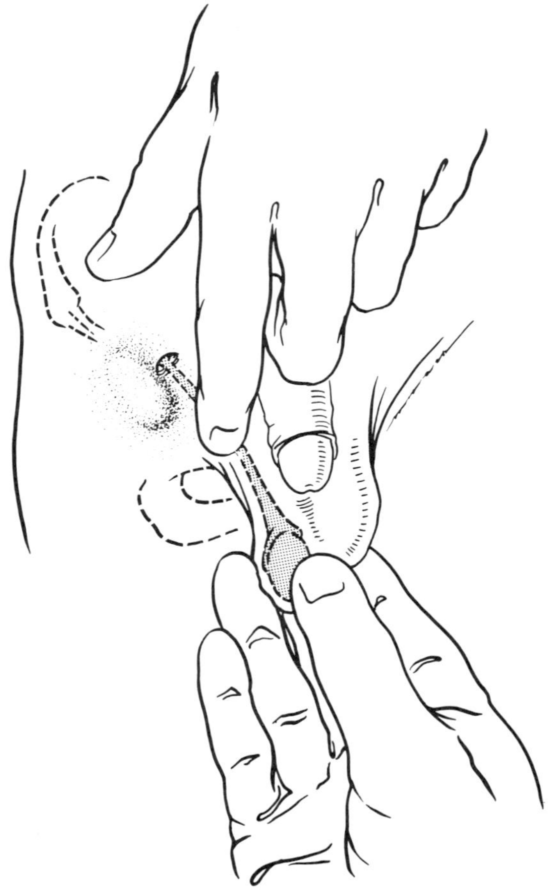

Figure 13-8. This mass is probably an enlarged lymph node.

If uncertainty persists concerning the possibility of an incarcerated hernia it is useful in an infant to perform a bimanual rectal examination. One index finger should be placed in the rectum to palpate the internal ring from inside the abdomen, and the second index finger should palpate the cord at the inguinal ring externally. If bowel is not palpated at the internal ring the mass is a hydrocele of the cord and not an incarcerated hernia. With an older child in whom a finger in the rectum cannot reach the internal ring an abdominal roentgenogram may be helpful in excluding bowel from the groin mass.

A groin mass that is clearly anteromedial to the cord on tension and that merges with the internal ring must be considered a bowel-containing hernia. (In such a case it will not be possible to palpate normal cord between the mass and internal ring [Fig. 13-10].)

If the scrotum is empty and a testis cannot be palpated in association with a mass as described previously, the testis is probably incompletely descended. This must be recognized during any attempt at reduction, because the hernia should be reduced separately to prevent en-masse reduction of the hernia, testis, and hernia sac with persistence of bowel entrapment. In addition, failure to recognize an undescended testis as part of the groin mass can result in damage or even rupture to the testicle during attempts at reduction.

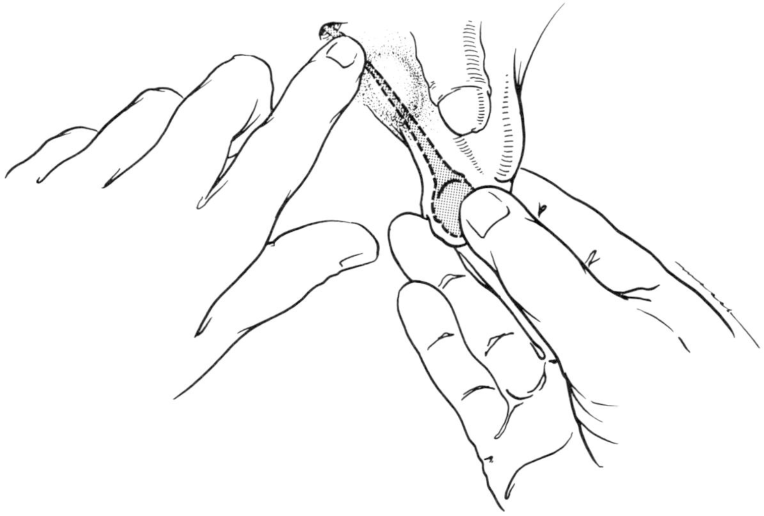

Figure 13-9. The groin mass here is a hydrocele of the cord.

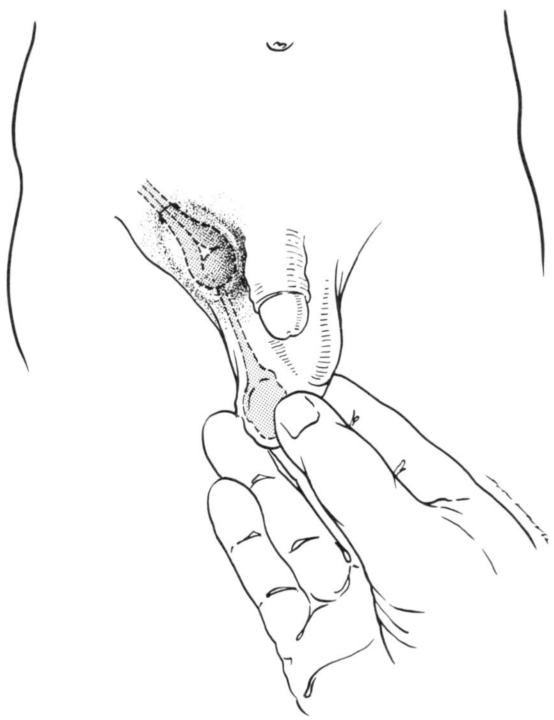

Figure 13-10. This groin mass that is clearly anteromedial to the cord on tension and that merges with the internal ring must be considered a bowel-containing hernia.

EVALUATION OF HERNIA IN FEMALES

The preceding statements regarding the examination of a groin mass apply to females as well, but examination is more difficult in a female because the round ligament cannot be placed on tension in the way the cord can be tightened by traction on the testis. Palpation at the inguinal ring in a female is still very useful in differentiating incarcerated bowel from an ovary incarcerated in the hernia sac. In the case of the ovary, the narrow vascular pedicle of the ovary will be palpable between the mass and the inguinal ring. When bowel is in the hernia the mass will merge with the inguinal ring, and the finger cannot be placed between the mass and the ring. Also, the bowel-containing hernia is much less movable than is the incarcerated ovary. Incarcerated bowel is an emergency, and the hernia must be reduced or the child taken to the operating room for surgical reduction of the hernia. An incarcerated ovary is not an emergency because the narrow vascular pedicle is rarely compressed by the ring, which is large enough to admit the larger ovary into the sac. A female with an incarcerated ovary should have hernia repair at the first convenient time.

REDUCTION OF AN INCARCERATED HERNIA

Almost all incarcerated hernias in children can and should be reduced outside the operating room. The reasons for preoperative reduction are as follows: (1) Reduction converts an emergency operation to an elective procedure. (2) Concern over bowel injury or infarction cannot be settled by operative exposure of the entrapped bowel. Reduction and time for recovery are necessary before the extent of bowel injury, if any, can be accurately assessed. (3) The standard inguinal incision for hernia repair is the wrong incision for bowel assessment, and extension of the hernia incision to permit intraperitoneal examination of the bowel damages the inguinal anatomy and jeopardizes the integrity of the hernia repair. (4) Hernia repair associated with acute incarceration involves dissection and suture of edematous tissues and increases the chance of hernia recurrence or cord injury.

The technique of reducing an incarcerated hernia, provided that the diagnosis is correct as evaluated by the previously suggested maneuvers, is simple and uniformly effective: (1) The thumb and fingers of the right hand are used to pull downward (rather than push upward) on the hernia mass. Downward traction converts the mass to an inverted cone based on the inguinal ring and facilitates manipulation of bowel and contents into the abdomen. The usual upward pressure, shown in Figure 13-11, creates a mushroom deformity of the sac over the ring and often prevents reduction. (2) The thumb and first two fingers of the left hand are placed on either side of the hernia neck at the inguinal ring to produce gentle compression of the afferent and efferent segments of bowel at the inguinal ring. Gentle and continuous pressure for 2 to 3 minutes will compress edema from the swollen bowel wall and mucosa. (3) Alternating release of pressure by the two fingers of the left hand (which are used to compress edema from the bowel mucosa trapped at the inguinal ring) synchronously with inward squeezing of the right hand over the apex of the hernia will first empty the obstructed bowel of its fluid content and then progressively return the empty bowel loops into the abdomen (Fig. 13-12).

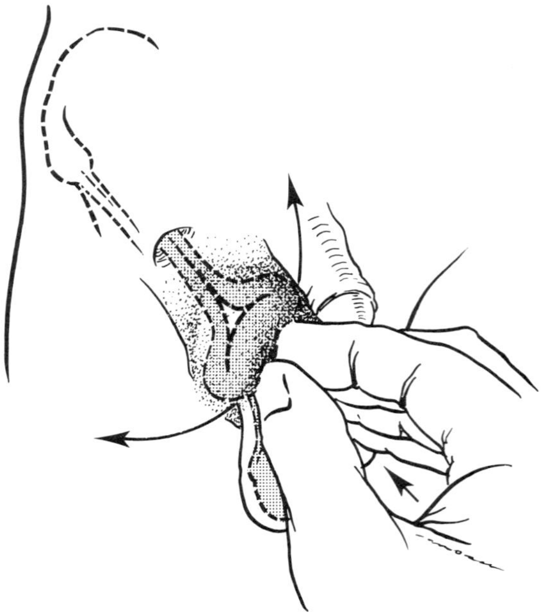

Figure 13-11. Simple upward pressure on an incarcerated hernia often creates a mushroom deformity and impedes hernia reduction.

Some surgeons have recommended sedation and elevation of the legs for hernia reduction. We do not favor this approach for three reasons. (1) Adequate sedation of an infant in pain from an incarcerated hernia may border on general anesthesia and is not safe in terms of respiratory depression. (2) A hernia that reduces easily with sedation and elevation can also be reduced easily by a few minutes of manipulation. (3) A hernia that is not reduced by sedation and elevation will require subsequent manipulation after a considerable delay and further possible compromise of blood supply to the bowel, testicle, or both. In some children with incarcerated hernia spontaneous reduction will occur during a bumpy ride in a car on the way to the doctor's office or the hospital. These hernias present no real problem, and hospitalization is not required for observation. A hernia that does require manipulative reduction should be observed in the hospital to make certain there has been no injury to the bowel.

If vomiting, distension, and signs of intestinal obstruction were present before reduction of the hernia, an abdominal roentgenogram should be obtained as a base line. Abdominal exploration should be undertaken if the obstruction does not resolve within 8 to 12 hours. Persistence of vomiting, leukocytosis, or fever or failure to pass stool are all common reasons to consider abdominal exploration following difficult manual reduction of an incarcerated hernia.

The majority of incarcerated hernias are reduced early by the previously described technique, and systemic symptoms subside and normal gastrointestinal function returns rapidly.

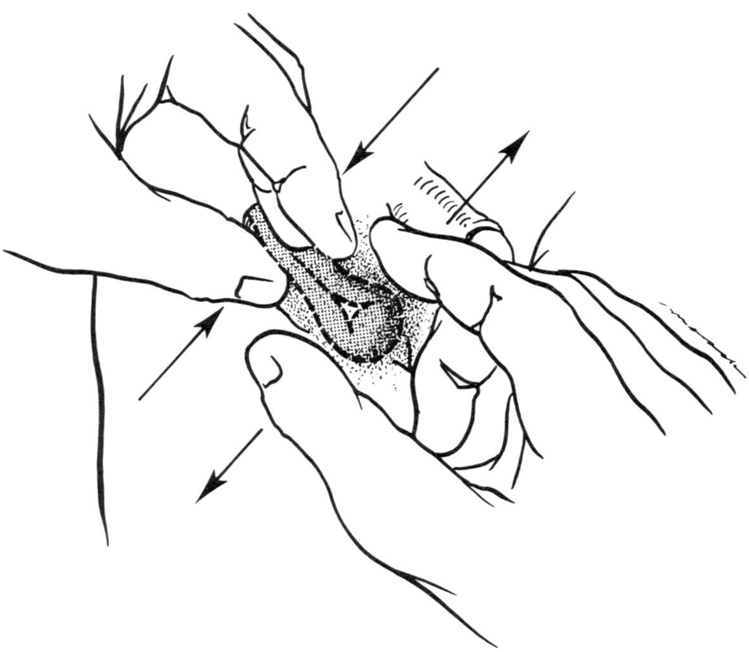

Figure 13-12. An alternating release of pressure by the two fingers of the left hand (which are used to compress edema from the bowel mucosa trapped at the ring) synchronous with an inward squeezing of the right hand over the apex of the hernia will first empty the obstructed bowel of its fluid content and then progressively reduce the empty bowel loops back into the abdomen.

Elective hernia repair is best done 24 to 72 hours following incarceration to allow resolution of edema and acute inflammation in the region of the internal ring. This waiting period eliminates uncertainty about bowel recovery, makes hernia repair technically simpler, and reduces the chance of recurrence of hernia from tears in edematous tissue.

OPERATIVE MANAGEMENT

The techniques of inguinal hernia repair are described in standard texts on pediatric surgery and will not be detailed here. Operative repair of inguinal hernia in infants and children is a hospital procedure and should not be attempted in an office or emergency room. However, for most pediatric hernias repair can be accomplished in the hospital on an outpatient basis without an overnight stay. Infants with a history of prematurity represent an outstanding exception. All infants born prematurely who are less than 46 weeks postconception should be monitored and observed overnight to avoid the risks of postanesthetic hypoventilation or apnea associated with the immature nervous system. In addition, those infants born prematurely who required ventilator support or treatment for apneic episodes may be at risk for periods beyond 46 weeks postconception, and it is wise to monitor them carefully before considering discharge on the day of operation.

Controversy still exists among surgeons concerning when to explore the opposite side in a child with a clinically evident hernia on one side only. A variety of arbitrary rules have been devised, depending on the surgeon's perspective and the particular set of statistics he happens to favor. Some surgeons explore the contralateral side in children under 1 year of age, others under 2 years, and others under 5. It is common to explore the contralateral side in females under 5 years, and more common to explore the contralateral side if the clinical hernia is on the left rather than the right. In our own practice we have found that 10% to 15% of patients will return for operation on the contralateral side when we operated only on the clinical side and think that the contralateral side is normal by examination. If we were to perform routine exploration we would be exploring roughly 80% to 85% of patients unnecessarily. Because we have excellent support from pediatric radiologists our own solution has been to utilize an inguinal herniogram in problem cases. A comparison of our clinical diagnoses with demonstration of a contralateral hernia by a herniogram (Fig. 13-13) reveals a 15% error in our clinical evaluation. This is almost precisely the same number of patients without herniograms who return for subsequent operation on the contralateral side. We are aware of the fact that demonstration of a patent processus vaginalis on a herniogram does not necessarily mean the patient will subsequently have a hernia. Adult autopsy specimens without clinical evidence of hernia have been shown to have a patent processus vaginalis in 15% to 37% of those examined. We do not operate on a minimally patent processus vaginalis, but we do operate on an unsuspected processus vaginalis that is large enough to admit bowel at some future time. An inguinal herniogram is useful only in the hands of an experienced radiologist who can minimize the possible complications from the procedure itself.

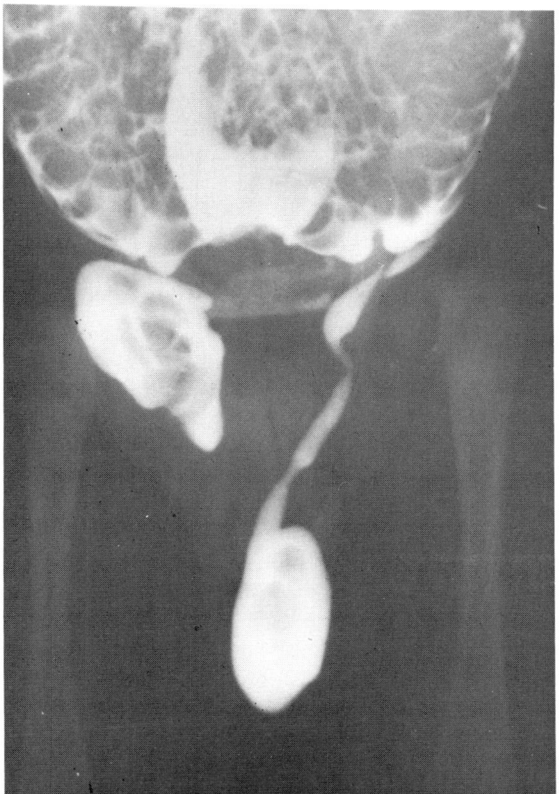

Figure 13-13. The inguinal herniogram confirms the clinical hernia on the right side in this patient but also demonstrates an unsuspected potential hernia on the opposite side.

ABNORMALITIES OF SCROTUM, GROIN, AND TESTIS

HYDROCELE

Hydrocele is a collection of fluid in the tunica vaginalis. The fluid may be limited to tunica vaginalis testis, in which case the hydrocele is in the scrotum only. The fluid may extend up the cord alone and be called a hydrocele of the cord. Inguinal scrotal hydrocele and hydrocele limited to the cord are usually associated with patency of the processus vaginalis at the internal ring sufficiently large to form a hernia in time. Many of these hydroceles communicate with the peritoneal cavity, and the mother will give a history that the hydrocele changes in size. It usually becomes smaller at night and enlarges during the daytime when the child is up and about. It is uncommon that one can decompress a hydrocele into the peritoneal cavity by direct pressure because the opening is usually very small and pressure simply kinks off the communication.

If there is no evidence of hernia by history or physical examination, there is no urgency in surgical correction of hydrocele. It is possible to have a residual hydrocele of the testis in the presence of a processus vaginalis testis that has closed at the internal ring. When this happens the hydrocele fluid resorbs spontaneously and progressively disappears over the course of 3 to 6 months. It is generally assumed that hydrocele of the testis present beyond 6 months of age must be associated with a peritoneal communication and that eventually a hernia will become manifest. This is certainly not true in every case, but most children over 6 months of age with persistent hydrocele of the testis will have evidence of a patent processus vaginalis on a herniogram. There is no indication for surgical repair of testicular hydrocele in a child younger than 6 months of age if there is no evidence of hernia. Some infants, however, have massive hydroceles that extend up along the cord and produce gross enlargement of the scrotum. These massive hydroceles rarely decrease in size spontaneously, and surgical excision along with herniorrhaphy is the appropriate treatment.

INGUINAL LYMPHADENOPATHY

Suppurative lymphadenitis of the groin occasionally presents as a mass that is confused with an incarcerated hernia. A careful history and examination will usually reveal a lesion of the extremity or perineum that will suggest a cause for lymphadenitis, and careful examination of the mass in relation to the spermatic cord or the normal inguinal structures, as detailed previously in the section on hernia, will differentiate a suppurative lymph node from an incarcerated hernia. The appropriate treatment of an incarcerated hernia is reduction and subsequent repair. The appropriate treatment for suppurative lymphadenitis is surgical incision and drainage if the lymph node is fluctuant. An occasional fluctuant lymph node can be treated by aspiration with a large-bore no. 14 cannula. One must be very certain of the anatomy and the diagnosis by physical examination before inserting a needle. Needle aspiration of an inguinal hernia is contraindicated.

TORSION OF THE TESTICLE AND TORSION OF THE APPENDIX TESTIS

Torsion of the testis typically presents with a painful, swollen hemiscrotum and with local edema and erythema as shown in Figure 13-14. The pain is usually gradual in onset but may be sudden and dramatic. In 20% to 25% of cases there is a prior history of trauma. The most common error in diagnosis is on the part of a physician who confuses the scrotal erythema and edema with signs of epididymitis or epididymo-orchitis. Acute epididymitis is seldom seen in prepubertal males, and it is rare even in late adolescence. Epididymitis, when it does occur in children, is almost always accompanied by urinary tract infection with symptoms of fever and pyuria. Diagnosis and treatment for torsion when epididymo-orchitis is present results in no harm to the patient. A mistaken diagnosis of epididymitis or epididymo-orchitis when in fact the patient has torsion may result in loss of the testicle through failure to correct the torsion surgically.

Torsion of the testis may occur at any age, but the peak incidence is from 12 to 18 years. Occasionally torsion is seen in a newborn, but almost always the torsion occurs *in utero* and the testis is already infarcted at the time of birth. Torsion may involve the cord above the tunica vaginalis testis, but more commonly it is within the tunica vaginalis testis because of a high insertion of the tunica vaginalis on the cord. This is the so-called clapper bell testis. Occasionally, torsion occurs between the tes-

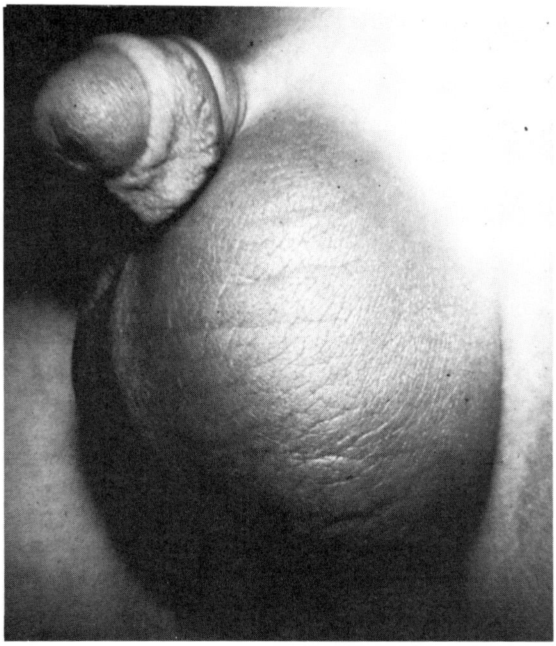

Figure 13-14. Torsion of the testis typically presents as a painful, swollen hemiscrotum with local edema and erythema.

tis and the attachment of epididymis within the tunica vaginalis testis.

Torsion may also involve the appendages of the testicle. There may be four small embryologic remnants called appendicular appendages, but the most common one is the appendix testis on the superior pole of the testicle. This is a small, pea-sized globular nodule that may twist on its pedicle and cause acute pain. If the patient is examined early the pain is localized to the superior pole of the testicle and can be defined very well with the rubber eraser of a lead pencil as portrayed in Figure 13-15. With torsion of the appendix testis the pain produces tenderness relative to the superior pole of the testicle. With torsion of the entire testicle the pain is diffused throughout the testis. If diagnosis is delayed, however, it is usually not possible to differentiate the two. Whenever there is doubt the situation should be treated as if the whole testis were twisted.

Appropriate treatment involves surgical exploration of the swollen scrotum with examination of the testis. If torsion of the testicle itself is present it should be reduced. If the viability of the testis is questionable, it should be removed to prevent impairment of spermatogenesis in the contralateral testis. This is a change from former practice that advocated preservation of a questionably viable testis for the sake of hormone function. One viable testis is more than adequate for hormone function, and long-term follow-up studies have shown atrophy in two thirds of the testes left behind and abnormalities of sperm volume, count, and motility in 80% to 90%, indicating bilateral dysfunction. In contrast, semen analyses have been normal in patients where the twisted testis was removed. The mechanism for this effect on spermatogenesis may be autoimmune, and it seems clear that the testis suffering significant ischemic injury should be removed.

If torsion of the appendix testis is present, the appendix is merely excised. If the process proves to be orchitis or epididymitis, no harm has been done. It may be helpful to make re-

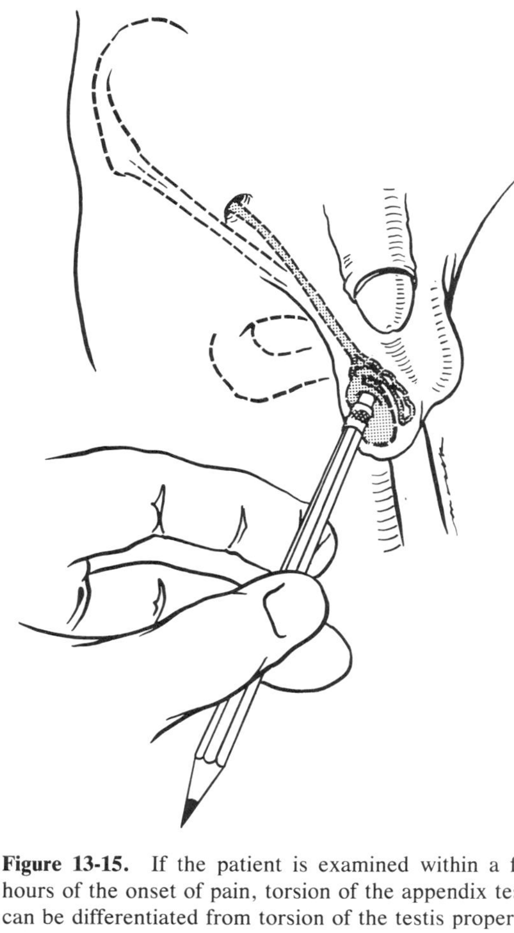

Figure 13-15. If the patient is examined within a few hours of the onset of pain, torsion of the appendix testis can be differentiated from torsion of the testis proper by point tenderness limited to the superior pole of the testicle.

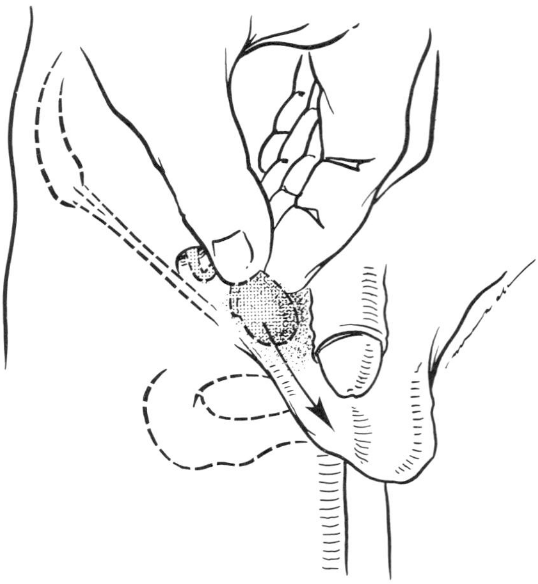

Figure 13-16. Differentiation of a retractile testis can be advanced into the scrotum by lateral, sliding pressure from the thumb and forefinger and can in this way be differentiated from a truly undescended testicle.

laxing incisions in the tunica albuginea to decompress the testicle for such an inflammatory process.

Whenever testicular torsion is present the contralateral testis should also be surgically fixed within the scrotum. Torsion is associated with a congenital abnormality of testicular fixation that affects both sides.

Two newer diagnostic aids are available for evaluation of testicular torsion. One involves the Doppler stethoscope to detect reduction of blood flow associated with torsion. Radioisotope imaging for the same purpose has also been used with sodium pertechnetate ^{99m}Tc and a gamma camera. Neither study should be performed if such studies require significant time delay in treating a possible torsion of the testis.

UNDESCENDED TESTICLES

A patient with an empty scrotum on one or both sides may occasionally come to the emergency room or the pediatric surgical clinic with a lump in the groin. The surgical management of undescended testicle is discussed in other textbooks of pediatric surgery and will not be detailed here. It is important to recognize the difference, however, between simple undescended testicle, undescended testicle associated with incarcerated hernia, and torsion of the testicle, whether descended or undescended.

The first approach to diagnosis is the maneuver described previously under examination of an inguinal hernia. An attempt should be made to place the testicle in the scrotum on traction while palpating the cord at the inter-

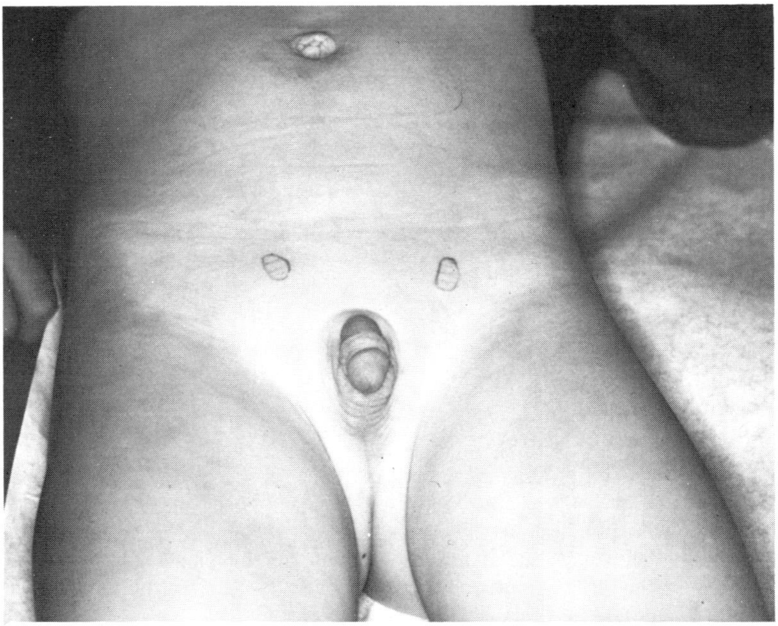

Figure 13-17. This child with bilateral groin masses and an empty scrotum was referred for therapy of suspected undescended testicles.

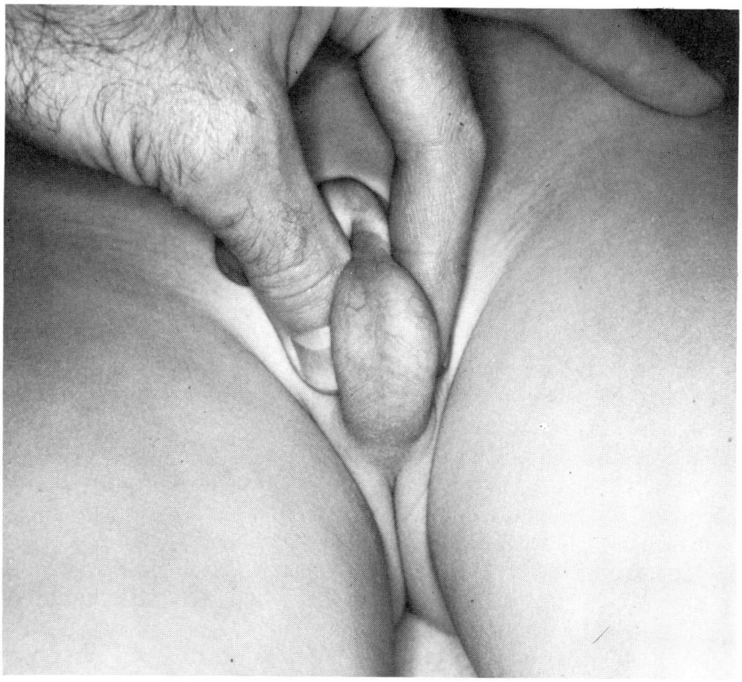

Figure 13-18. Both testicles in the child in Figure 13-17 were easily manipulated into the scrotum with lateral, sliding pressure, proving the diagnosis of retractile rather than undescended testicles. Such children require no specific therapy. The testes will rest normally in the scrotum at puberty with the endogenous hormonal influence of increased testicular weight and relaxation of the cremaster muscles.

nal ring. If the mass in the groin is an undescended testicle, it will be somewhat movable and can be pushed in the direction of the scrotum by pressure from the thumb and forefinger placed lateral to the mass as shown in Figure 13-16. If the testicle moves all the way into the scrotum it is not undescended but merely retractile. Retractile testes, demonstrated in Figures 13-17 and 13-18, are a normal variant and need no specific therapy. The testes will rest normally in the scrotum at puberty with the endogenous hormonal influence of increased testicular weight and relaxation of the cremaster muscles. If a definite undescended testicle can be palpated along with a mass anteromedial to the testis, it is an undescended testicle with an associated hernia. If the testicle itself is extremely tender and swollen, there is the possibility of either torsion of an undescended testis or compression of the testicular vessels by associated incarcerated hernia. If the anatomy at the inguinal ring is consistent with an associated hernia, the hernia should be reduced to relieve pressure on the vessels. If this cannot be accomplished, the testicular torsion or the incarcerated hernia, as the case may be, should be reduced surgically. For hernia associated with an undescended testis, orchiopexy must be included with herniorrhaphy to prevent entrapment of the undescended testis in the healing herniorrhaphy wound.

ABNORMALITIES OF THE HEAD AND NECK

LYMPHADENITIS

Enlarged cervical lymph nodes are frequently found in children between the ages of 6 months and 4 years. Neoplasia must always be considered a possible cause, but by far the majority of enlarged lymph nodes in this age group are due to pyogenic infection associated with a previous or present infection of the pharynx. Palpably enlarged and moderately tender lymph nodes at the angle of the mandible are a very common finding in most children of this age group. The situation becomes of more concern, however, when there develops a sudden increase in swelling, tenderness, and firmness of the mass with loss of the discrete character of the lymph nodes. Acute infectious lymphadenitis goes through a period of tenderness and often erythema. Because these nodes are beneath the deep cervical fascia, however, there may not be erythema of the overlying skin. In most situations children with this problem are administered antibiotics because of pain and fever, and by the time the surgeon examines the child the acute tenderness may have diminished. With suppurative cervical lymphadenitis the lymph node is not discrete, but there is a definite tense mass beneath the cervical fascia. It is often not possible to feel fluctuation, and it is a mistake to wait so long that fluctuation is obvious or that the skin starts to break down.

Initial management of a tender mass that appears suddenly in the neck of a child and appears to be associated with the lymph nodes involves culture of a specimen from the pharynx, antibiotic therapy, and application of local heat to the mass. If heat is applied with a warm Turkish towel four times a day, sufficient to increase circulation but not sufficient to burn the skin, the majority of these masses will resolve without need for surgical drainage. If the mass is still present 1 week later, it is unlikely it will resolve with heat and antibiotics alone. Continuation of antibiotic therapy for prolonged periods often results in chronic enlargement and inflammation of the node, which does not break down and suppurate but which does not resolve. Needle aspiration with a large-bore no. 14 cannula is usually the quickest way to resolve suppurative lymphadenitis. If the offending agent is a staphylococcus or streptococcus, the pus is often so thick it will not come through a smaller needle. Aspiration of the center of a necrotic node will usually effect prompt resolution of the swelling and provide precise information concerning diagnosis. It is important to reemphasize that most suppurative lymph nodes in the neck will appear tense and nonfluctuant because they are deep to the cervical fascia. Aspiration will often reveal pus even though the node feels tense rather than spongy from the surface. It is almost always necessary to repeat the aspiration once or twice at 4- to 6-day intervals. After each aspiration the swelling usually subsides, but the residual node undergoes further liquefaction and must be aspirated. The majority of suppurative lymph nodes treated in this way will resolve without open incision and drainage. This is a great advantage for the child and the parents. There is no draining wound or cumbersome dressings, resolution is faster, and there is no residual cosmetic deformity, that is, a scar on the face or neck. Occasionally, an infectious process is so far advanced that it will not respond to simple aspiration, and it must then be incised and drained. The aspiration technique is nearly always worthwhile first, because most of the time it is all that is needed.

Differential diagnosis for the swollen mass in the neck includes the acute appearance of a cystic hygroma, granulomatous lymphadenitis, cat-scratch disease, fungal lymphadenitis, or neoplastic processes. The neoplastic processes are usually not tender; they develop more slowly and are chronic. Viral lymphadenitis, as with cat-scratch disease, may arise fairly rapidly, but it rarely suppurates and is usually more distinct to palpation than the bacterial infections of lymph nodes. Aspiration of such nodes does not reveal pus. The same is true of granulomatous lymphadenitis, and in each case these lesions are generally best handled by excisional biopsy in the operating room. Occasionally, a cystic hygroma will first become manifest with obstruction and hemorrhage into the abnormal lymphatics that have preexisted. These masses are tender if hemorrhage is involved, but the location is often different from that of suppurative lymphadenitis, and the findings on palpation are usually characteristic of lymphangioma. The masses are more movable and more globular and clearly cystic. If doubt exists, aspiration will reveal brownish hemorrhagic fluid rather than pus from the lymph node. From lymphangioma the culture will be negative. Subsequent excision is necessary in this case rather than repeat aspiration.

One must always be aware that cervical tuberculosis is still a possibility, in which case lymph nodes are chronically enlarged, and they are more discrete and less tender than the bacterial infections. The appropriate skin testing should be done prior to any surgical manipulation. It is more common now to see infections with atypical mycobacteria, and the therapy for these is usually surgical excision in the operating room.

CYSTS AND SINUSES OF THE NECK

The most common cysts and sinuses in the lateral area of the neck are related to the embryologic development of the branchial arches and pharyngeal pouches. The most common remnants in children are thought to be related to the first and second branchial clefts and pouches. A variety of skin tabs, cartilaginous remnants, and preauricular cysts and sinuses may be found in relation to the tragus of the ear, and these lesions are thought not to be related to the branchial arches. The preauricular sinuses often are very short and end blindly and do not connect internally to the external auditory canal or the eustachian tube. Preauricular cysts occasionally become infected and require drainage. Following resolution of the infection, excision is a simple matter.

In *cysts related to the first branchial cleft* there are swellings in front of, behind, or below the lobe of the external ear or in the submandibular area. The external openings are usually below the mandibular area. The external openings are usually below the mandible and above the hyoid bone. Recurrent bouts of inflammation are the rule. Spontaneous or surgical drainage of infection with subsequent resolution is necessary before formal excision in the operating room. Radiographic studies using contrast material are useful preoperatively, and dye staining of the tract at the time of excision is very useful in the operating room.

The most common lateral cervical sinus occurs at the midportion of the anterior border of the sternocleidomastoid muscle as depicted in Figure 13-19. *These sinuses are thought to be related to the second branchial cleft.* They routinely connect with the pharynx, and they routinely drain mucoid material or obstruct and become infected. An infected lateral neck cyst should be drained surgically as an outpatient procedure. Once the acute inflammation has subsided, the patient should be admitted to the operating room for complete excision. It is preferable, of course, to excise these congenital sinus tracts prior to a bout of significant infection. Preoperative studies incorporating injection of radiopaque contrast material are useful to determine full extent of the sinus tract.

The most common midline cervical neck masses include thyroglossal duct cyst, midline dermoid cyst, and midline submental lymph node. *Submental lymph nodes* may mimic a thyroglossal duct cyst, but physical examination reveals they are higher than the hyoid and are not attached to the central portion of the hyoid bone. Careful examination and palpation within the mouth may reveal a source for the submental lymphadenopathy such as an abscessed tooth or a gum infection. This problem can usually be handled by local application of heat and antibiotics. A *midline dermoid cyst* is seldom infected and is not attached to the hyoid bone. The dermoid cyst may lie in a position very similar to a thyroglossal duct cyst, but it is usually more movable and it is seldom tender or infected. It is often not possi-

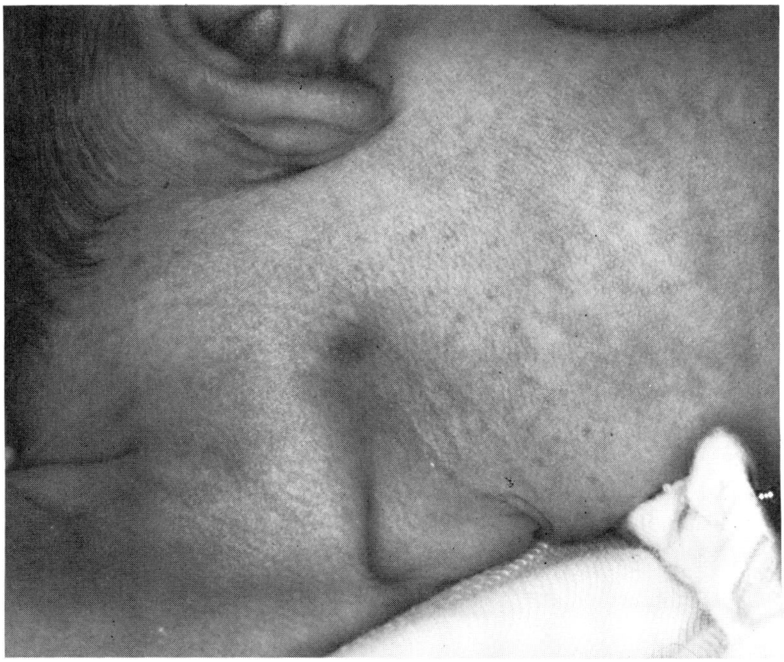

Figure 13-19. The most common of the branchial cleft sinuses presents as a small, draining punctum at the anterior border of the midportion of the sternocleidomastoid muscle.

ble to differentiate the two, however, because the dermoid cyst may appear to be fixed because of its position beneath the strap muscles.

A *thyroglossal duct cyst* is an embryologic remnant of the developing thyroid as an outpouching from the pharynx. The thyroglossal duct maintains its communication with the pharynx at the base of the tongue at the foramen cecum, and this communication is the source of the inevitable infection that appears in thyroglossal duct cysts and sinuses. The thyroglossal duct cyst does not spontaneously communicate with the skin, but an infected cyst may eventually rupture through to the skin and drain spontaneously. This should be avoided by appropriate incision and drainage when it is apparent that a midline cyst is infected and does not subside with local heat and antibiotics. The thyroglossal duct passes through the central portion of the hyoid bone, and the cyst is therefore attached to the hyoid on palpation. This is an important diagnostic point. Most of the thyroglossal cysts make their appearance after the second birthday, and over 50% are clinically apparent by the tenth birthday. Approximately 1% of the cysts are lateral to the midline, but they still have the connection to the hyoid bone.

An infected cyst that does not respond to local heat and antibiotics may often be controlled with needle aspiration and a large-bore no. 14 cannula to remove the infected contents from the cyst. The advantage of this method is simply avoidance of an unsightly drainage incision in the midneck with the unpleasantness of purulent dressings. A badly infected cyst will require open drainage until the infection resolves. Elective excision in the hospital must then be performed to include removal of the central portion of the hyoid and the entire tract down to the base of the pharyngeal mucosa to prevent recurrence.

Epidermal inclusion cysts occur on the head overlying cranial sutures. A common location is at the lateral aspect of the eyebrow. These lesions usually produce saucerization of the anterior table of the cranium but do not extend through both layers. Intracranial extension is possible but is extremely rare. For this reason it is common to obtain skull films, although for lesions in typical locations this is a nonproductive study. Dermoid cysts of the scalp appear fairly fixed because of their attachments to the pericranium, but they shell out easily and can be excised on an outpatient basis. They rarely become infected and are not emergencies.

TORTICOLLIS

Congenital torticollis, or wryneck, is fairly common in infants, being reported as frequently as 0.4% of all births. There are many causes of torticollis in childhood, and one must consider the possibility of cervical hemivertebrae, cervical adenitis, acute fasciitis, and imbalance of ocular muscles. The most common type of torticollis in pediatric practice, however, and particularly in infants, is the result of fibrosis in the sternocleidomastoid muscle. The cause is unknown. The rotational deformity of the neck is secondary to endomysial fibrosis and deposition of collagen and fibroblasts around individual muscle cells that undergo atrophy in the sternocleidomastoid muscle. The infant subsequently develops a rotational deformity of the head, and in 60% of the infants a "tumor" develops in the midportion of the body of the sternocleidomastoid muscle (Fig. 13-20). The tumor makes it appearance sometime between 14 and 21 days after birth. The reason for the delayed development of the tumor is unknown. Such children are often referred with suspicion of a neoplasm in the neck. Examination reveals the tumor mass to be part of the sternocleidomastoid muscle. Confusion with a rhabdomyosarcoma is possible, but this tumor has not been reported in this location in young infants.

Management is almost entirely nonsurgical. Gentle rotational exercises performed three or four times daily will restore full range of motion and cause spontaneous resolution of the mass over a period of weeks or months. Surgical division of the sternocleidomastoid muscle is indicated only for progressive facial deformity secondary to pressure effects associated with the torticollis and the failure to rest on both sides of the head. A condition called concordant plagiocephaly develops with flattening of the cranium and downward sagging of the cheek and facial structures if the infant continues to rotate the head to one side only. In addition to rotational exercises the infants are positioned during feeding and sleeping so that they must lie on the opposite side of the face. If surgical division of the muscle become necessary to arrest the progress of the cranial facial deformity, postoperative rotational exercises are important to ensure a good result.

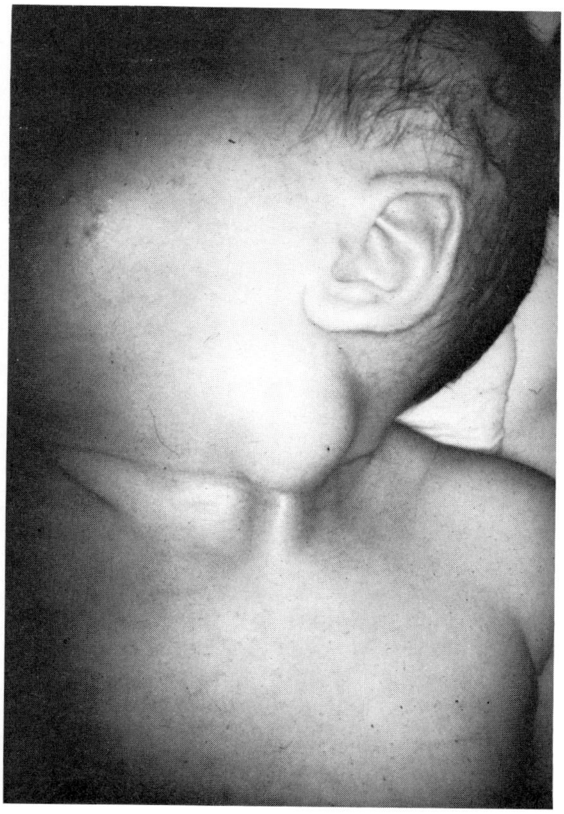

Figure 13-20. Congenital torticollis.

There is difference of opinion concerning the extent of surgery indicated. In most cases the tumor mass should not be excised. Simple division of the muscle is all that is required, and this should be accomplished through the smallest and most cosmetically acceptable incision.

LYMPHANGIOMAS OF THE HEAD AND NECK

The most common cystic lesions of the head and neck are associated with congenital malformations of the lymphatic system that form multilocular subcutaneous cysts. When located in the neck in infants these lesions are called cystic hygromas, but they may occur in the neck, axilla, thorax, or mouth and tongue. Lesions in all of these locations require hospitalization and formal surgical excision. Occasionally, small cystic accumulations may occur suddenly in the apparently normal neck of an older child. These represent hemorrhage and obstruction in previously abnormal but undiagnosed lymphatic malformations.

Lymphangiomatosis of the tongue is a complicated lesion that may require resections of the tongue. Occasionally, a simple sublingual cyst associated with a sublingual salivary gland can be treated with an outpatient surgical procedure under general anesthesia. These salivary cysts, also called ranula, can be managed successfully by marsupialization of the cyst with drainage into the oral cavity.

ANKYLOGLOSSIA INFERIOR

Ankyloglossia inferior or tongue-tie is a common problem in infancy that often disappears spontaneously with sucking and normal tongue movements. In some severe cases in which mobility of the tip of the tongue is limited, release can be obtained by a simple maneuver of elevating the tip of the tongue with a grooved director. The frenulum is allowed to slip between the slot of the grooved director and is then cut transversely as it is exposed as a thin membrane. Gentle pressure will usually stop any bleeding, and this can be done as an office procedure. If the child is older, however, it may be necessary to do this in the hospital with electrocautery under anesthesia.

BREAST MASSES

Bilateral breast enlargement in the subareolar area is common in infants 1 to 2 weeks of age, and this often precipitates a visit to a physician's office. The breast enlargement is presumed to be a result of hormonal influences from the mother, either through a direct effect of residual maternal estrogen and prolactin still circulating or secondary stimulation of the infant's hypophysis due to withdrawal of these maternal hormones. The stimulated infant breast may produce a thin secretion called witch's milk by the layman, and attempts at manual expression of this fluid from the infant's breast will cause secondary mechanical stimulation and continuation of the secretion. If mechanical stimulation is terminated the breast hypertrophy will subside spontaneously. In an occasional infant mastitis will develop, either secondary to the mechanical stimulation or perhaps spontaneously. The mastitis is due to pyogenic organisms, and if it does not clear with antiobiotic therapy and if it becomes fluctuant, it must be drained through a small circumareolar incision.

Hypertrophy of the breast tissue beneath the areola at the time of puberty is common for both males and females, and it usually occurs asymmetrically so that the plaque of breast tissue beneath the nipple on one side becomes firm and tender before the other side develops. This gives rise to considerable concern among young males who fear they are being feminized, and when this premature thelarche develops it may also cause concern in young females. Its occurrence is usually considerably before the onset of puberty. If the development of mass beneath the areola is symmetric and if the characteristics of the mass are consistent with developing breast tissue, one should not perform surgical biopsy. Excision of a quadrant of this tissue will remove a quadrant of the future breast and leave the child with a significant cosmetic deformity.

Older girls in their teens occasionally do have benign tumors of the breast such as fibroadenomas, and carcinomas of the breast in both female and male children have been reported but are extremely rare. The vast majority of breast swellings in both male and female preadolescents are simply the developing normal breast, and biopsy should not be done.

UMBILICAL LESIONS

The umbical cord of the newborn infant often heals unevenly. The natural sequence is for the cord to dry up and separate, leaving the stump of the umbilical vein and umbilical arteries to close and epithelialize over the surface. Occasionally, this process does not proceed normally, and the infant develops some granulation tissue that progresses to a polypoid mass resembling a fleshy tumor (Fig. 13-21). These umbilical granulomas will either bleed or seem to weep a watery secretion that causes the mother great concern.

In evaluating such a problem at the umbilicus one must be certain not to overlook the possibility of a communication with the intestinal tract, as in the case of a patent omphalomesenteric duct or a persistent omphalomesenteric cyst (Fig. 13-22). A second possible lesion at the umbilicus is a persistent urachal remnant that allows leakage of urine from the umbilicus. If one carefully inspects and probes the umbilicus for these possibilities and rules them out, the umbilical granuloma can be handled by simple ligation of its base with an absorbable suture such as Dexon or catgut. No anesthesia is required for this. Another approach for this small granuloma is simple application of silver nitrate to cauterize the granulation tissue. If the polyp is not small, the ligature at its base is more effective.

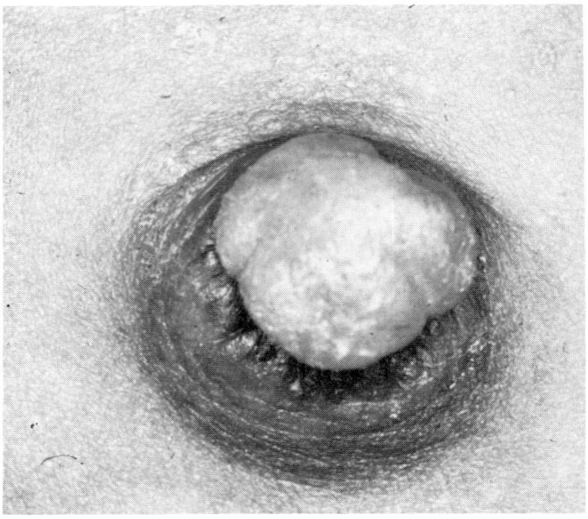

Figure 13-21. Polypoid granuloma of the umbilical cord.

UMBILICAL HERNIA

Persistent circular defects in the abdominal wall fascia at the site of the umbilicus are very common. Ordinarily, the abdominal fascia contracts down around the regressing umbilical vein and arteries to eliminate the defect in

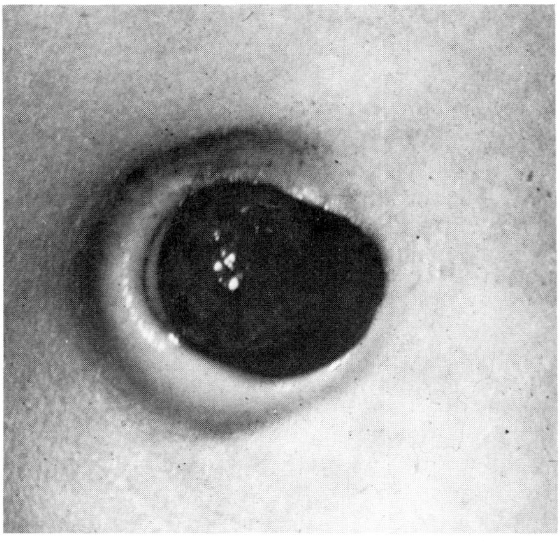

Figure 13-22. A persistent omphalomesenteric duct presents as a mucosally lined structure connecting to the umbilicus. Such lesions usually leak intestinal content.

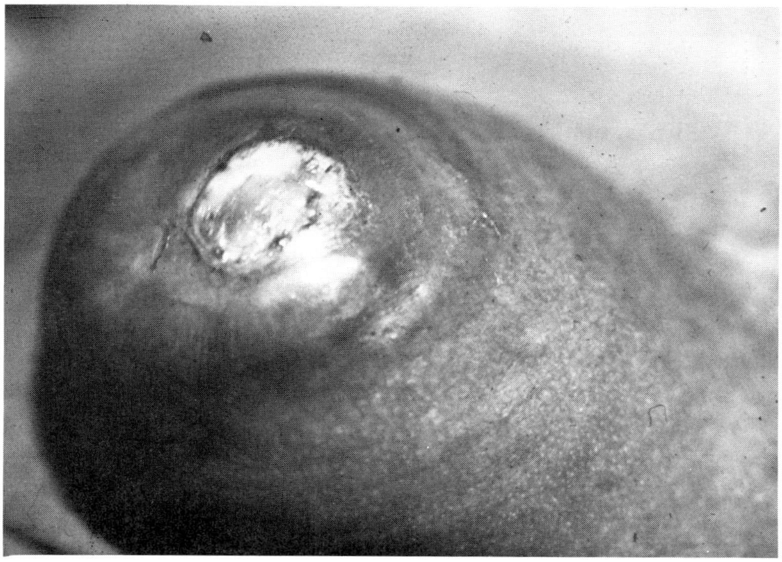

Figure 13-23. Ulceration of the skin overlying an umbilical hernia.

the abdominal wall. In many infants, however, this process is slow. An umbilical defect in the fascia that admits an index finger is very common. Occasionally, these lesions are large enough to admit two or three fingers and allow palpation of the internal abdominal viscera.

The size of the umbilical defect in a small infant is not well correlated with its ability to close spontaneously. At least 90% of the umbilical hernias that are round and limited to the umbilical area will close spontaneously by the age of 5 or 6 years. The extent of the skin protrusion is not correlated with the ability of the fascial ring to contract, and even some of the apparently large hernias will undergo spontaneous closure. Unless there is some specific complication requiring surgical repair, it is rarely indicated to perform umbilical herniorrhaphy as a single procedure in a child under 2 years. Our own policy is to wait for spontaneous closure, until the child is 5 or 6 years of age. If a female still has a small umbilical defect at 6 years, this should be closed surgically because the chance of subsequent closure is greatly diminished. Females should not be left with an umbilical defect and the threat from bowel incarceration during a subsequent pregnancy.

Special circumstances that might indicate surgical closure before 5 or 6 years of age include:

A history of incarceration. Umbilical hernias rarely incarcerate bowel, and when this does happen it seems justified to believe there is something different about the anatomy and that this hernia should be closed to prevent recurrent incarceration.

Skin ulceration (Fig. 13-23). Any sign of skin ulceration is an indication to repair the hernia and prevent possible peritonitis.

Asymmetry. An asymmetric defect in the fascia with extension upward in the midline is unlikely to close spontaneously, and this should be closed as an elective procedure.

Emotional inability of the parents to cope with an umbilical hernia that produces a large skin protrusion. If such a protrusion causes embarrassment to the 2- or 3-year-old in the local swimming club, it seems reasonable to proceed with repair. Two of our male patients confused the protruding skin at the umbilicus with the penis and presented problems with toilet training. These children would urinate on the floor as they directed the protruding skin of the umbilicus toward the toilet.

The old-fashioned remedy of taping an umbilical hernia or placing a coin in the umbilicus beneath the tape is ineffective in maintaining reduction and may cause harm through irritation of the overlying skin.

ABNORMALITIES OF THE ANUS AND RECTUM

ANORECTAL BLEEDING

The patient's age and the character of the bleeding from the rectum are most important factors in evaluating diagnostic probabilities and deciding whether the problem can be managed on an outpatient basis. The passage of tarry black material that tests positive for blood signifies upper gastrointestinal bleeding. Blood from the esophagus or stomach has been broken down by gastric acid to produce the black character. Occasionally, newborn infants with hemorrhagic disease of the newborn caused by vitamin K deficiency will pass tarry to dark red material per rectum. It is also possible for an infant who has swallowed maternal blood to pass tarry stool transiently.

Bright red blood on the outside of the stool originates from the region of the anus or rectum, and the diagnostic probabilities include anal fissure or rectal polyp. In a newborn infant bright red blood on the outside of the stool would signify anal trauma secondary to a vigorous digital examination. Bright red or maroon blood mixed in with the stool comes from the midintestinal tract and is usually associated with infectious diarrhea. Newborn infants with necrotizing enterocolitis may pass maroon to red blood, and older infants with Meckel's diverticulum pass dark red to maroon blood mixed with the stool. Older infants with intussusception often pass bloody stool described as current jelly. Except for anorectal fissures, rectal polyps, and rectal prolapse, most of the other causes of rectal bleeding require hospital admission and work-up.

ANORECTAL FISSURE

Acute anal fissure is fairly common in infants and children and represents a split in the anal mucosa associated with the forceful passage of a large, hard stool. The condition may be multiple, and most of the time the fissures heal rapidly. In small infants the pain from the fissure causes anal sphincter spasm, which in turn leads to constipation, hard stool, and recurrence of the fissure when the large stool is finally passed and recracks the healing anal mucosa.

Diagnosis can usually be made by simple examination of the anus with the buttocks spread apart. Insertion of a speculum or a sigmoidoscope is usually not necessary. If the child has bleeding, however, examination of the anorectal canal is necessary. The bleeding is nearly always characterized as bright red and on the outside of the stool and small in quantity. On occasion in a child 2 years of age or older a polyp in the rectal ampulla rather than a fissure may be the cause of the bleeding. For this reason, digital examination and possibly sigmoidoscopy are important to rule out the presence of polyp. Some of the low rectal polyps can be prolapsed through the sphincter with a finger and simply ligated with a stitch ligature.

Management of anorectal fissure is nearly always nonsurgical in infants and children. The key to successful therapy is lubrication and cleansing of the anorectal canal and softening of the stool. An increase of carbohydrate in the stool and the addition of stool softeners such as Metamucil or Colace are important components of management. For the small infant it is useful for the mother to lubricate the anus with petrolatum and gently dilate the sphincter by massage when the infant starts to strain at stool. Following defecation the anorectal area should be cleansed carefully and lubricated with petrolatum, and the surrounding anorectal skin should be protected with a standard preparation for diaper rash. Complete healing with resolution of symptoms may take several weeks. Sphincter massage with lubrication is one of the most important components of treatment, but lubrication of the stool and reduction of its bulk are also important.

ANAL POLYPS

Mucus-retention polyps are a common cause of rectal bleeding in children over 2 years of age. The bleeding may appear on the outside of the stool if the polyp is low or may be mixed in with the stool for high polyps. Routine work-up includes sigmoidoscopy, which can be done on an outpatient basis. Sedation is usually helpful for sigmoidoscopy of children, but general anesthesia is virtually never necessary.

An air-contrast barium enema study is usually the next procedure utilized to search for polyps at a higher level. In the case of extensive multiple polyposis, either familial or nonfamilial, the barium study would confirm this diagnosis and further therapy could be planned. Flexible colonoscopy is probably more precise in making the diagnosis of colon polyps, but the procedure is more difficult for a child and usually is not necessary.

Most polyps in children are mucus-retention polyps that in time cause temporary bleeding and usually undergo subsequent spontaneous slough. Adenomatous or premalignant polyps are extremely rare in children, and the barium enema screening study is probably sufficient to rule out the more serious problems. If bleeding persists from a higher polyp or if the barium study suggests some unusual nature relative to a higher polyp, colonoscopy should be performed.

PERIANAL ABSCESS

The majority of perianal abscesses in the adult population are enteric in origin. Surgical drainage of a perianal abscess in an adult results in a chronic anal fistula in at least half of the cases. In contrast, infants and children may develop perianal subcutaneous abscess associated with diaper rash and organisms that are not enteric. Simple drainage of these lesions does not necessarily result in a chronic fistula, and perianal fistula develops perhaps 25% of the time following external drainage of a perianal abscess in an infant.

If a chronic draining fistula does develop, the internal opening must be located in one of the infected anal crypts. Appropriate therapy involves anal fistulectomy with complete excision of the tract from the internal opening to the external opening. This is a hospital procedure.

RECTAL PROLAPSE

External protrusion of rectal mucosa or full-thickness of bowel in small infants is not uncommon and is distressing to mothers. This often begins to appear in small toddlers as they assume the upright position. At this stage of development the sacrum has not developed its full concavity, and the configuration of the bowel is almost straight downward. The levator at this stage does not seem to cause enough angulation of the bowel to prevent prolapse. The mucosa or, more often, full-thickness bowel will extrude with straining at stool.

The most effective therapy is simple manual reduction of the prolapse by the mother following defecation. This maneuver may be required for many months, but as the child grows the prolapse tends not to recur and the problem resolves spontaneously.

A variety of surgical procedures have been tried for rectal prolapse in infants, but the majority of these are not indicated. Some success has been reported with perirectal injection of sclerosing solutions, the safest being 30% saline. One method involves the subsacral approach to the posterior rectal wall for fixation to the sacrum either with a temporary gauze pack or by direct suture of the rectum. In extreme cases these procedures can be useful. For the vast majority of cases of prolapse, however, simple reduction of the prolapse at the time of defecation will contain the problem until nature provides a cure.

BIBLIOGRAPHY

Committee on Accident and Poison Prevention: Revised first aid for the choking child. Pediatrics 78:177, 1986

Matlak ME: Foreign bodies. In Mayer T (ed): Emergency Management of Pediatric Trauma, Chap. 31. Philadelphia, WB Saunders, 1985

Nixon GW: Foley catheter method of esophageal foreign body removal: Extension of applications. Am J Radiol 132:441, 1979

Standards of Guidelines for Cardiopulmonary Resuscitation (CPR) and Emergency Cardiac Care (ECC). JAMA 255:2905, 1986

Welch KJ et al: Pediatric Surgery, 4th ed. Chicago, Year Book Medical Publishers, 1986

14 Scalp, Face, and Salivary Glands

CLIFFORD C. SNYDER AND PRESTON N. RICHARDS

SCALP

OPERATIVE ANATOMY

The scalp is the soft tissue that blankets the skull, extending from the supraorbital ridges anteriorly to the external occipital protuberance posteriorly and blending bilaterally with the temporalis fascia. The scalp is layered, which is quite important to the patient and profoundly advantageous to the surgeon. The outermost layer of the five strata is the *skin* (Fig. 14-1), which is unequaled in thickness anywhere else in the human body. The skin is so firmly adherent to the next two underlying layers, the superficial fascia and the galea aponeurotica, that surgically the three must be considered as one. This intimate soft-tissue intertexture is responsible for the limited gaping of superficial scalp wounds and the restricted spread of infections, whereas the infinitesimal degree of blood vessel retraction from these wound edges and the prolonged patency of the severed blood vessel ends are to blame for the profuse hemorrhaging from simple scalp lacerations.

The second layer, or *superficial fascia*, is remarkably inelastic because it is composed of short fibrous septa that hold it firmly to the skin above and the galea below. Any swelling immediately below this dense layer, such as hematoma, exudate, or edema, becomes incarcerated and compresses the adjacent sensory nerves, inducing aggravating pain. If the material becomes offending, it must be released externally.

The *galea aponeurotica*, the third layer of the scalp, is the conjoined aponeurosis for the scalp muscles. The glistening helmet of fibrous protection is loosely attached to the periosteum by an intervening subaponeurotic layer.

The fourth layer, or *subaponeurotic layer*, consists of loose areolar connective tissue. The surgeon should consider this stratum the danger layer, because it contains the emissary veins, which empty into the venous sinuses of the cranial hemispheres. Lacerations involving this scalp stratum are surgical emergencies, as they gape widely, remain open, and afford direct portals for bacteria to the meninges and intracranial sinuses. These wounds should be cleansed thoroughly, debrided, and closed loosely.

The fifth and deepest scalp layer is the *periosteum*, which is surprisingly thin to be such a tenacious structure. One can strip it easily from the skull merely with the finger, except where it attaches to the dura mater at the suture lines. Bone in any part of the body needs coverage, and the skull bone is similar in this respect. Therefore the periosteum, being the last line of defense for the skull, should remain intact. Split-thickness skin grafts take well on periosteum but live with difficulty on bare bone.

The vascular anastomoses of the scalp are so profuse that fresh wounds heal readily, and serious infections are rare when proper surgical care is provided (Fig. 14-2). Hinge and trapdoor scalp flap wounds produced by trauma usually remain viable because of the abundant circulation supplied by the temporal, supraorbital, supratrochlear, posterior auricular, and occipital blood vessels. Unfortunately, hematomas are common because of this vascular abundance, but usually they are confined to a single skull bone by the adherent periosteum at the suture lines.

Most of the venous tributaries of the scalp terminate in the external jugular veins, but the emissary vessels empty into the superior sagittal sinus, and the frontal and supraorbital veins contribute to the cavernous sinus via the ophthalmic veins. The lymph drainage of the

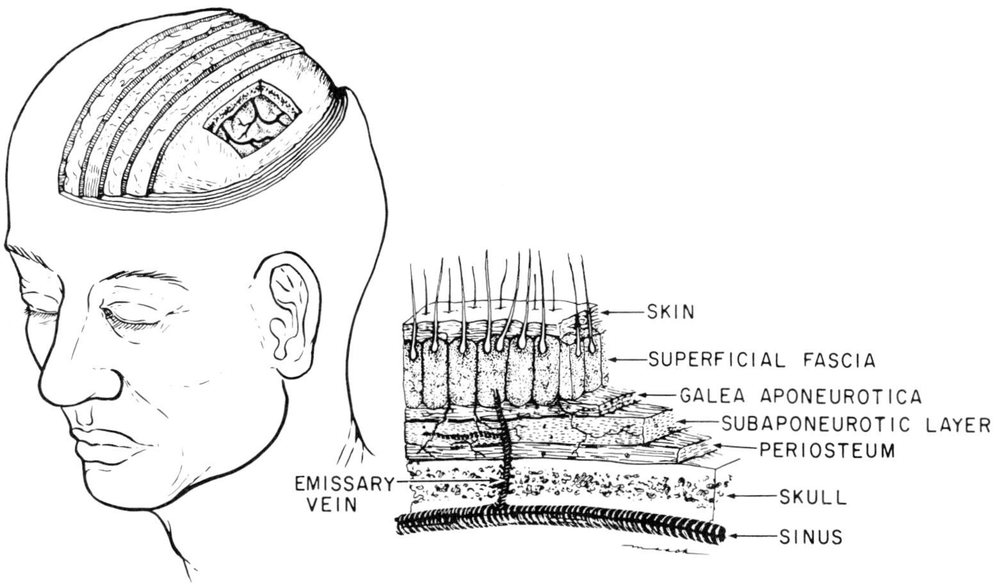

Figure 14-1. Anatomy of scalp.

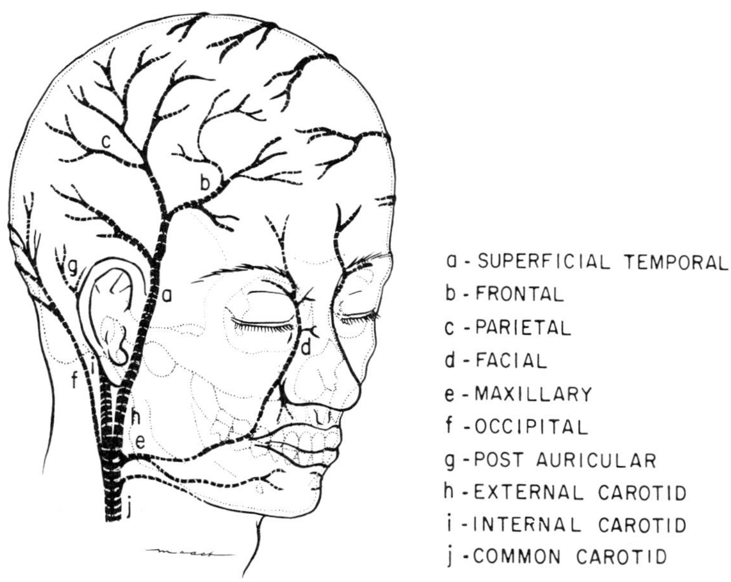

Figure 14-2. Arteries of scalp and face.

scalp is important both in acute and chronic disease and should be inspected with each examination of the patient. The frontal scalp lymphatics empty into the submaxillary modes, the posterior scalp vessels into the occipital nodes, and the lateral scalp channels into the posterior auricular nodes. Knowledge of these lymph pathways becomes important when examining malignant tumors of the head.

LACERATIONS

All cranial trauma, regardless of the extent, demands neurologic evaluation. This may be achieved quickly but must be noted in the patient's chart.

Local infiltration of 0.5% lidocaine (Xylocaine) with epinephrine suffices for shaving, cleansing, debridement, and wound closure. If scalp hemorrhage is a problem, the superficial

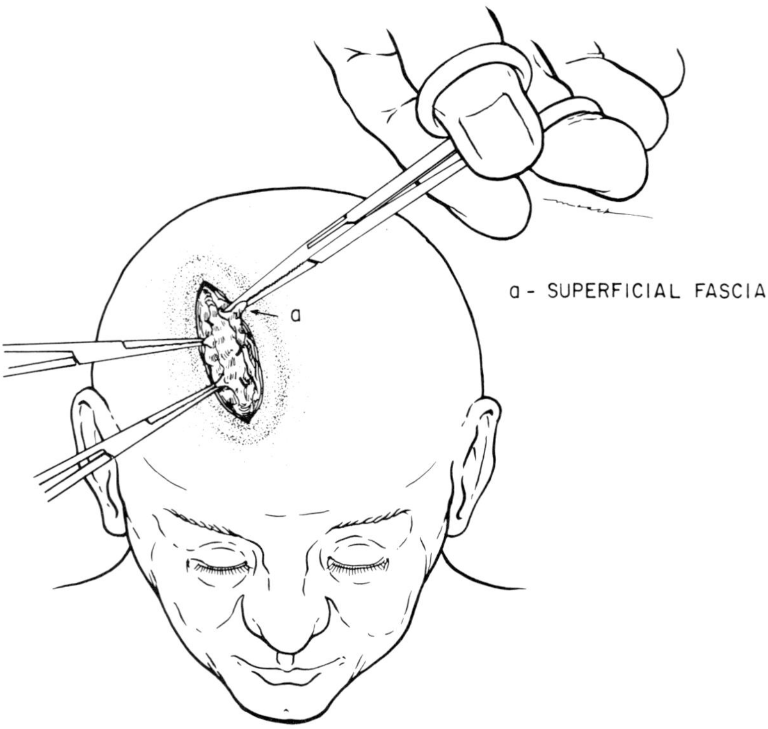

Figure 14-3. Control of hemorrhage from scalp wounds.

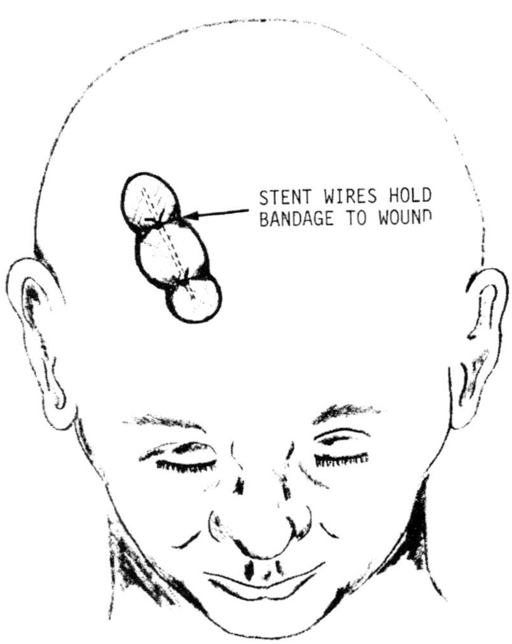

Figure 14-4. Stent wire sutures.

fascia is grasped with hemostats and pulled over the bleeding vessels temporarily (Fig. 14-3). The wound edges are debrided of nonviable tissue in such a manner that the margins can be approximated without tension. Then stent sutures of medium-sized stainless steel wire are positioned and the scalp edges coapted. The stent-wire sutures are tied over a bandage as though around a package (Fig. 14-4). When the wound is too large for primary closure, parallel relaxing incisions may be indicated (Fig. 14-5). The open donor sites may be grafted or left to granulate. Surgical alternatives to this closure are a variety of local skin flaps; scalp arteries are always used as a nutritive source. Partial avulsion of the scalp occurs daily in industry, on the highways, and on the ski slopes.

INFECTIONS

All traumatic wounds of the scalp must be considered contaminated, because bacteria accompany the traumatizing agent and pieces of dirty skin and clothing into the wound. If the wound margins become devitalized, a favorable medium for the bacteria is furnished,

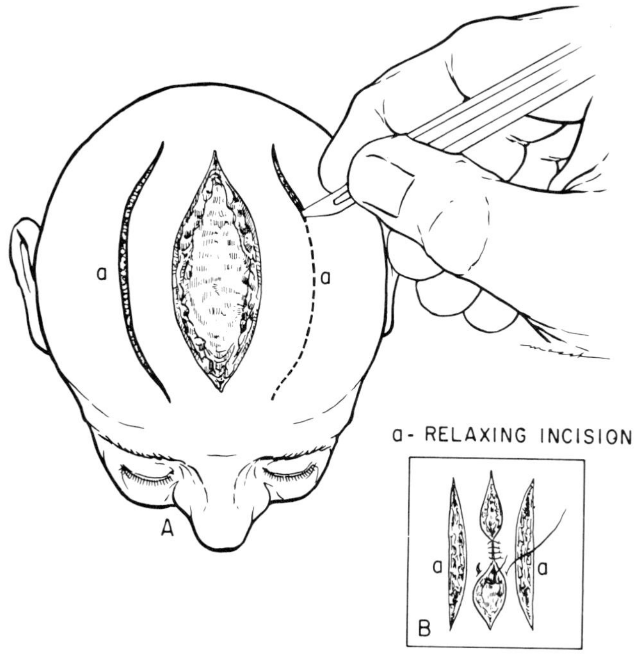

Figure 14-5. Parallel relaxing incisions.

thus permitting a contaminated wound to become an infected wound. As long as only the wound is contaminated—that is, the bacteria remain on the skin surface—prevention of infection is possible by cleansing with soap and water combined with surgical debridement. Once the wound is infected by penetrating bacteria, cleansing and excising may result in the sacrifice of vital structures. Obviously, the period of contamination (preinfection period), which averages 6 to 8 hours after trauma, is the ideal time to treat a wound. Determinants that alter the period of contamination are the patient's general condition, the type of wound (clean incision, laceration, contusion, puncture), circumstances at the time of injury, and efficacy of the first-aid treatment. In the treatment of all potentially infected wounds it is essential to remember that the healthy living cell is the best of all antiseptics and better than any antibiotic; therefore as many living cells must be saved as possible for better wound healing.

CELLULITIS

Diffuse inflammation of the scalp usually begins as a local infection (folliculitis, puncture, or abrasion), and initial attention should be focused on this primary lesion with fomentations, incision, or excision. The secondary reaction, consisting of erythema, edema, and pain, is given the usual hygienic care. If a definite organism is responsible, and this is substantiated, it is treated with specific antibiotic therapy. Circumscribed purulent lesions such as furuncles are shaved of surrounding hair, incised, and drained. Invasive furuncles, such as carbuncles and subaponeurotic abscesses, are treated more vigorously because of the possibility of extension of the infection into intracranial venous sinuses. The causative organism is determined, and the infection is treated locally as well as systemically. Local therapy includes liberal incision and debridement of necrotic tissue, packing with iodoform gauze, and use of a rubber tissue drain or continuous wet dressings with an antibiotic solution. A systemic broad-spectrum antibiotic is administered orally or parenterally.

DISSECTING CELLULITIS

Dissecting cellulitis of the scalp, also known as perifolliculitis chronica abscedens et suffodiens, is similar to hydradenitis suppurativa in that multiple epithelial-lined cysts that are chronically infected invade the scalp. Conservative management should be attempted; however, the majority require excision of the infected tissue with subsequent split-thickness skin graft or local scalp flap for coverage.

ALOPECIA

Surgical management of alopecia may be indicated for patients with hair loss due to disease, trauma, or hereditary conditions such as male pattern baldness. Three main techniques have been devised to transplant or autograft hair. Hair plugs, which are most commonly used for male pattern baldness, are 4 mm to 5 mm in diameter and are full-thickness plugs of scalp that are harvested from a hair-bearing region of the scalp. These are placed in a recipient bed created with a skin biopsy punch instrument approximately 0.5 mm to 1 mm smaller than the donor plug. The angle of the hair shaft is aligned to match existing hair. Plug-type grafting is performed in two to four stages, depending on the size and nature of the defect, so that the non–hair-bearing skin between the plugs can be replaced. Most donor sites do not require suturing and will contract to an acceptable-sized scar.

Full-thickness strip skin grafts, which are 0.5 cm to 1 cm wide from the temporal and occipital scalp, can be grafted to the anterior scalp to re-create the frontal hairline. These offer a greater number of hair follicles but have a greater incidence of graft failure. The area posterior to the hairline can then be filled in with hair plugs as previously described.

Scalp flaps, both random delayed multistage and flaps based on arterial blood supply, can be rotated from the temporal region to the frontal hairline. The width of these flaps is determined by the ability to close the donor defect primarily. These larger skin flaps are much more demanding for both the surgeon and the patient.

DERMOID CYSTS

Dermoid cysts are congenital and may be seen at birth, although 60% are diagnosed between the ages of 15 and 40 years. They are found at various suture lines but are most common at the lateral end of the supraorbital ridge (Fig. 14-6) and the frontonasal plate (50% of cases). They are also seen in the palate and the floor of the mouth (25%) and the ventral–dorsal body midline (15%). The dermoid cyst appears as a painless, round, encapsulated mass, deep to the skin and attached at its base to the skull suture line or adjacent tissue. When it is removed and examined its wall is found to be thick and lined with a skinlike membrane-containing hair follicles, sweat and oil glands, and squamous cells, but the layers are in reverse order, the horny layer being toward the center. The cyst contains a caseous matrix of dead epithelium, hair, sebum, and, occasionally, vestigial remnants of other germ layers (bone, cartilage). Dermoid cysts of the floor of the mouth may simulate cystic hygroma, thyroglossal duct or branchial cyst, lipoma, mucocele, or salivary gland tumor. It makes little difference because all these lesions are treated identically—surgically. Sialograms are useful in establishing a diagnosis. Dermoid cysts should be removed because they interfere with function, may cause deformity, undergo infection, and occasionally become malignant (1% to 3%). In infants, when the stalk is connected intracranially, surgery may be delayed until after puberty, as sometimes skull growth obliterates the opening. In older children, or in the event of intervening infection before puberty, the cyst may be incised, drained, and later removed. When elective surgery is done, the skull opening, if present, may be closed by a splinter bone plug, rotating a small peristeal flap, or cauterizing the foramen.

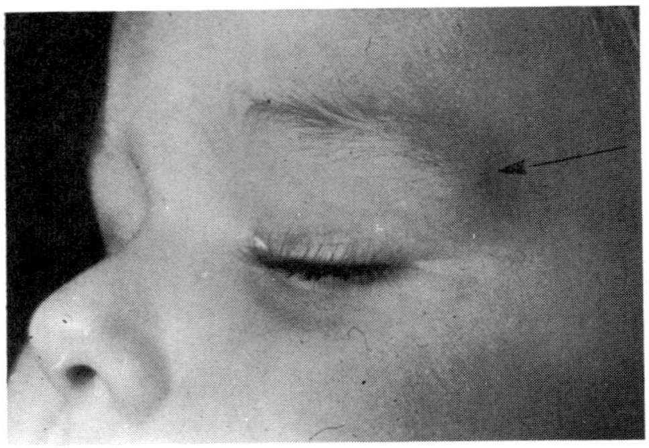

Figure 14-6. Dermoid cyst of supraorbital ridge.

For removal of dermoid cysts, general anesthesia or local infiltration anesthesia may be used. An incision is made over the cyst; for supraorbital cysts, incisions are made in the eyebrow; cysts in the floor of the mouth (Fig. 14-7) are enucleated through incisions in the gingivobuccal sulcus; and for other cysts, inci-

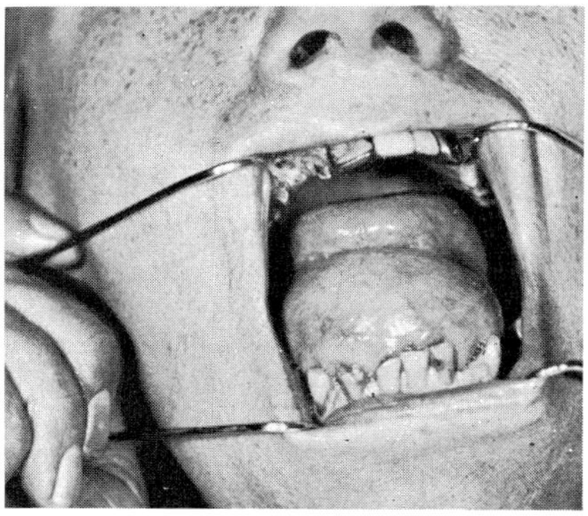

Figure 14-7. Dermoid cyst in the sublingual area. (Shore BR: Ann Surg 108:305 1938)

sions are made in the flexion creases of the skin. When the cyst is behind the ear, excision is best performed through an incision parallel to the cephalic border of the ear. A cleavage line is established, and the cyst is excised by blunt dissection. Sometimes it is necessary to incise the cyst wall and empty the contents so the cavity lining will reveal the extent of the lesion. With a finger or an instrument in the cavity, the lesion is easily removed by dissecting close to the external wall of the cyst. To inhibit recurrence the entire cyst should be extirpated. The wound is closed with stent sutures.

SEBACEOUS CYSTS

Because oil glands are numerous in the scalp and face, sebaceous cysts are common in this area.

Surgical intervention is achieved under local anesthetic infiltration between the cystic mass and adjacent tissues. After the area of the cyst has been shaved and prepared, an elliptic incision is made in the skin surrounding the duct orifice, and this island of tissue is elevated with a skin hook. The cyst is freed along a cleavage line by combined sharp and blunt dissection. After the lesion has been removed the wound is closed by stent and skin sutures, the former tied over a cotton bolus to obliterate dead space, eliminate hematomas, reduce edema, and fix the bandage without tape, gauze, or collodion. If the sebaceous cyst is on the face, the treatment of choice is to excise the ductal orifice through an elliptic incision, empty the contents by digital expression, grasp the cyst wall with a mosquito hemostat, and deliver it through the skin incision. The wound is closed with one stent and one or two skin sutures. Multiple adjacent sebaceous cysts behind the ears should be excised as a group and the skin closed. Less than 1% of sebaceous cysts become malignant.

FACE

OPERATIVE ANATOMY

Like the scalp, the cheeks are composed of five layers. The outermost is the skin, and the next is a superficial fascia layer; a modest muscular layer follows, and the inner layers are the submucosa and mucosa. The remaining portions of the face lack the last two layers. The facial skin contains sweat and oil glands and hair follicles. The epidermis follows the ducts of the glands and the shafts of the hair deep into the dermal area. This is a most important anatomic feature, because when the skin is burned or the top layer is abraded, these downgrowths of epithelium furnish islands of new epidermal replacement. Hair shafts grow at an angle, and when transplanting hair follicles for eyebrows, it is necessary to design the surgical incisions respecting this angle. The skin is composed of reticular fibrous bundles containing elastic tissue fibers that keep the skin in a state of tension and also facilitate construction and transfer of surgically formed skin flaps. It is this same elastic tissue that on degeneration releases the skin tension. This skin hypotonicity, associated with aging and shrinking of the underlying musculature, produces excessive skin folds that are commonly known as wrinkles (Fig. 14-8). Successful surgical closure of a large defect is dependent on separating or undermining the superficial skin from the underlying short facial muscles and on stretching the remaining elastic fibers.

In 1861 Langer punctured the skin of a freshly deceased human body with an auger and watched the round holes become elliptic, the long axis of the puncture wound being parallel to the lines of skin tension. Wounds that are parallel to the lines of tension (flexion creases) tend to become narrower and to heal readily, whereas wounds at right angles to the lines of tension tend to gape open and to heal

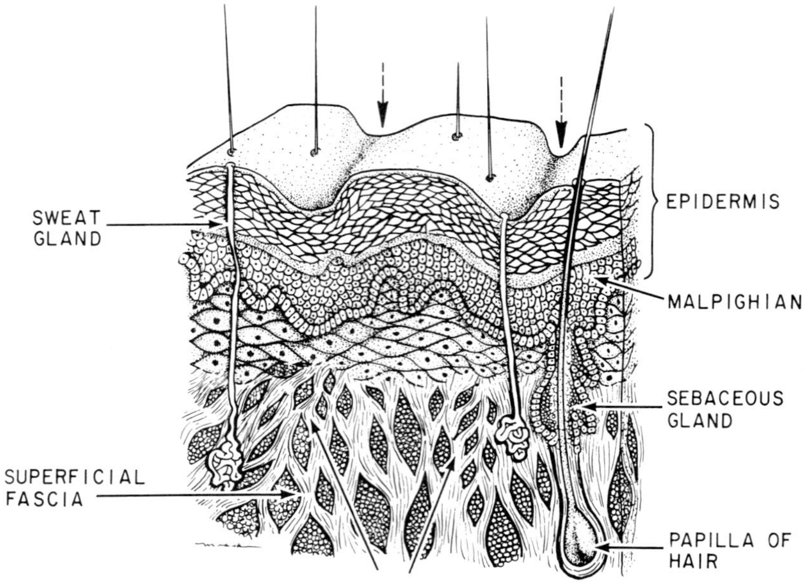

Figure 14-8. Anatomy of skin. Shrinking of underlying musculature produces skin folds (wrinkles).

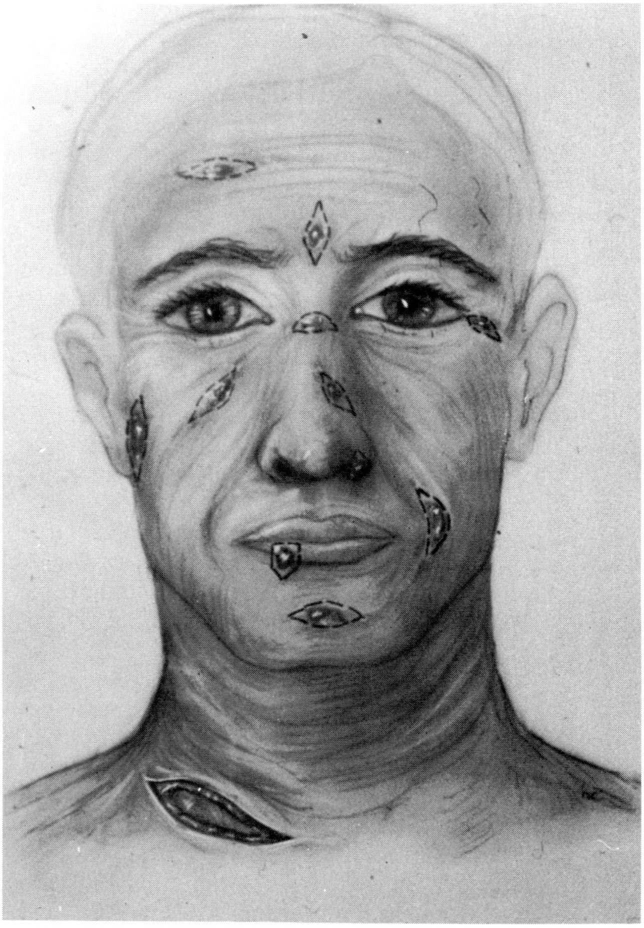

Figure 14-9. Excision of flexion creases.

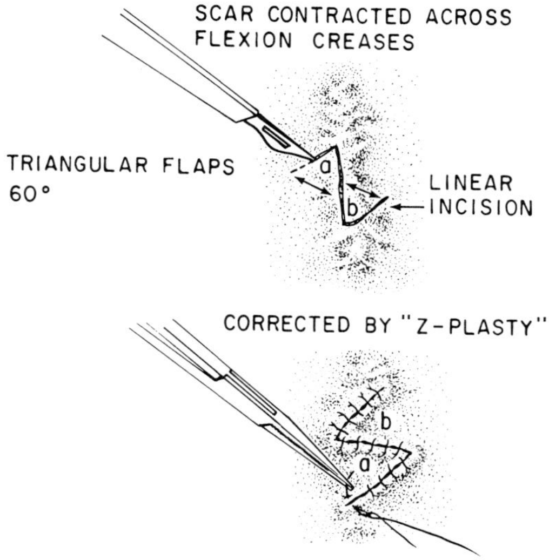

Figure 14-10. Z-plasty. The angles at the apices (*a* and *b*) of the triangular flaps should be about 60 degrees. If they are less than 60 degrees the vascularity of the flap is endangered, and if they are more, the rotational mobility becomes less. All the incisions should be through the depth of the scar and should include a portion of subcutaneous fat.

slowly, with formation of heavy scars. Elective incisions should be positioned parallel to these lines of tension for fast healing and less scarring (Fig. 14-9). When a scar has contracted across a flexion crease it may be released and corrected by Z-plasty (Fig. 14-10).

The blood vessels of the face form a network that is abundant everywhere but in the avascular epidermis. The vascular mesh is particularly dense in the lips, auricle, and nasal mucosa membrane. The larger blood vessels are the basis for designing skin flaps (Fig. 14-11). Branches of the external carotid artery, such as the occipital, external maxillary, and superficial temporal arteries, will maintain satisfactory vascularization to a variety of skin flaps. As the matching of skin color on the face is the difference between a good and a superb result, skin flaps from the face to the face are preferred.

SOFT-TISSUE INJURIES

Soft-tissue wounds are corrected as early as possible. Washing the wounded area with a mild soap and irrigating with sterile saline or water is less damaging to the exposed wound depth than the use of tinctures or strong antiseptics. A local nerve block, or infiltration with an anesthetic, permits clamping of bleeding vessels, debridement, and repair. While this is being done, the nurse or attendant should administer antitetanus therapy as described elsewhere (see Chap. 6).

PRIMARY REPAIR OF LACERATIONS

After the wound is free of contaminants and devitalized tissue, stent sutures of 5-0 stainless steel wire are positioned to obliterate

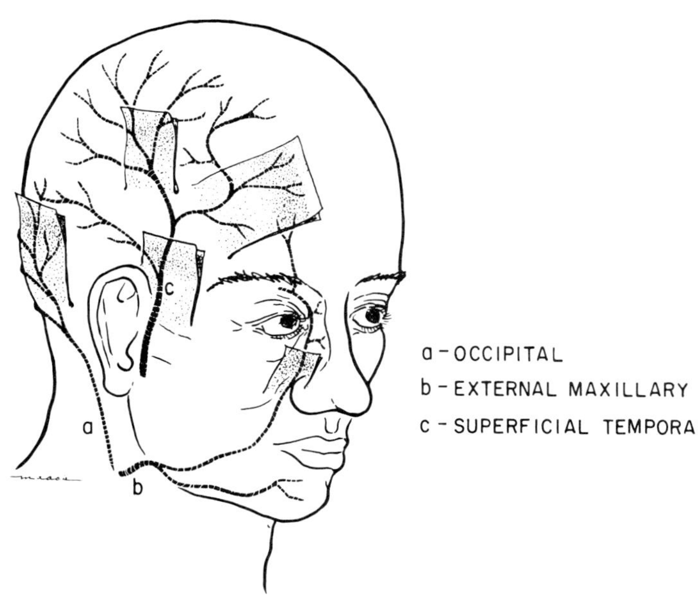

Figure 14-11. Satisfactory vascularization to a variety of skin flaps.

dead space, render hemostasis, reduce edema, decrease tension on the wound edges, and hold the bandage to the wound (see Fig. 14-4). Subcutaneous sutures of 5-0 clear nylon, either as a continuous pullout or interrupted subcuticulars, are used to coapt the dermis. An occasional skin suture of the same size nylon, or paper adhesive strips, will complete the epidermal closure. The steel stent sutures are then tied over a bandage. This eliminates taping and head bandages.

PRIMARY REPAIR OF AVULSIONS

Early skin replacement by means of free grafts or attached flaps is possible because of the abundant network of facial blood vessels. That wound surgical judgment is necessary before initiating repair is axiomatic, and this is dependent on experience. All completely detached skin parts are inspected, and if they are not macerated severely, they are transformed into full-thickness grafts by resecting the adipose tissue and replanting the skin over the cleaned wound. Tie-over sutures of nylon immobilize the bandage over the skin graft (Fig. 14-12). If the avulsed soft tissue remains attached to the host by a pedicle it deserves defatting, revising, and replacement into the recipient bed (Fig. 14-13). Half-buried mattress sutures of 5-0 nylon reattach the dermal flap.

Eyebrow trauma is common in facial injuries. Lacerations through the eyebrow need approximation and on occasion may benefit from Z-plasty (Fig. 14-14). There are instances when a whole eyebrow or parts of an eyebrow must be reconstructed, and the procedures used differ with the individual patient. The hair-bearing free graft is taken from the scalp in an area where the hair follicles are plentiful and the hair shafts are parallel. The free graft must be thick enough to include the follicles and wide enough to incorporate three rows of hair shafts. The eyebrow graft is sutured into its bed with fine nylon, and a light compressive bandage is applied. There is usually shedding of the shafts during the next 2 months, but regrowth takes place. Sometimes a second free graft must be added to achieve the desired result. The superficial temporal artery flap ensures complete brow restoration as well as surgical satisfaction. It is an island flap attached to the branches of the superficial temporal vessels. It is tunneled subcutaneously through the scalp to its recipient supraorbital area (Fig. 14-15).

FACIAL NERVE INJURY

Whenever facial lacerations are deep the wound should be inspected for injuries to nerves and to Stensen's duct. Any severed portion of the facial nerve may be satisfactorily repaired if the two cut ends can be brought together. The monosuture technique (Fig. 14-16) is adaptable to small peripheral branches. A 5-0 black nylon suture is introduced through a small button of fascia from the wound (or a

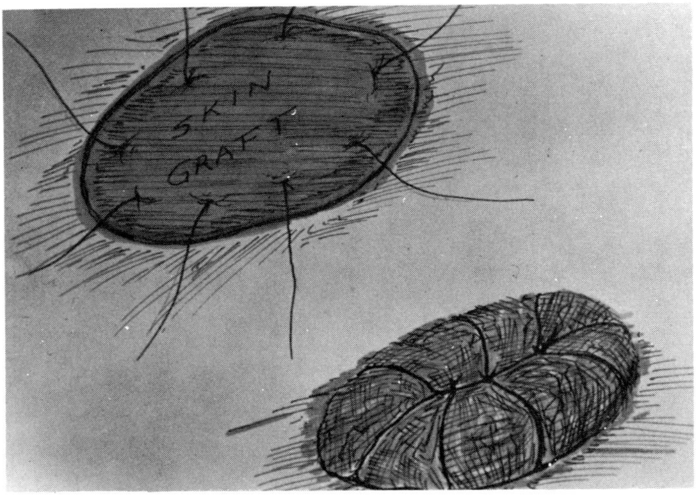

Figure 14-12. Stent tie-over bandage.

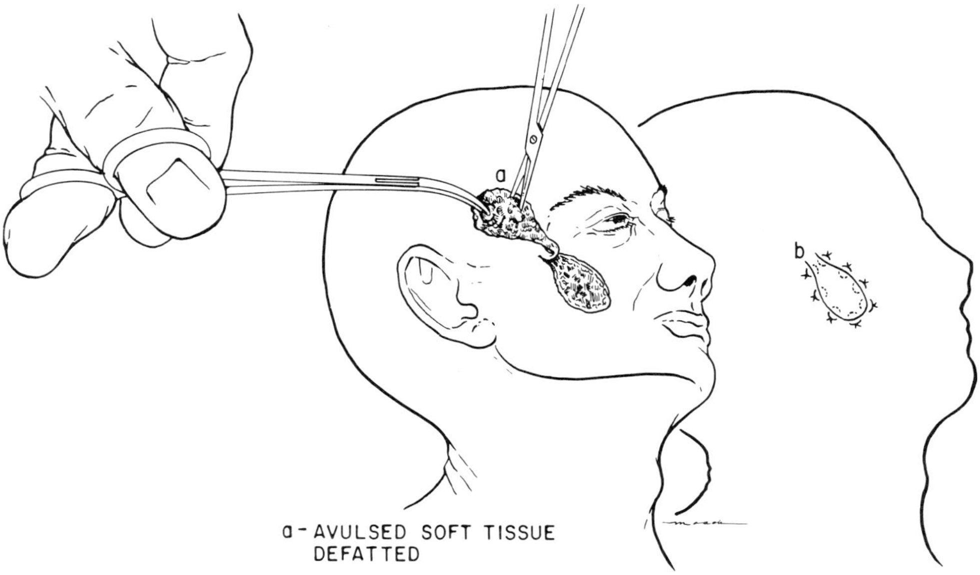

Figure 14-13. Primary repair of avulsions.

piece of silicone) and then is passed intraneurally through both cut nerve ends. The nerve is reefed for approximation, and the suture is tied over another button of fascia. Larger severed nerves are repaired by the epineurial cuff method (Fig. 14-17). The two cut nerve ends are placed end to end, and on end is pared, saving the epineurium, the most tenacious part of a peripheral nerve. The epineurium is pulled over the other cut nerve end and sutured. This enhances an approximated covered repair. A silicone wrapping for further protection may be added if desired.

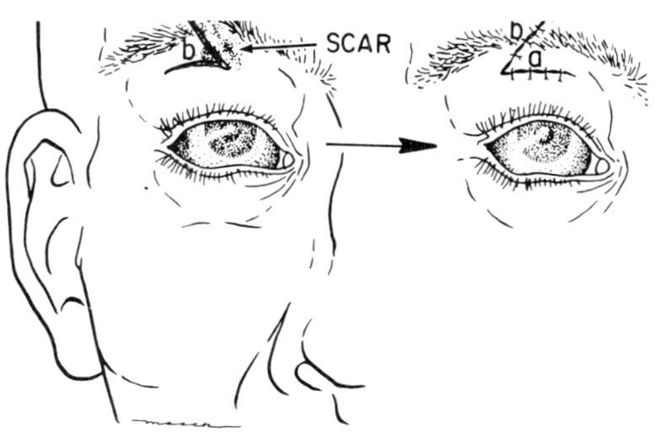

Figure 14-14. Repair of lacerations through the eyebrow (Z-plasty).

STENSEN'S (PAROTID) DUCT INJURY

Stensen's duct is located in the vicinity of the intersection of a straight line drawn from the middle of the upper lip to the auricular tragus with an oblique line parallel to the anterior border to the masseter muscle (Fig. 14-18). The buccal branch of the facial nerve crosses Stensen's duct as it exits from the parotid parenchyma. The syndrome of facial injury, scar, swollen face, and numbness is pathognomonic of leaking Stensen's duct or parotid gland laceration. The various treatments for early duct injury are (1) direct anastomosis, (2) ligation of the proximal end, or (3) creation of a mucosal fistula with the proximal end. Repair is facilitated by threading a polyethylene catheter through the duct ends (Fig. 14-19). The catheter should remain in the duct for a week and then be retrieved.

TEMPOROMANDIBULAR JOINT DISLOCATION

The temporomandibular joint is one means by which the mandible is attached to the skull. The only one other joint in the primate similar to it is the sternoclavicular joint. Acute lux-

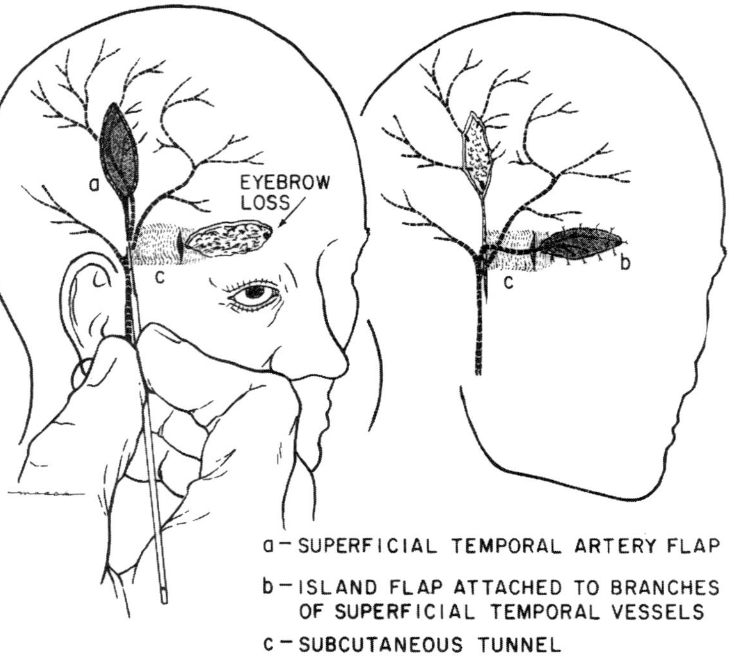

Figure 14-15. Island flap for repair of laceration of eyebrow.

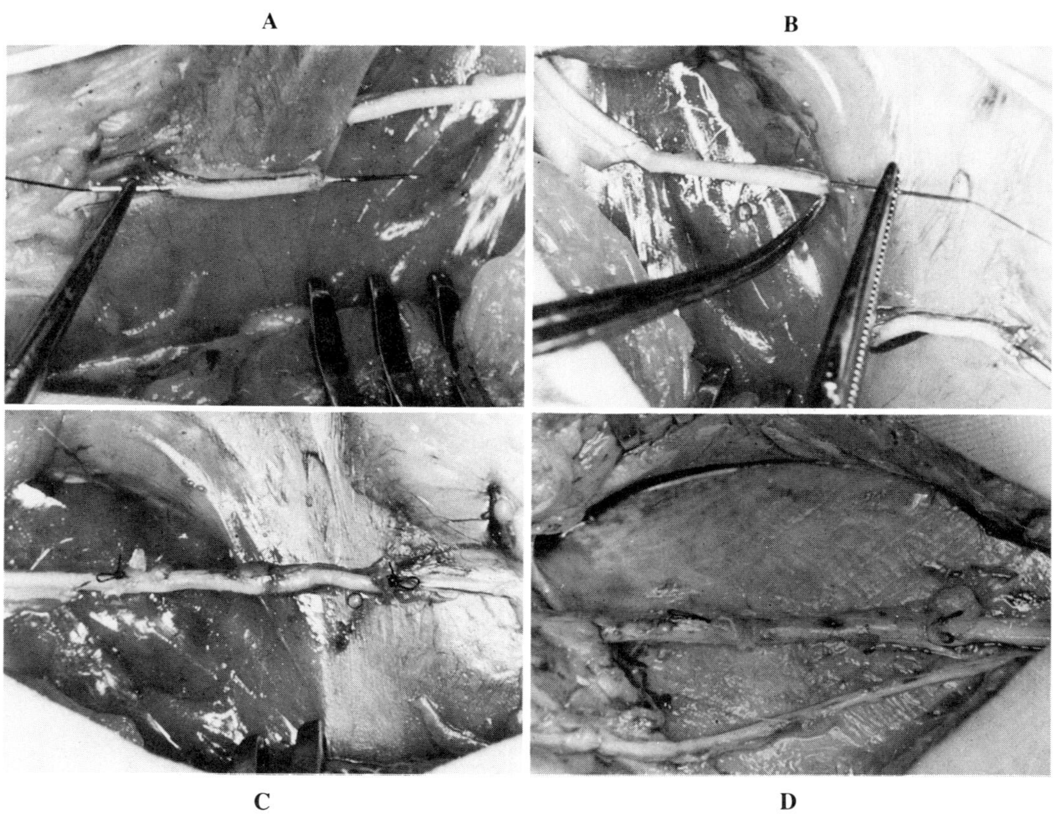

Figure 14-16. Monosuture neurorrhaphy. (*A*) Single intraneural suture through the proximal nerve end. (*B*) Continuation of single suture through the distal nerve end. (*C*) Nerve ending reefed for approximation, and single suture tied over a small piece of fascia. (*D*) Appearance 8 weeks postoperatively.

A

B

C

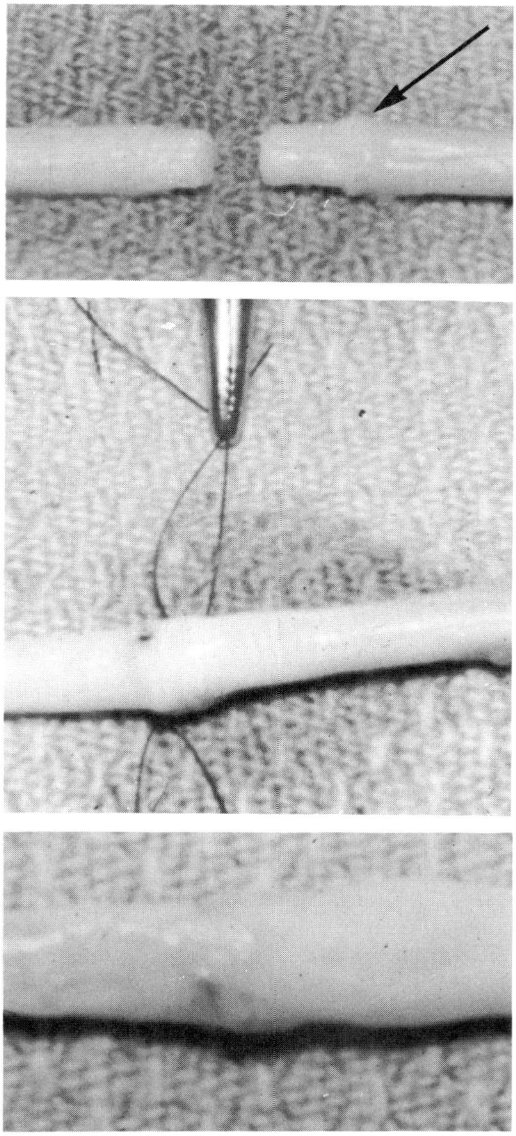

Figure 14-17. Epineurial cuff neurography. (*A*) The epineurial cuff is on the right; a single suture is in place. (*B*) The epineurial cuff is turned back over the apposed nerve ends. Interrupted fine sutures are in the epineurium only. (*C*) The anastomosis is complete; silicone sheeting is wrapped around the suture line.

ation of the condyle is usually anterior; if it luxates medially or laterally there generally is an associated fracture. Failure to reduce the dislocated condyle results in a chronic problem due to deformity and poor function. To treat an acute dislocation the physician stands either in front or in back of the patient, who is sitting. The thumbs are positioned bilaterally on the molar area, and the remaining fingers grasp the mandible extraorally. Thumb pressure is exerted downward and finger pressure upward. This allows the condyle to glide over the tubercle and into the glenoid fossa of the temporal bone. If infiltration of a local anesthetic into the joint capsule does not afford muscle relaxation, then the reduction should be accomplished under general anesthesia. The patient always feels better if a head–jaw bandage is used to hold the mandible closed and a small ice pack is placed over the temporomandibular joint area.

NOSE

OPERATIVE ANATOMY

The surgical approach to nasal trauma, infections, and tumors is through a thorough knowledge of anatomy. The nose is the most prominent and conspicuous part of the face and is a common recipient of violence. The skin covering the root or base of the nose is thin and loose and offers itself for easy repair. However, the skin over the remaining nose is thick, taut, and adherent and contains many sebaceous glands, all factors challenging the physician. When sections of nasal tissue are lost from the distal half, as a result of avulsion or surgical removal, repair by primary closure is difficult. Infected lesions of the nasal skin do not swell much but are exquisitely tender and painful from pressure on the nerves. The nasal *mucosal lining* is extremely vascular and intimately attached to the cartilage and bone; therefore most nasal fractures are compound.

The *circulation* to the nose is through the internal and external maxillary and the ophthalmic arteries, which end as plexuses in the skin and mucosa. The blood vessels of the skin communicate freely with those of the mucosa. These anastomoses are responsible for the spread of infectious processes from the nasal fossa to the skin and are also the reason external nasal surgery must be delayed until internal inflammations subside. Yet this abundant vessel network affords the advantages of prompt healing, less danger of tissue slough, and less conspicuous scarring.

Innervation to the nose is mainly sensory, as the only motor supply needed is a branch of the facial nerve to the alar muscles. The supra-

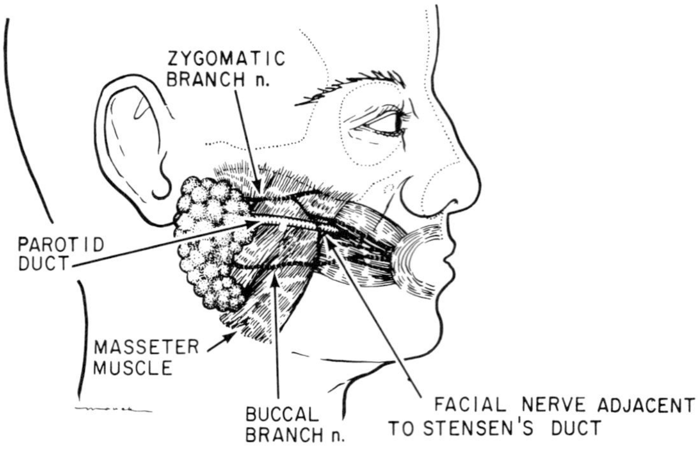

Figure 14-18. Location of Stensen's duct.

trochlear nerve supplies sensation to the nasal root; the external nasal branch of the opthalmic, to the nasal tip; and the infraorbital branch of the superior maxillary, to the sides of the nose. The mucosa is furnished sensation through the nasopalatine, olfactory, and anterior ethmoidal nerves. Complete anesthesia of the entire nose is easily achieved by injecting less than 8 ml of lidocaine (Xylocaine) into the circles as diagramed (Fig. 14-20). The sphenopalatine ganglia may be blocked with a lidocaine or cocaine intranasal pack.

The osseous scaffolding of the nose comprises two nasal bones: the perpendicular plate of the ethmoid and the vomer. The remaining architecture is cartilaginous and includes the superior and inferior lateral cartilages, occasional alar or sesmoid cartilages, and the septal cartilage.

FRACTURES

The mosaic pyramid of bone and cartilage that constitutes the nose is more subject to trauma than are neighboring solid facial structures. Through direct or glancing blows the bones lend themselves to unilateral, bilateral, linear, comminuted, depressed, or superimposed fractures—which are nearly always compound (Fig. 14-21). Unfortunately, fractures of the nose usually receive trivial care by attendants who are not acquainted with the

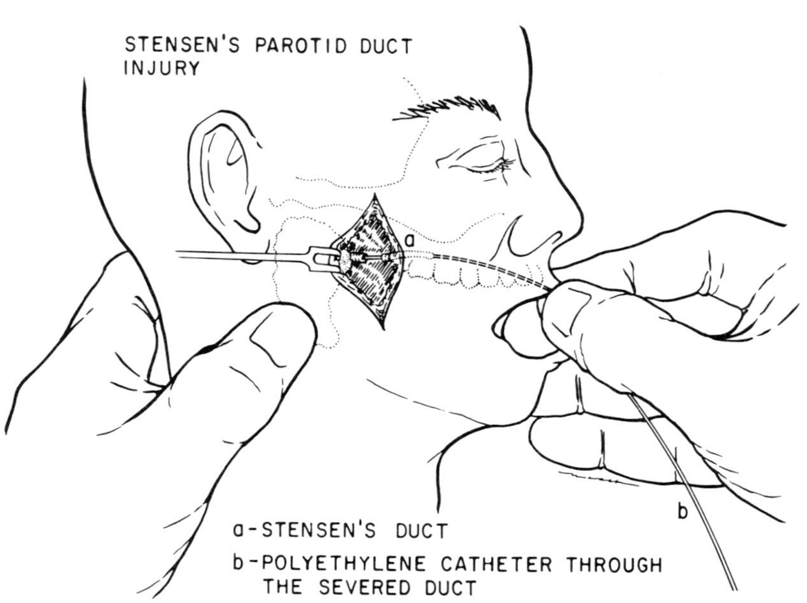

Figure 14-19. Repair of Stensen's duct with a polyethylene catheter.

A

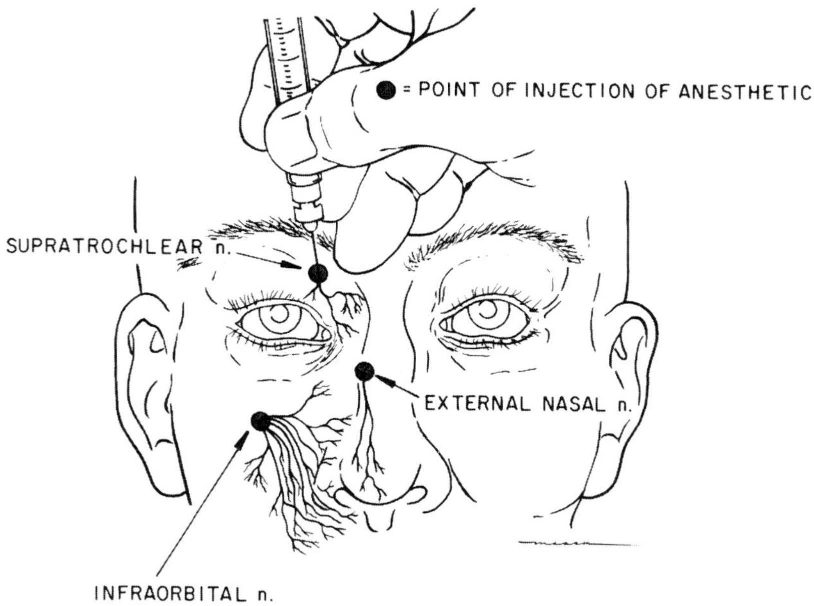

B

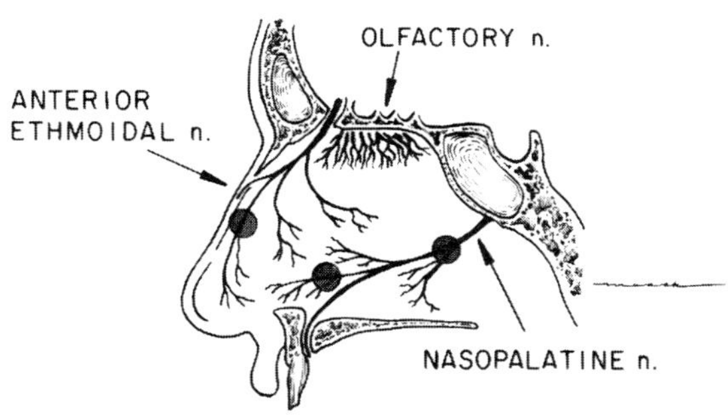

Figure 14-20. (*A*) Extranasal points of injection of anesthetic solution. (*B*) Intranasal points of injection.

anatomy or who are too busy to devote the necessary attention, and severe complications ensue. Diagnosis may be difficult, but there is always a history of trauma and, usually, epistaxis, orbital ecchymosis, pain, crepitation, deformity, and swelling; x-ray films reveal the break. The two most frequently observed fractures are the bony tip fracture and the lateral in–out fracture. In the former the fractured tip is either depressed or elevated. The lateral in–out type exhibits a concavity on the side of impact and a convexity on the contralateral side. Roentgenograms sometimes are unsatisfactory; a lateral view is more demonstrative than an anteroposterior film. When a definite diagnosis is in question, treat the injury as a fracture regardless, because of the serious sequelae that may result. Because of the excellent vascular supply, fractured nasal bones ossify very rapidly; within 2 weeks a strong callus has united the broken edges, and in another week they are solid. Therefore displaced nasal fractures should be corrected as soon as possible.

First-aid attention is focused on control of the hemorrhage, which usually is arrested by ice, digital pressure, or intranasal tampon; 1% lidocaine (Xylocaine) with epinephrine is used for anesthesia and also assists in hemostasis. Fracture reduction is better accomplished when the patient is free of pain and the area is tidy.

Nonimpacted fractures may be successfully treated with closed reduction by simple digital force. If this cannot be achieved, then an Asche, Walshom, or Kelly forceps serves well. The forceps blades are padded with gauze or rubber tubing, and, with one blade on

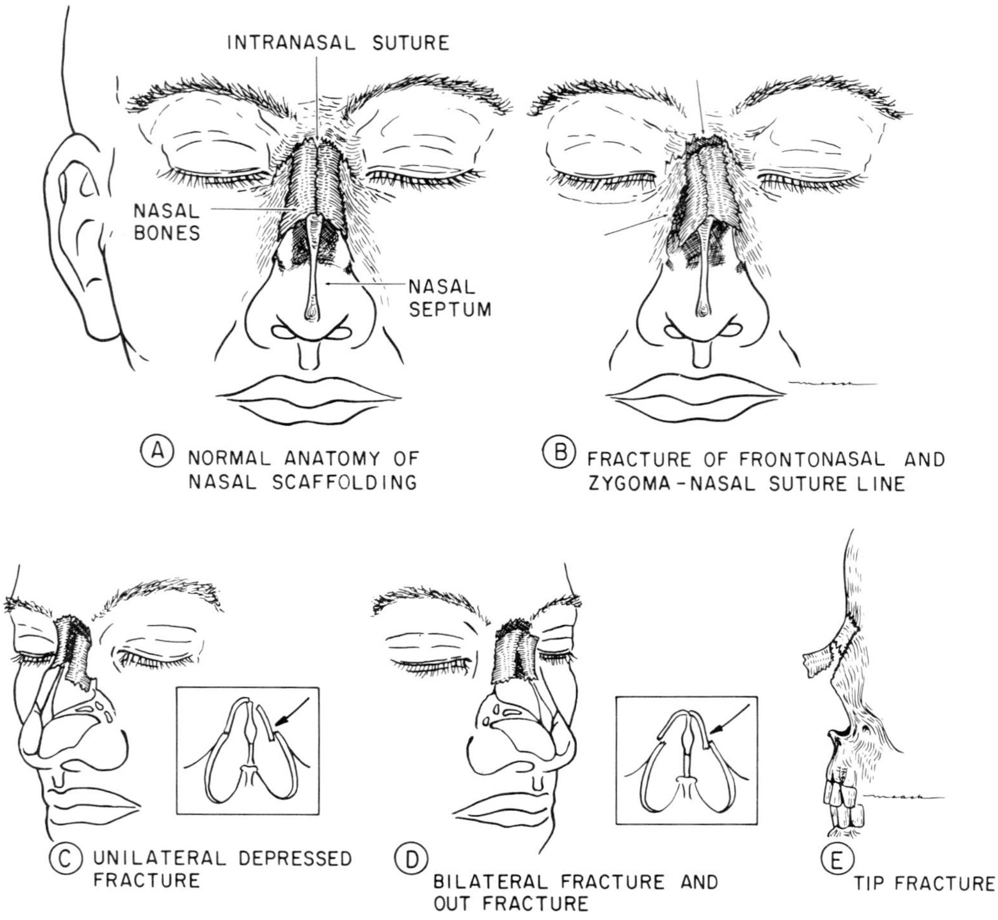

Figure 14-21. Fractures of nose.

the inside and the other on the outside, the fracture is elevated and repositioned. Nasal-tip fractures are corrected with a blunt instrument and force (Fig. 14-22). Unlike long bones, nasal bones are not influenced by muscle action (flexion and extension), yet it is necessary that immobilization be used. Immobilization for at least 4 days is required to prevent hemorrhage, hematoma, and edema and to protect the patient from accidentally reinjuring the nose. An intranasal packing of petrolatum gauze enclosed in a Surgicel wrapping is inserted, and counterpressure is applied externally by means of a splint of dental compound or metal and adhesive strips (Fig. 14-23). Ice packs made with a wash cloth, ice chips, and rubber bands are used postoperatively on the eyes and nose (Fig. 14-24). The splint and intranasal packings may be removed in 2 to 7 days, depending on the patient's original trauma and his convalescent progress.

FOREIGN BODIES

Children are the common recipient of foreign bodies in the form of peas, beans, beads, small coins, buttons, and various types of insects. If the object is not too large, a cotton applicator or hemostat may be used to push it into the posterior pharynx, from which it is easily retrieved. Objects that are fixed in the mucosa and that will not budge may be retrieved by a skin or dural hook or by splitting the object into small portions. It is not inconceivable, when other methods fail, to fenestrate the septum or surgically separate the ala for more room. Neosynephrine or ephedrine nasal drops will shrink the mucosa, which helps open the passageway. Although syringe

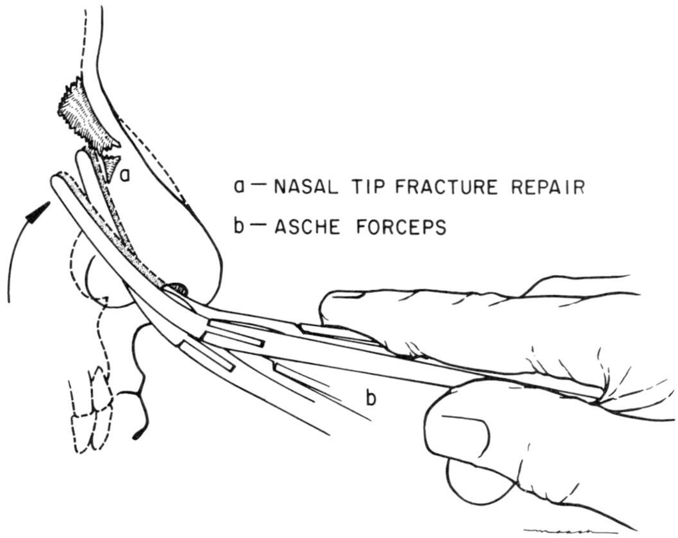

Figure 14-22. Repair of nasal tip fractures.

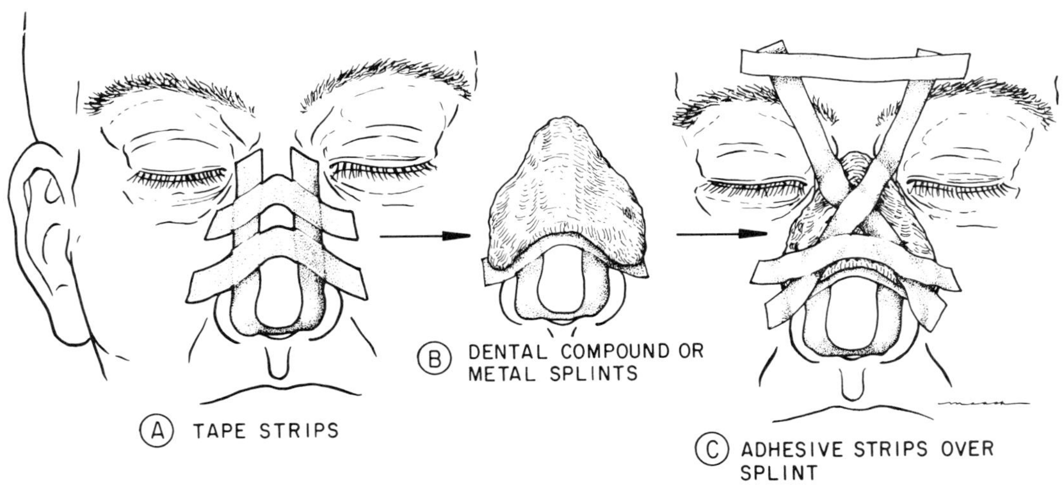

Figure 14-23. Immobilization of fracture of nose.

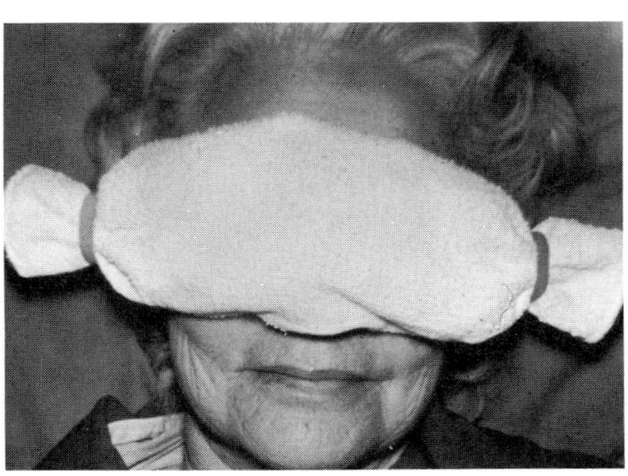

Figure 14-24. Ice pack in place.

irrigation is contraindicated in the treatment of foreign bodies in the nasal vestibule, this is a choice method of removing objects from the ear canal.

EAR

FOREIGN BODIES

Mismanagement of foreign objects in the ear may lead to deafness, and because these emergencies occur frequently, good judgment is important. These foreign bodies may be alive and very active, or they may be inanimate.

The former group includes ants, flies, gnats, bees, and larvae; the latter includes peas, beans, hairs, pieces of matches, toothpicks, pencils, and chips of stone or metal.

The object of therapy is to remove the offending agent, and there are various approaches. It may be advisable to use a general anesthetic in small children. If the offender is an active insect it should be killed promptly by instilling into the ear a nonirritating oil, such as olive oil, followed by syringing with boric acid, salt, or any mildly antiseptic solution. If this method is unsuccessful, a small forceps, a metallic hook, or a wire loop should be used to retrieve it. Sometimes a cotton applicator with glue on the end will adhere to the foreign body and retrieve it. If all other approaches have been unsuccessful, it may be necessary to detach the external auricle and cartilaginous canal partly through a posterior approach, allowing the object to be removed from the edematous passage.

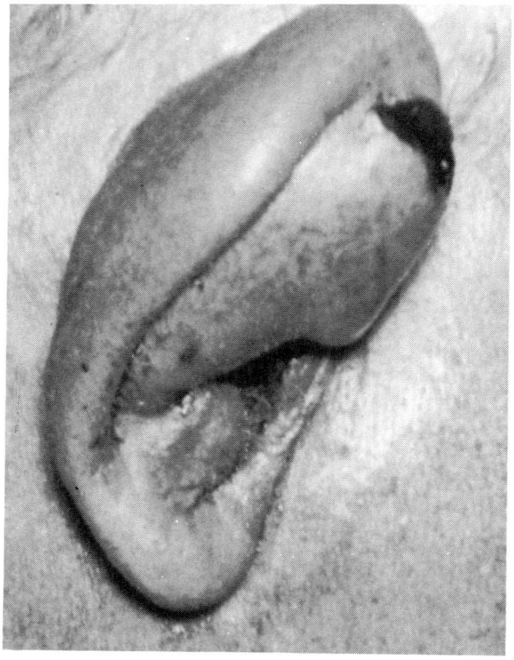

Figure 14-25. Hematoma of ear.

LACERATIONS

Injuries that expose the ear cartilage should be treated as soon as possible to prevent chondritis and suppuration. The exposed cartilage should be trimmed sufficiently to afford satisfactory skin approximation. The wound edges are coapted with 5-0 nylon sutures, loosely enough to permit drainage of serum. The dressing should not be tight but should be occlusive and absorptive. Such dressing should be inspected in 24 hours and allowed to remain in place another 4 days, unless local pain or other evidence of infection makes redressing imperative.

HEMATOMAS

Hematomas of the ear occur daily in athletes such as boxers and wrestlers, although they are also observed as a result of contusions from any cause (Fig. 14-25). The fluctuant swelling that appears beneath the skin on the anterior surface of the ear, if untreated and not infected, undergoes organization and secondary fibrosis. The ear becomes noticeably thickened and misshapen, resembling a cauliflower; hence the terminal deformity in cases of repeated hematomas is spoken of as a cauliflower ear.

The treatment of auricular hematoma is early drainage of the blood and serum found between the skin and the cartilage; this is best performed within 24 to 48 hours after the injury. Although it is enticing to aspirate the liquid collection by introducing a large needle through a wheal of local anesthesia, it is better judgment to make a small incision at the most dependent part of the hematoma and provide a drain to inhibit recurrence. A moderate-pressure dressing must be applied immediately, using a sponge, gauze padding, or a stent suture tied over a bolus of cotton. The dressing is held in place by a circular bandage involving the head and the ear. This dressing may be left in place for 5 to 6 days, when it may be removed without danger of recurrence of the hematoma.

Occasionally, a patient with an old hematoma of the ear may wish to have the deformity removed. In such cases the fibrous tissue producing the deformity may be excised under local anesthesia. The skin is separated from the underlying scar tissue along one of the natural creases of the ear, and the excessive fibrous tissue is excised down to normal cartilage. The skin then is replaced in its normal position, and the wound is sutured with fine nylon. A mold of wet cotton is fitted to the ear to form the future normal contour, and a pressure bandage is applied.

CONGENITAL PREAURICULAR SINUS

Congenital preauricular sinus is an anomaly seen in the helix, in front of the helix, and as far medially as the cheek. It results from faulty closure of the first branchial cleft and consists of a sinus tract, composed of squamous epithelium, hair follicles, and other elements of normal skin, that leads to a blind pouch lined with columnar epithelium. The sinus opening may become occluded, and abscess formation then results; this requires incision and drainage. The noninfected preauricular sinus requires careful dissection and excision of the entire sinus tract. The optimum time to operate is before infection appears, and the operation is usually performed under local anesthesia.

EARLOBE PUNCTURE

Puncture of the earlobes for the wearing of earrings is commonly requested. It is performed under local anesthesia after symmetric points in the centers of the earlobes have been marked. A 20-gauge hypodermic needle is used to make the tunnel. The purpose is to form an epithelial-lined tract through the lobe. A wire of gold, silver, or steel is placed through the puncture wound and is moved back and forth the next few days. The earlobe is cleaned daily with alcohol. All patients, but especially blacks, must be warned of the possibility of keloid development.

MOUTH AND TONGUE

MUCOCELES

A mucocele is a retention cyst of the mucous glands within the mouth. It is commonly found on the inner surface of the cheek, in the line of occlusion of the teeth. It may even occur on the dorsum of the tongue. Distension of the ducts of the glands of Blandin beneath the tip of the tongue may cause swelling of considerable size. This cyst occurs most frequently on the lower lip and appears as a soft, regular, bluish swelling, which frequently varies in size, periodically discharging its contents into the mouth (Fig. 14-26). It produces symptoms due to its presence on the lip, causing a thickness and protrusion, and not infrequently it is bitten inadvertently by the patient. It causes no pain and almost never becomes infected. The only indications for treatment are the inconvenience and the disfigurement it produces.

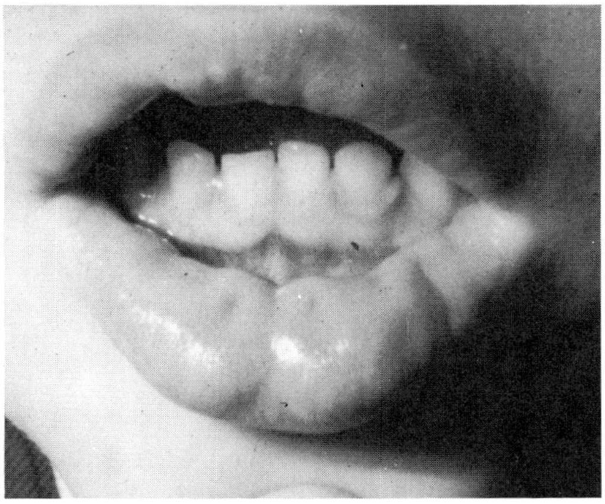

Figure 14-26. Mucocele of lower lip.

Treatment

A mucocele is treated by excision, and the operation is performed under local anesthesia.

After the area around and underneath the cyst is infiltrated with 0.5% procaine–epinephrine solution, an assistant everts the lip and holds it firmly on each side between the thumbs and index fingers. An incision is made over the surface of the cyst, and the mucous membrane is dissected without cutting the cyst wall. Skin hooks are placed on the mucous membrane on each side of the incision, and the cyst wall is separated from the surrounding tissues by gentle dissection. The deeper portions of the cyst are somewhat more adherent to surrounding structures, but by careful dissection the cyst may be removed intact. The wound may be left open, since it heals in a few hours, or may be closed with one or two absorbable sutures.

TONGUE LACERATIONS

Lacerations of the tongue may occur as a result of tooth penetrations incidental to convulsions, contact sports, or falls. Suturing is rarely necessary except to control severe bleeding. As a rule, simple lacerations that do not pass entirely through the tongue or do not tear the margin of the tongue leaving a flap of tissue may be treated conservatively. Through-and-through lacerations involving the edges of the tongue, producing a flap of tongue substance, are best treated by suture. The sutures may be inserted after infiltration with procaine-epinephrine solution. They are placed with curved smooth-edged needles and should include half of the thickness of the tongue. Absorbable sutures are the choice, and in spite of the abundant bacterial flora of the mouth, wounds of the tongue usually heal primarily. Mouthwashes are useful during the first few post-trauma days.

TONGUE-TIE

Congenital shortening of the frenum of the tongue is a rather uncommon but easily treated abnormality. This deformity is usually noted in infancy or childhood. The parents become aware of it because of inability of the child to stick out the tongue or because of a speech impediment.

On examination the short lingual frenum is at once apparent. Often the tongue cannot be protruded beyond the teeth, and during efforts to extend it, the tip is pulled down, and the body bulges upward in the mouth.

Treatment

Treatment of tongue-tie is incision of the shortened frenum. This operation may be performed in infants without anesthesia, but in older children local infiltration anesthesia is advisable. The infiltration should be made toward the floor of the mouth. Using the broad end of an ordinary grooved director as a retractor, the frenum may be slipped into its central slot and so isolated as to make it easily visible. It is then divided with scissors, care being taken not to carry the incision too far backward because of the danger of injuring the frenal artery. The small amount of bleeding that occurs usually stops without active treatment.

EXOSTOSES

Exostoses, or dense bony excrescences, are found in both jaws.

Torus Palatinus. Torus palatinus is an exostosis of the hard palate in the midline, which presents as hard oval swelling that varies in size and may be smooth or nodular. It is often mistaken for an osteoma. It is present normally in a certain percentage of people, most of whom never know it is there. It is painless, does not grow, and should be removed only when it interferes with the fitting of a denture or when the overlying mucous membrane becomes irritated.

Torus Mandibularis. Torus mandibularis is an exostosis found on the lingual surface of the mandible, usually bilaterally, in the region of the canines and the premolars. The indications for its removal are similar to those in the case of torus palatinus.

Exostoses may be found frequently in the region of the tuberosities of the maxilla and occasionally in other areas. If removal is indicated, the bone may be trimmed away with bur and chisel under a mucoperiosteal flap.

LEUKOPLAKIA

Leukoplakia, white patches in the mucous membrane resembling white enamel paint, is a very common precancerous lesion of the mouth (Fig. 14-27). It represents a piling up of the outer layers of the epithelium and is almost invariably caused by excessive use of tobacco. It may be smooth in the early stages, but in more severe cases it becomes very thick and rough, with fissures and induration at the base.

Treatment

The application of any irritants to these lesions is contraindicated. Smoking should be prohibited and the lesions watched at regular intervals. If they become hard and fissured, they should be excised with an electrosurgical

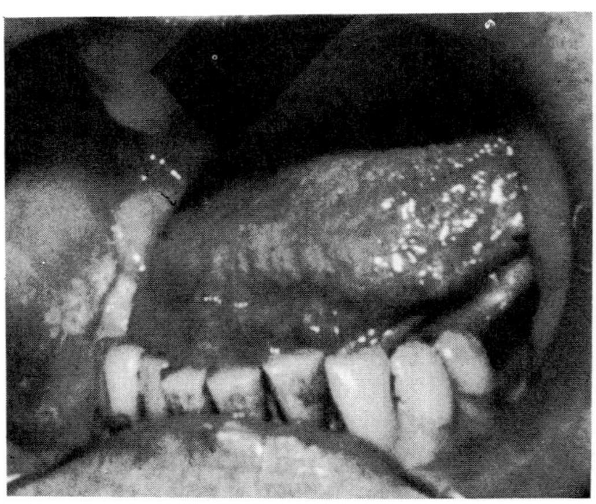

Figure 14-27. Leukoplakia of mouth.

knife or with actual cautery, and the tissue should be examined under the microscope. Otherwise they should be left alone. They may disappear following removal of the cause, or they may remain dormant and harmless.

It should be recognized that leukoplakia is definitely a premalignant lesion, and when there is not a definite tendency to regression or when the patient cannot be observed frequently, excision is the safer treatment. Leukoplakia and carcinoma in situ of the lip are removed by a lip shave and, possibly, wedge resection, which is actuated by excising the mucosal surface and replacing it by advancing the labial mucous membrane to the skin margin (Fig. 14-28).

CARCINOMAS OF THE TONGUE

Most carcinomas of the mouth arise from the pavement epithelium of the buccal cavity. They are called epitheliomas or epidermoid carcinomas. They appear much more frequently in men than in women, and this is believed to be due largely to the frequency of smoking in males.

Etiology

It is estimated that 50% to 75% of carcinomas of the tongue could be prevented by vigorous elimination of precancerous conditions. Leukoplakia is believed to account for 35% of a buccal cancer. Destruction of these areas is probably the most important single prophylactic measure against lingual cancer. Papillomas, ulcers, and fissures are other premalignant lesions of the tongue. These are usually overlooked or disregarded by the patient or by the examiner who sees them at this stage. Nevertheless, vigorous early treatment may prevent subsequent development of cancer. Many of these lesions may be excised, either with a knife or with an electric needle, during the precancerous stages, and in most in-

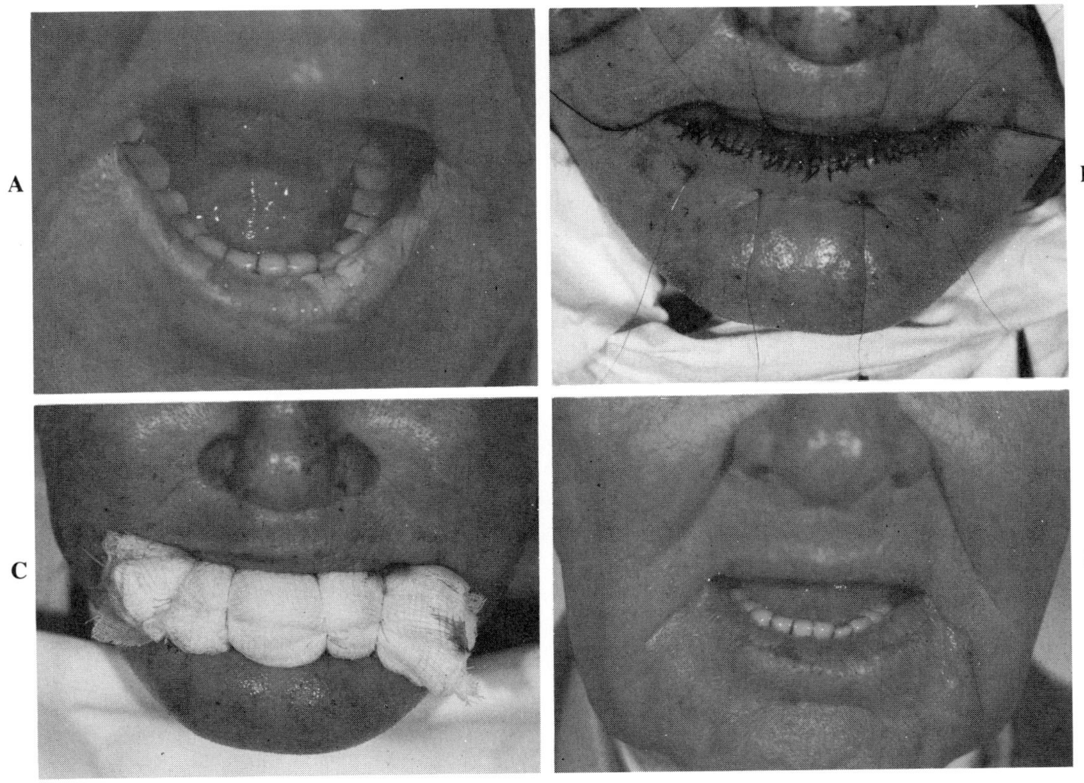

Figure 14-28. (*A*) Several areas of leukoplakia on the lower lip. (*B*) The surface of the lip has been removed by sharp dissection and the raw surface covered with mucous membrane of the mouth advanced to the anterior edge of the lip by undermining the buccal mucosa. (*C*) A roll of gauze is tied in place by four steel wires placed through the lip. This gives firm pressure. (*D*) The lip 10 days later.

stances the operation may be performed under local anesthesia in the ambulatory patient.

Diagnosis

At times there is doubt as to the nature of a lesion that appears on the tongue or in the mouth. The diagnosis often can be made on simple inspection and palpation if it is borne in mind that most malignant diseases of the buccal mucosa are characterized by an indurated ulcer. Sometimes the growth may be more papillary in character, and occasionally it appears as a hard nodular growth that involves the mucous membrane secondarily. An exfoliative cytologic smear is useful as a diagnostic method before biopsy.

Usually a correct diagnosis can be made clinically, but at times it may be difficult to distinguish between carcinoma and a luetic lesion, either gumma or sclerosing glossitis. This is especially true if a history of syphilis or a positive Wassermann reaction is obtained. The important differential point is that carcinoma usually occurs as a single lesion, situated most often at the border of the tongue, whereas in gumma there are multiple lesions, which may be at any site on the tongue. Furthermore, the carcinomatous ulcer is usually painful and bleeds easily, whereas the gumma is not particularly painful, nor does it bleed readily.

Tuberculosis of the tongue is seen occasionally, and this also must be distinguished from carcinoma. The tuberculous lesion appears almost invariably in an individual who has pulmonary tuberculosis. It may occur as a superficial or a fairly deep ulcer, and it usually appears at the tip of the tongue. The lack of induration surrounding the ulcer is a diagnostic point.

Biopsy is perhaps the most conservative method of making a diagnosis. This can be accomplished very frequently in ambulatory patients. A topical application of cocaine solution, 10% to 20% is used; it is held in place on a pledget of gauze for 1 to 3 minutes. Excision biopsy, with a knife, a biopsy punch, or the loop electrode, may be done using this type of anesthesia (Fig. 14-29). In biopsy it must be remembered that the tissue at the edge of the

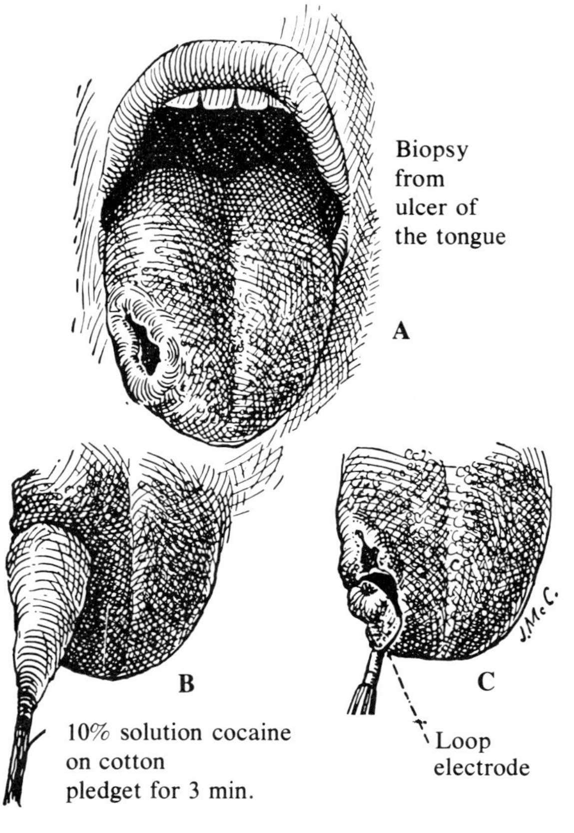

Figure 14-29. Biopsy of an ulcer of the tongue following local application of 10% cocaine solution. The cutting current with a loop electrode is an excellent method of removing a specimen.

ulcer gives the most characteristic appearance under the microscope. The necrotic, fungating material at the base of the ulcer may be nothing but chronic granulation tissue or necrotic cells and of no help in diagnosis.

Treatment

For treatment of carcinoma of the mouth, especially of the tongue, hospitalization is advised. However, in some instances, irradiation may be carried out with the patient ambulatory throughout the period of treatment. Irradiation is the treatment of choice for the invasive posterior group, whereas surgery plus irradiation benefits the great number of patients with cancer of the anterior tongue.

CARCINOMAS OF THE LIP

Almost all that has been said concerning carcinoma of the tongue may be repeated with regard to the lip. There is, however, a characteristic difference between these two tumors: Carcinoma of the tongue is a rapidly growing lesion that is fatal because of early metastasis to regional lymph nodes. Carcinoma of the lip is a comparatively slow-growing ulcer with a fairly good prognosis if it is seen in the early stages. It appears almost invariable as an ulcer and most frequently in the lower lip (Fig. 14-30). Many believe that chronic irritation is a definitive factor in its causation. The ulcer refuses to heal, and this is a diagnostic point in differentiating it from other ulcerative lesions of the lips. Any ulcer that persists and does not show progress in healing in a period of 2 weeks should be strongly suspected to be carcinoma.

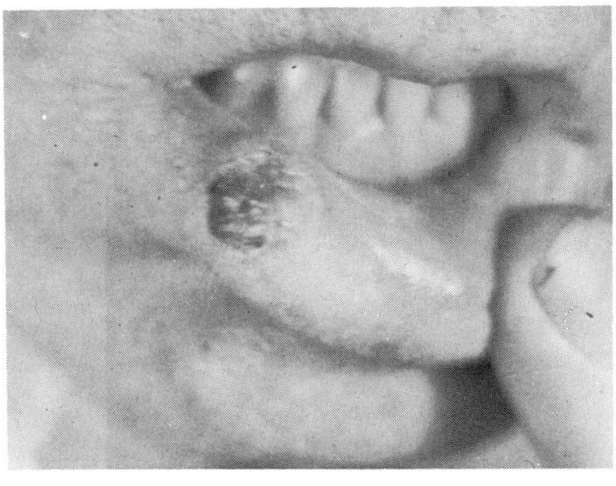

Figure 14-30. Squamous cell carcinoma of the lip.

Treatment

The treatment of carcinoma of the lip has progressed greatly with the advent of new methods of irradiation. A combination of surgical excision and irradiation is used in many clinics. No attempt will be made here to outline the therapy, since this is not an area for ambulatory surgical care.

SALIVARY GLANDS

ANATOMY

The major salivary glands of surgical concern are the sublingual (smallest), the submaxillary (submandibular), and the parotid. All of these are involved in a variety of traumatic, inflammatory, and neoplastic conditions, of which many respond best to surgical management. A working knowledge of the anatomy and pathology is important, because a lack of such may terminate in facial paralysis or recurrence of the initial disease. The sublingual glands are positioned immediately behind the mandibular symphysis, one on each side of the midline, covering the mylohyoid muscle, and excrete saliva onto the floor of the mouth by several minor ducts and one large duct. The submaxillary salivary glands are larger and are situated posteriorly and laterally and fold around the mylohyoid muscle. (Fig. 14-31). Their excretion empties into the mouth by a relatively long (Wharton's) duct. By elevating the tongue, the openings of both the submaxillary and the sublingual ducts on each side of the lingual raphe are noted.

RANULAE

The term *ranula* (frog) is rather loosely applied to all forms of retention cysts that appear on the floor of the mouth beneath the tongue, yet some surgical pathologists limit it to a retention cyst of the sublingual salivary gland. Most observers believe that it occurs from an obstruction of the sublingual duct, although some believe that it is due to myxomatous degeneration of a mucous gland. Wharton's duct is not involved in ranula, and on sialography, may often be seen as an opaque strand near the cyst. In true ranula this duct is always pa-

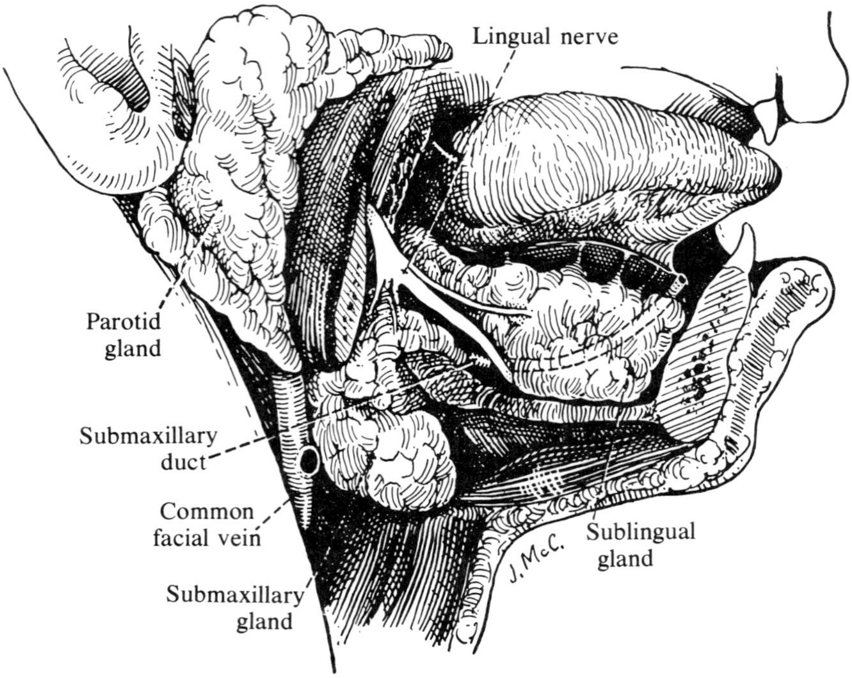

Figure 14-31. Anteroposterior section of the floor of the mouth as viewed from within. Note the relation of the sublingual gland to the mucous membrane of the mouth and the position of the submaxillary gland as it folds around the mylohyoid muscle. The submaxillary duct is long and extends forward, mesially, and upward.

tent, and there is no swelling of the submaxillary gland.

DIAGNOSIS

The cyst begins as a small, domelike swelling in the floor of the mouth beneath the anterior surface of the tongue. The mucous membrane is stretched tightly over the cystic swelling, which is soft and filled with a viscid fluid (Fig. 14-32). The cyst gradually increases in size and elevates the tongue. It is invariably unilateral, but it may extend to the opposite side by expansion. There is absence of any inflammatory symptoms, and the swelling is painless unless it assumes considerable size, when it may become annoying. The larger cysts are apt to interfere with speech. Not infrequently, the obstruction within the duct may be intermittent, and the ranula may therefore vary in size, with a salty, mucouslike material appearing in the mouth as it empties periodically.

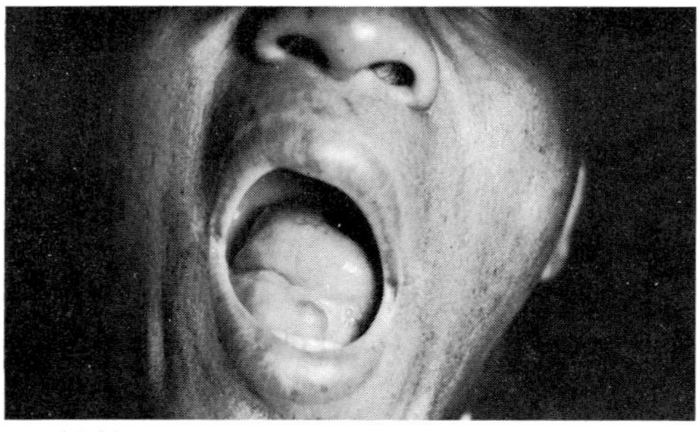

Figure 14-32. Ranula. Excision and marsupialization are the treatment of choice.

TREATMENT

The treatment of a small ranula is excision and closure. If the lesion recurs or is very large, it may necessitate marsupialization, excision of the enlarged duct, or, occasionally, excision of the duct and the sublingual gland. Simple incision or insertion of a seton in a large ranula to permit drainage of the contents almost invariably results in recurrence.

Marsupialization may be performed as an ambulatory procedure under local anesthesia.

After local infiltration with procaine–epinephrine solution around the cystic swelling, the mucous membrane is incised and retracted gently with surgical-gut traction suture to expose the dome of the cyst. When the dissection has been carried downward to the level of the floor of the mouth, the projecting portion of the cyst is excised. A thick, mucuslike material will escape from the cyst. It is well, in excising the dome of the cyst, to catch the lining membrane with several fine surgical-gut sutures that pass through the cyst wall and the adjacent mucous membrane of the floor of the mouth. The entire circumference of the cyst wall thus is sutured to the mucous membrane bit by bit as the projecting portion of the cyst is excised. Sutures are placed about 3 mm apart, and they should be left long in order to serve as tractors until all the sutures have been placed and then are severed. During the operation a small suction apparatus is of great help in keeping the field free of blood and saliva. Usually little bleeding is encountered, and the only postoperative care necessary is the use of saline mouthwashes.

The prognosis must be guarded, even in cases in which a large opening seems to have been left after marsupialization, for recurrence is frequent.

SALIVARY CALCULI

INCIDENCE

Calculi do not occur with equal frequency in the various salivary glands; 80% are found in the submandibular, 19% in the parotid, and 1% in the sublingual gland. Minor salivary gland calculi occur quite infrequently. Calculi are multiple in only 25% of cases and are almost always confined to a single gland.

Most calculi are composed of calcium phosphate; however, the portion of calcium varies between the different glands, resulting in 90% of submaxillary and only 10% of parotid calculi being radiopaque.

Calculi occur frequently in the submaxillary gland ducts (Wharton) but less so in those of the parotid (Stensen) and the sublingual gland ducts. Calculi may be present in both the gland and the duct. The cause of the calculus formation has been ascribed to inflammation or infection. Parotid calculi are usually preceded by an inflammatory response. Submaxillary calculi usually form around a nidus of mucus because it is more alkaline with a higher concentration of calcium phosphate. The duct is longer and the flow of fluid is against gravity.

SYMPTOMS

The symptoms of a stone in the submaxillary duct are typical and characteristic, but in spite of this, the patient is often treated for long periods for toothache, lingual neuralgia, lymphadenitis, or even cancer. The presence of the stone causes intermittent, or often complete, obstruction of the duct. The result is a painful swelling in the region of the submaxillary gland just below the angle of the jaw (Fig. 14-33). The symptoms are most marked at mealtimes, when physiologic engorgement occurs and back pressure on the gland increases. Pain may also be elicited by lemon juice or a pickle. When the obstruction is intermittent, the patient often notes discharge of a salty material into the mouth, with subsequent relief of pain in the gland.

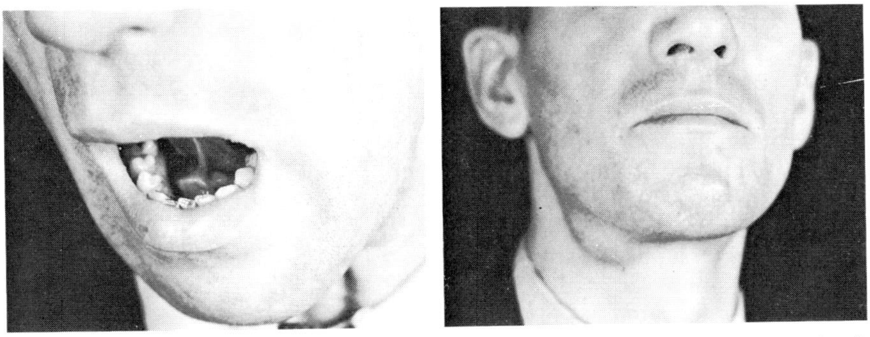

Figure 14-33. (*A*) Calculus of the submaxillary gland. (*B*) Note swelling beneath angle of the jaw.

On examination during an acute attack a tender, edematous swelling may be noted along the course of Wharton's duct on the involved side. At times the stone may be associated with a purulent infection of the duct. In such cases the outlet of the duct may be reddened, and pus may be expressed from it.

DIAGNOSIS

In the majority of cases the stone lies in the anterior two thirds of the duct, and usually it may be palpated along the course of the duct with one finger in the mouth and another under the chin. In a few cases the stone may be found presenting at the orifice of the duct. If the stone cannot be palpated, roentgen examination frequently reveals its presence and location. Occlusal bite films show stones in the submaxillary duct to best advantage, whereas stones in the gland proper are shown by lateral films.

TREATMENT

The treatment of a submaxillary calculus is removal. This is a relatively easy procedure if the stone is large and lies in the distal two thirds of the duct. Several ambulatory procedures may be followed.

Under local infiltration or mandibular or lingual block anesthesia, the oral mucous membrane is incised over the calculus, exposing the duct lumen and permitting removal of the calculus. When the stone is small and movable, insertion of a fine silk suture around the duct behind the calculus prevents the calculus from slipping back toward the gland during its retrieval. The suture is removed after it has served its purpose. The duct may be immobilized by inserting two silk traction sutures through its orifice. These may be held by an assistant, or they may be hooked between the patient's teeth so as to convert the duct orifice into a fairly large entrance. The duct is then slit open from the orifice until the stone is reached. This technique is most valuable for stones in the distal third of the duct.

After removal of the stone the mucous membrane may be closed with fine gut sutures or it may be left open. Usually no sutures are inserted if there has been associated infection of the duct, but postoperative oozing may temporarily need a small pack in the wound. Postoperatively, saline mouthwashes are of value for several days. For the first 24 hours a sedative may be necessary, although usually relief of pain and discomfort is almost immediate after removal of the calculus obstruction.

When the calculus lies in the proximal third of Wharton's duct or at its junction with the gland, hospitalization is advised because usually the gland, as well as the calculus, must be removed through an external incision. It is a more formidable procedure because of the important anatomic sutures surrounding the gland.

Dilatation of the duct is another method of treament. Ballon and Ballon have reported cases in which they are able to dilate the submaxillary duct enough to allow the calculus to be extruded through its orifice. They recommend this procedure when for some reason operation is inadvisable or will not be permitted by the patient.

PAROTID GLAND INFECTIONS

ACUTE PYOGENIC PAROTITIS

Etiology and Symptoms

The gland becomes infected through the ascending spread of resistant strains of organisms along Stensen's duct. The condition known as surgical parotitis (*acute pyogenic parotitis*) nearly disappeared a few years ago, but there has been an increase of this suppurative type recently, apparently due to resistant strains of *Staphylococcus aureus*. This type of parotitis, which is frequently observed in postoperative patients, is now commonly found in patients with debilitating conditions and associated with malnutrition, poor oral hygiene, decreased parotid excretions, and chronic cardiohepatorenal diseases.

The onset is rapid with pain, tenderness, redness, and swelling of the involved parotid gland. If nothing is done, sepsis develops and 40% to 50% succumb. Treatment is prophylactic in not allowing the condition to exist and progress, but if such could not be prevented, intervention with type-specific antibiotics is next. It may be necessary to incise and drain the affected areas.

Chronic recurrent parotitis is sialadenitis characterized by episodes of swelling of the parotid gland with pain lasting several days or weeks. In some instances the swelling may be present in the morning and disappear after eating. The excretion from the gland may not be altered, although some patients may occasionally note excessive discharge of pus and saliva. Often the discomfort occasioned by the swelling may be relieved by pressure over the gland or the duct. There is usually no febrile reaction and no impairment of the general health.

Apparently, there is no definite cause for this chronic parotitis, although cases are reported that would suggest that dental infection, tonsilitis, sinusitis, calculi, stricture, or inadequate cleansing of dentures may be predisposing causes. The most common organism found is *Streptococcus viridans* (O-hemolytic).

Diagnosis

On examination the involved gland is found to be enlarged, firm, often nodular, and usually slightly tender to pressure. Pressure along the duct or over the gland may often produce a discharge of cloudy saliva, a mass of thick mucus, fibrin, or even pus. It is important to be sure that no stone is obstructing the duct. The diagnosis of calculus may easily be made by sialography.

Treatment

Treatment of chronic recurring parotitis consists in attempting to obtain a free flow of saliva by stimulation of the glands and by gentle dilatation of the ducts. In addition, attention must be paid to eradication of any focal infection in the mouth. Infected teeth and tonsils should receive appropriate treatment. Antibiotics control most of these complications. In most cases simple massage of the gland and stimulation of the salivary flow by mastication or by taking a small amount of lemon juice in the mouth will be sufficient to alleviate obstruction of the duct and to produce subsidence of the symptoms. In most cases dilatation of the ectatic ducts is advisable. This may be accomplished by insertion of small filiforms of gradually increasing size. The cheek is grasped with gauze, and the orifice of Stensen's duct is located opposite the upper second molar. A filiform then is inserted through the meatus into the duct until it is stopped by the edge of the masseter muscle. If the cheek then is pulled forward, the duct straightens out and the filiform can pass backward to the gland. By the use of large filiforms the duct is dilated gradually. Usually little pain is caused by this maneuver. Other types of treatment have been irradiation of the gland and total parotidectomy.

Other conditions, such as Mikulicz's disease (inflammation of all the salivary glands) and Sjögren's syndrome (inflammatory disease of all the salivary glands and the lacrimal glands), may be associated with parotitis, but they are treated in similar fashion.

MUSCLE, MYOCUTANEOUS, AND FREE FLAPS

Where there exists a defect of the head or neck region that may be so deep or devastating that a skin graft or skin flap will not accomplish the desired result, a muscle flap alone or accompanied by skin, fat, fascia, and bone may be the choice of reconstruction. The blood and nerve supply to the designated muscle are left intact. The repair may be achieved in one surgical maneuver or may necessitate secondary operations, depending on the contemporary problem. Muscle flaps are not new to the surgeon. Portions of the sternocleidomastoid muscle have been used as a protection cover for the common carotid artery, the subclavius muscle with the clavicle bone to reconstruct the mandible and floor of the mouth, and the temporalis muscle used to substitute for facial muscle functions. The myocutaneous flaps have been popularized through the efforts of our present generation of surgeons, and John B. McCraw should be given credit for rediscovering this technique, although Desprez, Hueston, Orticochea, Owens, and many others historically contributed to this significant advancement (Fig. 14-34).

Free flaps or free tissue transfers are relatively new involving microvascular and microneural anastomoses. This concept of reconstructive surgery has improved tremendously and the vessel-patency has increased to the extent that the method is used universally. Commendations are in order to Harry Buncke for initiating the current standards and enticing the Ohmori's, Harii, O'Brien, and so many others in developing techniques for free tissue transfer. The most accommodating free flap for head and facial reconstruction is the temporalis muscle or fascia flap. The superficial temporal vessels are large and afford the sur-

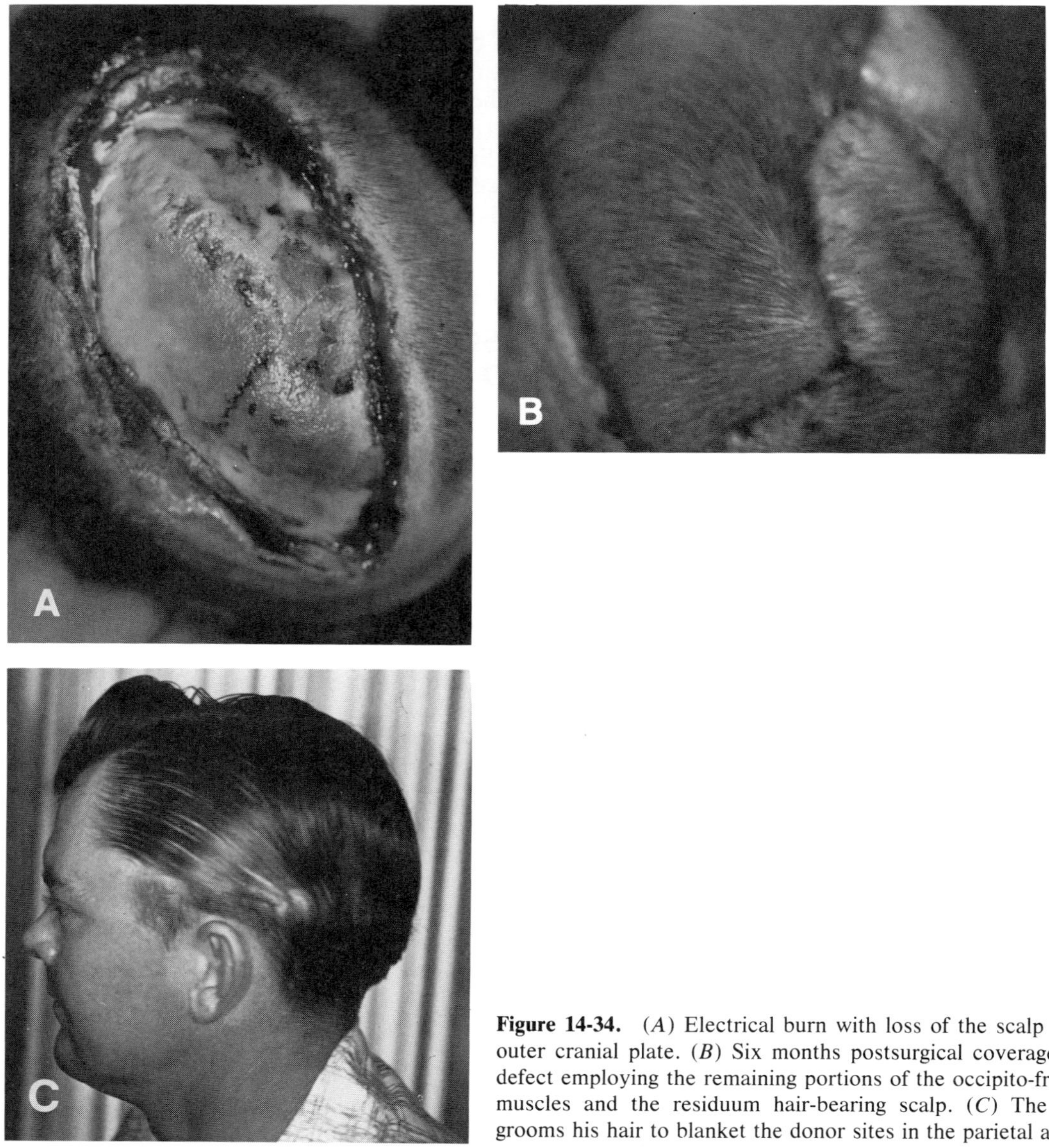

Figure 14-34. (*A*) Electrical burn with loss of the scalp and the outer cranial plate. (*B*) Six months postsurgical coverage of the defect employing the remaining portions of the occipito-frontale's muscles and the residuum hair-bearing scalp. (*C*) The patient grooms his hair to blanket the donor sites in the parietal area.

geon accessibility and amenability for transfer with very good success.

TISSUE EXPANSION

Large defects of the scalp, face, or neck present challenging problems that hair plugs, skin grafts, and skin flaps are unable to satisfy. Gradual spreading of tissue adjacent to the defect by an inserted expanding silicone elastomer affords the surgeon a satisfactory method of covering and closing defects with similar tissue to the original pretrauma skin, and eliminating the necessity to close the donor site. The inflatable soft-tissue expander has been a revelation to the trauma surgeon. The expanders are available in all sizes and contours. There is a small catheter attached to the expander and connected to a reservoir or hollow button with a valve. Fluids are injected through the skin into the reservoir, which permits the fluid to advance into the expander but not to return to the reservoir. Prescribed amounts of fluid are injected at intervals into the expander, stretching the overlying skin to the needed amount to cover the pending body defect. The expander is then retrieved in 6 to 8

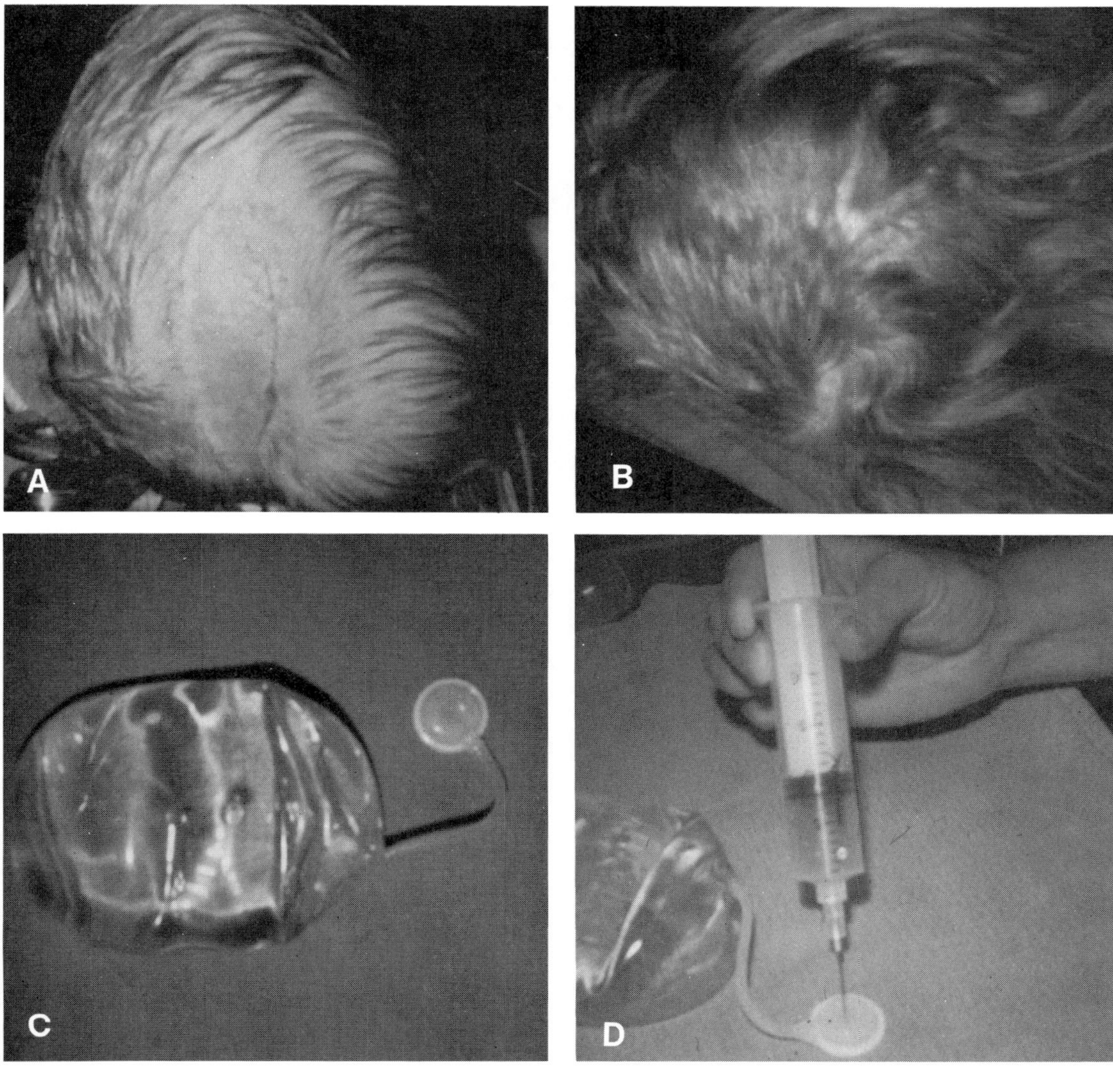

Figure 14-35. (*A*) Fifteen-year-old male with alopecia of the scalp. Note the imbedded expander (*arrow*). (*B*) Stretched hair-producing scalp advanced camouflaging the excised burn scar. (*C*) Silicone expander with attached catheter and metal-backed induction button (reservoir). (*D*) Syringe with needle introducing fluid into the expander via the button and catheter.

weeks and the expanded tissue advanced over the resected defect (Fig. 14-35). Tissue expansion is a valuable adjunct in head and neck reconstruction where color match, skin texture, and possibly hair-bearing tissue are indispensable.

BIBLIOGRAPHY

Scalp

Warwick R, Williams PL: Gray's Anatomy. Philadelphia, WB Saunders, 1973

Alopecia

Devine JW, Howard PS, Norstrom REA: Treatment of male pattern baldness: Update. In Habal et al (eds): Advances in Plastic and Reconstructive Surgery. Chicago, Year Book Medical Publishers, 1987

Unger WP: Hair Transplantation. New York, Marcel Dekker, 1979

Dermoid Cysts

Demis DJ, Crounse RG, McGuire J, Dobson RL: Clinical Dermatology. Hagerstown, MD, Harper & Row, 1972

Zarem HA, Lorincz AL: Benign growths and generalized skin disorders. In Grabb, Smith (eds): Plastic Surgery. Boston, Little, Brown, & Co, 1979

Soft-Tissue Injuries

Meaglier SW: Human factors engineering: A primer for the surgeon's participation in industrial injury prevention. Contemp Orthop 8:73, 1984

Snyder CC: Trauma to the lips and chin. In Stark RB (ed): Plastic Surgery of the Head and Neck. New York, Churchill Livingstone, 1987

Tenta LT, Keyes GR: Biogemetry: The logic in the process of selection, siting, design, construction, and transfer of flaps. Clin Plas Surg 12:423, 1985

Tongue

Gifford GH: Ankyloglossia, glossoptosis, macroglossia, cleft tongue, and medial palatal cyst. In Plastic Surgery of the Head and Neck. New York, Churchill Livingstone, 1987

Posnick JC: Tongue flaps in closure of end stage palatal fistulae. In Plastic Srugery. New York, Churchill Livingstone, 1987.

Ranulae

Cataldo E, Mosadomi A: Mucoceles of the oral mucous membrane. Arch Otolaryngol 91:360, 1970

Lore JM: An Atlas of Head and Neck Surgery, 2nd ed. Philadelphia, WB Saunders, 1973

Parotitis

Beahrs OH: The surgical anatomy and techniques of parotidectomy. Surg Clin North Am 57:477, 1977

Conley J: Search for and identification of the facial nerve. Laryngoscope 88:172, 1978

Woods JE: Parotidectomy: Points of technique for brief and safe operation. Am J Surg, 145:678, 1983

Muscle, Myocutaneous, and Free Flaps

McCraw JB: The recent history of myocutaneous flaps. Clin Plast Surg 7:3, 1986

Tobin GR: Myocutaneous and muscle flaps: Refinements and new applications. Curr Prob Surg 1986

Webster MHC, Soutar DS: Practical Guide to Free Tissue Transfer. London, Butterworths, 1986

Tissue Expansion

Argenta LC, Marks MW, Pasyk KA: Advances in tissue expansion. Clin Plast Surg 12:154, 1985

Chang TS, Jim YT: Application of tissue expansion in the treatment of post-burn skin contractures and alopecia. Eur J Plast Surg

Cohen M: Tissue expansion: A new technique in reconstructive surgery. Contemp Orthop 13:58, 1986

Radovan C: Tissue expansion in soft tissue reconstruction. Plast Reconstr Surg 24:482, 1984

15 Otolaryngology

JAMES L. PARKIN AND LELAND P. JOHNSON

EAR

FOREIGN BODIES

A foreign body in the external auditory canal can usually be removed with simple instruments and without anesthesia. An impacted foreign body may require complicated operating room procedures. Dried vegetable matter can absorb moisture and result in firm impaction. It is important to remember that the tympanic membrane, middle ear ossicles, and inner ear structures are very delicate (Fig. 15-1). The inner ear is capable of sensing motion in the magnitude of the diameter of a hydrogen atom. This delicate structure should not be traumatized during removal of a foreign body from the external auditory canal. Grasping instruments should not be used since they can result in pressure and trauma to the tympanic membrane and ossicles before the foreign body can be successfully grasped.

Removal of foreign bodies is best accomplished by development of a force medial to the foreign body that pushes the foreign body laterally without pressure against the tympanic membrane. This force is best accomplished by passage of a small right-angle hook medial to the foreign body. The hook is then rotated 90 degrees and pulled laterally, dragging the foreign body in front of it. This concept is illustrated in Figure 15-2. Irrigation, suction, or both may also be helpful. It is advisable not to attempt to remove a foreign body from a struggling patient. If the patient cannot be firmly secured, it is best to provide some form of anesthesia or tranquilization to prevent unexpected movement during the procedure.

The presence of cerumen in the external auditory canal is the most common reason for inadequate ear examination. The cerumen can be carefully removed from the external canal with a curette, a right-angle hook, suction, or water irrigation. If irrigation is to be used, it is important that the water be body temperature to avoid vestibular stimulation. The physician should not irrigate if the tympanic membrane is perforated or thin and monomeric. The force of the irrigating fluid should be directed above or below the cerumen so that the water flows behind the cerumen and pushes it laterally for removal.

TRAUMA

Physical trauma to the auricles in a contact sport is a common cause of laceration or hemotoma formation (Fig. 15-3). Hematoma of the auricle should be treated by incision and drainage and application of a pressure dressing. Frequent reassessment is necessary to prevent repeat hematoma formation, which can ultimately lead to cauliflower ear. Lacerations of the auricle should be closed carefully in a layered fashion and a mastoid type of pressure dressing applied. Frostbite and thermal injuries can also involve the auricle and require specific treatment.

The external auditory canal is frequently traumatized in attempts to clean the canal with cotton swabs, bobby pins, screwdrivers, paper clips, and the like. Serious injuries to the ear canal and tympanic membrane can result. The ear canal should be carefully cleaned of all blood, cerumen, and debris. The integrity of the tympanic membrane is assessed, and topical antibiotic–steroid solution may be utilized for several days to treat the secondary infection or prevent secondary infection from developing.

Mandibular fractures can result in ear canal lacerations and fractures when the mandibular condyle is forced posteriorly into the ear canal at the time of trauma. Severe lacerations of the external auditory canal require careful debridement and repair. Topical antibiotics are used for prevention of infection. In many of these cases stent formation is required to prevent stenosis of the external auditory canal.

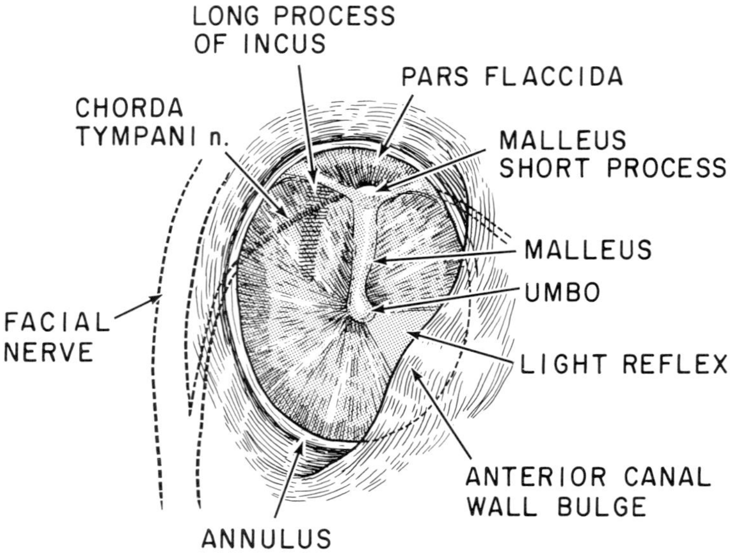

Figure 15-1. Normal anatomy of the right tympanic membrane.

A direct blow to the ear can generate sufficient force to rupture the tympanic membrane. An acute perforation usually has an angular appearance because flaps of tissue are folded under, whereas chronic perforations tend to be circular or kidney shaped (Fig. 15-4). Water sports such as skiing and high diving are also frequent causes of perforations of the tympanic membrane. The flow of water into the middle ear space at the time of rupture of the tympanic membrane increases the risk of infection. The majority of traumatic perforations heal spontaneously; however, the healing rate may be enhanced by proper emergent treatment of the traumatic rupture. The tympanic membrane is anesthetized, and the flaps of the membrane are restored to their original position. A small piece of cigarette paper is placed over the ruptured tympanic membrane to hold the flaps in place until healing occurs.

Severe head trauma with fracture can result in disturbances of all functions of the temporal bone structures, including the facial nerve, the cochlea, and the vestibular apparatus. Rotatory vertigo, peripheral facial nerve paralysis, profound hearing loss following head injury are strong indicators of the presence of tempo-

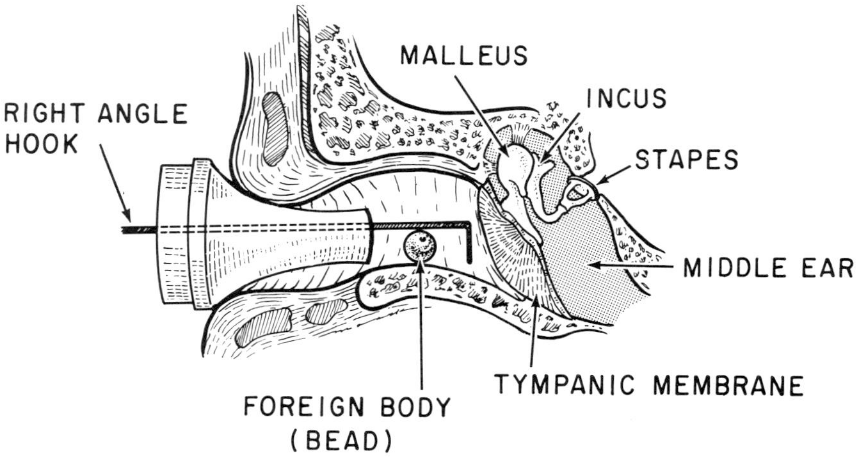

Figure 15-2. Removal of a foreign body from the external auditory canal with a right-angle hook.

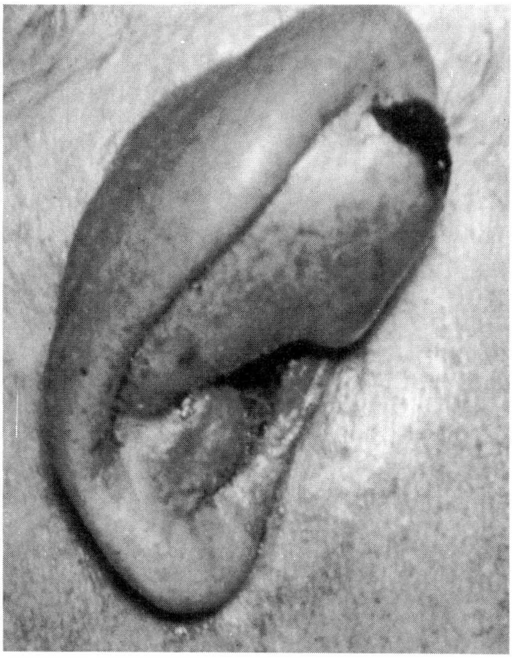

Figure 15-3. Hematoma of auricle.

ral bone fracture. If the facial nerve paralysis is of sudden onset, surgical exploration and grafting of the nerve are often required. Temporal bone trauma can also affect middle ear ossicles, with resultant ossicular discontinuity and conductive hearing loss. A fracture line extending through the temporal bone may result in cerebral spinal fluid leakage, causing a clear discharge from the ear if the tympanic membrane is not intact, or a clear postnasal discharge of fluid from the eustachian tube if the tympanic membrane is intact. These cerebrospinal fluid leaks require mastoid surgery for repair if the leak has not ceased spontaneously within 2 to 3 weeks following the trauma.

INFECTION

Ear infection is a frequent reason for patient visits to ambulatory care offices and centers. Infections of the external auditory canal are most frequently seen in the summertime, particularly in association with swimming in polluted waters, hence the designation *swimmer's ear*. *Staphyloccus aureus* and *Pseudomonas aeruginosa* are common pathogens in otitis externa. The ear canal is tender and swollen and seeping clear to mucopurulent material. It is often hard to differentiate otitis externa from otitis media with a ruptured eardrum because of difficulty in examining the tympanic membrane. The treatment of otitis externa should include careful cleansing of the external auditory canal. A cotton or cellulose wick is placed in the ear canal. Topical antibiotic or acetic acid solutions (2%) are then applied four times daily. The patient should return frequently for follow-up and for cleaning of debris from the external canal until resolution has occurred. The wick is removed in 5 to 7 days.

Acute otitis media results in loss of sleep for many patients, parents, and physicians. It usually occurs in association with respiratory infection leading to eustachian tube obstruction, middle ear effusion, and middle ear suppuration. The first symptoms often appear in

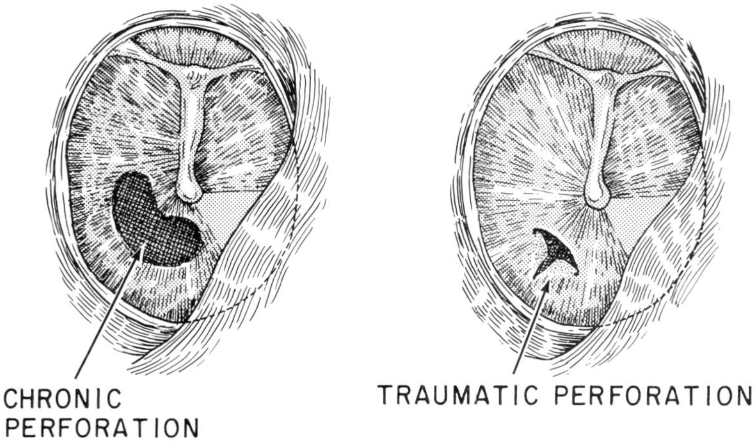

Figure 15-4. Perforations of tympanic membrane.

the middle of the night. When an individual is supine, venous engorgement in the head is increased, making eustachian tube obstruction occur more easily, with the resultant chain of events leading to middle ear infection. Should spontaneous perforation of the tympanic membrane occur with the infection, the pain is usually relieved. This is an important fact. In otitis media a discharging ear is often painless, whereas in otitis externa or myringitis bullosa a discharging ear is usually associated with pain.

The most common pathogens involved in otitis media include *Hemophilus influenzae, Streptococcus pneumoniae,* β-hemolytic streptococcus, and *Staphylococcus aureus*. Gram-negative organisms may be present in a child less than 1 year of age and in patients with other complicating illnesses such as leukemia, diabetes mellitus, and carcinomatosis.

In acute otitis media the tympanic membrane generally first becomes erythematous around the annular margin and down the long process of the malleus. As the infection progresses, the pars flaccida becomes diffusely erythematous and bulging. The pars tensa then becomes similarly involved. If the tympanic membrane has perforated, a specimen carefully obtained from the perforation is helpful in deciding on proper antibiotic therapy. Myringotomy can be utilized in evaluation and treatment of acute otitis media. Any patient with a complication, that is, facial nerve paralysis, vertigo, significant decrease in hearing, or meningismus, should undergo myringotomy and aspiration of middle ear contents to be certain that antibiotic therapy is appropriate. Myringotomy can also be utilized to relieve severe pain and to obtain a specimen for culture in cases refractory to treatment. Myringotomy is most safely performed in the anterior inferior quadrant (see Fig. 15-1). In an emergency situation the posterior inferior quadrant is sometimes utilized. The posterior superior quadrant should be avoided because of the possibility of damage to the auditory ossicles.

Early eustachian tube obstruction is an important part of the pathophysiology of otitis media, and decongestants have been used to relieve eustachian tube obstruction. However, controlled studies have not substantiated that decongestants play a significant therapeutic role. Antihistamines may be useful in decreasing the recurrence rate of otitis media. In acute otitis media antibiotics that will provide coverage for most common organisms should be used. Since the advent of antibiotics, complications from acute otitis media have decreased dramatically. Complications can be seen from the direct involvement of temporal bone structures and include meningitis, brain abscess, and lateral sinus thrombosis. Death may occur. Roentgenograms of the mastoid obtained during the early course of acute otitis media usually show fluid accumulation in the mastoid air cells. This occurs because the air cells are in continuity with the middle ear space, and the effusion will involve the mastoid air structures. Surgical mastoiditis usually develops 10 days to 2 weeks following the initial symptoms of acute otitis media. Roentgenograms obtained at this time reveal a breakdown and coalescence of the mastoid air-cell system. Coalescent mastoiditis frequently requires surgery.

Inner ear infections can be considered a complication of suppurative middle ear disease. Bacterial infection of the cochlea usually results in total, irreversible hearing loss and loss of unilateral vestibular function. Viral disease of the inner ear may affect the vestibular system and the cochlea separately or together. Cochlear symptoms include sudden sensorineural hearing loss, which is frequently reversible. Rotatory vertigo occurring in an epidemic fashion and termed acute vestibular neuronitis or acute labyrinthitis may occur as a result of viral labyrinthine infection. Treatment of this condition is mainly symptomatic.

Idiopathic facial nerve paralysis is believed by many to represent viral infection of the intratemporal course of the facial nerve. It is important in evaluation of sudden onset of facial nerve paralysis to remember that other disease processes can result in facial paralysis. Bell's palsy is a diagnosis by exclusion of these other causes.

TUMORS

The auricle is a frequent site for the occurrence of basal cell carcinoma in the elderly and in individuals with a history of much sun exposure. Ulcerative and other suspicious lesions of the auricles should have biopsy. Preferred treatment includes wide local resection with appropriate reconstruction. Tumors of the ear canal and middle ear are less common. Malignant tumors of the middle ear are rare.

The most common middle ear tumors include cholesteatoma and glomus tumors. These are also best treated surgically.

NOSE

SURGICAL ANATOMY AND EXAMINATION

The external nose is maintained by the superior bony and inferior cartilaginous pyramids. The bony pyramid is composed of the paired nasal bones, the frontal processes of the maxillae, and the nasal process of the frontal bone. The cartilaginous pyramid is composed of the lower alar cartilages, the upper lateral cartilages, and the cartilaginous nasal septum (Fig. 15-5). Anteriorly the quadrilateral cartilage and posteriorly the vomer bone and the perpendicular plate of the ethmoid bone comprise the major portion of the nasal septum (Fig. 15-6). Transition from stratified squamous epithelium covering the external nose and nasal vestibule to respiratory epithelium occurs at the junction of the upper and lower lateral cartilages in the nasal cavity.

Sensory innervation of the external and internal nose is derived from branches of the first and second divisions of the trigeminal nerve. Internal maxillary and facial branches of the external carotid artery and the anterior and posterior ethmoid branches of the ophthalmic branch of the internal carotid artery provide the blood supply for the nose.

Examination of the external nose requires no special equipment. For examination of the nasal cavities a source of illumination (a head mirror or a headlight) and a nasal speculum are required. Availability of a nasal suction and bayonet forceps allows removal of blood and crust for better examination. Additional visualization can be obtained by shrinking the nasal mucous membranes with a vasoconstrictor such as 1% phenylephrine HCl solution or 5% topical cocaine solution. Cocaine is a potentially toxic medication, especially when used in excessive amounts. A safe total topical cocaine dose should not exceed 5 mg/kg to 7 mg/kg. A 5% solution contains 50 mg/ml of cocaine; hence, a 70-kg man should not receive more than 7 ml to 10 ml of a 5% solution.

EPISTAXIS

The nose is second only to the uterus as a source of spontaneous hemorrhage.[1] Blood loss can be minimal or massive enough to produce hypotension, shock, and death. Because there is so little submucosal tissue to protect the underlying vessels, minor trauma or drying can result in vessel disruption and epistaxis.

The anterior nasal septum is the most common site of epistaxis. The anterior nasal septum is a point of anastomosis of the ethmoid, internal maxillary, and facial arteries forming Kiesselbach's, or Little's, area. Bleeding sites in the superior third of the nasal cavity are

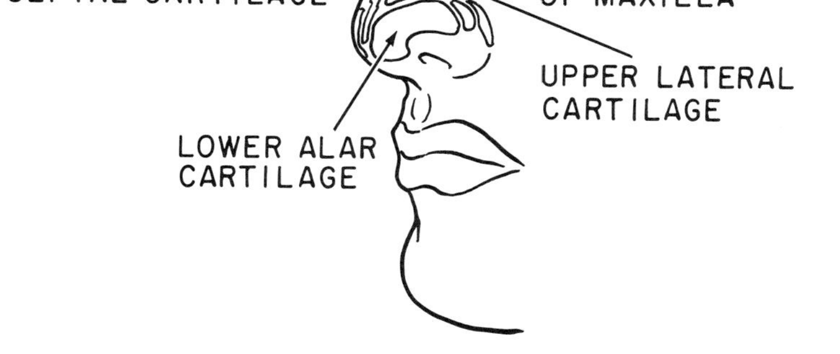

Figure 15-5. Anatomy of the external nose.

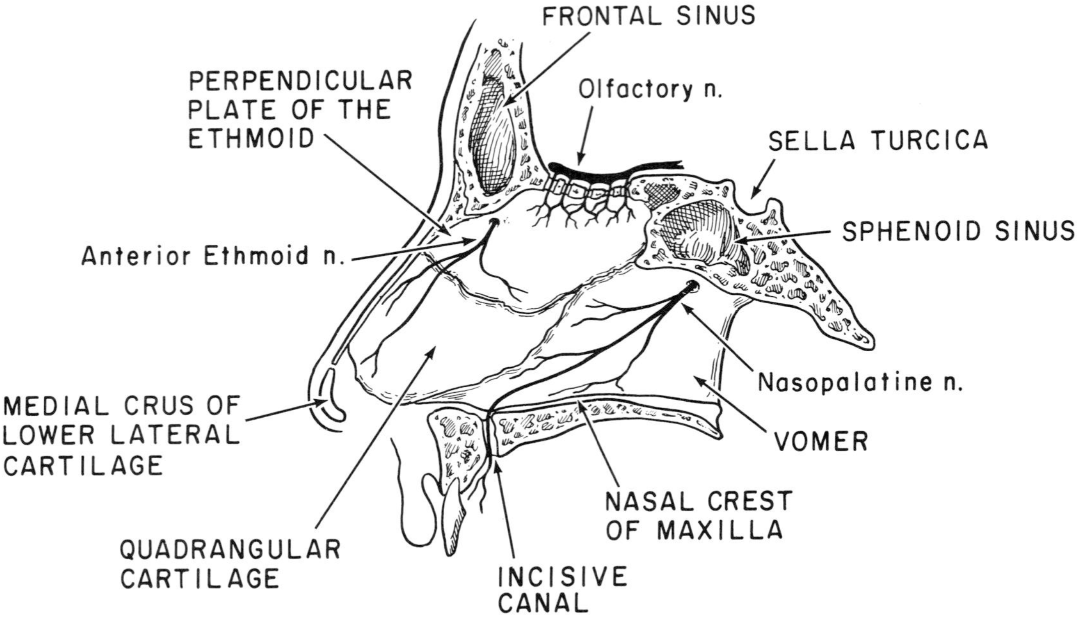

Figure 15-6. Anatomy of the medial nasal wall.

supplied by the anterior and posterior ethmoid arteries. Branches of the internal maxillary artery supply the majority of bleeding sites in the remainder of the posterior and inferior nasal cavity.

Following is a list of possible causes of nosebleed:

Trauma
- Mucosal drying and fissuring secondary to low humidity, medications, fever
- Nasal fracture
- Postsurgical
- Nose picking

Inflammation
- Acute and chronic rhinitis, sinusitis, or both
- Granulomatous disease (i.e., syphilis, tuberculosis, Wegener's)

Circulation
- Hypertension, atherosclerosis, or both
- Hereditary hemorrhagic telangiectasia
- Coagulopathies (i.e., due to anticoagulants, aspirin, leukemia, clotting-factor and platelet disorders)

Neoplasia
- Malignant tumors of nose, sinuses, or nasopharynx
- Angiofibroma
- Benign tumors (i.e., papilloma, granuloma, polyps)

Miscellaneous
- Foreign body
- Chemical irritants
- Septal perforations

The initial evaluation in epistaxis should include a brief history and estimation of the amount of blood loss. A more detailed historical investigation should be delayed until the bleeding is controlled. If there is evidence of marked blood loss either from the history or vital signs, an intravenous line should be established and a blood sample obtained for typing and crossmatching and appropriate studies. Definitive measures should then be initiated to control the epistaxis.

The nasal cavity should be cleaned of blood and blood clots. This can be accomplished with suction or by having the patient blow his nose. Examination of the nasal cavities may then allow identification of the bleeding site. Topical anesthesia should be promptly supplied with intranasal packs or sprays utilizing cocaine, lidocaine, or tetracaine. Vasoconstriction is accomplished with cocaine solution or by the addition of phenylephrine hydrochloride to other topical anesthetics. Topical vasoconstriction may slow or stop the bleeding and make identification of the bleeding site easier. In most children and young adults the site will be the anterior septum. Posterior bleeding sites are more often encountered in older patients and those with systemic diseases.

Control of bleeding is accomplished by cauterization, packing, or vessel ligation, alone or combined. When the bleeding site is localized to the anterior septum, chemical or electric cauterization can be performed. Injection of the anterior nasal septum with local anesthetic is beneficial, especially when electric cauterization is utilized or when the cautery site will extend to the squamous-epithelium-lined portion of the nasal vestibule. A supplemental anterior pack of petrolatum gauze or a piece of oxidized cellulose may be necessary to reinforce the area of cautery. The patient is more comfortable if the bleeding can be controlled successfully without the use of packing.

Epistaxis from a posterior site is often more difficult to control, and blood loss is greater than initially appreciated because of drainage into the posterior pharynx. A distinct bleeding site is also more difficult to identify in posterior epistaxis. Injection of 2 ml 1% lidocaine HCl into the pterygomaxillary space via the greater palatine foramen of the hard palate can often slow or stop posterior bleeding by a compression effect on the sphenopalatine artery (Fig. 15-7). (Epinephrine should not be utilized in this injection because of the delayed rebound effect on the vessel.) A 25- to 27-gauge needle is used; it should be bent at an angle of approximately 45 degrees. The length of the needle from the tip to the angle should not exceed 2.5 cm so that the tip of the needle will not enter the orbit. This same injection will also block the second division of the trigeminal nerve and result in anesthesia of the nasal cavity, facilitating placement of a posterior pack if bleeding is not controlled.

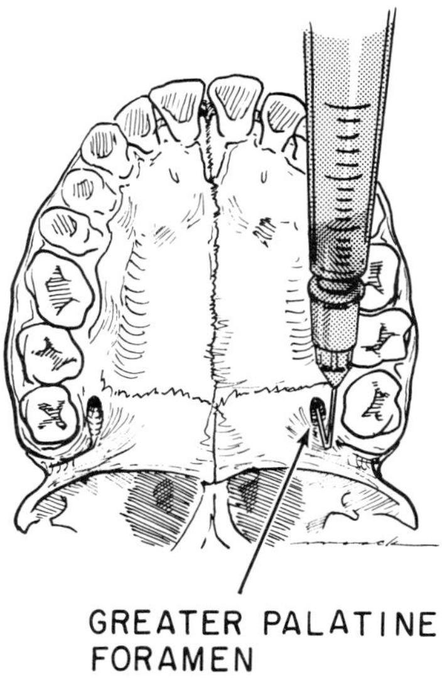

Figure 15-7. The greater palatine foramen is injected for control of posterior epistaxis, anesthesia of the area supplied by the second division of the trigeminal nerve, or both.

Nasal packing is often necessary to control epistaxis. Anterior nasal packing is accomplished by layering in a continuous petrolatum gauze strip (Fig. 15-8). It is important not to simply stuff the strip into the nose because the posterior end can work its way into the pharynx. The patient will then swallow the packing, allowing the bleeding to resume.

Placement of a posterior pack is illustrated in Figure 15-8. The posterior pack applies pressure in the posterior choanae and posterior nasal septal area. It also acts as a platform to support the anterior pack. The posterior pack can be fashioned from a gauze sponge folded in quadrants or from a tonsillectomy sponge. An alternative to the posterior pack illustrated in Figure 15-8 is the use of a Foley cathether with a 30-ml balloon, filled with 10 ml to 15 ml of water. The Foley cathether is secured anteriorly by tying it to dental rolls or over a platform of gauze sponge to prevent pressure to the nasal ala. Several inflatable devices with both anterior and posterior balloons are available that can also control posterior epistaxis effectively. A patient who requires posterior packing can experience a decrease in arterial PO_2; such a patient frequently has some other systemic illness such as hypertension, diabetes, renal disease, leukemia, or coronary artery disease; and it is important that he be hospitalized, have frequent monitoring or arterial blood gases, and receive supplemental oxygen. Use of antibiotic ointment on the pack and systemic use of antibiotics decrease the degree of bacterial growth in the nose and the incidence of sinusitis that can develop from the obstructed sinus ostia.

When packing cannot control the epistaxis or when bleeding occurs following removal of the packing, the specific bleeding vessels should be ligated. Ligation of the anterior or posterior ethmoid arteries is accomplished by means of a medial orbital incision. Ligation of the internal maxillary artery is performed

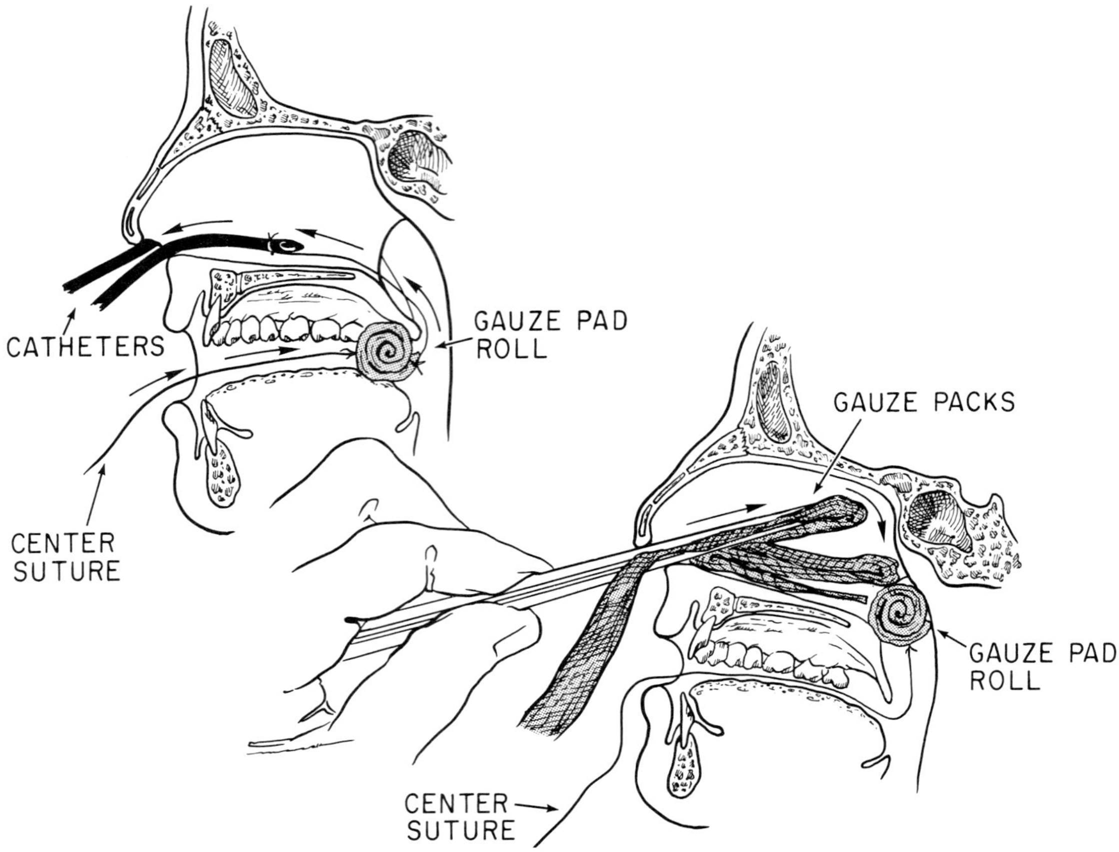

Figure 15-8. Anterior and posterior nasal packing. A red rubber catheter is directed through each anterior nares into the posterior pharynx, where the catheters are grasped with a clamp and brought out through the mouth. A heavy silk suture attached to the posterior pack of rolled 4 × 4 gauze pad is then tied to the end of each catheter. The catheters are then pulled out through the nose to advance the pack into the nasopharynx, while a finger of the opposite hand directs the pack around and above the soft palate. The pack is then secured anteriorly to the nose by tying the silk suture over dental rolls at the nares. The other end of the silk suture coming from the mouth is taped to the cheek to use as a traction stitch for lateral removal of the pack.

Anterior packing of Vaseline gauze is then layered in front of the posterior pack.

through the maxillary sinus. Ligation of the external carotid artery is rarely indicated.

Techniques for embolization of the bleeding vessels with occlusive materials under angiographic control have also been utilized for difficult cases. In a patient with a coagulopathy, fresh blood or blood-component transfusions are often needed for control even with adequate nasal packing. An extensive work-up for the detection of underlying conditions is indicated in a patient with severe or recurrent episodes of epistaxis.

TRAUMA

The nasal bones are the most commonly fractured bones of the facial skeleton. Associated nasal injuries include lacerations and septal fractures, dislocations, and hematomas. Nasal fractures can be open or closed and unilateral or bilateral.

Historically, the mechanism of injury, change of external appearance, change in nasal airway, and epistaxis are important facts. Most nasal fractures result in intranasal mucosal tears so that the absence of epistaxis makes a fracture highly unlikely. If a patient with a nasal fracture is seen early, before significant edema and ecchymosis have developed, comparison with photographs (e.g., driver's license) can distinguish recent from remote nasal deformity. A history of associated injuries or loss of consciousness warrants additional evaluation. The possibility of cervical spinal injuries should not be overlooked in a patient with facial trauma.

On examination, nasal fractures are manifested by deformity of the nasal dorsum, a palpable fracture line, or crepitus of the nasal bones on side-to-side palpation. Marked tenderness over the fracture site and periorbital ecchymoses are often present. Dislocation of a fracture of the septum is detected on intranasal examination and palpation of the septum after topical anesthesia. Many septal deformities are remote, and lack of movement on palpation will make this distinction. The presence of clear nasal drainage in addition to the expected bleeding should suggest associated fracture of the cribiform plate with resultant cerebrospinal rhinorrhea.

Photographic recording of the nasal trauma is valuable for postreduciton as well as potential medical–legal comparisons. Roentogenograms are often obtained for evaluation of nasal trauma, but because the age of the nasal fracture is difficult to determine by this means, the physical findings mentioned previously are more reliable for the diagnosis of acute nasal fractures.

After associated injuries are either ruled out or stabilized, reduction of the nasal fracture is accomplished with use of local anesthesia in most adults or general anesthesia in children. If the patient is seen early, that is, before edema and ecchymosis makes appreciation of the nasal profile difficult, reduction can be accomplished at this time. After edema develops, ice packs and elevation of the head are utilized. Reexamination in 3 to 5 days will determine the appropriate time for fracture reduction.

Local anesthesia for closed reduction of nasal fractures is accomplished by topical application and specific injections. The nasal mucosa is anesthetized by means of a spray or saturated packing; 5% cocaine, 2% tetracaine, or 4% lidocaine solution may be utilized. Injection of 1% lidocaine with epinephrine to block the specific branches of the first and second divisions of the trigeminal nerves is illustrated in Figure 15-9. The adequacy of anesthesia is then determined by palpation of the nasal dorsum and septum. Anesthesia is less effective if much edema is present.

Displaced nasal fractures require simultaneous elevation and rotation to accomplish reduction. The Asche forceps is designed for reduction of such fractures. One blade is placed on either side of the nasal septum under the nasal bones. Reduction of the fracture is accomplished with upward motion to elevate the fragment at the same time the fingers of the opposite hand replace the reposition of the

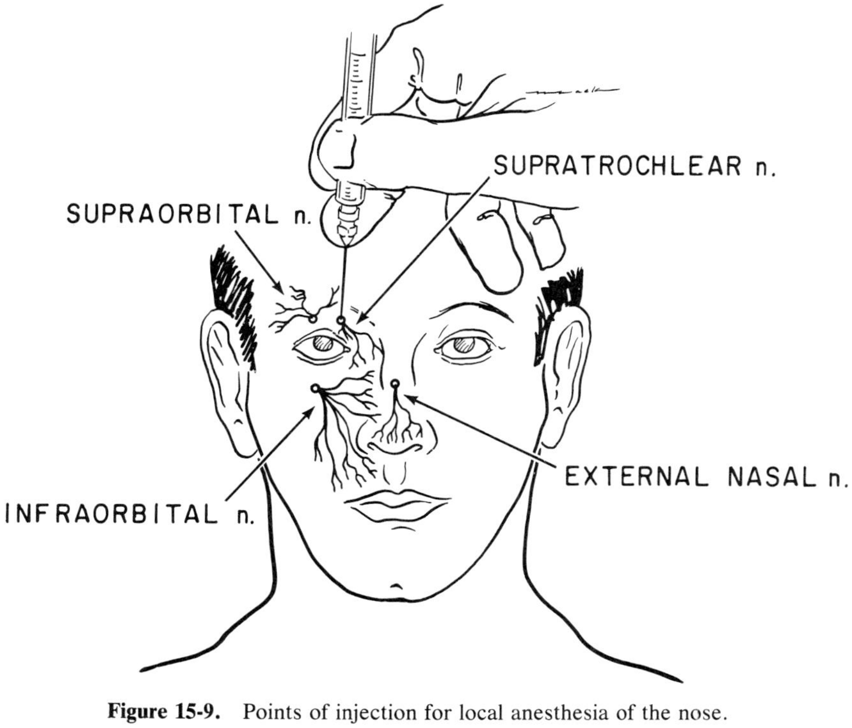

Figure 15-9. Points of injection for local anesthesia of the nose.

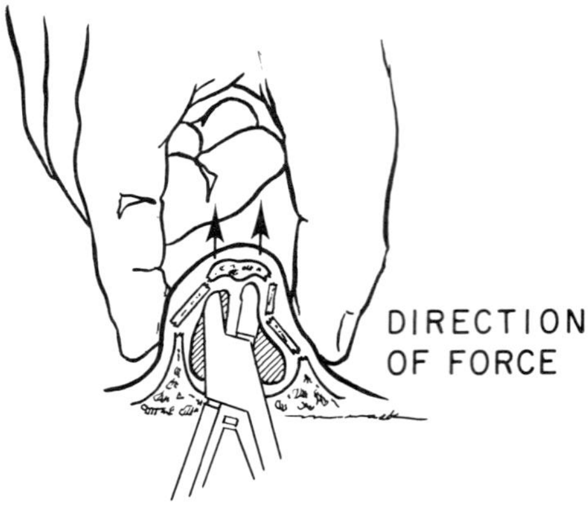

Figure 15-10. Reduction of nasal fracture with upward force and movement of fracture fragments to midline.

dorsum in a midline position (Fig. 15-10). Similarly, an empty scalpel handle can be placed in the nasal cavity underlying the nasal bone for the elevation and reduction. Fractures of the nasal septum can also be reduced with the Asche forceps, the blades being positioned on either side of the septum and the septum manipulated into the midline position.

Early diagnosis and treatment of a complicating septal hematoma is important. Blood accumulates beneath the perichondrium of the septum. An unrecognized hematoma can result in aseptic necrosis of the septal cartilage. The hematoma can become infected and produce a septal abscess, which also results in necrosis of the cartilaginous nasal septum and eventual saddle-nose deformity. Treatment is accomplished by making an incision through the septal mucosa overlying the hematoma and placing a drain or an anterior nasal pack to prevent hematoma reaccumulation.

Following reduction of a nasal fracture, bilateral anterior nasal packing is usually necessary to support the fragments. Petrolatum gauze impregnated with an antibiotic ointment is commonly used for this purpose. An external splint fashioned from five layers of cast plaster or available aluminum splints (Fig. 15-11) should be worn for 2 to 3 weeks to prevent displacement of the fracture fragments. This splint can then be worn at nights for an additional 2 weeks to prevent displacement of the fragments during sleep.

A patient with a nasal fracture should be cautioned that although all efforts have been made to restore external configuration and septal position, residual deformity may require additional nasal surgery later.

CEREBROSPINAL RHINORRHEA

Nasal and facial fractures involving the cribriform plate, base of the skull, paranasal sinuses, or temporal bone may result in cerebrospinal rhinorrhea. The clear nasal drainage is positive when tested for glucose. Most cases of cerebrospinal rhinorrhea stop spontaneously. Management includes elevation of the head and avoidance of nose blowing, nasal packing, and heavy exertion. Persistent cerebrospinal rhinorrhea or development of men-

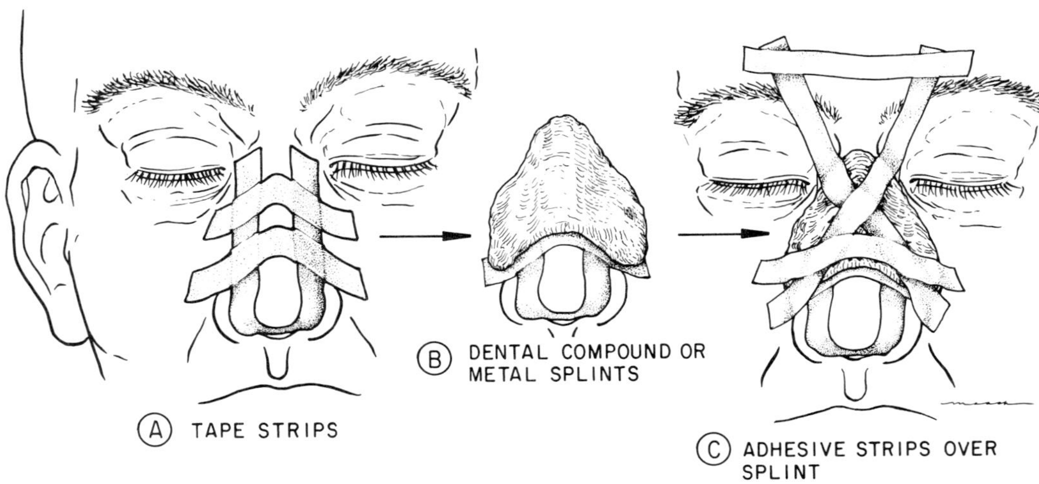

Figure 15-11. Splinting after reduction of a nasal fracture.

ingitis requires additional surgery for closure of the leak. Prophylactic use of antibiotics in these cases is controversial.

FOREIGN BODIES

A foreign body in the nasal cavity is common in children. Unilateral purulent rhinorrhea in a child suggests this diagnosis. Removal of a foreign body can usually be accomplished with topical intranasal anesthesia and appropriate instrumentation. In addition, small children usually require restraint; a papoose board is useful for this.

A blunt right-angled hook or wire cerumen loop can be maneuvered to engage the posterior end of the foreign body and drag it to the anterior naris for removal. Small grasping forceps can be used for removal when the presenting edge of the foreign body is visible and lends itself to grasping. Another way of removing a foreign body is to use suction or magnets. A bean or similar vegetable inserted in a nostril can swell on exposure to moisture and require general anesthesia for removal. After removal of a nasal foreign body it is important to check the opposite nostril to be certain all foreign bodies have been removed.

NEOPLASMS

The allergic polyp is the most common benign intranasal neoplasm. Removal can be accomplished following topical intranasal anesthesia and the use of polyp snare. A squamous papilloma can involve the skin of the nasal vestibule and anterior septum. Surgical removal can be performed with use of local anesthesia. Cryosurgery has also been utilized for this purpose. The papilloma should be sent for pathologic examination. Inverting papilloma is an intranasal neoplasm capable of malignant degeneration. Squamous cell carcinoma is the most common malignant neoplasm of the nasal cavity.

A dermoid cyst or sinus may present as a midline mass of the nasal dorsum. Complete removal must take into account a path that can pass through the nasal bone and into the nasal cavity. Infants and children may have a midline external nasal or intranasal mass consisting of neural tissue, that is, glioma or encephalocele. Clinical suspicion of one of these lesions warrants hospitalization and consultation with a neurosurgeon. Malignant lesions of the external nose, including basal cell carcinoma and squamous cell carcinoma, are discussed in Chapter 14.

PARANASAL SINUSES

The paranasal sinuses are air-containing cavities within the bones of the skull and facial skeleton lined by ciliated respiratory epithelium similar to that found in the nose. The paired paranasal sinuses include the maxillary, ethmoid, frontal, and sphenoid. The most common symptoms involving these structures result from bacterial infections.

Any process that compromises the ventilation or drainage of the paranasal sinuses can result in infection. Common causes include upper respiratory viral infections, allergic rhinitis, deviated nasal septum, nasal polyp, nasal foreign body, and the nasal congestion associated with pregnancy.

Pain develops early in the course of bacterial sinusitis, directly over the involved sinus or referred to other areas of the skull. Sphenoid sinusitis characteristically refers pain to the vertex of the head. Maxillary sinusitis is often associated with pain in the maxillary teeth due to the proximity of the dental roots to the sinus floor. The pain of sinus infection is often increased when the head is in a dependent position. Sinus pain is characteristically more severe after the patient has been recumbent. Purulent nasal or posterior pharyngeal drainage and nasal obstruction also accompany acute sinusitis. In adults the maxillary sinus is most commonly infected, followed by the ethmoid, frontal, and sphenoid. Young children most frequently develop ethmoid sinusitis.

INFECTIONS

The skin lining the nasal vestibule is subject to furunculosis or a more general infection, vestibulitis, which requires treatment with a topical antibiotic ointment such as neomycin. Systemic antibiotics may also be required. Incision and drainage may be necessary in the management of a furuncle. Nasal septal abscesses also require incision, drainage, and appropriate antibiotics. Since *Staphylococcus aureus* may be the causative organism, as determined by culture, a penicillinase-resistant penicillin should be utilized. The venous drainage pattern of the superior nasal cavity makes the complication of cavernous sinus thrombosis possible in nasal infections.

ALLERGY

Nasal mucous membrane is the target tissue for multiple allergens. Nasal congestion, sneezing, and clear rhinorrhea of seasonal allergy or hay fever are well known. Medical management consists of avoidance of the allergens, systemic antihistamine–decongestant preparations, or topical intranasal use of steroids as the initial line of control. With increasing or persistent symptoms not controlled by these measures, systemic use of steroids or allergic evaluation with desensitization may be necessary. The formation of nasal polyps has been associated with chronic nasal allergies and chronic nasal infections.

The distinction between the more common symptoms of nasal obstruction and clear rhinorrhea associated with allergic rhinitis and upper respiratory tract viral infection from symptoms of acute sinusitis is important. The combination of facial pain and tenderness overlying the anatomic location of the sinus, purulent nasal drainage, abnormal transillumination of the involved sinus, or sinus roentgenograms demonstrating an air–fluid level or sinus opacification differentiates acute sinusitis from allergic rhinitis or upper respiratory viral infections.

Initial treatment of acute sinusitis with antibiotics is based on the organism most commonly encountered in these infections. Most common causative organism include *Diplococcus pneumoniae, Hemophilus influenzae,* β-hemolytic streptococcus, and *Staphyloccus aureus*. Gram-negative organisms and anaerobic organisms can play a role in chronic sinusitis. The causative organisms should be confirmed by culture to determine appropriate antibiotic therapy. In a patient not allergic to penicillin, ampicillin is currently the initial antibiotic of choice for acute sinusitis. Because of an ever-increasing incidence of β-lactamase producing *Hemophilus influenzae,* the initial use of trimethoprim-sulfa or cefaclor is also appropriate. Systemic or topical decongestants and humidification are also beneficial.

With failure of resolution of acute sinusitis or for symptomatic relief of sinus pain, apsiration and irrigation of the maxillary sinus can be performed. After topical anesthesia of the inferior meatus, a trocar is inserted into the maxillary sinus through its bony medial wall. Material can be obtained for culture and the purulent sinus contents can be irrigated. This procedure is analogous to incision and drainage of an abscess, and it will often provide marked pain relief. Failure of conservative management in the treatment of frontal, ethmoid, or sphenoid sinusitis usually requires hospitalization and surgical treatment.

Facial fractures commonly involve the paranasal sinuses, and reduction of these facial fractures will restore the continuity of the sinuses. Traumatic compromise of the frontonasal duct can result in formation of a secondary mucocele with progressive, extensive local destruction and secondary infection. Maxillary and frontal fractures require hospitalization with appropriate reduction and fixation.

Negative intrasinus pressure that develops with descent in air travel or in scuba diving can result in intense facial pain overlying the involved sinus. Barotrauma of this type usually involves the maxillary or frontal sinuses. The intrasinus pressure differential will cause tearing of the mucous membrane lining from the bony sinus wall with resultant hemorrhage and hematoma formation. This hemorrhage can be visualized on roentgenograms of the sinus as an air–fluid level similar to that seen in acute sinusitis. Barotrauma may resolve with only topical and systemic use of decongestants. Severe barotrauma requires surgical drainage of the involved sinus with equalization of intrasinus pressures.

CHOANAL ATRESIA

Choanal atresia is an anomaly in the newborn in which the communication of the nasal cavity with the nasopharynx is blocked by a persistent membrane at the posterior nares. Because the newborn is an obligate nose breather, bilateral choanal atresia results in immediate airway distress, which is relieved by crying or establishment or an oral airway. Confirmation of choanal atresia is made by inability to pass a catheter from the anterior nares to the posterior pharynx. Contrast x-ray studies can also be utilized to establish the diagnosis. For bilateral choanal atresia, early surgical correction is needed.

ORAL CAVITY

ANATOMY

The vestibule and mouth are the two components of the oral cavity. The vestibule is the space between the lips anteriorly, the cheeks, and the teeth. The mouth is then bounded by the teeth, gums, palate, and oropharyngeal inlet.

TRAUMA

Lacerations

Lacerations within the oral cavity less than 1 cm in length may not need repair. Those greater than 1 cm are reapproximated with absorbable suture. Through-and-through lacerations of the cheek require repair of the oral mucosa in addition to reapproximation of the skin of the face. The most dependent extent of the mucosal laceration may be left open for drainage because of the wound contamination from intraoral organisms. Lacerations of the tongue greater than 1 cm in length or on the free edge of the tongue require surgical repair. Because of the tendency for the traumatized tongue to develop marked edema, tight approximation is not indicated.

Fractures

Dental fractures require evaluation by a dentist to determine viability of the teeth and whether they can be preserved. Avulsed teeth can be replaced in the dental socket with a fair chance of survival, especially in children. Consultation with a dental surgeon is appropriate.

Mandibular fractures can be isolated or they can be associated with other facial fractures in a patient with multiple trauma. Of facial bones fractured, the mandible is second in frequency only to the nasal bones. Following injury development of pain and swelling at the fracture site, pain on chewing, and change in the bite due to altered dental occlusion indicate a mandibular fracture. Physical examination may reveal a palpable step-off at the fracture site, intraoral mucosal laceration over the fracture, abnormal dental occlusion, and associated dental injuries. A bilateral mandibular fracture can allow posterior displacement of the tongue and suprahyoid structures to produce acute airway obstruction. This is relieved by forward displacement of the mandibular fragment or by tracheostomy.

Fracture management includes reduction and fixation for approximately 6 weeks in the adult. Fixation is achieved by placement of arch bars onto the teeth or denture for maxillomandibular stabilization. An unfavorable mandibular fracture is one in which muscle pull may displace the fragments (Fig. 15-12). For unfavorable fractures open reduction is necessary with wire or plate fixation of the fragments. Management of a mandibular fracture should await examination for associated injuries, especially those of the cervical spine.

Subluxation of the Temporomandibular Joint

The temporomandibular joint is a combination gliding and hinge joint. Extreme opening or protrusion of the mandible, as in yawning or laughing, can result in subluxation of the mandibular condyle anterior to the articular tubercle of the temporal bone. The patient is unable to close the mouth and has an open bite.

Treatment involves reduction of the mandible by placement of the thumb intraorally over the mandibular molars and the fingers over the angle of the mandible. Initial downward pressure is slowly exerted to overcome spasm of the muscles of mastication and to depress the mandibular condyle first below and then posterior to the articular tubercle. At this point the condyle usually slips back into the mandibular fossa. With marked muscle spasm not allowing reduction, injection of local anesthetic into the area of the temporomandibular joint or intravenous administration of diazepam preceding the reduction is helpful. Many times the problem is recurrent, and the patient can be instructed in the method of reduction. In an extreme case of recurrent dislocation, surgical removal of the articular tubercle can provide relief.

Inflammation or arthritis of the temporomandibular joint can result in a myriad of symptoms—from ear, face, scalp, or neck pain, the most common, to tinnitus. With the original pain developing in the temporomandibular joint, muscle spasm involving pterygoid muscles and the muscles of the scalp and neck can result in extension of facial pain patterns. Changes in dental occlusion from recent dental work, poorly fitting dentures, current dental disease, and tooth grinding are the most

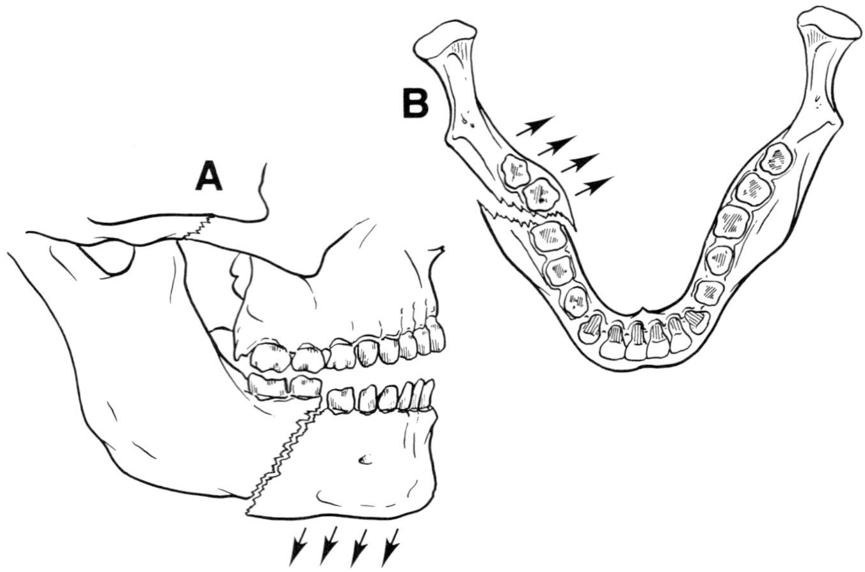

Figure 15-12. Unfavorable mandibular fractures in which muscle pull results in distraction: (*A*) in the vertical plane; (*B*) in the horizontal plane.

common causes of temporomandibular joint syndrome. Diagnosis is somewhat by exclusion in eliminating ear or pharyngeal origins for referred pain. On examination there is often tenderness over the involved temporomandibular joint with crepitus. Roentgenograms are usually normal except in cases with longstanding symptoms.

Treatment most importantly involves dental consultation to correct any underlying occlusal abnormalities. Acute pain is managed with a soft diet, local heat, and antiinflammatory analgesic agents such as aspirin. Resolution of symptoms may require time and consultation with a dentist familiar with this syndrome who can build intraoral appliances that can be helpful for treatment. Surgery is seldom necessary except in cases of posttraumatic temporomandibular joint syndrome when the articular cartilage of the joint has been damaged.

CARCINOMA OF THE ORAL CAVITY AND TONGUE

Squamous cell carcinoma is the most common malignant neoplasm (85% to 90%) of the oral cavity and tongue. The etiologic role of smoking and alcohol has been established.

Chronic irritation of the oral mucous membrane from many agents, including smoking, alcohol, and poorly fitting dentures or jagged teeth, can result in leukoplakia. This is a white plaque or patch that can occur in a discrete area or be extensive in the oral cavity. Only microscopic examination can determine those areas of leukoplakia that show atypia and may be considered premalignant squamous cell carcinoma; 2% to 5% of these leukoplakic lesions are premalignant, but erythroplasia, which is a more velvety, thickened, red area of the mucous membrane, is more often premalignant (80%).

Management of areas of leukoplakia involves biopsy to exclude carcinoma in situ or invasive squamous cell carcinoma. Biopsy is commonly done as an outpatient procedure, using topical anesthesia, 5% cocaine, or 2% tetracaine with additional injection of 1% lidocaine hydrochloride. Planning the biopsy to include an area of normal mucosa adjacent to the lesion in question makes the procedure more informative (Fig. 15-13).

Removal of known mucosal irritants can result in resolution of leukoplakia. Periodic observation is needed to determine any suspicious areas of induration or ulceration in the mouth or tongue.

A mass or area of induration or ulceration that remains for more than 2 weeks also warrants biopsy to determine if it is malignant. Again, biopsy is conducted using local anes-

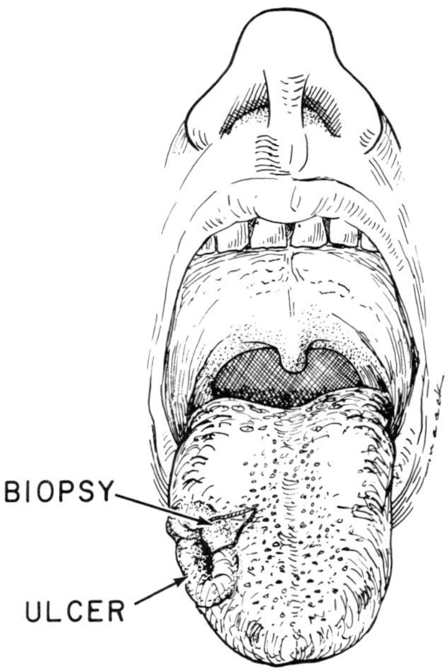

Figure 15-13. Design of biopsy to include a portion of adjacent tissue as well as the lesion.

thesia and includes adjacent normal mucosa and avoids a specimen from the midst of the ulcer crater or necrotic tissue.

Evaluation of cervical adenopathy in an older patient should always include examination of the head and neck and indirect laryngoscopy and pharyngoscopy to determine a primary site. The areas of highest risk for development of squamous cell carcinoma in the oral cavity are the lateral margins of the anterior two-thirds of the tongue, the floor of the mouth, soft palate, and anterior tonsillar pillar complex. The nasopharynx, piriform sinuses, larynx, and postcricoid region are more common sites of silent primary carcinoma.

Both surgery and radiation therapy are used individually or in combination for treatment of squamous cell carcinoma of the oral cavity and tongue, depending on the extent of the primary lesion and evidence of cervical node metastases.

ANKYLOGLOSSIA OR TONGUE-TIE

Ankyloglossia, or tongue-tie, is abnormal shortness of the lingual frenulum that limits protrusion of the anterior portion of the tongue. This is usually noted in infants if difficulty in nursing is encountered. Generally, if the tip of the tongue can contact the inner surface of the maxillary incisors, there is no difficulty with articulation.

Infrequently, tongue-tie is marked enough to require surgical division of the short lingual frenulum. After adequate local anesthesia a thin lingual frenulum is divided toward the floor of the mouth, caution being taken to avoid the frenular artery and submandibular duct. A thick frenulum or recurrent ankyloglossia requires plastic repair under general anesthesia.

SALIVARY GLANDS

Salivary glands are classified as major (parotid, submandibular, and sublingual) or minor (those scattered throughout the mucosa of the oral cavity). The major salivary glands are paired and discharge saliva through ducts. The parotid or Stensen's duct opens through a papilla on the buccal mucosa adjacent to the second maxillary molar. The submandibular gland drains into the floor of the mouth via Wharton's duct lateral to the lingular frenulum. Sublingual glands open into the duct of the submandibular gland or directly into the floor of the mouth.

INFLAMMATION

Sialadenitis can be acute, chronic, or recurrent and viral, bacterial, or allergic. The most common infectious disease of the salivary glands is that produced by the mumps virus. Bacterial infection results in sialadenitis characterized by pain, erythema, gland swelling, and expression of pus from the duct draining the involved gland. These symptoms are often increased with meals and any stimulation of salivation. Suppurative parotitis is usually seen in a dehydrated, debilitated patient. Treatment by rehydration, antibiotics, and occasionally incision and drainage is required. *Staphylococcus aureus* is often the responsible organism and a penicillinase-resistant penicillin is the initial antibiotic of choice.

Children can experience recurrent inflammation of the parotid gland, which often resolves by adolescence. The cause of this inflammation is not known.

A salivary duct stricture or a salivary duct stone can cause sialadenitis. Salivary calculi are most commonly encountered in the submandibular duct (70% to 80%) and are radiopaque in 75% to 80% of x-ray examinations. The stone may be palpated in the floor of the mouth by bimanual techniques or demonstrated on x-ray studies.

If the stone is in the portion of the duct in the floor of the mouth, removal can be accomplished under local anesthesia, often with rapid resolution of symptoms. Local anesthesia described previously can be used, followed by placement of a suture around the duct proximal to the stone both to produce traction and prevent retrograde displacement of the stone toward the gland. An incision is then made over the stone to open the duct. The duct can be left open or the lining sutured to the oral mucosa to marsupialize the duct. Dilatation of the duct will sometimes allow a stone to be removed more readily. Stones in the posterior third of the duct or at the junction of the gland and the duct often require surgical removal of the gland after control of the acute symptoms with analgesics and antibiotics.

Obstruction and dilatation of a sublingual salivary gland duct or the duct of a minor salivary gland can result in a cystic mass known as a ranula. Symptoms are produced by the mass effect on tongue function rather than by pain or inflammatory manifestations. Treatment consists of marsupialization, usually as an outpatient procedure. After local anesthesia is attained the mucosa over the cyst is excised to expose the cyst wall. A portion of the cyst wall is removed. The cyst wall lining is approximated to the oral mucosa membrane to eventually create a large communication of the cyst with the floor of the mouth. The cyst can also be excised. Recurrence of a ranula is not uncommon.

A pyogenic granuloma is a mass composed of granulation tissue and inflammatory cells resulting from chronic inflammation and irritation of the oral mucosa or tongue. The most common site is on the gingiva. These lesions can be confused with squamous cell carcinoma. Excision and microscopic examination are required for differentiation. Recurrence is possible if the source of irritation—for example, jagged teeth or biting—is not corrected.

NEOPLASMS

Mass lesions of salivary gland origin usually represent a tumor. The majority, 80% to 90%, of salivary gland tumors, arise in the parotid. Of parotid gland tumors, 80% are benign and 20% are malignant. In the submandibular gland, 40% to 50% of tumors are malignant. In sublingual and minor salivary glands the malignancy rate is up to 75%. Mixed tumor (pleomorphic adenoma) is the most common benign tumor of the parotid. Warthin's tumor is the next most common benign parotid gland tumor. Malignant salivary gland tumors are mucoepidermoid carcinoma, adenoid cystic carcinoma, and squamous cell carcinoma; 25% of all salivary gland tumors are malignant. Symptoms of malignant parotid tumors include rapid increase in size, pain, and facial nerve paralysis.

Surgical treatment of benign parotid tumors consists of either superficial or total parotidectomy with facial nerve identification and dissection. The recurrence rate in benign mixed tumors is high if the tumor is only enucleated without removal of surrounding salivary gland tissue. Treatment of malignant salivary gland tumors involves surgical excision with or without sacrifice of the seventh cranial nerve for parotid tumors, possible neck dissection, and radiation therapy.

TRAUMA

Soft-tissue facial trauma in the area of the parotid gland can involve the peripheral branches of the facial nerve and the parotid duct. Exploration of these two structures is required if laceration is lateral to a line dropped at the outer canthus of the eye. Facial nerve branches can be identified by a nerve stimulator, and any severed branch should be reapproximated by microsurgical techniques. Parotid duct injury can be identified by observing saliva in the wound and by retrograde passage of a polyethylene catheter via Stensen's duct to the area of injury. Reapproximation of the duct over a stent left in the duct is the indicated primary treatment. Diversion of the proximal end of Stensen's duct into the mouth or ligation of the proximal end of the duct has also been utilized to manage salivary duct injury and fistula.

PHARYNX

INFECTIOUS DISEASE

Pharyngeal abscess formation usually follows acute tonsillitis or pharyngitis and is commonly caused by β-hemolytic streptococ-

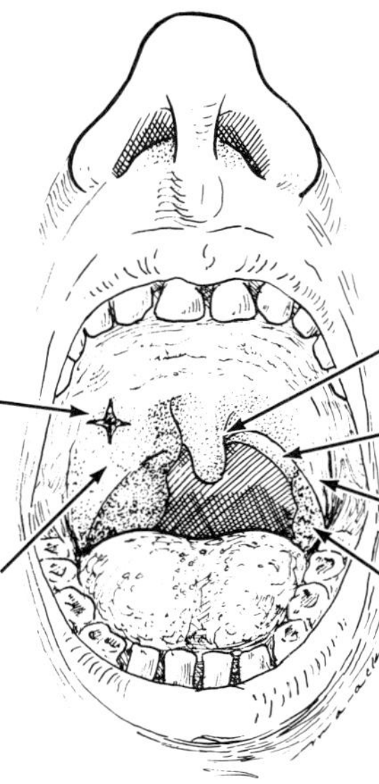

Figure 15-14. Site for incision and drainage of peritonsillar abscess.

cus or anaerobic organisms. It is often manifested first as a peritonsillar or a retropharyngeal abscess.

Historically, these patients have had antecedent pharyngitis or tonsillitis and then develop increasing throat pain, odynophagia, and symptoms of systemic toxicity. A peritonsillar abscess can result in inability to handle oral secretions and muffling of the voice. A retropharyngeal abscess can result in upper airway obstruction. Peritonsillar abscess is characterized by marked asymmetry between the two tonsillar fossae with the tonsil being displaced inferiorly and medially on the involved side. In retropharyngeal abscess a lateral roentgenogram of the neck shows that the posterior pharyngeal wall is thickened or there is increased soft-tissue thickness of the retropharynx.

Treatment requires incision and drainage of the abscess and initiation of systemic antibiotic therapy. Aspiration of the peritonsillar abscess with a large-gauge needle can be an alternative to incision and drainage. For peritonsillar abscess an incision is made in the upper outer quadrant or the most prominent portion of the abscess (Fig. 15-14). Interval tonsillectomy has been recommended following incision and drainage, or tonsillectomy has followed a 24-hour period of systemic antibiotic administration. This accomplishes drainage of the abscess and often results in marked pain relief. Drainage of a retropharyngeal abscess requires hospitalization and general anesthesia.

After tonsillectomy a patient may come to the emergency room with a complaint of increasing throat pain or of bleeding. The crust in a postoperative tonsillar fossa has a gray-white shaggy appearance. After tonsillectomy most bleeding occurs either within the first 24 hours or approximately 7 to 10 days postoperatively when the crust comes free from the tonsillar fossa. Management of delayed bleeding is somewhat similar to that for epistaxis; adequate illumination and suction are needed. Topical anesthesia of the posterior pharynx with 2% tetracaine spray prior to instrumentation, or injection of the tonsillar fossa with 1% lidocaine can make control of bleeding more comfortable for the patient. Any blood clot in the tonsillar fossa is removed and the bleeding site controlled by pressure in the fossa with a folded 4-in. × 4-in. sponge, silver nitrate cautery, or cautery with a tannic acid solution. If these methods fail, a suture may be placed in the fossa to control the bleeding vessel. It is important to assess the blood loss to determine need for blood replacement.

LARYNX

INFECTIONS

Infections of the larynx resulting in airway obstruction are medical emergencies. Acute epiglottitis in a child should be distinguished from laryngotracheal bronchitis or croup (Table 15-1).

TABLE 15-1. Signs and Symptoms of Laryngotracheobronchitis and Epiglottitis

LARYNGOTRACHEO-BRONCHITIS	EPIGLOTTITIS
1–3 yr of age	2–5 yr of age, rare under 1 yr
Viral	Bacterial, *Hemophilis influenzae*
Croupy cough	Absence of cough
Inspiratory and expiratory stridor	Inspiratory stridor
Area involved is below level of true cord—normal lateral roentgenograms of neck	Involved supraglottic larynx with abnormal lateral roentgenogram of neck
More gradual onset of symptoms	Rapid progression of symptoms and airway obstruction
	Child avoids supine position to maintain airway
Absence of drooling	Drooling due to pain on swallowing

In a child with epiglottitis airway obstruction develops rapidly; in an adult the same process is more gradual but just as dangerous. The incidence of epiglottitis in adults is higher than appreciated. Sore throat, fever, cough, marked pain on swallowing, gagging, vomiting, and stridor in an adult should arouse suspicion of epiglottitis. Indirect laryngoscopy should be performed to rule out epiglottiditis. Lateral films of the neck can help to demonstrate the thickened supraglottic area and narrowed airway. The patient requires hospitalization for administration of antibiotics, adequate humidification, and observation. Use of steroids is advocated by some. This treatment will be effective in approximately 75% of adult patients, with 25% requiring endotracheal intubation or tracheostomy to maintain an adequate airway.

In a child with epiglottitis, establishment of an airway is mandatory. When adequate nursing supervision is available, nasotracheal intubation is most commonly used today, although tracheostomy is an alternative. Examination of a child to detect epiglottitis should be done in the operating room with the assistance of an anesthesiologist and with bronchoscopes and equipment ready for intubation or tracheostomy. Most of the immediate post-tracheostomy complications can be avoided by this preparation. Because epiglottitis in a child is most often caused by *Hemophilus influenzae* type B, concurrent treatment with ampicillin or chloramphenicol is necessary.

Indirect laryngoscopy is an important technique in evaluation of epiglottitis, laryngeal foreign body, and upper airway obstruction. The method is easy to learn with fiberoptic laryngoscopes. Use of a head mirror and laryngeal mirrors is also a well known technique but is more difficult to learn. The technique and equipment are illustrated in Figure 15-15.

TRACHEOSTOMY

The technique of endotracheal intubation or tracheostomy for emergency establishment of an airway is important for any physician to know. Tracheostomy should be performed with a secure airway established with either an endotracheal tube or a bronchoscope and in an operating room if possible. The majority of immediate tracheostomy complications result when these precautions are not taken.

Technique

Following infiltration of local anesthesia with 1% lidocaine with 1 : 100,000 epinephrine, a horizontal incision is made overlying the second to third tracheal ring. A horizontal incision is much more acceptable cosmetically. Deep to the skin all dissection is done in a midline plane with a blunt technique to localize the trachea. The thyroid isthmus is often present in the field, and if it is not possible to retract it away from the anticipated tracheostomy site it should be divided. At this point, midline sharp dissection may be necessary to divide the pretracheal fascia to expose the cartilaginous rings of the trachea. If the procedure is being done with use of local anesthesia, injection of additional anesthetic into the tracheal lumen will anesthetize the tracheal mucosa prior to creation of the tracheotomy. All bleeding should be controlled before the trachea is entered. Various tracheal incisions have been described in the area of the second to third tracheal rings. A simple vertical midline incision through rings two and three is adequate. An inferiorly based tracheal flap is shown in Figure 15-16. Tracheal cartilage has been removed to create the tracheostomy opening, but this should never be done in a child because of the increased incidence of subsequent tracheal stenosis and collapse. A tracheostomy tube with a cuff (previously tested) is then placed within the tracheal lu-

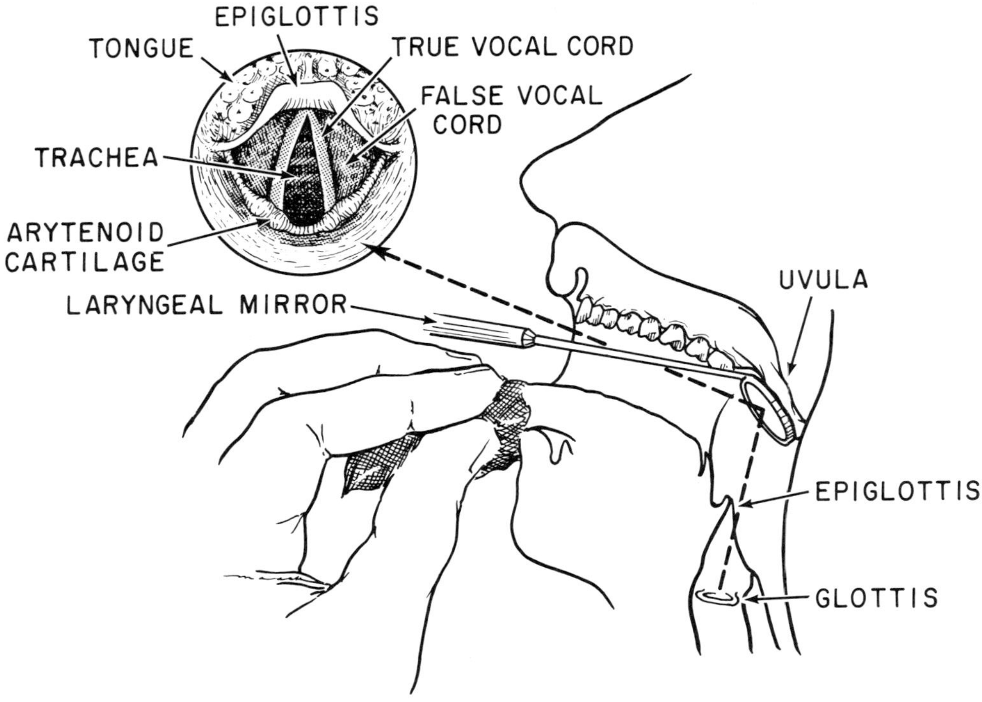

Figure 15-15. Normal laryngeal anatomy and indirect laryngoscopy.

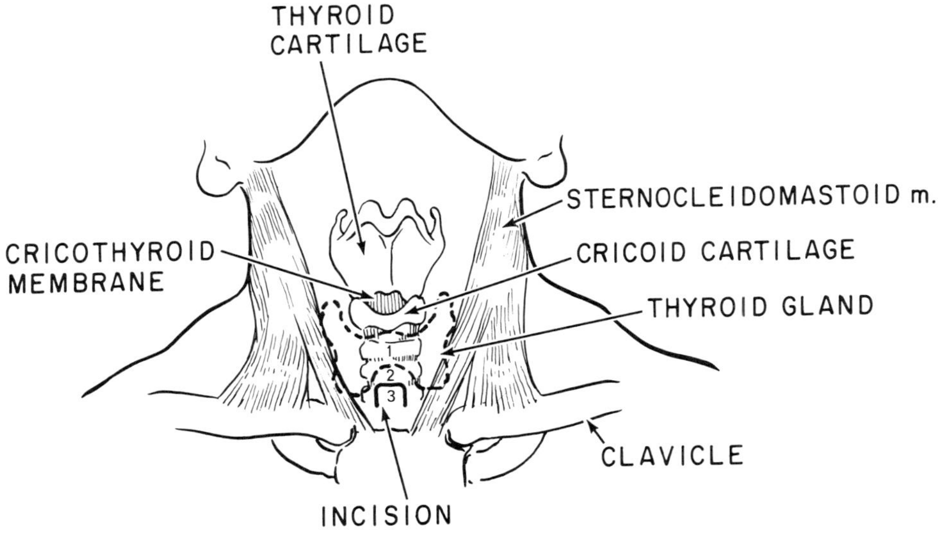

Figure 15-16. Anatomy and location of incision for tracheostomy.

men. The wound is closed only loosely, and gauze dressing applied. A post-tracheostomy chest film is obtained to check tube placement and pneumomediastinum or pneumothorax.

Post-tracheostomy Care

Tracheostomy removes the warming and humidifying functions of the nose and upper airway and presents relatively dry air to the tracheal mucosa. The use of a humidifier to provide this moisture is important for at least the first 2 weeks after tracheostomy. Suction of the tracheostomy tube using sterile technique is needed as secretions develop. It may be necessary every few minutes or hours, but the frequency will decrease with time as the amount of mucus produced is decreased.

The possibility of formation of a mucus plug in the tracheostomy tube or stoma should be considered with development of any increased stridor or shortness of breath. The tracheostomy tube should be removed and examined for such a plug and replaced with a clean tube. An obstructing crust can develop in the tracheal stoma. If a postlaryngectomy patient comes to an emergency room with difficulty in breathing or noisy respiration, such crusts should be suspected and removed.

TRAUMA

A patient with a laryngeal injury will have shortness of breath, neck pain, voice change, or aphonia and subcutaneous emphysema of the neck. A laryngeal injury is often a component of multiple trauma. Emergency tracheostomy is required with further laryngeal exploration and repair of the laryngeal fractures and mucosal lacerations when the patient's condition is stabilized. Endotracheal intubation is often difficult but can be attempted prior to emergency tracheostomy. When more limited laryngeal trauma results in hematoma, intubation or tracheostomy is often necessary prior to resolution of the hematoma.

FOREIGN BODIES

After aspiration of a foreign body into the larynx or pharynx a history to determine the nature of the foreign body, roentgenography of the neck, and indirect laryngoscopy are required. In an adult, some foreign bodies can be removed in the ambulatory clinic using instrumentation and indirect visualization following topical anesthesia. For a partially obstructive foreign body or foreign body in a child, removal should be accomplished in the operating room with general anesthesia. For acute laryngeal obstruction due to a foreign body the Heimlich maneuver can dislodge the foreign body and be lifesaving. Management of esophageal and tracheobronchial foreign bodies is discussed in Chapter 25.

BIBLIOGRAPHY

Applebaum EL, Bruce DL: Tracheal Intubation. Philadelphia, WB Saunders, 1976

Dingman RO, Natvig P: Surgery of Facial Fractures, Chap 9. Philadelphia, WB Saunders, 1964

Hawkings DB et al: Acute epiglottitis in adults. Laryngoscope 83:1211–1220, 1973

Otolaryngologic and Head and Neck Emergencies. ENT Clin North Am 12:May 1979 (entire volume)

Sessions RB: Nasal hemorrhage. The nasal cavities. ENT Clin North Am 6:727–744, 1973

16 Ambulatory Care of the Breast

J. M. McGREEVY

The female breast is a dynamic organ. It is constantly changing as a result of monthly fluctuations in sex hormones. Because of this continual change, the female breast can develop many conditions that result in consulting an ambulatory surgical facility: a *breast lump, breast pain,* an *abnormal mammogram,* and *nipple disorders*. These conditions will be discussed by presenting a different diagnosis for each complaint. Two additional areas that will be considered in this chapter are *postoperative problems* and the *male breast*. Emphasis will be placed on the management of each diagnosis in an ambulatory care setting. The purpose of this chapter is to provide the reader with a manual-style reference that provides succinct guidelines for the management of common breast complaints.

BREAST LUMPS

Breast lumps create a level of patient anxiety that is unique. Nearly every patient who seeks consultation for a breast lump suspects cancer. The physician has two responsibilities to these patients: (1) to spend enough time with the patient, because informative discussion often lessens the fear of malignancy, since the large majority of breast lumps are benign, and (2) to pursue a diagnosis in every breast lump even though the majority are benign.

DIAGNOSIS

An interview and physical examination are conducted to gather as much information as possible that may explain the presence of the breast lump. During this interview process the examiner should explain the reason for each question and examination maneuver. If the patient is informed during the interrogation, she will frequently discover, along with the doctor, that there is little reason to suspect a malignancy. If she is misinformed or uninformed during the consultation, her anxiety will increase.

Of the many conditions that may be associated with an increased risk of breast cancer, only a few are established: a history of breast cancer in an immediate relative, a history of previous breast cancer in the patient, age, and nulliparity.

The use of estrogen-containing medication (contraception, estrogen replacement) is associated with fibrocystic disease, since the hormone stimulates and supports breast hypertrophy. Recent studies do not support an association between estrogen therapy and breast cancer. Cyclic breast pain and enlargement also suggest fibrocystic disease. Breast feeding may be associated with breast abscess. And because this problem can be recalcitrant, a history of breast abscess suggests that the breast lump is another abscess. A history of trauma suggests contusion, hematoma, or fat necrosis.

On physical examination, the following findings are signs of malignancy: bloody nipple discharge, skin dimpling, a firm mass with indistinct margins, a fixed mass, bulky axillary adenopathy, and painlessness. Breast tenderness suggests infection or fibrocystic disease. Erythema is usually present with a breast abscess, although it can be the hallmark of the particularly aggressive inflammatory carcinoma. The erythema of an abscess is usually localized, whereas that associated with inflammatory carcinoma commonly involves the entire breast.

Once a clinical impression has resulted in a working diagnosis, that diagnosis can be tested in a variety of ways: (1) operative biopsy, (2) needle aspiration for fluid, (3) needle aspiration for cells, (4) observation and reexamination after a 3- to 4-month interval, and (5) mammography.

The simplest test of the working diagnosis is an aspiration for fluid. This is effective, cheap, easy, and pain-free. Because of these advantages, aspiration with a large needle should be done on every breast lump. If nonbloody fluid is found on aspiration, the work-up can frequently be terminated. Since cysts do not always feel like cysts on examination, it is worthwhile to aspirate all lumps.

TECHNIQUE FOR CYST ASPIRATION

The skin over the lump is cleansed with an alcohol swab. Next, the lump is immobilized between two fingers of one hand. The skin over the lump is anesthetized with a small amount (0.5 ml to 1.0 ml) of 1% lidocaine without epinephrine. If too much local anesthetic is used, the lump may be obscured. An 18-gauge needle on a 10-ml syringe is passed through the skin and is directed to the lump (Fig. 16-1). Palpation with the nonaspirating hand that is immobilizing the lump will confirm penetration of the mass. With the needle in place, aspiration will determine whether or not fluid is present. The amount of fluid may vary from less than 1 ml to over 15 ml. It can be various colors, most often greenish brown. If it is bloody, a biopsy must be performed. Another indication for biopsy after aspiration is the persistence of a palpable mass. The fluid may be sent for cytologic examination. Since the frequency of breast cancer in this setting (viz., a mass that disappears after aspiration of nonbloody fluid) is less than 0.5%, the cost–benefit ratio for routine cytologic examination of the aspirated fluid will be very low. The patient is asked to return for a reexamination in 1 month. If the mass has recurred, a biopsy should be performed.

If the mass is solid on aspiration, a choice between observation and excisional biopsy must be made. A benign-appearing mass in a low-risk, young patient may be followed through several menstrual cycles. If the mass persists after the predetermined observation period (2 to 4 months), it should be removed. A suspicious-feeling mass in an older or high-risk patient should be biopsied immediately.

Two tests can help in this decision: mammography and needle aspiration for cytology. Mammography has a limited role in the evaluation of a palpable breast mass. It may help to confirm a clinical suspicion that a lump is benign and reinforce the decision to follow it. However, breast cancer may look benign on mammography. So any lump that persists after an observation period must be biopsied regardless of its mammographic appearance. There have been cancers that were followed for months and years because of a nondiagnostic report from the mammographer.[1]

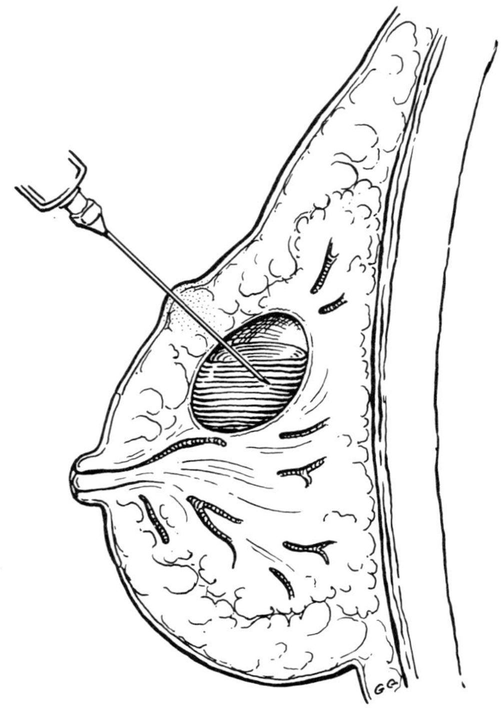

Figure 16-1. Needle aspiration of a discrete breast cyst.

Another popular test that may be useful in the evaluation of a palpable mass is a needle aspiration for cytologic examination.

TECHNIQUE FOR CYTOLOGIC ASPIRATION

The technique for cytologic aspiration is similar to the previously described large-needle aspiration for fluid. A smaller (21-gauge) needle is passed into the mass several times while negative pressure is applied with a 10-ml syringe. The needle and syringe are sent immediately to the cytology laboratory, where the harvested cells are washed from the needle. The subsequent evaluation of these cells by an experienced cytopathologist can be highly accurate for malignancy if there is no sampling error. Most breast cancers are accompanied by dense scarring. Therefore this test is limited by the question of adequate sampling. If the cytology report is positive for malignancy, it is useful in preoperative planning. The diagnosis must be confirmed by conventional biopsy before undertaking cancer therapy. If the report from the cytologist reads "no malignant cells seen," additional work-up will be necessary because the needle aspiration may have missed the malignant area of the mass. This test is extremely useful when it is positive for malignant cells because the false-positive rate is very low. On the other hand, the false-negative rate is high, so a benign report is less useful.[2]

If observation is chosen, the mass must be carefully described in the medical record. When the patient returns after 2 or 4 months, this description is read prior to the reexamination. If the breast lump is still present, a biopsy should be done.

TECHNIQUE FOR BREAST BIOPSY

Breast biopsy is commonly done in an ambulatory care setting under local anesthesia. There is no longer a need to perform a definitive procedure (viz., mastectomy or wide excision and axillary dissection) on the day of the biopsy. An interval of 2 weeks is acceptable between diagnosis and treatment. This allows for second opinions and adequate preoperative counseling.

Breast biopsy is a minor procedure that occasionally becomes demanding. The rich blood supply of the breast can provide brisk bleeding that always seems to occur at the bottom of a deep wound. The wound is usually oblique and narrow because of the common use of the cosmetically superior circumareolar incision. For this reason the operation should be performed in a fully staffed and fully equipped facility. This includes a registered nurse, proper lighting, electrocautery, suction, blood pressure and ECG monitor, and capability to deliver complete ACLS cardiopulmonary resuscitation.

The patient may require preoperative sedation. Midazolam (2 mg to 4 mg) given intravenously has been superior to intramuscular diazepam. It provides more sedation and less recall of unpleasant events. An intravenous line and oxygen (2 liters/min to 3 liters/min by nasal cannula) are standard therapy during breast biopsy.

The choice of incision depends on the preoperative diagnosis and the position of the lesion. If cancer is suspected, an incision is planned such that the entire biopsy site can be removed with the subsequent cancer operation. If the lesion is close to the nipple, a circumareolar incision can be made. If the distance from the areola is greater than 10 cm, an incision directly over the mass in the lines of Langer is easier on the patient and the surgeon.

After infiltration with at least 10 ml of 1% lidocaine without epinephrine, the incision is made through to the subdermal fat. Care should be taken to avoid a bevel in the skin edge. The mass is palpated through the incision. The wound is developed directly to the mass with palpation as a guide. Before the mass is seen, an Allis clamp is placed on the tissue that surrounds the lump. The lump is then dissected free of the surrounding breast with sharp dissection. If the lump is small (<2 cm), it should be removed in its entirety with adequate adipose to assure negative margins. If it is large, the mass should be visualized and a part of it removed. This leaves a cavity that is more easily encompassed by the later resection (mastectomy or lumpectomy) if it is a malignant tumor.

The resected specimen should be examined with a frozen section. This allows preservation of tissue for estrogen receptor analysis. It also provides valuable information for immediate patient counseling. Making the patient wait for 2 days while the slides are processed is cruel and unnecessary. The patient can be informed of the probable diagnosis at the time of the biopsy. Prior to closure, the wound is everted by placing an Allis clamp at the base. The sides of the biopsy cavity are inspected with the aid of a headlight. All bleeding points are cauterized to minimize the chance of hematoma formation. The wound can be closed in a single layer with an absorbable subcuticular suture. Deeper sutures are ineffective in eliminating dead space, and they may not control bleeding. They do cause dimpling of the skin, which can be cosmetically unacceptable.

The patient is advised to wear a firmly fitting bra, both day and night, for 5 days. The wound should be kept dry for the same period of time. There are no limitations on normal activity after breast biopsy, but serious exertion (e.g., contact sports) should be avoided for 2 weeks.

BREAST BIOPSY RESULTS
IN 110 PATIENTS

44%	fibrocystic disease
25%	cancer
10%	fibroadenoma
6%	normal breast
4%	recurrent cancer
4%	duct ectasia
3%	lipoma
4%	other lesions
	Fat necrosis
	Intraductal papilloma
	Lactating adenoma

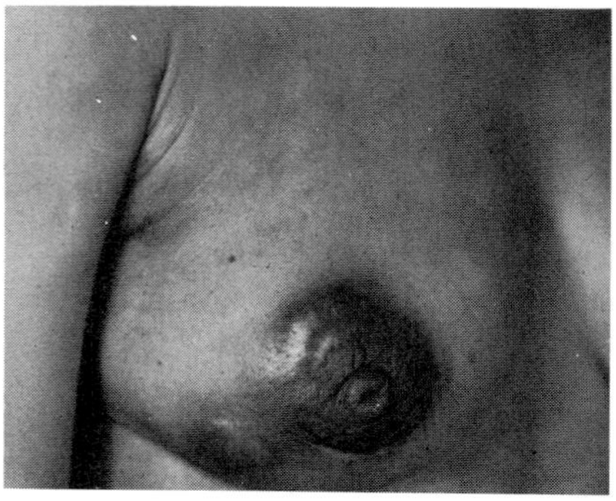

Figure 16-2. Superficial abscess of the breast. In this case there are two abscesses; one subareolar and one subcutaneous.

In a typical practice, the majority of breast biopsies result in a benign diagnosis. The figures listed under "Breast Biopsy Results in 110 Patients" show our recent experience; the most frequent diagnosis is fibrocystic disease.

Breast masses that require special consideration are abscess, Mondor's disease, duct ectasia, intraductal papilloma, cystosarcoma phyllodes, and masses that occur in pregnant patients.

MANAGEMENT OF BREAST ABSCESS

Breast abscesses are less common than they were several years ago; this may be due to better perinatal care for the nursing mother. The majority of abscesses are minor and subareolar in location (Fig. 16-2). These small abscesses can usually be handled with local anesthesia. The area is cleansed and draped with sterile technique. A field block with 1% lidocaine is placed around the perimeter of the abscess. The abscess itself should not be infiltrated with the anesthetic. The pH of the abscess contents inactivates the lidocaine. In addition, injection can result in increased pressure in the cavity, causing more pain and bacterial dissemination. A large needle (18-gauge) is used to locate the cavity. With the needle as a guide, an incision is made into the cavity. The purulent fluid is cultured. Once the cavity has been found, the incision is enlarged to allow free drainage (Fig. 16-3). A recurrence of this problem is frequent and persistent. To prevent recurrence, the drainage incision in the skin must be wide. Passive drainage of the cavity with a soft rubber drain through a narrow skin incision will promote recurrence. The incision should be wide enough to allow packing with 0.25-inch gauze. With daily packing changes, the wound is debrided and kept clean. Antibiotics should be used. Dicloxacillin (250 mg q 6 hr) can be given until the culture results are available. The wound is allowed to close by secondary intention.

Recurrence of a subareolar abscess may indicate the presence of a mammary duct fistula.[3] This condition is a communication between an abnormally enlarged lactiferous sinus, lined with squamous epithelium instead

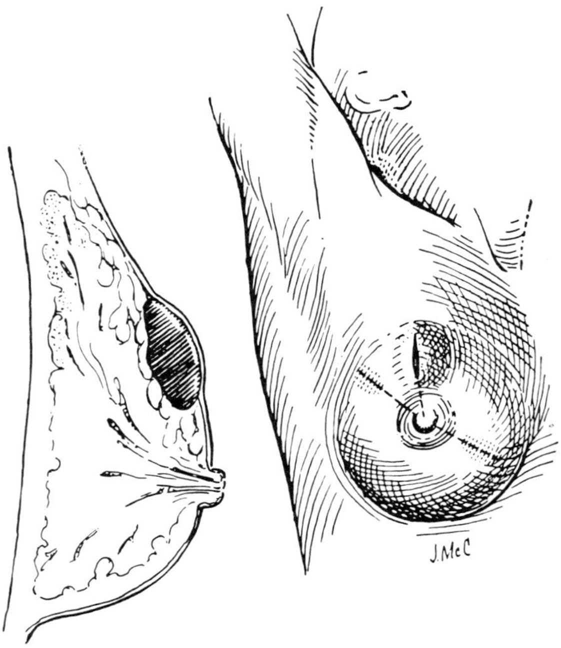

Figure 16-3. Superficial abscess of the breast. Note the line of incision radiating from the nipple over the fluctuant area.

of the usual columnar, and the abscess. In order to prevent recurrence, this fistula must be excised. The fistula may be located by exploring the inside of the recurrent abscess with a lacrimal duct probe. The fistula is identified by passing the probe into the lactiferous sinus and out of the duct orifice at the nipple. The fistula is treated by cutting through the nipple down to the probe. Once the fistula tract has been opened, the metaplastic lining is excised sharply or destroyed with the electrocautery. The wound is allowed to heal secondarily.

If the abscess is deeper than subareolar (submammary or intramammary), effective and comfortable treatment cannot be given under local anesthesia (Figs. 16-4 and 16-5). This deeper location may be discovered during the attempted drainage. In this case the procedure is terminated and the patient is prepared for a general anesthetic. Deeper abscesses should be debrided and drained to prevent recurrence. Large and deep abscesses mimick inflammatory cancer; a biopsy is necessary to make the distinction.

MANAGEMENT OF MONDOR'S DISEASE

The problem of Mondor's disease (thrombosis of the thoracoepigastric vein) is almost always evident on physical examination. The mass is in a characteristic location along the lateral aspect of the breast. It is linear, long, thin, and just under the skin (Fig. 16-6). It is tender and may be associated with skin retraction because of the subcuticular location. Biopsy is rarely necessary. If the mass persists after 2 or 3 weeks of observation, biopsy should be performed. During observation, symptomatic relief can be obtained with local heat, mild oral analgesia, and a firmly supporting bra. Anticoagulation is not necessary.

MANAGEMENT OF INTRADUCTAL PAPILLOMA

A mass in the subareolar or periareolar position raises the suspicion of an intraductal papilloma, especially if there is bloody discharge from the nipple. In this situation, a galacto-

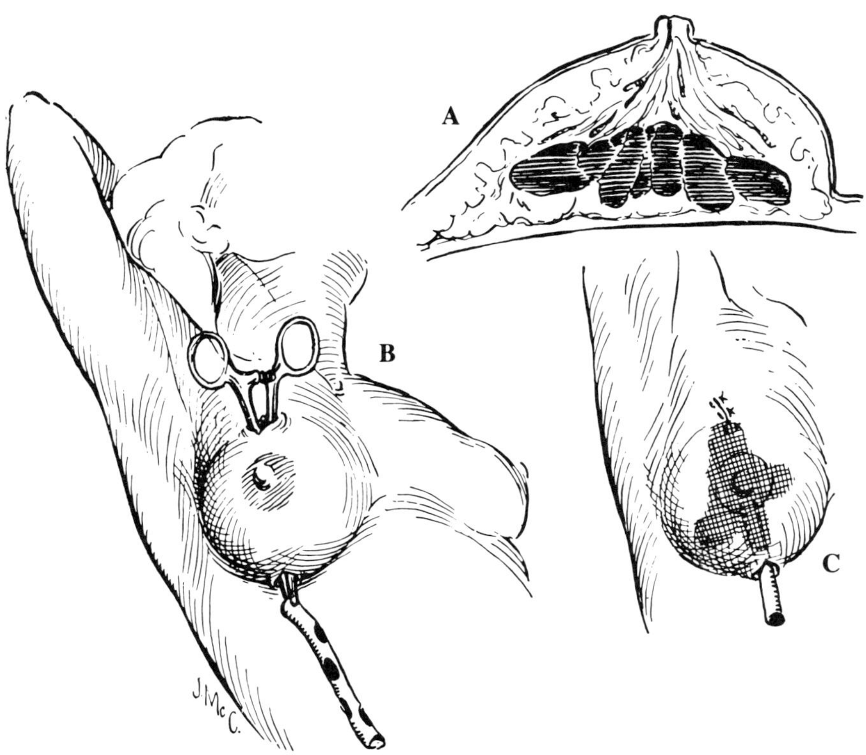

Figure 16-4. Method of draining intramammary abscess with through-and-through tube insertion.

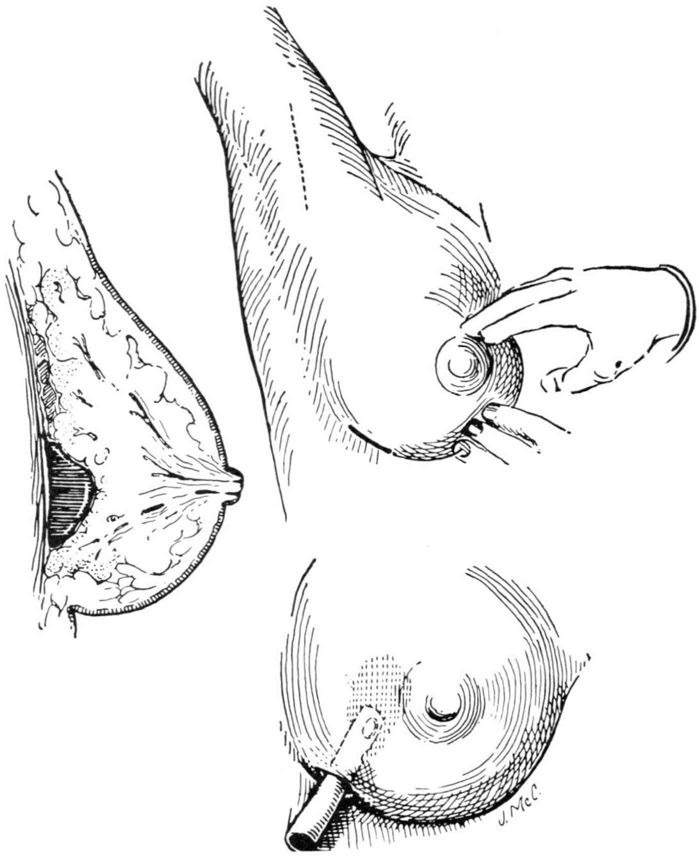

Figure 16-5. Retromammary abscess diagrammatically shown underneath the breast. Note the line of incision in the fold of the breast and the method of drainage by tubes.

gram can be helpful. If the location of the papilloma is known, a circumareolar incision can frequently be used. The nipple is raised as a flap off of the subareolar complex. The duct system that contains the papilloma is usually dilated and filled with blood. That duct is excised with sharp dissection. If a mass is not palpable and the operation is done for bloody nipple discharge, a wider duct excision with the galactogram as a guide is needed. If a mass is not palpable and a galactogram cannot be done, the entire duct system including the nipple orifice must be included in the excision. This is done by producing the discharge and identifying the involved duct. A wedge-shaped incision is made with the apex in the nipple such that the opening of the involved duct is excised. A wide segment of the subareolar tissue is removed along with the wedge of nipple and areola. The areola is reapproximated carefully with subdermal sutures so that the margins are well aligned.

MANAGEMENT OF MAMMARY DUCT ECTASIA

Mammary duct ectasia is usually a problem in older women. It results from dilation and obstruction of the lactiferous sinuses in the subareolar region. The ducts become filled with cellular debris and a lipid material. At the early stages, a nipple discharge may be the only physical sign of duct ectasia. With progression of the problem, the ducts become fibrotic, shortened, thickened, and surrounded with an inflammatory reaction. At this stage, the patient may complain of pain and a subareolar mass. In its late stages, mammary duct ectasia may produce an irregular mass associated with nipple retraction. The symptoms of duct ectasia are rarely severe enough to require excision. But the physical signs produced by duct ectasia are often indistinguishable from cancer such that excision of the subareolar mass is necessary to exclude the presence of a malignancy. The procedure is

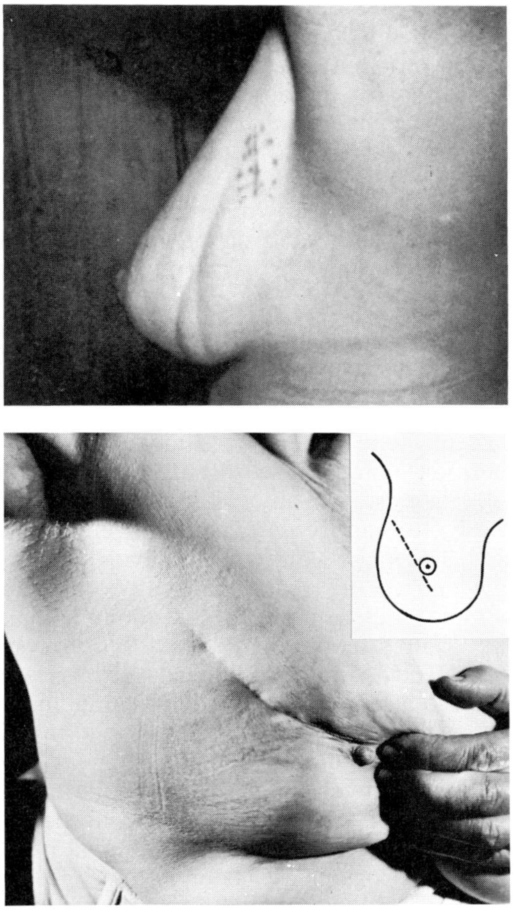

Figure 16-6. Subcutaneous phlebitis of the breast (Mondor's disease). (*Top*) Four weeks after excision of benign breast mass. Note characteristic skin retraction. (Honig HC, Rado R: Ann Surg 153:589, 1961) (*Bottom*) Note method of demonstrating cordlike vein with depressed skin line due to inflammatory shortening of the skin. (Musgrove JE: Can Med Assoc J 85:34, 1961)

similar to that of a breast biopsy. A circumareolar incision is used. The nipple is raised off of the subareolar complex as an attached skin flap. The entire subareolar complex is removed so that the palpable mass is surrounded with a margin of normal tissue. The nipple is then replaced with a running, subcuticular absorbable suture. Deeper sutures are avoided because they cause dimpling of the nipple.

MANAGEMENT OF CYSTOSARCOMA PHYLLODES

Cystosarcoma phyllodes is a rare breast tumor (0.3% to 0.5% of all breast tumors). It is considered to be a variant of fibroadenoma with more stromal hypertrophy. Its epithelial elements can develop malignant potential, although there are no histologic or clinical clues to predict which of these tumors will behave in a malignant fashion. Cystosarcoma phyllodes usually presents as a rapidly growing tumor that may stretch the overlying skin. Size is not related to malignant potential. The gross appearance of the tumor is similar to that of a fibroadenoma, the microscopic evaluation is diagnostic. Only 8% to 13% of patients with this tumor die of their disease; death is due to distant disease as the tumor spreads through the blood and not the nodes. Wide local excision is usually curative. If the tumor is large, the excision should be a mastectomy with immediate reconstruction. Since this tumor does not spread through the nodes, an axillary dissection is not usually recommended. The 5-year survival in those patients with tumors that show obvious malignant changes (10% to 30% of all cystosarcoma phyllodes) is 80% with operative therapy.[4]

MANAGEMENT OF THE PREGNANT PATIENT WITH A BREAST LUMP

The pregnant patient with a breast mass should be managed in a similar fashion to nonpregnant patients. Even though breast cancer is uncommon in child-bearing years, it does occur. Therefore a mass that presents in the first two trimesters should be biopsied under local anesthesia. A mass presenting in the third trimester may be biopsied or observed until the completion of the pregnancy when intravenous sedation can be used. Breast biopsy in the pregnant or lactating breast is more difficult due to the hypertrophy and vascularity of the stimulated breast. So it is even more important in this situation to have an adequate environment (lighting, electrocautery, monitoring, etc.) for the biopsy.

Mammography in the pregnant patient is not helpful due to the radiographic density of the stimulated breast.

Lactating adenomas occur in the pregnant breast and can grow to a large size. They are a variant of tubular breast adenomas. Rather than a predominant stromal pattern as seen in a fibroadenoma, tubular adenomas are composed of numerous tubular structures that are indistinguishable from breast ductules. With the hormonal environment of pregnancy, these tubular adenomas can enlarge, so that by the second or third trimester, they are 2 cm to 6 cm, firm, movable, nontender, and well demarcated. Such a mass may be observed through the pregnancy, since they usually occur late. If the mass persists after childbirth, it should be removed.

BREAST PAIN

Breast pain and tenderness is a common complaint. Slightly more than 50% of randomly sampled women reported cyclic breast pain, yet only 0.4% of the sample missed work because of the pain.[5] Most women who seek consultation for breast pain do so because the pain is new to them and they fear cancer. Reassurance that a malignancy is not present is the only treatment required in up to 85% of patients.[6]

The most common pathologic diagnosis associated with breast pain is fibrocystic disease. Other, less common causes are abscess, mastodynia, hormone changes, cancer, and chest wall disorders. Abscess has been covered in the section on breast lumps. If no abscess is present, the diagnosis and management of breast pain consists of (1) exclusion of cancer and (2) management of the mastodynia.

DIAGNOSIS AND MANAGEMENT OF FIBROCYSTIC DISEASE

Fibrocystic disease is an imprecise yet popular term used to describe a variety of histologic and clinical conditions. To a pathologist, it means microcysts, macrocysts, adenosis, apocrine change, fibrosis, fibroadenoma or ductal hyperplasia.[7] These histologic findings, however, have no correlation with the severity of the pain. In fact, some patients with pain have normal biopsies, and some patients with severe histologic changes on biopsy have no pain. Pathologists are now discouraging the use of the term *fibrocystic disease* for every breast biopsy that does not show cancer. They now prefer to describe breast abnormalities in terms that have more descriptive and clinical meaning.[8] The majority of biopsies (70%) show lesions with no proliferative activity. This includes mild hyperplasia, cysts, epithelia-related calcification, and fibroadenoma. Patients with this finding do not have an increased risk for developing breast cancer. The remaining biopsies show proliferative activity; these are divided into those with (4%) and without (26%) atypia. Proliferative lesions are associated with an increased risk for developing breast cancer, especially the proliferative changes with atypical hyperplasia.[9]

To the clinician, fibrocystic disease means tender lumps in a woman's breast. These lumps are flat and disk-shaped rather than three-dimensional. They can come and go between office visits. They usually vary in size and tenderness with the menstrual cycle. And the condition can worsen when the female hormone environment is changing, such as with the addition of oral contraception, estrogen replacement therapy, or menopause. This condition is not a disease but rather the normal response of an endocrine organ, the breast, to endogenous and exogenous steroids. The majority of women have a "physiologic lumpiness" that is clinically significant only inasmuch as it obscures a dominant mass that requires biopsy. Patients with fibrocystic disease and a dominant lump should be treated the same as patients who have a lump and no fibrocystic disease. If the mass is solid to needle aspiration, it is likely to disappear after two or three cycles. This is especially true in those women who have dramatic fibrocystic symptoms. A reduction or withdrawal of exogenous estrogen may hasten this change. The minimum daily dose of estrogen to prevent osteoporosis is 0.625 mg. If the patient is already on this low dose, the addition of a progestational agent may diminish pain and lumpiness. Medroxyprogesterone acetate (Provera; 5 mg/day to 10 mg/day) may be given on the last 5 to 10 days of the cycle to oppose the effects of the estrogen. Another alternative is to stop the estrogen replacement for 3 months and then reexamine the breasts. If the symptoms have abated, then the estrogen may be restarted at 0.625 mg/day. A dominant lump that persists in a fibrocystic breast after an appropriate observation period (2 to 4 months) should be biopsied.

Mammography can help to confirm the clinical impression of fibrocystic disease. The film may show patterns suggestive of cysts, fibrosis, enlarged ducts, and microcalcifications within fibroadenomas. Ultrasound can confirm that the patterns seen on mammogram are cystic. Neither of these tests, however, should delay the biopsy of a dominant mass in a fibrocystic breast, even if the imaging study suggests no malignancy. There have been several instances of treatment delay for a breast cancer due to a benign appearance on mammography.[1]

MANAGEMENT OF MASTODYNIA

Patients with lumpy, painful breasts and no dominant lump should be reassured first that they do not have a malignancy. If the patient is not assured with a normal physical exam and if she is over 35 years old, a mammogram should be done. The American Cancer Society recommends that all women over 35 have a baseline screening mammogram. The x-ray may also support the clinical diagnosis of fibrocystic change and no malignancy. The majority of patients will require no other treatment beyond this reassurance. Patients who continue to have pain can be managed with one or several of the following measures:

Support bra. An athletic support bra worn day and night when symptomatic frequently provides sufficient relief of pain.

Dietary restrictions. Removal of methylxanthines (coffee, tea, cocoa, cola) may benefit some patients with mild symptoms. Since there is little risk, a 4-week period should be tried. The effectiveness of this measure seems to depend on a high baseline intake of these substances.

Vitamins. Vitamins E, B, and C have been advocated.[10] As long as these are not ingested in toxic doses, there is little risk in a trial of vitamin therapy. They may benefit patients with mild symptoms.

Hormone therapy. Since the basis of this problem is estrogen stimulation, some patients benefit from an alteration in their replacement therapy or an interruption in their natural cycle. As discussed previously, patients may benefit from a reduction in their estrogen dose to 0.625 mg/day. This amount still provides protection against osteoporosis. If the patient is already on this dose, elimination of the replacement estrogen for 3 months may help. And finally, addition of medroxyprogesterone acetate (Provera; 5 mg/day to 10 mg/day) to the estrogen regimen on the last 5 or 10 days of the cycle often provides relief of pain. For patients who also desire pregnancy protection, oral contraceptives may diminish breast tenderness. This probably works by restoring a more normal balance between estrogen and progesterone. On the other hand, it is not unusual for a woman to develop breast tenderness after beginning oral contraceptives. If this problem does not respond to a reduction in the dose, the pill may need to be stopped to relieve the breast pain.

Hormone inhibitors. Danazol completely relieves the pain and tenderness in 70% to 80% of patients.[6] The dose is 200 mg/day to 400 mg/day. The drug may take up to 3 months to work, and it has some side-effects. Patients may develop weight gain (17%), acne (8%), flushes (5%), hair and skin oiliness (4%), headache and nausea (3%) while on danazol.[11]

Surgery. Mastectomy may be offered to the rare patient who has not responded to other measures to control breast pain. Women should be selected very carefully for operation. A chest wall source for the pain should be sought (intercostal neuritis, costochondritis) with trigger point injections and nerve blocks. A minimum of 6 months of diet and hormone-inhibitor therapy is mandatory. Ideal candidates are those with a high risk for cancer, and whose breasts have been distorted by multiple biopsies. When operation is undertaken, the patient should understand that the pain may persist after mastectomy.[6] A total mastectomy should be done, as opposed to a subcutaneous mastectomy. This operation, which removes all of the breast tissue instead of most of it, has the best chance of relieving the pain.

ABNORMAL MAMMOGRAM

Screening mammography is beginning to catch hold in the minds of primary practitioners and patients alike. Radiologic imaging of the asymptomatic breast may detect early cancer in up to 45% of women screened. Breast cancer discovered by screening mammography in an asymptomatic woman is most frequently Stage I disease (negative axillary lymph nodes). The accuracy of mammography is variable. Nationally, the reported rate of malignancy in mammographically suspicious lesions averages 25%. This incidence can vary widely, however, and in actual practice may be only 10%. This low true-positive rate is partially due to the manner in which some mammographers report the test. If every abnormality is described as "possibly malignant," then an operative biopsy cannot be avoided. With increasing experience, radiologists and surgeons should be able to identify those abnormalities associated with a higher probability of malignancy. This type of qualitative interpretation will decrease the number of biopsies for an abnormal mammogram due to benign disease.

There are three responsibilities in the management of this problem: (1) to reassure the patient that the likelihood of cancer may be 10% or less, (2) to evaluate the mammograms with a knowledgeable radiologist who is informed of the pertinent clinical information, and (3) to carefully examine the breast that harbors the radiographic abnormality.

DIAGNOSIS AND MANAGEMENT

The initial evaluation of the patient with an abnormal mammogram is similar to that for the woman with a breast lump. An interview is conducted with specific attention to the presence of risk factors for breast cancer. Next, a careful physical examination is done. The mammogram should be reviewed prior to the exam so that the suspicious areas can be evaluated with more care. If a lump is found, it should be managed as any other breast lump. This may include needle aspiration and possibly operative biopsy. If the lump is in the area of the mammographic abnormality, a biopsy is necessary. If no dominant lump is found in the breast, then the mammogram should be evaluated by a second radiologist who will interpret the mammogram in a qualitative fashion. This should be done jointly by the radiologist and the surgeon. The pertinent clinical information (estrogen therapy, previous biopsies, radiation exposure, cancer risk, etc.) can influence the interpretation of the x-ray. In addition, it is helpful for the surgeon to understand the reasons that the x-ray is abnormal. This cooperation between the radiologist and the surgeon will facilitate the operative localization and biopsy of mammographic abnormalities. In our experience, this critical reevaluation of mammograms that have been called suspicious can prevent a biopsy 50% of the time. In the past 3 years we have evaluated 88 patients for an abnormal mammogram. On examination, 11 patients had a palpable mass. All of these were biopsied. The remainder were biopsied if the mammogram demonstrated one of the following criteria: (1) more than five microcalcifications within 1 cm, (2) microcalcifications in an irradiated breast (regardless of the number), (3) circumscribed and dense masses with indistinct margins, (4) masses that increase in size, or (5) architectural distortion of the contralateral breast. Based on these criteria, 32 of the 88 patients had a localized breast biopsy; two cancers were found. Forty-three patients were followed with repeat mammography. None have developed a malignancy or criteria for biopsy. This high sensitivity and low selectivity of mammography demands close cooperation between the radiologist and surgeon to prevent unnecessary biopsies and to assuage the anxious patients.

TECHNIQUE FOR MAMMOGRAPHIC BREAST BIOPSY

The surgeon should be present for the localization. This is the best opportunity to obtain a three-dimensional concept of the lesion in its relationship to topographical landmarks. If the surgeon cannot be present, the films should be reviewed and discussed with the radiologist. We have been using a wire with a barb on the end to identify mammographic lesions. This wire is inserted through a hypodermic needle directed toward the lesion. The wire usually enters the breast directly above the lesion to minimize dissection. Occasionally, the wire can be placed adjacent to the areola so that a circumareolar incision can be used. After placement, the wire is taped securely to the skin; the patient is taken directly to the operating room on a stretcher to avoid dislocation of the wire.

Since a wire-directed breast biopsy can be more difficult than the biopsy of a palpable lump, the surgeon may choose general anesthesia. We have been satisfied with local anesthesia supplemented with intravenous midazolam. The surgeon must have an idea of the orientation of the wire in the breast as the biopsy is begun. The skin incision is made through the hole that contains the wire. This is developed to the subcutaneous fat. Then a core of breast tissue is removed around the wire down to a depth of approximately 2 cm beyond the wire or the lesion (whichever is deepest). Depending on the size of the lesion, the diameter of the biopsy core may be increased as the end of the wire is approached. Ideally, the wire and the lesion are not seen during the operation. Many patients with abnormal mammograms have small lesions that are ideal for breast-conservation treatment. This newer approach, which avoids mastectomy, requires negative margins on the original biopsy. Once the biopsy core and the wire have been removed, a specimen mammogram is done. If there are no microcalcifications, specimen mammography may be omitted as it is difficult to identify lesions that are suspicious for architectural distortion. Lesions that have calcifications, however, can be identified by mammography of the specimen. Two views of the specimen are obtained with a 90-degree rotation. These films are reviewed by the radiologist who performed the localization. If the abnormality is in the biopsy, the specimen is taken to the pathologist for a frozen section. An immediate evaluation of the biopsy is justified because it allows provision of material for estrogen receptor assay and it permits early treatment planning if the lesion is malignant.

If the specimen mammogram does not demonstrate the lesion, an additional biopsy is taken. Before this is done, the films are reviewed again by the surgeon and the radiologist together. An attempt is made to identify the relationship of the tip of the localizer wire to the lesion. The second biopsy is made in the base of the wound in the area of the breast that contained the lesion, medial or lateral and cephalad or caudad. If this second "blind" biopsy does not contain the lesion, we quit and close the wound. A repeat mammogram is obtained in 4 to 6 months to see whether the microcalcifications were removed and just not evident on specimen mammography. If the lesion is still present, a second localization biopsy is scheduled. The miss rate for wire-directed biopsy of mammographic abnormalities is 10%.

NIPPLE DISORDERS

The nipple abnormalities that most often arouse patient concern are discharge and erosion. Secretion from the nipple is almost always a benign condition. Erosion and crusting, however, are serious symptoms that require prompt attention.

DIAGNOSIS

Secretion from the nipple is a common occurrence in a menstruating woman. The many causes of this discharge are listed under "Causes of Nipple Secretion."

The goal in the management of the patient with nipple discharge is twofold: (1) to establish that no malignancy is present and (2) to remove the cause if the secretion becomes persistent and bothersome.

Cancer should be strongly suspected in a woman over 60 who has bloody discharge from a single duct, especially if there is an associated mass. Malignancy is less likely if the patient is young and menstruating, if the discharge is nonbloody, bilateral, and present in several ducts in the same breast. Bloody breast secretion during pregnancy is considered normal. It is probably related to the vascular engorgement that occurs with pregnancy. If there is no mass in the breast, evaluation should be deferred until the pregnancy has been completed. If the discharge persists in the postpartum period, then it should be evaluated.

Several tests are helpful in the evaluation of the patient with persistent nipple discharge. Mammography can detect malignant and benign neoplasms that cause nipple discharge. It can also show the large, dilated ducts of subareolar abscess, duct ectasia, or intraductal papilloma. The x-ray may suggest fibrocystic disease that can cause secretion of the same

CAUSES OF NIPPLE SECRETION

- Etiology outside of the breast
  - Hyperprolactinemia
  - Primary hypothyroidism
  - Cushing's syndrome
  - Chest wall trauma
  - Drugs (phenothiazines, tricyclic antidepressants, oral contraceptives)
  - Mechanical stimulation
- Etiology within the breast
  - Intraductal papilloma
  - Malignancy
  - Fibrocystic disease
  - Chronic subareolar abscess
  - Duct ectasia
  - Breast trauma

type of fluid that is found in breast cysts: greenish-brown to dark brown, clear or cloudy. A galactogram is useful if the duct producing the fluid can be identified. The opening of the duct is dilated by the radiologist and intubated with a small catheter. Contrast is placed into the duct and x-rays are taken. This study can demonstrate detailed ductal anatomy. It is especially useful when an intraductal papilloma is present. Cytologic examination of the nipple secretion can be very helpful if malignant cells are found because the incidence of a false positive is very low. If no malignant cells are found, however, the diagnosis should still be pursued because the incidence of false negatives is high.

Nipple crusting or erosion should be treated as Paget's disease until proved to be otherwise by biopsy. Paget's disease may also appear as thickening, redness, or roughness in the nipple. The patients frequently complain of an associated itching or burning. The incidence of Paget's disease is low (1% to 4% of all breast cancers), so a delay in diagnosis is typical, as the patient is usually treated for eczema. The origin of the Paget cell has been argued. It may be a malignant cell invading the epidermis of the nipple and arising from an underlying intraductal malignancy. Or it may be an epidermoid cell that is transformed in situ by the same influences that cause the growth of a malignancy in the ducts below the nipple. Whatever the source, Paget's disease is associated with intraductal or invasive malignancy nearly all the time. If a mass can be felt under the nipple, the presence of a cancer is certain. This occurred in 58% of a large series of patients with Paget's disease of the nipple.[12] There have been reports of cases in which no cancer has been found under the nipple once it had been removed for Paget's disease.[13] These cases may represent an early stage of the disease or failure to find a small focus of malignancy. Several of these cases have developed a subsequent recurrence in the same breast, suggesting that the original tumor had been missed.

Regardless of the uncertainties with respect to this disease, any nipple erosion, crusting, redness, or thickening should be managed with a full-thickness skin biopsy immediately. The incidence of axillary metastasis in women with Paget's disease and skin changes only is between 5% and 18%. When a mass is also present at the time of presentation, 50% to 68% of patients will have axillary nodal disease.[14]

MANAGEMENT OF NIPPLE DISCHARGE

The initial step in the management of nipple discharge is dictated by the presence or absence of a mass. If a mass can be felt in the breast with the discharge, it should be biopsied without additional testing or delay. If no mass is present, a decision is made to evaluate the patient or observe them based on the probability that a malignancy is present. Factors that increase the likelihood of cancer being associated with the discharge include the following: age over 60, concurrent mass on examination, bloody discharge, persistent and spontaneous discharge, discharge from a single duct, and nonmenstruating status. If the risk factors are low, the patient can be observed. Evaluation and biopsy may be done in the future if the discharge persists for 3 to 6 months. If the risk factors are high, an evaluation should be done to identify the cause of the discharge. This may include cytologic examination of the fluid, mammogram, and/or galactogram. If the work-up identifies the lesion, it should be excised. Malignant diagnoses based on cytology should be confirmed with a formal biopsy before recommending treatment. If the work-up does not identify the lesion, then an operative procedure should be done for diagnosis. The type of procedure depends on the ability to localize the breast segment that contains the pathology. The breast should be compressed around the areola. If pressure on one segment consistently produces secretion, then a wedge excision of the nipple, areola, and underlying nipple–areolar complex can be done. If the duct cannot be localized, then the nipple should be raised as a flap by incising 180 degrees of the circumference. The nipple and areola are sharply dissected off of the underlying central duct complex. A cylinder of tissue is then removed with the same diameter as the areola and a height of at least 4 cm. If a large duct is identified during the dissection, it should be completely removed. Once the biopsy and duct excision are done, the nipple is replaced with a single running suture in the subcuticular layer of the skin and areola. If the specimen shows duct ectasia or an intraductal papilloma, the procedure should be curative. If a cancer is found, additional treatment will be needed.

MANAGEMENT OF NIPPLE EROSION

Nipple erosion is a condition that should not be observed. A biopsy of full-thickness skin should be done through the involved areas of the nipple. The biopsy should include some normal-appearing skin. If Paget's disease is found, modified radical mastectomy is usually recommended. This results in the following 10-year survival:[12]

Noninvasive, intraductal carcinoma	100%
Invasive carcinoma, skin changes only	80%
Invasive carcinoma, palpable mass	70%
Invasive carcinoma, mass and involved nodes	30%

Since the incidence of Stage II breast cancer (positive axillary lymph nodes) is between 5% and 18% in patients with skin changes and no mass, modified radical mastectomy is a reasonable approach. Recently, an alternative approach has been advocated for patients with no mass and a normal mammogram. Six patients with biopsy-proved Paget's disease had their nipple and subareolar complex removed. If there was no underlying carcinoma in the specimen, they did not receive a mastectomy. All are alive and well with an average follow-up of 50 months.[15]

If the nipple biopsy demonstrates inflammation and no Paget's cells, treatment can be directed toward the symptoms. If there is no resolution within 4 weeks, a dermatologic evaluation is indicated.

POSTOPERATIVE PROBLEMS

Most postoperative complications after breast surgery are managed in an ambulatory care setting. Most of the minor outpatient procedures carry a low morbidity rate, so the majority of problems that develop in the postoperative period occur after major procedures, especially mastectomy. The topics that will be addressed in this section are infection, hematoma, seroma, arm swelling, frozen shoulder, skin flap necrosis, and local recurrence.

INFECTION

Infection is a rare occurrence after breast biopsy or mastectomy. A hematoma is more common after breast biopsy than infection, so a mass in the operative site is not enough evidence to begin treatment for infection. Pain, redness, and fever are present when the mass is due to postoperative infection. A hematoma can cause tenderness and skin redness also, so equivocal cases should be resolved with a diagnostic aspiration. The skin is prepped with an alcohol swab. Then the mass is penetrated with an 18-gauge needle on a 10-ml syringe. A small amount of 1% lidocaine without epinephrine can be used for patient comfort prior to the aspiration. Some surgeons feel that the lidocaine causes more discomfort than the needle; others place the needle through the healing scar where there is no sensation. If the aspirate is purulent, the wound is opened enough to allow daily packing with 0.25-inch plain gauze. There is no need for systemic antibiotics once the wound has been drained. The packing continues until the wound closes spontaneously. If the needle aspirate is bloody, a gram stain and culture should be done to make the diagnosis. A positive culture indicates an infected hematoma that should be drained and packed. Antibiotic therapy will not sterilize an infected hematoma.

Wound infection after mastectomy can be more serious and may require hospitalization. A seroma under the skin flaps is more common than infection after mastectomy, however the two problems have common features that can make the initial management difficult. Wound infection after mastectomy will present with swelling, redness, and fever. All of these signs can occur in a patient with partial necrosis of the skin flaps; ischemia of the skin flaps will look exactly like the erythema of a wound infection. In these cases, a wound aspiration through normal skin should guide therapy. If no fluid is obtained, or if the fluid that is obtained is sterile, then the wound should be examined by the surgeon every 3 to 5 days. Infection after mastectomy is handled by opening the incision wide enough to allow packing of the entire abscess cavity. If the cavity is small, this can be managed on an ambulatory basis. Antibiotics are not necessary once the abscess has been drained. When the infection involves the entire operative site such that wound care would be difficult at home, the patient should be admitted for wide drainage and packing until the wound becomes smaller. Other reasons for admission are systemic sepsis and infection in a patient with neutropenia from adjuvant chemotherapy. In these situations, intravenous antibiotics are needed.

Antibiotics may also be useful in the patient with erythema from skin flap necrosis or ischemia. These problems are often surrounded by a mild cellulitis that can be bacterial colonization of the defective skin. Since this cellulitis is usually due to staphylococcus or streptococcus, oral dicloxacillin (500 mg q 6 hr) is useful.

Delayed infection in the wounds from axillary dissection has been common when radiotherapy is used as the primary treatment for breast cancer. These have been occurring 2 or 3 weeks after operation. Since the wound is in the radiation field, these wounds are slow to heal. They should be managed with packing just like other breast infections. If there is a lymphatic leak, the packing should be changed two or three times a day.

HEMATOMA

Hematomas are a common occurrence after breast biopsy. They usually cause a minor lump in the area of the biopsy. In this case, the only treatment necessary is to inform the patient that the mass will slowly resolve. Hematomas from breast biopsies do not cause symptoms unless they become very large. This problem is usually prevented by carefully examining the wound for arterial bleeding before closing. Slow oozing into the wound stops with the pressure provided by a firmly fitting bra; arterial bleeding continues until the wound is tensely packed with blood. Deep sutures in the breast parenchyma do not prevent either form of bleeding; they do cause deformity of the breast with skin dimpling. Large hematomas are usually painful. For this reason, and because they are less likely to resolve completely, they should be evacuated. This may require a general anesthetic. The wound is opened entirely. The clot is removed and the cavity irrigated. A careful search is made for the bleeding vessel; occasionally, none is found. The skin closure is done in a running, subcuticular fashion with a small, absorbable suture. A drain is usually unnecessary unless the cavity is very large.

Hematomas after mastectomy are uncommon because large drains are frequently placed under the skin flaps to evacuate the blood. As with breast biopsies, minor hematomas may be left. Large, symptomatic hematomas, however, should be evacuated in the operating room. This requires a general anesthetic so that the wound can be searched thoroughly. The vessel responsible for large hematomas after mastectomy is usually in the axillary area or on the chest wall where the branches from the internal mammary artery perforate the pectoral muscle. Hematomas requiring operative intervention occur in the immediate postoperative period. Late fluid collections after mastectomy are almost always due to seromas.

SEROMA

Seromas result from an accumulation of lymph and interstitial fluid after mastectomy. This complication is seen in obese women more frequently than in women with a thin subcutaneous fatty layer. Seromas are usually asymptomatic until the skin flaps are placed under tension. When this happens it is advisable to drain the seroma for patient comfort and to improve perfusion of the skin flaps. Smaller, asymptomatic seromas can be left alone; they will gradually resolve. Repeated aspiration of postmastectomy seromas may result in contamination of the seroma with bacteria. This converts the seroma into a large abscess of the chest wall. In order to prevent this problem, aspiration should be done only when necessary and with careful sterile technique. The patient is placed in a supine position. Local anesthetic is usually unnecessary due to denervation of the skin flaps. An 18-gauge needle is placed on a three-way stopcock. A 60-ml syringe is connected to one outlet; the remaining outlet is fixed to a segment of iv tubing that drains into a collecting pan. This arrangement allows aspiration with a single needle puncture rather than repeated ones. The site of the needle puncture is in a dependent part of the wound, usually in the lower skin flap. The needle should not be placed through the incision, as this area may contain poorly perfused skin with bacterial colonization. Once the wound has been punctured, the needle is left in place while the syringe is filled and evacuated through the iv tubing. After complete aspiration of the seroma, the patient should be encouraged to return to normal activity. Immobilization of the arm and binding the chest do not prevent reaccumulation of the fluid.

ARM SWELLING

Arm swelling occurs much less frequently than in the past. The primary reason for its disappearance is the popularity of a less complete axillary node dissection at the time of mastectomy. In the absence of gross axillary disease, a lower-level dissection that yields ten nodes is sufficient for staging purposes. This type of axillary dissection virtually never causes arm swelling unless the axilla is irradiated. Minor lymphedema of the upper extremity can be managed with a compressive garment that is worn at night. More severe swelling may require that the garment be worn during the day as well. Compressive pumps are available that "milk" the lymphatic fluid from the arm with waves of pressure that begin at the fingers and travel centrally. Some patients prefer to use the pump for several hours at night and then be free of the compressive arm stocking. Advanced lymphedema is a serious problem that may have no solution. Some success has been reported with a microvascular anastomosis of enlarged lymphatics to subcutaneous veins in the arm. This approach has a 50% success rate.

FROZEN SHOULDER

Frozen shoulder occurs in patients who do not move their shoulders after mastectomy. This is usually due to fear more than pain as the discomfort after mastectomy is not severe. Once the shoulder contracture has occurred, it becomes painful and reinforces the patient's desire to hold her arm at her side. The patient should be encouraged to use the arm in everyday tasks, such as hair care, brushing teeth, reaching overhead to library shelves, and so on. Two exercises are useful for this problem. The first involves "walking" two fingers up a wall. The patient should mark the height attained and attempt to surpass it three times a day. The second exercise consists of bending at the waist, allowing the arm to fall straight down, and then spinning the arm in ever-widening circles. This is also done three times a day. If the patient is unable to work out the shoulder contracture, a physical therapy consultation should be obtained.

SKIN FLAP NECROSIS

Skin flap necrosis can vary from discoloration of the edges of the flap to necrosis and subsequent ulceration. The wound should be followed on a regular basis as the amount of nonviable tissue becomes evident. During this time the wound should be washed two or three times a day with warm, soapy water. It is covered with a dry dressing and kept clean. As the skin necrosis is established, the dead skin is cleaned away with sharp debridment until bleeding is seen in the margins of the wound. Once an ulcerated wound occurs, it is dressed with gauze moistened in saline after each cleansing session (warm, soapy water, three times a day). If the ulcerated wound is small, it may be allowed to close. If it is large, a skin graft may be needed for closure once the ulcerated bed is clean and the surrounding skin is well perfused.

LOCAL RECURRENCE

Local recurrence usually presents as a small lump under the incision scar or under the skin flap. Any firm nodule in these areas, or in the axilla, should be managed with an incisional biopsy. The biopsy should be small so that the entire wound can be removed with the recurrence if the biopsy is positive. This may be done with a small needle aspiration for cytology that avoids a skin incision altogether.

MALE BREAST

The male and female breast are identical prior to puberty. The male breast does not develop like the female breast, but it retains the rudimentary, simple ducts of childhood. These ducts can respond to hormonal, drug, and other stimuli, resulting in hypertrophy of the stroma and ducts (gynecomastia). These ducts can also give rise to every histologic type of breast cancer that is found in women. Gynecomastia is more common than breast cancer in men. Fortunately, the two problems are usually easily distinguishable on physical examination.

DIAGNOSIS

Male breast cancer is not common. It occurs only once for every 100 female breast cancers. The peak age incidence is between 60 and 65 years. The most common presenting symptom is a painless mass (75% to 95%). One third of patients have nipple involvement, and skin or fascial fixation. One half present with axillary metastasis. The small volume of the male breast and patient procrastination contribute to the larger percentage of cases that present in an advanced stage compared with female breast cancer. Stage for stage, however, male breast cancer has the same survival outlook as female breast cancer. The other causes for a breast lump in a male are gynecomastia, sarcoma, metastatic cancer, and such benign tumors as lipomas. The most common of all these is gynecomastia.

"Comparison Between Gynecomastia and Male Breast Cancer" contrasts cancer and gynecomastia; the two are almost always easily distinguishable[16]:

COMPARISON BETWEEN GYNECOMASTIA AND MALE BREAST CANCER

Carcinoma

Increases with age
Nontender
Unilateral
Hard
Irregular
Fascial fixation
Associated with
  Discharge
  Axillary nodes
  Ulceration

Gynecomastia

Any age, higher in young and very old
Tender
Many bilateral
Firm to soft
Well-defined, discoid
May adhere to areola
Associated with
  Other medical conditions—liver disease, heart disease, and endocrine disorders
  Drugs—estrogens, corticosteroids, cimetidine, digitalis, thiazides, reserpine, phenothiazines, marijuana

(Adapted from Strombeck J, Rosato F [eds]: Surgery of the Breast. New York, Georg Thieme Verlag, 1986)

MANAGEMENT OF GYNECOMASTIA

Tender buttons of breast tissue can usually be ignored in the teenage years. Enlargement of the male breast is very common during puberty and almost always regresses within two years of onset (Fig. 16-7). If there are ominous signs on physical exam, such as nipple fixation, nipple erosion, or stony firmness, the enlarged breast tissue should be removed regardless of the patient's age. Breast enlargement that occurs in later life is more likely to be malignant, so operative management is prudent. The procedure of choice for this disorder is subcutaneous mastectomy (Fig. 16-8). This

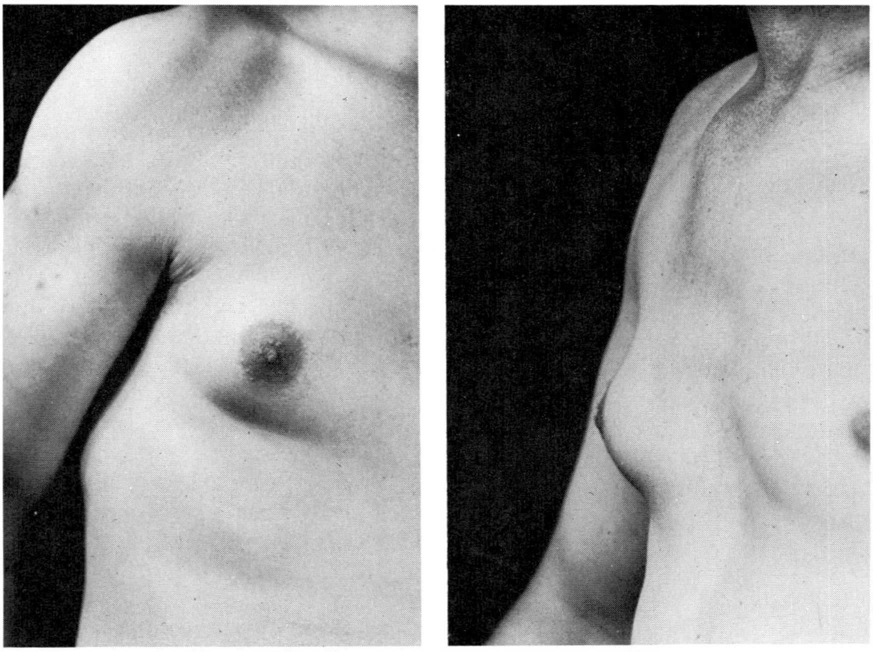

Figure 16-7. Gynecomastia in an 18-year-old boy.

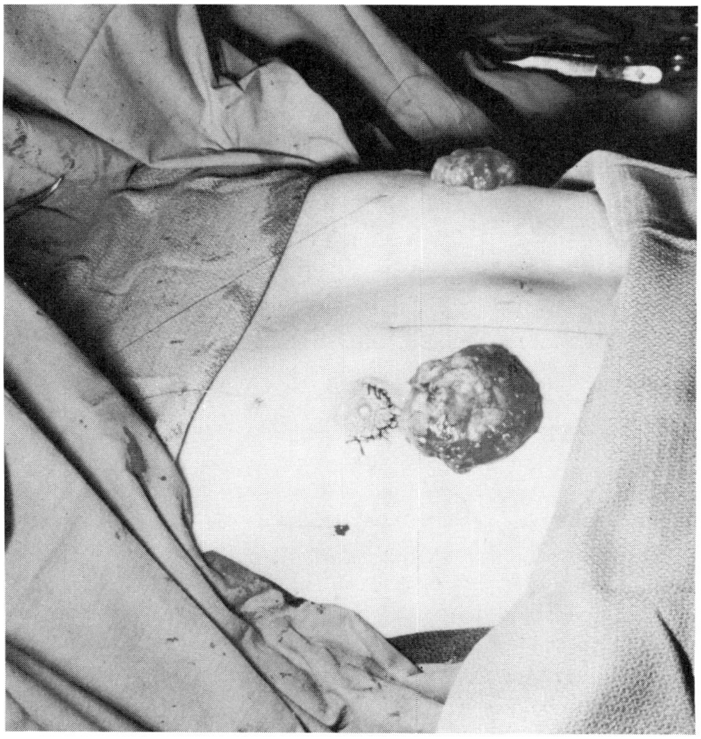

Figure 16-8. Bilateral gynecomastia treated by removal of tissue through a circumareolar incision. (Note removed specimens lying near closed incisions.)

is done under local anesthesia, supplemented with intravenous midazolam. All the routines outlined for biopsy of the female breast are followed, including intravenous access, cardiac monitor, nasal cannula oxygen, and so on. Because of the size of the field block, 0.5% lidocaine with no epinephrine is used. The dermis under the nipple is infiltrated, then a spinal needle is used to infiltrate the skin around the nipple that overlies the palpable breast tissue. A circumareolar incision is used. The nipple is raised off of the underlying breast tissue. Next, the skin is elevated off the chest wall with sharp and blunt dissection in the subcutaneous plane (Fig. 16-9). There should be a layer of fat left with the skin that is at least a centimeter thick. The skin should be elevated circumferentially so that the enlarged breast tissue can be felt completely within the wound. An Allis clamp is placed on the edge of the breast tissue for traction. Then the breast mass is excised in its entirety by sharply dissecting in a plane between the mass and the pectoralis fascia. The wound should be carefully inspected for hemostasis after the mass has been removed. All bleeding is stopped with the electrocautery to prevent the formation of a hematoma. If the right amount of subcutaneous fat is left with the skin flaps, there will be little or no depression under the nipple when the wound is closed. No drain is needed. The wound is closed with a running, subcuticular, small (4-0 or 5-0) absorbable suture. Sutures are not placed in the subcutaneous layer because they do not effectively eliminate dead space and they usually cause unsightly skin dimpling. Steri-Strips are placed in a radial fashion to complete the closure.

MANAGEMENT OF BREAST CANCER

If the mass in a male patient's breast has the characteristics of a malignancy, then a small incisional biopsy should be done instead of a subcutaneous mastectomy. Aspiration of the mass for cytology is a good alternative to incisional biopsy. Even though a malignant diagnosis by cytology should be confirmed with incisional biopsy, the certainty of a positive cytologic report allows preparation to proceed with definitive treatment at the time of incisional biopsy. The biopsy should be done directly over the mass so that the entire biopsy wound can be removed with the subsequent mastectomy specimen. Since the male breast has a small volume, and since male breast cancer frequently invades skin, nipple, and/or

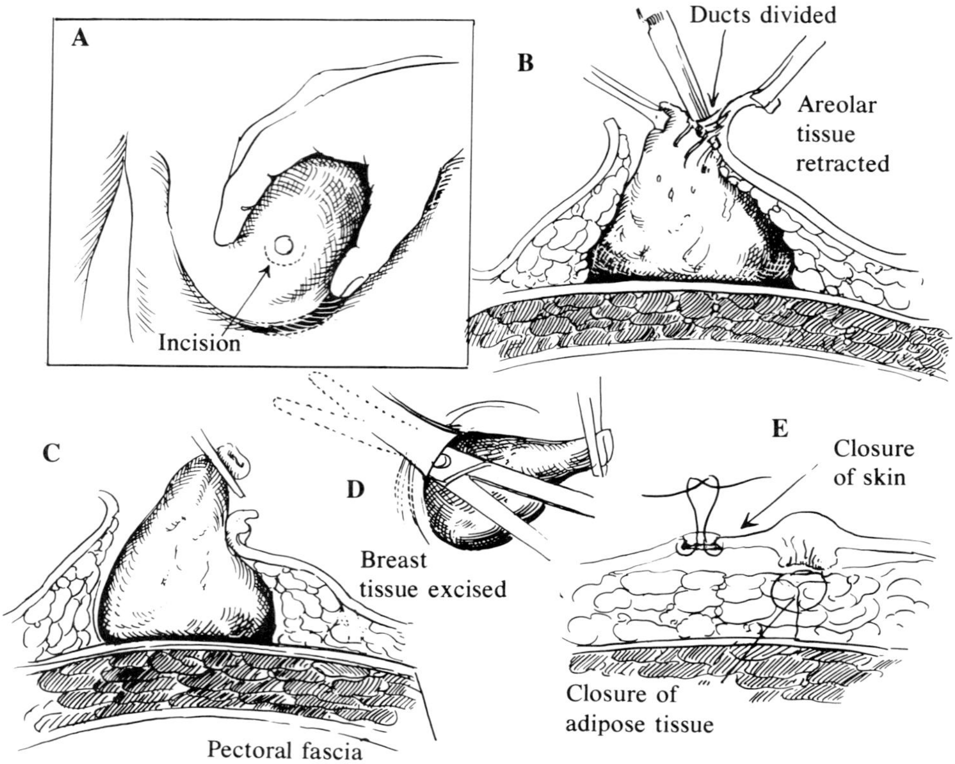

Figure 16-9. Technique of operation for gynecomastia through an incision at the edge of the areola. (Lynch RC: Plast Reconstr Surg 13:412, 1954)

muscle fascia, a formal radical mastectomy with skin grafting is usually recommended.

REFERENCES

1. Mann B, Giuliano A, Bassett L et al: Delayed diagnosis of breast cancer as a result of normal mammograms. Arch Surg 118:23–24, 1983
2. Millis R: Needle biopsy of the breast. Monogr Pathol 25:186–203, 1984
3. Johnsen C: Inflammatory lesions of the breast, Chap 6. In Strombeck J, Rosato F (eds): Surgery of the Breast. New York, Georg Thieme Verlag, 1986
4. Vorherr H, Vorherr U, Kutvirt D, Key C: Cystosarcoma phyllodes: Epidemiology, pathohistology, pathobiology, diagnosis, therapy and survival. Arch Gynecol 236:173–181, 1985
5. Campbell B, Trachtenbarg D, Barclay A: Cyclic breast pain. J Fam Pract 19:549–550, 1984
6. Pye J, Mansel R, Hughes L: Clinical experience of drug treatments for mastalgia. Lancet ii(8451):373–377, 1985
7. Rosai J: Ackerman's Surgical Pathology. St Louis, CV Mosby, 1981
8. Love S, Gelman R, Silen W: Fibrocystic "disease" of the breast—A nondisease? N Engl J Med 307:1010–1014, 1982
9. Dupont W, Page D: Risk factors for breast cancer in women with proliferative breast disease. N Engl J Med 312:146–151, 1985
10. Leis H: Symposium—Fibrocystic disease. Contemp Surg 23:97–126, 1983
11. Brookshaw J: Danazole treatment of benign breast disease: A survey of USA multicenter studies. Postgrad Med J 55(Suppl 5):52–58, 1979
12. Kister S, Haagensen C: Paget's disease of the breast. Am J Surg 119:606–609, 1970
13. Ashikari R, Park K, Huvos A et al: Paget's disease of the breast. Cancer 26:680–685, 1970
14. Rosato F, Boova R: Nipple discharge and Paget's disease, Chap 16. In Strombeck J, Rosato F (eds): Surgery of the Breast. New York, Georg Thieme Verlag, 1986
15. Lagios M, Westdahl P, Rose M, Concannon S: Paget's disease of the nipple—Alternative management in cases without or with minimal extent of underlying breast carcinoma. Cancer 54:545–551, 1984
16. Messerschmidt W, Rosato F: Male breast carcinoma, Chap 30. In Strombeck J, Rosato F (eds): Surgery of the Breast. New York, Georg Thieme Verlag, 1986

17 Abdomen

LAYTON F. RIKKERS AND JON S. THOMPSON

The emergency or outpatient physician is seldom called on to provide definitive treatment for intra-abdominal disorders. However, his skill in early diagnosis and initiation of therapy, especially of emergent conditions, may make the difference between eventual success and failure. This chapter deals with diagnosis and management of abdominal pain, gastrointestinal bleeding, and abdominal wall hernias. Emphasis will be placed on those aspects of the work-up and therapy that are frequently performed or initiated in the emergency room or physician's office.

ABDOMINAL PAIN

Abdominal pain is a completely subjective complaint that may herald the presence of a wide spectrum of intra-abdominal disease—from lesions that cause death within minutes if left untreated to benign functional disturbances secondary to overeating. The sudden appearance of abdominal symptoms in a previously asymptomatic individual has been referred to as "acute abdomen," a term that implies that a surgical disease is usually, but not always, present. Diagnosis is frequently difficult because few of the diseases that present as so-called acute abdomen have pathognomonic physical or laboratory findings. It is a major challenge, therefore, to the outpatient physician, utilizing the history, physical examination, and appropriate laboratory and roentgenographic studies, to determine in any individual with abdominal pain if (1) hospitalization is required, (2) operative therapy is necessary, and (3) *immediate* surgery is required to salvage life. There are few abdominal conditions in which delay of diagnosis and treatment by minutes or hours will compromise eventual outcome, but these entities should always be considered, if only briefly.

The essentials to diagnosis of abdominal pain are the history, physical examination, and laboratory and radiologic evaluations. Space does not allow a comprehensive consideration of all these factors, so certain aspects, which we feel are particularly valuable in differential diagnosis of acute abdominal conditions, are emphasized. Finally, three conditions that require urgent diagnosis and surgical therapy and four common causes of the acute abdominal state are discussed.

HISTORY

Possibly the most significant information gained from the history is the character and mode of onset of abdominal pain:

- Rapid and severe
  - Mesenteric thrombosis
  - Perforated viscus
  - Common duct stone
  - Ureteral stone
  - Myocardial infarction
- Gradual and steady
  - Appendicitis
  - Acute cholecystitis
  - Diverticulitis
- Intermittent and colicky
  - Mechanical bowel obstruction

Severe pain that develops suddenly is usually indicative of surgical lesions, such as mesenteric thrombosis or visceral perforation. However, medical illnesses, such as myocardial infarction and pulmonary embolism, may present in a similar way, and surgery is obviously contraindicated in these situations. It takes an astute clinician to differentiate among these entities. Abdominal pain that develops over several hours and is constant usually reflects an underlying inflammatory process such as appendicitis or diverticulitis, whereas intermittent, crampy pain is suggestive of small-bowel obstruction. Vomiting occurs in most patients with significant abdominal pain. If pain precedes vomiting the underlying disease will most likely require surgery. If vomiting occurs prior to the onset of abdominal pain, the patient probably has a medical disorder such as gastroenteritis.

PHYSICAL EXAMINATION

A major objective of the physical examination is to determine if the patient with abdominal pain has peritonitis, as most lesions resulting in peritoneal inflammation require surgical management. However, it must be remembered that some disorders that necessitate urgent surgery—for example, mesenteric ischemia and ruptured aneurysm—do not initially present with evidence of peritonitis. Generalized peritonitis, as that resulting from a perforated duodenal ulcer, is usually easy to diagnose. The patient appears acutely ill and lies still because any movement results in pain. The abdomen is rigid, sometimes boardlike, and bowel sounds are absent. Localized peritonitis, signaling underlying appendicitis, acute cholecystitis, or diverticulitis, is often subtle in presentation. The patient may report localized abdominal pain aggravated by sudden movements, such as those during a bumpy ride to the hospital. This pain may be elicited by the examining physician if the patient is asked to cough or to drop suddenly to his heels after standing on his toes. Prior to these maneuvers the abdomen is carefully examined, beginning with gentle light percussion to localize the area of tenderness. Next, gentle palpation is used to determine if involuntary guarding, a very sensitive indicator of underlying peritoneal inflammation, is present. The test for rebound tenderness, which often startles even patients without significant abdominal disease, is seldom useful. The most significant finding resulting from this examination is a localized area of tenderness with involuntary spasm of overlying abdominal muscles. A cooperative patient can often *point* to this maximally tender spot. Such a finding is almost always indicative of the need for surgical therapy.

LABORATORY EVALUATION

In general, laboratory findings help confirm impressions gained from the history and physical examination but seldom make or exclude diagnoses on their own. Complete blood count and differential count, urinalysis, and serum amylase determination should be ordered on nearly all patients presenting with significant abdominal pain. If vomiting or diarrhea has been a prominent symptom, serum electrolyte and blood urea nitrogen values should also be obtained. The white blood cell count is usually increased in inflammatory disease of the abdomen, and the differential count generally reveals a shift to more immature forms. However, a normal count does not exclude any of the disorders that present as an acute abdominal condition. In borderline cases repeated white blood cell counts at the time of abdominal reexaminations may be helpful. A high hematocrit may reflect decreased plasma volume secondary to protracted vomiting or loss of fluid into a third space secondary to inflammation. White blood cells or bacteria in the urinary sediment are indicative of urinary tract sepsis, whereas red blood cells signify the presence of a ureteral stone or a renal infarct. Gram stain and culture of the urine are important because pyuria without bacteria may reflect an adjacent inflammatory process such as acute appendicitis. The serum amylase must be considered carefully. Acute pancreatitis may result in elevation of the serum amylase level, but so may a variety of other abdominal disorders, including intestinal perforation or infarction, acute cholecystitis, and ruptured ectopic pregnancy. Likewise in severe hemorrhagic pancreatitis with necrosis of the majority of pancreatic tissue, the serum amylase value may be normal or low.

Examination of peritoneal fluid for white blood cells, red blood cells, bacteria, and amylase may be helpful in elderly, obtunded, or chronically ill patients in whom it is impossible to perform a meaningful abdominal examination or in whom intra-abdominal inflammation may not result in typical signs and symptoms. Simple aspiration of the peritoneal cavity may yield a positive result, or peritoneal lavage, as described elsewhere in this text, may be utilized. More than 500 WBCs/mm^3 or 100,000 RBCs/mm^3 or bacteria on Gram stain constitute a positive lavage.

RADIOLOGIC EVALUATION

Assessment of posteroanterior and lateral films of the chest and flat plate, left lateral decubitus, and upright views of the abdomen is frequently helpful in evaluating acute abdominal pain. Chest roentgenograms are essential because several thoracic illnesses, including pneumonia, pulmonary embolus, and empyema, may initially present with abdominal pain. Likewise, certain infradiaphragmatic inflammatory processes, such as pancreatitis, may be associated with alterations on a chest roentgenogram. The left lateral decubitus abdomen and the upright, PA view of the chest are the best films for detection of free intraperitoneal air (Fig. 17-1).

Abdominal films must be inspected systematically to gain maximum information. First, the outlines of the solid organs and psoas muscle are identified. Obliteration of one psoas shadow in the appropriate clinical setting may suggest a retroperitoneal inflammatory process. Next the gas patterns of stomach, small bowel, and colon are examined. Distended loops of small bowel with air-fluid levels and the absence of colonic gas are suggestive of complete, mechanical small-bowel obstruction (Fig. 17-2). Dilated small and large bowel, often with air–fluid levels, is more indicative of ileus secondary to an abdominal inflammatory process. Presence of gas outside the intestinal lumen is always abnormal. Air in the biliary tree indicates either a communication between bile ducts and intestinal lumen, such as gallstone ileus, or infection of the biliary tract with gas-forming organisms. Air beneath the diaphragms or outlining the falciform ligament is suggestive of intestinal perforation, although there are several nonsurgical causes of intraperitoneal air (Fig. 17-1). A speckled gas pattern, similar to that seen with feces but not overlying colon, is suggestive of intra-abdominal abscess. Finally, the films are inspected for abnormal calcifications; 10% of gallstones and 90% of ureteral stones are radiopaque and may represent the cause of abdominal pain. Calcifications in a transverse pattern across the upper abdomen are indicative of chronic pancreatitis (Fig. 17-3). Abdominal aortic aneurysms and splenic aneurysms are frequently calcified and therefore visible on plain films of the abdomen.

Ultrasonic examination, especially of the upper abdomen, has been useful in evaluating

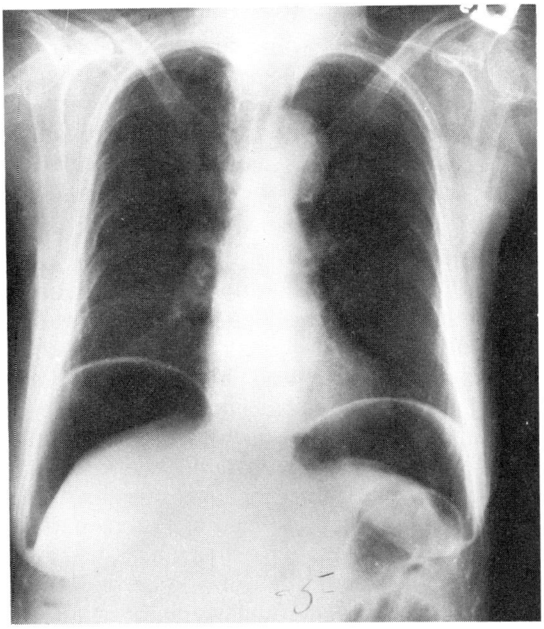

Figure 17-1. Free intraperitoneal air secondary to perforation of a duodenal ulcer.

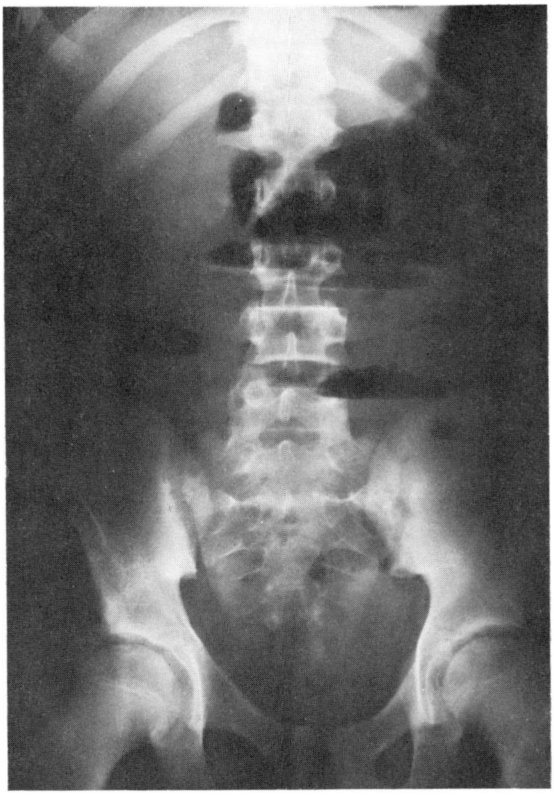

Figure 17-2. Mechanical small-bowel obstruction, rather then adynamic ileus, is indicated by air–fluid levels in the small bowel and a paucity of colonic gas in this upright abdominal film.

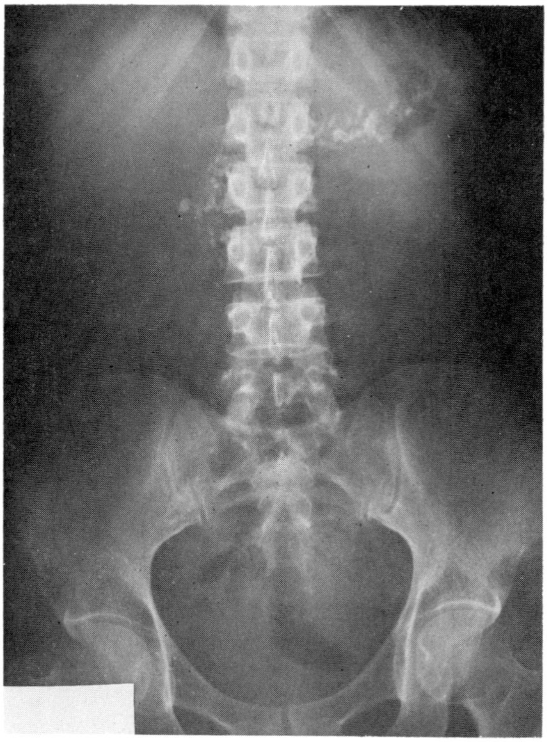

Figure 17-3. Pancreatic calcifications. Transversely situated calcifications across the upper adbomen are indicative of chronic pancreatitis.

patients with abdominal pain. Gallstones, biliary sludge, dilated intrahepatic and extrahepatic ducts, pancreatic pseudocyst, and abscesses can be reliably detected with this technique. Visceral angiography should be utilized when mesenteric ischemia is suspected or the site of intra-abdominal bleeding, such as ruptured adenoma of the liver or delayed rupture of the spleen, needs to be defined. In difficult cases a diatrizoate meglumine (Gastrografin) swallow may be required for diagnosis of lower esophageal (Boerhaave's syndrome), gastric, or duodenal perforation. Barium enema is likewise occasionally indicated to rule out colon obstruction or to make the diagnosis of acute appendicitis.

IMMEDIATE LIFE-THREATENING CAUSES OF ABDOMINAL PAIN

The following entities require prompt diagnosis and surgical therapy if patient salvage is to occur.

Massive Intra-abdominal Hemorrhage

Hemorrhage into the peritoneal cavity or into the retroperitoneum may result from spontaneous or delayed rupture of the spleen, spontaneous rupture of a hepatic neoplasm, rupture of an abdominal aortic aneurysm, ectopic pregnancy, or rupture of a visceral arterial aneurysm (abdominal apoplexy).

History. Free bleeding into the peritoneal cavity is usually associated with the acute onset of diffuse abdominal pain often rapidly followed by circulatory collapse. Hemorrhage into the retroperitoneum results in back pain, sometimes mimicking that commonly seen with degenerative disease of the spine. A pathologically enlarged spleen, as found in infectious mononucleosis, leukemia, and myelofibrosis, may rupture spontaneously or following minimal trauma. A subcapsular hematoma of the spleen may rupture into the peritoneal cavity at a time distant from the trauma causing the original splenic injury. Initial symptoms are usually left upper quadrant and left shoulder pain. Hepatic adenomas, which have increased in incidence since the introduction of oral contraceptives, cause right upper quadrant pain following rupture. Most abdominal aortic aneurysms are asymptomatic until they rupture, causing intense abdominal or low back pain. Abdominal apoplexy, though rare, is most frequently secondary to rupture of a splenic artery aneurysm. There is usually sudden, severe abdominal pain rapidly followed by circulatory collapse. Pelvic pain and symptoms of hypovolemia in a sexually active female with menstrual irregularity makes one suspicious of ectopic pregnancy.

Physical Examination. The most prominent findings on physical examination are abdominal tenderness and impending or overt circulatory collapse, manifested by pallor, cold sweat, tachycardia, and hypotension. This constellation of physical findings should lead the examiner immediately to diagnostic paracentesis, which will be productive of nonclotting blood if the hemorrhage is intraperitoneal. Shock may be absent if bleeding is retroperitoneal, as in aortic aneurysm, and therefore careful palpation of the aorta is an essential part of the physical examination in all patients with abdominal pain. It should be noted that peripheral pulses are often normal in patients with ruptured aortic aneurysm. In ectopic pregnancy pelvic examination often reveals uterine enlargement, an adnexal mass, and pain on cervical motion. Since pelvic inflammatory disease and ovarian cysts often present with similar findings, the correct diagnosis is frequently made by aspiration of nonclotting blood during culdocentesis.

Laboratory Findings. The hematocrit may be normal or decreased, depending on the time of onset and rapidity of hemorrhage. The pregnancy test utilizing human chorionic gonadotropin B subunit is positive in 90% of patients with ectopic pregnancy.

Radiologic Findings. In general, radiologic procedures are contraindicated. Immediate laparotomy is essential for maximal patient salvage.

Mesenteric Ischemia and Infarction

Mesenteric ischemia or infarction may result from arterial occlusion by thrombosis or embolus, venous thrombosis, or, most frequently, nonocclusive, intestinal low blood flow state.

History. Nonocclusive intestinal ischemia usually occurs in elderly patients, often with chronic congestive heart failure treated with digitalis, a potent splanchnic vasoconstrictor. Onset of symptoms is frequently precipitated by mild hypovolemia secondary to diuretic therapy or dehydration from diarrhea or vomiting. Mesenteric arterial thrombosis is generally confined to older patients with advanced atherosclerosis, whereas embolic disease occurs in individuals with atrial fibrillation or following myocardial infarction. Intestinal venous thrombosis may afflict individuals with a hypercoagulable state or have no apparent cause. The most constant symptom with all forms of intestinal ischemia is severe, diffuse abdominal pain, often unresponsive to even large doses of narcotics. A minority of patients, especially those in the older age groups, may present with mild nonspecific abdominal discomfort.

Physical Examination. The hallmark of intestinal ischemia is pain out of proportion to physical findings. In the early stages bowel sounds may be normal or even hyperactive, and tenderness to abdominal palpation is difficult to elicit. When infarction occurs the typical findings of peritonitis are present. Paracentesis is productive of peritoneal fluid, which is the color of port wine. Rectal examination may produce bloody stool secondary to mucosal hemorrhage.

Laboratory Findings. Loss of fluid into the peritoneal cavity or intestinal lumen may result in hemoconcentration. Leukocytosis is usually impressive. The serum electrolyte profile may reveal a decrease in bicarbonate secondary to metabolic acidosis. The intestinal isoenzymes of alkaline phosphatase, LDH, and CPK may be elevated when intestinal infarction occurs. Serum amylase and phosphate may also be increased.

Radiologic Findings. Plain abdominal films usually display nonspecific findings such as an ileus pattern and a thickened bowel wall. More specific findings, such as gas intramurally or in the portal venous radicles, occur late in the course of the disease. Visceral angiography should be performed promptly whenever mesenteric ischemia is suspected. Although the angiographic pattern in nonocclusive ischemia may be nondiagnostic, in occlusive disease the obstructed vessels and the alternatives for arterial reconstruction can be defined.

Perforated Duodenal or Gastric Ulcer

History. The major symptom of a perforated duodenal or gastric ulcer is sudden generalized abdominal pain. The patient can often give the exact minute or hour of pain onset. There may or may not be a history of intermittent epigastric pain in the past, indicating chronic peptic ulcer disease. Occasionally, the colon and omentum partially wall off an anterior perforation, directing the escaped luminal fluid into the right paracolic gutter and right lower quadrant. In this case the patient may present with both epigastric and right lower quadrant pain, and differentiation from appendicitis may be difficult or impossible.

Physical Examination. Introduction of acidic gastric contents into the peritoneal cavity results in a peritoneal burn and subsequent sequestration of fluid. Thus, depending on how long after perforation the patient is evaluated, signs of hypovolemia such as rapid pulse and decreased blood pressure may be present. The cardinal abdominal finding is generalized peritonitis evidenced by absence of bowel sounds and a rigid, boardlike abdomen. In a minority of patients free peritoneal air may be detected as tympany on percussion over the liver in the midaxillary line.

Laboratory Findings. If third spacing has occurred, the hematocrit may be increased secondary to hemoconcentration. The white blood cell count and serum amylase may be increased.

Radiologic Findings. The most specific x-ray finding is free air beneath one or both diaphragms on upright chest or abdominal films (see Fig. 17-1). The left lateral decubitus abdomen and posteroanterior chest films are the most sensitive ones for detection of free air, and the x-ray technician should be instructed to position the patient upright for at least 5 minutes prior to taking the films, so that the intraperitoneal air has time to collect beneath the diaphragms or the right abdominal wall. The left lateral decubitus film of the abdomen should be obtained in patients too ill to maintain an upright posture. Despite these considerations free air cannot be detected in 25% of patients. In these individuals an upper gastrointestinal series with a water-soluble contrast agent such as diatrizoate meglumine (Gastrografin) may reveal the site of perforation.

COMMON CAUSES OF ACUTE ABDOMINAL STATE

The following entities frequently occur as causes of the acute abdominal state. Although prompt diagnosis and treatment are not as essential as in those diseases discussed previously, undue delay in diagnosis may result in increased morbidity and even mortality.

Acute Appendicitis

Because of the variable anatomic locations of the appendix, inflammation of this organ can simulate most other causes of the acute abdominal state.

History. In classic right lower quadrant appendicitis the onset usually consists of vague, periumbilical discomfort and nausea, sometimes followed by emesis. A variable time later the pain shifts to the right lower quadrant. In retrocecal and pelvic appendicitis progression of symptoms may be similar, but the pain is less well localized, tending toward the right upper quadrant in the former and the lower midline in the latter.

Physical Examination. The most characteristic and diagnostic physical finding in acute appendicitis is localized tenderness. If asked to cough the patient can usually place his finger on a single painful area. Likewise, a careful examiner can locate the same point by one-finger palpation or gentle percussion of the abdomen. Localized tenderness is so characteristic in appendicitis that its absence often argues against the diagnosis. Exceptions, however, are retrocecal and pelvic appendicitis, which may have unimpressive anterior abdominal finding. Rather, maximal tenderness can be elicited by rectal examination (pelvic appendicitis) or stretching the right psoas muscle by extending the upper leg (retrocecal appendicitis).

Laboratory Findings. In more than 90% of patients the white blood cell count exceeds 10,000, usually with a shift to the left. An inflamed retrocecal or pelvic appendix overlying the right ureter may cause sterile pyuria.

Radiologic Findings. Most frequently a flat plate of the abdomen is normal, but it may occasionally show a calcified fecalith, obliteration of the right psoas margin, indentation of a gas-filled cecum, or localized ileus. Patients who are particularly difficult to examine, such as young children, may benefit from a carefully performed barium enema examination. Positive findings include lack of appendiceal filling, partial filling, and a cecal impression.

Acute Cholecystitis

Acute cholecystitis results from obstruction of the cystic duct by a gallstone in over 98% of cases. Cystic duct obstruction then leads to a sequence of events, initially chemical inflammation of the gallbladder wall, usually followed in 24 to 48 hours by bacterial invasion, that produce signs and symptoms of right upper quadrant peritonitis.

History. The typical symptom is the rather sudden onset of right upper quadrant pain with radiation to the scapula following a meal. The pain is usually severe and constant and frequently accompanied by nausea and vomiting.

The majority of patients have had previous, intermittent symptoms of biliary colic.

Physical Examination. The temperature is usually mildly elevated to 38°C to 39°C, and evidence of toxicity, such as a rapid pulse, may be present. In contrast to other biliary diseases such as chronic cholecystitis and choledocholithiasis, localized peritonitis can be detected in the right upper quadrant over the typical position of the gallbladder. Voluntary and involuntary guarding, as well as inability to take a deep breath during palpation beneath the right costal margin (Murphy's sign), is usually present. In 25% to 50% of patients a tender, enlarged gallbladder can be palpated. Signs of chronic liver disease, such as spider angiomas, liver palms, and gynecomastia, should be looked for because patients with alcoholic hepatitis, who frequently also have gallstones, may present with similar physical findings. Mild scleral icterus may be detected in a small proportion of patients with acute cholecystitis.

Laboratory Findings. Moderate leukocytosis (10,000/mm^3 to 15,000/mm^3) is a frequent finding. Serum bilirubin, alkaline phosphatase, and the hepatocellular enzymes SGOT and SGPT are often mildly increased. Before a decision is made for surgery, liver enzymes should be measured in all patients with right upper quadrant pain to exclude the possibility of acute hepatitis.

Radiologic Findings. Approximately 10% of gallstones are radiopaque and can be seen on plain films of the abdomen. The most valuable diagnostic aid is ultrasonic examination of the right upper quadrant. If gallstones are detected in an individual with typical symptoms, physical signs, and laboratory findings of acute cholecystitis, no additional radiologic examinations are necessary. This technique can also exclude other pathologic processes, such as liver abscess and diverticular abscess of the transverse colon, which can mimic acute cholecystitis. If signs and symptoms are confusing and demonstration of cystic duct obstruction is necessary to confirm the diagnosis, a ^{99m}Tc-HIDA scan should be obtained. If this isotope appears in the common bile duct but not in the gallbladder within 1 hour of intravenous injection, the study is diagnostic of cystic duct obstruction.

Acute Pancreatitis

The term *acute pancreatitis* is somewhat misleading, as it covers a wide spectrum of pathologic processes from very lethal hemorrhagic pancreatitis to benign acute exacerbations of chronic pancreatitis. Although there are exceptions, acute pancreatitis is generally not a surgical disease. However, its clinical manifestations may closely mimic other abdominal conditions that require surgical management. If these other diseases cannot be ruled out in an individual patient, exploratory laparotomy is mandatory.

History. The patient usually complains of the abrupt onset of fairly severe, constant epigastric pain following eating. Radiation of the pain straight through to the back and nausea and emesis are prominent associated symptoms. The patient may relate a history of alcoholism or of biliary colic.

Physical Examination. In hemorrhagic pancreatitis or in advanced edematous pancreatitis the patient may present with signs of shock secondary to hypovolemia resulting from the retroperitoneal burn. In such cases abdominal examination reveals diffuse epigastric tenderness with evidence of peritonitis and absence of bowel sounds. In milder forms, however, physical findings may be subtle because inflammation is confined to the retroperitoneum. Careful percussion or palpation over the left flank may elicit tenderness, as may deep palpation in the epigastrium and left upper quadrant.

Laboratory Findings. The hematocrit may be either increased because of third-spacing of fluid or decreased because of retroperitoneal hemorrhage. The latter finding is a grave prognostic sign. The white blood cell count is usually normal or mildly increased. Serum amylase is increased in 90% of cases, but its magnitude does not correlate with severity of the disease. As discussed previously, serum amylase can also be increased in several other acute abdominal disorders and therefore is not diagnostic unless markedly increased (>1500 units/100 ml). Elevation of both serum lipase and amylase suggests that acute pancreatitis is present. Serum calcium may be depressed and generally correlates with the severity of the pancreatitis. Liver function tests may reflect cholestasis with an elevated bilirubin and alkaline phosphatase levels. Arterial blood gases may show hypoxemia.

Radiologic Findings. Patients with acute exacerbations of pancreatitis on a background of chronic, alcoholic pancreatitis frequently have pancreatic calcifications on plain films of the abdomen. More common findings in acute pancreatitis are an isolated loop of gas-filled jejunum (sentinel loop) in the left upper quadrant and sudden transition in the transverse colon of a distended right colon to an airless left colon (colon cutoff sign). Ultrasound generally reveals an enlarged, edematous pancreas. This examination is particularly valuable in detecting complications of acute pancreatitis such as pancreatic pseudocyst and pancreatic abscess. Severely ill patients with suspected pancreatitis should undergo abdominal CT scan so that a pancreatic abscess can be detected early in its course.

Intestinal Obstruction

Mechanical intestinal obstruction results most frequently from an extrinsic lesion, that is, adhesive band. Ileus refers to failure of intestinal transit because of disordered propulsive activity of the bowel. This is an important distinction, since the latter may be a harbinger of a more serious intra-abdominal condition. Simple mechanical obstruction may progress to strangulation obstruction if the mesenteric vessels become occluded. When both afferent and efferent ends of an intestinal segment are obstructed (i.e., close-loop obstruction), there is a greater propensity for strangulation to occur.

History. Simple mechanical obstruction presents as abdominal pain, vomiting, and failure to pass gas or stool per rectum. Initially, there is a poorly localized cramping, peristaltic pain with intervening quiescent periods. The period between painful attacks is shorter with high intestinal obstruction. When simple obstruction is not relieved and progresses to strangulation, there is more constant, generalized dull pain. Vomiting of feculent material occurs shortly after obstruction develops and is more severe with high obstruction. Failure to pass gas or stool per rectum occurs with complete obstruction, whereas gas and diarrhea may pass with partial obstruction. Gas and feces distal to the obstruction may pass within a few hours after obstruction occurs.

Physical Examination. Vital signs are initially unremarkable. Abdominal distension results from long-standing obstruction involving the distal small intestine. Guarding and abdominal tenderness occur during attacks of pain. Auscultation reveals loud, high-pitched bowel sounds occurring in bursts and rushes during attacks of colic. Bowel sounds are infrequent with adynamic ileus. When obstruction persists and progresses to strangulation, abdominal distention and dehydration occur, rebound tenderness develops and the abdomen becomes silent. Fever and tachycardia precede shock, which is the eventual outcome if the obstruction is not treated.

Laboratory Findings. Extracellular fluid losses result in dehydration with an initial increased hematocrit, BUN, and urine specific gravity. Either metabolic alkalosis or acidosis may occur, depending on the level of obstruction and presence or absence of strangulation. The white blood cell count is mildly elevated in simple obstruction, whereas strangulation obstruction is associated with more marked leukocytosis ($>15{,}000/mm^3$) and a shift to the left. Serum amylase levels may be elevated with intestinal obstruction.

Radiologic Findings. Abdominal x-rays reveal air–fluid levels in a ladder pattern (Fig. 17-2). There is a paucity of air in the colon unless the obstruction is partial. Air–fluid levels also occur with ileus, but air is diffusely present throughout the large and small intestine. A persistently dilated single loop of intestine may occur with strangulation. Instillation of contrast material above the obstruction may help differentiate between mechanical obstruction and ileus. Contrast materal is rapidly diluted, which makes visualization difficult with distal obstruction.

Gastrointestinal Bleeding

Gastrointestinal bleeding may manifest itself in many ways, from occult blood detected in the stools by chemical means to massive, exsanguinating hemorrhage. This discussion emphasizes diagnosis and early management of patients with acute blood loss from the gastrointestinal tract. The approach to these patients has been fairly well standardized and consists of four steps: (1) resuscitation (repletion of intravascular volume), (2) identification of the level of bleeding, (3) visualization of the bleeding lesion, and (4) control of hemorrhage. The task of the physician who first comes in contact with the patient is to ensure that the work-up proceeds in an orderly fashion. This can best be accomplished by enlisting and coordinating a team of physicians that includes a gastroenterologist, surgeon, and radiologist soon after the patient arrives in the emergency department.

Resuscitation. It is essential that all diagnostic procedures be deferred until intravascular volume has been restored and vital signs are stable. Early emphasis on diagnosis may result in cardiac arrest during endoscopy or in the radiology department. If the systolic blood pressure is less than 100 or the pulse is greater than 100, the patient has probably lost 20% or more of his blood volume. Even if vital signs are stable but blood pressure decreases on assumption of the erect position (orthostatic hypotension), major acute blood loss has occurred. In such patients the initial step in management is insertion of two large-bore intravenous lines (preferably 16 gauge) into the upper extremities. After obtaining blood for a complete blood count, typing and cross matching and coagulation studies, infusion of an isotonic salt solution at a wide open rate is begun and continued until vital signs are restored. A useful method of assessing adequacy of cardiac output is hourly monitoring of urinary output with a Foley catheter.

General Diagnostic Measures. HISTORY. A carefully obtained history can be helpful in determining approximate volume of blood lost, general level of bleeding, and etiology. If syncope followed the bleeding episode, it can be assumed that more than 20% of blood volume was lost. Rarely an observant patient or family member can estimate the quantity of bloody vomitus or stool passed. Hematemesis generally localizes the bleeding lesion above the ligament of Treitz. Likewise, melena usually indicates that the source of hemorrhage is proximal to the ileocecal valve. Unfortunately, there are occasional exceptions to both of these generalizations (e.g., small-bowel obstruction causing hematemesis with a distal lesion and colonic stasis resulting in melena from a right-colon bleeding site). In addition, massive upper gastrointestinal hemorrhage from duodenal ulcer may present as bright red rectal bleeding and not result in hematemesis. If emesis precedes gastrointestinal bleeding, a Mallory–Weiss tear at the gastroesophageal junction is suggested. However, in some series less than 50% of patients with this lesion give such a history. A history of chronic or recent-onset abdominal pain suggests a mucosal inflammatory lesion such as duodenal or gastric ulcer, esophagitis, or gastritis. Individuals with esophageal varices, diverticulosis, or arteriovenous malformation as the bleeding source usually have no antecedent abdominal pain. A history of ulcerogenic drug use or alcohol abuse may also be helpful in establishing the etiology of gastrointestinal hemorrhage.

PHYSICAL EXAMINATION. A careful examination of the skin may give clues to the etiology of gastrointestinal bleeding. The presence of spider angiomas, erythema over the thenar and hypothenar eminences (liver palms), and distended veins over the abdomen suggest chronic liver disease and portal hypertension. Multiple pigmented areas over the lips may be associated with intestinal polyposis (Peutz–Jegher syndrome), which sometimes leads to bleeding. Small hemangiomas of the lips and oral cavity may be associated with similar potential bleeding lesions throughout the gastrointestinal tract (Osler–Weber–Rendu disease). In a patient with suspected portal hypertension abdominal examination may reveal splenomegaly, ascites, or hepatomegaly alone or in combination. Rectal examination should be performed to detect rectal carcinoma or hemorrhoids, both of which may cause lower gastrointestinal hemorrhage.

Specific Diagnostic Techniques (Fig. 17-4). NASOGASTRIC TUBE. Nasogastric intubation should be the first diagnostic technique performed in patients who are suspected to be actively bleeding from the gastrointestinal tract. The presence of fresh or old blood in the stomach indicates that the bleeding lesion is probably proximal to the ligament of Treitz. A guaiac-negative gastric aspirate suggests a more distal site of bleeding, but occasionally even a massively bleeding duodenal ulcer will fail to reflux blood into the stomach.

UPPER GASTROINTESTINAL ENDOSCOPY. Endoscopy is the key means for visualization of bleeding lesions in the esophagus, stomach, and duodenum. This technique is successful in

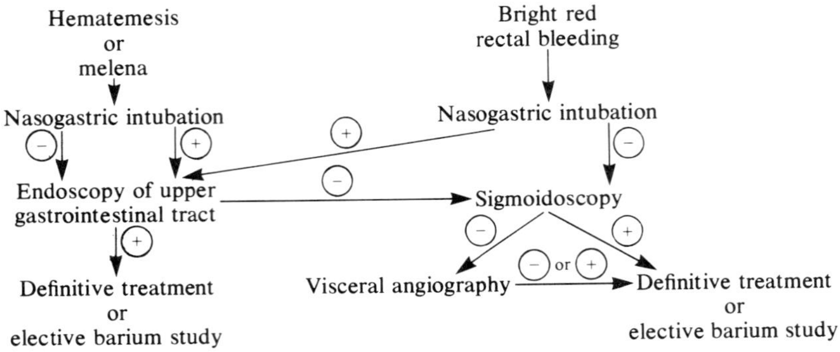

Figure 17-4. Diagnosis of acute gastrointestinal hemorrhage.

diagnosing the site of bleeding in 75% to 95% of cases as compared with a 25% to 50% success rate with barium sites. Even if upper-gastrointestinal disease is known to be present, endoscopy is essential to determine if the previously diagnosed lesion or some other unexpected condition is responsible for the present bleeding episode. For example, in individuals with known esophageal varices who have acute bleeding episodes, the varices are the confirmed site of bleeding only 50% of the time.

Prior to performance of endoscopy, a large-bore tube such as an Ewald tube is inserted to evacuate clots from the stomach. As previously mentioned, it is essential to establish hemodynamic stability before any diagnostic procedures are carried out. Although the actual bleeding lesion is usually identified, occasionally the diagnosis is made by exclusion. For example, if the patient is not actively bleeding at the time of endoscopy but a proximal site is suspected because of old blood in the stomach or prior hematemesis, the presence of a duodenal ulcer and the absence of other lesions indicates that the ulcer was most likely the source of hemorrhage.

In recent years several therapeutic techniques have been adapted for use through the endoscope. In certain centers a variety of bleeding lesions have been temporarily or permanently controlled with electrocautery, lasers, heater probes, and injection of sclerosants. As these methods become more refined they may eliminate the need for emergency surgery in these high-risk patients.

LOWER GASTROINTESTINAL ENDOSCOPY. Sigmoidoscopy should be performed in all patients with bright red rectal bleeding. Although this examination usually reveals that the blood is coming from a lesion proximal to 25 cm, occasionally the bleeding site is identified in the rectum or rectosigmoid colon. Because of the difficulty of visualization in a colon filled with blood, colonoscopy has not been established as a useful diagnostic procedure in acute lower gastrointestinal hemorrhage, but it can be quite valuable in the evaluation of intermittent or chronic bleeding.

RADIONUCLIDE SCANS. Radionuclide imaging has emerged as an accurate, minimally invasive method of detecting gastrointestinal bleeding. Both ^{99m}Tc sulfur colloid and ^{99m}Tc-labeled erythrocytes have been used. Although accuracy and sensitivity are similar to those of visceral angiography, the bleeding site cannot be localized as well. ^{99m}Tc-labeled erythrocytes can be detected for up to 24 hours, which is an advantage in the identification of an intermittent source of bleeding. Radionuclide imaging should be performed prior to angiography, since angiography is likely to be unrevealing if no bleeding is identified by nuclear scans.

ANGIOGRAPHY. Visceral angiography is an effective means of diagnosing the site of bleeding when the rate of blood loss exceeds 0.6 ml/min. Because endoscopy and barium studies are so ineffective, angiography is the primary diagnostic technique for establishing the site of bleeding in the lower gastrointestinal tract. The main limitation of this method is the around-the-clock availability of a well-trained angiographic team. It is important to defer barium studies until angiography is performed because barium may obscure extravasation of the vascular contrast agent into the intestinal lumen. Angiography is occasionally useful in patients with upper gastrointestinal hemorrhage, especially when a rapid rate of bleeding makes endoscopic interpretation difficult. However, variceal hemorrhage can rarely be localized by angiography.

Visceral angiography also has a therapeutic potential. Infusion of vasoconstrictors such as vasopressin into the artery supplying a bleeding lesion has been very effective in arresting hemorrhage. This technique has been especially useful in high-risk patients with lesions, such as hemorrhagic gastritis, that are not very amenable to surgical therapy. Transcatheter embolization can also be employed to decrease blood flow to a site of gastrointestinal bleeding.

BARIUM CONTRAST STUDIES. Although the upper gastrointestinal series and barium enema studies were primary diagnostic techniques for gastrointestinal hemorrhage in the recent past, these methods now play only a secondary role. In fact, injudicious use of barium studies may prevent subsequent utilization of more effective methods such as angiography and endoscopy. However, barium studies may be useful after stabilization of the patient and performance of endoscopy or angiography or both to delineate more fully the extent of the pathologic process or possibly to detect lesions not seen with the initial diagnostic procedures.

Abdominal Wall Hernia

An abdominal wall hernia can be defined as the protrusion of properitoneal fat or intraperitoneal contents through a defect or weakness in the fascia investing the abdominal cavity. The fascial defect may be either congenital (indirect inguinal hernia) or acquired (incisional hernia). Chronically elevated intra-abdominal pressure as from straining at stool, urinary obstruction, or ascites may lead to fascial attenuation and subsequent herniation or aggravate a preexisting hernia.

The most common site of hernia formation is the groin. Of all abdominal wall hernias, indirect inguinal hernias comprise 50%; direct inguinal hernias, 25%; and femoral hernias, 5%. Other frequent sites of herniation are operative incisions, the umbilicus, and the linea alba between the xiphoid and umbilicus (epigastric hernias).

A hernia is reducible if its contents can be replaced within the peritoneal cavity. Incarceration refers to a trapping of the herniated structures by the fascial defect, preventing their easy reduction without operative intervention. A strangulated hernia is one in which entrapment by the fascial ring is so tight that blood supply to the contents of the sac is compromised. Emergency surgery of strangulated hernias is necessary to prevent ischemic necrosis. Because it is often difficult to clinically differentiate incarceration alone from incarceration with strangulation, incarcerated hernias generally should not be reduced except under direct vision during an emergency operation. This principle prevents the reduction of gangrenous structures into the peritoneal cavity. Small fascial defects with firm edges, as often present in femoral, umbilical, and indirect inguinal hernias, frequently lead to incarceration and strangulation. Diffuse areas of fascial weakness such as most direct inguinal and incisional hernias rarely cause incarceration. If the incarcerated contents include small intestine, signs and symptoms of small bowel obstruction frequently, but not always, develop. In fact, after postoperative adhesions, hernia is the second most common cause of small bowel obstruction. Therefore it is essential to examine all potential sites of herniation in persons who present with obstruction of the small intestine. It is this complication that results in the morbidity and occasional mortality secondary to hernias and that makes the elective repair of incarceration-prone hernias mandatory.

Umbilical Hernia. An umbilical hernia represents a true congenital fascial defect and is common in infants, especially among blacks. Most umbilical hernias close spontaneously, and operative repair is not indicated during the first 2 years of life unless complications supervene. In contrast, an umbilical hernia in the adult is prone to incarceration and strangulation and should be repaired when diagnosed. Local anesthesia may be utilized for small, uncomplicated umbilical hernias, but general or spinal anesthesia is advisable for all others.

Epigastric Hernia. Epigastric hernias protrude through the linea alba above the umbilicus and are frequently multiple. They generally become symptomatic when they incarcerate properitoneal fat or omentum. Because these hernias almost never entrap small or large bowel, repair is indicated only to relieve symptoms. Single defects can easily be repaired under local anesthesia, whereas general anesthesia is indicated for multiple hernias.

Incisional Hernia. Incisional hernias develop because of inadequate wound healing. Common etiologic factors, frequently present in combination, are malnutrition, obesity, postoperative wound infection, improper wound-closure technique, midline incisions, and postoperative pulmonary complications. These hernias are often large and sometimes require synthetic mesh for successful repair. Incisional hernias are an inpatient problem and should always be repaired under general anesthesia.

Indirect Inguinal Hernia. An indirect inguinal hernia passes through the internal inguinal ring into a congenitally patent processus vaginalis peritonei within the spermatic cord. These hernias are common early in life, and virtually all groin hernias in infants are of the indirect inguinal variety. Indirect inguinal hernias frequently do not become clinically apparent until later in life, when chronically elevated intra-abdominal pressure may force abdominal contents through a dilated internal inguinal ring into a patent peritoneal sac that has been present since birth. Except in the elderly, the indirect inguinal hernia is the most common type of groin hernia in all age groups and in both sexes. Inguinal hernias are often asymptomatic and first discovered on routine physical examination, although it is not unusual for them to produce chronic pain in the groin. Rarely, the first evidence of a groin hernia is the onset of symptoms and signs of small bowel obstruction.

Physical examination for inguinal hernia consists of careful observation and palpation of the groin area while the patient voluntarily increases intra-abdominal pressure. A bulge can usually be seen with moderate and large hernias. Smaller hernias can be detected by invaginating the scrotum and inserting the examining finger through the external inguinal ring into the inguinal canal. As the patient "bears down," a palpable bulge becomes evident. It is very difficult to differentiate indirect from direct inguinal hernias on physical examination with the single exception that large indirect hernias are often present in the scrotum because they travel with the cord contents. Preoperative distinction is not essential, however, because the initial operative approach to both direct and indirect inguinal hernias is the same, and precise diagnosis can be made intraoperatively.

Direct Inguinal Hernia. A direct inguinal hernia protrudes through a weakness in the floor of the inguinal canal medial to the epigastric vessels. The transversalis fascia, the most important component giving strength to the inguinal canal floor, may become attenuated, especially in older men, and allow diffuse herniation to develop. Therefore these hernias seldom incarcerate or strangulate. An important exception is a direct inguinal hernia of the funicular type that passes through a small, well-circumscribed fascial defect. Detection of direct inguinal hernias by physical examination is the same as that for indirect hernias. Because direct hernias are separate from the spermatic cord, they infrequently pass into the scrotum.

Femoral Hernia. Femoral hernias pass through the femoral canal beneath the inguinal ligament and medial to the femoral vein. It is the least common variety of groin hernia and is much more common in women than in men. Because of its relative rarity, femoral hernias still comprise only one third of groin hernias in women, the remainder being mostly indirect inguinal hernias. Femoral hernias usually protrude inferior to a line between anterior inferior iliac spine and pubic tubercle (inguinal ligament). Unfortunately, some femoral hernias dissect subcutaneously to a position superior to the inguinal ligament and are difficult to differentiate from other groin hernias. The fascial defect producing these hernias is usually very narrow and therefore femoral hernias are frequently not discovered until incarceration or strangulation has developed.

Repair of Groin Hernias Under Local Anesthesia. Most inguinal hernias can be safely and effectively repaired under local anesthesia during an outpatient visit or a brief hospitalization. The major advantages of this technique are safer anesthesia for most patients and an economic savings of up to 80%. Nearly all uncomplicated indirect and direct inguinal hernias in adults can be repaired utilizing local anesthesia. Surgery for recurrent hernias, incarcerated or strangulated hernias, and hernias in infants and children and in uncooperative adults is probably better performed under general or spinal anesthesia.

TECHNIQUE. If outpatient surgery is to be done, a complete evaluation including history, physical examination, and appropriate laboratory tests is performed in the physician's office or in the clinic preoperatively. The patient is asked to report to the outpatient surgery area with an empty stomach approximately an hour and a half prior to the anticipated procedure. Intravenous fluids are started and premedication, consisting of 50 mg meperidine, 25 mg hydroxyzine hydrochloride, and 0.5 mg atropine sulfate is administered intramuscularly. The patient is taken to the operating suite and electrocardiographic monitoring is begun while the groin area is shaved, prepared, and draped in the usual manner. If the patient becomes restless during the procedure, small intravenous doses of diazepam are used to supplement the premedications.

We prefer the local anesthesia technique described by Chang and Farha (Figs. 17-5 and 17-6). The local anesthetic used is a solution of 50 ml of 0.5% lidocaine and 50 ml of 0.25% bupivacaine. Because it might contribute to postoperative bleeding, epinephrine is omitted from the local anesthetic solution. Using a 25-gauge spinal needle, the proposed line of skin incision and underlying subcutaneous tissue is infiltrated. The ilioinguinal nerve is blocked by injecting 1 ml to 2 ml of anesthetic beneath the

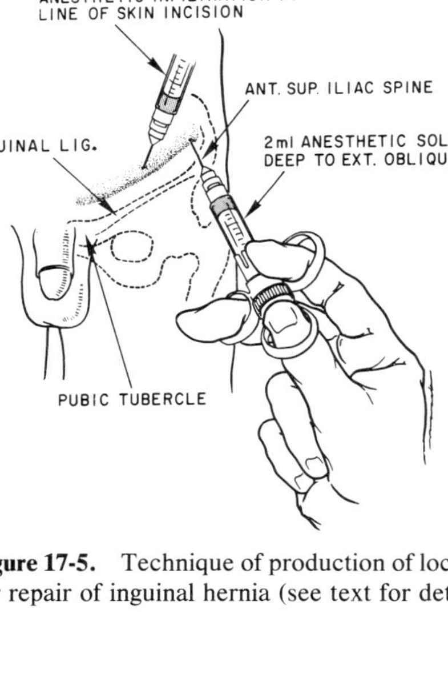

Figure 17-5. Technique of production of local anesthesia for repair of inguinal hernia (see text for details).

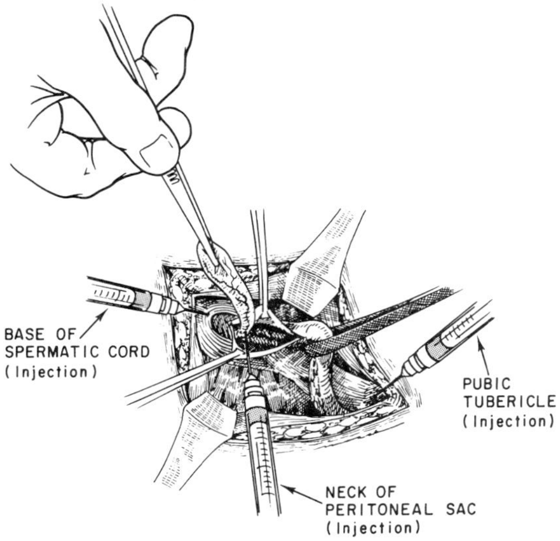

Figure 17-6. Technique of production of local anesthesia for repair of inguinal hernia (see text for description).

external oblique aponeurosis approximately 2 cm medial to the anterior inferior iliac spine at the lateral limit of the skin incision. After the incision is made down to the external oblique aponeurosis, this fascial layer is infiltrated under direct vision and opened, exposing the inguinal canal and its contents. Prior to mobilizing the spermatic cord, the pubic tubercle, the inguinal ligament, and the base of the spermatic cord are injected with anesthetic solution.

The spermatic cord is mobilized at the pubic tubercle and dissected back to the internal ring. At this point the patient is asked to bear down to determine the area or areas of herniation. The spermatic cord is then explored at its anteromedial aspect in search of a peritoneal sac. If an indirect hernia is found, the sac is dissected from surrounding cord structures and infiltrated at its exit from the internal ring prior to ligating it. If the peritoneal sac is small and the internal ring competent, high ligation of the sac is sufficient. If the internal ring is patulous, it is tightened to admit the tip of a finger by suturing the transversalis fascia superior to the inguinal ligament inferiorly by the method of Bassini.

If a direct hernia is discovered the inguinal canal floor is incised from internal ring to pubic tubercle. A Cooper's ligament repair, as described by McVay, is then performed by suturing transversalis fascia superiorly to Cooper's ligament inferiorly. It is not necessary to infiltrate Cooper's ligament with anesthetic solution. The lateral part of the repair is completed by apposing transversalis fascia to inguinal ligament over the femoral vessels. For all repairs utilizing Cooper's ligament, a relaxing incision should be made in the fascia overlying the rectus muscle after infiltration with anesthetic solution.

After completion of the hernia repair the patient is again asked to bear down. In this way the adequacy and strength of repair can be observed. The external oblique aponeurosis, Scarpa's fascia, and skin are then closed in sequence to complete the operation.

BIBLIOGRAPHY

Acute Abdomen

Botsford TW, Wilson RE: The Acute Abdomen, 2nd ed. Philadelphia, WB Saunders, 1977

Cope Z: The Early Diagnosis of the Acute Abdomen, 16th ed. London, Oxford University Press, 1983

Dunn JT, Halls JM, Berne TV: Roentgenographic contrast studies in acute small bowel obstruction. Arch Surg 119:1305–1308, 1984

Roh JJ, Thompson JS, Harned RK, Hodgson PE: Value of pneumoperitoneum in the diagnosis of visceral perforation. Am J Surg 146:830–833, 1983

Sarr MG, Bulkley GB, Zuidema GD: Preoperative recognition of intestinal strangulation obstruction. Am J Surg 145:176–182, 1983

Gastrointestinal Bleeding

Dent T: Evaluation of the bleeding patient. Surg Gynecol Obstet 151:817–820, 1980

Fleischer D: Endoscopic therapy of upper gastrointestinal bleeding in humans. Gastroenterology 90:217–234, 1986

Himal HS, Perrault MD, Mizabi R: Upper gastrointestinal hemorrhage: Aggressive management decreases mortality. Surgery 84:448–454, 1978

Hussey KP: Vasopressin therapy for upper gastrointestinal tract hemorrhage: Has its efficacy been proven? Arch Intern Med 145:1263–1267, 1985

McKusick KA, Froelich J, Callahan RJ et al: $^{99}T_c$ red blood cells for detection of gastrointestinal bleeding: Experience with 80 patients. AJR 137:1113–1118, 1981

Rahn NH, Tishler JM, Hau SY, Russinovich NAE: Diagnostic and interventional angiography in acute gastrointestinal hemorrhage. Radiology 143:361–366, 1982

Abdominal Wall Hernias

Bowen JB, Thompson WR, Dorman BA et al: Change in the management of adult groin hernia. Am J Surg 135:564, 1978

Chang FC, Farha GJ: Inguinal herniorrhaphy under local anesthesia. Arch Surg 112:1069, 1977

Flanagan L, Bascom JU: Repair of the groin hernia—outpatient approach with local anesthesia. Surg Clin North Am 64:257–267, 1984

18 Endoscopic Approach to Diagnosis and Surgery of the Colon

KENNETH N. BUCHI AND JOHN A. DIXON

The works of Hippocrates contain the first known reports of attempts to visualize the rectum by means of a speculum.[1] The roots of modern proctocolonoscopy, however, date back only about two centuries. Bozzini first utilized an anorectoscope with a candle light source in 1795.[2] Desornaux utilized a similar instrument with an alcohol lamp as the light source in the mid-1800s.[3] Following the turn of the century, rigid proctoscopes utilizing incandescent bulbs as light sources were developed by Tuttle[4] and Kelly.[5] Although these advances made the examination much more effective, and undoubtedly much more reassuring to the patient, visual examination remained limited to the distal 20 cm to 25 cm of the bowel, and treatment was limited to the distal rectum.

Flexible fiberoptic sigmoidoscopes were developed in Japan beginning in the late 1950s,[6] but early clinical applications were difficult and mostly unsuccessful.[7–10] By 1969 several reports of successful insertion into and through the sigmoid colon appeared.[11–13] In that same year Wolff and Shinya began to apply the technique on a large scale, using fluoroscopic guidance and progressively longer instruments to ultimately reach the ileocecal valve and terminal ileum. By 1971, electrocautery was being used for removal of polyps through the colonoscope.[14]

Over the subsequent 15 years rapid advances have been made in both the instrumentation and the applications of the technique. This chapter outlines some of these developments and acquaints the student, resident, and primary care physician with some of the current knowledge regarding the capabilities and the shortcomings of modern colonoscopy. Specific objectives are to assist the reader with information concerning equipment, indications, contraindications, complications, and results of the use of diagnostic and therapeutic endoscopy of the colon. A detailed description of the techniques of colonoscopy is beyond the scope of this discussion. For this purpose the reader is referred to any of several excellent reports in the recent literature.[15–17]

Routine diagnostic colonoscopy is an ambulatory procedure. In some instances overnight hospitalization may be necessary prior to or following the procedure. Very elderly or frail patients or those with severe associated disease are usually admitted prior to the procedure to prepare the patient under close observation. These same patients may require overnight observation following the procedure. Most simple therapeutic procedures, such as biopsies or excision of small polyps, can also be performed routinely on an outpatient basis. The decision to admit a patient for observation following a procedure is based on the complexity or difficulty of the procedure, the occurrence of known or suspected complications (medication reactions, prolonged pain, etc.), as well as the ability of the patient to follow instructions and their proximity to medical care should delayed complications occur. Most authors recommend overnight observation following multiple polypectomies or following removal of large (>2 cm) polyps.[16]

COLONOSCOPY

INDICATIONS

Any colonic symptom or sign may be an indication for colonoscopic evaluation. Indications have been expanding as expertise and technology have made the procedure safer and easier to perform. There are several specific indications on which there is general agreement:[16–19]

- An abnormal or equivocal finding seen on barium enema—to confirm or disprove the presence of pathology and to obtain biopsies
- Evaluation of symptoms or lower gastrointestinal bleeding when barium studies do not show a source of the problem
- The presence of polyps—for snare excision and to look for synchronous lesions
- Evaluation of the extent and nature of inflammatory bowel disease and of such complications as strictures or polyps
- Follow-up and surveillance in patients who have undergone prior polypectomy or resection of colon cancer
- Detection and removal of foreign bodies
- Therapy of bleeding lesions with electrocoagulation, photocoagulation, or thermal coagulation

Indications continue to expand, and recent reports have suggested that colonoscopy may be of value in the reduction of sigmoid or cecal volvulus and in decompression of colonic ileus (Ogilvie's syndrome).

CONTRAINDICATIONS

Contraindications to colonoscopy can be classified as absolute or relative. Absolute contraindications mostly encompass situations in which perforation of the bowel is likely. Relative contraindications pertain more to an increased risk of the procedure and must be carefully balanced against the potential benefit to the patient.

- Absolute contraindications
  - Acute fulminant inflammatory bowel disease, including ischemic or radiation-induced
  - Toxic megacolon
  - Acute diverticulitis
  - Suspected bowel perforation or presence of peritonitis
  - Recent (<1 week) bowel surgery
  - Uncooperative patient
- Relative contraindications
  - Partial or complete obstruction
  - Presence and severity of associated medical conditions
  - Chronic radiation colitis
  - Significant pelvic or abdominal adhesions
  - Inadequate bowel preparation

PREPARATION OF THE PATIENT

It is absolutely essential that proper bowel preparation be carried out prior to colonoscopy. Residual liquid fecal material can be aspirated through the colonoscope, but particulate material causes difficulty for the endoscopist and increases the possibility of overlooking lesions such as vascular malformations or small polyps.

There are many ways to cleanse the colon. Most are based either on a liquid diet followed by laxatives (usually castor oil or magnesium citrate) and enemas[16,17,19] or on an electrolyte lavage method using several liters of normal saline or Golytely solution given over a 1- to 3-hour period shortly before the procedure.[16,17,20,21]

One current regimen consists of 24 hours of a clear liquid diet followed by 4 liters of Golytely taken orally over 1 hour either the morning of the procedure or the evening prior, allowing at least 2 to 3 hours after the purge for the colon to empty. A second effective method is to have the patient on a clear liquid diet for 48 hours with 2 ounces of castor oil given orally on the evening prior to the procedure. Tap water enemas are then given the morning of the procedure until all particulate fecal matter is cleared.

Whichever method is used, it is important to individualize the preparation to the patient. Time spent detailing the instructions to the patient will be rewarded by an increased number of adequately cleansed colons. Oral metoclopramide given at the beginning of an electrolyte purge may increase patient tolerance and minimize the side-effects of nausea or vomiting. Elderly or frail patients may not tolerate the 48-hour clear liquid diet. In these patients a 48-hour low-residue formula diet may still result in adequate preparation of the colon.[22,23] Special circumstances may dictate either a more vigorous or a less vigorous preparation, such as in patients with chronic constipation, partial bowel obstruction, or diarrheal diseases. Finally, patients at risk for bacterial endocarditis should be considered for antibiotic prophylaxis as part of their preparation for colonoscopy, especially if polypectomy or other surgical procedures are contemplated.[24]

PREMEDICATION

Most endoscopists routinely use premedication to minimize discomfort to the patient. The majority prefer an intravenous analgesic and narcotic regimen. The amount of medication required varies considerably from patient to patient and should be administered slowly over a period of 2 to 3 minutes until the desired state of mild somnolence is achieved. Meperidine (Demerol) 25 mg to 75 mg and diazepam (Valium) 2.5 mg to 15 mg are commonly used in combination. Glucagon (1 mg) is occasionally useful as an antispasmodic agent but should be used with caution and ideally only when withdrawing the colonoscope.

An intravenous drip is routinely used for all patients in whom polypectomy or other surgical procedures are anticipated and may also be useful in selected patients for diagnostic procedures.

INSTRUMENTATION

Since their introduction in the late 1960s colonoscopes have undergone changes in design, length, image resolution, and adaptability, and they continue to do so. The basic design is similar for all the major manufacturers of endoscopic equipment in the United States (Fig. 18-1): American Cystoscope Makers, Inc. (ACMI); Fujinon Optical, Inc.; Machida America, Inc.; Olympus Corporation of America; Pentax Precision Instrument Corporation; and Welch Allen, Inc. Current models all have four-directional tip control provided by two concentric control knobs, which can be locked to stiffen or hold the tip in place. Trumpet-type valves provide for air or carbon dioxide insufflation, suction, and lens washing.

Colonoscope flexibility varies with each manufacturer. Most have differential flexibility built in, with greater flexibility at the tip and less in the body shaft. Pediatric instruments are designed to have maximal flexibility throughout. Tip and shaft diameter varies from 11 mm to 15 mm, and length varies from 105 cm to 185 cm.

Colonoscopes have a channel through which devices can be passed for brushing or biopsying lesions or for irrigating and suctioning bowel contents. Operating colonoscopes have a single large (up to 4.2 mm) channel or two separate channels to facilitate instrumentation and allow for simultaneous irrigation or suction.

Devices to pass through the channels are seen in Figure 18-2. A number of variations

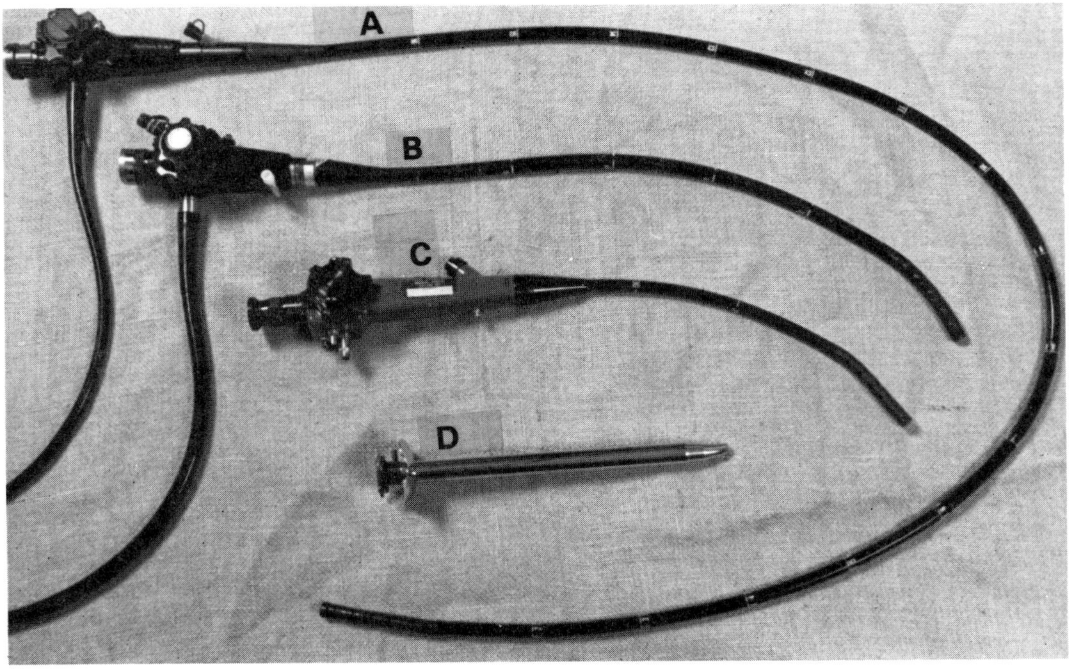

Figure 18-1. Flexible fiberoptic endoscopes. (*A*) 170-cm colonoscope, Pentax Precision Instrument Corporation; (*B*) 65-cm sigmoidoscope, Fujinon Optical, Inc.; (*C*) 35-cm sigmoidoscope, Olympus Corporation of America; (*D*) 25-cm rigid sigmoidoscope, Welch Allen, Inc.

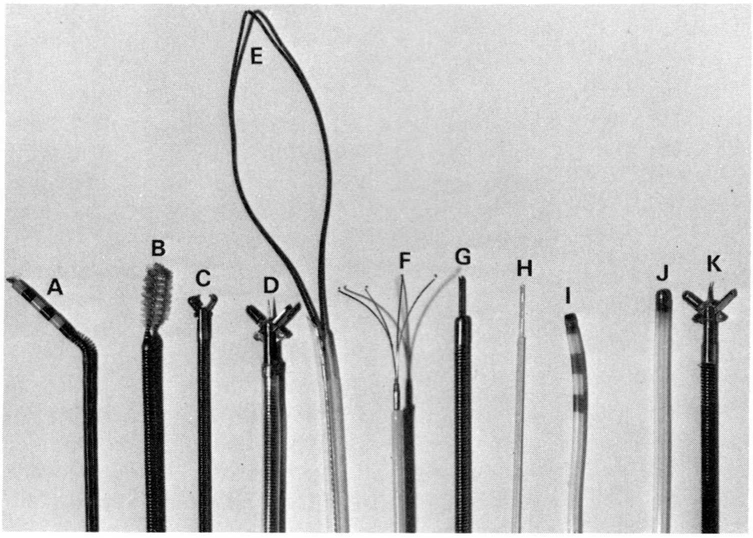

Figure 18-2. Endoscopic devices for use through endoscope channels. (*A*) Measuring device; (*B*) brush; (*C*) toothed grasping forceps; (*D*) biopsy forceps; (*E*) polypectomy snare; (*F*) four-pronged grasping forceps; (*G*) flat-blade forceps; (*H*) bare laser fiber; (*I*) cannulation catheter; (*J*) irrigation catheter; (*K*) large biopsy forceps.

are available and allow for such maneuvers as biopsy, polypectomy and retrieval, foreign body removal, measurement, irrigation, laser or thermal treatment of lesions, and so on.

A light source is required for the colonoscope, generally also containing suction apparatus, appropriate switches for direct viewing, still or video photography, and a reservoir for irrigating fluid.

TECHNIQUE

Safe and successful colonoscopy depends largely on the technical skill and experience of the operator. There is no substitute for "hands-on" experience under direct supervision to attain that skill. Such training is strongly advised for anyone contemplating the use of colonoscopy in their practice.

Actual techniques vary between colonoscopists and are difficult to describe. Nevertheless, there are a few basic technical aspects that are used regularly, and these are covered briefly here. Excellent detailed descriptions of colonoscopic techniques are available in the literature.[15–17]

Colonoscopy is performed on an examination table. The patient lies on the left side with the knees and thighs flexed. The endoscopist sits or stands behind the patient. The assistant is free to move about to check the patient or handle accessory equipment.

Prior to insertion, the anus is inspected and a digital rectal exam is performed, both to identify unsuspected pathology and to increase the ease of insertion by lubricating and relaxing the anal sphincter. The index finger is then laid parallel to the tip of colonoscope, and the lubricated tip is inserted gently by finger pressure tangentially.

Throughout most of the examination the operator holds the head of the instrument in the left hand, controlling the directional reels with the left thumb and the suction–irrigation valves with the index or middle finger. The right hand is used along the shaft to insert, withdraw, or rotate the colonoscope in conjunction with the directional tip control of the left hand.

Insofar as possible the colonoscope is advanced under direct vision with a clear view of the lumen ahead. Occasionally, however, the mucosal slide-by technique may be utilized. In this maneuver the instrument is advanced without direct visualization of the lumen, watching always that pink mucosa is "sliding by" the tip of the colonoscope. The maneuver must be stopped if the endoscope does not advance easily or if the mucosa turns white or pale, representing undue pressure and compression of mucosal blood flow.

Passage of the colonoscope through the sigmoid colon may occasionally be a problem in elderly patients with redundant sigmoid loops. In such cases the operator may elect to perform an alpha maneuver. This is accomplished by rotating the colonscope in a counterclockwise direction while advancing to the sigmoid–descending colon juncture. This will change the configuration of the sigmoid colon to a loop resembling the Greek letter α, which then permits easier passage of the colonoscope through the sigmoid colon. When the splenic flexure is reached, the alpha loop can be removed by locking the tip over the flexure and withdrawing the instrument slowly while rotating it clockwise. This will usually straighten the sigmoid colon and allow further advancement into the transverse colon.

Passage through the transverse and ascending colon may be facilitated by palpation of the abdomen by the assistant to prevent reformation of sigmoid loops or to straighten the transverse colon as the instrument is advanced.

Fluoroscopic observation may be useful to assist with some of the preceding maneuvers but becomes less necessary as technical skill improves with experience. Other means to identify progress and localize lesions consist of observing the point at which the endoscope light is visible on the abdominal wall, or one-finger abdominal palpation, which will indent the colon and be visible to the operator.[15,25]

The cecum is identified by its characteristic junction of the three teniae and identification of the ileocecal valve or appendiceal opening, in addition to seeing light in the right lower quadrant.

COMPLICATIONS

Diagnostic colonoscopy has a reported complication rate ranging from 0.3% to 2% and a mortality rate of 0.01% to 0.06%.[17,19,26–28] When polypectomy is performed, the morbidity rate ranges from 1% to 4.9%, with a mortality rate of 0.01% to 0.03%.[17,19,28,29] The chief complication is perforation, which occurs in 0.1% to 0.4% of diagnostic colonoscopies and 0.4% to 1.9% of polypectomies. Hemorrhage is seen rarely in diagnostic procedures, even with biopsy, but occurs in 0.7% to 2.5% of patients following polypectomy. Hemorrhage may be seen immediately or it may occur from 1 to 14 days following the procedure.

Other significant complications include arrhythmias, drug reactions or overdose, vasovagal reactions, splenic tears, and colonic gas explosion.[17,19,26–28]

Complication rates vary considerably with the skill and experience of the endoscopist—underscoring the need for adequate training, particularly before performing therapeutic maneuvers.[27,30] Perforations occur more frequently in association with pelvic adhesions or prior pelvic surgery, and the risk increases with the size and number of polyps removed at polypectomy.[17,28]

Overall, the complication rate for diagnostic colonoscopy is low in experienced hands. While higher for polypectomy, it still remains within acceptable limits and less than that for transabdominal polypectomy.

LIMITATIONS

It is theoretically possible to visualize the entire colon in every patient. In practice, excessive colon redundancy, stenoses, uncooperative patients, and a variety of other factors make a complete examination impossible in some patients. Experience also has a large impact on the length of colon visualized, as might be expected. One study reported that among a group of colonoscopists with varying degrees of experience, the hepatic flexure was reached in only 22% of patients, and the cecum in 13%.[31] Experienced operators should reach the cecum in 90% to 95% of procedures.[32,33]

The preparation of the colon makes a great difference in the degree of mucosal detail visible and in the ability to detect small lesions. Nevertheless, even with good preparation there are certain relatively blind areas where lesions may be missed by an experienced colonoscopist. These include the sigmoid, splenic, and hepatic flexures; portions of the cecum; and the distal rectum.[16,19]

THERAPEUTIC PROCEDURES

BIOPSY

Biopsy of suspicious areas or colonic lesions is a routine part of a complete colonoscopy. Numerous types and sizes of forceps are available (Fig. 18-2D,K). The forceps are passed through the biopsy channel until they are visible 1 cm to 2 cm beyond the tip of the colonoscope. Small lesions may be removed completely by several bites of the forceps. Larger lesions should be sampled at any suspicious areas, as well as centrally and at the margins. Brushing or washing may also be performed for cytologic specimens (Fig. 18-2B,J).

POLYPECTOMY

Colonoscopic polypectomy, first introduced in 1969, is now a widely used procedure.[14,17,30,34–36] Although pedunculated polyps are ideally suited for removal, many sessile ones can also be excised. Removal is accomplished with a braided wire snare, with varying shaped loops that can be advanced out of a Teflon tube (Fig. 18-2E). The snare is passed through the endoscope channel in the closed position. When the end of the Teflon tube is in the colonoscopic field of view, the snare loop is advanced out of the Teflon sheath, maneuvered over the polyp, and gently closed around the stalk of the polyp. The polyp is then tented toward the lumen, with care not to touch the opposite wall with its head, and coagulation current is applied through the snare to coagulate and transect the stalk. The polyp is removed for histologic examination by means of the snare, by the use of grasping forceps (Fig. 18-2C,F), or by applying suction to trap the polyp against the tip of the endoscope and withdrawing them together.

Polypectomy increases the risk of colonoscopy. It must be emphasized that polypectomy and other therapeutic procedures should be attempted only after the operator has adequate training and experience with diagnostic colonoscopy. A thorough understanding of the principles of electrocautery and electrical currents is also essential.[37,38]

THERMAL COAGULATION

The development of flexible delivery systems for laser energy in the early 1970s raised the possibility that laser energy could be transmitted through endoscopes to treat gastrointestinal lesions. The possibility became reality through the pioneering work of Fruhmorgen and his colleagues[39,40] and Dwyer and associates,[41] who utilized the argon laser to control gastrointestinal bleeding in humans. Dixon and colleagues expanded the applications by using endoscopic argon laser to ablate upper and lower gastrointestinal polyps,[42,43] and Keifhaber and co-workers added the neodymium : YAG (Nd : YAG) laser to the therapeutic armamentarium.[44]

The 1980s have seen increasingly widespread use of endoscopic laser technology, with more centers using lasers and more reports of utility, efficacy, safety, and other aspects of use appearing in the literature. Several reviews are now available in the literature.[45–48]

Neodymium : YAG laser photoablation of colorectal tumors is now an accepted therapeutic procedure in selected patients.[49–51] The therapy is primarily palliative, for control of bleeding or to prevent or relieve bowel obstruction. Ideal patients are those in whom extent of disease or associated medical illnesses preclude surgery or those who refuse surgery. As experience continues to accumulate, laser therapy may prove useful as primary or adjunctive rather than palliative therapy in some patients.

Although the use of laser palliation cannot be expected to improve survival in these patients when compared with surgery or radiation therapy, it does have several important advantages: It can usually be performed on an outpatient basis with minor or no sedation. This avoids the risks of general anesthesia and major surgery as well as reducing the costs of prolonged hospitalization. It can be applied on a repetitive schedule, with no limiting cumulative dose. Finally, although there are definite risks involved, systemic side-effects are few, thus increasing patient acceptance of the therapy.

Colonoscopic laser therapy also has become an accepted tool for the treatment of vascular malformations of the lower intestinal tract when they are known to be responsible for blood loss on a chronic or recurrent basis. Although the Nd : YAG and argon lasers are both effective, the argon laser may prove to be safer because of its shallow depth of penetration in tissue and its preferential absorption by hemoglobin.[52–55]

The Nd : YAG laser has been used by several groups for the ablation of rectal villous adenomas.[56–58] The results have been encouraging, particularly with small adenomas, but caution must be employed because of the premalignant nature of these lesions. Snare electrocautery removal of these lesions, when possible, remains the therapy of choice. It allows complete histologic examination of the polyp and resection margins, which cannot be done when using laser ablation.

Additional reports have described the use of endoscopic laser for successful incisional enlargement of postoperative intestinal stenosis.[59,60]

Other thermal options available for use

through the colonoscope include monopolar electrocautery, the bipolar electrocoagulation unit, and the heater probe. These techniques have been evaluated primarily for the endoscopic control of upper gastrointestinal bleeding.[61] They have also been reported in a few small series to be effective treatment for colonic vascular malformations.[47,62,63] All three modalities appear to be equally effective, although the greater and less predictable depth of injury from monopolar electrocautery would appear to increase the risk for perforation, particularly in the right colon and cecum.

FLEXIBLE SIGMOIDOSCOPY

The standard 25-cm rigid sigmoidoscope has been used routinely for the evaluation of colorectal disorders for many years and has proved to be an effective screening tool for colorectal polyps and cancer in asymptomatic individuals.[64,65] The procedure has several disadvantages, however. First, even in experienced hands the average depth of insertion is only 16 cm to 19 cm.[66] The procedure is not used on a widespread basis because of poor patient and physician acceptance, so the benefits are more potential than real.[67] Finally, although colorectal cancer historically has been more frequent in the distal colon, recent studies indicate the disease is moving proximally, with up to two thirds of colon cancers now found above the reach of the rigid sigmoidoscope.[68,69]

These factors inspired a need for an instrument that would be longer and more flexible than the rigid sigmoidoscope but that could still be employed routinely in the physician's office without the need for extensive prior bowel preparation. The need resulted in the development of the flexible sigmoidoscope, now available in lengths of 60 cm to 70 cm from most endoscope manufacturers (see Fig. 18-1). More recently, a 30-cm instrument has become available to confuse the picture further.[75–78]

Several centers have reported on the utility and effectiveness of these instruments, but considerable controversy remains regarding their ultimate role in patient care.[67,70–74] These reports have established that flexible sigmoidoscopy (long or short) has several advantages over rigid sigmoidoscopy. The increased length of colon visualized results in a two- to three-fold increased yield of pathologic findings.[70,71,73] Interestingly, there is little overall increase in yield with the 60-cm over the 30-cm instrument.[75–77] Patient tolerance is consistently better for flexible versus rigid sigmoidoscopy, especially with the 30-cm instrument.[72,75,77] Disadvantages include the increased cost of the equipment, both initial and maintenance, and the increased training and experience necessary for safe and effective use of the flexible instruments.[76,77,79]

INDICATIONS

Considerable disagreement still exists about the indications for flexible sigmoidoscopy. It has gained wide acceptance for screening the asymptomatic individual for colon cancer or polyps.[67,70,71,77] The length of the instrument used should be commensurate with the experience of the operator; the 30-cm endoscope is ideal for the general internist, surgeon, or family practitioner, whereas the longer instrument can be used by the trained gastroenterologist or surgeon.[75,77,78]

Other, but less well established, indications include[71,72]

Polyp surveillance
Monitoring inflammatory bowel disease
Symptom resolution
Cancer follow-up
Anastomosis inspection
Confirmation of x-ray findings
Preoperative bowel clearance

Contraindications to flexible sigmoidoscopy are the same as those for colonoscopy. Flexible fiberoptic sigmoidoscopy should not be used to supplant colonoscopy in patients with multiple polyps or at high risk for development of colon cancer. Nor is it adequate as the sole investigation of lower gastrointestinal bleeding or in other symptomatic disorders where evaluation of the more proximal colon or terminal ileum is essential.

PREPARATION OF THE PATIENT

In most cases a single tap-water or Fleet enema prior to the procedure is sufficient to allow adequate visualization. More extensive preparation negates one of the primary reasons for the procedure, which is the ability to perform it on short notice or as part of the routine screening physical examination.

Premedication is generally not required, since patient tolerance of flexible sigmoidoscopy is excellent.[72,75,77] In the apprehensive patient, intravenous diazepam (5 mg to 10 mg) may be used.

INSTRUMENTATION

Flexible sigmoidoscopes are available in either 60-cm to 70-cm or 30-cm to 35-cm lengths (see Fig. 18-1). Controls are similar to those of colonoscopes, with four-directional tip control provided by two concentric control knobs. Valves provide for air insufflation or suction. Some models also have valves for irrigation, whereas others rely on irrigation via a syringe through the channel. Operating channels range from 2.6 mm to 3.8 mm in diameter.

TECHNIQUE

The procedure is performed with the patient in the left lateral decubitus position with the knees and thighs flexed. The operator sits or stands behind the patient. Following a digital rectal examination, the instrument is introduced into the rectum and advanced into the sigmoid colon under direct visualization. The flexible sigmoidoscopes are generally somewhat stiffer than colonoscopes. This allows the operator to use rotational torque to maneuver the instrument into and through the sigmoid colon. Thus the alpha maneuver and mucosal slide-by technique are rarely required.

The complete examination by an experienced operator will take about 10 to 15 minutes for the 60-cm instrument, and somewhat less than half that for the 30-cm instrument.[70,75,77]

Any of the therapeutic procedures performed through the colonoscope also may be done through the flexible sigmoidoscope. Brushing and biopsy of suspicious areas or lesions may be performed readily. Small polyps can be removed with biopsy forceps, and palliative tumor ablation with the laser may be accomplished.

Polypectomy or monopolar electrocautery should not be performed routinely through the flexible sigmoidoscope, however. There are two major reasons for this restriction. First, in the absence of a complete bowel preparation, the possibility of gas explosion is increased during the use of electrocautery. Second, if biopsies reveal a polyp to be adenomatous, a total colonoscopy will be necessary to search for synchronous lesions, and polypectomy is best performed at that time.

COMPLICATIONS

The major complications of flexible sigmoidoscopy are the same as those for colonoscopy: perforation and hemorrhage. The perforation rate with the 65-cm instrument is reported to be about 1 in 1000 to 5000 procedures. The frequency of bleeding is slightly less.[71,76] These would be expected to increase if therapeutic procedures are performed, but thus far no such series has been reported. There have been no major complications reported with the use of the 35-cm sigmoidoscope.[76]

REFERENCES

1. Milne JS: Surgical Instruments in Greek and Roman Times, pp 149–150. Oxford, Clarendon Press, 1907
2. Schinder R: Gastroscopy, Chicago, University of Chicago Press, 1937
3. Clark ES: History of gastroenterology. In Paulson M (ed): Gastroenterologic Medicine. Philadelphia, Lea & Febiger, 1969
4. Tuttle JP: A Treatise on Diseases of the Anus, Rectum and Pelvic Colon. New York, Appleton, 1905
5. Kelly HA: Instruments for use through cylindrical rectal specula, with the patient in the knee–chest position. Ann Surg 37:924, 1903
6. Matsunaga F, Tsushima H, Kuboto T: Photography of the colon. Gastroenterol Endosc 1:58, 1959
7. Kanazawa T, Tanaka M: Endoscopy of colon. Gastroenterol Endosc 7:398, 1965
8. Oshiba S, Watanabe A: Endoscopy of the colon. Gastroenterol Endos 7:400, 1965
9. Turell R: Fiberoptic sigmoidoscopes. Am J Surg 113:305, 1967
10. Niwa H, Utsumi Y, Kaneko E et al: Clinical experiences of colonic fiberoscope. Gastroenterol Endosc 2:163, 1969
11. Overholt BF: Flexible fiberoptic sigmoidoscope. CA 19:81, 1969
12. Dean ACB, Shearman DJC: Clinical evaluation of a new fiberoptic colonoscope. Lancet 1:550, 1970
13. Fox JA: Retrograde colonoscopy. Endoscopy 4:182, 1969
14. Wolff WI, Shinya H: Colonofiberoscopy. JAMA 217:1509, 1971

15. Sugarbaker PH, Vineyard GC, Peterson LM: Anatomic localization and step by step advancement of the fiberoptic colonoscope. Surg Gynecol Obstet 143:457, 1976
16. Cotton PB, Williams CB: Colonoscopy. In Cotton PB, Williams CB: Practical Gastrointestinal Endoscopy, 2nd ed, pp 99–141. Oxford, Blackwell Scientific Publications, 1982
17. Shinya H: Colonoscopy: Diagnosis and Treatment of Colonic Diseses. New York, Igaku-Shoin, 1982
18. Wolff WI: Colonoscopy updated. Adv Surg 13:145–168, 1979
19. Schrock TR: Fiberoptic colonoscopy. In Sleisenger MH, Fordtran JS (eds): Gastrointestinal Disease, 3rd ed, pp 1617–1626. Philadelphia, WB Saunders, 1983
20. Goldman J, Reichelderfer M: Evaluation of rapid colonoscopy preparation using a new gut lavage solution. Gastrointest Endosc 28:9, 1982
21. Ernstoff JJ, DeGrasia A, Howard JB et al: A randomized, blinded clinical trial of a rapid colonic lavage solution (Golytely) compared with standard preparation for colonoscopy and barium enema. Gastroenterology 84:1512, 1983
22. Gutwein I, Baer J, Holt PR: The effect of a formula diet on preparation of the colon for barium enema examination. Arch Intern Med 141:993, 1981
23. Kruss DM, DeBartolo M, Livak AP, Serlovsky R: Explosion-safe, enema-free, nutritious colonoscopy preparation using a prepackaged formula diet. Gastrointest Endosc 31:18, 1985
24. Kaye D: Prophylaxis for infective endocarditis: An update. Ann Intern Med 104:419, 1986
25. Waye JD: Colonoscopy. Surg Clin North Am 52:4, 1972
26. Rogers BHG, Silvis SE, Nebel OT et al: Complications of flexible fiberoptic clonoscopy and polypectomy: An analysis of the 1974 A/S/G/E survey. Gastrointest Endosc 22:73, 1975
27. Macrae FA, Tan KG, Williams CB: Towards safer colonoscopy: A report on the complications of 5000 diagnostic or therapeutic colonoscopies. Gut 24:376, 1983
28. Gilbert DA, Hallstrom AP, Shaneyfelt SL, Mahler AK, Silverstein FE: The national ASGE colonoscopy survey—complications of colonoscopy. Gastrointest Endosc 30:156, 1984
29. Overholt BF: Colonoscopy. Gastroenterology 68:1308, 1975
30. Johnson SM: Colonoscopy and polypectomy. Am J Surg 136:313, 1978
31. Abrams JS: A hard look at colonoscopy. Am J Surg 133:111, 1977
32. Gaisford WD: Fiberendoscopy of the cecum and terminal ileum. Gastrointest Endosc 21:13, 1974
33. Waye JD: Colitis, cancer, and colonoscopy. Med Clin North Am 62:211, 1978
34. Wolff W, Shinya H: Polypectomy via the fiber colonoscope. N Engl J Med 288:329, 1973
35. Panish JF: State of the art. Management of patients with polypoid lesions of the colon. Am J Gastroenterol 71:315, 1979
36. Shinya H., Wolff WI: Morphology, anatomic distribution and cancer potential of colonic polyps. An analysis of 7,000 polyps endoscopically removed. Ann Surg 190:679, 1979
37. Barlow DE: Endoscopic applications of electrosurgery: A review of basic principles. Gastrointest Endosc 28:73, 1982
38. Brandt LJ: Electrosurgery. A review of various characteristics of electrical currents and risks attending their use. Endosc Rev 1:22, 1984
39. Fruhmorgen P, Reidenbach HD, Bodem F et al: Experimental examinations on laser endoscopy. Endoscopy 6:116, 1974
40. Fruhmorgen P, Bodem F, Reidenbach HD et al: Endoscopic laser coagulation of bleeding gastrointestinal lesions with report of the first therapeutic application in man. Gastrointest Endosc 23:73, 1976
41. Dwyer RM, Yellin AE, Craig J et al: Gastric hemostasis by laser phototherapy in man. JAMA 236:1383, 1976
42. Richey GD, Dixon JA: Ablation of atypical gastric mucosa and recurrent polyps by endoscopic application of laser. Gastrointest Endosc 27:224, 1981
43. Dixon JA, Burt RW, Rotering RH, McCloskey DW: Endoscopic argon laser photocoagulation of small sessile colonic polyps. Gastrointest Endosc 28:162, 1982
44. Keifhaber P, Nath G, Moritz K: Endoscopic control of massive gastrointestinal hemorrhage by irradiation with a high power neodymium YAG laser. Prog Surg 15:140, 1977
45. Fleischer D: Lasers and gastroenterology. AM J Gastroenterol 79:406, 1984
46. Buchi KN, Brunetaud JM: Endoscopic gastrointestinal laser therapy. In Dixon JA (ed): Surgical Application of Lasers, 2nd ed, pp 95–118. Chicago, Year Book Medical Publishers, 1987
47. Fleischer D, Jensen D, Bright-Asare P (eds): Therapeutic Laser Endoscopy in Gastrointestinal Disease. Boston, Martinus Nijhoff, 1983
48. Buchi KN: Endoscopic gastrointestinal laser therapy. West J Med 143:751, 1985
49. Fleischer D: Endoscopic laser therapy for gastrointestinal neoplasms. Surg Clin North Am 64:947, 1984
50. Brunetaud JM, Mordon S, Maunoury V et al: Laser treatment of benign and malignant rectal neoplasms. In Brunetaud JM, Jensen DM (eds): Lasers in Endoscopy. Amsterdam, Martinus Nijhoff, (in press)
51. Bowers J: Laser therapy of colonic neoplasms. In Fleischer D, Jensen D, Bright-Asare P (eds): Therapeutic Laser Endoscopy in Gastrointesti-

nal Disease, p 139. Boston, Martinus Nijhoff, 1983
52. Waitman AM, Grant DZ, Chateau F: Argon laser photocoagulation treatment of patients with acute and chronic bleeding secondary to telangiectasia. Gastrointest Endosc 28:153, 1982
53. Jensen D, Machicado G, Tapia J, Beilen D: Endoscopic treatment of hemangiomata with argon laser in patients with gastrointestinal bleeding. Scand J Gastroenterol 17(Suppl 78):182, 1982
54. Hunter JG, Bowers JH, Burt RW et al: Lasers in endoscopic gastrointestinal surgery. Am J Surg 148:736, 1984
55. Rutgeerts P, Van Gompel F, Geboes K et al: Long term results of treatment of vascular malformations of the gastrointestinal tract by neodymium YAG laser photocoagulation. Gut 26:586, 1985
56. Lambert R, Sabben G: Laser therapy in colorectal tumors: Early results. Gastroenterology 84:1222, 1984
57. Brunetaud JM, Mosquet L, Houcke M et al: Villous adenomas of the rectum. Results of endoscopic treatment with argon and Nd:YAG lasers. Gastroenterology 89:832, 1985
58. Mathus-Vliegen EMH, Tytgat GNJ: Nd:YAG laser photocoagulation in colorectal adenoma: Evaluation of its safety, usefulness, and efficacy. Gastroenterology 90:1865, 1986
59. Chen PC, Wu CS, Chang-Chien CS, Liaw YF: YAG laser endoscopic treatment of an esophageal and sigmoid stricture after end-to-end anastomosis stapling. Gastrointest Endosc 30:258, 1984
60. Sander R, Posl H, Spuhler A: Management of non-neoplastic stenoses of the GI tract—a further indication for Nd:YAG laser application. Endoscopy 16:149, 1984
61. Fleischer D: Endoscopic therapy of upper gastrointestinal bleeding in humans. Gastroenterology 90:217, 1986
62. Rogers BHG: Endoscopic diagnosis and therapy of mucosal vascular abnormalities of the gastrointestinal tract occurring in elderly patients and associated with cardiac, vascular, and pulmonary disease. Gastrointest Endosc 26:134, 1980
63. Jensen DM, Machicado GA: Bleeding colonic angioma: Endoscopic coagulation and follow-up. Gastroenterology 88:1433, 1985
64. Browne DC, McHardy G: An evaluation of routine proctosigmoidoscopy. South Med J 41:372, 1948
65. Gilbertsen VA, Nelms JM: The prevention of invasive cancer of the rectum. Cancer 41:1137, 1978
66. Nivatvongs S, Fryd D: How far does the proctosigmoidoscope reach? A prospective study of 1,000 patients. N Engl Med 303:380, 1980
67. Crespi M, Weissman GS, Gilbertsen VA et al: The role of proctosigmoidoscopy in screening for colorectal neoplasia. CA 34:158, 1984
68. Tedesco F, Waye J, Avella J: Diagnostic implications of the spatial distribution of colonic mass lesions: A prospective colonoscopic study. Gastrointest Endosc 26:95, 1980
69. Rosato FE, Marks G: Changing site distribution patterns of colorectal cancer at Thomas Jefferson University Hospital. Dis Colon Rectum 24:93, 1981
70. Winnan G, Berci G, Panish J et al: Superiority of the flexible to the rigid sigmoidoscope in routine proctosigmoidoscopy. N Engl J Med 302:1011, 1980
71. Marks G, Boggs HW, Castro AF et al: Sigmoidoscopic examinations with rigid and flexible fiberoptic sigmoidoscopes in the surgeon's office: A comparative prospective study of effectiveness in 1,012 cases. Dis Colon Rectum 22:162, 1979
72. Lewis M (ed): Flexible fiberoptic sigmoidoscopy: Its use and misuse. A/S/G/E National postgraduate Endoscopy Course II Symposium. Gastrointest Endosc 29:122, 1983
73. Bohlman TW, Katon RM, Lipshutz GR et al: Fiberoptic pansigmoidoscopy: An evaluation and comparison with rigid sigmoidoscopy. Gastroenterology 72:644, 1977
74. Schapiro M: Flexible sigmoidoscopy or short colonoscopy? Why settle for half a loaf? Gastroenterology 77:1156, 1979
75. Zucker GM, Madura MJ, Chmiel JS, Olinger EJ: The advantages of the 30-cm flexible sigmoidoscope over the 60-cm flexible sigmoidoscope. Gastrointest Endosc 30:59, 1984
76. Sanowski RA, Groveman HS, Klauber M: Training primary care physicians in flexible sigmoidoscopy: Performance evaluation of 17,167 procedures. Gastrointest Endosc 31:149, 1985
77. Dubow RA, Katon RM, Benner KG et al: Short (35-cm) versus long (60-cm) flexible sigmoidoscopy: A comparison of findings and tolerance in asymptomatic patients screened for colorectal neoplasia. Gastrointest Endosc 31:305, 1985
78. Griffin JW: Editorial: Flexible fiberoptic sigmoidoscopy—longer may not be better for the "nonendoscopist." Gastrointest Endosc 31:347, 1985
79. Bowman MA, Wherry DC: Training for flexible sigmoidoscopy. Gastrointest Endosc 31:309, 1985

19 Anorectum

J. PRESTON HUGHES

PROBLEMS OF THE RECTUM AND THE ANUS

SYMPTOMS

The treatment of anorectal problems requires an adequate diagnosis, which is possible only with an adequate history and a careful examination of the involved area. In the history of a patient with anal difficulties, four symptoms are of major importance, and inquiry should be made about them.

The first and most important of these symptoms is bleeding. The appearance of bright red blood in the stool signifies an ulceration or trauma to the lower bowel or the anus. Bright red blood on the tissue paper is distinguished from dark or wine-colored blood mixed with mucus.

The second symptom to be inquired about is pain. It is important to know whether the pain is constant or appears only with bowel movement. Usually constant pain signifies an inflammatory lesion. A knifelike, cutting pain with the bowel movement is significant when associated with a touch of blood in patients with a fissure. An aching, heartbeatlike pain follows the bowel movement. Nearly always pain signifies a lesion of the ectodermal portion of the anal canal; that is, the area supplied by somatic nerves. Strangulated internal hemorrhoids probably produce pain because of the associated edema and inflammatory reaction that appear in the adjacent skin. Pain of acute onset with marble-sized swelling in the anal area is often a thrombosed external hemorrhoid. Constant pain indicates an abscess.

Prolapse or protrusion or painless bleeding internal hemorrhoids can be differentiated by the patient's history.

The author is particularly grateful to the following people for their assistance: Theresa Setze, for her assistance in editing; Bonnie Jean Darling, for her typing; and Dr. William A. Shaver, for his original chapter.

The third symptom to inquire about is itching, which indicates perianal irritation.

The fourth symptom about which inquiry should be made involves the bowel habits of the patient: Has there been any change in the character and the number of bowel movements, has there been any abdominal pain associated with them, or has any increase in the amount of laxatives been necessary?

With this information one may obtain a fair idea of the nature of the lesion and whether it is located in the anus or in the rectum.

EXAMINATION OF THE PATIENT

No matter how much information is obtained from the history of a patient with an anal lesion, a diagnosis cannot be made without a thorough examination. Diagnosis of anal lesions without an examination is inexcusable negligence because the examination is one that can easily be performed in any office. If a thorough examination is to be made the patient should cleanse the lower bowel with an enema at least 2 hours before coming to the office. Inspection of the anal canal is possible without preparation, but since an adequate examination usually includes inspection of the lower bowel through the proctoscope, enema preparation is imperative. An enema can be given in the office if for some reason it was not taken earlier.

POSITION OF THE PATIENT

For examination of the anal region the patient should be in one of three positions. For older people and pregnant women the most satisfactory one is probably the lateral, or Sim's, position (Fig. 19-1A). The patient lies on the left side with the left leg extended; the right knee is flexed, and the patient is draped to expose the anal region.

The knee-chest position is perhaps more

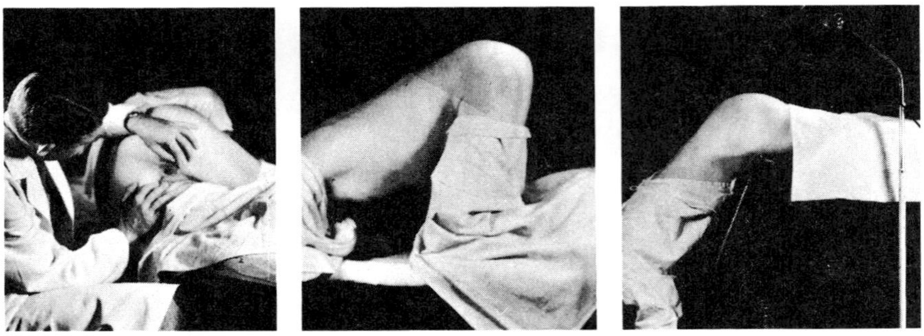

Figure 19-1. (*A*) Lateral, or Sim's, position for examination of the anal region and the lower rectum. (*B*) Knee–chest position for examination of the anal canal and the lower rectum. (*C*) Position on the proctoscopic table for examination of the anal canal and the lower rectum.

convenient (Fig. 19-1B) for examination and proctoscopy. The thighs should be perpendicular to the table, the feet extending over the end of the table. It is a difficult position for older patients, and for that reason the lateral position is more often used in examining them.

The most satisfactory position for examination and treatment of anal lesions is that obtained on the proctoscopic table (Fig. 19-1C). In this position the patient leans over the table, which is so tilted that the buttocks and the anal region are easily seen.

The examination should be done in an orderly manner: first, inspection of the anal orifice and the perianal region; second, digital examination of the anal canal and the lower rectum; and third, examination with anoscope and proctoscope of the anal canal, the rectum, and the rectosigmoid.

Inspection of the anal orifice and the perianal region is best done by spreading the buttocks apart, using small pieces of gauze to hold the skin under the fingers. The digital examination of the anal canal and the lower rectum is performed with the finger covered with a well-lubricated examining glove or finger cot. If there are painful lesions of this area the finger should be introduced against the opposite anal wall. In this way pressure is avoided and pain is reduced to a minimum. Examination should include first the region of the anal canal. The finger can then be advanced to palpate the rectum, the coccyx, and, in male patients, the prostate. Two things to look for in palpation of the anal canal and the lower rectum are areas that are tender on pressure and masses.

After thorough inspection and palpation, instrumental examination is best made with a lighted anoscope. In its introduction due regard must be taken for painful lesions of the anal canal, and the well-lubricated anoscope should be passed along the anal wall away from the painful lesions. The anoscope permits inspection of the structures of the anal canal.

All the foregoing examinations may be made without any particular preparation of the patient and without anesthesia. For the examination of patients with painful lesions, 2.5% lidocaine (Xylocaine) ointment reduces the pain of the examination.

To complete the examination proctosigmoidoscopy should be performed. This entails insertion of a lighted tube through the rectum and rectosigmoid for inspection of the wall of the lower bowel (Fig. 19-2). For this examination the bowel must be free of fecal material. Occasionally, it is possible to make the examination without previous preparation, but as a rule, the bowel should be emptied 1 or 2 hours before by a cleansing enema.

A Fleet enema (a solution of 16 g sodium biphosphate and 6 g sodium phosphate in a 4.5-fluid-ounce plastic squeeze bottle with lubricated tip) can be given during the office visit if the bowel has not been prepared previously.

Proctosigmoidoscopy is facilitated considerably by the use of an aspirator to remove liquid fecal material and mucus. In addition, long cotton swabs should be at hand for cleansing as necessary.

At times, after a thorough examination of the rectum and the anus, no cause of the patient's symptoms is found. Adjacent organs may be pressing on the rectum, thus causing symptoms referred to that area. For this rea-

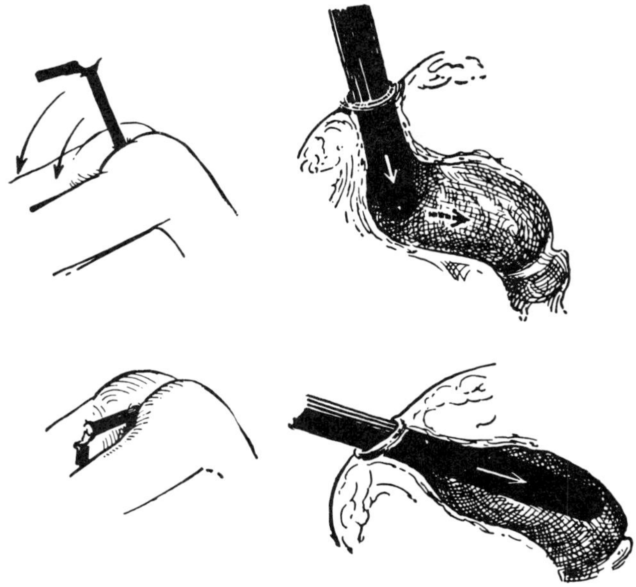

Figure 19-2. Insertion of the proctoscope. When the patient is in the jackknife supine position, the well-lubricated proctoscope is inserted. After having passed through the anal canal the outer end of the proctoscope is directed toward the patient's feet and then advanced into the rectum.

son a pelvic examination is important, especially in female patients in whom rectal pain and discomfort may be due to pressure of a myoma or retroflexed uterus.

DISEASE OF THE PERIANAL REGION

CONDYLOMA ACUMINATUM (VENEREAL WART)

Anal warts appear in the perianal skin, skin of the anal canal, and rectal mucosa (Fig. 19-3). They arise from the papillary layer of the skin and consist of a connective-tissue stalk containing blood vessels and covered with stratified squamous epithelium. One type looks like the usual verruca vulgaris, a wart-like growth in the perianal skin; the other and more common type is often spoken of as a venereal wart. They are often seen in homosexuals.

Hidradenitis is a suppurative disease that causes abscesses and fistula. It, along with Bowen's disease, Paget's disease, and squamous cell carcinoma, is sometimes confused on inspection.

Etiology and Diagnosis

Anal warts are caused by papovaviruses. They may be found associated with hemor-

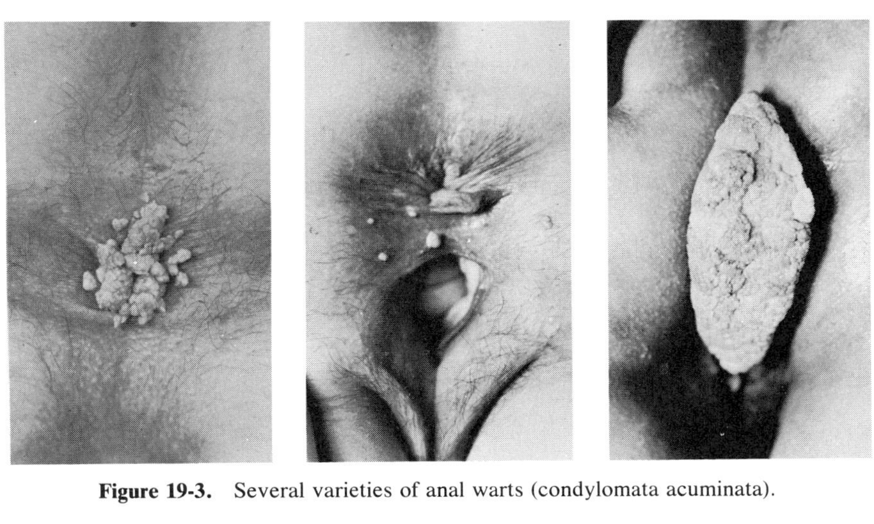

Figure 19-3. Several varieties of anal warts (condylomata acuminata).

rhoids or proctitis. In female patients they may be due to leukorrhea. They appear as pointed, cauliflowerlike growths, which frequently surround the anal orifice and may extend upward in the anal canal. Usually they are small, but they may attain a very large size. The warts are soft and pale and bleed readily when traumatized.

Symptoms

Anal growths cause irritation of the anal area, with itching, moisture, and excoriation of the perianal skin. Bleeding may be a symptom, and pain may occur.

Treatment

The treatment of anal condylomas by electrocoagulation under local anesthesia has been a tedious, time-consuming, and not always adequate process. Culp and Kaplan suggested local application of a 25% suspension of podophyllin in mineral oil to the condylomas. A local reaction, with some edema and inflammatory change in the tissues, is produced at the site of application. The condylomas blanch and slough off on the second and third days after application of the podophyllin, and on the fourth or fifth day the tissues return to normal without ulceration or scarring.

If recurrent or new growths appear they may be treated in the same way. At least a week should be allowed for recovery from one application before another is given. Repeated applications are usually necessary. The CO_2 laser has been used to destroy the warts of recurrence.

PRURITUS ANI

Itching of the perianal region and anal orifice is one of the most troublesome conditions a physician is called on to treat. This symptom complex is not uncommon.

Symptoms

Itching usually begins in a relatively mild form, and the patient tries various proprietary and home remedies in an effort to obtain relief. Lack of success with this therapy may result in more vigorous efforts to obtain relief by the use of anesthetic ointments or other local applications. Sleeplessness and worry add to the patient's irritability and increase the severity and the prominence of the local symptoms so that a vicious cycle is established, and the distressing symptoms become almost intolerable.

Etiology

In spite of voluminous literature on the subject, the cause of pruritus ani has never been well established. Itching is believed to be a subpain sensation, traveling over the same nerve paths that transmit pain. The impulses of itching arise in the epidermis, and itching is absent when the epidermis is removed or destroyed. Scratching stops the itching by causing a distinct painful sensation that the cerebral cortex can interpret. With these facts in mind, one can easily see how minor lesions of the anal canal or of the anal orifice, such as skin tabs or cryptitis with edema of the adjacent papillae, serve as sites of an original irritation, which can be increased and spread by scratching.

Many believe that in every case some local pathologic process of the anal canal or of the perianal region can be found to explain the origin of the itching. Others explain the perianal itching as being due to moisture in the perianal region between the buttocks.

Another factor that is often cited as the cause of pruritus is local uncleanliness. Paradoxically, excessive scrubbing with soap can cause pruritus. In the more marked cases, however, it is believed by some that there is sensitization to the bacteria of the stool and the rectal secretions. Epidermophyton that causes ringworm of the feet and toes is often a primary or secondary invader.

There is evidence that venous congestion may cause mild edema of the skin at the anal orifice that produces secondary itching.

Finally, there is a large group of patients in whom no etiologic factor is demonstrable. These are usually the patients with the most severe pruritus, who are therefore the most difficult to treat.

Inability to find a local cause and the fact that the itching may follow ingestion of certain foods have suggested an allergic basis for the itching. Alcohol, tea, coffee, colas, caffeine, chocolate, and scented toilet paper may bring it on. A marked neurogenic factor in the production of pruritus is shown by the fact that during periods of stress and strain patients may suffer exacerbation or recurrence of their itching.

Examination

On examining the patient complaining of pruritus, one may find any of several types of local pathologic processes, depending on the duration and the severity of the disease. The skin around the perianal region appears to be thickened and is grayish pink. The normal radiating folds of the skin at the anal orifice are thickened into rugae, between which may be found deep sulci containing shallow linear ulcers (Fig. 19-4). At times the surface of the skin is thick and sodden. Most commonly the linear ulcerations are seen in the gluteal fold in the posterior midline. Sometimes there is an acute process characterized by intense redness of the perianal tissues. The skin is evidently edematous, and the process is one of acute dermatitis. In other instances the skin may be thin and shiny, evidently atrophic.

Treatment

The treatment of any disease with such ill-defined etiology as pruritus is at once difficult and unsatisfactory. A carefully taken history may disclose that itching is related to fatigue or nervous upsets or to the use of alcohol, coffee, colas, or chocolate. Local lesions of the anal canal and the lower rectum should be carefully sought and eradicated. Local anal deformities, such as sentinel piles, fissures, hypertrophic skin tabs, or hypertrophic anal papillae, should be removed as sources of local irritation. If hemorrhoids are present, they should be treated. Irritating discharges from anal fistulas or, in female patients, cervical discharges should be given appropriate treatment.

After eradication of all apparent local causes—and in many cases there are no causes to be discovered—many patients continue to have itching. This is probably due to changes in the skin of the perianal region itself, and therefore the itching is no longer initiated by the anal lesion.

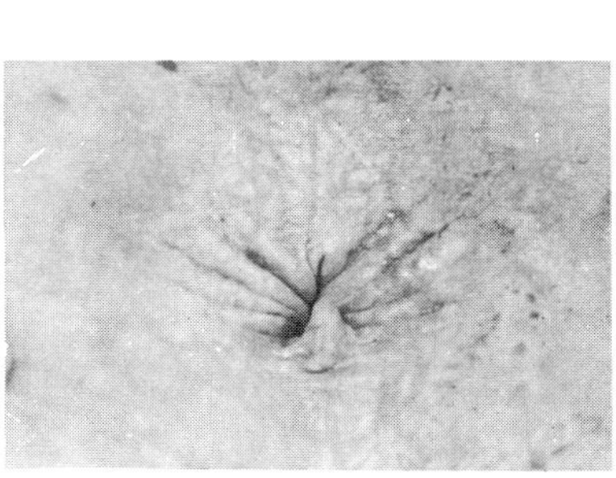

Figure 19-4. Pruritus ani, showing the thickened perianal skin with deep fissures and furrows between the perianal folds. Note the excoriation due to scratching.

The first important measure is to prevent further irritation. This means no further scratching or rubbing of the perianal skin. The patient must recognize that scratching and rubbing with toilet paper increase the perianal irritation and so prolong the itching. Therefore use of toilet paper should be avoided. Instead, moist, warm cotton may be used for cleansing.

The next therapeutic step is an attempt to return the perianal skin to normal. Application of moist heat is the most effective measure. This may be accomplished best by the use of hot sitz baths. Plain hot water is used in the bath. Sufficient water should be used to cover the perineum. The bath should last about 20 minutes, after which the perineum is dried by blotting it with dry cotton or a hair dryer. Instead of using toilet paper the patient should take a sitz bath after each bowel movement. After the sitz bath the perianal skin is protected with a mild antipruritic ointment. Icthammol (Ichthyol) (3% in zinc oxide) ointment is effective in about 90% of the cases of mild inflammation.

In cases with more intense inflammation or with lichenification, crude coal tar ointments (crude coal tar 8 g, zinc oxide powder 8 g, cornstarch 60 g, and petrolatum 60 g) can be used. Ointments prevent maceration of the skin. If this plan of therapy is followed conscientiously, it will permit the skin to return to its normal texture.

In those cases in which the perianal skin has a moist, soggy appearance, with deep fissures between the rugae, the Trichophyton is frequently a secondary factor, and various types of fungicidal ointments may be used. Half-strength Whitfield's ointment often gives relief in such cases. The patient should be warned of some smarting or burning following its application. This is not intolerable, however.

With the advent of adrenal steroids a new method of therapy for pruritus ani has become available. Hydrocortisone acetate applied locally in a 1% or 0.5% cream apparently has some local antipruritic effect. Sarner and better results with the use of fluocinolone acetonide cream, 0.025% (Synalar). The skin is blotted dry, and a pea-sized dab of hydrocortisone cream is applied with the finger. This routine is followed in the morning and after bowel movements and at night before retiring. A favorable response should be obtained within 24 to 48 hours. When complete relief of itching is obtained, the treatment may be reduced to once daily for 1 week.

A normal-residue diet, without stimulants, is prescribed. If any relationship has been found between itching and the ingestion of any specific foodstuff or of coffee, the offending substance should be eliminated from the diet. Tranquilizers and sedatives, especially trimeprazine (Temaril), are of value.

There is some reason to believe that in some cases pruritus may have an allergic basis. Hydroxyzine pamoate (Vistaril) or hydroxyzine hydrochloride (Atarax) may be helpful.

Scratching is interdicted, since little improvement in pruritus can be expected as long as it is continued. If the patient scratches during sleep, cotton gloves should be worn to bed. Instead of toilet paper for cleansing, cotton moistened with warm water should be used. In no circumstances should there be any vigorous rubbing of the perianal skin. Finally, some provision should be made to ensure the patient's obtaining a good night's rest. Diphenhydramine hydrochloride (Benadryl) 50 mg at bedtime helps to prevent scratching during sleep and is a mild, effective sedative. Barbiturates may be necessary during acute exacerbations of pruritus.

DISEASE OF THE ANAL CANAL

HYPERTROPHIED ANAL PAPILLAE

The dentate (mucocutaneous) line in the anal canal is marked by small conical projections from the skin margin. These are called papillae. Normally they are soft and tend to flatten as the anal canal is dilated by the passage of the stool mass.

Etiology

Papillae often become hypertrophied as a result of trauma produced by evacuation of a large, hard stool or by repeated spasm of the sphincter in diarrhea. Infectious inflammation plays a significant role in hypertrophy of papillae, which is associated with cryptitis and fissure. When hypertrophy occurs the papillae may easily be identified by palpation as hard nodules on the wall of the anal canal. They enlarge, becoming two or three times their normal size, and may even assume the proportions of true polyps (Fig. 19-5). Occasionally, a hypertrophied papilla has enlarged to a polypoid prolapsing tumor. Sometimes they are confused with polyps and have been called *medical polyps*.

Symptoms

Hypertrophied papillae produce varied symptoms. Frequently they are the cause of pain at the time of bowel movements due to a drag or pull as the stool mass passes over them. Often bleeding is associated. They cause anal discomfort by prolapsing during exercise. They may be one of the causes of anal irritability, spasm, and itching.

Diagnosis

The diagnosis is made by palpation and inspection of the anal canal. If the external sphincter is relaxed, papillae often appear in the anal orifice when the patient strains and the canal is everted by the examiner's fingers. The characteristic nodules are easily recognized by palpation with the finger. They are found within the anal canal.

Treatment

The hypertrophied papillae are removed when they produce symptoms. After local infiltration at the base and base placement of a chromic suture, the papillae are excised with a cautery or with scissors. The resulting wounds are often painful for a few days.

When hypertrophied papillae occur in association with fissures, cryptitis, or hemorrhoids, they may be taken care of at the time of treatment of the other lesion (Fig. 19-6).

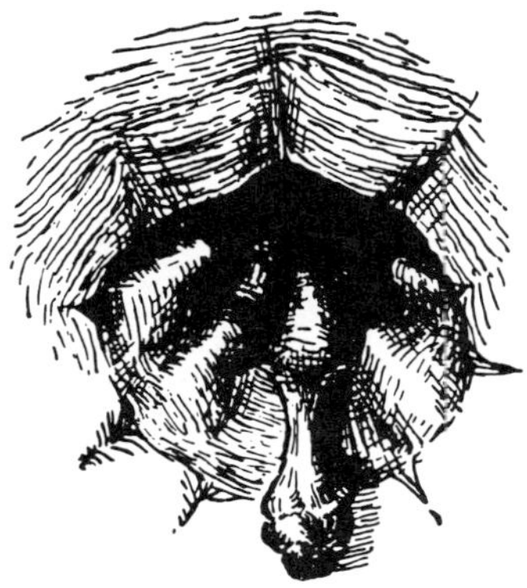

Figure 19-5. Hypertrophied anal papillae.

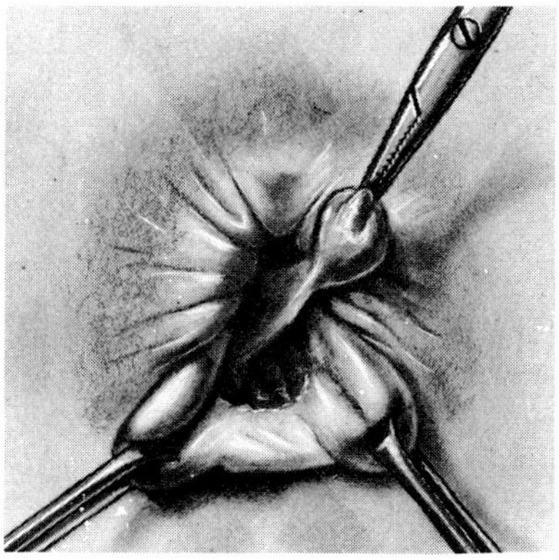

Figure 19-6. Hypertrophied anal papillae. These are often associated with an anal fissure, and both the fissure and papillae should be looked for.

PYOGENIC INFECTIONS OF THE ANAL CANAL

Almost all pyogenic infections of the anal canal may be considered to have a common origin in the crypts of Morgagni. These crypts, which may be deep pockets, lie above the dentate line, or mucocutaneous junction. They are lined by mucous membrane, and deep tortuous glands extend from them into the submucosal tissues. In addition, there are patches of lymphoid tissues that lie underneath the mucosa. An infection may extend from the crypt pockets to these glands and the lymphoid tissue, giving no symptoms until it reaches the adjacent skin tissue.

When an infection in the anal crypts progresses by burrowing, it may extend between the sphincter muscles as an abscess, or it may perforate and thus form an ischiorectal abscess.

CRYPTITIS

ETIOLOGY

Normally, the pockets lying between the columns of Morgagni flatten out during the passage of the stool mass. They are formed by the puckering action of the sphincter muscles and are absent in the cadaver where the muscle tone is lost. Trauma incidental to evacuation of large, hard stools in constipation, or in diarrhea, permits infecting organisms to gain entrance into the tissues. The relatively deep crypt may not drain spontaneously, and the inflammation extends to the lymphoid tissue and the glands underlying its surface. The crypts most often involved lie in the posterior half of the anal ring and, in the majority of cases, at the posterior commissure.

SYMPTOMS

When confined to the mucous membrane and the submucosal tissue the infection may produce no symptoms. When, however, the inflammation extends to the adjacent papillae, producing an edematous swelling of this sensitive tissue, anal pain and spasm become prominent symptoms.

DIAGNOSIS

The diagnosis of cryptitis can be made by anoscopic examination. Usually the edematous, hypertrophied papilla can be palpated, and pressure over the affected crypt gives marked pain. When an anoscope is inserted the crypt may be entered with a hooked probe (Fig. 19-7). As a rule, except for the edema of the skin edge, few inflammatory signs may be seen. However, insertion of the probe into the crypt usually causes definite pain.

TREATMENT

Treatment of anal cryptitis should err on the conservative side. It does not seem logical to expect any very intense relief from topical applications in the crypt, although many have been recommended. The objective is to hasten the subsidence of the inflammation or, if the inflammation continues because of its deep lo-

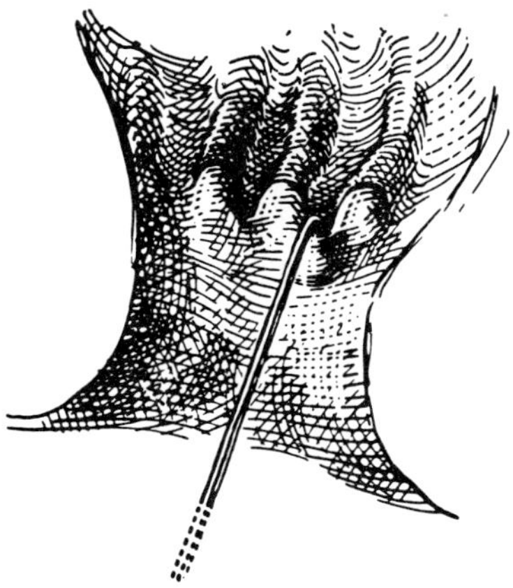

Figure 19-7. Hooked probe inserted into an anal crypt.

cation, to produce adequate drainage. As an aid in reducing the inflammation, warm rectal instillations are beneficial in keeping the parts clean and the crypts empty. Sitz baths may also be used as a method of applying heat.

When infection has begun to burrow, so that the exploring probe hooks into a deep opening overhung by the tissues at the dentate line, the treatment indicated is adequate drainage. With a speculum inserted into the anal canal the pocket of the infected crypt can easily be identified with the hooked probe. The tissues beneath the hook are excised with narrow scissors, and in this way the deep pocket is converted into an open wound. Bleeding is usually slight and can be controlled by insertion of plain or petrolatum gauze into the anal canal for a few hours. Frequently there is postoperative discomfort lasting for 24 hours, which can be relieved by hot sitz baths and anesthetic ointments. After 48 hours there is little discomfort except at the time of bowel movements.

PERIANAL ABSCESS

When the infection of an anal crypt extends deeply to the perianal lymphatic tissue and then burrows caudally between the mucous membrane and the anal muscles, an abscess forms that can be found at the anal orifice. This is called a perianal abscess. This type of lesion appears most often at the midline posteriorly as a painful, reddened swelling.

DIAGNOSIS

The history given by the patient may often be misleading as to the true course of the infection. There is often a period of several days during which the patient has noted slight discomfort and soreness in the anal canal. The pain then becomes severe and, at the time of bowel movements, almost intolerable. Usually it is sufficient to keep the patient awake at night. The systemic reaction is slight. On digital examination, an indurated, rounded tender mass may be palpated just outside the anal wall, usually in the posterior half of the anal canal and on either side of the midline. The abscess may be situated at the level of the infected crypt. When the buttocks are pulled apart, pus may be seen to escape from the anal orifice. An anoscope can be introduced gently without pain if pressure is maintained away from the area of the abscess. The infected crypt can then be identified by the drainage of pus from it, and the hooked probe will extend through it into the abscess cavity (Fig. 19-8).

TREATMENT

The treatment of such an abscess is relatively simple and may be done without admitting the patient to a hospital. The result is almost immediate relief of pain and discomfort. With the speculum in place and the hooked probe in the infected crypt, anesthesia is produced by infiltration with 1% procaine or 1% mepivacaine (Carbocaine) solution. Usually it is best to infiltrate at the crypt opening first, because edema may obscure this area if the anesthetic is first introduced over the swelling of the abscess cavity. No effort is made to obtain deep anesthesia. The mucous membrane overlying the abscess is anesthetized from the infected crypt to the farthest extent of the abscess cavity at the anal orifice.

A single incision is then made to drain the cavity and to remove the purulent material by suction or gentle sponging. The cavity is then gently packed with petrolatum or narrow iodoform gauze.

The operation as described earlier is not absolutely painless, but it may be performed with a minimum of discomfort. Sponging of the unanesthetized abscess cavity and insertion of packing are the procedures that cause pain. If the patient is warned beforehand, and if gentleness is used, little difficulty is experienced.

As a rule, incision of the abscess causes almost immediate relief of pain, but it is good to provide the patient with two or three tablets of a potent analgesic to be taken by mouth every 3 hours if needed for relief of pain during the first night after operation. Sitz baths of warm water once or twice daily and after each bowel movement are an easy and efficient method of keeping the wound macroscopically clean during the healing process. The ordinary sanitary napkin makes a convenient and an easily obtainable dressing after the wound begins to granulate on about the fifth or sixth day. This wound is not and never can be considered sterile, but ordinary cleanliness suffices. Occasionally, drainage from the wound causes excoriation and chafing of the buttocks. A thick layer of zinc oxide ointment at the site of

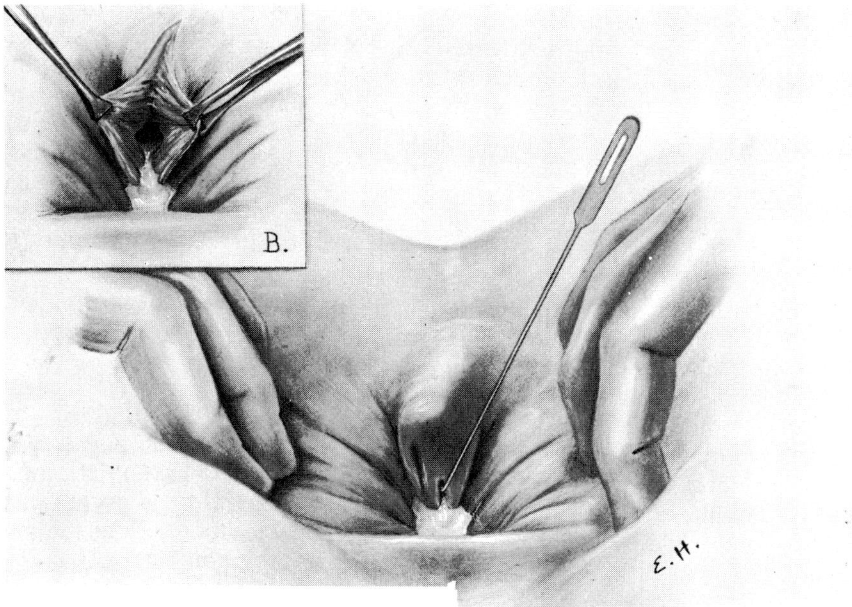

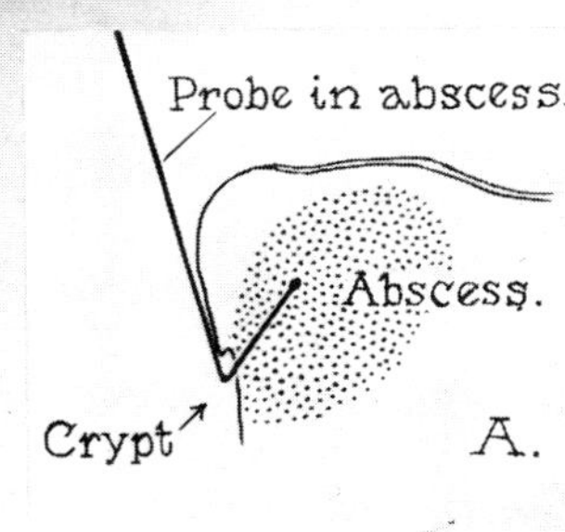

Figure 19-8. Incision and drainage of a perianal abscess. The infected crypt is identified with a hooked probe (*A*), and, after line infiltration with local anesthesia, an incision is made over the dome of the abscess into its cavity. The lips of the wound are held apart by Allis forceps while the pus is removed with soft cotton or an aspirating tip (*B*).

irritation will give relief in 24 hours. The passage of a formed stool is more to be desired than numerous soft or liquid stools. No laxatives are given unless indicated for reasons other than the operative wound.

ISCHIORECTAL ABSCESS

When infection from a crypt burrows laterally, it may pass between the sphincters or through the fibers of the external sphincter to enter the ischiorectal fossa. This pyramidal space lying between the anal canal and the tuber ischii is filled chiefly with fatty tissue, which offers little resistance to the progress of an infection. Therefore the abscess may rapidly extend upward along the wall of the rectum of laterally around the anal canal into the fossa of the opposite side.

SYMPTOMS

The rapid necrosis of the fatty tissue does not permit a walling off of the infected process so that a temperature elevation and other systemic changes often result. On local examination, a tense, red area may be seen to the side of the anal orifice. On palpation, either in the anal canal or over the reddened area, acute tenderness is elicited. The area is usually so tender that demonstration of fluctuation is impossible. It is often difficult, even impossible, to demonstrate the infected crypt without general anesthesia. In ischiorectal abscess, as in perianal abscess, there is often no previous history. Nevertheless, the almost inevitable development of a secondary fistula after the drainage of an ischiorectal abscess indicates that the origin of the infection is cryptoglandular.

TREATMENT

Because of the rapid progress of an infection in the fat of the ischiorectal fossa, incision and drainage at the earliest moment are the indicated treatment. As a rule, general, low spinal, or caudal block anesthesia is required, and hospitalization is advised. Simple incision of the abscess may be performed under local infiltration anesthesia in ambulatory patients, with the knowledge that a secondary fistula will probably result. With the patient in the supine or lithotomy position, infiltration with 0.5% procaine or 1% mepivacaine (Carbocaine) is made carefully over the dome of the abscess. When making the infiltration, one must remember that pressure on an abscess wall, by increasing the tension of the abscess, causes definite increase in pain. The lines of infiltration should be radial and long enough to permit an incision that will open the entire extent of the abscess. A radial incision permits more complete drainage and closure of the wound does not occur too soon. Local anesthesia does not permit a completely painless operation, but the relief of tension immediately following the incision gives such relief to the patient that this type of anesthesia may be used.

The skin and subcutaneous tissues are cut through with sweeping strokes of the knife, and the abscess cavity is entered. Frequently, the foul-smelling pus spurts out under considerable pressure. In smaller abscesses the knife is guided toward the abscess cavity by the finger in the anal canal. In deeper, smaller abscesses it may be necessary to make deeper infiltration of the subcutaneous fat to obtain anesthesia.

The wound is then held open with Allis forceps or rake retractors while it is cleaned gently with an absorbent gauze sponge or irrigated with sterile saline. The cavity is then packed with plain or iodoform gauze. Dressings are applied and are held in place by a T binder. Postoperative care is similar to that mentioned for perianal abscess. After removal of the packing, the wound edges are held apart by insertion of a simple gauze dressing. Warm sitz baths keep the area clean. Healing usually requires 2 to 3 weeks.

ANTIBIOTICS AND ANAL INFECTIONS

Antibiotics are not of great value in the treatment of perianal and ischiorectal infections. These lesions are rarely seen until they are in the abscess stage, and in that stage, antibiotics are no substitute for incision and drainage. If adequate drainage is provided, the need for antibiotics is slight and their value is negligible. Rosser believes that they "slow the process and change the clinical picture, at times sufficiently to confuse the diagnosis or give a false sense of security."

FISTULA IN ANO

ETIOLOGY

Fistula in ano is a tubular tract, lined with infected granulation tissue, that extends from the infected crypt outward to the skin surface at either side of the anal orifice. This infected tract may appear as a sequel of an ischiorectal abscess. The abscess, drained by an incision, still leaves the infected crypt and the infected tract. As a result of the incision, the abscess cavity heals by granulation up to and around the drainage tract, which extends to the skin surface at the site of the incision. Sometimes the abscess may heal entirely by granulation, and the wound breaks open some time later, with the appearance of a fistulous opening. Sometimes the fistula appears without preexisting acute ischiorectal abscess. In such cases the organism may be of lower virulence or the tissues of higher resistance. In any event the infection extends from the anal crypt across the inner part of the ischiorectal fossa to form a small subcutaneous abscess. This usually ruptures spontaneously and a fistula remains.

Frequently, the posterior fistulous tract is tortuous, and secondary fistulous openings may appear on the skin surface. The infection burrows through the wall of the original fistulous canal and the rectum. Almost always, however, these numerous tracts arise from a single infected crypt.

SYMPTOMS AND DIAGNOSIS

The symptoms of a fistula in ano are diagnostic. The patient states that he notices a drainage of thick malodorous material from the fistulous opening. The drainage is sufficient to soil the clothing and requires a pad between the buttocks. For a time, as the scar tissue at the skin opening contracts, the drainage may lessen. Eventually, the external opening may close entirely, and the patient may consider his fistula healed. Gradually, however, the infected material of the tract produces a small subcutaneous abscess at the site of the former cutaneous opening, and recurrent pain and soreness develop. In 2 or 3 days the abscess ruptures at the scar of the cutaneous opening of the fistula. The pain is relieved, but the drainage becomes apparent again. This continuous infection produces a fistulous tract lined by infected granulation tissue with a wall of dense fibrous tissue. In a longstanding fistula the cutaneous opening is easily recognized by its raised circle of scar tissue, from which a drop or two of pus may easily be expressed. By palpation the fistulous tract may often be identified as a firm, fibrous cord extending toward the anal canal.

A frequently cited means for locating the internal opening has been found to be useful: An imaginary line is drawn between the tubera ischii so as to bisect the anal orifice transversely (Fig. 19-9A). If the primary external opening of the fistula lies anterior to this line, the internal opening is usually in an infected

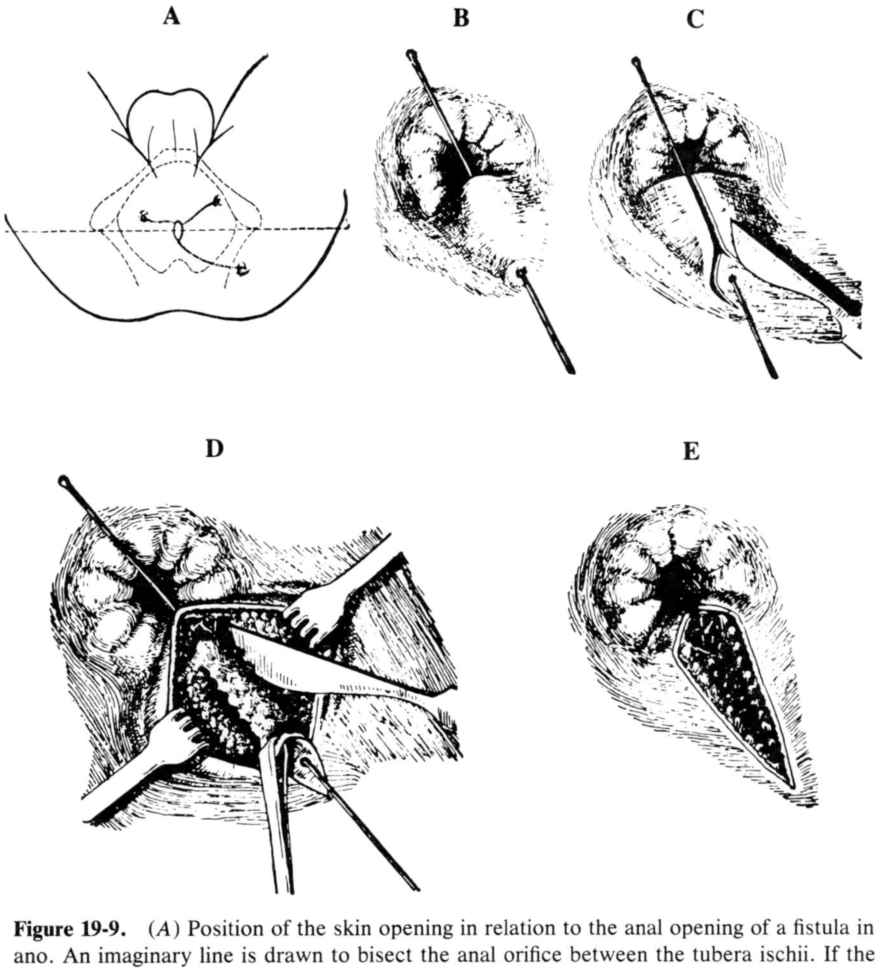

Figure 19-9. (*A*) Position of the skin opening in relation to the anal opening of a fistula in ano. An imaginary line is drawn to bisect the anal orifice between the tubera ischii. If the cutaneous opening of the fistula lies posterior to this line, the anal opening is almost invariably at a crypt in the posterior midline. If the cutaneous opening lies anterior to this line, the tract courses in a radial direction to the anal canal.

(*B*) Short fistula in ano identified with a probe inserted from the cutaneous opening to the infected crypt. Procaine 1% containing epinephrine is infiltrated along the line of the fistula and around the cutaneous opening.

(*C*) Skin incision for excision of a short fistula in ano.

(*D*) Excision of fibrous fistulous tract as a cylinder on the identifying probe.

(*E*) Wedge-shaped wound resulting from excision of the fistulous tract is packed with plain or iodoform gauze. Healing by granulation is permitted.

crypt on a straight line drawn from the external opening to the anal orifice. If the external opening of the fistula lies posterior to this line, the fistulous tract usually is curved and has its origin in an infected crypt at the midline posteriorly.

TREATMENT

The treatment of fistula in ano is incision of the fistulous tract from the infected crypt to all the cutaneous openings. When the skin opening of the fistula lies close to the anal orifice and when the tract can be identified easily by palpation or by gentle insertion of the probe along its course, it is possible to incise the fistula under local anesthesia. The patient may be ambulatory throughout the period of treatment.

With the anoscope in the anal canal, a probe is introduced through the fistulous tract to emerge at the infected crypt. The end of the probe is then advanced slowly until it appears at the anal orifice. Although this may cause the patient slight discomfort, it is much better to insert the probe before injection of a local anesthetic has caused distortion of the tract. A local anesthetic is then injected into the tissues above and around the probe. First, the skin is infiltrated adequately. As a rule, it is best to begin the infiltration at the anal end of the fistula. The tissues are then incised down through the fistulous tract. With sharp rake retractors or Allis forceps the edges of the wound are pulled apart, and the incision is carried down through the exposed tract.

The incision is carried down to the probe and the fistulous tract is laid open. Postoperative care is similar to that described for perianal abscess.

When the fistulous tract opens at some distance from the anal orifice, the patient is usually hospitalized and operated on under low spinal, caudal, or general anesthesia. With the patient in the supine position the anal canal is visualized with a Hill–Ferguson retractor. With a hooked probe the infected crypt that marks the internal opening of the fistulous tract is identified (Fig. 19-9B). The probe is held in the crypt. In long and tortuous fistulas it is not always possible to insert a probe throughout the entire length of the tract. It is imperative that the infected crypt that marks the anal opening of the tract be identified early in the operation. The most important part of the operation is the incision of the crypt. Recurrences are frequently due to the fact that the infected crypt was not laid open at the first operation.

In cases of deep fistulas it is frequently wise to leave the portion that passes under the sphincter muscle. When this type of operation has been chosen, a probe or a grooved director is inserted into the fistulous opening as far as it will pass without force. An incision is then made in the direction of the probe, and the skin and subcutaneous tissues are divided down to the tract (Fig. 19-9C). The skin incision is carried around the fistulous opening. The tract may be dissected out intact down toward the anal canal (Fig. 19-9D).

As the dissection progresses, the fistulous tract is held taut on the probe with a hemostat. Usually the probe can be passed without any effort along the tract. It is dissected free and emerges in the anal canal at the crypt previously identified by the hooked probe. When the dissection has been carried down to the anal musculature, the freed portion of the fistula is cut off and drawn off the probe. A fistulotomy often suffices rather than excising the fistula.

The lateral edges of the wound are sutured with a running locking chronic suture for hemostasis. The iodoform packing is removed on the second postoperative day. Warm sitz baths relieve much of the pain.

Sometimes a rubber band seton is placed around the muscle tissue. The rubber band seton is tightened by pulling on the ends. A silk suture is tied near the muscle. The resulting tension on the band cuts through the muscle. This is done 2 to 3 weeks following the operative procedure, when the wounds have healed solidly up to the seton. This second stage can be done in the ambulatory patient.

FISSURE IN ANO

ETIOLOGY

A painful ulcer of the anal canal is called a fissure in ano. Most often this ulceration appears as a splitting or tearing of the skin tissues at the anal orifice by the passage of a large, hard stool. Because of the direction of the anal canal in relation to that of the lower rectum, the stretching and the tearing of the thin skin at the anal margin most often occur posteriorly. There may be a slight amount of oozing incidental to the injury, but in the majority of cases healing takes place without complication. In those cases in which the tear becomes an ulcer, infection occurs, with resulting inflammation of the wound and of the surrounding tissues. The inflammatory reaction frequently produces edema of the papilla.

SYMPTOMS

The symptoms produced by a fissure (Fig. 19-10) are tearing, cutting, pain, bright red blood, and aching in the anal canal after the bowel movement. The pain occurs characteristically with defecation, and usually it persists for a half-hour to 2 or 3 hours after defecation. Usually the amount of bleeding is small and noticed only on the toilet paper. The trauma to the ulcer due to the bowel movement stretches the tissues, causing intense pain, followed by a spasm of the sphincter muscle. This spasm further traumatized the ulcer and prolongs the pain. Defecation is such a painful procedure for these patients that it is often avoided as long as possible. The stool mass becomes larger and harder as the water is more completely absorbed from it, and the following movement is more painful than ever. The dread of a bowel movement and of the consequent severe pain results in constipation.

Scar tissue forms at the edges of the ulcer with edema and secondary fibrosis—a sentinel pile (Fig. 19-11). This pile can easily be seen and almost 90% of the time is at the posterior midline. With the passage of time and the deposit of fibrous tissue in and around the fissure, the symptoms change to those of chronic fissure in ano. The chief symptom is a duller, prolonged pain that occurs at the time of bowel movement. The pain in this case is due to the stretching of the ulcer and the underlying fibrosis. In addition, there may be marked pain due to pulling on a hypertrophied papilla at the upper limit of the ulcer.

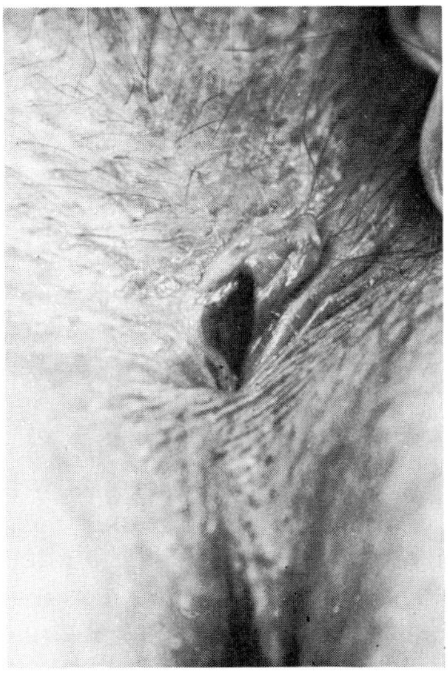

Figure 19-10. Acute fissure at the usual site at the posterior midline of the anal orifice.

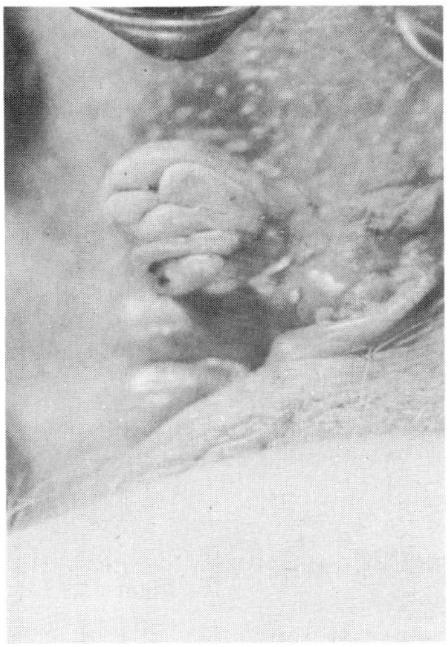

Figure 19-11. Chronic fissure. Note the hypertrophic tissue commonly designated as a sentinel pile.

DIAGNOSIS

The diagnosis of anal fissure may frequently be made from the history alone. The pain associated with and persisting after defecation and the appearance of small amounts of bright blood are quite typical. However, one should not rely on the history; the anal area must be examined. The fissure usually can be seen if the buttocks are separated, but such an examination may cause considerable discomfort. Lidocaine (Xylocaine) ointment (2.5%) has also been used on the gloved finger, providing some relief. If the fissure can be seen, the rectal examination can be delayed until later with less pain.

When no anesthesia is used the index finger should be inserted and pressure should be made away from the fissure. The finger may then be turned and the area of the fissure palpated. The ulcer is felt as a depression with dense fibrosis on either side of the fissure, of-

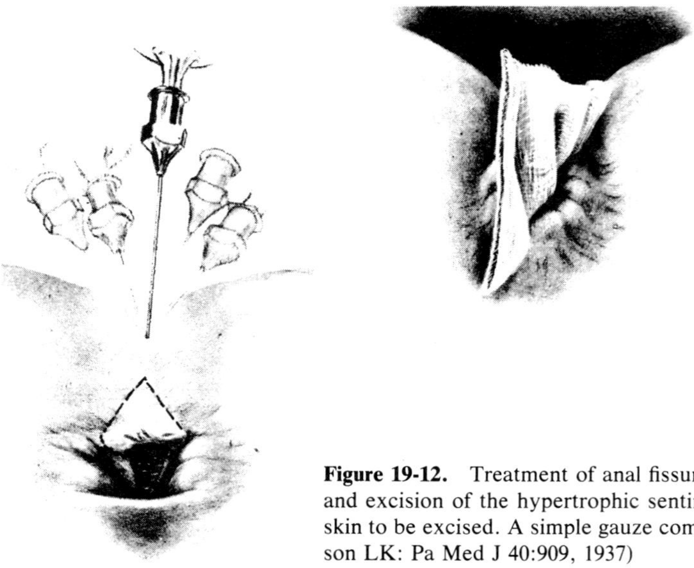

Figure 19-12. Treatment of anal fissure by a perianal injection of a local anesthetic and excision of the hypertrophic sentinel pile. The dotted lines indicate the area of skin to be excised. A simple gauze compress dressing is all that is necessary. (Ferguson LK: Pa Med J 40:909, 1937)

ten producing an almost shelflike constriction of the posterior part of the anal canal. Frequently, an edematous and fibrosed papilla at the upper margin of the fissure can be palpated as a small, tender, round, smooth mass. The fissure may be seen with the aid of an anoscope.

TREATMENT

The treatment of acute fissures may be either conservative or operative. When the fissure is only a recent tear at the anal orifice, stool softeners and hot applications or sitz baths may produce healing. Anesthetic ointments may help.

When the fissure is really an anal ulcer with a flat grayish pink base, sharply demarcated by edema of the surrounding rim of transitional epithelium, conservative treatment should be abandoned. The left lateral subcutaneous anal internal sphincterotomy is the procedure of choice. The internal sphincter white muscle fibers are divided through a small skin incision over the intersphincteric groove at the anal verge. Local anesthesia with bupivacaine (Marcaine) or etidocaine (Duranest) is used with intravenous sedation.

When the fissure is chronic, with a well-marked sentinel pile and a polypoid hypertrophied papilla at its upper margin, a more extensive procedure may be necessary to effect a cure. In such cases it is necessary to inject a local anesthetic in a wedge-shaped area around the sentinel pile and underneath the fissure. A wedge-shaped excision of skin extending from 0.5 inch to 0.75 inch from the anal orifice is carried toward the anal canal. The sentinel pile and the fissure are removed with the hypertrophied anal papilla (Fig. 19-12). A strip of Telfa is placed in the anal canal for a few hours as a dressing with a fluff gauze on the outside. After a sitz bath the Telfa is moist enough to permit removal without much discomfort. Simple superficial dressings are then all that are required, the area being kept clean by sitz baths four to six times a day.

HEMORRHOIDS

DEFINITION

Hemorrhoids are protruding vascular tissue in the anal canal and at the anal verge. They are spoken of as external when they lie distal to the dentate line and are covered with the modified skin or squamous tissue of ectodermal origin. They are called internal when they originate above the dentate line and are covered by mucous membrane of endodermal origin. When the hemorrhoidal tissue extends throughout the length of the anal canal, it is a mixed hemorrhoid of both external and internal hemorrhoids.

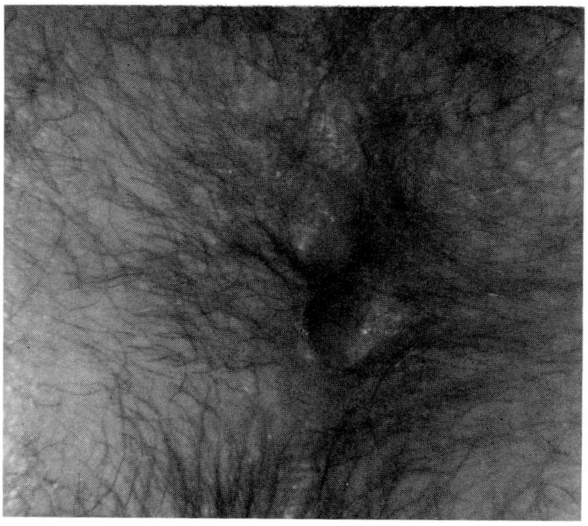

Figure 19-13. External hemorrhoids.

ANATOMY AND ETIOLOGY

Under normal conditions there are two venous plexuses at the anal orifice and in the anal canal. These lie in the subcutaneous and submucosal tissues and are loosely supported by the overlying tissues. The upper plexus drains into the middle and superior hemorrhoidal veins. The lower plexus drains into the inferior hemorrhoidal vein. The two plexuses are united by numerous anastomotic branches, and it is not unusual to find that both are involved in the same pathologic process.

Most commonly, the cause of hemorrhoids is straining at stool, because of constipation or diarrhea. Less commonly, straining associated with physical exertion may be an etiologic factor. The venous stasis produced by pregnancy and childbirth is frequently the cause of hemorrhoids in women. Many female patients date the onset of their hemorrhoidal symptoms from the birth of their first or second child (Fig. 19-13).

EXTERNAL HEMORRHOIDS

ETIOLOGY

Dilation of the external hemorrhoidal plexus is accompanied by stretching and edema of the skin. When venous stasis is produced by straining, the plexus becomes distended. It is most frequently noticed by the patient as swollen tissue at the anal verge.

SYMPTOMS

The only symptom produced by external hemorrhoids is the feeling of swelling at the anus after straining, which rarely demands treatment. Sometimes, however, the veins of the external hemorrhoidal plexus become thrombosed, adding the symptom of pain to the swelling.

The severity of pain in a thrombosed external hemorrhoid varies. In a large majority of cases, only one or two small veins become thrombosed. These appear as firm, rounded, purplish masses at the anal orifice (Fig. 19-14). They are tender on pressure and give pain when traumatized by bowel movements or by standing for long periods. If untreated, the smaller thrombi may undergo organization, and the hemorrhoidal mass will remain as a tab of skin overlying an area of fibrosis. Larger thrombosed external hemorrhoids may slowly progress to ulceration of the skin overlying the thrombosed vein. Bleeding in small amounts then develops. The blood is dark and necessitates a protective dressing. Eventually, the clot is discharged through the ulcer, and healing takes place by granulation. Many

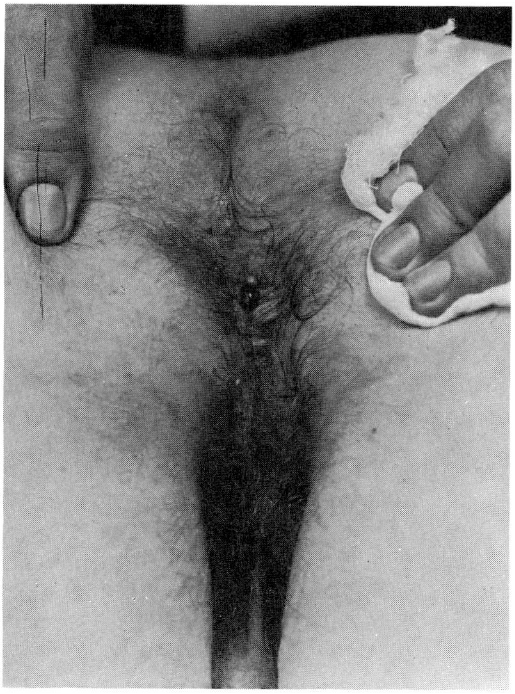

Figure 19-14. Thrombosed external hemorrhoid seen as a mass at the anal orifice.

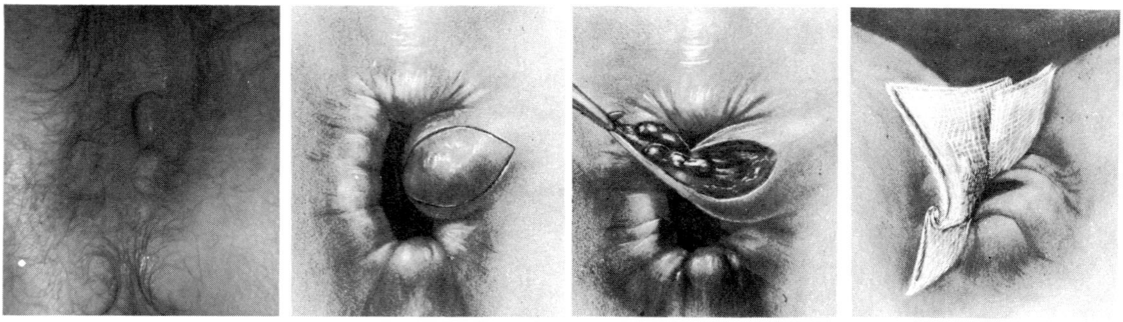

Figure 19-15. Excision of a thrombosed external hemorrhoid. The area under and around the thrombosed mass is infiltrated with 1% procaine hydrochloride containing epinephrine. An elliptical incision is made over the thrombosed mass, and the point of the ellipse is picked up in a hemostat or Allis forceps. The incision is then carried downward to remove the thrombosed vein with the overlying skin. A gauze compress is inserted into the anal canal to lie in the wound. No further dressing is necessary. (Ferguson LK: Pa Med J 40:909, 1937)

small thrombosed points scattered throughout the area of diffuse edema may be a problem.

TREATMENT

Uncomplicated external hemorrhoids rarely demand treatment.

Thrombosed External Hemorrhoids

When thrombosis occurs in the external hemorrhoidal plexus, the patient usually seeks the help of a physician because of the pain experienced. Almost immediate relief can be given in those cases in which the thrombosis is confined without marked edema. In such cases the pain seems to be due to distension in the area of thrombosis, and relief is obtained by excision of the thrombosed segment of the vein. With the patient in position on the proctoscopic table, the area about the thrombosed vein and the overlying skin is infiltrated with a local anesthetic (Fig. 19-15). With tension on the skin away from the anal orifice, an elliptical incision is made around the thrombosed vein. The flap of skin is then picked up with forceps to expose the underlying thrombosed vein, which is excised with the skin. The corner of a small square gauze compress, 3 × 3 inches, is placed on the wound. Hemostasis is achieved and no further dressing is required. The gauze is left in place for a few hours. The patient is told to expect a slight amount of pain when the effect of the anesthetic disappears. This pain may easily be relieved by a potent oral analgesic.

This method of unroofing a thrombosed hemorrhoid by the use of an elliptical incision gives better results than the simple single incision and evacuation of the clot.

The treatment of a thrombosed external hemorrhoid associated with marked edema is much less simple. Occasionally, conservative treatment with hot, moist dressings produces a gradual decrease in the inflammatory symptoms, so that the previously described procedure of unroofing the hemorrhoid is not necessary. More often, however, the thrombosis is not confined to a few large segments of veins but is diffuse. In such cases it may be necessary to excise the inflammatory mass, which is treated more satisfactorily in the hospital. Occasionally, however, it may be possible to excise the hemorrhoidal masses under local anesthesia in an ambulatory patient.

INTERNAL HEMORRHOIDS

ETIOLOGY AND SYMPTOMS

Dilatation of the upper hemorrhoidal plexus is associated almost invariably with looseness of the mucous membrane just above the dentate line or mucocutaneous junction. A question not yet settled is whether the dilatation of the hemorrhoidal vessels causes stretching and looseness of the overlying mucous membrane or whether loose attachment of the mucous membrane offers such poor support for the underlying venous plexus as to permit it to become dilated. In any event, because of straining at stool, there is distension of the internal hemorrhoids, which bulge into the lumen of the anal canal. The passage of a hardened stool mass or the frequent straining in diarrhea traumatizes the protruding mucous membrane and causes it to bleed. Frequently, the loose mucosa is dragged downward with passage of the stool, so that it prolapses through the external sphincter. In extreme cases the mucosa of the entire upper portion of the anal canal may be everted as a crimson rosette outside the anal sphincter. The bleeding is bright red and frequently appears in spurts. It may continue as long as the prolapse exists and even after the mucous membrane is replaced inside the anal canal. This troublesome symptom is most often seen in patients whose external sphincter is relaxed. The symptoms of internal hemorrhoids, therefore, are painless bright red bleeding and prolapse.

Thrombosis of internal hemorrhoids occurs less frequently than thrombosis of external hemorrhoids. When thrombosis of internal hemorrhoids is seen, the hemorrhoids are usually of the mixed type and are not the simple internal variety. However, thrombosis does occur in internal hemorrhoids. These hemorrhoids are palpated as along the wall of the upper anal canal. As a rule, they are not as hard and firm as most thrombosed external hemorrhoids.

DIAGNOSIS

The diagnosis of internal hemorrhoids may often be suspected if a careful history is taken. Even the finding of internal hemorrhoids should not deter the physician from making a careful examination of the entire lower bowel. Other lesions, such as a rectal polyp and carcinoma, may cause bleeding from the rectum.

Internal hemorrhoids may be suspected on digital palpation, but one can be certain of their pressure only on visual examination. If the patient has large hemorrhoids associated with a relaxed external sphincter, by pulling the buttocks apart as the patient strains, one can often see the mucous-membrane-covered hemorrhoidal tissue presenting at or prolapsing through the anal orifice.

Most often internal hemorrhoids can be seen on the right side posteriorly at the 2 o'clock position, and anteriorly at the 5 o'clock position; and on the left side, laterally at the 9 o'clock position (Fig. 19-16). These sites correspond to the positions of the venous radicals that drain upward from the rectum.

More definite knowledge can be obtained by examination with a lighted anoscope. With this instrument in place the hemorrhoids can be seen and become more apparent as the patient strains. Often, as the hemorrhoids are distended, bleeding appears.

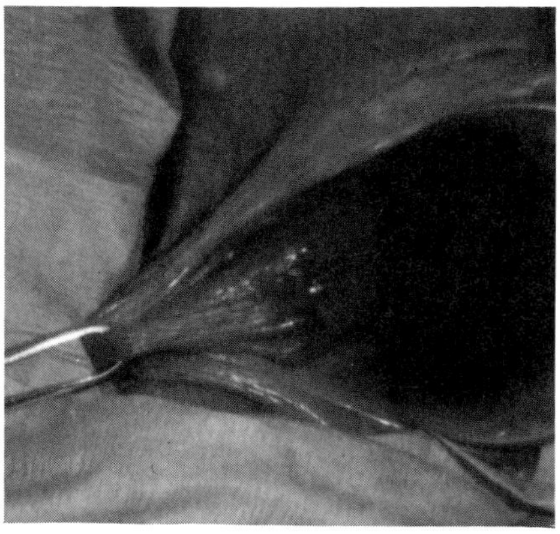

Figure 19-16. Combined prolapsed hemorrhoids.

TREATMENT

Occasionally, bleeding from internal hemorrhoids may be associated with constipation or diarrhea. Often in such cases regulation of the patient's bowel habits entirely relieves the condition. When the bleeding appears at frequent intervals in spite of well-regulated bowel habits, some more active form of therapy must be employed.

Ligation

Internal hemorrhoids have few innervating pain fibers. If one stays at least 3 mm proximal to the mucocutaneous line, there is little or no discomfort. Therefore prolapsing and often bleeding internal hemorrhoids may be treated by ligation with no anesthesia. Many methods have been and are being used. A technique now popular is the rubber band method. Corman describes his technique.

> With an anoscope in place an alligator forceps is passed [Fig. 19-17].
>
> The most prominent hemorrhoid is treated first. It is grasped and pulled through the drum of the ligator which has also been inserted through the anoscope. If the patient experiences pain, a point slightly more proximal is selected and the step is repeated. The tissue is drawn into the drum until it is taut and the trigger is released, expelling two rubber rings [Fig. 19-18].

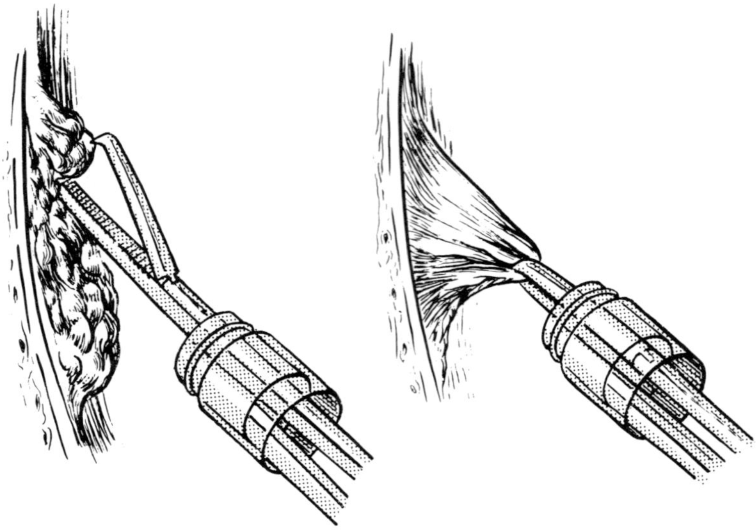

Figure 19-17. Ligation of internal hemorrhoid. (Corman ML: Rubber band ligation of hemorrhoids. Arch Surg 112:1257, 1977)

Two rings are used in case one breaks. The anoscope is then withdrawn.

The patient rarely experiences such pain that it is necessary to remove the rubber rings, but this can be done easily if necessary. They should be snapped off with a hemostat rather than cutting them with a knife or scissors because this may cause bleeding. More than one hemorrhoid site can be treated during each visit, depending on the patient's tolerance.

After the procedure, the patient should use a stool softener and take sitz baths once or twice daily. A mild analgesic is prescribed. There may be some slight bleeding when the bands cut through in 4 to 8 days. Complications include delayed hemorrhage when the rings cut through, slippage of the ligature, anal ulceration and severe pain. The procedure is a reasonable alternative to surgical hemorrhoidectomy.

Hemorrhoidectomy. Internal hemorrhoids that severely prolapse and bleed are best treated by excision. The operation is done with caudal or general anesthesia in the operating room. The patient is placed in the prone or jackknife position with the buttocks taped apart laterally. A Hill–Ferguson retractor is used for visualization of the anal canal and hemorrhoids.

A 2-0 chromic suture is placed above the prolapsing mucosa and hemorrhoids and ligated. An elliptical incision is made around the hemorrhoids as they are held up with Allis clamps. The hemorrhoids are dissected down

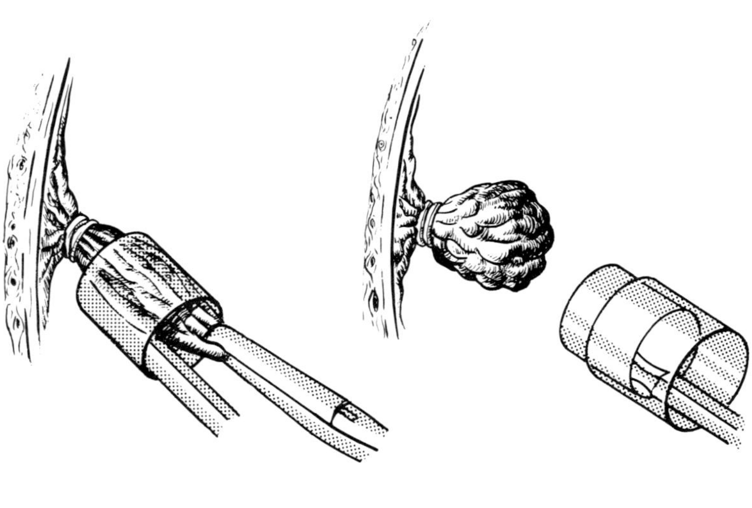

Figure 19-18. Ligation of internal hemorrhoid. (Corman ML: Rubber band ligation of hemorrhoids. Arch Surg 112:1257, 1977)

to the chronic suture and excised. The suture is used to close the surgical incision. A strip of Telfa and fluff gauze is used as dressing. Intravenous fluids are limited and the patient only sips water as needed postoperatively to help prevent urinary retention.

Cryosurgery. In cryosurgery the hemorrhoidal tissue is frozen with a liquid nitrogen or nitrous oxide probe, but the technique is not used much anymore.

Dilatation of the Anal Canal. The treatment of vigorous dilatation of the anal canal under general anesthesia, followed by regular postoperative outpatient dilatation, was described by Peter H. Lord in 1969. This procedure has the advantages of being quick, requiring only a short hospital stay, and causing less pain than surgery. The disadvantages are that there may be fecal incontinence and the patient still has the hemorrhoidal masses. This technique is not used often.

MANAGEMENT OF THE PATIENT AFTER HEMORRHOIDECTOMY

The patient who has had a hemorrhoidectomy should be examined a week after discharge from the hospital and again in a month. A digital examination is not necessary to evaluate the state of healing. If skin tags are a problem, they may be excised under local anesthesia.

Taking a hot sitz bath after each bowel movement and at least three or four times daily is the best method of keeping the area clean and of relieving the discomfort that comes from anal spasm. These baths should be continued as long as there is an open wound. At times there is some excoriation and irritation of the perianal skin. The best dressing is the easily available sanitary napkin.

Regulation of the bowels should aim for one formed stool daily. This is best accomplished by an adequate water intake. Coffee and tea should not be taken in excess. The diet should include such high-bulk and high-fiber foods as bran cereals, whole-grain cereals, and bread. If it is thought that some bulk laxative is necessary, one of the hydrophilic psyllium preparations (Effersyllium, Metamucil, Konsyl) may be used. In about 2 weeks the patient should be able to return to work and have bowel movements without discomfort.

RELIEF OF PAIN AFTER ANAL OPERATIONS

Various methods have been suggested for relief of pain after anal operations. These apply to ambulatory patients following excision of thrombosed external hemorrhoids, fissure operation, hemorrhoidectomy, and incision and drainage of an acute inflammatory perirectal abscess. Topical applications of ointments containing local anesthetics, such as lidocaine (Xylocaine) and dibucaine (Nupercaine), have been used with rather mediocre results.

Postoperative pain due to adherent clotted dressings may be largely avoided by soft strips of Telfa inserted into the wound before the fluff gauze dressing is applied. This not only results in a less painful wound but is also hemostatic.

Pain is due to traumatic irritation at the operative site. This irritation may be held to a minimum if approximation of mucosal or skin edges can be effected. The traumatic irritation of the wound site causes secondary spasm of the anal sphincter. This is most marked at the time of bowel movement. The sphincter spasm grasps and squeezes the wound and prolongs the pain after bowel movement. Applications of moist heat (hot compresses or hot sitz baths) are the most effective way to relax anal spasm and relieve anal pain. They should be used after each bowel movement and at least two times daily.

There is a general idea that the softer the stool, the less pain the patient experiences after anal operations. Greater trauma and a worse inflammatory reaction in the operative wound are caused by soiling from frequent loose or watery stools than are caused by a firm formed stool. One formed stool per day should be the aim. Usually a cathartic is not advisable, but the hydrophilic stool softeners are useful.

DISEASE OF THE RECTUM

All patients with anal, rectal, and bowel symptoms require proctosigmoidoscopy. Flexible fiberoptic sigmoidoscopes and colonoscopes and their use are discussed later. The proctosigmoidoscope should have an airtight window and a bulb-type insufflator for distending the bowel during the examination. A tube for suction, about 4 inches longer than the proctosigmoidoscope, is useful to remove liquid bowel contents.

In an endoscopic examination of the bowel the instrument should be advanced only when a lumen is seen. By manipulating the sigmoidoscope and inflating the bowel under direct vision the lumen can usually be seen. This is especially important when using the flexible fiberoptic sigmoidoscope. A proctoscopic examination should be a painless procedure. If pain is produced it usually indicates that the bowel is fixed in a position that does not allow it to be straightened out on the sigmoidoscope, and the examination should be discontinued.

The position on the table for the proctoscopic examination should be tolerable for the patient.

POLYPS OF THE RECTUM

Small polyps of the rectum are not uncommon. Most frequently they are nodules half the size of a pea. They arise from the mucosal surface of the bowel. They give no symptoms, but their prophylactic removal is recommended because they may become larger and may undergo carcinomatous change.

TREATMENT

Their removal with basket-type biopsy forceps or with a coagulating electrode is a simple matter. The tissue thus obtained should be sent for histologic examination. Hemostasis may be obtained by pressure with a swab soaked in epinephrine or by electrocoagulation.

PEDUNCULATED POLYPS OF THE RECTUM

Pedunculated rectal polyps may vary from masses the size of marbles to those so large as to encroach materially on the lumen of the rectum. They may have broad or narrow peduncles attached to the rectal wall at a relatively broad base. They may be on digital examination.

SYMPTOMS

Pedunculated polyps are subjected to the trauma of peristalsis and of the passage of the fecal mass over them. The initial symptom is frequently bleeding with the bowel movement.

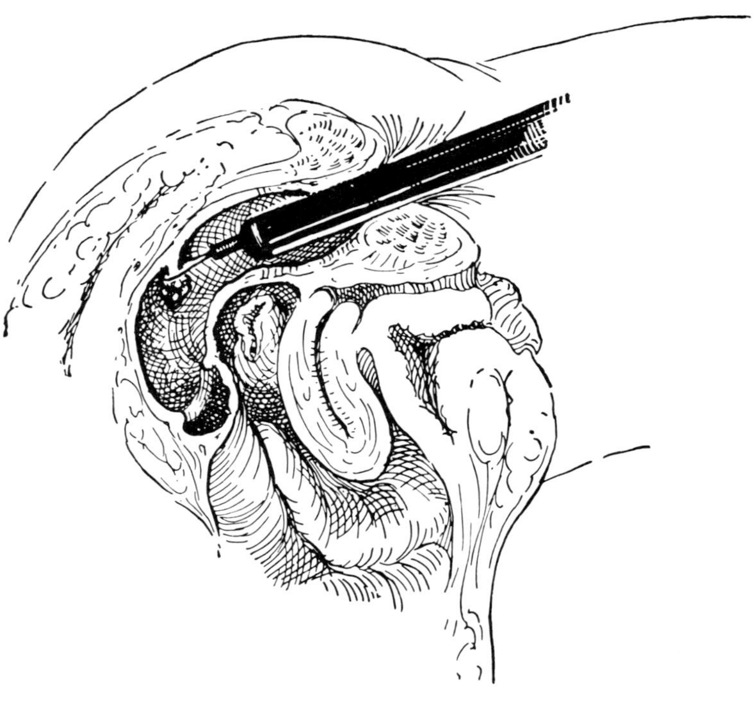

Figure 19-19. Excision of a pedunculated rectal polyp through a proctoscope; an electrocoagulating snare is being used.

Patients may complain of a dragging sensation in the rectum at the time of bowel movements, and if the polyp is large there is the constant sensation of incomplete evacuation. Occasionally, a polyp in the lower rectum may prolapse through the anus. The cause of the bleeding is easily discovered on proctoscopic examination. The bleeding may be sufficient to cause clots to form in the rectum. Most of the time the blood is bright red and mixed with mucus.

TREATMENT

It is thought that small polyps (less than 1 cm in diameter) are true adenomas and rarely have malignant potential. Large polypoid growths, however, may be small, early carcinomas. It is important, therefore, that all these growths be subjected to pathologic examination. In some cases biopsy is done before excision. In others the polyp itself is removed and is used as the specimen.

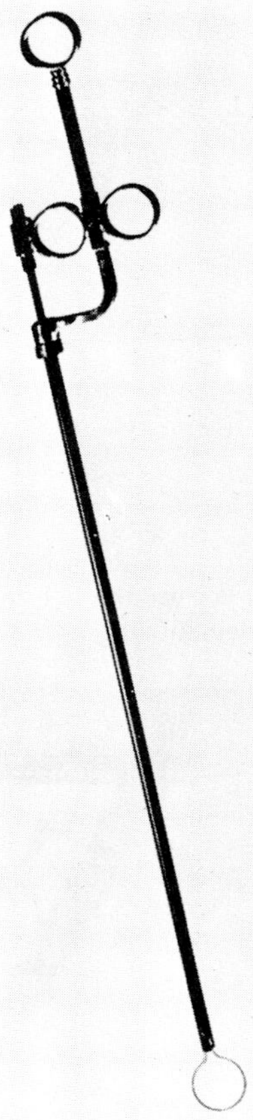

Figure 19-20. Snare for the endoscopic removal of rectal and sigmoidal polyps by electrodesiccation. (Coles Electronic Corp.)

The polyp is seen through the proctoscope. With a snare attached to an electrocoagulating current, it may be removed at its base without bleeding (Fig. 19-19 and 19-20), or it may be destroyed by electrodesiccation at one or two sittings. No anesthesia is required.

Usually no specific aftercare is required. The ulceration resulting from removal of the polyp heals in about 2 weeks, leaving a small scar. This area should be examined after 6 months and a year.

DIAGNOSIS AND BIOPSY OF RECTAL CARCINOMA

The symptoms of rectal cancer are a change in bowel habits, passage of blood, mucus, or both in the stools, crampy abdominal pains relieved by the passage of gas, extremely foul-smelling stools, passage of ribbonlike stools, and a feeling of fullness in the rectum.

This diagnosis can be made in most cases by an examination performed on an ambulatory patient. With the patient in the knee–chest or proctoscopic position, a digital examination may disclose a soft fungating mass, a deep ulcer crater with heaped-up edges, or a hard constriction of the rectal lumen. The diagnosis can be made on proctoscopic examination, by visualizing the lesion that has produced the findings of digital examination. To confirm the diagnosis a specimen is removed for biopsy.

The specimen can be obtained with a long-handled biopsy forceps (Fig. 19-21), which is introduced through the proctoscope. With the lesion under direct vision a piece of the tumor is snipped off and placed in a bottle of formalin. To control the bleeding that usually occurs, electrodesiccation may be used. The long-handled electrode with a suction attachment for smoke removal is excellent for this purpose (Fig. 19-22).

PILONIDAL CYSTS AND SINUSES

ETIOLOGY

Cysts and sinuses that develop in the sacrococcygeal area are common lesions that frequently require surgery. The origin of these

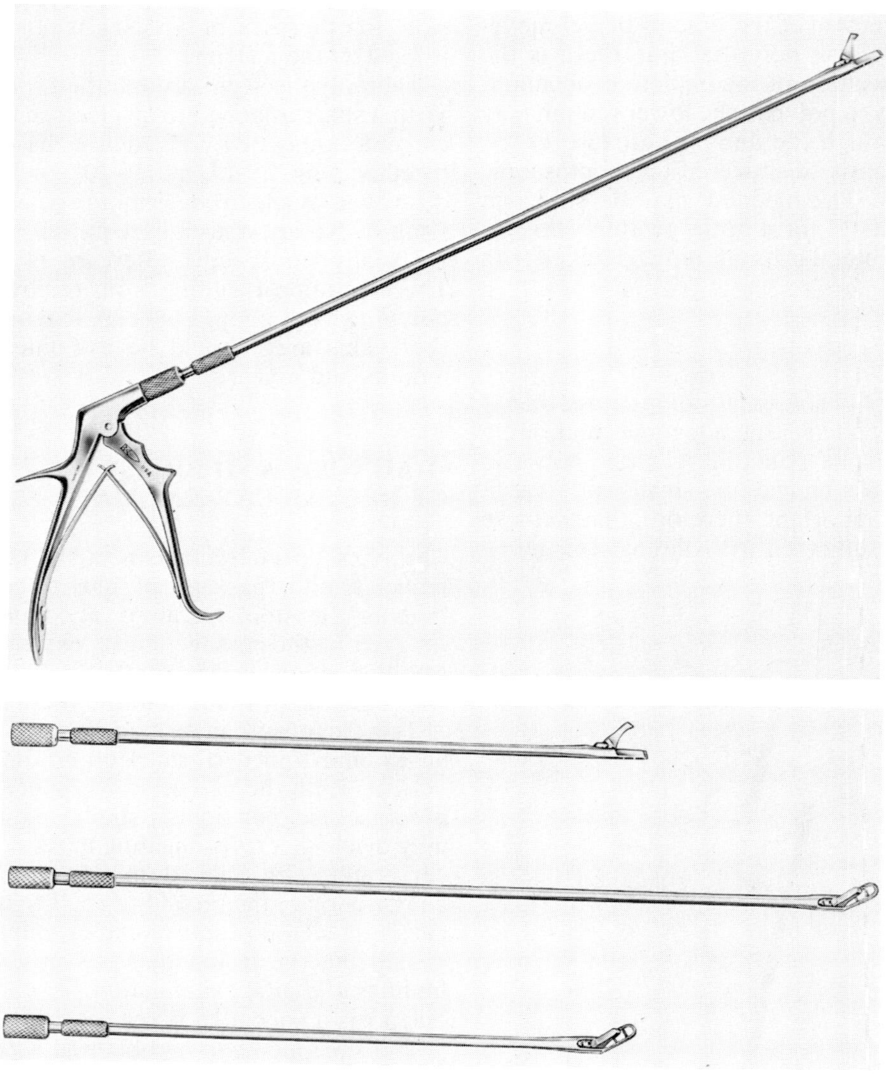

Figure 19-21. Biopsy forceps with interchangeable cutting heads for use through the protoscope to obtain specimens of rectal and sigmoidal lesions. (Welch Allyn)

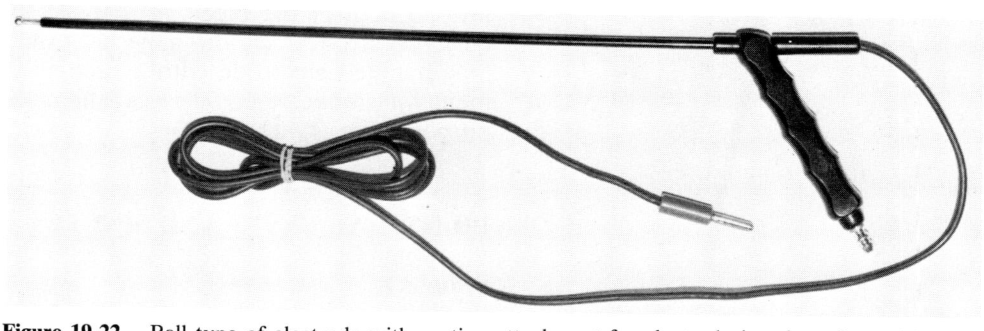

Figure 19-22. Ball type of electrode with suction attachment for electrodesiccation of rectal lesions through the proctosigmoidoscope. This instrument is often used to destroy polyps and to control bleeding after biopsy of rectal lesions (carcinomas). (Coles Electronic Corp.)

cysts has not been well established despite much embryologic and pathologic research. However, the evidence is that the lesion is primarily a typical foreign-body (hair) granuloma.

CLINICAL MANIFESTATIONS

Whatever the true etiology of these cysts and sinuses, the clinical symptoms are constant. In almost all cases there are from one to several tiny openings in the midline of the intergluteal cleft over the lower portion of the sacrum. Hairs often protrude from these openings, and there is frequently a discharge sufficient to keep the skin moist and sometimes macerated. Less commonly, there are no openings on the skin but simply a mass in the midline over the lower sacrum. As a rule, the sinuses are not noticed by the patient until early adult life, and the first symptoms are the presence of moisture, maceration, itching, and sometimes burning in the region of the sinuses.

The usual reason for treatment of a pilonidal cyst is secondary infection. The infection may be relatively mild and may subside spontaneously by the drainage of pus from the tract for a few days. Often secondary fistulous openings appear, usually at either side of the midline. These secondary fistulas may be numerous and may be some distance from the original cyst opening (Fig. 19-23).

When infection produces an abscess, a tender, red swelling appears in the midline over the lower sacrum. The patient complains of pain and tenderness, and on examination, the abscess is easily demonstrated. Frequently, pus appears at the sinus openings or following the removal of hairs that protrude from one of the sinus tracts.

TREATMENT

The treatment of pilonidal sinuses must be divided into treatment of an acutely infected pilonidal cyst or sinus and treatment of a quiescent sinus or cyst.

INCISION AND DRAINAGE

When an acute infection appears in a pilonidal cyst, it is unwise to attempt to do anything more than drain the purulent material and permit the acute inflammation to subside. It is inadvisable to attempt radical extirpation of the cyst or the sinus at this time because of cellulitis, edema, and inflammation of the surrounding tissues.

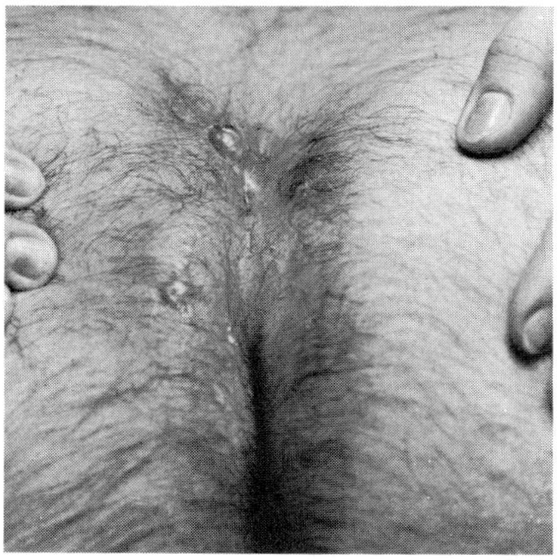

Figure 19-23. Pilonidal cyst with secondary sinus opening.

Treatment of an acute inflammation therefore consists of drainage of the purulent material and application of hot, moist dressings. This can be accomplished under local infiltration anesthesia in the ambulatory patient. The anesthetic solution is injected intradermally in the line of the proposed incision. If a suction apparatus is available, the pus in the abscess cavity may be aspirated without discomfort to the patient. Antibiotic therapy appears to aid in controlling the infection, although the inflammatory process will subside promptly without it if adequate drainage is provided.

After removal of the packing at the first dressing, the wound is searched for hair collections or deep pockets. The hairs are removed with forceps. The edges of the wound are kept apart with gauze until the wound cavity begins to fill with granulation tissue. The wounds are allowed to heal, and no further surgery is attempted in such cases for a period of 2 to 3 months.

In a very few cases there will be no recurrence after simple incisions. This is especially true if the incision has been wide and adequate drainage has been obtained. More commonly, however, recurrence can be expected unless the sinus tract is excised.

EXCISION AND PRIMARY SUTURE

In a pilonidal sinus that has healed following incision for acute infection or in a chronic draining pilonidal sinus without marked inflammatory reaction, excision of the tract and primary suture of the wound are a good method of treatment.

Procaine with epinephrine is injected around and under the sinus tract and cyst. The incision is then begun in the midline over the sinus tract and continued downward to surround the sinus opening. With sharp rakes as retractors, the incision is deepened to isolate the sinus opening entirely. An Allis forceps is then applied to close the sinus orifice and to serve as a tractor on the tissue to be removed. With the tissue constantly on tension, the dissection is then carried upward, isolating the sinus and the cyst. The line of separation from the fascia overlying the sacrum is easily recognized. When there are secondary sinus openings they are dissected out.

After removal of the cyst and the sinus, a clean wound remains with normal fatty tissue on the sides and sacral fascia in the base. Closure is effected with two layers of sutures. The first layer of four or five interrupted sutures is placed so as to include the fatty tissue on each side of the wound and the sacral fascia at its base. These sutures are all inserted before any are tied, because partial closure of the wound makes it difficult and even impossible to insert the last two sutures. This layer of sutures obliterates dead space in the base of the wound. The skin edges are approximated, and dead space is further obliterated by the use of mattress sutures of monofilament nonabsorbable material like Prolene tied over gauze rolls. Often these mattress sutures are placed first so that the deep portion of each suture includes all the layers of the wound, including the sacral fascia. The superficial portions of the mattress sutures are not placed until the buried fine sutures have been introduced and tied. Usually several interrupted sutures of fine wire are used to aid in approximation of the skin edges. A pyramidal pressure dressing of gauze is applied and held in place with firm adhesive strips.

When primary closure cannot be effected without too much tension, the skin edge is sewn to the sacral fascia or to the base of the cyst as recommended by Buie.

Most of the patients with pilonidal cyst are of the hairy type. The hairs on each side of the gluteal cleft often grow downward and act as a bristle brush on the fresh scar tissue of the healed pilonidal wound. If this healed scar is not protected, it is often traumatized by the hairs on each side of the wound, and a new ulceration appears. To avoid this complication, the area around the wound should be repeatedly shaved.

BIBLIOGRAPHY

Fistula in Ano

Dunphy JE, Pikula J: Surgery for fistula in ano. Surg Clin North Am 35:1469, 1955

Hanley PH: Anorectal supralevator abscess—fistula in ano. Surg Gynecol Obstet 148:899, 1978

Hanley PH, Ray JE, Pennington EE et al: Fistulae in ano: A ten year follow-up study on horseshoe abscess fistulae in ano. Dis Colon Rectum, 19:507, 1976

Hanley PH: Anorectum. In Hardy JD (ed): Rhoads Textbook of Surgery: Principles and Practice, 5th ed, pp 1259–1279. Philadelphia, JB Lippincott, 1977

Fissure in Ano

Arabi Y, Alexander-Williams J, Kaghley MRB: Anal pressures in hemorrhoids and anal fissure. Am J Surg 134:608, 1977

Bengt F, Rietz KA: Treatment of fissure in ano. Acta Chir Scand 128:312, 1964

Blaisdell PC: Pathogenesis of anal fissure—implication as to treatment. Surg Gynecol Obstet 65:672, 1957

Graham-Stewart CW, Greenwood RK, Loyd-Davies RW: A review of 50 patients with fissure in ano. Surg Gyecol Obstet 113:445, 1961

John N, Weinstein MA: Acute anal fissure: Treatment by lateral subcutaneous internal anal sphincterotomy. Am J Surg 136:277, 1978

Ray JE, Penfold JCB, Gathright JB Jr, Roberson SH: Lateral subcutaneous internal and sphincterotomy for anal fissure. Dis Colon Rectum 17:139, 1974

Pruritus Ani

Alexander RM, Manheim SD: The effect of hydrocortisone acetate ointment on pruritus ani (preliminary and short report). J Invest Dermatol 21:223, 1953

Buie LA: Anal pruritus. J Iowa Med Soc 29:185, 1939

Sarner JB: Etiology, diagnosis and therapy of pruritus ani. Clin Med 70:75, 1963

Condyloma Acuminatum

Abcarian H: Immunotherapy for anal condyloma acuminatum. JAMA 237:760, 1977

Culp OS, Kaplan IW: Condyloma acuminatum: 200 cases treated with podophyllin. Ann Surg 120:251, 1944

Hemorrhoids

Anscombe AR, Hancock BD, Humphreys WV: A clinical trial of the treatment of hemorrhoids by operation and the Lord procedure. Lancet ii:250–253, 1974

Barron J: Office ligation of internal hemorrhoids. Am J Surg 105:563, 1963

Barron J, Fallis LS: Nonoperative treatment of internal hemorrhoids. Can Med Assoc J 90:910, 1964

Bartigal J, Slosberg PA: An alternative to hemorrhoidectomy. Arch Surg 112:534, 1977

Corman ML: Rubber band ligation of hemorrhoids. Arch Surg 112:1256, 1977

Eisenhammer S: Internal anal sphinceterotomy plus free dilatation versus anal stretch with special criticism of the anal stretch procedure for hemorrhoids. Dis Colon Rectum 17:493, 1974

Ferguson JA, Heaton JR: Closed hemorrhoidectomy. Dis Colon Rectum 2:176, 1959

Goliger JC: Cryosurgery for hemorrhoids. Dis Colon Rectum 19:213, 1976

Khubchandani IT, Trimpi HD, Sheets JA: Closed hemorrhoidectomy with local anesthesia. Surg Gynecol Obstet 135:956, 1972

Kratzer GL: Improved technic in hemorrhoidectomy. Dis Colon Rectum 7:177, 1964

Polyps of the Rectum and Colon

Colcok BP: Relation of polyps to carcinoma of the colon and rectum. In Mulholland JH (ed): Current Surgical Management, Vol II, pp 45–53. Philadelphia, WB Saunders, 1960

Spratt JS Jr, Ackerman LV: Treatment of polyps of the colon as benign lesions. In Mulholland JH (ed): Current Surgical Management, Vol II, pp 37–41. Philadelphia, WB Saunders, 1960

Spratt JS, Ackerman LV, Moyer CA: Relationship of polyps of the colon to colonic cancer. Ann Surg 148:682, 1958

Pilonidal Disease

Abrahamson DJ: A simple marsupialization technic for treatment of pilonidal sinus: Long-term follow-up. Ann Surg 151:261, 1960

Abramson DJ: Excision and delayed closure of pilonidal sinuses. Surg Gynecol Obstet 144:205, 1977

Cherry JK: Primary closure of pilonidal sinus. Spring Gynecol Obstet 126:1263, 1968

Culp CE: Pilonidal disease and its treatment. Surg Clin North Am 47:1007, 1967

Hardaway RM: Pilonidal cyst—neither pilonidal nor cyst. Arch Surg 76:142, 1958

Heifetz CJ: Pilonidal disease: A study of fifty consecutive cases treated successfully by excision and primary closure. Am J Surg 96:405, 1958

Hirshowitz B, Mahler D, Kaufmann-Friedman K: Treatment of pilonidal sinus. Surg Gynecol Obstet 131:119, 1970

Kluge DN: Hospital versus outpatient treatment of pilonidal sinus. Surgery 57:244, 1965

Maurice BA, Greenwood RK: A conservative treatment of pilonidal cysts. Br J Surg 51:510, 1964

Notaras MJ: A review of three popular methods of treatment of postanal (pilonidal) sinus disease. Br J Surg 12:886, 1970

Pyrtek LJ, Bartus SA: Excision of pilonidal cyst with simplified partial wound closure. Surg Gynecol Obstet 118:605, 1964

Waddle RO: Ambulatory pilonidal cystectomy. J Am Osteopath Assoc 75:1066–1089, 1975

Warren JC: Abscess, containing hairs on the nates. Am J Med Sci 28:113, 1954

20 Diseases of the Vascular System

PETER F. LAWRENCE

ARTERIAL DISEASE

CHRONIC ARTERIAL OCCLUSIVE DISEASE

The development of atherosclerotic plaques in large and small arteries is a normal part of the aging process. However, this process is accelerated in smokers and persons with hypertension, diabetes, and hyperlipidemia.[1] Often, relatively few clinical symptoms appear until the atherosclerotic process is advanced, but it can be assumed that patients with localized symptoms have generalized atherosclerosis in many other vessels as well. Treatment of patients with peripheral arterial occlusive disease include palliation of localized symptomatic disease and the search for disease of other vital organs (heart, brain, kidneys, bowel) that can be life-threatening as well as disabling.

Arterial occlusive disease often begins in the abdominal aorta or any point distal to it (Fig. 20-1) and usually causes symptoms in the lower extremities. The most common location of disease is the distal superficial femoral artery as it passes through Hunter's canal.[2] Symptoms usually begin with fatigue (claudication) of the large muscles of one or both legs, thighs, or hips, which occurs with exercise and is usually relieved quite rapidly (in several minutes) by rest. Claudication occurs when the diameter of the artery supplying the symptomatic extremity is narrowed at least 50% to 60%;[3] although blood flow is adequate at rest, an increase in metabolic rate in the exercising muscle cannot be met by an adequate increase in blood flow because of the arterial narrowing. The muscle, therefore, becomes ischemic, and the patient develops fatigue. The more the atherosclerotic process narrows the lumen of the artery, the shorter the exercise time before the onset of claudication. In some patients the artery becomes so narrow that there is not even enough blood flow at rest, and the symptomatic extremity becomes painful, usually in the toes and forefoot. At this point, when the leg is chronically ischemic, the tissue is highly susceptible to injury or infection, and the blood flow is not adequate to meet the metabolic demands of these problems. Patients may then develop ischemic ulcers or infection that they are unable to heal unless blood flow to the extremity is increased.

With progressive narrowing of the lumen, there is an increasing pressure gradient across the stenosis,[4] which results in slow enlargement of preexisting blood vessels on each side of the stenosis. These blood vessels begin to carry an increasing amount of the blood around the stenosis, resulting in collateral circulation. Although it is possible for these small collateral vessels to carry the entire flow to the extremity, many vessels are needed, since flow within a blood vessel is proportional to the fourth power of its radius.[5] Therefore the total flow in the extremity and severity of symptoms are determined by the degree to which the collateral circulation can compensate for the narrowing of the major artery.

PHYSICAL EXAMINATION

The physical examination of a patient with arterial occlusive disease should involve more than merely palpation of pulses. The search for generalized diseases is an important part of the evaluation of these patients. Vital signs should be measured on all patients, including blood pressure measurements in both upper extremities to determine whether there is coexisting hypertension or upper-extremity arterial occlusive disease. A careful funduscopic

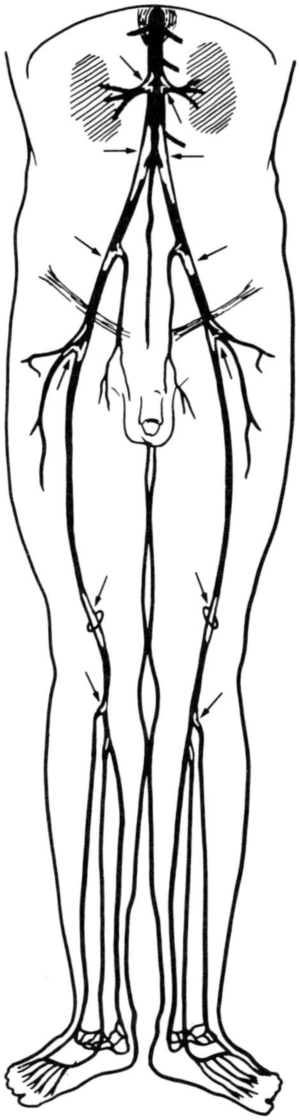

Figure 20-1. *Arrows* indicate the most common sites of atherosclerotic involvement of the abdominal aorta and its branches.

exam should be performed, searching for findings of diabetes, hypertension, or emboli to branches of the retinal artery (Hollenhorst plaques or Fisher platelet-fibrin plugs). Carotid pulses should be auscultated to identify the presence of carotid artery stenoses. The aorta and all peripheral lower-extremity pulses should also be both auscultated for bruits and palpated. Palpation can be used to grade the pulses (1–4+), to determine the presence of aneurysms, and to assess the quality of the vessel (calcified versus compliant). The feet should also be examined to determine whether trophic changes (thickened nails, thin skin, muscle atrophy) are present that indicate chronic poor tissue perfusion. In addition, rubor of the toes in the dependent, foot-dangling position and pallor on elevation of the feet above the heart both indicate poor tissue perfusion at rest. Last, capillary refill may be measured in the supine position. A delay in refill (>3 sec) indicates inadequate perfusion at rest. At the completion of the physical examination, the examiner should have an indication about the presence of generalized atherosclerotic disease, the level of arterial disease, and the degree of impairment of blood flow to the extremities.

VASCULAR LABORATORY

Since the symptoms of arterial occlusive disease usually progress slowly, careful monitoring of these symptoms can help to predict future impairment of and risk to the limb. A vascular laboratory examination, an extension of the physical examination, can provide objective documentation of the patient's condition.[6] Although most experienced vascular surgeons can accurately evaluate the degree of impairment without the aid of a laboratory, less experienced physicians may find the laboratory useful to confirm or modify their clinical impressions. Also, the vascular laboratory can be used in patients with atypical or confusing symptoms and to document changes in symptoms, which indicate the effectiveness of the therapy.

For most patients adequate assessment can be made with blood pressure cuffs, a Doppler velocity-flow detector, and a treadmill. The entire evaluation lasts 30 to 60 minutes and can be performed on an ambulatory basis. Documentation of pulses by palpation should be confirmed with a Doppler probe. Segmental arterial blood pressures are then measured by placing the Doppler probe distal to an appropriately sized blood pressure cuff. A fall in blood pressure between two cuffs of more than 30 mm Hg is evidence that a hemodynamically significant lesion is present between the cuffs.[7] The patient may then be exercised on a 10% graded treadmill at 2.25 mph until symptoms of claudication occur. Segmental blood pressures are measured again immediately after exercise. Criteria for intermittent claudication include reproducible symptoms of claudication, a maximal walking time of less than 5 minutes, and a fall in ankle segmental blood pressure to less than 60 mm Hg.[8] Treadmill testing should not be used without cardiac monitoring in patients with evidence of ischemic heart disease.

After completing the physical examination and vascular laboratory examination, a physician should be able to determine whether the patient has hemodynamically significant arterial occlusive disease and whether there is an absolute indication for surgery. Absolute indications for surgery include gangrene, an ischemic ulcer, or ischemic pain in the extremity at rest. A relative indication is disabling claudication, which prevents a patient from working or severely restricts life style. When relative indications are present, the decision about therapy should be made based on the location of disease, risks of surgery, and likelihood of short- and long-term success.

OUTPATIENT ANGIOGRAPHY

Outpatient cerebral and peripheral angiography are routine procedures. Vast experience since the 1970s has shown the safety of these techniques, but only in the past few years have they been done by large numbers of radiologists, due mainly to the use of smaller 5 French catheters. Digital subtraction arteriography (a computerized image) led to the popularity of these smaller catheters, but standard cut-film techniques can also be obtained in outpatient settings using these catheters. In fact, one does not need digital subtraction equipment to perform outpatient angiograms.

We perform the outpatient angiogram on nonhypertensive (or controlled hypertensive) patients and keep the patient 4 to 5 hours following removal of the femoral artery catheter. In more than 1000 outpatient examinations we have had to admit only three patients because of rebleeding or hematoma occurring during the 4-hour waiting period. A responsible family member or friend must always accompany the patient home and stay with the patient overnight. We instruct patient and family on compression techniques but have not had to resort to their use.

Outpatient intravenous digital subtraction angiography (DSA) was popular in the early 1980s but has fallen in popularity because of poor-quality studies in 30% of the patients. Outpatient arterial studies using the femoral or brachial routes have largely replaced IV DSA angiography. We prefer and recommend the femoral route, when possible, since 10% of patients develop decreased pulses (usually without symptoms) when the brachial artery approach is used.

A few institutions in the United States, and a larger number in Canada, are performing outpatient angioplasty for iliac arterial occlusive disease with minimal complications. However, in most institutions superficial femoral artery angioplasty and renal arterial balloon dilation require hospitalization for 48 to 72 hours.

NONOPERATIVE THERAPY

In patients who do not require surgery, nonoperative therapy usually is successful at slowing the progression of disease and reducing disability. The physiologic effect desired in all nonoperative therapy is increased blood pressure distal to the lesion through increased collateral flow, reduced resistance peripheral to the lesion, and increased delivery of red cells and oxygen to the tissue. To achieve these effects the following forms of nonoperative therapy are available:

Discontinuation of smoking is an initial and extremely important step for any patient with arterial occlusive disease. This has an immediate effect of decreasing the vasospasm due to nicotine absorption. A long-term benefit is prevention of the accelerated atherosclerosis associated with smoking.

Exercise conditioning is the mainstay of all nonoperative therapy[9] and should be prescribed for most patients. Each patient should be given a regular exercise program that consists of walking, at least three times a day, to the point of claudication. The patient should be taught to increase the number of times walked to claudication per day in a slow, progressive program. Exercise conditioning probably causes an increase in the size of the collateral blood vessels[10] and may change muscle metabolism and increase pain threshold.

The one drug that appears to effectively increase a patient's walking distance is *pentoxyfilline,* a xanthine derivative that becomes incorporated into the red blood cell membrane and increases the flexibility of the red blood cell. This allows more red cells to deliver oxygen to the tissue, and consequently exercise tolerance may increase. The usual dose of 400 mg t.i.d. is rarely associated with side-effects. It takes 6 to 8 weeks for the drug to be incorporated into enough red cells for a therapeutic effect to be seen clinically. *Transluminal angioplasty,* originally described by Dotter and Judkins in 1964,[11] did not achieve acceptance until developments in instrumentation reduced the complication rate.[12,13] The technique consists of passing a catheter to the level of the stenosis or occlusion and then forcibly dilating the artery. Angioplasty appears to be most useful in patients with iliac artery stenoses, although it is also effective in patients with more peripheral short segment stenoses or occlusions (Fig. 20-2). Long-term comparative studies show comparable results to surgery for the most favorable lesions. Angioplasty should be performed only by experienced practitioners.

ACUTE ARTERIAL OCCLUSION

Acute arterial insufficiency occurs suddenly and is due to obstruction of an artery by thrombus or embolus; early diagnosis and therapy are critical to salvage an extremity, which can usually tolerate complete ischemia for only 4 to 6 hours.[14] Although this problem is not managed on an outpatient basis, the physician who deals with ambulatory patients should be able to recognize it and initiate steps necessary for immediate management. The common findings in patients with acute ischemia are frequently referred to as the six p's: pain, paresthesia, pallor, paralysis, pulselessness, and poikilothermia. Not all these findings are present to the same degree in each patient, but their existence should alert the physician that the patient needs immediate therapy. While treatment is arranged, the is-

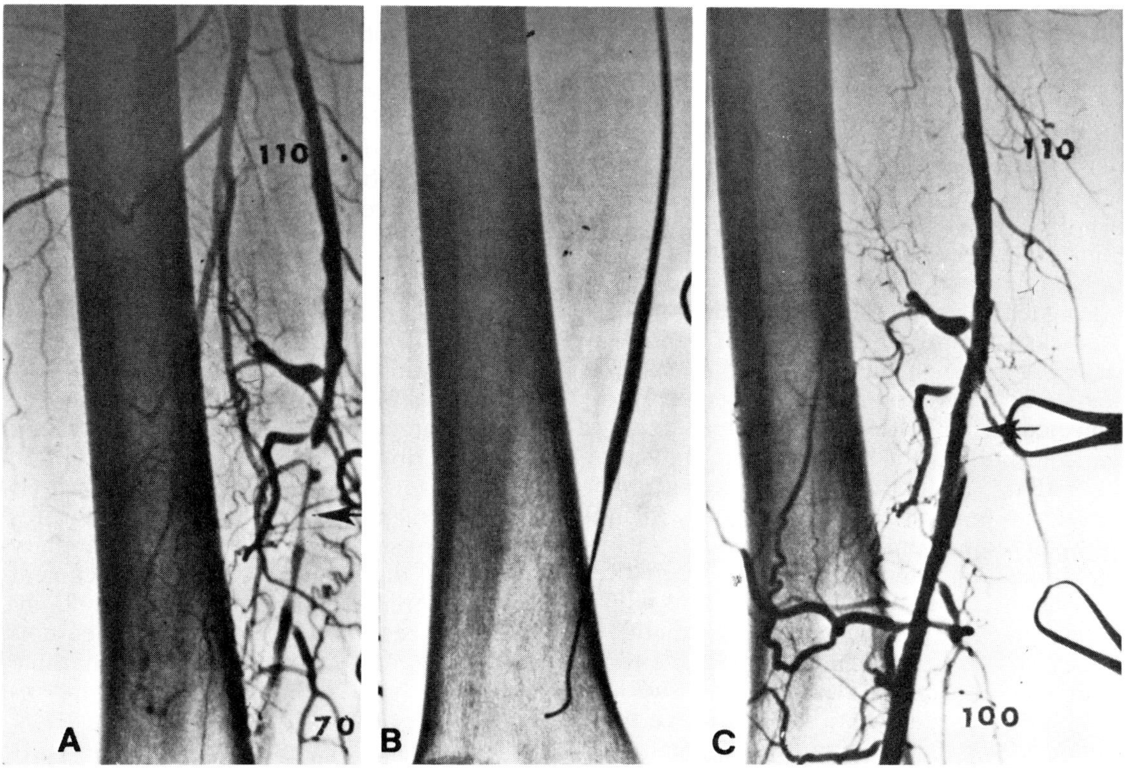

Figure 20-2. (*A*) Angiogram of a patient with rest pain in the foot, showing a gradient of 40 mm Hg across an occlusion (*arrow*) of the superficial femoral artery. (*B*) A Gruntzig balloon catheter that has been passed through the occlusion is shown inflated. (*C*) Angiograms after dilation demonstrate recanalization (*arrow*) of the artery and reduction of the pressure gradient to 10 mm Hg.

chemic limb, which is quite susceptible to injury, should be protected from excessive heat or cold. If immediate revascularization cannot be accomplished, systemic anticoagulation should be started with therapeutic doses of heparin to prevent distal propagation of thrombus.[15] If there is evidence of dehydration, fluid volume should be restored to improve the blood flow to marginal tissue. Angiography is sometimes necessary to locate the level of embolus or thrombosis, although patients without preexisting atherosclerotic disease, whose site of clot can be localized, do not necessarily need an angiogram.

ACUTE PERIPHERAL ARTERIAL INJURIES

In the civilian population, arterial injuries due to blunt and penetrating trauma are increasing as a result of motor vehicle accidents and urban violence. Early recognition of primary and associated arterial injury should lead to prompt and successful management of many of these patients. Some patients with a penetrating or blunt injury of the extremity can be managed on an ambulatory basis unless an arterial injury is suspected. The following findings suggest arterial injury:

Proximity of the injury to a major artery
Large or expanding hematoma
Absence of or reduced distal pulse
Bruit at the site of injury
Injury to a nerve adjacent to an artery

Frequently, exploration or angiography is necessary to verify the presence of arterial injury.[16] A common misconception is that patients with an arterial injury always have a diminished distal pulse; patients may have a palpable pulse with severe intimal injury or disruption.[17] A diminished pulse signifies that an arterial injury is hemodynamically significant and requires immediate attention. All patients in whom arterial injury is suspected require admission to the hospital. Patients with a penetrating injury to the extremity without evidence of a vascular injury should have thorough debridement of devitalized tissue and tetanus immunization prior to discharge from the hospital. Reexamination after 24 hours but sooner than 48 hours for further evidence of devitalized tissue, infection, or arterial ischemia due to edema and extrinsic compression is important.

RAYNAUD'S SYNDROME

Vasospasm of the distal arteries of an extremity exists in two forms, one idiopathic (Raynaud's disease) and one associated with an underlying connective tissue disorder (Raynaud's phenomenon). Vasospasm may occur secondary to many stimuli, but cold and anxiety are the most common. The hands typically undergo a progression of color changes from white to blue to red, because of the interruption of arterial flow followed by vasodilation. Patients with Raynaud's disease are often young women who have no organic obstruction of the digital arteries and in whom the disease rarely progresses to ulceration of digits and autoamputation. Those with Raynaud's phenomenon and an underlying disease frequently have organic obstruction of the artery,[18] and the disease may progress to digital ulceration and autoamputation.

DIAGNOSIS

Most patients have a history of cold sensitivity associated with characteristic changes in temperature and color of the hand on cold immersion. If the disease is bilateral and occurs in an otherwise healthy individual, the most likely cause is idiopathic Raynaud's disease.[19] Patients with digital ulceration or unilateral symptoms probably have an underlying disease, and a careful search should be made for this. The following work-up should be considered in patients with unilateral symptoms or tissue loss:

Careful physical examination and search for skin or joint abnormalities and signs of carpal-tunnel or thoracic outlet syndrome
Chest roentgenography to determine whether cervical ribs are present
Noninvasive laboratory studies, including (1) measurement of segmental blood pressures and plethysmography from upper extremity to distal digits, which help to document fixed arterial occlusive disease; (2) cold immersion tests with temperature measurement (patients with Raynaud's syndrome typically have prolonged temperature recovery)[20]
Laboratory work-up, including lupus erythematosus preparation, antinuclear antibodies (ANAs), complement (C3), Coombs' test, platelet count, erythrocyte sedimentation rate

Angiography to help define the location of arterial disease in patients with tissue loss, unilateral Raynaud's symptoms, or evidence of arterial occlusive disease. This should include an arch study for proximal disease and angiography of the upper extremity with detailed films of the hand. If vasospasm is noted, priscoline may be infused to vasodilate the vessels and differentiate fixed occlusive from vasospastic disease.

Nerve conduction studies in patients with symptoms of carpal tunnel or thoracic outlet syndrome

THERAPY

The treatment of vasospasm should be tailored to the patient and determined by the degree of cold sensitivity. All therapy has as its goal a reduction in vasospasm, usually by reducing sympathetic tone. Nonoperative therapy is successful in most patients, particularly those with Raynaud's disease. Most patients with Raynaud's syndrome will have mild symptoms and require only education about the need to avoid cold contact with the hands. All smokers should be encouraged to discontinue tobacco use. In patients who have symptoms in spite of cold avoidance, drugs that reduce sympathetic tone are frequently used. Orally administered norepinephrine-depleting drugs (guanethidine 10 mg/day to 30 mg/day) and α-adrenergic blocking agents (phenoxybenzamine 20 mg/day to 30 mg/day) benefit 80% to 90% of patients and should be tried in all symptomatic patients.[21] Nifedipine (30 mg/day) has also been successful in many patients. Biofeedback, a behavioral conditioning technique, trains patients to warm the distal extremities prior to cold contact.[22] In our experience this technique has high patient acceptance and frequently allows patients to discontinue other drugs.

ACCESS ROUTES FOR HEMODIALYSIS

Over the past 20 years the increased availability of hemodialysis machines has allowed most patients with chronic renal failure to undergo long-term dialysis. With the increased use of hemodialysis for patients with acute and chronic renal failure, procedures to achieve access to the circulation have become extremely common. In fact, at some hospitals, vascular access procedures are among the most commonly performed. Because of the limited number of sites for easy vascular access, the timing, location, and technique in performing an access procedure are of critical importance in making the dialysis comfortable for the patient and in reducing the number of subsequent surgical procedures necessitated by access site failure.

PREOPERATIVE ASSESSMENT

All patients who are to undergo an angioaccess procedure must be carefully evaluated preoperatively to determine the optimal site for initial placement of the access route. In patients with chronic renal failure it is important to make decisions regarding the location and type of access prior to the development of end-stage renal failure. In this way only one procedure is necessary to establish vascular access. Also, it is useful to know who will be performing the dialysis procedure, since technicians who have had experience in hemodialysis are more adept at the handling and puncture of all access sites. Patients undergoing dialysis at home without a technician may need a large superficial fistula to reduce the difficulty of performing the procedure. The access site is also important in patients with reversible renal failure; however, the location is not as critical because the catheter will be removed within months, and often no further access site will be needed. In patients with either irreversible or chronic renal failure, future access sites must be protected from repeated venous or arterial puncture. We have found it useful to mark the arm with indelible ink to dissuade inexperienced or desperate blood drawers from sticking the site selected for a future fistula.

PHYSICAL EXAMINATION

In many patients a careful physical examination is all that is necessary to determine the optimal location of an access site. Examination of the extremity should consist of a search for evidence of chronic arterial or venous insufficiency, active infection, and superficial or deep thrombophlebitis. The adequacy of an artery frequently can be determined by palpation; the optimal artery is soft with an adequate pulse. Diabetics may have medial sclerosis of the artery, which creates the feeling of a rigid pipe; although not optimal, this artery can be used if it has an adequately sized lumen with satisfactory blood flow through it. After palpation of the artery, an attempt should be made to determine the physiologic consequences of the angioaccess procedure. Allen's test helps to determine if the deep arch is patent and if there is adequate collateral blood flow to perfuse the distal extremity when one vessel is occluded (Fig. 20-3).

The recipient vein can be assessed by placing a tourniquet on the proximal extremity and occluding venous outflow. The ideal vein runs adjacent to the donor vessel, distends easily to a large caliber, has few side branches, and lies in a superficial position. Frequently, we must accept a less than ideal vein and make plans to correct it in the operating room.

NONINVASIVE VASCULAR LABORATORY

Sometimes it is difficult to determine by physical examination alone whether a particular site has an adequate artery and vein for placement of a shunt or fistula. Many patients have previously been subjected to multiple venous and arterial punctures, which have resulted in thrombosis of these vessels. Also, those who require hemodialysis often have diabetes, hypertension, and atherosclerosis in addition to uremia, all of which are associated with a high incidence of arterial occlusive disease. Rather than exploring an extremity blindly, hoping to find an adequate artery or vein, it is far better to predict preoperatively the best site for angioaccess.

The vascular laboratory can help assess the patency of arteries, determine the adequacy of collateral circulation distal to a donor artery, and assure the patency of recipient veins. We find that the vascular laboratory examination is particularly helpful in a patient who has had a prior access procedure.

We would suggest that the following be included in a routine vascular laboratory examination:

All arteries in the limb should be assessed with a Doppler probe. Normal arteries have a Doppler signal with three components[23]; characteristics of the Doppler wave form that indicate arterial obstruction include widening and decreased amplitude of the forward flow component and absence of reversed flow.

Segmental limb pressures can determine whether a hemodynamically significant lesion is present in the limb.[24] With a Doppler probe placed over the artery just distal to an appropriately sized blood pressure cuff, in a normal patient blood pressure in the distal limb is equal to or 10% higher than blood pressure in the proximal limb. If a hemodynamically significant lesion is present, the distal blood pressure will be at least 20 mm Hg to 30 mm Hg lower than the proximal pressure. In diabetic and nondiabetic patients with medial sclerosis of the vessels, segmental blood pressures may be falsely elevated because of "stiff arteries."[25]

Collateral compression tests, such as a modified Allen's test (Fig. 20-3), can help determine the presence of collateral circulation, particularly when the standard Allen's test is equivocal.

Determination of the patency of small superficial recipient veins can be difficult for an inexperienced examiner, but all veins (superficial or deep) have characteristic sounds when patent.[26] Venous sounds are low pitched and may be heard best with the 5-MHz Doppler. To locate normal veins it is helpful to compress the extremity distal to the Doppler, causing an increase in venous return (compression augmentation). Respiratory cycling—that is, alterations in venous return with changes in intrathoracic pressure—can normally be heard in the larger proximal veins. The absence of respiratory cycling and compression augmentation is indicative of obstructive venous disease. To reduce observer error when evaluating the venous system, the extremity should be compared with the contralateral side.

ANGIOGRAPHY–VENOGRAPHY

Although noninvasive studies are helpful in determining the adequacy of the artery and vein for an arteriovenous (AV)-fistula, it is sometimes difficult to determine the location of an adequate vein. Rather than exploring the vein in the operating room, we often use preoperative venography, particularly in obese patients with deep subcutaneous veins, patients with multiple small veins, or those who have had previous access procedures. We rarely find it necessary to perform arteriography to determine the adequacy of the donor artery.

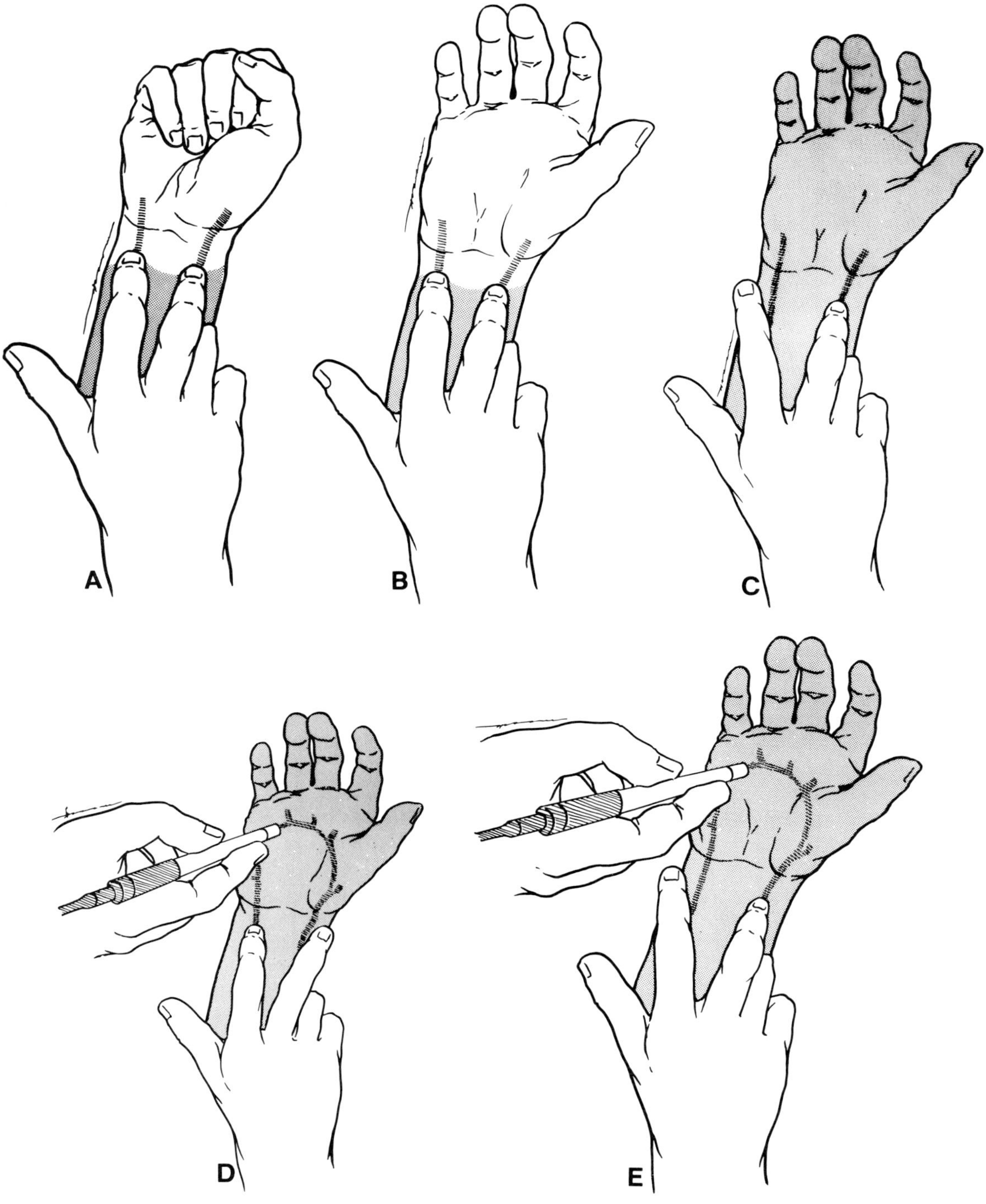

Figure 20-3. Allen's test of patency of the ulnar artery, radial artery, and deep arch. (*A*) While the patient's fist is clenched the examiner occludes the radial and ulnar arteries simultaneously. (*B*) Paleness of the hand on opening of the fist confirms that the pressure is adequate to occlude the arteries. (*C*) On releasing of the ulnar (or radial) artery normal color will return to the hand within 3 to 5 seconds if the artery and deep arch are patent.

When the standard Allen's test is equivocal a modified test is performed: while the radial artery (*D*) or ulnar artery (*E*) is occluded the examiner listens with the Doppler detector over the deep palmar arch; if the vessel and arch are patent, normal arterial sounds should be heard with the Doppler detector.

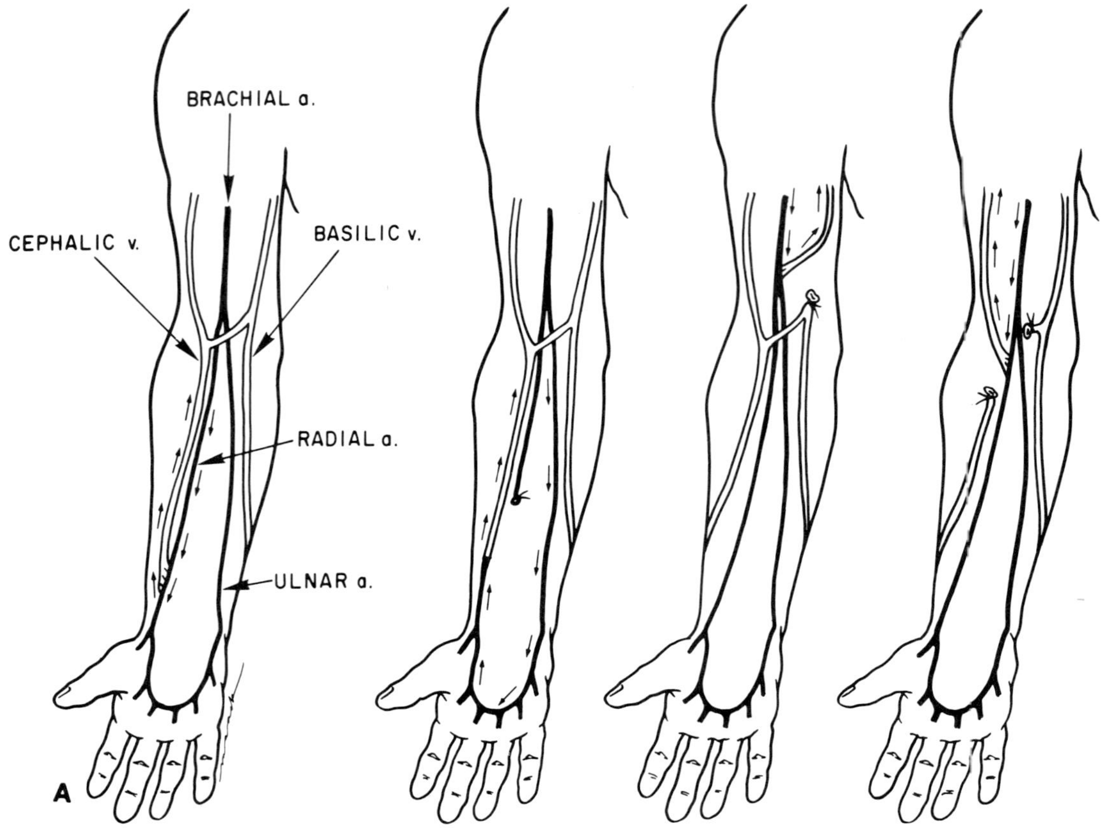
BRACHIAL a.
CEPHALIC v.
BASILIC v.
RADIAL a.
ULNAR a.
A

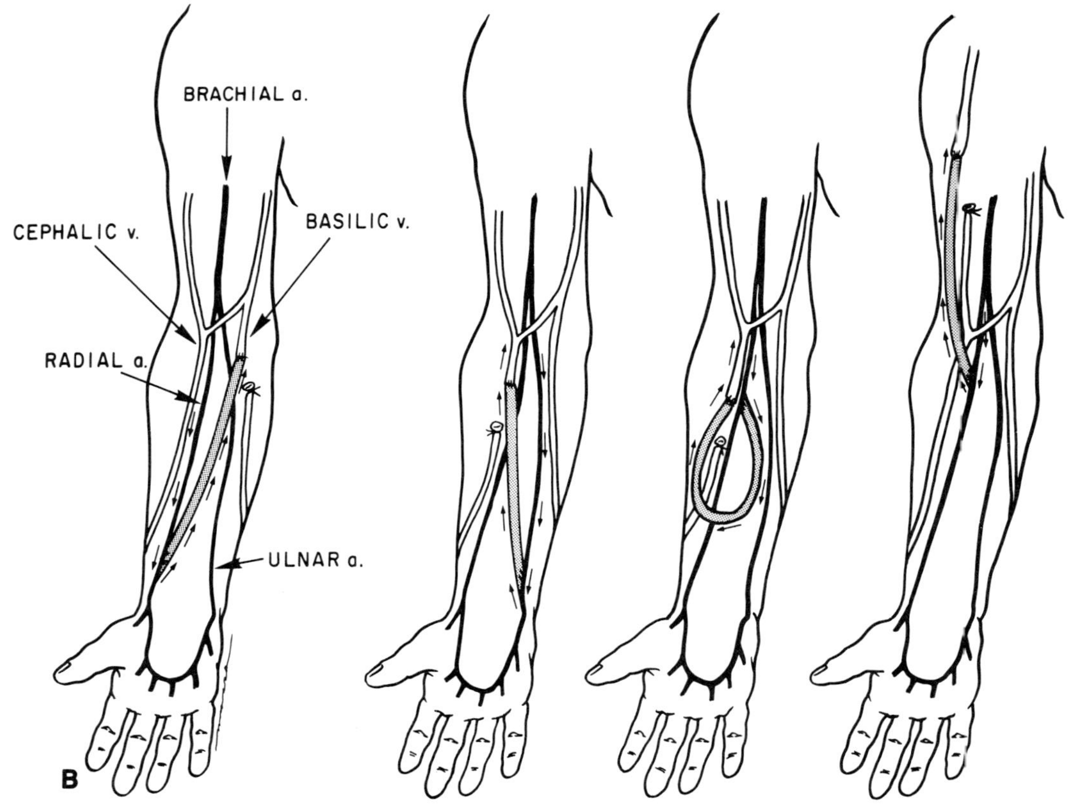
BRACHIAL a.
CEPHALIC v.
BASILIC v.
RADIAL a.
ULNAR a.
B

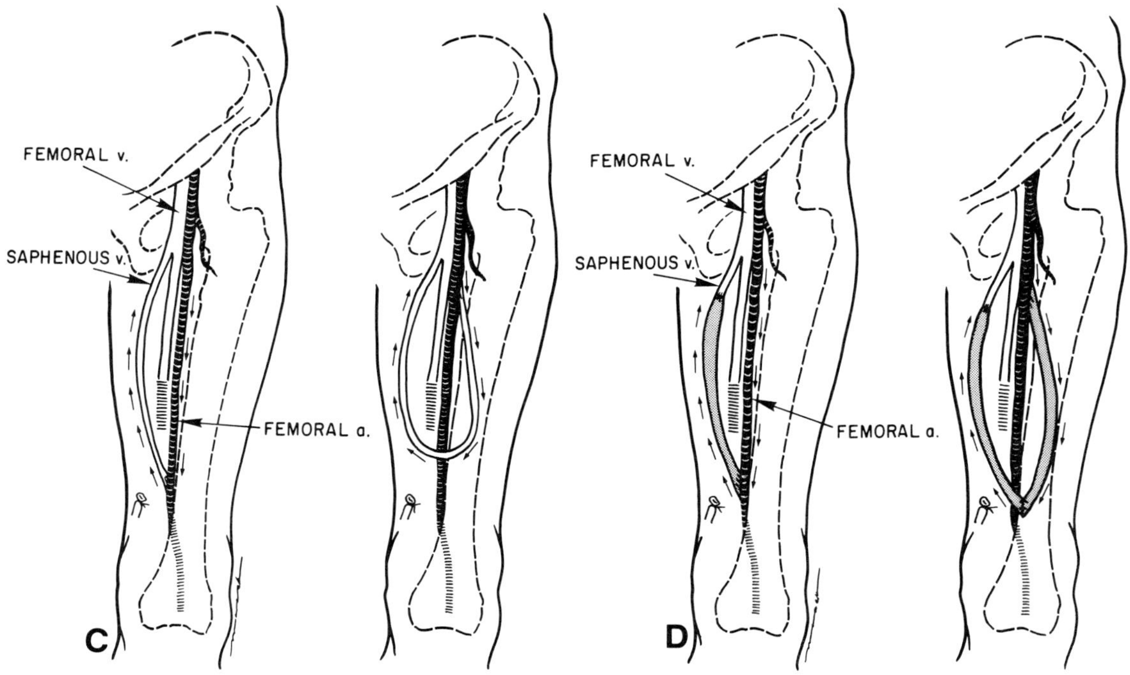

Figure 20-4. Potential sites of arteriovenous fistulas: in the upper extremity using (*A*) native veins and (*B*) a graft material; in the lower extremity using (*C*) native veins and (*D*) a graft material.

ACCESS FOR ACUTE HEMODIALYSIS

In situations in which the need for hemodialysis develops suddenly, a temporary site may need to be used to provide immediate access for hemodialysis. The subclavian dialysis catheter has replaced the external Scribner shunt as the most commonly used device to provide immediate access. The subclavian catheter can be placed percutaneously and used immediately for hemodialysis. The catheter frequently remains patent for months, while another permanent access site for hemodialysis is developed.

ARTERIOVENOUS FISTULA

Once it has been decided that a patient will require long-term hemodialysis, it is preferable to use an internal AV fistula, which has a higher patency rate than an external shunt or subclavian catheter, is associated with fewer complications (i.e., infection, dislodgment), and allows the patient to lead a more normal life style (e.g., bathing).

The more careful the initial assessment of artery and vein, the higher the likelihood of success when preforming an AV fistula. Unfortunately, the one factor that cannot be predicted accurately from any preoperative test is the capacity of the vein to dilate to a diameter that makes fistula puncture and adequate flow (200 ml/min to 350 ml/min) possible.

Although a variety of sites has been suggested for initial placement of an internal AV fistula (Fig. 20-4), we feel that a systematic approach is associated with a combination of the highest patency rate, lowest incidence of complications, and most conservative use of potential access sites that may be needed in the future. Our plan is generally as follows:

1. Construct a fistula between the most distal adequate artery and vein in the nondominant forearm.
2. If this fails or a site is unavailable, move proximally up the nondominant forearm, again using the most distal artery and vein available. If there is a distance between these vessels, vascular graft (expanded polytetrafluoroethylene) should be used.
3. If the fistula fails in the forearm, the upper arm is the next available site.
4. After access sites have been used on one upper extremity, the same progression should be used in the other extremity. If

preferred, one may instead alternate between the upper extremities, using the most distal available site.

5. Lower-extremity fistulas should be considered in patients in whom upper-extremity AV fistulas have failed, although the complication rate is higher with these fistulas.
6. In patients who are obese, have poor superficial veins, or present special problems, the best artery and vein available should be used initially.

Although we generally prefer an AV fistula of the Brescia–Cimino type, there are advantages and disadvantages to all types of internal fistulas[27,28] and graft materials[29] (Table 20-1), and the approach should be based on the experience of the surgeon and individualized to the patient's needs.

Technique for Arteriovenous Fistula at the Wrist

Either local infiltration or axillary block anesthesia is used. The radial artery and the cephalic vein are mobilized to free 3 cm to 5 cm of both artery and vein so that no tension exists at the suture line and no excessive angulation of the vessels is produced.

The vein is carefully dissected free of all surrounding tissue to permit its dilatation once arterial flow is established. The artery is likewise carefully freed, and all small branches are ligated. Wrapping both artery and vein for 5 to 10 minutes with a gauze sponge soaked in a 1% papaverine solution helps reduce spasm. Blood flow is controlled by plastic tourniquets placed proximally and distally on the artery and vein. After these tourniquets are tightened, an incision is made in the artery. If necessary, the vein is spatulated to fit the longitudinal artery.[30] Prior to construction to the anastomosis, 5F and 8F infant-feeding tubes filled with heparinized saline solution are passed up the vein to the elbow, with the solution being used to dilate the vein gently. The ability to pass an 8F feeding tube ensures that the vein is of adequate caliber and has been shown to correlate closely with development of an adequately sized AV fistula.[31]

The anastomosis is created with a running 6-0 or 7-0 double-armed atraumatic nonabsorbable suture (Fig. 20-5). Great care in suture placement is necessary to assure catching all layers of both vessels. Be sure to place sutures carefully at both corners. If a palpable thrill is not present at the completion of the anastomosis, the likelihood of fistula failure is high (95%), and the fistula should be revised. A light dressing is applied and great care is taken to prevent compression or kinking. To increase flow through the fistula, the patient is instructed to exercise the arm by squeezing a rubber ball repeatedly at least three times a day.

Postoperative Evaluation

In most patients a postoperative physical examination is adequate to evaluate the functioning of an AV shunt or fistula. A thrill can usually be felt just proximal to the anastomosis of a fistula. If the thrill is not palpable, auscultation usually reveals a bruit secondary to turbulent flow.

At times palpation or auscultation may be difficult because of swelling around the wound. In these situations the Doppler can be useful in assessing the patency of the AV fistula. Although it is not possible to dialyze through a fistula that is audible but not palpable, the presence of a Doppler signal demonstrates that the fistula is still functioning and may develop a palpable thrill. The successful, mature AV fistula shows characteristic changes of normal or increased segmental blood pressures and increased diastolic Dop-

TABLE 20-1. Common Graft Materials

MATERIAL	EARLIEST USE	POST-OPERATIVE CELLULITIS	% 1-YR PATENCY	INTIMAL HYPERPLASIA (1 YR)	INFECTION (1 YR) (%)	THROMBOSIS (1 YR) (%)	ANEURYSM (1 yr) (%)	COST OF GRAFT
Autogenous vein in situ (Brescia–Cimino)	3–6 wk	Rare	≈95	Develops slowly	Rare (1)	Rare (5)	Rare (1)	Free
Expanded PTFE	1-4 wk	Common	≈75	Develops moderately fast	Rare (5)	Uncommon (8)	Rare (1)	Expensive

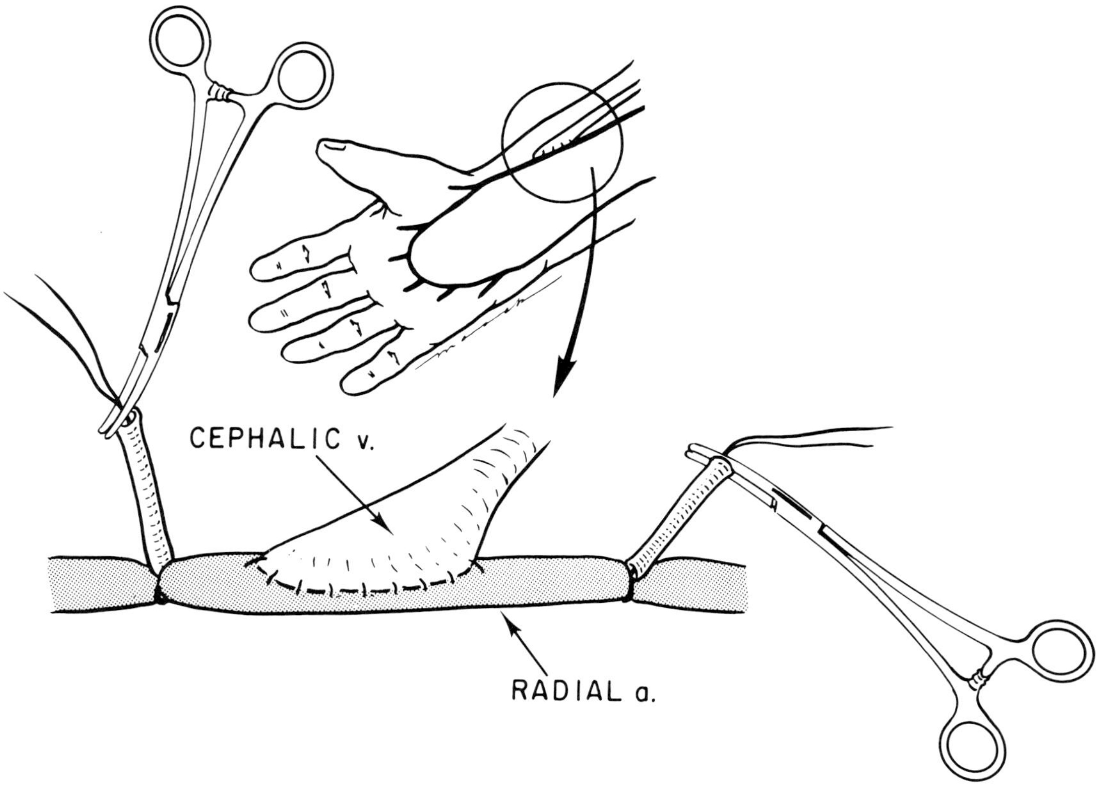

Figure 20-5. Meticulous technique must be used with the arteriovenous anastomosis so that there is no narrowing of the bell-shaped vein.

pler velocity proximal to the fistula, with normal to decreased values distally.[32] The vascular laboratory also can be quite useful in evaluating numerous complications of an AV fistula or shunt, including narrowing of the fistula and imminent failure, distal steal, arterial insufficiency, and distal venous hypertension.

Venous fistulography can be extremely useful in examining a malfunctioning AV fistula that still has a palpable thrill.[33] It is possible with this technique to evaluate both decreased arterial inflow to the fistula and high venous resistance or obstructed outflow. When there is malfunction of an AV fistula, we suggest that this technique be performed early rather than allowing the fistula to thrombose. The technique is quite simple and involves placing a 19-gauge scalp vein needle into the proximal portion of the AV fistula, occluding all flow to the arm with a proximal arm cuff of 250 mm Hg and injecting 20 ml angiographic contrast material while performing serial radiography. Filming starts 0.5 sec before the end of the injection and continues at a rate of two/sec, and the cuff is released after the third film. If any question remains about differentiating arteries from veins, the fistula can be occluded first proximal and then distal to the needle during injection of contrast material.

Complications of an Arteriovenus Fistula

Thrombosis. The most frequent cause of fistula failure is thrombosis; common causes of initial failure are poor surgical technique with anastomotic narrowing, inadequate venous runoff or venous spasm, and external compression from a tight bandage. If the fistula fails after having functioned adequately, common causes include hypovolemia, intimal flaps from fistula puncture, perifistula hematoma with compression, hypercoagulability during general anesthesia, and intimal hyperplasia around the suture line.[34] Impending failure of an AV fistula should be suspected when there is a reduction in flow or a progressive increase in venous pressure during dialysis. When a previously functioning fistula begins to fail, it is critical that the situation be rapidly evaluated, usually by fistulography, to determine the site of and reason for failure. Although surgical revision of a narrowed fistula is frequently successful, we have had excellent results using the Grüntzig balloon catheter to dilate narrowed segments of the fistula.[35]

Aneurysm. A common complication due to repeated fistula punctures at the same site is a fistula aneurysm.[36] Once an aneurysm is noted, this site should not be used for any more punctures. Frequently, the aneurysm stabilizes at a small size and does not require excision. Indications for excision include expansion, skin erosion, and infection. Usually the same fistula can be used for hemodialysis after the aneurysm is excised.

Undeveloped Fistula. An inadequate fistula for dialysis is a common problem, particularly when distal fistulas are created. Three to 4 weeks are usually necessary to allow the fistula to mature. If it does not have adequate flow at this time, a search should be made for branches of the vein that may be carrying a large volume of blood and not allow the main vein to dilate. These can easily be ligated under local anesthesia. Fistulography is indicated for any fistula that does not have adequate flow for dialysis.

Arterial Insufficiency. The uncommon problem of arterial insufficiency occurs in patients with a high-flow AV fistula or underlying arterial occlusive disease.[37] To reduce the risk of this complication, careful preoperative evaluation should identify patients with inadequate collateral blood flow. Also, if fistulas are limited to less than 8 mm in anastomosis length and grafts of 6-mm diameter or less are used, then the risk of a high-flow steal will be reduced. Fistulas constructed to large proximal arteries should have tapered graft placed to reduce the risk of a steal syndrome. If arterial insufficiency occurs, the effect of fistula occlusion on segmental blood pressures should be determined and the fistula revised or ligated to improve peripheral flow. Also, ligation of the distal radial artery can be helpful in patients with radial artery steal syndrome.

Venous Hypertension. Venous hypertension should not occur if an end-vein-to-side-artery AV fistula is constructed and major venous branches are ligated. If venous hypertension does occur, manual compression of venous branches, fistulography, or both can help determine which branches should be ligated.

Infection. Infection in fistulas is uncommon compared with its incidence in shunts. It usually responds to antibiotics, but if sepsis or infection of a graft occurs, excision of the fistula and/or graft material may be necessary.

Congestive Heart Failure. Occurring mainly in patients with AV fistulas greater than 8 mm in diameter with flows of more than 400 ml/min to 500 ml/min, congestive heart failure, although an uncommon problem, may necessitate narrowing or ligation of the fistula.

VENOUS DISEASE

Although venous problems remain one of the most common causes of morbidity among the general population, they rarely cause mortality and therefore are sometimes relegated to a secondary priority by many physicians. The lack of an effective treatment or "cure" for many venous disorders also discourages some physicians from an aggressive therapeutic approach. Yet recently there has been considerable progress in treating certain venous disorders, such as proximal venous obstruction.[38] In order to recognize patients with venous disorders who might benefit from these newer forms of therapy, it is important to diagnose and classify accurately all venous disease. Venous disease can conveniently be divided into two general categories: primary varicosities or varicose veins (i.e., abnormal enlargements of the superficial veins) and the clinical sequelae of deep vein thrombophlebitis (secondary varicose veins and the postphlebitic leg).

ANATOMY AND FUNCTION OF THE VENOUS SYSTEM

Venous blood is returned to the heart from the extremities by two sets of veins, the deep and the superficial (Fig. 20-6). The deep veins run below the muscular fascia and usually are adjacent to major arteries; below the knee and elbow these veins are paired (venae comitantes). All deep veins have thin, slightly muscled walls, since they are externally supported by the bones, muscles, and fascia. The superficial system is much more variable in its location, although major branches (greater

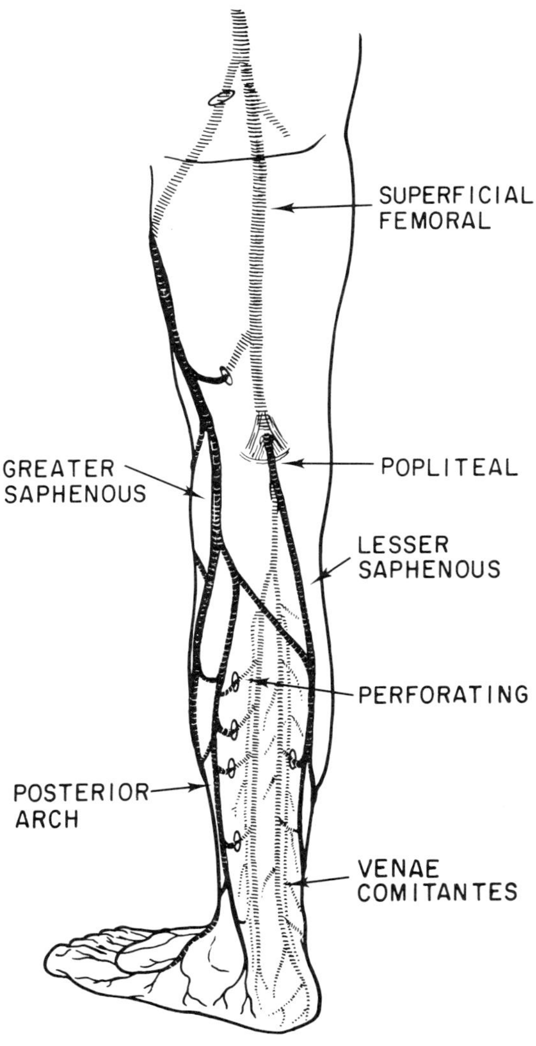

Figure 20-6. Normal venous anatomy of the lower extremity. Note the perforating venous connections between the superficial and deep systems.

and lesser saphenous veins) tend to have a predictable course. Since there is minimal external support, these veins possess a thicker muscular wall, which is thickest in the most dependent part of the leg. Connections between the superficial and deep systems, called perforating veins, occur at numerous sites along the leg and arm.[39] It should be noted that these "perforators" often do not originate from the major subcutaneous veins; this has great clinical significance, since removal of the major vein may not correct perforator disease. Bicuspid valves are present in the superficial, perforating, and deep veins, directing the blood flow from superficial to deep and toward the heart. Competent valves are critical to the efficient return of blood to the heart.[40] When a muscle contracts, raising venous pressure up to 200 mm Hg, venous blood is propelled toward the heart. As the muscle relaxes, competent venous valves prevent the backflow of venous blood to its former position. Other forces that contribute to venous flow include capillary pressure and negative intra-abdominal pressure with respiration. In addition to their function as conduits of blood, veins have major thermoregulatory and capacitance functions.[41]

VARICOSE VEINS

The attitude of some physicians toward the normal and varicosed (abnormally enlarged) superficial veins of the lower extremity has been somewhat cavalier in the past, since these veins, which carry only 15% to 20% of the venous return from the legs, were felt to be of little value to the patient. With the use of the normal saphenous vein for peripheral vascular reconstruction and coronary artery bypass, it has become increasingly important that normal portions of this vein are left in situ. It has also been recognized that these veins dilate not only as a result of disease in the superficial venous system (primary varicosities), but from pressure transmitted through diseased deep and perforating veins (secondary varicosities; Fig. 20-7).[42] Recognition of this difference between primary and secondary varicose veins is critical to the successful management of these patients.

Etiology

Primary varicose veins are due to either congenital or acquired dilatation of the superficial vein associated with incompetence of the valves. Although there is a familial predilection to primary varicose veins, reports suggest that these varicose veins may also be related to environmental and dietary factors.[43] Many conditions that increase intra-abdominal pressure, such as pregnancy, are associated with a higher incidence of varicose veins. Congenital defects in valves, particularly at the saphenofemoral junction,[44] may dilate the proximal saphenous vein and cause subsequent dilatation of the other previously competent valves.

Secondary varicose veins occur when there has been damage and incompetence of the

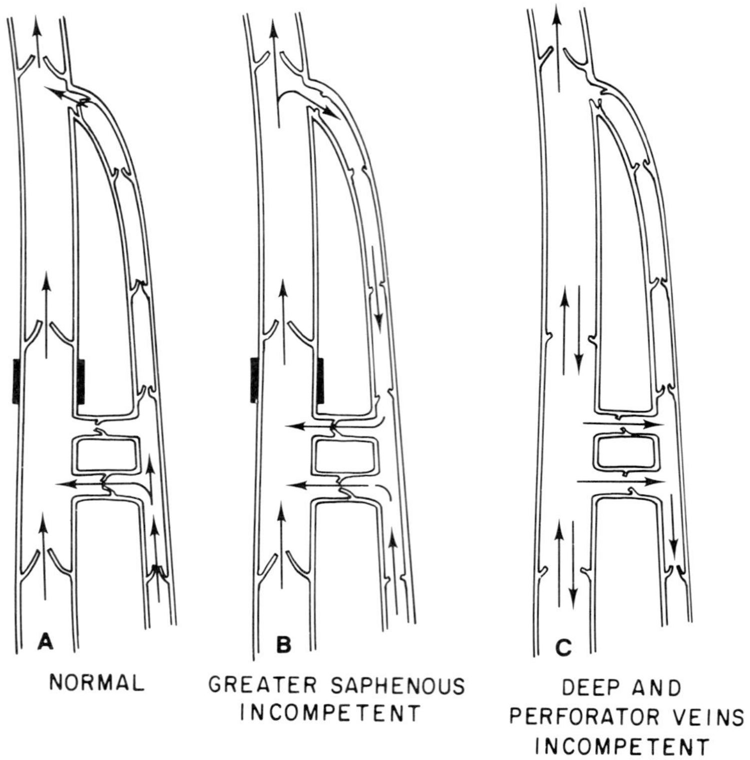

Figure 20-7. Varicosities can occur as a result of incompetence of the values of the (*B*) great saphenous vein—primary varicose veins—or (*C*) perforating veins—secondary varicose veins. The normal state is depicted in (*A*).

valves of the perforating and deep veins so that pressure in the deep venous system is transmitted to the superficial system (Fig. 20-7).

Clinical Findings

In most patients primary varicose veins are asymptomatic and cause minimal functional disability. In others varicose veins cause a sensation of heaviness and fatigue, which usually occurs after prolonged standing and slowly resolves with elevation. The slight ankle swelling that frequently accompanies these symptoms resolves overnight. Nocturnal calf and foot cramps are frequently associated with symptomatic varicose veins. Primary varicose veins rarely, if ever, cause stasis ulcers or skin pigmentation, although these veins are susceptible to trauma and may rupture as well as thrombose.

Findings on physical examination of the patient with primary varicose veins are usually limited to the dilated superficial system. Examination of the patient should be performed with the patient standing on a low platform and the extremities undressed. Tests for valvular incompetence can be helpful to differentiate primary varicose veins from secondary varicose veins. The vein can usually be identified by the Schwartz or percussion test, which is performed by palpating the medial aspect of the thigh while tapping the saphenous vein in the calf (Fig. 20-8). After the greater saphenous vein is localized, its competence can be evaluated by tapping the proximal vein and palpating distally for a fluid wave. The saphenofemoral junction can be evaluated next by the Trendelenburg test (Fig. 20-9): Elevate the leg to collapse the veins, then stand the patient up while compressing the saphenofemoral junction. If the varicose veins do not immediately reappear, but instead slowly fill from the ankle, it can be assumed that the varicose veins originate from an incompetent saphenofemoral junction. This can be demonstrated by releasing the saphenofemoral junction and watching the vein rapidly fill. If the veins fill rapidly to a specific level while the saphenofemoral junctions is being compressed, it can be assumed that this blood is passing from the deep to the superficial system by incompetent perforating veins; that is, the patient has secondary varicose veins. To document the actual site of an incompetent perfo-

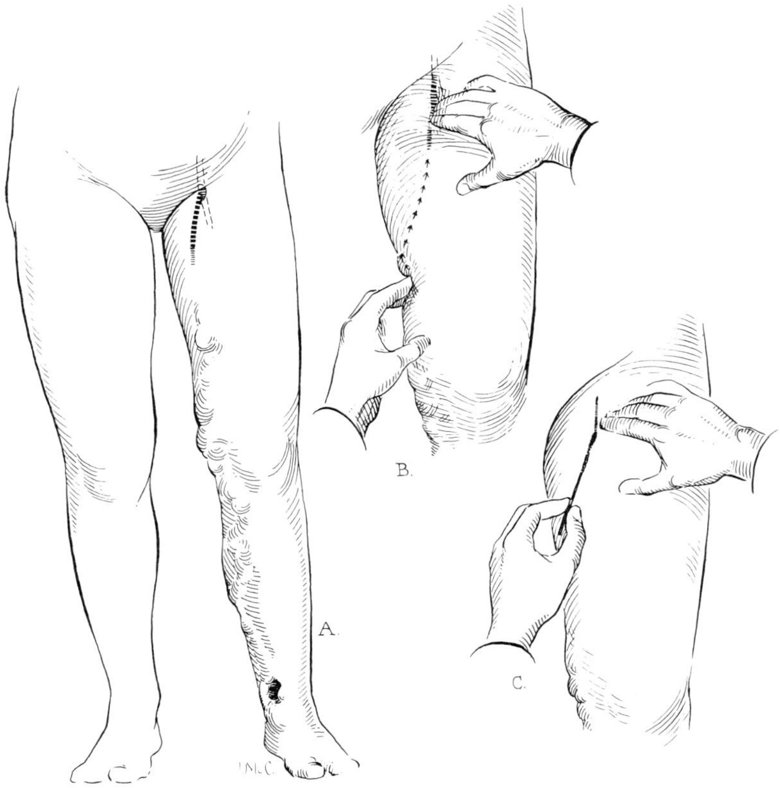

Figure 20-8. The Schwartz, or percussion, test. (*A*) The patient stands with the weight distributed equally on both feet. (*B*) For examination of the left leg, the right hand is placed in the region of the groin, and the vein is percussed gently with the left hand. A percussion wave, palpated at the upper portion of the saphenous vein, gives the examiner an accurate idea of the location of the vein. (*C*) To prepare the patient for ligation a colored antiseptic solution is used to mark the course of the vein on the skin.

rating vein, the leg or thigh is palpated at the site where the saphenous vein became distended. Frequently, a defect can be palpated in the fascia, and pressure through this defect will prevent the veins from rapidly distending after the saphenous vein has been elevated and emptied.

In all patients with evidence of secondary varicose veins the deep venous system should be elevated, since underlying perforator and deep venous disease often coexist. A careful history of symptoms of deep vein thrombophlebitis should be taken, and the degree of function of the deep veins determined. The Perthes test can be used to document complete obstruction of the deep venous system: Place a tourniquet around the proximal aspect of the thigh to occlude only superficial venous return and then have the patient exercise. If the deep venous system is obstructed, the patient often complains of a bursting sensation in the calf as the superficial veins become distended. Unfortunately, this test does not always identify partial deep venous obstruction and therefore is limited in clinical usefulness.

Noninvasive Vascular Lab

The equipment that is found in a vascular laboratory is frequently useful in evaluating venous as well as arterial disease. Doppler auscultation of varicose veins can be used to determine the path of the vein and competence of the valves. In addition, perforators are easily identified with Doppler auscultation. The patency and valvular function of the deep venous system can also be evaluated with a combination of Doppler auscultation and plethysmography. In addition, venous

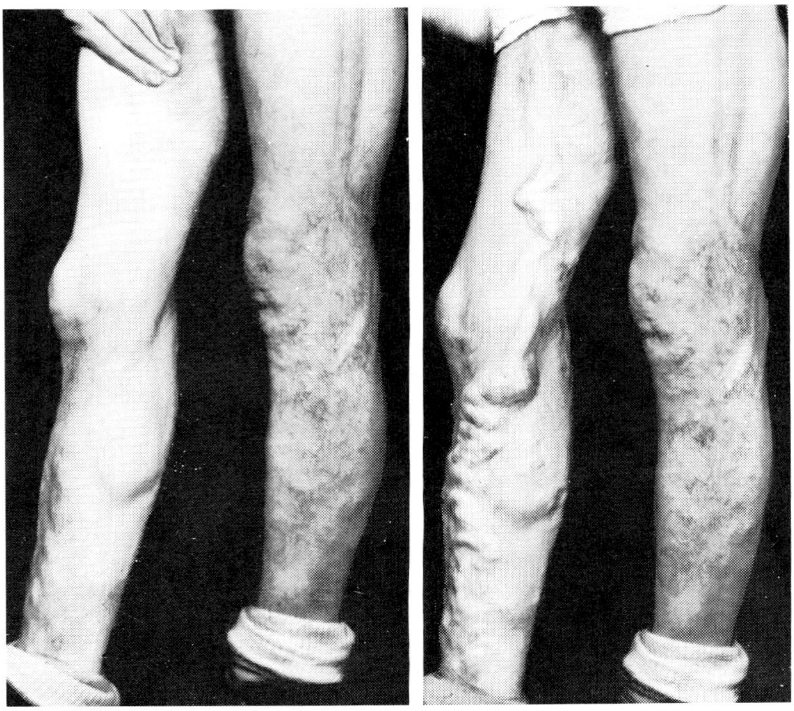

Figure 20-9. After the blood has been emptied from the superficial veins of the leg while the patient is on the examining table, pressure is applied with the hand over the uppermost portion of the saphenous vein. Then with the patient standing the veins are not apparent while the pressure is maintained (*A*), but as soon as the hand is removed the veins fill rapidly from above (*B*). This is a positive Trendelenburg test.

pressure studies can be used to separate the contributions of deep venous obstruction from valvular incompetence. Recently, the deep veins have also been imaged with a duplex scanner to examine for fresh thrombus, chronic occlusion, and normally patent deep veins.

Phlebography remains the "gold standard" against which noninvasive lab tests are compared to determine their diagnostic valve. In addition, when the noninvasive lab studies are equivocal, phlebography should be used to demonstrate the anatomy precisely.

Treatment of Primary Varicose Veins

For most patients treatment is aimed at alleviating the chronic symptoms caused by varicose veins. The forms of therapy include the following:

Compression with well-fitting support stockings (25 mm Hg to 40 mm Hg pressure) frequently relieves symptoms in patients with varicose veins. If compression with stockings or elastic bandages does not relieve symptoms, the symptoms may not be due to the varicose veins. Compliance with this treatment is poor, since many patients find these stockings unattractive and cumbersome.

Compression sclerotherapy, as popularized by Fegan,[45] can be used for patients with primary varicose veins, although it is more frequently applied to patients with secondary varicosities and incompetent perforating veins.

Surgery for varicose veins has been the standard approach in the United States; most surgeons require that patients have symptoms as well as cosmetically displeasing veins. It is imperative that true varicose veins be identified, since many patients request surgery for vague symptoms, and nonvaricosed veins might be needed later in life for a coronary bypass procedure. Indications for surgery include symptomatic varicose veins, recurrent ruptured superficial varices (which may necessitate emergency procedures), and recurrent episodes of superficial phlebitis.

Surgical Procedures. Many surgical procedures can be performed in an ambulatory setting for patients with primary varicose veins. Although ligation without removal of the varicosities is advocated by some surgeons, once a vein or its valves are damaged, complete removal of the vein provides the only absolute assurance that the varicosity will not recur. Also, since primary varicose veins rarely cause complications, only the portion of the vein that is varicosed or has abnormal valves needs to be removed. Frequently, removal of the upper or lower portion of the greater saphenous vein is acceptable, leaving the normal nonvaricosed vein with normal valve function in place.

A thorough knowledge of anatomy is critical in performing the procedure under local anesthesia or regional anesthesia. It is helpful to mark out the course of the dilated vein with indelible ink while the patient is standing, since the veins collapse and are difficult to locate when the patient is in the supine position. Removal or stripping of the greater saphenous vein begins with thorough preparation of the patient and draping from the inguinal ligament to the toes so that the vein can be removed without contaminating the field. The proximal and distal ends of the varicose veins are then identified and, if local anesthesia is used, injected with 1% lidocaine without epinephrine. We prefer transverse incisions in the skin lines for ease of dissection and cosmetic reasons. If the saphenofemoral junction is the proximal limit of the varicosities, care must be taken to ligate the saphenous vein as it enters the fossa ovalis to prevent future varicosities of the numerous branches in this area. The distal vein is then dissected from the surrounding tissue and a traction suture is passed around it. Care must be taken to avoid injury to the sensory nerves (saphenous and sural), which parallel the veins in the lower leg. Injury to a nerve may result in trading uncomfortable symptoms of the veins for sensory nerve symptoms. After both ends of the vein have been isolated, the entire path of the vein should be infiltrated with lidocaine. After the suture is tied on the distal vein, the vein is incised and an internal stripper passed up the vein to the proximal incision. After the stripper is passed out of the vein, the bullet-shaped head is attached to the stripper and the vein is tied tightly to the stripper with a 2-0 silk suture. The stripper is then pulled slowly from the distal incision and the vein is removed. If a large branch prevents the stripper from moving, a small incision is made and the branch is ligated. This prevents troublesome bleeding from the avulsed branch. The path of the vein is then firmly compressed with towels for at least 5 minutes to thrombose small avulsed branches. After the major vein has been removed, other marked branches can be removed or ligated. The incisions are then closed; dressings are placed over the path of the vein; and the leg is wrapped from the toes to the groin with rolled, soft gauze and elastic bandages. The patient is instructed to walk but not to sit for prolonged periods of time for at least 2 days. Nonabsorbable sutures can be removed in 7 days, although elastic bandages should be used for at least 2 weeks. Medication is usually necessary for pain for 2 to 4 days. If the patient walks as advised, deep vein thrombophlebitis is uncommon.

VENOUS THROMBOSIS AND ITS SEQUELAE

Thrombosis of the deep or superficial veins of the leg may be related to trauma, infection, autoimmune disease, hypercoagulability, or underlying congenital venous anomalies, although most commonly the etiology is unknown.[46] Determining the location of thrombus is critical to the effective management of the patient, since superficial phlebitis is a self-limited low-risk disease, whereas deep vein thrombophlebitis frequently has severe acute and long-term complications.[47]

Superficial Venous Thrombosis (Phlebitis)

Superficial venous thrombosis (phlebitis) usually occurs in the lower extremities and rarely necessitates hospitalization. Because of the small caliber of veins and intense inflammatory reaction, thrombi rarely embolize to the deep venous system and lungs.[48] The involved vein becomes tender, warm, and surrounded by a streak of erythema. There is no tenderness in other areas of the extremity and no swelling of the leg to suggest deep vein thrombosis. Treatment is directed at the symptomatic relief of the inflammatory reaction, which usually subsides with antiinflammatory drugs (aspirin 600 mg orally four times daily) and compression with elastic bandages. The patient should be instructed to continue ambulation, since bed rest may lead to deep venous thrombosis. The major sequelae of superficial phlebitis are valvular destruction and varicose veins. Although compression may help sclerose the phlebitic veins, patients frequently need acute vein stripping or long-term management of the developing varicose veins.

Deep Venous Thrombophlebitis

Deep venous thrombophlebitis is a common disease that can cause serious immediate and long-term effects and that should be managed very carefully. Although most patients with deep vein thrombosis of the upper or lower extremities should be hospitalized, a selected group of patients may be candidates for ambulatory management.[49]

A patient with deep vein thrombosis of the lower extremities frequently notices swelling of the calf or thigh and deep muscle pain from walking. Although patients may have deep vein thrombosis with no clinical findings, most have swelling, edema, dilated superficial veins, pain on motion of the foot, and warmth of the entire leg or thigh.

With deep venous system thromboses, outflow of blood from the leg is carried by deep collateral veins and superficial veins. The thrombus is initially loosely adherent to the intima of the vein, but slowly there is organization of the thrombus, ingrowth of fibroblasts, and firm adherence to the wall.[50] During this phase the fragile bicuspid valves are damaged or destroyed. Over months the vein may slowly recanalize, although in areas such as the iliac vein this does not always occur.[51] The end result of this pathologic process is damage to the deep venous walls, destruction of valves in the deep and perforator systems, and variable stenosis or occlusions of the venous segment or both.

It is imperative that the clinician make every attempt to document objectively the presence of deep vein thrombosis with noninvasive testing or venography, since the clinical diagnosis is frequently in error[52] and since treatment involves long-term hospitalization and anticoagulation.

The Doppler venous examination and duplex scanning can be quite helpful when an obstructing thrombus is present, since the obstruction causes characteristic changes in the venous sounds.[53] These include absence or decrease of compression augmentation and respiratory cycling. Plethysmography also demonstrates reduction in segmental venous capacitance and slowing of maximal venous outflow. Duplex scanning can frequently visualize clot in the deep venous system. If the results of the noninvasive vascular laboratory testing are equivocal, phlebography remains the "gold standard" for diagnosis of deep vein thrombosis[54] and can be performed rapidly and with little risk. When the diagnosis of deep vein thrombosis is established, anticoagulation therapy with heparin should be utilized to prevent pulmonary embolus and further destruction of the deep veins and valves. Thrombosis localized below the popliteal vein has a low risk of pulmonary emboli but can lead to chronic venous insufficiency. Deep vein thrombosis of the upper extremity has been recognized for many years, although the frequency of occurrence and recognition may be increasing.[55] Diagnosis and management are similar to those for deep vein thrombosis of the lower extremity, although early surgical venous thrombectomy has been advocated by some surgeons.[56] The inpatient treatment of deep vein thrombosis will not be covered in this text.

Sequelae of Deep Vein Thrombosis

Although the immediate risk of pulmonary embolus to the patient with deep vein thrombosis may be life threatening, it is the chronic sequelae of deep venous thrombosis that cause most of the morbidity. Many patients with chronic venous insufficiency have little recollection of a prior episode of deep vein thrombosis, although it presumably occurred.

Chronic Venous Insufficiency. Chronic venous insufficiency is caused by destruction of deep venous and perforating valves, with resulting inability to move blood effectively toward the heart against gravity. The high pressure in the deep venous system is then transmitted through incompetent perforating valves to the superficial veins, causing ambulatory superficial venous hypertension and secondary varicose veins.[57]

Long-standing superficial venous hypertension caused edema and fibrosis due to transudation of fluids, hyperpigmentation due to extravasation of blood cells, and subcutaneous ischemia due to increased AV shunting. If this highly susceptible tissue is injured, an ulcer may develop. Usually ulcers occur in the area of maximal superficial venous hypertension and skin changes, referred to as the "gaitor zone" around the ankle (Fig. 20-10).

It has been recognized that in some patients with deep vein thrombosis, the veins never recanalize and that, consequently, chronic venous obstruction develops in addition to venous insufficiency.[58] The clinical symptoms include severe edema as well as venous claudication (gradual onset of a bursting sensation in the calf with exercise, which is relieved by prolonged rest and elevation). Stasis ulcers in these patients tend to be more difficult to heal until the obstruction is relieved.

DIAGNOSIS OF THE POSTPHLEBITIC LEG. Management of a patient with skin ulceration presumed to be due to chronic venous insufficiency begins with evaluation of the location of the ulcers, assessment of the site of incompetent perforating veins, and documentation of the location and degree of arterial occlusive disease. Also, a careful search should be made for evidence of venous obstruction, often manifested by a swollen, edematous limb. Noninvasive vascular examinations using a Doppler over the femoral vein will demonstrate reduced respiratory cycling and compression augmentation in a patient with proximal chronic venous obstruction. If obstruction is suspected, venography and femoral venous pressure studies will help determine whether hemodynamically significant venous obstruction is present.[59] If significant venous obstruction is found, the patient may benefit from a venous bypass procedure, and the condition should be evaluated for surgery.

TREATMENT OF THE POSTPHLEBITIC LEG. Initially, patients with chronic venous insufficiency may be managed nonoperatively. Those with a history of deep vein thrombosis but no stasis changes or ulcers need to be educated about the pathophysiology of chronic venous insufficiency and the need to continuously wear compression stockings of 40 mm Hg to prevent the ulcers and chronic changes in the legs. If a patient develops stasis ulcers in the legs, three forms of therapy are available.

Nonoperative therapy is usually successful in reducing the local skin complications of this disease. Stasis dermatitis often follows edema and can be due to excoriation of pruritic areas around the ankle or maceration of skin from dressings and bandages. The cellulitis responds rapidly to antibiotics, and the edema can be reduced with a short course of diuretics. Dermatitis usually clears with locally applied steriod cream. At night, after the cream has been applied, the leg may be covered with a sheet of cellophane to facilitate penetration.

The main effort for patients with chronic

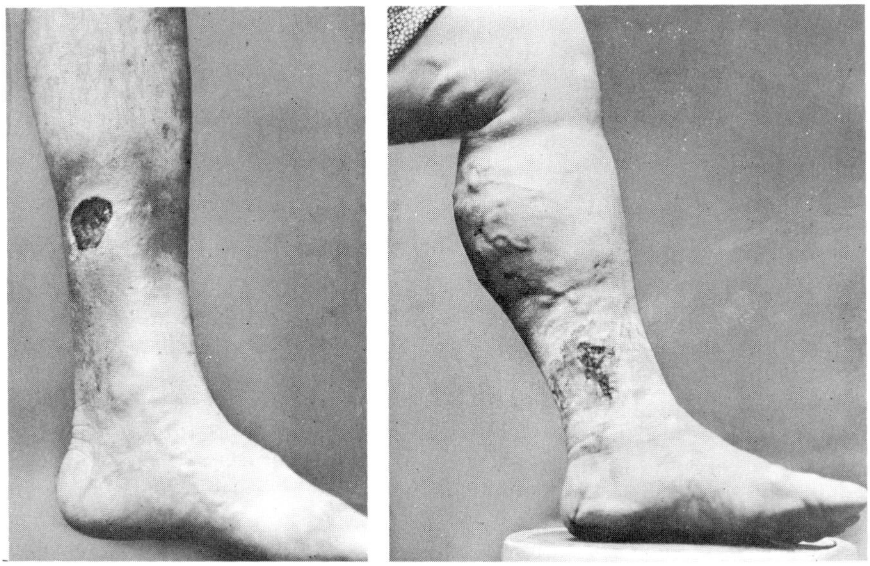

Figure 20-10. Leg ulcers. (*A*) Stasis ulcer with surrounding hyperpigmentation. (*B*) Stasis ulcer in the typical location. Note the contraction of subcutaneous tissue.

stasis ulcers should be directed at reduction of superficial venous hypertension and edema. Ulcers usually heal quite rapidly when the edema and venous hypertension are eliminated. Unna's paste boot causes compression of the subcutaneous tissue when the medicated gauze is wrapped like a soft cast around the foot and leg. The boot then prevents superficial venous hypertension, edema, and weeping from the ulcer when the patient stands. To prepare a leg for application of an Unna boot the patient should be scheduled to see the physician after a 12- to 18-hour period of elevation. If the ulcer has a clean base, a tight boot may be applied directly onto the foot and ulcer. The patient is then instructed to walk as desired. The boot often needs to be changed in the first 3 to 4 days as exudate seeps through the dressing, but the frequency between changes can be lengthened up to 14 days as the ulcer heals.

If the ulcer is infected or contains nonviable tissue, it is usually advisable to debride the wound and treat the patient at home with wet to dry dressings and elevation of the legs for at least 1 week prior to applying the Unna boot.

Compression sclerotherapy attempts to reduce venous hypertension by obliterating the perforating veins that connect the superficial and deep systems.[60] Deep venous hypertension is then not transmitted to the subcutaneous tissue. Incompetent perforators are localized by physical examination and marked with ink. The legs are then elevated to collapse distended veins. After the vein has been emptied, it is compressed approximately 1 cm proximal and distal to the site of the perforator. The needle is introduced into the vein, blood aspirated, and a solution of 1 ml to 5 ml of 3% sodium tetradecyl sulfate (or 30% NaCl and 50% glucose) injected. Care must be taken not to inject the solution into the surrounding tissue, since this may result in tissue slough. Results of therapy seem to be better when the vein is compressed with an elastic bandage for 3 to 4 weeks following injection. The solution causes endothelial injury and destruction when placed in the lumen of the vein and will completely obliterate the lumen if the vein remains collapsed. Otherwise, there may be gradual recanalization of the vein and recurrence of varicosities.

Technical factors may make compression sclerotherapy unsuccessful in some patients, particularly those with obese thighs and saphenopopliteal or saphenofemoral incompetence, since all of these varicosities are difficult to compress.

Surgical ligation of incompetent perforating veins is indicated in patients with stasis dermatitis and ulceration who have not responded to the preceding forms of therapy or in whom skin ulceration recurs. Also, some patients have skin fibrosis that is so firm that identification of perforating veins is difficult; in these patients, if venography confirms incompetent perforators, then they should be ligated surgically. It should be understood that the principle in ligation is exactly the same as that in compression sclerotherapy, namely, preventing transmission of the high pressures in the deep venous system to the superficial veins.

LYMPHEDEMA AND THE SWOLLEN LIMB

THE SWOLLEN LIMB

A swollen edematous limb is a common ambulatory problem that may cause significant morbidity.[61] To treat the patient with edema appropriately, the physician must determine the cause of the swelling. Edema has several possible causes:

Systemic disease: congestive heart failure, hepatic failure, renal failure, hypoproteinemia, idiopathic cyclic edema
Venous disease: deep vein thrombosis, chronic venous insufficiency, proximal venous occlusion (extrinsic and intrinsic), AV fistula (chronic)
Lymphatic disease: primary lymphedema, secondary lymphedema
Trauma: burn, soft tissue injury
Infection

Early determination of the etiology of edema is especially important because a variety of systemic diseases may require immediate therapy. Patients who have unilateral swelling can be assumed to have a local problem due to lymphatic or venous hypertension or trauma, and a search for systemic disease need not be made. In patients who have no systemic disease and no history of tissue injury, the differential diagnosis is between lymphedema and venous disease. This differential diagnosis often can be made from a careful history and physical examination (Table 20-2), particularly in the late stages of these diseases. Patients with lymphedema cannot relate the swelling to previous trauma or to an episode of deep vein thrombosis. The leg is rarely painful, and swelling, which involves the dorsum of the foot, is only slowly improved with elevation. With time the leg becomes more swollen and tissue more fibrotic, but never with the development of stasis pigmentation or ulceration. Although episodes of cellulitis may occur, the infection rarely leads to chronic skin ulceration. In contrast, the leg with chronic venous insufficiency develops secondary varicose veins, pigmentation in areas of maximal venous hypertension around the ankles, and often ulcers around the medial and lateral malleolus. With progression of the disease, *contraction* and fibrosis of the tissue around the ankle occur.

When the etiology of edema cannot be clearly determined by history and physical examination, attempts to document the source of the problem should be made. The noninvasive venous examination of the lower extremity is the first and simplest test to be performed (see the section entitled "Venous Disease"). An attempt should be made to document incompetence of the superficial, perforator, and deep vein valves as well as obstruction of the deep venous system. If results of this examination are equivocal or abnormal, we routinely perform venography to document the location and extent of disease. When the noninvasive venous examination and venography are normal, and systemic causes of edema have been eliminated, it can be assumed that lymphedema is the cause of the swollen leg.

To document clearly that lymphatic obstruction is the cause of the edema, lymphangiography may be performed by injecting contrast material into the lymphatics on the dorsum of the foot.[62] Although not always necessary for appropriate therapy, a lymphangiogram will document the location of lymphatic disease and help to determine whether primary lymphedema is due to aplasia, hypoplasia, or varicosities of the lymphatic system.

LYMPHEDEMA

Lymphedema is a relatively uncommon cause of swelling in the extremities. Although there are multiple causes of lymphedema, they all result in high pressure in the lymphatics, removal of less fluid and protein, and increased tissue pressure.

Primary lymphedema, a condition in which there is no history of trauma or infection, is due to a congenital anomaly of the lymphatic system, with the age of onset of symptoms closely related to the degree of functional impairment.[63] Lymphedema congenita is present shortly after birth and is associated with aplasia of the lymphatics. In lymphedema praecox, the most common form of lymphedema, onset occurs before the age of 35 years and is caused by lymphatic hypoplasia. The onset of lymphedema tarda occurs after 35 years of age and the lymphatics frequently show only varicosities.

Secondary lymphedema is due to injury to previously normal lymphatics. Although the most common cause of lymphedema worldwide is filariasis due to the nematode *Wuchereria bancrofti,* this disease is relatively uncommon in the United States. In the United States the common causes of secondary lymphedema are surgical removal of the lymphatics (e.g., mastectomy) and neoplastic obstruc-

TABLE 20-2. Differentiation Between Venous and Lymphatic Causes of Edema

VENOUS	LYMPHATIC
History of trauma and deep vein thrombosis	No history of trauma or phlebitis
Swelling stops at ankle, pigmentation changes present, ulcers frequently present, varicose veins present	Swelling includes dorsum of foot, no pigmentation, no ulcers, no varicose veins
Late changes include fibrosis and contraction of tissue	Late changes include fibrosis and expansion of tissue
Elevation reduces edema rapidly	Elevation reduces edema slowly
Venogram and noninvasive venous examination abnormal	Venogram and noninvasive venous examination normal
Lymphangiogram normal	Lymphangiogram abnormal

tion of the lymphatics that drain an extremity. Other common causes include recurrent lymphangitis and postirradiation lymphatic obstruction. Tuberculosis and syphilis may also be causes.

In patients with lymphedema it is important to document the severity of impairment in activity, frequency of infection (cellulitis and lymphangitis), and any history suggestive of secondary lymphedema, particularly neoplastic. Palpation of lymph nodes in the proximal limb is particularly important in detection of adenopathy; all patients with lower-extremity lymphedema should have a rectal or pelvic examination or both to determine if a pelvic neoplasm is obstructing the lymphatics.

When lymphedema has been diagnosed, therapy should be directed at treating the underlying cause of lymphatic obstruction (e.g., rectal carcinoma), if one exists, reducing the edema, and preventing infection in the lymphedematous limb. In most patients therapy cannot totally eliminate the edema, and the goal should mainly consist of enabling the patient to function normally. Therapy is usually nonoperative;[64] edema may be reduced by prolonged and repeated elevation of the extremity, external compression with an elastic stocking, and intermittent compression with a mechanical compression device. Patients should be fitted with a stocking at 40 mm Hg pressure after the edema has been reduced by prolonged elevation. They need to be instructed that the edema will persist for life and may worsen if the limb becomes infected.

To avoid infection, injury to the extremity with foreign body puncture and drying of the skin should particularly be avoided. If infection does occur, the patient should be hospitalized and treated with intravenously administered antibiotics effective against the most common organism (streptococcus)[65] and edema in the extremity reduced by elevation and administration of diuretics. Some patients with recurrent cellulitis may benefit from long-term oral use of penicillin.[66]

Surgical procedures for lymphedema have limited success, require extensive tissue dissection, and often have poor cosmetic results[67–69]; therefore they are reserved for severe disability or recurrent infection of the limb. Long-standing lymphedema is associated with an increased risk of lymphangiosarcoma,[70] so all patients should be examined at regular intervals.

REFERENCES

Arteriovenous Disease

1. Gordon T, Kannel WB: Predisposition to atherosclerosis in the head, heart, and legs: The Framingham study. JAMA 221:661, 1972
2. Haimovici H: Patterns of atherosclerotic lesions of the lower extremity. Arch Surg. 95:918, 1967
3. May AG, Vande Berg L, De Weese JA, Rob CG: Critical arterial stenosis. Surgery 54:250, 1963
4. Sumner DS: The hemodynamics and pathophysiology of arterial disease. In Rutherford RB (ed): Vascular Surgery, pp 25–46. Philadelphia, WB Saunders, 1977
5. Strandness DE, Sumner DS: Physics of arterial blood flow. In Strandness DE, Sumner DS: Hemodynamics for Surgeons, pp 73–95. New York, Grune & Stratton, 1975
6. Raines JK, Darling RC, Ruth J et al: Vascular laboratory criteria for the management of peripheral vascular disease of the lower extremities. Surgery 79:21, 1976
7. Strandness DE Jr, Bell JW: Peripheral vascular disease: Diagnosis and objective evaluation using a mercury strain gauge. Ann Surg 1612 (Suppl 4):1, 1965
8. Sumner DS, Strandness DE: The relationship between calf blood flow and ankle blood pressure in patients with intermittent claudication. Surgery 65:763, 1969
9. Fitzgerald DE, Keates JS, MacMillan D: Angiographic and plethysmographic assessment of graduated physical exercise in the treatment of chronic occlusive arterial disease of the leg. Angiology 22:99, 1971
10. Strandness DE Jr, Sumner DS: Therapy of occlusive arterial disease. In Strandness DE, Sumner DS: Hemodynamics for Surgeons, pp 290–341. New York, Grune & Stratton, 1975
11. Dotter CT, Judkins MP: Transluminal treatment of arteriosclerotic obstruction: Description of a new technique and a preliminary report of its application. Circulation 30:654–670, 1964
12. van Audel GJ: Percutaneous Transluminal Angioplasty (the Dotter-Procedure). Amsterdam, Excerpta Medica, 1976
13. Gruntzig A: Percutaneous transluminal recanalization with the double lumen dilatation catheter. In Percutaneous Vascular Recanalization, pp 17–23. New York, Springer-Verlag, 1978
14. Hardy JD, Conn JH, Fain WR: Nonatheroslcerotic occlusive lesions of small arteries. Surgery 57:1, 1965
15. Allen VE, Brown GE: Raynaud's disease: A critical review of minimal requisites for diagnosis. Am J Med Sci 183:1875, 1932

16. Wagner O, Piza F, Lechner G: Indications and late results of Palmas venous bypass in chronic pelvic vein thrombosis. Vasa 2:347–352, 1973
17. Cockett FB: The pathology and treatment of venous ulcers of the leg. Br J Surg 43:260, 1955
18. Porter JM, Snider RL, Bardana EJ: The diagnosis and treatment of Raynaud's phenomenon. Surgery 77:11, 1975
19. Abboud FM, Eckstein JW, Lawrence MS: Preliminary observations in the use of intra-arterial reserpine in Raynaud's phenomenon. Circulation 35:49, 1967
20. Porter JM, Snider RL, Bardana EJ: The diagnosis and treatment of Raynaud's phenomenon. Circulation 35:49, 1967
21. Rich NM, Spencer FC: Vascular Trauma, pp 75–105. Philadelphia, WB Saunders, 1978
22. Drapanas J, Hewitt RL, Weichert RF, Smith AD: Civilian vascular injuries: A critical appraisal of three decades of management. Ann Surg 172:351, 1970

Access Routes for Hemodialysis

23. Yao JST: Arterial survey with the Dopplar ultrasonic velocity detector. In Rutherford RB (ed): Vascular Surgery, pp 87–95. Philadelphia, WB Saunders, 1977
24. Carter SA: Role of pressure measurements in vascular disease. In Bernstein EF (ed): Noninvasive Diagnostic Techniques in Vascular Disease, pp 216–287. St. Louis, CV Mosby, 1978
25. Lazarus HM, Albo D, Welling D, Hutto W: Doppler ankle pressures and stiff arteries. In Diethrich EB (ed): Noninvasive Cardiovascular Diagnosis: Current Concepts, p 1227. Baltimore, University Park Press, 1978
26. Sumner DS: Evaluation of the venous circulation using the ultrasonic Doppler velocity detector. Rutherford RB (ed): Vascular Surgery, pp 179–189. Philadelphia, WB Saunders, 1977
27. Giacehiuo JL, Geis P, Buckingham JM et al: Vascular access: Long-term results, new techniques, Arch Surg 114:403–409, 1979
28. Zerbino VR, Tice DA, Katz LA, Niudus BD: A 6 year clinical experience with arteriovenous fistulas and bypasses for hemodialysis. Surgery 765:1018–1023, 1974
29. Tellis VA, Kohlberg WI, Bhat DJ et al: Expanded polytetrafluorethylene graft fistula for chronic hemodialysis. Ann Surg 189:101–105, 1979
30. Paruk S et al: Arteriovenous fistulas for hemodialysis in 100 consecutive patients. Am J Surg 131:552–555, 1976
31. Mansberger AR: Acute renal failure. In Hardy JD (ed): Rhoads Textbook of Surgery: Principles and Practice, 5th ed, p 107. Philadelphia, JB Lippincott, 1977
32. Rutherford RB, Fleming PW, McLeod FD: Vascular diagnostic methods for evaluating patients with arteriovenous fistulas. In Diethrich EB (ed): Noninvasive Cardiovascular Diagnosis: Current Concepts. Baltimore, University Park Press, 1978
33. Anderson CB et al: Venous angiography and the surgical management of subcutaneous hemodialysis fistulas. Ann Surg 187:194–204, 1978
34. Stehbeus WE, Karmody AM: Venous atherosclerosis associated with arteriovenous fistulas for hemodialysis. Arch Surg 110:176–180, 1975
35. Lawrence PF, Miller F: Percutaneous vascular recanalization. Unpublished results
36. Byrne JP et al: Advantages of surgical arteriovenous fistulas for hemodialysis. Arch Surg 102:359, 1971
37. Fee HJ, Golding AL: Lower extremity ischemia after femoral arteriovenous bovine shunts. Ann Surg 183:42–45, 1976
38. Guyton AC: The systemic circulation. In Guyton AC (ed): Textbook of Medical Physiology, p 246. Philadelphia, WB Saunders, 1977
39. Ludbrook J, Jamieson G: Disorders of systemic veins. In Sabiston D (ed): Textbook of Surgery, pp 1808–1827. Philadelphia, WB Saunders, 1981
40. Fegan G: The clinical pathology of venous insufficiency of the lower limb. In Fegan G (ed): Varicose Veins, p 38. Springfield, IL, Charles C Thomas, 1967
41. Burkitt DP: Varicose veins, facts and fantasy. Arch Surg 111:1327–1332, 1976
42. Raivio E. Untersuchungen über die Venen der unteren Extremitaten mit besonderer Beruck-sichtigung der gegenseitigen Verbindungen zwischen den oberflachigen and tiefen Venen. Ann Med Exp Fenn 26:1948
43. Fegan WG: Treatment of varicose veins by injection compression: A method practiced in Eire. In Hobba JT (ed): The Treatment of Venous Disorders, pp 99–112. Philadelphia, JB Lippincott, 1977
44. Kakkar VV, Jouhar AJ: Thromboembolism: Diagnosis and Treatment. Edinburgh, Churchill Livingstone, 1972
45. Gjores JF: The incidence of venous thrombosis and its sequelae in certain districts of Sweden. Acta Chir Scand (Suppl)206, 1956
46. Roberts GH: Venous thrombosis in hospital patients: A postmortem study. Scott Med J 8:11, 1963
47. Stillman RM et al: A ten year study of heparin therapy for thrombophlebitis for ambulatory patients. Surg Gynecol Obstet 145:193–197, 1977
48. Ludbrook J, Jamieson GG: Disorders of systemic veins. In Sabiston D (ed): Textbook of Surgery, pp 1808–1827. Philadelphia, WB Saunders, 1981
49. Bergvall U, Hjelmstedt A: Recanalization of deep venous thrombosis of the lower leg and thigh. Acta Chir Scand 134:219, 1968

50. Browse N: Deep vein thrombosis: Diagnosis. Br Med J 4:676, 1969
51. Barnes RW: Doppler ultrasonic diagnosis of venous disease. In Bernstein EF (ed): Noninvasive Diagnostic Techniques in Vascular Disease, pp 344–350. St. Louis, CV Mosby, 1978
52. Pavlov H et al: Simplified outpatient lower extremity venography. Radiology 126:525–527, 1978
53. Prescott SM, Tikoff G: Deep venous thrombosis of the upper extremity: A reappraisal. Circulation 59:350–355, 1979
54. DeWeese JA, Adamns JT, Gaiser DL: Subclavian venous thrombectomy. Circulation (Suppl 2)16:158, 1970
55. Fegan G: The clinical pathology of venous insufficiency of the lower limb. In Fegan G (ed): Varicose Veins, pp 38–39. Springfield, IL, Charles C Thomas, 1967
56. Mavor GE, Galloway JMD: Collaterals of the deep venous circulation of the lower limb. Surg Gynecol Obstet 125:561, 1967
57. Rigas A et al: Measurement of the femoral vein pressure in edema of the lower extremities. J Cardiovasc Surg 12:411, 1971
58. Sigg K: Treatment of varicose veins by injection-sclerotherapy: A method practiced in Switzerland. In Hobbs JT (ed): The Treatment of Venous Disorders. Philadelphia, JB Lippincott, 1977

Lymphedema and the Swollen Limb

59. Dale WA: The swollen leg. Curr Probl Surg, pp 1–66, September 1973
60. DeRoo T: The value of lymphography in lymphedema. Surg. Gynecol Obstet 124:755, 1967
61. Kinmonth JB: The Lymphatics: Diseases, Lymphography and Surgery. Baltimore, Williams & Wilkins, 1972
62. Bauchman HH, Lewis SR: The treatment of lymphedema. Plast Reconstr Surg 54:64–69, 1974
63. Freeman RM et al: Streptococcal gangrene in an infant with congenital lymphedema. South Med J 66:830–832, 1973
64. Babb RR: Prophylaxis of recurrent lymphangitis complicating lymphedema. JAMA 195:871–873, 1966
65. Kinmonth JB, Patrick JH, Chilvers AS: Comments on operations for lower limb lymphedema. Lymphology 8:56, 1975
66. Thompson N: Buried dermal flap operation for chronic lymphedema of the extremities: Ten year survey of results in 79 cases. Plast Reconstr Surg 45:541, 1970
67. Goldsmith HS: Long-term evaluation of omental transposition for chronic lymphedema. Am Surg 180:847, 1974
68. Laskas JJ, Shelley WB, Wood MG: Lymphangiosarcoma arising in congenital lymphedema. Arch Dermatol 111:86, 1975

BIBLIOGRAPHY

Ahearn DJ, Maher JF: Heart failure as a complication of hemodialysis arteriovenous fistula. Ann Intern Med 77:201, 1972

Coffman JD, Mannick JA: Failure of vasodilator drugs in arteriosclerosis obliteraus. Ann Intern Med 76:35, 1972

Delphia EAS: Swelling of the hand after arteriovenous fistula for hemodialysis. Am J Surg 132:373–376, 1976

Malan E, Tattoni G: Physio- and anatopathology of acute ischemia of the extremities. J Cardiovasc Surg 4:2, 1963

21 Gynecology

JAMES C. WARENSKI

Gynecologic operative procedures of short duration and low risk and requiring little postoperative care are easily performed in an ambulatory surgical care setting. With comparatively minor modifications an examining room in a physician's office, outpatient clinic, or emergency room can be suitably equipped for the minor surgical procedures that are commonly performed with use of either local infiltration anesthesia, transvaginal nerve block, or no anesthesia at all. However, the patient's needs and the degree of risk should be basic considerations, and those procedures that require general anesthesia or more complex conduction anesthesia should be performed only in facilities that are adequately equipped and staffed.

PELVIC EXAMINATION

A thoughtfully elicited history and carefully performed physical examination with emphasis on abdominal, pelvic, and rectal findings are most important in the diagnosis of disorders of the female reproductive tract. Only in this way can special office procedures useful in the differential diagnosis of common gynecologic complaints (pain, bleeding, discharge, mass) be logically and efficiently utilized.

To carry out an adequate pelvic examination, the patient is placed in the lithotomy position on a comfortable examining table with the buttocks brought over the edge of the table and the stirrups properly adjusted. A good light and warm instruments are essential (Fig. 21-1). The examination is made easier if the patient is relaxed and has an empty bladder and bowel.

After a systematic check of the external genitalia, an appropriate-sized speculum is inserted obliquely through the introitus toward the vaginal vault. It is slowly rotated and advanced with downward pressure to avoid pain against the rigid pubic symphysis and urethra. The speculum is then opened and adjusted and the vagina and cervix inspected. Specimens are obtained for cultures and a Papanicolaou test. A scraping with a wooden spatula is obtained from the squamocolumnar junction of the cervix, and the material is smeared on a glass slide that is fixed immediately to prevent air drying and distortion of the cells. A second smear is obtained from the endocervical canal by bulb aspiration or with cotton-tipped applicator and placed on a second slide. After removal of the speculum, a gentle bimanual examination is carried out to evaluate the condition of the uterus, fallopian tubes, and ovaries. A complete gynecologic examination requires a rectovaginal examination.

VULVA AND PERINEUM

BIOPSY

Patients with vulvar lesions may be asymptomatic but often complain of chronic irritation, itching, or discharge. In many instances there is an unfortunate delay of months or years from the onset of symptoms to the diagnosis of vulvar carcinoma due to procrastination on the part of the patient or prolonged symptomatic therapy by the physician. Because diagnosis by inspection and palpation alone is notoriously inaccurate, any ulcerated, indurated, or chronic vulvar lesion warrants biopsy and microscopic examination.

Local infiltration anesthesia with 1% lidocaine solution in a small syringe using a 25-gauge needle is very effective. The small Keyes dermal punch biopsy instrument is useful for most simple biopsies of the vulva (Fig. 21-2). However, a standard no. 15 Bard–Parker blade is also satisfactory, particularly for excisional biopsies (Fig. 21-3). To select the most severely involved area, it is helpful first to wash the vulva with a 1% solution of acetic acid followed by an aqueous solution of

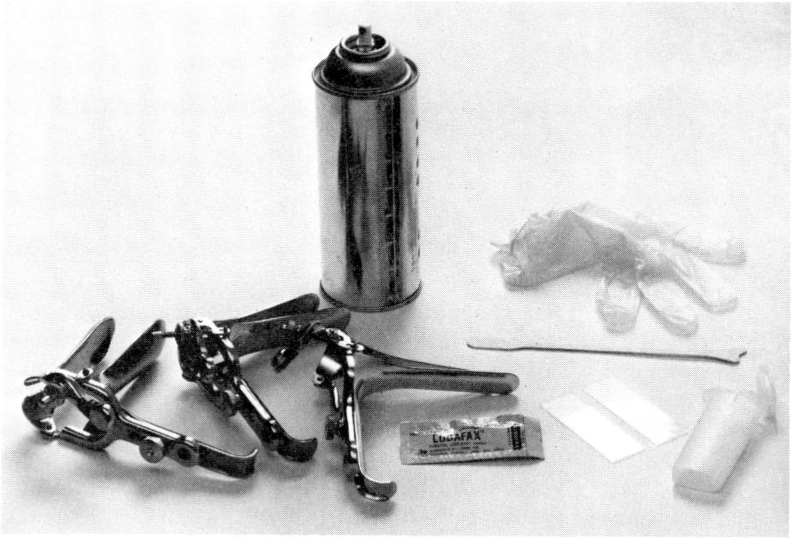

Figure 21-1. Minimal equipment for pelvic examination includes a proper-sized speculum, lubricant, gloves, and slides, fixative, and a wooden spatula for cervical cytology.

1% toluidine blue. The dye is then removed by sponging again with the acetic acid solution; a blue stain remains in skin areas that have abnormal nuclear activity or malignant potential. An elliptic incision following natural skin lines is preferred for larger excisional biopsies. Interrupted or subcuticular running sutures of 4-0 chromic surgical gut swaged on a small cutting needle do not require a return visit specifically for suture removal. Small bleeding areas are easily controlled by topical application of a silver nitrate stick, Monsel's solution (subferrous sulfate), or electrocoagulation. If required, more extensive vulvar anesthesia can be achieved by transvaginal pudendal nerve block with 5 ml to 10 ml of 1% lidocaine.

CONDYLOMA ACUMINATA

Condyloma acuminata (venereal warts) are initially benign genital growths caused by several subtypes of the human papilloma virus

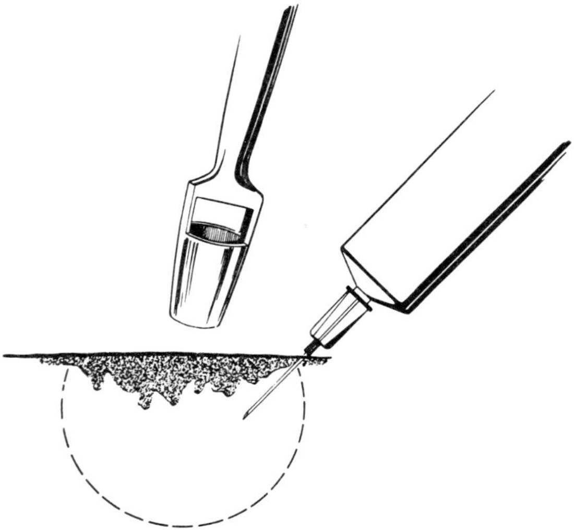

Figure 21-2. The punch, used like an apple corer, is slightly twisted and bored down to the depth desired. After withdrawal of the punch the separated core is picked up with a small forceps and the base cut across with a fine scissors. (Friedrich EG: Vulvar Disease. Philadelphia, WB Saunders, 1983)

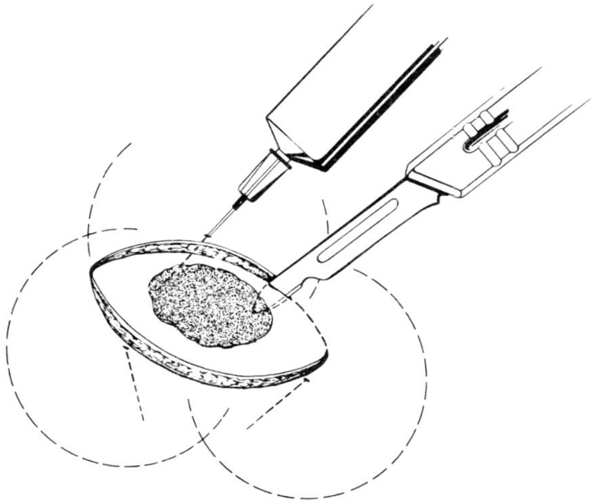

Figure 21-3. Elliptical excisional biopsy done under local anesthesia. (Friedrich EG: Vulvar Disease. Philadelphia, WB Saunders, 1983)

(Fig. 21–4). Although most frequently presented by the patient as warty vulvar lesions, they commonly involve the vagina and cervix as well. Particularly in the latter location, they may have a flat growth form and be visible only after application of acetic acid, which reveals the appearance of a white plaque. The causative viruses are sexually transmitted, and recently it has been appreciated that certain subtypes play an important role in the induction of vulvar, vaginal, and cervical cancer. Therefore it is essential that patients treated for condylomata be carefully screened by clinical and cytologic examination for malignant or premalignant lesions. Furthermore, although their typical appearance is ordinarily sufficient for diagnosis, condylomata of pigmented or other atypical appearance, or persisting after therapy, must be biopsied.

Vulvar condylomata localized to small areas may be treated satisfactorily by the application of 25% podophyllum in tincture of benzoin, which is left on for 4 to 6 hours and then washed off. Treatment is repeated weekly as necessary. Systemic absorption from treating too large an area of the vulva at one time can lead to severe toxicity. For this reason as well, treatment of mucosal surfaces (vagina and cervix) should not be attempted, and use of podophyllum at any site in pregnancy is contraindicated. Application of trichloracetic acid to vulvar lesions, repeated as necessary, is also effective and may be used in the pregnant patient. Normal surrounding skin should be protected with petrolatum jelly and vaginal and cervical lesions should not be treated with this agent. 5-Fluorouracil (5% Efudex) has been used successfully in treatment of condylomata involving the vaginal mucosa but should not be used during pregnancy.

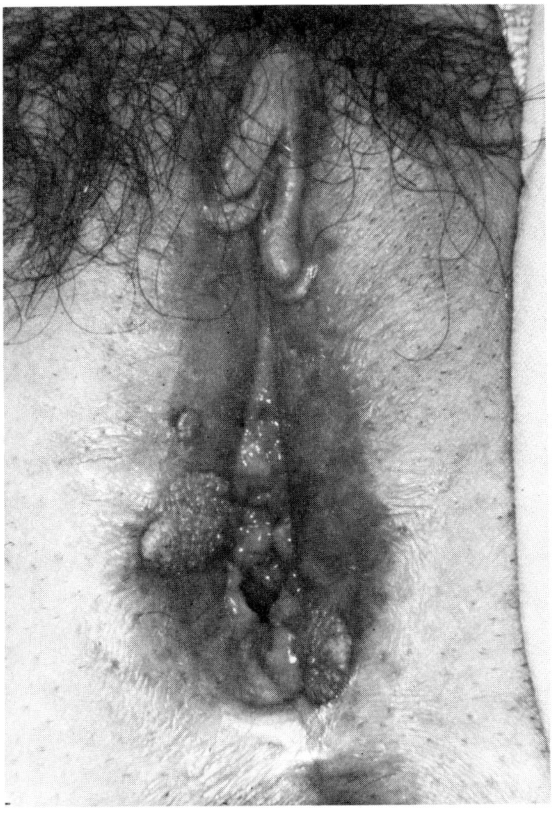

Figure 21-4. Vulvar condylomata acuminata.

For large or recurrent condylomata, including those presenting in the pregnant patient, surgical excision, fulguration, or electrodissection with adequate regional or general anesthesia may be required. Cryotherapy, either with liquid nitrogen or a cryoprobe, has been disappointing in treating vulvar or vaginal condylomata because of the high recurrence rate. However, regional cryotherapy of the cervix in treating condyloma-associated dysplasia is an effective approach. Where the specialized equipment and an operator trained in its use are available, the CO_2 laser has proved highly effective in treating condylomata at all genital sites.

In treating condylomata it is essential to treat any underlying vaginitis productive of increased discharge. Indeed, this treatment alone may at times cause regression of the lesions. In recalcitrant cases discontinuing oral contraceptives may be necessary. Examination and concomitant treatment of the sexual partner may be required, with use of condoms advisable.

BARTHOLIN'S CYSTS

Bartholin's glands are bilateral compound racemose glands with a single excretory duct located at the junction of the upper two thirds and lower one third of the vulvovaginal ring. Infection of these glands occurs frequently, and a cyst or abscess may result if the excretory duct remains obstructed. Small asymptomatic cysts require no treatment, and an acute abscess with extensive surrounding inflammatory response may require direct incision and drainage with local infiltration or topical anesthesia. However, most recurrent abscesses

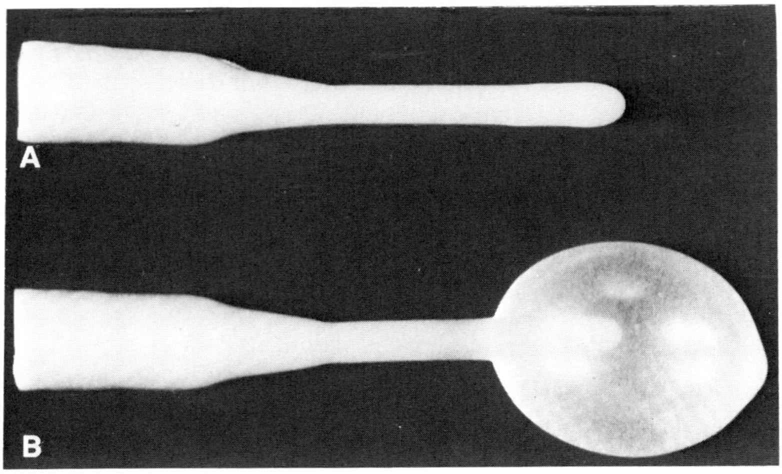

Figure 21-5. The Word catheter as inserted (*A*) and inflated (*B*). (Friedrich EG: Vulvar Disease. Philadelphia, WB Saunders, 1983)

and symptomatic cysts are best treated by marsupialization to avoid subsequent recurrence. Marsupialization can be accomplished either with a Word catheter (Fig. 21-5) or by a suturing technique. The incision should always be made in the mucous membrane just outside the hymenal ring, centered on the location of the normal orifice of the gland. With the Word catheter, an incision adequate for drainage is made, pus is cultured if present, and, after probing with a Kelly clamp, the catheter is inserted into the cavity and left in place for several weeks until a permanent sinus tract forms as epithelialization occurs around the catheter.

With marsupialization by suture fixation, a

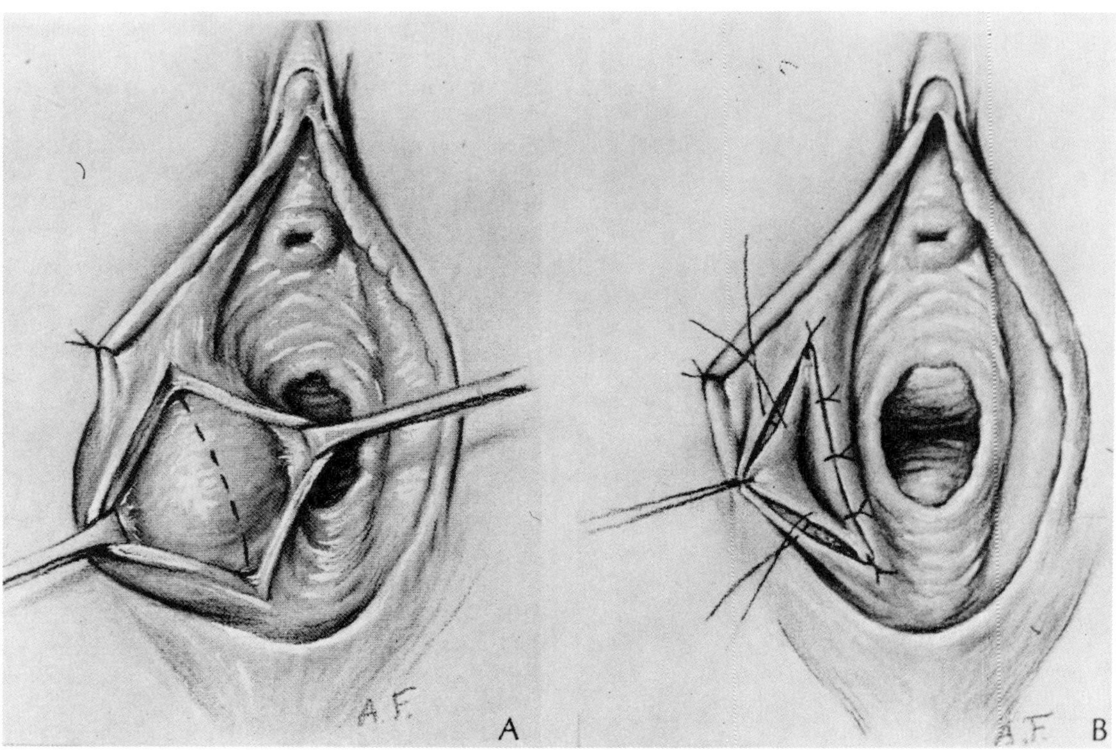

Figure 21-6. (*A*) Incision for marsupialization. (*B*) Marsupialization. (Tancer ML, Rosenberg M, Fernandez D: Obstet Gynecol 7:609, 1956)

generous linear incision is made over the cyst or abscess along the mucocutaneous junction of the vagina and vulva, and an eliptic piece of cyst wall and skin is removed with small scissors or scalpel. The incision is enlarged vertically until one finger can be inserted into the cyst cavity. The edge of the cyst lining is then sutured to the adjoining skin edge with interrupted 3-0 chromic catgut sutures (Fig. 21-6). Drains and packs are not necessary, but frequent sitz baths are advised for several days. The patient should be seen in 48 to 72 hours to ensure that the edges of the incision are not agglutinated. Resolution of the cyst is usually complete within a few weeks. Marsupialization by either technique is simple, involves minimal blood loss, can be done safely in the presence of infection, and can be undertaken with local infiltration of pudendal block anesthesia. Excision of a cyst and the associated glandular tissue should be reserved for patients who are postmenopausal or in whom the mass is solid. If excision is to be performed, a hospital setting is advisable because of the risk of bleeding from branches of the pudendal artery.

LACERATIONS AND HEMATOMAS

Traumatic lesions of the perineum are often seen in the emergency room or office. In children these are frequently straddle injuries. Unless a child is old enough to cooperate, general anesthesia is usually necessary for thorough evaluation and repair. In adults recent superficial injuries can be repaired by debridment and closure under local anesthesia. However, if the trauma is extensive, examination and repair, including evacuation of large hematomas, should be carried out with the use of general anesthesia with more extended postoperative observation.

VAGINA

INFANTS AND CHILDREN

The most common cause of vaginal discharge in young girls is a foreign body in the vagina. Often these can be palpated on rectal examination, but adequate visualization of the vagina is usually necessary both to establish a diagnosis and to remove the object. If the child is apprehensive, a mild sedative given in a recommended pediatric dosage is useful. Visual examination of the vaginal canal with the patient in the lithotomy or knee–chest position is accomplished by gently inserting a nasal speculum or pediatric cystoscope. Material for cultures is obtained, and any foreign body can usually be extracted with a small forceps or removed by irrigating with warm water.

VAGINAL CYSTS

Cystic lesions in the vagina are of two general types. The first is an inclusion cyst that has formed in the posterior distal area of the vagina or perineum following a previous laceration or episiotomy repair. Most inclusion cysts require no treatment, but if the cyst becomes large and symptomatic, it can be excised under local anesthesia. The second, Gartner's duct cyst, is a remnant of the wolffian duct typically found along the anterolateral aspect of the vaginal wall. Excision is indicated if they achieve sufficient size to cause discomfort or interfere with intercourse.

Solid vaginal lesions should be excised or biopsy should be done primarily to rule out malignancy. Because of difficulty in achieving adequate pain relief with local anesthesia, inaccessibility of some lesions without adequate retraction and assistance, and unexpected problems in controlling bleeding, it is often preferable to perform these procedures in the operating room.

STRESS INCONTINENCE

Stress incontinence is the involuntary loss of urine through an intact urethra secondary to a sudden increase in abdominal pressure without voiding action. Although the surgical correction should be performed in the hospital, much of the preoperative evaluation for this condition can be accomplished in an outpatient facility.

A detailed medical history is of utmost importance in documenting true stress incontinence as well as in ruling out other problems that tend to be confused with this condition. One should determine the amount of urine lost with coughing, sneezing, laughing, running, or change in position. Surgical treatment is indicated when loss of urine is significant enough to result in social embarrassment, wearing of protective pads, or chronic vulvar irritation, and when careful evaluation verifies the diagnosis of stress incontinence.

It is important to document the amount of anatomic derangement present at the time of pelvic examination. The degree of descent of the bladder base and detachment of the urethra under increased intra-abdominal pressure are the most important factors. Descensus uteri and cystourethrocele or rectocele will be evident by simply inserting a speculum into the vagina, having the patient bear down, and slowly withdrawing the speculum. However, this observation alone does not mean that the incontinence is due to the anatomic defect.

The urinary stress test is an easily performed screening test. The patient is asked to empty her bladder, a catheter is inserted, and any residual urine is measured and submitted for culture. The bladder is then filled with normal saline, and the patient notes the first sensation of bladder fullness (150 ml to 200 ml) and the point at which she feels her bladder can hold no more (500 ml to 700 ml). The urge to void with much smaller volumes suggests a primarily contracted bladder, and the ability to hold extremely large volumes may indicate an atonic bladder. In either case, further urologic investigation such as cystoscopy, urethroscopy, and quantitative urodynamic studies should be undertaken before any pelvic surgery is performed. With approximately 250 ml of saline in the bladder, the catheter is removed and the patient is urged to cough. If stress incontinence is not demonstrated while the patient is supine, the process is repeated in the upright position. If urine leaks immediately with coughing, and the anatomic findings are consistent with loss of support of the bladder neck, one of the surgical procedures for bladder neck support is indicated.

CULDOCENTESIS

Direct sampling of peritoneal fluid via the posterior cul-de-sac is comparable to the peritoneal tap often used as a diagnostic aid in evaluation of acute upper abdominal disorders. This procedure can be done readily in an outpatient setting and is particularly useful in the diagnosis of ruptured ectopic pregnancy.

Following a bimanual examination to be sure there is no mass in the cul-de-sac, a speculum inserted into the vagina is opened widely with the set screw on the speculum handle. The posterior lip of the cervix is elevated with a tenaculum to visualize the cul-de-sac (Fig. 21-7). Ordinarily, no anesthesia is required, although local anesthetic may be injected first at the puncture site. A 3.5-inch, 20-gauge needle attached to a 10-ml syringe filled with 2 cc of air is advanced through the cul-de-sac with a single deliberate thrust. The patient usually experiences a sudden but brief pain when the needle traverses the peritoneum. The air in the syringe is injected to ensure a free flow, and any fluid in the cul-de-sac of Douglas is then aspirated.

The fluid obtained, depending on its nature,

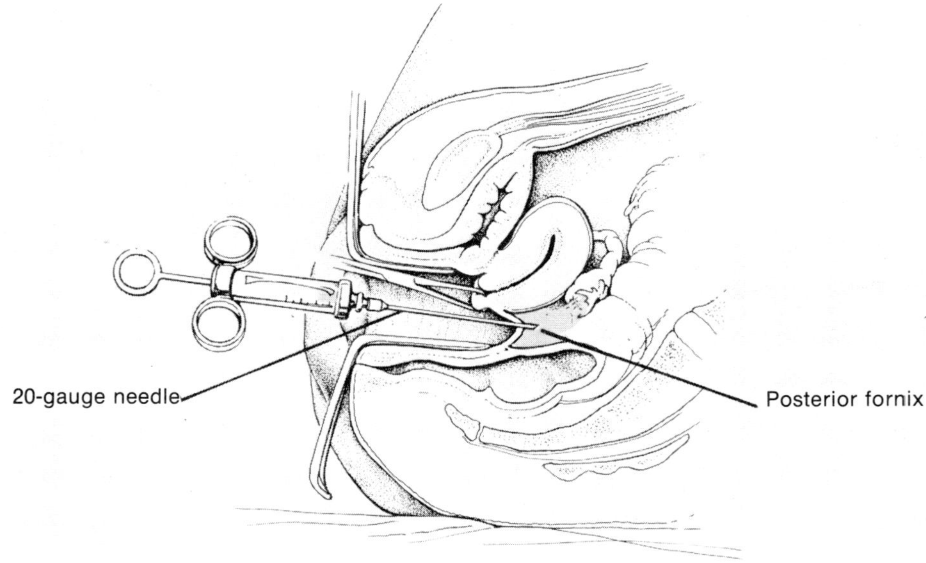

Figure 21-7. Technique for culdocentesis.

may suggest the following: (1) scant, clear, or straw colored—a normal pelvis; (2) turbid or purulent—pelvic inflammatory disease; (3) copious blood-tinged and serous, usually with a hematocrit less than 10%—a ruptured ovarian cyst; (4) bright blood that does not clot—a recently ruptured ectopic pregnancy. Hemoperitoneum warrants surgical exploration to determine the source of intra-abdominal bleeding. Inadvertent puncture of the sigmoid colon or a loop of small bowel during culdocentesis has proved to be of no clinical consequence.

CERVIX

BIOPSY

Although the Papanicolaou smear is an excellent screening method for the cytologic diagnosis of cervical cancer, it cannot replace other techniques for the definitive diagnosis of this disease. Cytologic methods are most useful when there are no visible cervical lesions. False positive Papanicolaou smears occur more frequently in the presence of invasive carcinoma and its associated inflammatory exudate. Cervical biopsy is relatively painless, and there are few contraindications. Following cytologic sampling, biopsies should be performed on any gross lesion of the cervix (Fig. 21-8) or when there is any departure from the normal-appearing cervix prior to any treatment. The use of Schiller's or Lugol's solution will facilitate selection of biopsy sites, as it will stain the normal glycogen-containing squamous epithelium a deep brown but will leave areas of columnar epithelium or abnormal epithelium unstained. A punch biopsy specimen should be obtained at a sufficient depth to contain enough stroma for differentiating invasive lesions. The tissue can be submitted to the pathology laboratory in separate labeled jars of formalin, or more than one specimen can be placed in the same container if each is individually wrapped in a piece of filter paper and labeled. To prevent blood from the first biopsy site from hampering vision from succeeding biopsies, biopsy specimens at the periphery of the cervix and on the posterior lip should be obtained prior to those from the external os or the anterior lip. If bleeding occurs, hemostasis can be achieved by applying Monsel's solution, silver nitrate, or placing a 2-0 chromic gut suture followed by the firm pressure with a sponge or cottonball.

In patients with abnormal cervical cytology, selection of biopsy sites by colposcopy is much more reliable (Fig. 21-9). Colposcopy requires both training and experience but establishes the location and extent of foci of abnormal epithelium. Colposcopic features such as color, opacity, vascular pattern, and surface contour are reliable indicators of the degree of histologic abnormality to direct biopsy. Endocervical curettage is combined with colposcopically directed biopsy for completeness of sampling and requires no anesthesia. The use of colposcopy in evaluating abnormal cervical cytology where a gross lesion

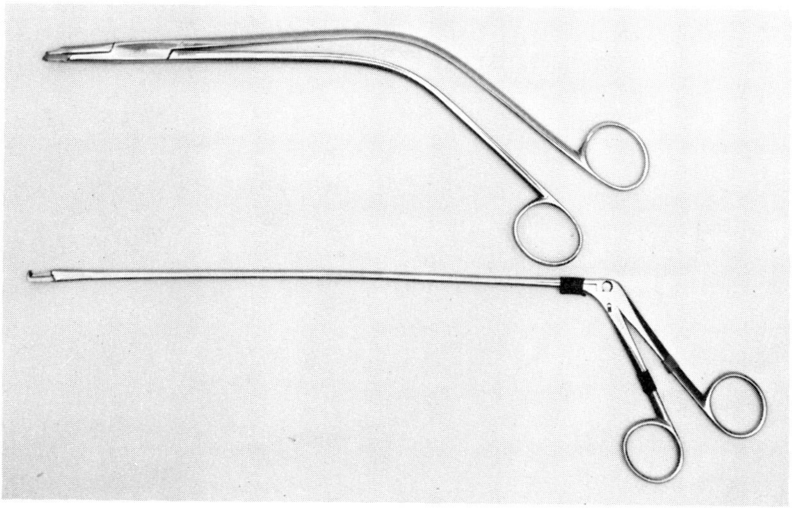

Figure 21-8. Instruments for punch biopsy of the cervix.

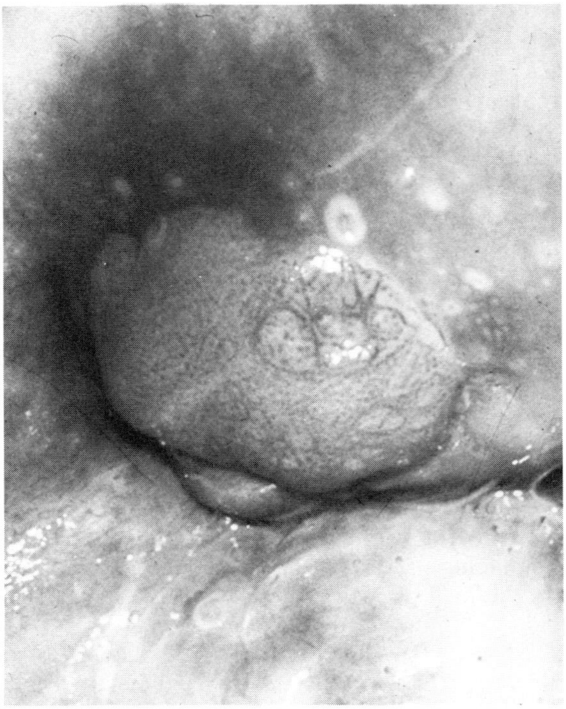

Figure 21-9. Colposcopic view of cervical lesion that was diagnosed as carcinoma by punch biopsy.

is not evident has reduced greatly the need for cervical conization. Direct resort to treatment is then permissible in most instances of cervical intraepithelial neoplasia (dysplasia and carcinoma in situ). However, if the total extent of the abnormality found on colposcopy is not visualized or if the histologic abnormality on biopsy does not explain the abnormal cytology, then conization biopsy remains essential for accurate diagnosis.

Endocervical polyps visible at the external os usually can be removed in the office by excisional biopsy. This is accomplished by grasping the base of the pedicle with a surgical clamp or ring forceps and twisting. Bleeding is usually minimal and can be treated by application of a silver nitrate stick when necessary. Although rarely malignant, polyps should be submitted for histologic study.

TREATMENT OF SUPERFICIAL CERVICAL LESIONS

It is important to reemphasize that an accurate diagnosis must be established and the possibility of a premalignant or malignant lesion be evaluated by appropriate biopsies and endocervical curettage before any therapy is performed. Large ectropions or cervicitis causing symptomatic vaginal discharge have often been treated with electrocautery. At present, cryotherapy is most often utilized for treatment of these conditions and is also an appropriate modality for treatment of properly evaluated cervical intraepithelial neoplasia (CIN). Since the cervix has no pain fibers that respond to temperature change, the procedure can be performed without anesthesia. The goal of treatment is regional destruction of abnormal tissue with minimal damage to the surrounding normal tissue.

The probe of the cryosurgery unit (Figure 21-10), chosen to cover the cervical lesion, is inserted into the cervical os. Lubrication of the tip with a thin layer of water-soluble jelly facilitates tissue cooling. The refrigerant is circulated through the probe, and the ice ball can be easily observed as it spreads laterally away from the circumference of the probe to a 4-mm to 5-mm margin. This process usually requires 2 to 3 minutes, the average length of a single freeze application using nitrous oxide or carbon dioxide as the cryogen. Once the diseased

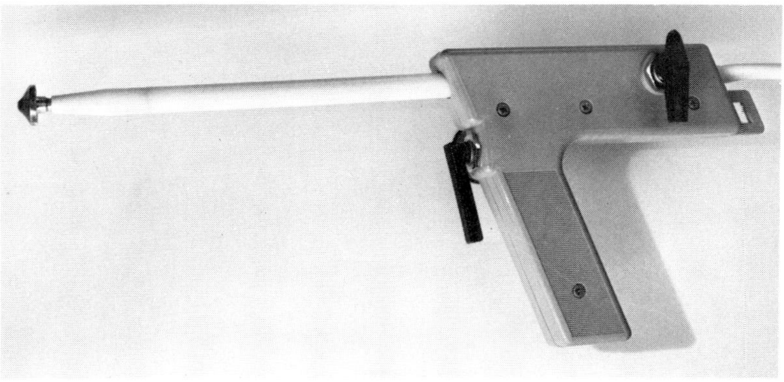

Figure 21-10. Typical cryosurgery unit with probe.

area has been frozen sufficiently, the probe is warmed and removed, although some operators prefer a second freeze cycle following a 5-minute thaw. The cervix is then carefully inspected to ascertain the extent of the ice ball and to make certain that the entire lesion has been frozen. The patient should be warned that she will develop a profuse, clear vaginal discharge beginning on the first postoperative day and lasting to 14 days. She should refrain from intercourse or douching during that time. Complete healing of the cervix is usual within 8 weeks of treatment, but reevaluation with cytology should be deferred until 4 months to avoid confusion with cellular changes of healing.

UTERUS

ENDOMETRIAL SAMPLING

Endometrial biopsy is a convenient office procedure that can be performed with only brief discomfort without anesthesia, but it is best tolerated with paracervical block anesthesia, particularly for more extensive sampling. It is a standard technique when timed in the luteal phase of the menstrual cycle to establish that ovulation has occurred with normal secretory endometrial histology. With perimenopausal and postmenopausal bleeding, endometrial biopsy is usually the advisable initial step in evaluation for possible endometrial cancer. A positive biopsy for malignancy obviates the need for dilatation and curettage in most cases, provided endocervical curettage and uterine sounding have been performed for staging of the disease. Although optimal techniques of endometrial biopsy have been more than 90% accurate in diagnosing endometrial cancer, it is still advisable to perform dilatation and full curettage when endometrial biopsy findings are negative in the situation of abnormal bleeding where endometrial cancer is suspect.

A variety of instruments and devices is available for endometrial sampling, but the Novak curette is the most widely used (Fig. 21-11). Prior to the biopsy, a bimanual examination is performed to determine the size and position of the uterus. The cervix is exposed with a speculum, and the cervix and upper vagina are cleaned with antiseptic solution. Traction is placed on the cervix with a tenaculum, and a cervical block may be employed by infiltration with 5 ml of 1% lidocaine at 1 cm depth near the junction of the cervix and vagina at the 4 and 8 o'clock positions. A 10-ml "control" syringe with a 22-gauge, 3.5-inch spinal needle serves well, and aspiration of the syringe is important to avoid intravascular injection in this highly vascular area. Several minutes should be allowed for anesthetic effect. If endometrial cancer is suspected, endocervical curettage with a small curette is per-

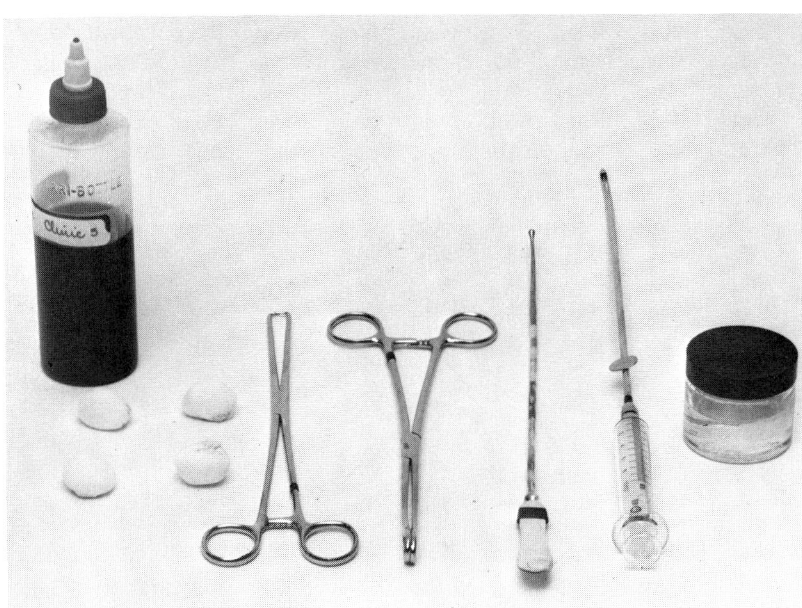

Figure 21-11. Minimal equipment for endometrial biopsy includes antiseptic solution, tenaculum, uterine sound, Novak curette attached to syringe, and fixative.

formed and the tissues are submitted separately. With moderate cervical traction the Novak curette, attached to a 10-ml syringe, is inserted through the endocervix so the curve of the curette conforms to the position of the uterine corpus. With suction on the syringe, strips of tissue are obtained as the curette is withdrawn. For ovulation evaluation one or two strips suffice. For diagnosis of endometrial lesions, circumferential sampling of the cavity with multiple strips is required. The biopsy specimens are expelled by flushing into a formalin solution. Since perforation of the uterus could occur, undue pressure should not be exerted when inserting the curette. If paracervical block anesthesia has been employed, then one may consider careful cervical dilatation with graduated dilators, as described later, in cases where the curette does not pass with ease. In addition to its use in endometrial sampling, the Novak curette can be used to retrieve a "lost" IUD when its string has retracted into the endometrial cavity.

Recently, the use of vacuum suction curettage has gained popularity as a reliable method of endometrial sampling (Fig. 21-12). This technique employs a small metal or plastic cannula of 4 mm diameter with a slightly curved tip. The small cannula diameter allows insertion through a narrow cervical canal and lessens the need for anesthesia. The cannula is connected to a plastic tube containing a cylindrical plastic filter for tissue retrieval. The apparatus is prepackaged in a sterile, disposable container, and the required vacuum force of approximately 60 cm of water can be provided either by a mechanical pump or faucet attachment.

Cervical dilatation and conventional uterine curettage can be done satisfactorily on an outpatient basis in most patients. It is often done under light general anesthesia in a "short-stay" facility, although in many cases it can be accomplished under paracervical block on an ambulatory basis (Fig. 21-13). The endocervix is first curetted, after which a small uterine sound is passed to measure uterine depth and to verify position of the uterine cavity. The cervix is then dilated, starting with small Hegar or Pratt dilators and progressing to a size 8 to 10. Perforation of the uterine wall by improper use of the dilator is usually due to lack of knowledge of uterine position. As resistance is felt with each larger dilator, steady pressure is carefully applied with the hand of the operator resting on the perineum to avoid a sudden thrust that results in perforation.

The uterine cavity is explored initially with a small stone forceps in search of an endometrial polyp as a cause of the patient's symptoms. A large, sharp curette is then inserted, and strips of endometrium are withdrawn, systematically sampling the entire uterine cavity and observing any irregular areas suggestive of a septum or submucous leiomyoma. The tissue collected on the piece of Telfa that had been inserted into the posterior area of the vagina is then placed in formalin solution.

Suction Curettage

For incomplete abortion, therapeutic abortion prior to 12 weeks' gestation, and evacuation of a hydatidiform mole, the classical curettage of the uterus has largely been replaced by suction curettage. The same techniques for preparation, local anesthesia, and cervical dilatation are utilized.

An appropriate-sized, plastic suction curette is inserted into the uterine cavity after it has been attached to the tubing of the suction

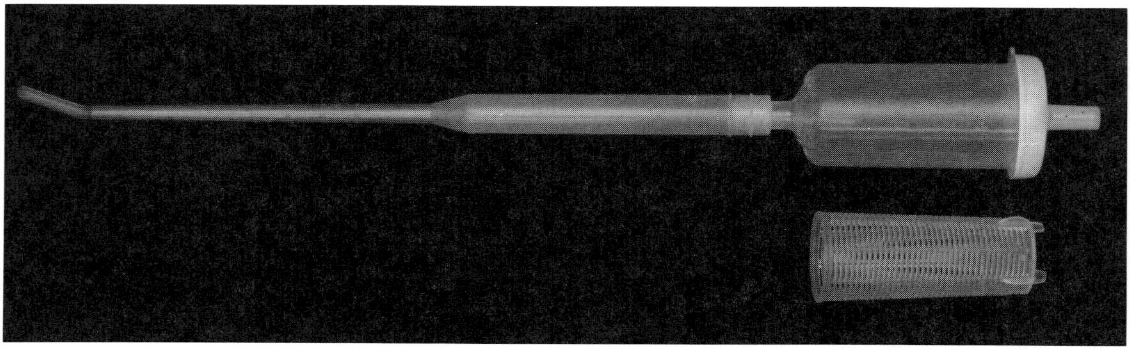

Figure 21-12. Disposable suction curettage apparatus (Vabra Aspirator) with tissue filter removed.

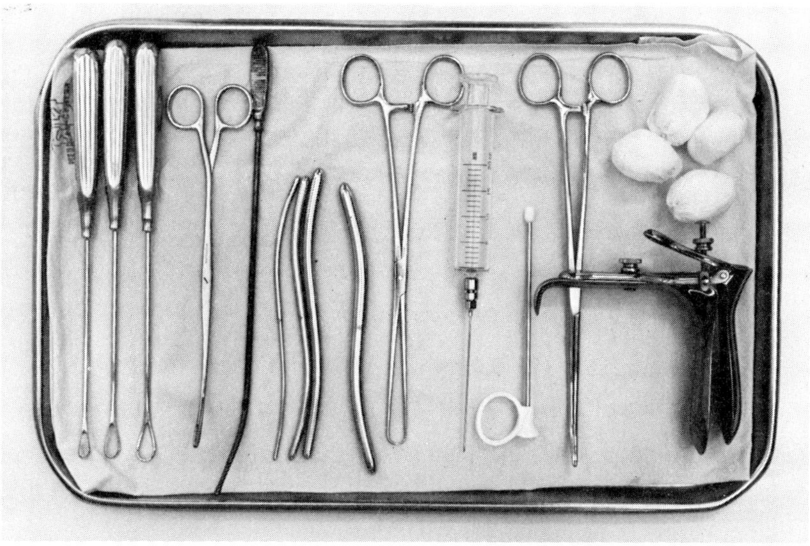

Figure 21-13. Standard set of instruments for outpatient dilatation and curettage.

machine (Fig. 21-14). The suction machine should also be checked prior to its use to determine that it is creating the proper negative pressure. By closing the escape valve, a vacuum of 50 cm Hg will be created. As curettage proceeds, tissue will be seen flowing into the curette and tubing. The curette is rotated 360 degrees clockwise as it is withdrawn, and the procedure is repeated in a counterclockwise direction. When a grating sensation is noted and no more tissue is obtained, the endometrial cavity is curetted gently with a sharp curette and followed by one brief suction curettage. At this point the evacuated material is examined.

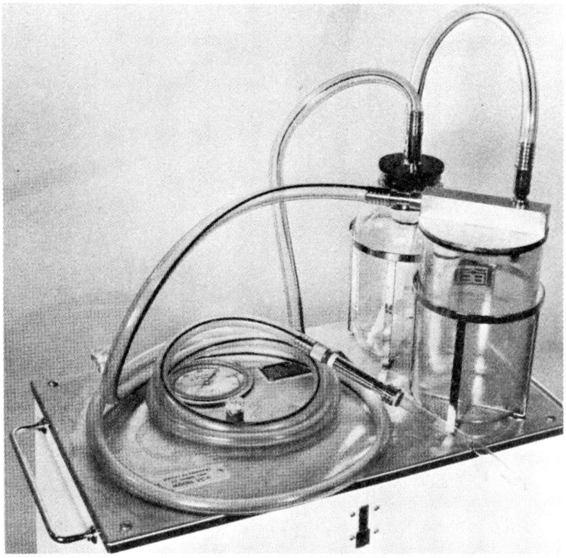

Figure 21-14. Electric suction apparatus with a swivel handle and plastic curette. (Mattingly RF: Te Linde's Operative Gynecology, 6th ed. JB Lippincott, 1985)

Blood typing should be done on every patient having a spontaneous or therapeutic abortion, and if her blood is Rh negative, Rh immune globulin should be given within 72 hours to protect her from Rh immunization. If no complications have occurred, the patient is discharged after 2 hours of observation. An appointment is made for examination within 2 weeks, but she is instructed to return earlier if any problems develop.

HYSTEROSCOPY

Hysteroscopy is a specialized technique with expanding usage in gynecologic diagnosis and therapy. The procedure is readily performed on an ambulatory or short-stay basis with either general or paracervical block anesthesia. Hysteroscopes are of either the contact or panoramic type. The latter type, which is in wider current use, is a modified cystoscope using fiberoptic illumination and permitting the introduction of biopsy and other instruments through an operating channel. Uterine distention is accomplished by dextran 32% solution or CO_2 gas. The technique is particularly useful in identifying symptomatic endometrial lesions that may have been missed by biopsy or curettage, such as polyps, submucous myomata, or a small focus of cancer.

Therapeutic uses have included resection of submucous myomata, location and retrieval of "lost" IUDs, diagnosis and treatment of intrauterine adhesions, and division of uterine septa (with concomitant laparoscopy).

FALLOPIAN TUBES AND OVARIES

HYSTEROSALPINGOGRAPHY

Uterotubal CO_2 insufflation (Rubin's test) at best can indicate only patency of one tube or occlusion of both tubes. Therefore the procedure has generally been abandoned in favor of hysterosalpingography, which permanently records any uterine abnormality and the presence or absence of tubal patency. Indications include infertility and habitual abortion. Acute inflammatory disease is a contraindication, and the test should be performed in the preovulatory phase of the menstrual cycle to avoid interfering with an early conceptus.

The patient is placed in the lithotomy position on the x-ray table and a speculum is introduced into the vagina. An insufflation cannula is introduced through the cervix by mechanically applying countertraction with a tenaculum on the cervix to maintain an airtight seal. The entire system should be filled with the dye from the attached syringe before insertion to eliminate air bubbles. One of the aqueous iodide media such as polyvinylpyrrolidone and sodium acetrizoate (Salpix) is employed; 1 ml to 2 ml of the medium is slowly injected into the uterus for optimum study of the uterine cavity under fluoroscopic visualization employing image intensification, and the first film is taken. A second injection of several more milliliters of the medium is slowly carried out to visualize both fallopian tubes and look for spill of the dye into the peritoneal cavity as evidence of tubal patency (Fig. 21-15). The patient may experience a discharge or spotting following the procedure, but no special treatment is necessary.

LAPAROSCOPY

Laparoscopy is a transperitoneal endoscopic technique that provides excellent visualization of the pelvic structures and permits the diagnosis of gynecologic disorders and limited surgery without laparotomy. To use the laparoscope safely and effectively, the physician needs thorough training and opportunity for extensive experience. Tubal coagulation is ideally suited to laparoscopy as an outpatient procedure, since the patient requesting surgical sterilization usually has a normal pelvis. However, when the possibility of subsequent laparotomy is significant (acute and chronic pelvic pain, infertility, "second look" in ovarian cancer patients), laparoscopy is best performed in a hospital setting.

Most basic laparoscopes are 10 mm in diameter and have a 180-degree viewing angle. The instrument has an effective length of over 25

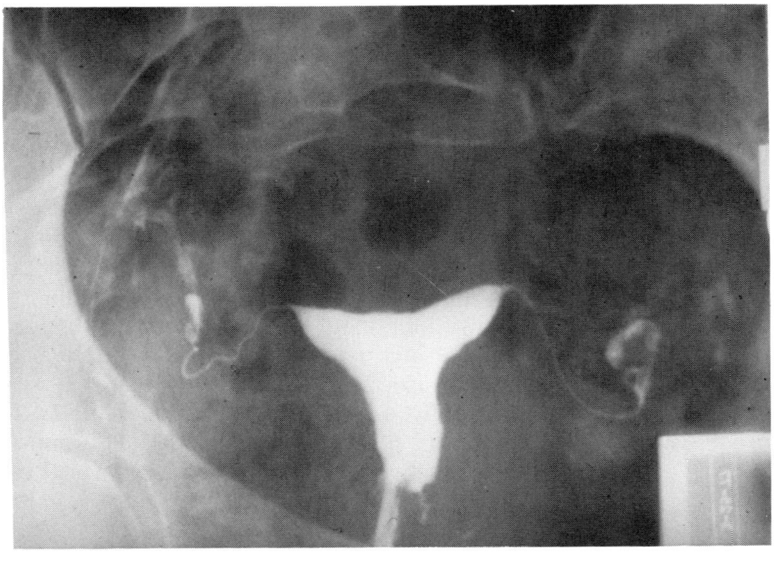

Figure 21-15. Hysterosalpingogram outlining normal uterine cavity and patent fallopian tubes, with spill of contrast material into peritoneal cavity.

cm and can be utilized with a standard fiberoptic light box supplying a 150-watt light source. In addition to the equipment used for observation, a variety of other instruments for biopsy, coagulation, aspiration, and manipulation can be passed through a separate cannula or inserted through the laparoscope.

Careful explanation of the contemplated surgery must be given to each patient and the operative permit signed. Preparation includes no solid food for at least 8 hours, no liquids for more than 6 hours preoperatively, a history and physical examination, routine blood studies, and urinalysis. Abdominal or perineal shaving or premedication is not necessary. General anesthesia with or without endotracheal intubation is usually used, but a periumbilical field block with 15 ml of 1% lidocaine can provide adequate pain relief in some patients.

The patient is placed in the dorsal lithotomy "frog-leg" position and draped after induction of anesthesia and preparation of the abdomen and perineum with povidone–iodine solution. If the patient has not voided just prior to surgery, the bladder is emptied by catheterization. After careful bimanual examination, a tenaculum is attached to the cervix and a tubal insufflation cannula is inserted into the cervical canal and fixed to the tenaculum so it can be used as a "handle" to maneuver the uterus. A 1-cm skin incision is made in the lower umbilicus through which the Verres needle is inserted into the peritoneal cavity. Approximately 2 liters of CO_2 should then be introduced and monitored by the pneumatic insufflator. The needle is withdrawn and the laparoscopic trocar and cannula inserted. After proper abdominal entry, the trocar is withdrawn and replaced with the fiberoptic laparoscope (Fig. 21-16). The examiner manipulates the intrauterine cannula so that the pelvic organs can be observed. Electrical coagulation forceps may be inserted through the operating laparoscope or through a second cannula inserted suprapubically under direct laparoscopic vision. Each fallopian tube is grasped in its midportion, moved to a safe position away from bowel and bladder, and electrocoagulated in two places. A thorough in-

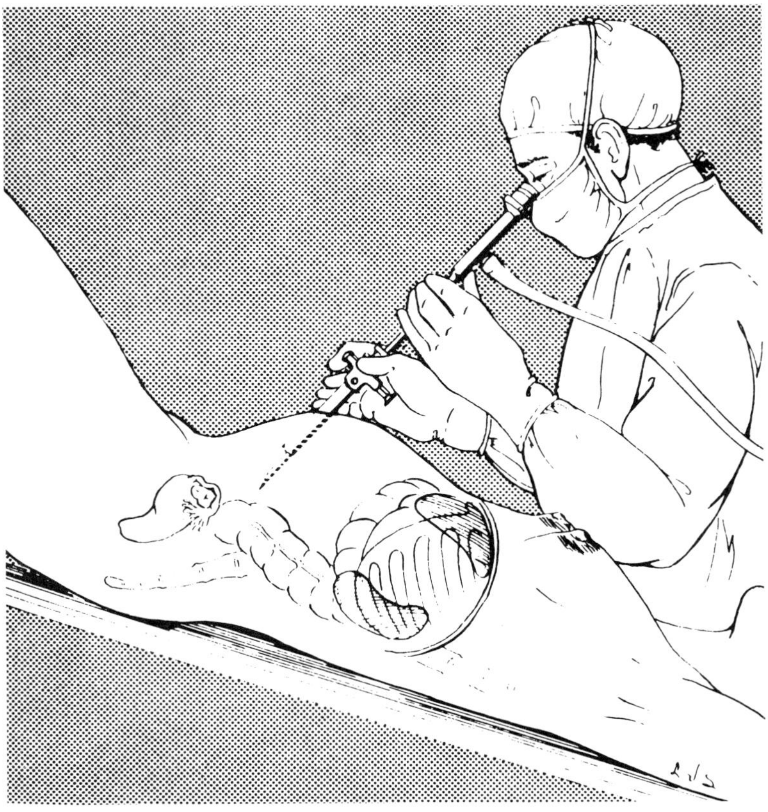

Figure 21-16. Laparoscope in place for visualization of pelvic structures.

spection for any bleeding points or pelvic disease should also be made. The laparoscope is then withdrawn, the trumpet valve is opened to evacuate the pneumoperitoneum, the trocar sleeve is withdrawn, and the skin incision is closed with a few 3-0 chromic surgical gut sutures. There is no need to perform any closure of the peritoneum, rectus fascia, or subcutaneous tissue. A bandage is applied and the patient is taken to the recovery room. She is discharged after several hours of observation and instructed on cleansing the incision and changing the bandage daily.

Relative contraindications to laparoscopy include previous intra-abdominal surgery that may have resulted in adhesions, peritonitis, and severe cardiac or pulmonary disease. The fact that the incidence of complications varies inversely with the amount of experience and training of the surgeon makes it clear that the procedure should not be undertaken by the occasional operator. Insertion of the Verres needle and trocar is a blind technique that could result in puncture of a blood vessel or injury to the gastrointestinal tract. Therefore the surgeon performing laparoscopy should be thoroughly familiar with abdominal and pelvic surgery, should a laparotomy become necessary.

A technique that may be considered in the patient where intraperitoneal adhesions are suspected is that of open laparoscopy. With this technique a 2-cm to 3-cm intraumbilical skin incision is carried through layers by visualized dissection to peritoneal entry. A modified cannula with a blunt trocar is inserted into the peritoneal cavity. Suture fixation of the fascia to the cannula allows a seal for pneumoperitoneum to be achieved by passing CO_2 through the cannula, after which the laparoscope is inserted. Following the procedure, the incision is closed in layers.

TUBAL STERILIZATION

In addition to tubal sterilization by laparoscopic technique, tubal ligation through either a mini-laparotomy incision or colpotomy incision is performed satisfactorily in a short-stay surgical facility. Mini-laparotomy appears to be the safest of female sterilization techniques and can be learned readily by an operator who has had basic surgical training. Although local abdominal wall and paracervical block anesthesia, combined with intravenous analgesia, provide satisfactory anesthesia for the procedure, general or spinal anesthesia are more often used in this country. The patient is placed in the dorsal lithotomy position ("knee rest" stirrups are preferred), and the lower abdomen and vagina are surgically prepared with povidine–iodine solution. Shaving only to the mons pubis is required. Insertion of a uterine manipulator to elevate the uterus to the incisional site is most helpful (Fig. 21-17). The Hulka tenaculum–sound is well suited for the purpose, but a Rubin's cannula or other similar instrument may be employed. The bladder is emptied with a catheter and a conventional vaginal speculum is inserted to expose the cervix. Sounding of the uterine cavity for depth and direction is carried out prior to securing the uterine manipulator to the cervix. Care must be exercised to avoid uterine perforation, and stabilizing the cervix by grasping the anterior lip with a single-tooth tenaculum can assist this process. With the patient in the Trendelenburg position, the uterus is elevated to slightly tent the abdominal wall, and a 4-cm skin incision is made over this site near the pubic hairline. A small Pfannenstiel incision is employed most often with only minimal elevation of the rectus sheath from the median raphe required. Peritoneal entry at the upper extent of exposure avoids the bladder. With the peritoneal cavity open, two "Army–Navy" retractors are inserted and the uterus is elevated to the operative site (Fig. 21-17). Rotation of the uterus in either direction successively exposes the fallopian tubes. After identifying each tube by tracing it to its fimbrial extremity, a Pomeroy ligation is accomplished by tying an elevated loop of the tube with plain catgut and excising the ligated knuckle (Fig. 21-18). Closure of the small abdominal wound is carried out in a routine fashion.

Colpotomy tubal ligation was performed more frequently prior to the advent of laparoscopic tubal ligation. For the experienced vaginal surgeon it remains an inviting choice in a multiparous patient with uterine retroversion. The colpotomy incision is closed in a single layer with a continuous locking technique using a delayed-absorbable (polyglycolic acid) suture. The higher failure rate with fimbriectomy makes a Pomeroy-type ligation a better choice in colpotomy sterilization. The prophylactic use of a single intravenous dose of a cephalosporin or other broad-spectrum antibi-

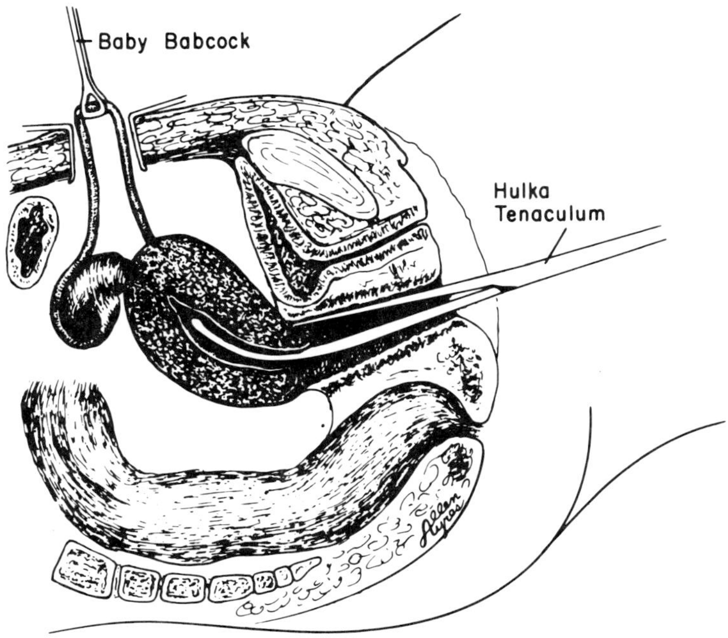

Figure 21-17. Minilaparotomy tubal ligation demonstrating the elevation of the fallopian tube through the abdominal wall. (Reprinted with permission from The American College of Obstetricians and Gynecologists. [Obstetrics and Gynecology, Vol 54, 1979, p 185])

otics is advised in this procedure, as in other transvaginal surgery.

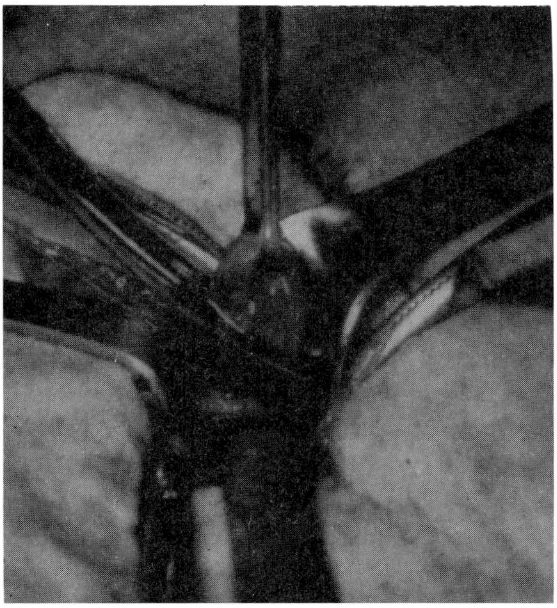

Figure 21-18. Excision of a knuckle of tube to complete a Pomeroy-type tubal ligation. (Reprinted with permission from The American College of Obstetricians and Gynecologists. [Obstetrics and Gynecology, Vol 54, 1979, p 185])

SEXUAL ASSAULT

Rape is defined as sexual intercourse by force or against the victim's will. Whether rape has occurred is a legal matter for court decision and is not a medical diagnosis. No conclusions, opinions, or diagnoses should be written in the record. It is the physician's responsibility to conduct the examination in such a manner that the objectively acquired evidence could be protective of either a real victim of sexual assault or a falsely accused defendant. If the patient alleges rape, there is usually a duty to report it immediately to designated officials.

The alleged victim should be given priority over nonemergent patients. A female chaperone should be present. Written and witnessed informed consent must be obtained before any examination is performed, photographs are taken, specimens are collected, or information is released to authorities. A thorough evaluation is greatly simplified by having available in the emergency room or clinic kits that contain an instruction sheet, a standard examination form, and specimen containers (Fig. 21-19).

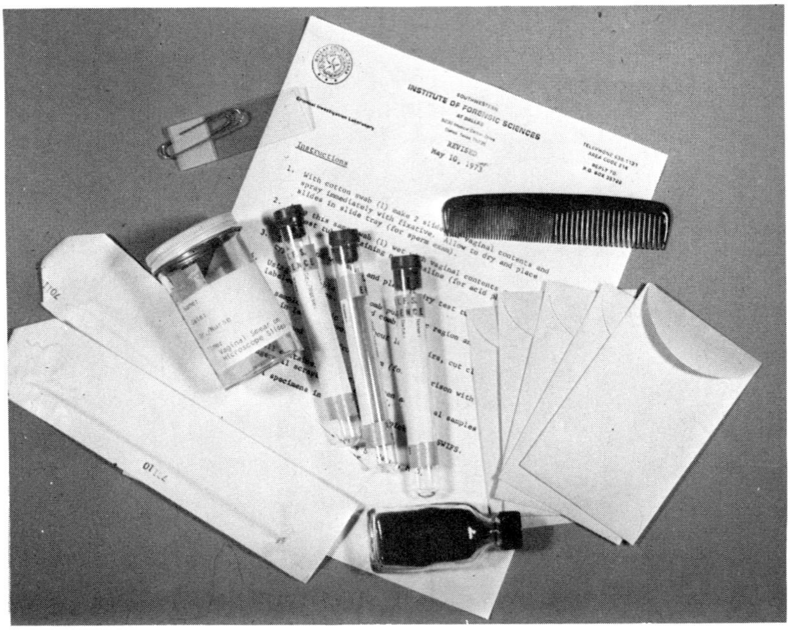

Figure 21-19. Equipment and specimen containers for collection of evidence in cases of alleged sexual assault.

HISTORY

The history should include the exact time and date the patient was examined and the time of the alleged offense; the patient's complaint should be recorded as a direct quotation. Details before, during, and after the alleged assault, last menstrual period, last intercourse prior to the event, and current contraceptive technique are all important. The patient should be specifically asked (1) "if the assailant's penis penetrated the vulva"; (2) if he experienced orgasm; (3) if he wore a condom; (4) if the patient has douched, bathed or showered, defecated, or urinated since the alleged assault.

PHYSICAL EXAMINATION

The emotional state should be noted, and the examination should include evaluation of the entire skin surface, with all bruises, contusions, and lacerations being noted on a drawing. The clothes should be examined for gross dirt, blood stains, and tears, and, if necessary, they should be retained and labeled or photographed for court evidence.

Pelvic examination should include a complete examination of the external genitalia for evidence of trauma and the state of the hymenal ring in terms of number of fingers or size of speculum easily inserted. The vaginal epithelium, particularly small mucosal tears, and the contents of the vagina should also be described.

LABORATORY SPECIMENS

The following laboratory specimens should be obtained: (1) blood for alcohol, toxicology, and baseline serology; (2) scraping and clipping of fingernails; (3) combings from pubic hair; (4) a sample of the patient's pubic hair; (5) loose hairs and scrapings of blood stains on the clothes and body; (6) saline washings from the vagina for sperm; (7) aspirate of vaginal fluid and secretions; and (8) culture of the cervix for gonococcus. A wet smear of the vaginal aspirate is examined microscopically by the physician for sperm and sperm motility. Four smears, two from the posterior vaginal fornix and two from the endocervix, are put on glass slides on which the patient's last name has been etched. Two of these smears are placed in a permanent fixative solution, and the other two are allowed to air-dry for later precipitin, acid phosphatase, and creatinine phosphokinase determinations. The collected specimens are kept under lock and key in a safe place until delivered to the pathologist. They should never be given to other hospital personnel to transport to the laboratory.

TREATMENT

The primary responsibility of the physician to a sexual assault victim is to treat her physical injuries, prevent unwanted pregnancy and venereal disease, and provide for her emotional needs. Lacerations should be repaired with fine catgut, and tetanus toxoid may be indicated, as these wounds may contain dirt particles and may become infected. Almost all adult women in whom sexual assault included coitus appreciate and should receive an antiseptic douche and shower as soon after the examination as possible.

Gonorrhea exposure is treated optimally at the time of examination. Administration of probenecid (Benemid) 1 g orally, followed by procaine penicillin 4.8 million units intramuscularly, is the treatment of choice. Patients at risk for pregnancy should be given two Ovral tablets initially and two additional tablets in 12 hours for pregnancy prophylaxis. This therapy should be instituted as soon as possible and no later than 72 hours after the exposure.

The physician should be aware that most women involved in assault episodes require comfort, understanding, and emotional support. These should be supplied initially by the physician; but in addition, many victims require the help of a crisis counselor, an appropriately trained social worker, or a psychiatrist. A repeat examination of the patient should be performed approximately 4 weeks after the episode. If a menstrual period has not occurred, a sensitive pregnancy test should be obtained, and abortion may be considered if the test is positive.

22 Urogenital Tract

RICHARD G. MIDDELTON AND DOUGLAS S. DAHL

URINARY INFECTIONS

GENERAL CONSIDERATIONS

Infection of the urinary systems of both sexes can be classified according to the site of the infection, the duration of the infection, and the causative organism. Serious infections of the urinary tract are uncommon in individuals with anatomically and physiologically normal urinary tracts. Natural protective mechanisms, including the continuous dilution of bacteria and continuous washout of the urinary tract by the flow or urine, resist infection of healthy transitional epithelium. Abnormalities of anatomic derangement, stasis of urine, decreased systemic resistance, and foreign bodies can usually be identified as etiologic mechanisms in most serious urinary tract infections.

The physician treating an infection of the urinary tract must search for underlying factors in the infected tract in addition to identifying the infectious agent and instituting treatment directed toward the infecting agent. When infected urine has been identified by the presence of WBCs and bacteria, bacterial cultures to identify the type and antibiotic sensitivity of the agent are merely the beginning of the evaluation. Urography, cystography, and cystoscopy are basic to the evaluation of the patient with an infection of the urinary system. These studies are particularly indicated when urinary infection recurs or persists. These investigations should be obtained in all but minor problems.

ACUTE CYSTITIS IN WOMEN

Acute cystitis in women is the most common urinary infection encountered in clinical medicine. When it occurs in the early months of marriage this infection has often been called honeymoon cystitis. Although the patient is acutely uncomfortable and may be very anxious, cystitis is not a serious illness and is easy to recognize and treat. Symptoms include burning, urinary frequency, urgency, lower abdominal cramps, and grossly bloody urine at times. Pain in the flank and fever are not a part of ordinary acute cystitis.

On bimanual pelvic examination the bladder is extremely tender. A catheterized urine specimen contains innumberable white cells, many bacteria, and often red cells. Cystoscopy should generally be avoided in acute cystitis. (The bladder mucosa is fiery red and edematous.) Usually urine culture reveals a high colony count of a gram-negative organism, most commonly *Escherichia coli*.

Treatment with sulfonamides, nitrofurantoin, trimethoprim-sulfamethoxazole, tetracycline, or ampicillin eases the symptoms promptly, and the infection will clear in several days. Sulfonamides and nitrofurantoin are generally effective and are recommended because they are inexpensive and cause few side-effects. Therapy for 5 to 7 days is sufficient, and therapeutic failure is uncommon. One-time treatment with increased doses of trimethoprim-sulfamethoxazole, amoxicillin, or tetracycline has been virtually as effective as more prolonged therapy. Flank pain, fever, or persistence of the infection for more than 5 to 7 days indicates the need for urologic investigation. However, urologic investigation in the woman with typical and periodic episodes of acute cystitis rarely reveals an anatomic abnormality.

Recurrence of symptoms in a woman who has received antibacterial treatment for acute cystitis nearly always proves to be a new infection with a different bacterial organism. Phenazopyridine hydrochloride (Pyridium) and other azo dyes are thought to soothe the irritated bladder slightly, but they are of dubious value in management of acute cystitis.

Traditionally, physicians have employed many schemes in the hope of preventing periodic acute cystitis in women. Regular urethral dilatation, urethrotomy, various bladder irrigations, and a variety of operations on the distal urethra have all been advocated and frequently performed. There is little scientific basis to relate acute cystitis in women to an abnormality of the urethra. Exceptions to this would be a patient with a urethral diverticulum or chronic infection in the periurethral glands.

URINARY INFECTION IN CHILDREN

The great majority of children never have a urinary infection, but a child with a urinary infection will usually develop further episodes of infection after the initial one is treated with an antibiotic. A child with repeated urinary infections is extremely likely to have a congenital abnormality of the urinary tract. It is reasonable to perform intravenous pyelography and cystography on any child who has had a urinary infection. Waiting for the second or third infection before carrying out investigation of the urinary tract increases the yield of abnormal findings but unnecessarily delays detection of serious urinary tract abnormalities at times. Certainly complete and prompt urologic investigation is vital in a child with a febrile urinary infection, an infant with a urinary infection, and a boy with any type of urinary infection.

ACUTE PYELONEPHRITIS

An acute bacterial infection of the upper urinary system (renal pelvis, calyces, and medulla) is characterized by fever, chills, flank pain, flank tenderness, pyuria, and bacteriuria. Pyelolymphatic and pyelovenous communication occurs readily; bacteremia is often present. Acute pyelonephritis is rare in a normal urinary system. The patient usually requires hospital admission, identification and treatment of the infection, and investigation of the urinary system. Urine and blood cultures and sensitivity studies should be carried out, but while the results are awaited treatment with a broad-spectrum antibiotic should be started.

An intravenous pyelogram is obtained as early as possible. A renal ultrasound study is a reasonable alternative. If hydronephrosis is detected by intravenous pyelogram or by ultrasound, prompt percutaneous nephrostomy is performed under ultrasonic control. The nephrostomy catheter provides drainage and decompression. A specimen of urine is also obtained for culture and sensitivity studies. Emergency passage of a ureteral catheter to the renal pelvis is an alternative to percutaneous nephrostomy. Surgical nephrostomy is rarely necessary in the acutely ill patient nowadays.

Infection behind an obstructed upper urinary system is dangerous and can lead to fatal septicemia if drainage is not accomplished.

When the patient with clinically acute pyelonephritis has no upper-tract obstruction by intravenous pyelogram or renal ultrasound study, vesicoureteral reflux should be considered. A cystourethrogram can be delayed until the infection is under control.

PYELONEPHRITIS OF PREGNANCY

"Physiologic" hydronephrosis and hydroureter are regularly seen in the later part of pregnancy. The degree of obstruction is nearly always greater on the right than on the left. In late pregnancy, therefore, the stasis of urine in the upper urinary system makes the woman vulnerable to pyelonephritis. The patient has high fever, chills and flank pain. There is often nausea, vomiting, and dehydration. Hospitalization is usually necessary. Intravenous fluids are administered. The bacterial organisms should be identified from a carefully obtained catheterized urine specimen. Broad-spectrum antibiotic treatment is begun, and the antibiotic may be adjusted when culture and sensitivity data are available. Treatment is similar to that of acute pyelonephritis in a nonpregnant woman. Most antibiotics can be given to a pregnant woman with urinary infection, but tetracycline and trimethoprim are generally to be avoided. After the acute episode is over it is desirable to maintain the patient on low-dose prophylactic antibiotic treatment for the balance of the pregnancy.

Occasionally, percutaneous nephrostomy drainage or cystoscopic passage of a ureteral catheter is useful when the acute pyelonephritis is not relieved by antibiotic treatment.

A clinical diagnosis is usually feasible without x-ray studies; however, limited intravenous pyelography is recommended unless a prompt response to antibiotics excludes a calculus. Improved renal drainage can sometimes be achieved if the patient lies on her side (affected side up) or assumes a knee–chest position.

CHRONIC PYELONEPHRITIS

A chronic bacterial infection of the upper urinary system may be characterized by variable flank pain or no flank pain at all. Fever is also variable. Persistent or recurring pyuria and bacteriuria are present, usually without symptoms of bladder irritability. A carefully obtained clean-catch specimen is helpful in a woman, but a catheterized urine specimen is more reliable. Thorough urologic evaluation is necessary; a search is made for obstruction, vesicourethral reflux, calculi, neoplasms, and tuberculosis. Some underlying anatomic disorder, congenital or acquired, and tuberculosis are major considerations.

MALE GENITAL AND LOWER URINARY TRACT DISEASE

GONORRHEA

Acute gonococcal anterior urethritis is extremely common and has reached epidemic proportions in many areas. Dysuria and profuse purulent urethral discharge begin within 7 days after coitus with an infected partner. The urethral discharge is thick and creamy and has a yellowish green tint. The diagnosis can be presumed on inspection of the typical urethral discharge, but demonstration of intracellular and extracellular gram-negative diplococci is necessary for definitive diagnosis. Specific culture media are available for gonococci but are rarely necessary to establish the diagnosis in men. Vaginal cultures for gonococci are valuable in women, in whom the infection may be insidious and asymptomatic.

Aqueous procaine penicillin G remains the preferred drug for treatment of gonorrhea. Its effectiveness has been somewhat diminished by emergence of strains partially resistant to penicillin. Since resistance is relative rather than absolute, the recommended dose of penicillin has increased somewhat in recent years. Probenecid enhances therapy by elevating and prolonging the blood levels of penicillin. The treatment recommended by the Centers for Disease Control in Atlanta is 1 g probenecid given orally 30 minutes prior to administration of 4.8 million units of aqueous procaine penicillin G, given in two intramuscular injections. An alternative treatment is the simultaneous oral administration of either 3.5 g ampicillin or 3 g amoxicillin with 1 g probenecid. When penicillin is ineffective or cannot be used because of allergy, an alternative treatment is tetracycline 0.5 g by mouth four times a day for 5 days (total dose 10 g).

Sexual intercourse should be completely proscribed until the infection has resolved. Anyone with whom the patient has had intimate contact should be examined, cultures should be obtained, and the individual should be treated. With adequate antibiotic treatment the urethral discharge and dysuria disappear completely over 2 to 4 days. Without treatment the discharge will continue for months and possibly several years. Untreated gonorrhea can result in gonorrheal prostatitis, epididymitis, late urethral stricture, and gonorrheal arthritis from hematogenous spread of this organism. Occasionally, after adequate treatment of gonorrhea, a watery, scanty discharge will linger for several weeks or longer. Cultures of this nonspecific discharge are almost invariably sterile. Gonorrhea is occasionally seen in the rectum and in the mouth in homosexuals and persons involved in unusual sexual practices.

NONSPECIFIC URETHRITIS

Nonspecific urethritis may be impossible to differentiate from gonococcal urethritis without laboratory studies. Purulent urethral discharge, dysuria, and urethral itching are common to both diseases. In nonspecific urethritis, however, the discharge is often mucoid, watery, or milky. The discharge in gonorrhea is generally profuse, purulent looking, and greenish yellow. Nongonococcal or "nonspecific" urethritis is commonly caused by organisms of the Chlamydia group. The incubation period after sexual transmission can be up to 4 to 6 weeks. The diagnosis is made by excluding gonorrhea on Gram stain of the discharge and on the basis of a negative culture for gonococci. Routine cultures of the discharge are generally negative. Laboratory testing methods for Chlamydia are now commonly available; these are culture and direct slide fluorescence tests. Tetracycline is the drug of choice in the treatment of nonspecific urethritis, whether or not Chlamydia are identified. Two or 3 weeks of treatment may be adequate, but at times up to 6 weeks of continuous treatment is needed.

HERPES SIMPLEX (HERPES PROGENITALIS)

Herpes progenitalis is an acute, localized inflammation occurring usually on the penis, but occasionally elsewhere on the genitalia. In women it is seen in the vulva and can occur in the urethra. Initially, there are pain, swelling, and erythema. Soon vesicles appear. Over the course of several days the vesicles dry up, and the process resolves spontaneously. The virus remains dormant between recurring episodes. Recurrences are common, and the triggering mechanisms are unknown. The infection probably is spread by sexual contact at times but is undoubtedly communicated in other ways too. Sexual intercourse should be avoided until the lesion is healed.

Acyclovir, an antiviral agent, has been advocated for the treatment of the acute herpetic eruption. Studies have shown that the administration of acyclovir by mouth will decrease the length of the acute inflammation. The use of this drug prophylactically in patients with recurrent eruptions and the use of other antiviral agents are under study. The inflammatory process will recede and disappear spontaneously.

Numerous topical agents have been suggested and used, and the placebo effect of any treatment is difficult to evaluate. There is no scientific basis for recommending any local agent at present.

CONDYLOMA ACUMINATUM (VENEREAL WART)

Condyloma acuminatum is a soft, bushy, papillary skin lesion occurring most often in young adults and located in moist areas—the external genitalia of the male, the vulva in the female, the groin, pubic area, and perianal area of both sexes. Commonly, the lesions are multiple. The usual sites in the male are on or underneath the foreskin and in the coronal sulcus. These lesions are caused by a virus similar to the one responsible for verruca vulgaris.

Local application of 25% podophyllin resin in tincture of benzoin is usually effective. Repeat treatment at intervals of 1 to 3 weeks may be necessary for complete disappearance of the lesion. Excision, fulguration, and the use of the YAG or CO_2 laser are also employed at times, but for small, multiple lesions, podophyllin in tincture of benzoin is simple and effective.

Occasionally, condylomata occur within the urethral meatus of the male, and they may extend proximally deeper into the urethra. Transurethral fulguration, laser treatment, or the use of fluorouracil cream are appropriate treatment for urethral condylomata.

ACUTE PROSTATITIS

Acute bacterial prostatitis may occur abruptly in a patient without prior urinary disease, probably as a result of hematogenous spread. More often it occurs in a patient with preexisting urinary infection. The patient with an indwelling Foley catheter, vesical calculi, urethral stricture, or residual bladder urine is a frequent victim of acute prostatitis. Generalized symptoms—myalgia, chills, fever, and anorexia—are accompanied by marked dysuria, frequency, perineal pain, and a weak urinary stream or even acute urinary retention.

The prostate is swollen, tense, and tender and may be very warm to palpation. Massage of the acutely inflamed prostate is risky and should be avoided; it is not necessary to make the diagnosis. The urine is loaded with white cells and bacteria, and urine cultures are usually positive.

Broad-spectrum antibiotics should be given until culture data are available, then specific antibacterial treatment can be employed. Narcotics may be necessary for pain. Aspirin is useful for the accompanying fever. Sitz baths may be soothing. Hospitalization is advised if the patient has a high temperature and is toxemic, or if he develops acute urinary retention. Acute epididymitis is common following acute prostatitis. If symptoms and fever persist despite antibiotic treatment the possibility of a prostatic abscess should be considered. When febrile prostatitis occurs in a patient requiring long-term catheter drainage, he should be treated by suprapubic cystostomy and removal of the urethral catheter. Cystostomy diverts the urine from the deep urethra and allows removal of the irritating foreign body from the urethra.

CHRONIC PROSTATITIS

Chronic prostatitis is a common condition in men of all ages, although it does not occur before puberty. Symptoms are mild burning, frequency, and urgency, often in association with aching in the groin, scrotum, perineum, and suprapubic and sacral areas. There may be a slight watery urethral discharge, often noted only in the morning on arising. Some patients describe a decrease in libido and a perineal ache after ejaculation. Bloody or brownish discoloration of the semen is also indicative of chronic prostatitis.

It is important on physical examination to exclude other diseases of the inguinal area, genitalia, and prostate. Hernia, hydrocele, epididymal cyst, and varicocele may give similar symptoms, as may prostatic cancer. In chronic prostatitis the prostate is often soft and boggy, and areas of softness and of fibrosis may be palpable in the same prostate. A three-glass test will reveal few white cells in the first glass, but many white cells are seen in the prostatic fluid or in the voided urine after vigorous prostatic massage. Prostatic fluid expressed by prostatic massage will generally contain more than 8 to 10 white cells per high-power field.

The urologic literature is full of speculations, opinions, and old-wives tales relating this condition to various sexual practices, diet, activity, local or distant infection, and trauma to the perineum. It is difficult to incriminate these factors scientifically, and often the urine and prostatic fluid are sterile on culture. Chronic prostatitis often seems to be a noninfectious swelling or congestion of the prostate.

Massage of the prostate yields fluid for microscopic examination and also seems to be therapeutic. Systematic stripping of the prostate from the base to apex by the gloved finger in the rectum relieves the symptoms and promotes resolution of the chronic prostatitis. Many patients benefit from one or two subsequent massages of the prostate at intervals of 1 to 2 weeks. Too frequent massage of the prostate and an indefinite course of prostatic massage are of doubtful value. Antibiotic treatment often seems helpful when there are increased numbers of white blood cells in the prostatic fluid, even when an organism cannot be found in the urine or prostatic fluid cultures. Trimethoprim-sulfamethoxazole has been effective treatment. Traditionally, the patient with chronic prostatitis is advised to alter the frequency of sexual intercourse (either increase or decrease the frequency) and avoid alcohol and spicy foods. The value of this advice is dubious.

BALANITIS–POSTHITIS

Balanitis is inflammation of the glans penis; posthitis is inflammation of the foreskin, but nearly always the undersurface. Balanoposthitis occurs almost invariably in an uncircumcised male and is induced by poor hygiene and phimosis. Beneath the foreskin is a warm, moist space with oily secretions and desquamated epithelial cells. This area provides a favorable site for nonspecific bacterial growth, and the result is localized dermatitis.

Balanoposthitis can be generally prevented by daily washing and careful drying of the penis with the foreskin fully retracted. When the inflammation is acute, frequent soap and water washing is helpful. Hydrocortisone cream is beneficial. Heat-lamp application to the area with the foreskin fully retracted is helpful several times a day. Circumcision is the definitive solution to the problem. If there is phimosis circumcision is strongly indicated.

ACUTE EPIDIDYMITIS

Acute inflammation of the epididymis is a common disease in adult males and very rare in preadolescent boys unless there is chronic urinary infection. There is pain and tenderness in one side of the scrotum with or without fever and dysuria. The pain is aggravated by all types of physical activity; it is dramatically relieved by lying flat. The involved epididymis is tender, tense, and swollen at first; it becomes progressively more indurated, and the junction between epididymis and testis ultimately becomes obliterated. Even with considerable induration, the epididymis is still very tender. A reactive hydrocele may develop. The urine is often infected, and infected urine passing down the genital tract to the epididymis seems to be the most common pathogenesis. Bed rest is important in treatment. Scrotal support and local heat application are helpful. A broad-spectrum antibiotic should be administered. If a urine culture discloses a pathogenic organism, sensitivity studies will dictate the ideal antibiotic for the epididymitis. Even with appropriate treatment resolution of the inflammatory process is slow. After relief of the acute symptoms the patient may regain moderate physical activity, but scrotal support and periodic heat application are still helpful.

At times epididymitis seems not to be caused by an infectious agent. Pain and swelling of the epididymis are seen at times after vigorous physical activity, and in the early months after vasectomy. In these instances, there is no fever, and the urine is free of infection. In such situations, bed rest, scrotal support, and local application of heat are helpful. Antibiotics are not indicated. If there is any doubt about the possibly infectious nature of the epididymitis, it is permissible to prescribe a course of broad-spectrum antibiotic.

PHIMOSIS–PARAPHIMOSIS

The normal prepuce is supple and can be retracted easily to expose the entire glans penis. When constriction or thickening of the leading edge of the prepuce prevents complete retraction the condition is termed phimosis. Unless the prepuce can be retracted easily, inflammation of the glans, or balanitis, is inevitable. Acute suppurative balanitis with phimosis causes bulbous inflammation of the distal penis, at times associated with fever, lymphadenopathy, and even urinary retention. An immediate dorsal slit allows drainage of pus, free voiding, and resolution of the infection (Fig. 22-1). When the inflammation has subsided, circumcision is advised. Paraphimosis results when the retracted prepuce becomes fixed proximal to the glans. With time, lymphatic and venous obstruction cause progressive swelling of the glans, resulting in ischemic necrosis in neglected cases. Manual reduction is possible early in the disease, but if reduction cannot be accomplished it is imperative that the constricting band be incised to permit reduction of the prepuce (Fig. 22-2). The area of constriction is recognizable as a blanched fibrotic ring. A local anesthetic is so instilled that a small wheal forms and the area is incised vertically, allowing the prepuce to slide forward. Circumcision is performed electively.

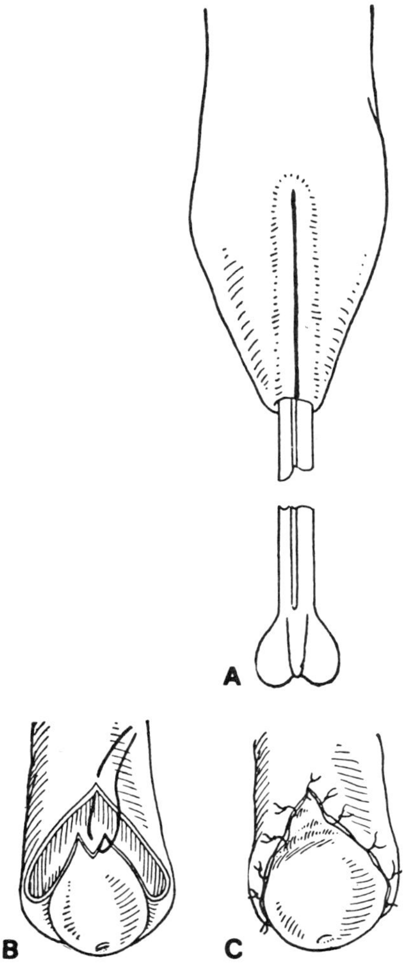

Figure 22-1. (*A*) A grooved director is inserted under the prepuce to the corona; then the prepuce is divided along the director with a pair of pointed scissors. (*B*) The edges of the dorsal slit are united with interrupted sutures of fine chromic catgut.

URETHRAL STRICTURE

Stricture of the male urethra causes decreased force, narrowing, splitting, and spraying of the urinary stream. Stricture often perpetuates nonspecific urethritis. In the past most strictures were due to gonorrhea; currently the common etiologic factors are inlying catheters, urethral instrumentation, and trauma.

A stricture is present when a lubricated 16 French catheter is arrested in the urethra. Definitive diagnosis requires a retrograde urethrogram, and urethral endoscopy is helpful. When the location, length, and caliber of a stricture are defined, proper treatment can be planned. Periodic urethral dilatation is acceptable treatment for many patients; however, urethroplasty is recommended for complicated strictures, those that require frequent dilatation, and strictures in young men. A patient who has experienced many dilatations can offer valid advice about the best instruments for his own case.

The following outlines the technique of urethral dilatation: The urethra is filled with 8 ml to 12 ml 4% lidocaine (Xylocaine), which is then retained in the urethra for 2 to 3 minutes

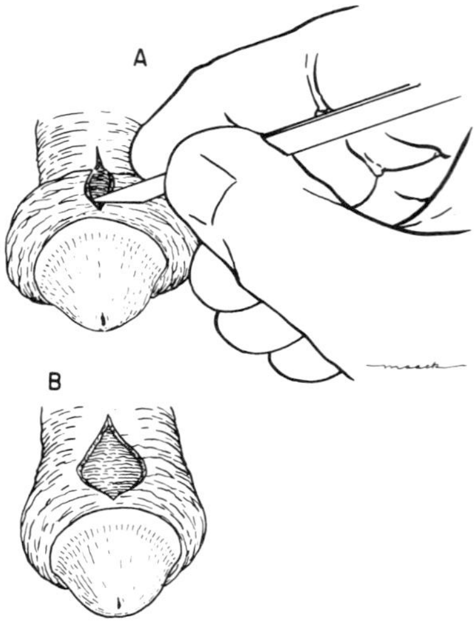

Figure 22-2. Dorsal slit for relief of paraphimosis. (*A*) Incision being made over edematous foreskin about 1–2 cm long. (*B*) The incision is allowed to remain open. This permits subsidance of edema and infection and permits the foreskin to be readily retracted. As edema subsides, secondary healing rapidly occurs.

by pinching the meatus. A well-lubricated no. 18 Van Buren sound is passed according to the diagrams in (Figs. 22-3 and 22-4). If the sound meets resistance and is gripped by the stricture, forceful passage is dangerous, and filiforms and following sounds or catheters should be substituted. The urethra is filled with a sterile, water-soluble lubricant instilled with a catheter-tipped syringe. Then a spiral-tipped filiform is introduced and advanced; if it reaches the bladder, a 16 French follower is screwed on and passed into the bladder. If the first filiform fails to reach the bladder it is left in the urethra and a second, third, and fourth are inserted and manipulated to and fro until one slips past the obstruction and enters the bladder (Fig. 22-5). Progressive dilatation with larger-caliber instruments is then possible by attaching them to the guiding filiform. As a rule, a 2 to 4 French enlargement of the urethral caliber at each dilatation is sufficient. Excessively vigorous dilatation aggravates the stricture and risks hemorrhage.

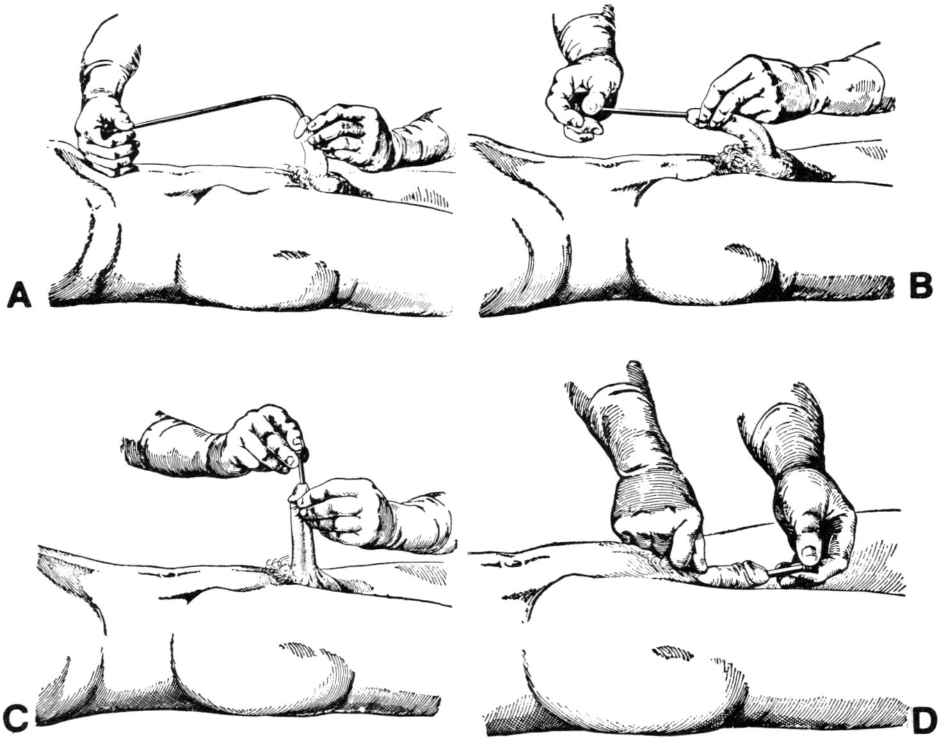

Figure 22-3. (*A*) While the penis is held steady with the left hand the tip of the sound is inserted into the meatus with the right hand. (*B*) The sound is advanced into the urethra as the penis is drawn up over the instrument. (*C*) Resistance is encountered by the sound at the bulbomembranous junction. (*D*) The handle of the sound is depressed slowly by the left hand. In this way the tip of the sound follows easily the curve of the posterior urethra. The right hand makes pressure downward over the root of the penis to relax the suspensory ligament.

A

B

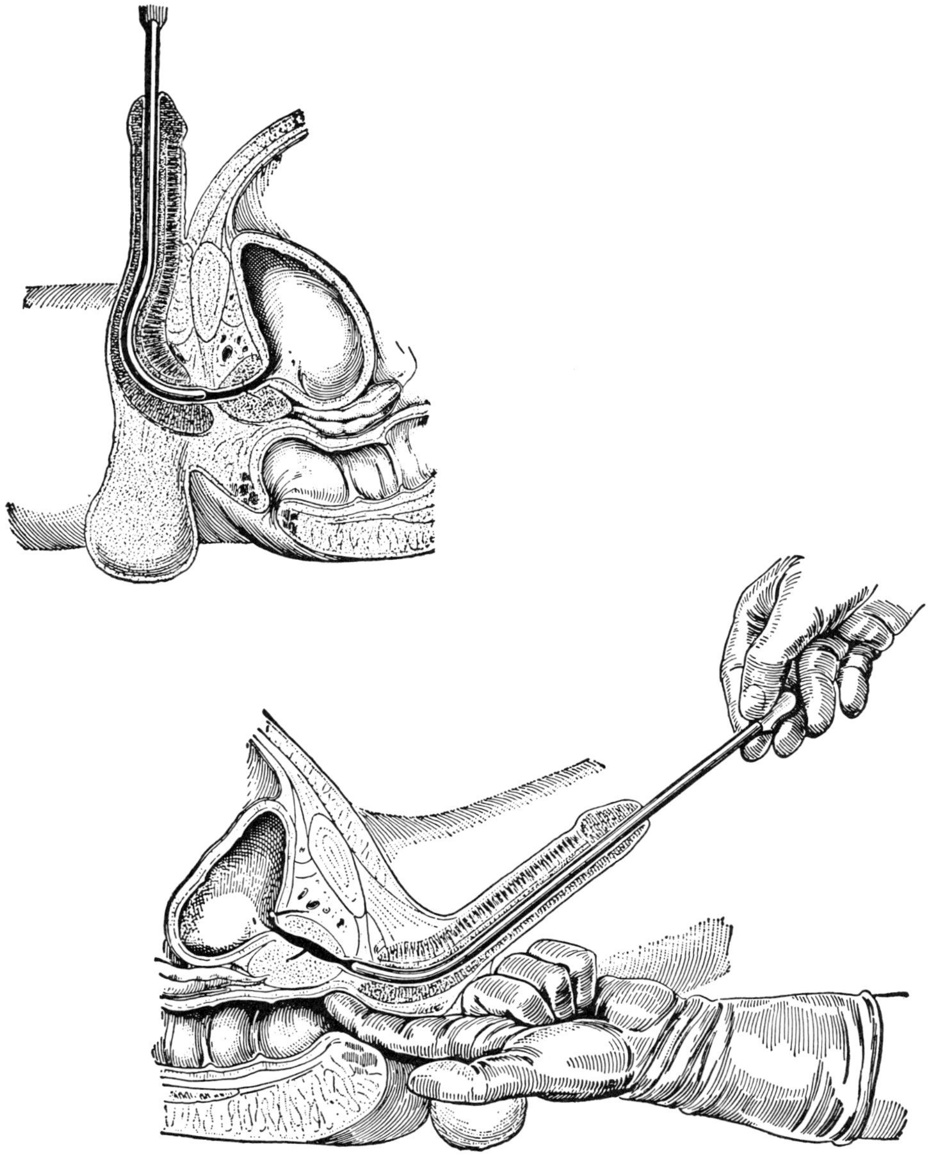

Figure 22-4. (*A*) Sagittal section shows the tip of the sound at the bulbomembranous junction (anterior layer of triangular ligament). (*B*) Passage of the sound may be aided by inserting the finger into the rectum to guide the instrument through the membranous and prostatic urethra.

Short strictures of the urethral meatus result from urethral instrumentation, meatal ulceration, and balanitis xerotica obliterans. The last is related to lichen sclerosus et atrophicus and produces atrophy and fibrosis of the glans and prepuce, with obliteration of the urethral meatus. Regardless of etiology meatal stenosis is treated by meatotomy. A local anesthetic is infiltrated at the ventral lip of the meatus, and this area is crushed with a hemostat. In the crushed area a sharp cut with a scissors is nearly bloodless. Then the mucosa is sutured to the skin with interrupted 4-0 chronic catgut sutures (Fig. 22-6).

URETHRAL FOREIGN BODY

Patients who have placed a foreign body into the urethra for autoeroticism or to support a flaccid penis during coitus present with bleeding, urethral pain, discharge, and, possibly, urinary retention. Plain x-ray films and

(*Text continues on p 346.*)

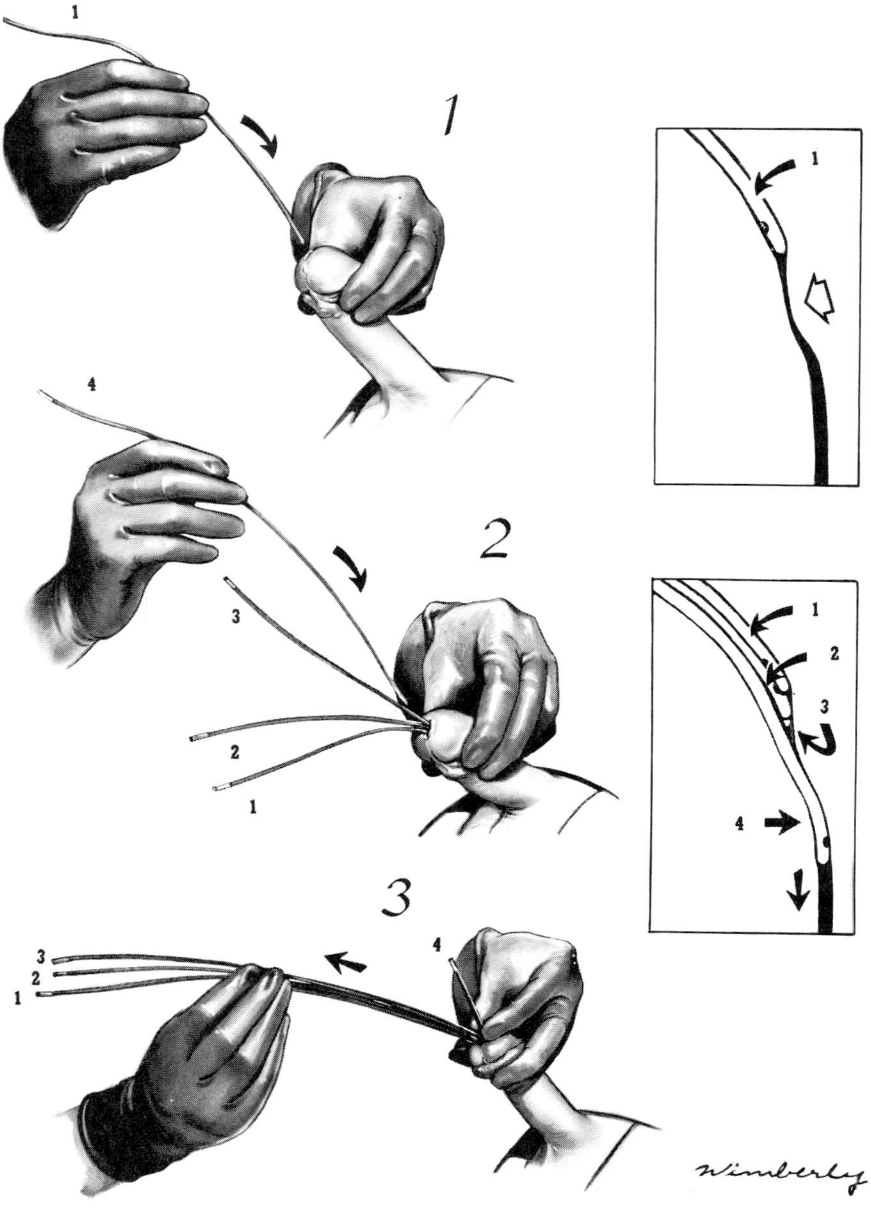

Figure 22-5. Dilatation of a stricture with multiple filiforms attached to a follower. (*1*) Introduction of a spiral-tipped filiform into urethra. (*2*) If the first filiform does not reach the bladder, additional filiforms are introduced. Eventually one filiform will be able to be passed into the bladder. (*3*) Manipulation of several filiforms in an effort to pass the stricture. The inserts show a side view of how insertion of several filiforms eventually will dilate the stricture, permitting one of them to pass into the bladder. (*4*) Once a filiform is passed into the bladder, a follower is attached by screwing it onto the filiform. It is guided by the filiform in the bladder past the stricture. (*5*) Urine drains from the catheter, now positioned in the bladder.

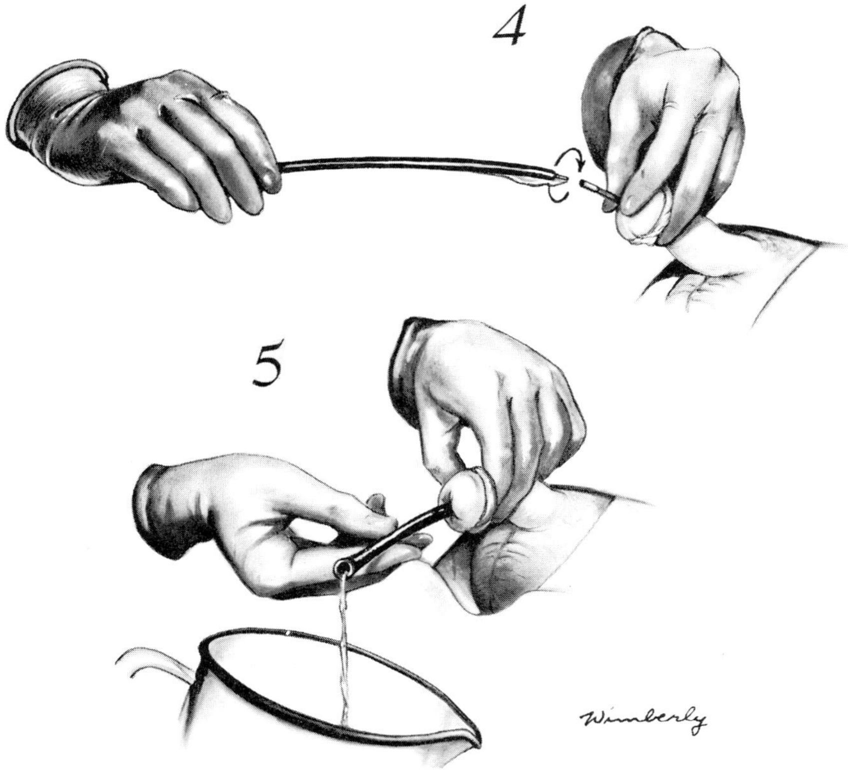

Fig. 23-5. *Continued*

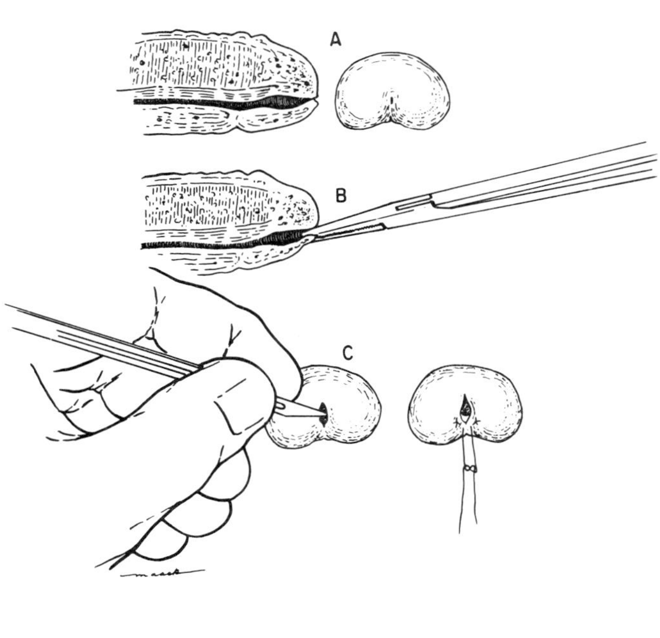

Figure 22-6. Meatotomy. (*A*) Short stricture of urethra meatus. (*B*) After infiltration with xylocaine the stricture area is crushed with a small straight hemostat. (*C*) A short cut with scalpel or scissors through crushed area is nearly bloodless. The mucosa of the urethra is now sutured to the skin on either side with interrupted 4-0 catgut sutures.

contrast urethrograms are useful to define the location of the foreign object. Pencils and swizzle sticks can be palpated and milked out of the proximal urethra after filling the urethra with lubricating jelly. Objects in the deep urethra and bladder demand hospitalization for surgical removal via cystotomy or urethrotomy.

HEMATURIA

No more than one or two red cells per high-power field are seen in normal urinary sediment. More than two red cells per high-power field in a centrifuged urinary specimen should be regarded as microscopic hematuria. Many more red cells are required to color the urine pink or red. The presence of reddish urine without red cells in the urinary sediment suggests hemoglobinuria or the ingestion of beets or azo dyes.

There are scores of causes of hematuria, such as tumors of the kidney, ureter, bladder, prostate, and urethra; caculi at all levels in the urinary tract; prostatic hypertrophy; strictures; and urinary infections (Fig. 22-7). Red blood cells are found in the urine in various types of glomerulitis (e.g., glomerulonephritis, lupus nephritis, and diabetic nephrosclerosis), but protein and casts, including red blood cell casts, will also be present. Hematuria occurs with various types of urinary tract infection; however, in infection the red blood cells are accompanied by white cells and bacteria.

A lesion of the kidney or ureter is suggested by hematuria associated with flank pain. Dysuria with hematuria, especially terminal hematuria, suggests a source of bleeding in the bladder, prostate, or urethra. Many common benign conditions produce hematuria, but one must suspect a malignant neoplasm in the urinary tract in any patient with hematuria, gross or microscopic. Virtually every instance of hematuria should be evaluated urologically by intravenous pyelography and cystoscopy. In the presence of gross hematuria prompt cystoscopy during the period of active bleeding is often helpful in identifying the source. One can often identify bloody efflux from the ureteral orifice at cystoscopy in instances of upper urinary tract bleeding. It is a common clinical mistake to assume that hematuria results from prostatic hypertrophy or an infection somewhere in the urinary system when an insidious neoplasm is the actual cause of the bleeding. Hematuria is a sign of serious disease until proved otherwise.

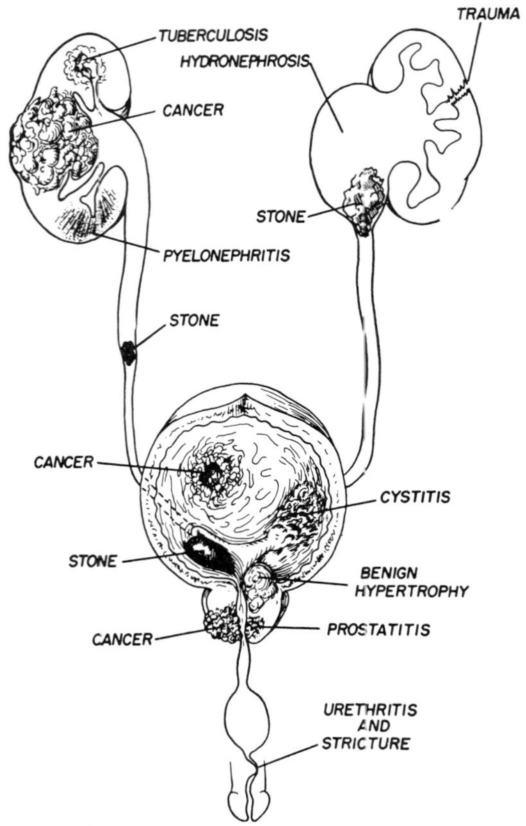

Figure 22-7. Common causes of hematuria. (Marshall VF: Textbook of Urology. New York, Hoeber-Harper, 1964)

ACUTE RENAL COLIC

Pain in acute renal colic is commonly very severe. It arises in the flank and extends into the ipsilateral lower abdomen, groin, and at times into the scrotum or labium majus. The patient moves about restlessly seeking a comfortable position, which he does not find. Characteristically, the pain is unrelated to position or physical activity, and it is not relieved by lying still. Nausea is common; vomiting is less common. Fever is rare. Having had a similar experience previously the patient with recurring renal colic recognizes the nature of his pain.

Hematuria is virtually always associated with acute renal colic—usually microscopic but occasionally gross. A catheterized urine specimen is mandatory in a woman who may be menstruating.

Intravenous pyelography should be performed promptly. This study not only establishes the diagnosis, but dictates the disposition of the case. A calculus in the lowest third of the ureter that is less than 5 mm in diameter, as measured on the x-ray film, will likely pass spontaneously within a few days. After initial control of the pain the patient can be sent home with oral narcotics and instructed to force oral fluids and strain the urine to recover the stone when it passes. A stone of greater size or higher in the ureter is less likely to pass. Urologic consultation is appropriate in such a situation.

Initial control of pain often requires a sizable parenteral dose of narcotics, such as intramuscular morphine sulfate 10 mg to 15 mg or meperidine (Demerol) 100 mg. After that oral narcotic agents are usually sufficient. At times, though, hospital admission is required for pain control or for intravenous administration of fluids.

If the patient with renal colic also has fever, prompt hospitalization is necessary, and urologic consultation is required. Antibiotic treatment is necessary, but relief of ureteral obstruction is also an urgent matter.

ACUTE URINARY RETENTION

Abrupt inability to void is painful. The patient experiences steadily increasing lower abdominal pain and progressive bladder distention with the passage of time. An elderly man with acute urinary retention is often in agony; drainage of his distended bladder with a catheter is a simple humanitarian act greatly welcomed by the miserable patient. The typical patient is a man over the age of 60 years who previously has had increasing symptoms of prostatism. Usually urinary retention is acute, but occasionally a man may have had retention for days, weeks, or even months, with marked frequency or continuous overflow urinary dribbling and a distended bladder. Rarely, a patient with "silent prostatism" has a distended bladder and a marked increase in residual urine and yet is unaware that his voiding pattern has changed significantly. Although some urologists advocate gradual withdrawal of urine from the distended bladder, it is safe and often easier to evacuate the bladder at once and completely with a catheter.

Generally urinary retention in an elderly man is caused by either benign prostatic hypertrophy or prostatic cancer. Acute retention in women is the result of neurologic disease, pelvic tumor, or drug abuse, or it is a psychologic phenomenon—often associated with unusual emotional stress.

Urinary retention in an elderly man is a prime indication for prostatic surgery and requires prompt admission to the hospital for preoperative evaluation and the procedure. If one simply evacuates the bladder and sends the patient home, the chances are great that he will return within a few hours, again with urinary retention. In managing a woman with acute urinary retention the following are important: evacuation of the bladder, bimanual pelvic examination, cessation of all anticholinergic and sedative drugs, and reassurance. Recurrence of retention in women is rare in the absence of neurologic disease or mechanical obstruction.

URETHRAL CATHETERIZATION

Types of Catheters (Fig. 22-8)

Straight, Soft-Rubber, or Plastic Catheter (Nélaton). The straight catheter is the one most commonly used for simple catheterization in a male or female; 16 or 18 French is appropriate and convenient for the adult patient of either sex.

Coudé-Tip Catheter. The coudé-tip catheter is more rigid than the ordinary soft-rubber catheter and is named for the fixed, upturned (coudé) tip of about 15 degrees. The single eye of this catheter is set back from the upturned tip. This catheter is extremely useful in a patient with prostatic enlargement and often passes readily into the bladder when a soft-rubber or plastic straight catheter buckles in the prostatic urethra. The slight angulation of the tip can often make a difficult catheterization in an elderly male patient a simple maneuver.

Metal Catheter. The metal catheter is a hollow metal tube, fashioned in the shape of a urethral sound, that provides maximum stiffness and can be used in catheterizing a man with prostatic hypertrophy. This catheter can

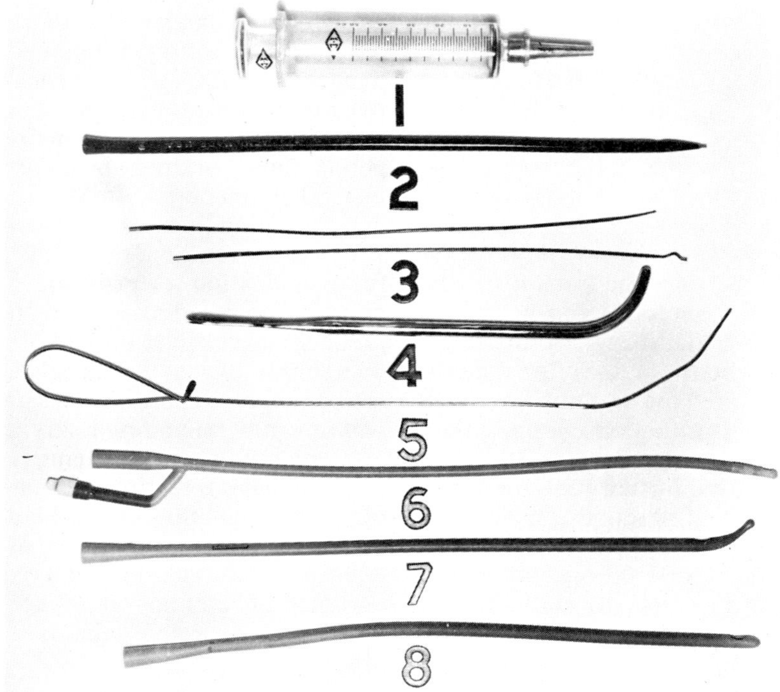

Figure 22-8. Common urologic instruments. Calibration of these instruments is on the French scale and is expressed in units, each unit equaling approximately 0.33 mm. For example, a 24 F instrument has a diameter of 8 mm. (*1*) Toomey syringe, (*2*) woven follower, (*3*) woven filiforms, (*4*) Van Buren sound, (*5*) catheter guide (mandrin), (*6*) Foley catheter, (*7*) olive-tip catheter with coudé curve, (*8*) straight, or Robinson, catheter.

cause great damage if not used carefully and properly and should be used only by an experienced physician when rubber catheters have failed.

Filiform and Woven Catheter Follower. A straight or corkscrew-shaped urethral filiform is used for probing a urethra that has stricture or is tortuous. Once the tract into the bladder has been negotiated, the woven following catheter is screwed firmly onto the filiform tip and is passed into the bladder.

Foley Catheter. A Foley catheter is a catheter with an inflatable bag near the tip. The inflated bag secures the catheter within the bladder.

Technique of Catheterization

Urethral catheterization requires proper positioning of the patient, cleansing of the urethral meatus, and use of sterile instruments. The catheter should be passed gently and with due consideration of the anatomy of the urethra. A male patient can be catheterized in the supine or the lithotomy position. A female patient can be catheterized satisfactorily only in the lithotomy position. In a male the foreskin must be retracted and the glans cleansed with an antiseptic solution. In a female the labia must be held widely apart to expose the urethral meatus for proper cleansing and for insertion of the catheter. Negotiating the female urethra is rarely difficult, but the male urethra regularly presents two problems: the angulation in the bulbous urethra and negotiation of the prostatic urethra and bladder neck. If a straight soft-rubber catheter will not pass through either of these problem areas, a coudé catheter should be tried next. A filiform and following catheter is the next resort. Rarely should one resort to a metal catheter. The catheter should be lubricated generously with a sterile water-soluble lubricant, and its passage should be gentle.

DISEASES OF THE FEMALE URETHRA

THE URETHRAL SYNDROME

The urethral syndrome of adult women is the combination of dysuria, suprapubic discomfort, frequency of urination, and a sensation of incomplete voiding attributed to nonspecific urethral inflammation. The symptoms mimic cystitis, yet urinary infection is absent.

Fatigue and anxiety accentuate symptoms. If the urethra is tender on bimanual examination, urethral dilatation may be helpful. Lidocaine (Xylocaine) or cocaine is applied topically to the urethra, following which the urethra is dilated to 30 to 36 French with steel sounds. More often, bimanual examination discloses tenderness in the area of the pubic symphyseal cartilage, and the symptoms seem related to mild inflammation of the symphyseal junction. Local heat, rest, antiinflammatory medications, and bladder antispasmodics are helpful.

URETHRAL CARUNCLE

Caruncles are polypoid, vascular, red lesions that protrude from the posterior urethral meatus. Benign but often tender, they may cause dysuria, postmicturition bleeding, and pain on sexual intercourse. Symptomatic lesions are treated by excision of fulguration after the application of 10% cocaine to the distal urethra. A simple method of removal is as follows: The lesion is stretched taut, the base is clamped with a hemostat, the lesion is excised, and the base is fulgurated before the clamp is removed.

MUCOSAL PROLAPSE

Mild degrees of prolapse of the urethral mucosa are common and do not require treatment. Extensive full-circle prolapse occurring in prepubertal girls and elderly women appears as a dramatic, violaceous, boggy, bleeding mass that obscures the meatus and is often mistaken for a neoplasm. The lesion is easily cured by applying a strangulating ligature over an inlying catheter. After 10% cocaine has been applied to the lesion, a 20 French Foley catheter is inserted through the urethra and the balloon is inflated. The prolapsed mucosa is drawn taught, and a 2-0 silk ligature is passed around the lesion and tied tightly over the catheter. After several days the necrotic lesion sloughs and the catheter can be removed.

CIRCUMCISION

Circumcision of an ambulatory patient can be performed painlessly by employing regional block anesthesia (Fig. 22-9). Premedication with diazepam (Valium), 10 mg by mouth, is helpful. The patient is instructed to shave the hair at the base of his penis and thoroughly wash his genitalia at home before the procedure.

Following skin preparation with povidone-iodine (Betadine), or a presurgical antiseptic (Ioprep or a similar solution), the penis is draped with sterile towels or an eye drape. The base of the penis is injected with 1% or 2% lidocaine (Xylocaine) in four separate spots, as follows: a small wheal of anesthesia is produced by subcutaneous injection at the 10-o'clock, 2-o'clock, 4-o'clock, and 8-o'clock positions. A 23-gauge needle is used. The needle is then passed through the wheal and through the fascia of the penis, slowly injecting as the needle is advanced. Approximately 2 ml is injected in each site. The prepuce will become insensitive shortly.

The tip of the prepuce is placed on slight tension, and a short transverse cut is placed at the level of the coronal sulcus. The penis is held upright, and short marking incisions are made on the ventral and lateral aspects of the skin of the penile shaft. An exact circumferential incision is made by connecting the marking cuts. The prepuce is then retracted to expose the glans. If the prepuce cannot be retracted because of phimosis, the edge of the prepuce is incised by making a dorsal slit to permit full retraction. A transverse incision is started in the precoronal skin and is extended circumferentially, perpendicular to the shaft. The incision must divide a full thickness of skin; this allows the edges of the incision to retract slightly. The free edge is lifted with forceps and is undermined with dissecting scissors. Hemostats are placed on a free edge and lifted, to permit further dissection. When

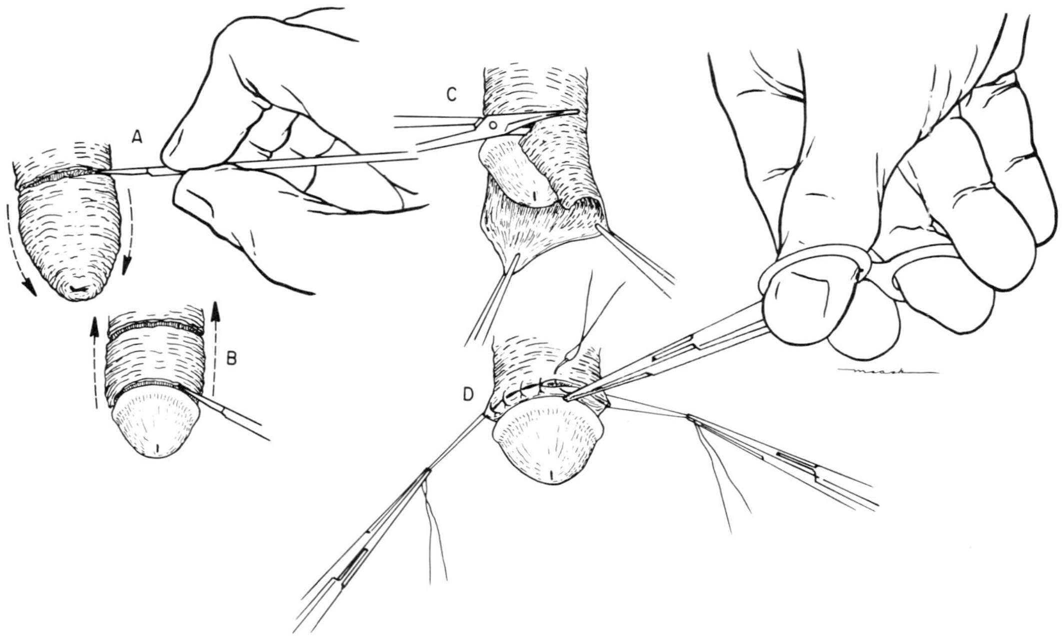

Figure 22-9. Circumcision.

the subcutaneous dissection has tunneled beneath the preputial skin to the first incision, a long hemostat is placed through the tunnel, and the blades are spread. A sharp cut is made in the groove of the open blades, and the free cut edges are clamped with hemostats. Dissection is continued in the loose subcutaneous tissue until the preputial skin is completely excised and discarded. Several veins are cut and must be clamped and ligated with fine plain gut. After the surgeon is certain that all bleeding points have been ligated or fulgurated, he can proceed. The skin of the penile shaft is united with the precoronal skin with 3-0 chromic sutures placed at the 12-o'clock, 3-o'clock, 6-o'clock, and 9-o'clock positions. The sutures are grasped with hemostats, providing traction that aids in further suturing. A suture is then placed in the center of one quadrant of the wound, and then in the center of one eighth of the wound, and so forth. Thus asymmetric closure, which can result in torsion of the penis, is avoided. Throughout the operation care is exercised to avoid roughly grasping the skin with tissue forceps. Careless handling results in postoperative pain and edema. After all of the sutures have been placed, the incised area is covered with a 1-inch strip of Telfa and wrapped snugly with 1-inch Kling. The dressing is removed in 48 hours, and the patient is allowed to bathe.

DISEASES OF THE SCROTUM AND SCROTAL CONTENTS

ACUTE SCROTAL SYNDROME

The triad of abrupt pain, swelling, and redness of the scrotum indicates either torsion of the testis or acute epididymitis. Differentiating between the two diseases is critical because torsion demands prompt surgical exploration to restore the testicular circulation, whereas epididymitis is treated by nonsurgical means. Epididymitis is rare before puberty; in mature males, however, epididymitis is more common than torsion. The acute scrotal condition in prepubertal males is usually due to torsion. Pyuria, when present, suggests epididymitis because of the frequent association of the latter with urinary infection. Although the patient's symptoms and the appearance of his scrotum may be similar in both diseases, a large tender epididymis is usually palpable in the early stages of epididymitis. In acute testicular torsion the structures in the scrotal mass cannot be differentiated. Often the twisted testis lies high in the scrotum; in contrast, acute epididymitis produces a mass involving the dependent scrotum. When the diagnosis of epididymitis is certain the patient is treated with rest in bed, elevation of the scrotum, local application of heat, and a broad-spectrum antibiotic. Treatment is continued until swelling and tenderness are markedly decreased and the patient can walk without pain. The patient must be examined repeatedly until there is complete resolution of the inflammation and a normal testis can be distinguished from the epididymis. When pyuria is present, urine culture is obtained and antibacterial treatment is based on the results of the sensitivity studies. Rarely, the acute scrotal syndrome is the result of insect bite, cellulitis, or viral orchitis. Viral orchitis does not occur before puberty, and in an adult male it is usually part of a generalized viral illness. Mumps orchitis is usually associated with mumps parotitis. Viral orchitis is treated by rest in bed, analgesics, scrotal elevation, and antiinflammatory agents. It is essential that surgical scrotal exploration be performed whenever the diagnosis of the acute scrotal condition is in doubt and testicular torsion is a possibility. Doppler study and a nuclear perfusion scan of the affected testicle can be helpful in making the diagnosis. Still, surgical scrotal exploration is mandatory when torsion is a clinical possibility.

SOLID LESIONS OF THE SCROTAL CONTENTS

An exact diagnosis of a solid scrotal mass should be made by the first physician consulted. Solid masses can be differentiated from cystic lesions by transillumination. The use of a fiberoptic light source in a dark room provides a high degree of accuracy. A nontransilluminating, solid mass of the testis must be considered a cancer and the patient hospitalized for inguinal orchiectomy. Scrotal ultrasound may be helpful in equivocal lesions. A "watch-and-wait" attitude toward testicular masses is unacceptable and inappropriate.

CYSTIC LESIONS OF THE SCROTUM

Cystic lesions of the scrotum include spermatocele (epididymal cyst), hydrocele of the cord, hydrocele of the testis, and communicating hydrocele, in which the processus vaginalis is patent from the peritoneal cavity to the testicle. Since all cystic lesions transmit light, transillumination is the first step in diagnosis. In the common hydrocele of the testis, a spherical mass obliterates all details of the testis and epididymis. In contradistinction, a spermatocele arises from the head of the epididymis and thus can be palpated distinctly above the testis. Often a spermatocele is considered a supernumerary testis by the layman.

Surgical repair of hydrocele is required only when it produces significant symptoms. Tapping a hydrocele is a temporary treatment that has little therapeutic value and carries a significant risk of infection. When a hydrocele prevents urethral instrumentation or obscures a testicular lesion, percutaneous aspiration is performed with a 14-gauge intravenous catheter or a trocar needle.

ACUTE PHEBLITIS OF THE SPERMATIC CORD

Varicocele, or varices of the pampiniform plexus, occurs in 10% to 20% of men and is confined to the left hemiscrotum. The varicocele becomes tense when the patient stands, and it feels like a bag of worms. Occasionally trauma or infection results in acute pheblitis of the varicocele. This painful lesion is identified by the presence of tender, indurated varices. General treatment consists of rest in bed, scrotal elevation, and local heat.

ACUTE DERMATITIS OF THE SCROTUM

The scrotum can be involved by many generalized dermatologic diseases that require the specialized care of a dermatologist; however, acute dermatitis, regardless of the underlying cause, can be treated effectively by the primary physician. Red, painful, weeping dermatitis is common on the crural areas and the scrotum. Obesity, diabetes, hot weather, and poor hygiene are predisposing factors. Chronic tinea cruris may have acute flare-ups when irritated by friction, heat, and sweat. Regardless of etiology, immediate palliative treatment consists of wet dressings soaked in Burow's solution (available in packets as Domeboro powder). Mix one packet in 1 pint of cool water. A piece of folded soft cotton sheeting is soaked in the solution, applied sopping wet, and changed frequently. Severe discomfort and anxiety should be treated with analgesics and sedatives. After the acute phase has subsided treatment is continued with a water-soluble steroid plus iodochlorhydroxyquin cream (Vioform-hydrocortisone ointment, 1% Domeform-HC cream).

VASECTOMY

THE OPERATION

Interruption of the vas deferens is performed to prevent recurrent epididymitis and for voluntary male sterilization. When epididymitis is the result of chronic prostatitis, vasectomy may prevent recurrence. In cases of chronic epididymitis with persistent epididymal thickening, epididymectomy is a more reliable operation.

The indications for voluntary sterilization encompass a myriad of ethical, moral, religious, and intellectual considerations. Sound judgment is required in patient selection. A thorough preoperative interview is necessary to be certain that the request for vasectomy is reasonable, that the result of vasectomy is clearly understood, and that alternative methods of birth control have been considered. Consultation with the family physician may also be helpful at times. Explicit, detailed, written consent should be obtained from the patient and also from his wife. Sample consent forms are available from several sources.

Vasectomy is easily performed in the outpatient operating room. The patient is required to shave his scrotum at home before the operation. Sedation with 5 mg to 10 mg diazepam (Valium) by mouth a half-hour before the procedure is helpful. With the patient supine the scrotal skin is prepared with povidone-iodine (Betadine), hexachlorophene (pHisoHex), or other nonastringent solutions. The field is draped with a three-towel triangular drape. The vas is grasped near the neck of the scrotum and is rolled between the thumb and forefinger, isolating it from other cord structures and fixing it directly beneath the skin. The scrotal skin and the tissues around the vas are infiltrated with 1% or 2% lidocaine (Xylocaine). An incision 1 cm long is made directly over the vas (Fig. 22-10). Spreading the incision with a small hemostat permits visualization of the vas deferens. An Allis clamp is gently closed about the vas, which is then lifted through the skin incision. Longitudinal, shallow cuts directly over the vas free it from its fascial envelope. The naked vas is further isolated by passing a hemostat beneath it. It is helpful to infiltrate the spermatic cord before proceeding with this step. The vas is stripped for 2 cm to 3 cm, and each end is crushed with a hemostat. A segment 1 cm to 3 cm long is removed, and the crushed ends are ligated with 2-0 chromic gut and are allowed to fall back into the wound. The ends may be doubled back on themselves and religated. The free ends of the vas may also be fulgurated. The skin is closed with a single mattress suture of 2-0 chromic gut. Sterile gauze is placed within a scrotal suspensory and allowed to remain in place for 48 hours.

Postoperative Care

The patient is urged to return home immediately and to lie in bed for 6 to 8 hours with an ice bag on his scrotum. Full activity is resumed in 24 hours. The scrotal suspensory can be discarded and bathing resumed after 48 hours. When vasectomy is done for sterilization, the patient must continue his usual birth control methods until his ejaculate contains no more sperm by microscopic examination. A clean-catch ejaculate is submitted for microscopic study after the tenth ejaculation or 1 month after vasectomy. Should any sperm remain, periodic semen examination is carried out till all sperm have disappeared from the semen.

Complications

Scrotal hematoma is an infrequent but distressing complication. A hematoma larger than a golf ball is best treated by incision and evacuation of the clotted blood. Aspiration has proved futile. Exploration can be performed in an outpatient operating room. The scrotum is thoroughly prepared with soap and an antiseptic solution. Sterile conditions are necessary. The scrotum is infiltrated with lidocaine (Xylocaine) along a 6-cm line over the hematoma. The skin is incised, and the edematous connective tissue is spread bluntly; usually this reveals a mass of "current-jelly" clots. Rarely, an active bleeding point can be identified and ligated. Penrose drains are placed in the wound, each end of the drain emerging at one of the extremities of the incision. The skin is closed with 2-0 chromic sutures. Any scrotal accumulation requiring drainage should be cultured for bacteria and treated with antibiotics empirically until results are available. A bulky gauze dressing

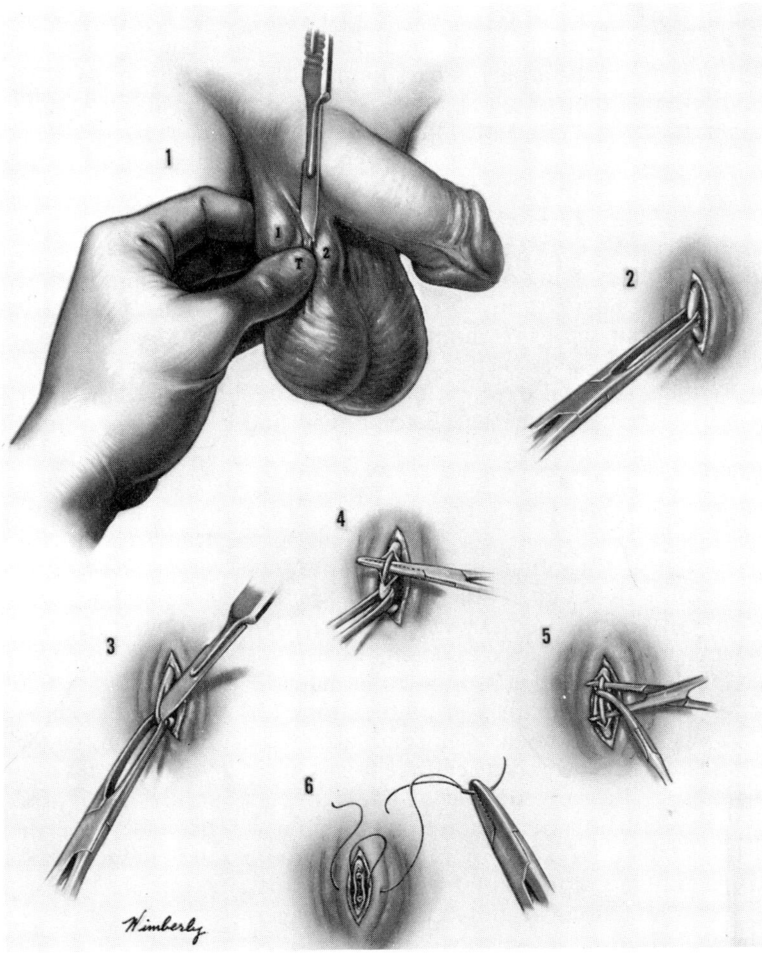

Figure 22-10. Steps in vasectomy. (*1*) The vas is grasped near neck of the scrotum and a 1.0-cm incision made through the skin directly over it. (*2*) After minimal blunt dissection with a small hemostat, the vas is grasped with an Allis forceps. (*3*) With the scalpel the vas is further freed from the surrounding fascial envelope. (*4*) The now completely "naked" vas is further isolated by passing a small hemostat beneath it. (*5*) By spreading this hemostat the vas is freed for 2–3 cm, at which point the bas is crushed at either end of this freed portion and a 1–3-cm segment of vas excised. The crushed ends of the vas are ligated with 2-0 chromic gut. (*6*) Skin closure is accomplished with a single mattress suture of 2-0 chromic gut.

and scrotal suspension are helpful. Usually the drains can be removed in 3 to 5 days. Smaller scrotal hematomas are managed with analgesics, local heat, and scrotal support.

Acute funiculitis and epididymitis have been observed weeks or months following vasectomy. The patient complains of unilateral or bilateral pain in the groin. A tender mass extends either proximally or distally from the point of ligature of the vas. Often the inflammation is due to spermatic granuloma. There may be pus in the urine or prostatic fluid. However, often no genitourinary infection is demonstrable. Empirically, broad-spectrum antibiotics, either tetracycline or ampicillin, and anti-inflammatory drugs are prescribed. The patient is instructed to apply a heating pad to the groin and to avoid vigorous activity until the inflammation has subsided.

GENITOURINARY TRAUMA

The following discussion of trauma of the genitourinary system is limited to injury confined to the urinary system or the male genital structures.

PENETRATING RENAL TRAUMA

Isolated renal trauma can result from penetrating missiles entering the upper part of the abdomen, the flank, and the lower part of the chest. Injuries to adjacent organs must be anticipated and excluded by chest and abdominal examinations. Wounds of entry or exit lying in the renal area should alert the physician to the possibility of renal damage. Excretory urography can be carried out with little additional effort during abdominal x-ray series. Urographic indications of renal injury include renal nonfunction, distortion and displacement of the calyces or renal pelvis, extravasation of contrast material into the perirenal tissues, and hydronephrosis. Gross hematuria is common, and microscopic hematuria is nearly inevitable. Frank renal bleeding may present through the wound site and may cause clot colic and bladder retention of urine due to intravesical clotting. The patient with any evidence of renal injury requires hospitalization and active monitoring of all vital signs. A CT scan or renal augiography is recommended in every case that shows pyelographic abnormalities. Nearly all cases of penetrating renal injury require surgical exploration—for the renal trauma but also to search for bowel and other injuries.

BLUNT RENAL TRAUMA

The degree of renal damage from blunt trauma often defies correlation with the nature and severity of the trauma. Any fall or blow to the flank may result in significant renal damage. Flank pain, flank guarding, colic, nausea, and specifically hematuria are indications for urography. Unequivocally normal urograms exclude the need for further investigation of the kidneys, but any degree of distortion or delay in excretion necessitates admission to the hospital, a CT scan or renal angiogram, and careful monitoring of the patient. Most cases of blunt renal trauma can be managed without surgery. However, severe injuries with massive destruction and hemorrhage require surgical treatment.

BLADDER TRAUMA

A patient with an isolated, penetrating bladder injury is unusual in an ambulatory surgical facility. However, such an injury may occur with gunshot, stabbing, or a fall on a sharp object. More commonly, bladder laceration and rupture occur with fracture of the pubic bones. The sharp spicules of the fractured pubis penetrate the adjacent bladder. There are pain and tenderness in the pubic and suprapubic areas. A suprapubic mass or sense of fullness may be detected. The injured patient may have difficulty initiating micturition, and the attempt to void can cause suprapubic pain and cramping. Grossly bloody urine or a bloody urethral discharge is common.

Cystography is performed by gravity filling of the bladder with a suitable contrast material; this will demonstrate bladder discontinuity in most cases. It is advisable to perform cystography even if a normal bladder shadow has been demonstrated on an intravenous pyelogram. A male patient with a pubic fracture may have laceration or complete disruption of the membranous urethra as well as bladder trauma. Retrograde urethrography is safer and preferred to passage of a catheter in such a patient. In general, most bladder perforations require surgical repair and cystostomy drainage. Cystostomy drainage is usually performed promptly for deep urethral trauma, although a urologist may, in favorable situations, repair a deep urethral injury primarily.

Although most bladder ruptures result in extraperitoneal urinary extravasation and hemorrhage, intraperitoneal rupture can occur as a result of a forceful, blunt blow to the lower abdomen when the bladder is full. This occurs at times in patients who are senile, confused, or intoxicated, and there may be no history or physical evidence of trauma. Diffuse abdominal pain, tenderness, paralytic ileus, erratic voiding, and an increase in BUN suggest this injury. Ileus and the increase in BUN occur because of urinary ascites. Surgical repair of the bladder and suprapubic cystotomy are appropriate treatment.

RUPTURE OF THE MALE URETHRA

Although bladder rupture is common with pelvic bone fractures, urethral rupture is more serious and requires skill in recognition and treatment. The disruption of the male urethra associated with pelvic fractures invariably occurs just above the level of the urogenital diaphragm where the membranous urethra is relatively fixed. Shearing of the membranous urethra accompanies fracture of the pelvic bones, allowing the bladder and prostate to rise from the urogenital diaphram and "float" away from the bulbous urethra. Partial urethral disruption can be inadvertently converted to complete disruption by urethral instrumentation; thus in a patient with a pelvic fracture retrograde urethrography should be done before urethral catheterization is attempted.

Pubic pain, tenderness, and suprapubic fullness are the rule. On rectal examination the prostate may be "floating," that is, displaced upward or cephalad. Much bogginess is often felt anterior to the rectum.

Generally, suprapubic cystostomy is appropriate primary treatment. Definitive deep urethral repair is carried out 3 to 4 months later electively.

GENITAL LACERATIONS

The scrotum and penis are often injured by falling on gravel, broken glass, wire fences, and the like. Initial evaluation requires gentle cleaning of the skin and removal of genital hair. Fragments of wood splinters, gravel, old paint, and so on require tedious flushing with sterile fluid and methodical exploration of each laceration. Penile urethral injury should be excluded as described later. After thorough and repeated cleaning and flushing, open lacerations can be sutured with use of local infiltration anesthesia and 3-0 to 4-0 catgut. Loose approximation of lacerations is adequate, and healing is usually rapid. After reapproximation of all lacerations greater than 1 cm in length, a fluffy compression dressing is paced beneath a large scrotal supporter. The wounds are potentially infected, and prophylactic antibiotic treatment with tetracycline, cephalosporins, or the like is recommended.

BLUNT GENITAL TRAUMA

Injury is usually due to a direct blow. Falling astride rafters, intentional assault with blunt instruments and accidental or intentional kicks to the genitals account for the mechanism of injury in most cases. Ecchymosis and hematoma are usual, and pain is often severe. Parenteral narcotic analgesia is often a prerequisite to definitive examination. Swelling, induration, and pain along the course of the urethra suggest urethral trauma, and a bloody discharge from the penis is definite evidence of urethral damage. (See next section, "Blunt Trauma to the Bulbous and Pendulous Urethra.")

When urethral trauma is excluded, the examiner should differentiate between superficial hematoma of the scrotum and injury to the testis. If one cannot definitely separate a mass in the scrotum from the testicle, the probability of testicular injury is great. A spherical mass filling the scrotum generally indicates damage to the scrotal contents, and surgical exploration of the scrotum is appropriate. A policy of exploring all patients with suspected testicular rupture based on the physical evidence of a definite intrascrotal hematoma has revealed a high incidence of repairable lacerations of the testis, avulsion of the epididymis, and hematoma within the epididymis. The relief of pain and rapid recovery from an injury after appropriate scrotal exploration contrasts dramatically with the painful, slow, disabling course after treatment by "conservative," nonsurgical methods.

BLUNT TRAUMA TO THE BULBOUS AND PENDULOUS URETHRA

Straddle injuries and direct blows to the urethra cause urethral bleeding, induration, and tenderness along the course of the urethra and may result in permanent disability if inappropriate, inadequate treatment is chosen. Retrograde urethrography is mandatory in any suspected urethral injury and should be done before urethral instrumentation. If possible, urethrography should be performed before the patient is allowed to void through a damaged urethra so as to avoid the additional injury due to urinary extravasation. Any case of urethral trauma demonstrated by retrograde urethrography should be evaluated by a urologist, although minor tears may require only urinary diversion by placement of a small urethral catheter and continuous urinary drainage for 7 to 10 days.

SCROTAL GANGRENE

Scrotal gangrene, a serious condition, is placed with the discussions of trauma because the patient often believes that the acute swelling, erythema, and pain are a result of minor trauma or insect bites. The process begins as a scrotal cellulitis, advances rapidly, and gives rise to gangrene, which also progresses. This disease is most common in the debilitated, the diabetic, and the alcoholic. The patient is often toxic and febrile. Prompt treatment with surgical debridement, massive parenteral doses of antibiotics, and careful monitoring are required to prevent extensive loss of scrotal skin and lethal sepsis.

SUPRAPUBIC CYSTOTOMY

INDICATIONS

Ideally, suprapubic cystotomy should be performed in a male patient who requires bladder drainage for several weeks to a number of months. Suprapubic cystotomy in such a case is preferred to prolonged drainage with a urethral catheter because urethral inflammatory trauma and its sequelae are avoided; the patient is spared epididymitis, prostatitis, urethral stricture, and periurethral abscess.

Suprapubic cystotomy is indicated in chronic urinary retention with dilation of the upper urinary system and impairment of renal function. Suprapubic cystotomy may be necessary in a patient with urinary retention who has significant medical disorders that make it necessary to delay prostatectomy. Suprapubic cystotomy is also employed when a catheter cannot be passed by way of the urethra into the bladder because of stricture or false passage in the urethra or when catheterization is contraindicated, as in acute urethritis, acute prostatitis, and epididymitis. The procedure is also employed at times in patients with neurogenic bladder dysfunction, but it is not suitable for permanent urinary diversion. Suprapubic cystotomy has other uses as part of operative procedures performed on the bladder or the urethra.

TECHNIQUE

Although general or spinal anesthesia is commonly used, local anesthesia will suffice. It is helpful to have the bladder full. A 3-cm to 4-cm suprapubic midline skin incision is made. A vertical incision is then made in the midline of the anterior rectus sheath (linea alba). Deep to this the rectus muscles are separated. The bladder wall is visualized and grasped with two Allis clamps or chromic catgut sutures. The bladder is opened for a distance of 2 cm, allowing the operator to feel the interior of the bladder. A Malecot or Foley catheter (22–26 French) is inserted with the tip lying about centrally in the bladder. The bladder incision is closed snugly around the catheter with 0 chromic catgut sutures. One or two 0 chromic catgut sutures are employed to fix the cystotomy site to the rectus sheath, to hold the area closely up against the abdominal wall. A Penrose drain is used in the prevesical space—especially if the urine is known to be infected. The fascial edges are closed with chromic catgut. The skin is closed with silk or nylon. The Malecot or Foley catheter should be firmly sutured to the skin edge and taped securely to the skin adjacent to closure.

CHANGING THE CATHETER IN AN ESTABLISHED SUPRAPUBIC CYSTOTOMY

Permanent suprapubic cystotomy provides urinary drainage and is a therapeutic elective in neurogenic bladder disease and prostatic obstruction in a poor-risk surgical candidate, and it is a stopgap procedure in other medical situations. Incrustation with urinary salts causes eventual catheter blockage, and thus a catheter must be changed periodically. A Malecot catheter is commonly inserted initially, but a Foley catheter is usually best and easiest to insert when changes are necessary. Often unexpected blockage or accidental withdrawal of the tube from the bladder necessitates cystotomy tube care from a physician unacquainted with the patient.

Even a well-established cystotomy fistula will contract rapidly if the catheter is withdrawn, so a relatively urgent problem is created when a cystotomy catheter is withdrawn from the fistula. Thus two different situations are related to inserting a cystotomy tube. The first, and easier, is when the tube lies in the established fistula and should be changed because of occlusion of the lumen. In this case the retaining bag is deflated if necessary, the substitute catheter readied for insertion, and the substitution is made, placing the new tube exactly in the position of its predecessor. If the tube has fallen out the site is prepared with antiseptic and the fistula stoma tentatively probed with a substitute catheter. Resistance to passage of a conventional size (22–26 French Foley) suggests contraction of the stoma, and one should use the largest catheter that can be inserted. The tract will dilate quickly to accept the accustomed size catheter.

After placing the new tube into the bladder and inflating the retaining balloon, prudent flushing of the catheter with sterile water is important to ensure successful placement and free return of liquid.

SUPRAPUBIC PERCUTANEOUS DRAINAGE

Although urethral catheterization is usually accomplished without difficulty, certain situations preclude urethral instrumentation (severe strictures, occlusive neoplasms of the bladder neck and prostate, giant prostatic hypertrophy, urethral false passage). Whenever a urethral catheter cannot be passed without fear of damage, excessive force, or pain, suprapubic percutaneous drainage is an alternative. Prepared commercial kits with trocar catheters and the needed accessories are available. The readily available angiocatheters and intracatheters are an acceptable short-term substitute.

Before suprapubic puncture drainage is resorted to, the diagnosis of total urinary retention with bladder distention must be confirmed with certainty by percussion and palpation. This procedure is dangerous in any patient with an incisional scar in the lower abdominal area. The skin of the suprapubic area should be shaved and cleaned with antiseptics. A wheal is raised with lidocaine 1% directly in the midline and exactly above the pubic symphysis. Gradual infiltration with a small-bore spinal needle will create an anesthetic tract, and aspiration of urine through the spinal needle will confirm the location of the bladder. After the depth of the bladder wall beneath the skin and the presence of urine are verified, the stylet-catheter is substituted. The catheter should be coiled within the bladder and securely taped to the abdominal skin. The bladder can be drained by suprapubic puncture for an uncertain period, so provisions should be made for more definitive drainage.

REPLACEMENT OF THE NEPHROSTOMY TUBE

Changing a nephrostomy tube is easy if the tube has been in place at least 6 weeks following the original surgery and if the tract into the renal pelvis is straight. The new tube should be ready for prompt insertion after removal of the old tube. A Malecot catheter must be inserted with a stylet, whereas a Foley catheter can usually be passed directly into the tract without a stylet. At times the catheter will not pass easily into the renal pelvis and may be impeded at the point where the tract penetrates the renal parenchyma. Forcing the tube often results in creation of a false passage and makes further attempts at inserting the catheter unsuccessful. Difficulty in replacing the tube is common if the previous tube has been out of the tract for several hours or longer. If difficulty is encountered, a smaller caliber coudé catheter is often successful. If the position of the tube is uncertain, injection of dye through the tube will identify its location. Surgical placement is occasionally necessary if the catheter cannot be replaced.

23 Initial Evaluation and Treatment of Major Trauma: Priorities and Algorithms for Emergency Department Management of Multiple-Injury Patients

BRUCE A. HOUTCHENS, MARK W. WOLCOTT, AND TERRY CLEMMER

For a number of years major trauma has been the fourth leading cause of death in the United States, surpassed only by heart disease, cancer, and cerebral vascular disease. It is the leading cause of death for individuals under 45 years of age. Recently in the United States there have been 140,000 to 160,000 trauma-related deaths annually, with about a third caused by motor vehicle accidents. Injury is the leading cause of physician contacts; more than a quarter of hospital emergency department (ED) visits are for the treatment of injuries. Injury is also a leading cause of short- and long-term disability: More than 3.5 million trauma patients are hospitalized annually, accounting for over 100 million hospital bed days. (This is more hospital occupancy than is needed for all cardiac patients, or for all babies born, and is four times the occupancy accounted for by all cancer patients.) The ratio of permanent disabilities to deaths from injuries is approximately 1 : 4. The annual societal costs of all injuries have been estimated conservatively at $75 billion to $100 billion. Clearly, trauma is a major health problem in the United States today.

Although major trauma is almost always an inpatient hospital problem, it is discussed in a text directed to ambulatory surgery and emergency medicine because the outpatient surgeon or emergency physician is most frequently the first hospital-based professional to encounter the severely traumatized patient, and the record would indicate that final outcome is often directly related to completeness and competency of the *initial* evaluation and management. In-hospital care of a patient with serious or critical multiple-systems injuries will almost always be assumed—either initially or on early transfer to a larger facility—by a general surgeon or critical-care physician, who should systematically reevaluate extent of injury and response to prior treatment. Yet if there is delay in urgently needed resuscitation immediately after arrival at the (first) hospital or if an injury is unrecognized during initial evaluation, progress is often adversely affected even hours or days later during the course of hospitalization. These are compelling reasons for outpatient surgeons and emergency-care physicians to be familiar with and able to apply currently accepted standards for initial evaluation and management of major trauma, regardless of the setting in which the critically injured patient is first seen.

STANDARDS OF TRAUMA MANAGEMENT: THE ALGORITHM-PROTOCOL APPROACH

Evolution of standards for evaluation and management of the critically injured patient seems to have paralleled that of the emergence of the critical-care physician as an identifiable specialist, the acceptance by the general surgeon of the role of "captain of the ship" in coordinating specialty teams in the care of multiple-organ-system injuries, and the development of major-medical-center trauma units. The critical-care physician and trauma surgeon have shown how to base decision making on specifically sought data rather than on conjecture. From the trauma units have come management protocols that have proved effective in earlier diagnosis of all injuries and increased salvage from severe injuries.

Key factors to be addressed are what information is needed, when and how to get it, how to organize and interpret it, how to act on it, how to evaluate the effect of intervention accurately, and how to provide immediate support while acquiring the data base.

With the critically injured patient, time is a significant factor influencing the approach. Dichotomous pressure, on the one hand, for swiftness and, on the other, for certainty and thoroughness is ever present. A given patient may tolerate neither delay nor error. Initial evaluation and management are not independent. There is a need to gain control and provide immediate support while, or even before, proceeding with multisystems evaluation. This implies the need to establish algorithms and priorities by which components of the evaluation of the problem and management of the trauma patient can be guided. It is important to sequence appropriately the various components of physical examination, laboratory and roentgenographic studies, and necessary support measures, so as to permit diagnosis and initiation of treatment of potentially life-threatening and permanently disabling conditions before time and attention are devoted to lesser, although perhaps more readily recognized, problems.

ORGANIZATION AND RESPONSIBILITY OF THE EMERGENCY DEPARTMENT TRAUMA TEAM

Local protocol should establish when the outpatient or ED team assumes responsibility for care of the trauma patient and when that responsibility is relinquished to inpatient physicians. Where emergency medical technician (EMT) and paramedic teams in the field communicate with an ED by radio, responsibility of the ED team often begins prior to arrival of the patient at the hospital. The ED team must be prepared to continue comprehensive care until the patient is moved to an operating room, admitted to an inpatient intensive care environment, or transferred to a larger facility or until the appropriate inpatient surgeon assumes responsibility for overall management. For multiple trauma most facilities have found that an effective system is to establish a call schedule of general surgeons with special interest in such patients, who can respond within a few minutes to direct evaluation and management while the patient is still in the emergency department.

It is of interest to note that delineation in *writing* of local protocols, policies, and responsibilities has been found to contribute both to enhancing efficiency of patient care and to *decreasing* exposure to potential medical-legal liability situations.

An "ideal" team from a standpoint of space–time efficiency for initial evaluation and resuscitation of most critically injured patients is two doctors and two nurses. When constant airway management is required, it is most helpful to include an anesthesiologist, nurse–anesthetist, or respiratory therapist as a fifth member at the head of the table. The presence of two doctor–nurse "subteams" allows initial attention to be simultaneously directed to airway and vascular access; and subsequent attention to be simultaneously directed to inserting the therapeutic and monitoring tubes and lines necessary to "gain control," while conducting (and documenting) a physical examination. The additional presence of one trained in monitoring ventilatory mechanics and operating suction apparatus and ventilatory support equipment allows both nurses to participate in removal of the patient's clothing, taking of vital signs, setting up and administering intravenous fluids and medications, and retrieving and opening equipment and supply packages, all of which must be accomplished with a compressed time frame, without neglecting frequent assessment of airway status. The "crash-cart" and "shock-room" concepts of prepositioning crucial supplies and support equipment can maximize efficient utilization of available personnel by reducing steps (and minutes) needed to gain control.

In most smaller community hospitals the constant presence of such a five-person team would represent an impractical luxury. In addition, the concept of priorities is less obvious when it is possible to accomplish many steps simultaneously. For these reasons it is more instructive to describe the general protocol from the standpoint of initial action by one doctor and one nurse.

GENERAL PLAN OF ACTION

The overall protocol for initial evaluation and management of a patient with critical injuries or multiple-systems injuries can usually be outlined by a series of steps the sequence of which is determined by priority of the action:

1. Control of airway and rapid hemorrhage; ventilatory support
2. Vascular access
3. Initial laboratory blood work
4. Assessment and replacement of blood loss
5. Physical examination and initial treatment of specific injuries
6. Special studies
7. Removal to operating room, intensive care unit, or larger facility

As the data base accumulates, the plan may need to be modified according to specific injuries and stability of the patient's course.

CONTROL OF RAPID EXTERNAL HEMORRHAGE

The first considerations in management of the severely injured are to ensure an adequate airway and to control brisk external hemorrhage. With transport from the scene of accident being effected by well-trained EMT and paramedic teams, it is unlikely a trauma patient will arrive in an emergency room without major external bleeding at least temporarily under control. Should this not be the case, arrest of brisk external hemorrhage should be the first priority because (1) by appropriate application of *pressure*, major bleeding can almost always be brought under control in seconds (oropharyngeal suction should also be accomplished immediately, if necessary, to prevent aspiration) and (2) if brisk external hemorrhage is allowed to continue during a several-minute "battle for the airway," several hundred milliliters of valuable oxygen-carrying capacity will be lost on the floor. Although the volume can rapidly be replaced, it will be the better part of an hour from time of arrival in the ED until type-specific, crossmatched blood is available for infusion.

In a critically injured patient external hemorrhage is best controlled initially by direct finger or hand pressure on the bleeding vessel or wound, followed by application of a sterile pressure dressing. Immediate application of a tourniquet in the ED is to be discouraged because (1) direct pressure is faster and just as certain when there is an extra hand to maintain it, (2) a tourniquet results in ischemia to all tissue distal to its location (since it occludes collateral flow as well as that through the injured vessel), (3) a tourniquet may cause severe pressure damage to underlying muscle and nerves, (4) improper application or slippage may result only in occluding venous outflow (which may actually *increase* bleeding), and (5) eventual release of the tourniquet may be complicated by a lactic acid "washout." Use of a tourniquet should be reserved for control of brisk limb bleeding that does not cease with application of a pressure dressing in a situation in which a single rescuer needs both hands to attend to other life-saving details. Immediate application of hemostats in the ED is also to be discouraged because of (1) uncertainty of quickly gaining proximal and distal control without adequate exposure and (2) high probability of causing permanent damage to vessels and adjacent nerves when nonvascular clamps are applied blindly in a bloody wound.

AIRWAY MANAGEMENT AND VENTILATORY SUPPORT

Airway management is the next (and usually first) immediate consideration. Aspiration of vomitus, blood, or both is a frequent cause of rapid death in unconscious or severely injured patients. When vomitus, blood, or excessive secretions are present in the posterior pharynx, frequent and vigorous suctioning is essential to prevent occlusion of the upper airway. Therefore a suctioning apparatus (>200 mm Hg continuous negative pressure), with connector tubing attached and with both nasopharyngeal catheters and tonsil sucker tips immediately available, must be in constant readiness if the airway is to be protected from the moment of arrival.

RAPID EVALUATION

Evaluation of the character of breathing and adequacy of airway begins when a member of the trauma team first sights the patient. Skin color, motion of the chest, and sound of fluid gurgling in the upper airway or air sucking in a chest wound are evident even before reaching the patient's side. At the patient's side, first-order priorities are (1) rapid visual inspection of the mouth and anterior neck, (2) simultaneous listening for breath sounds with an ear at the patient's mouth while palpating the carotid pulse and tracheal alignment with a finger and observing if chest motion is symmetric, and (3) bilateral auscultation of the chest with a stethoscope, with the patient's upper body clothing opened.

DECISION FOR CARDIOPULMONARY RESUSCITATION

If the pulse is not palpable and breathing is not spontaneous, it must immediately be decided whether cardiopulmonary resuscitation (CPR) is indicated. Such a decision must be influenced by the transport personnel's estimate of the probable interval without cerebral perfusion. When resuscitation efforts are successful in the absence of direct injury of the head or spinal cord, the infrequency of significant neurologic deficit in long-term survivors is surprising. Thus when there is doubt about the status of a young trauma victim, an all-out effort is usually indicated. In any case, if CPR is to be initiated, it should be done immediately and maintained continuously until resuscitation is achieved or it is decided to terminate the procedure.

If there is reason to believe arrest is due to airway obstruction or tension pneumothorax, correction of those problems (see also the section entitled "Chest Injury") combined with closed-chest CPR in accordance with advanced cardiac life-support standards of the American Heart Association may be successful. However, if arrest is due to exsanguination with hypovolemic shock or to cardiac tamponade, it will not be possible to resuscitate an empty heart or a tamponaded heart with closed-chest massage. In this situation a left thoracotomy and direct cardiac massage (with cross-clamping of the supradiaphragmatic aorta to maximize use of what vascular volume remains), or direct release of the tamponade, offers the best chance of salvage (see description of ED thoracotomy in the section entitled "Chest Injury").

Heroic resuscitation efforts in apparently mortally injured patients are frequently unsuccessful, expensive, and emotionally draining for both trauma teams and families. For example, at our institution, there has been a single survivor of blunt trauma (out of hundreds) when it has been necessary to initiate CPR at the scene or en route to the hospital. Clearly, it would be of value to have a means by which to predict "certainty" of fatality from multiple trauma with the same accuracy now accorded to the 95% burn. In an effort to achieve this goal, a number of scoring systems have been developed. Of these, two so far appear promising in civilian trauma management: the physiologically oriented trauma score and the anatomically oriented injury severity score. The physiologic status of the patient is most rapidly definable in the ED setting; therefore the trauma score, or some modification thereof, is the likely current candidate for a standard by which emergency physicians might feel comfortable in terminating efforts in "hopeless" cases. (Recent reports suggest that there is negligible survival associated with trauma scores of 3 or 4; yet in the heat of the action in the ED, it has been difficult for physicians to cease efforts for young trauma victims or to withhold efforts long enough to confirm accuracy of the score.)

IMMEDIATE VENTILATORY ASSISTANCE

In accordance with advanced cardiac life support standards, in the absence of adequate spontaneous breathing, *immediate* ventilatory assistance and preintubation oxygenation should be temporarily provided by use of mouth-to-mouth, pocket-mask, or bag-valve-mask techniques (unless facial injury precludes obtaining the necessary seal). With any of these techniques the cross-sectional area of the upper airway can be improved by placing the head in the so-called sniffing position: finger pressure applied in an anterior direction at the angle of the mandible or chin will thrust the jaw forward, thus pulling the base of the tongue away from the posterior pharyngeal wall and opening the upper airway. This position also facilitates intubation by improving the angle between the upper and lower airway.

A common error in airway management is to place the head in a flopped-back position over the edge of a litter or bed: When the horizontal plane of the occiput is below that of the back of the shoulders and the chin is not forward, the channel between upper and lower airway is *narrowed*. In a trauma patient who has not had a neurologic evaluation, posterior extension at the neck carries significant risk of aggravating a cervical spinal injury.

TRACHEAL INTUBATION

Usually the most rapid and effective way to gain definitive control of the airway is by endotracheal (ET) intubation with a cuffed tube so that positive-pressure ventilatory assistance can be provided and aspiration around the tube prevented. Indications for intubation include: (1) inadequate pulmonary toilet (inability to spontaneously clear the upper airway of secretions and aspiration), (2) inadequate ventilation (due to depressed central drive or impaired mechanics of breathing that may be related to thoracoabdominal injury) evidenced by high PCO_2 and low pH, and (3) inadequate oxygenation (due to pulmonary shunting and diffusion defects related to lung contusion, aspiration, or acute respiratory disease syndrome) evidenced by low PO_2 and hemoglobin saturation fraction. The timing of tracheal intubation will therefore depend on whether ventilation and oxygenation are spontaneous and on the patient's level of consciousness and combativeness. A patient combative enough to require sedation for intubation is usually alert and strong enough for ventilation to be spontaneous, provided that the airway is clear. Immediate blood gas measurement can confirm the ventilatory state.

After insertion of an endotracheal tube, the cuff should be inflated (pressure sufficient to seal the airway but not so tight as to occlude capillary circulation to the tracheal mucosa), the airway suctioned through the tube, and several breaths delivered by means of a bag connected to 100% oxygen. The position of the tube in the trachea should be confirmed immediately: Proper position is indicated by bilateral inspiratory expansion of the chest while breath sounds are heard by means of a stethoscope over each hemithorax (the stethoscope is also used over the upper abdomen to detect absence of air movement in the stomach) and later by location of the end of the tube on a chest roentgenogram. After the proper position of the endotracheal (ET) tube is confirmed, the tube may be secured by a strap around the patient's head or (in the absence of prohibitive facial injury) by taping to the patient's cheeks. (If time and facial injury permit, cleansing the face of blood and preparing the skin with benzoin will facilitate keeping the tube in place.)

Unless the reason for tracheal intubation is strictly pulmonary toilet and maintenance of an open airway, positive-pressure ventilatory assistance will usually be provided immediately by use of a bag-valve device or a mechanical ventilator. Appropriate starting tidal volume, ventilatory rate, and fraction of inspired oxygen (FiO_2) must therefore be estimated. Reasonable initial values are tidal volume, 10 ml/kg to 15 ml/kg; ventilatory rate, 15/min to 20/min; FiO_2, 40%. If the patient has sustained a period of hypoventilation and hypoxia (not uncommon), hyperventilation (30 breaths/min) with 100% FiO_2 should be provided for 5 to 10 minutes. Accuracy of these estimations then is assessed by measurement of the ventilation (PCO_2, pH) and oxygenation (PO_2, O_2 saturation) parameters of an arterial blood gas sample obtained 15 to 20 minutes after initiation of ventilatory assistance.

Tracheal intubation and intravenous fluid replacement probably represent the two most important life-saving procedures in early management of the major-injury patient. Yet, as with many procedures and manipulations utilized in emergency and critical care, tracheal intubation presents a distinct opportunity to harm, as well as to help, the patient. Several potential complications related to emergent ET intubation deserve consideration:

1. As previously mentioned, in the trauma patient whose neurologic status has not yet been evaluated, manipulation of the neck involves risk of *aggravating a cervical spinal cord injury*. Should ventilatory insufficiency appear so immediately life threatening as to necessitate tracheal intubation in a patient with probable cervical spine injury, it would be well to avoid hyperextension of the neck, position the chin forward the minimum amount needed to visualize the cords while also applying some cephalad axial traction at

the angle of the jaw, and try not to let the patient "buck" while the tube is being inserted. Nasotracheal intubation or cricothyroidotomy may be considered as alternatives to orotracheal intubation.

2. *Vomiting with aspiration*, prevention of which is one of the reasons for intubation, may be induced during attempted intubation of a patient with a vigorous gag reflex. Aspiration before the airway is secure in a patient whose ventilation is already markedly compromised can obviously be life threatening. It is important to be ready to suction the airway before, during, and after tracheal intubation.

3. *The tube may be placed in the esophagus, resulting in positive-pressure inflation of the stomach, compromise of diaphragmatic motion, and subsequent difficulty in inflating the lung.* This possibility can be reduced by properly positioning the mandible to open the airway, suctioning the upper airway sufficiently to permit clear visualization of the cords, and auscultating breath sounds over the chest (and abdomen) immediately after intubation.

4. *The tube may be inserted too far, resulting in selective intubation of the right main-stem bronchus (which has a more oblique angle with the trachea than the left), or it may slip into the right main-stem bronchus after initial positioning at the carina.* This causes high-grade obstruction of the airway to the left lung. In the trauma patient in whom the extent of pulmonary injury has not yet been determined and who may have severe right lung damage, even brief obstruction of the airway to the left lung may be life threatening. Obstruction of the airway to the left lung should be suspected if, immediately following intubation, breath sounds are audible over the right hemithorax but not over the left. The tube should then be withdrawn 1 cm to 2 cm at a time until breath sounds are audible bilaterally. (The position is confirmed later by chest roentgenogram.)

5. In the trauma patient in whom the extent of pulmonary injury has not yet been determined, *application of positive-pressure ventilation following intubation may convert pneumothorax to tension pneumothorax.* If the original pneumothorax is the result of a lung laceration or bronchial tear, delivery of only a few tidal volumes may generate sufficient pressure in the hemithorax to impair cardiac function and constitute an immediate threat to life. Rapid recognition and treatment of this problem are crucial, as will be subsequently described.

Once tracheal intubation is accomplished, the vocal cords cannot be closed to create sufficient airway pressure and flow for effective cough. Without the protective mechanism of a cough, the patient is dependent on suctioning to clear the airway. Once a ventilatory assist device is placed over an endotracheal tube, *a common error is to become so busy with other details that frequent suctioning of the airway is neglected.* It is surprising how quickly relocation of previously aspirated material or continuing hemorrhage from pulmonary injury can reocclude the airway below the endotracheal tube, with rapid deterioration of ventilation and oxygenation parameters.

Although orotracheal intubation is the procedure with which most physicians are more familiar (and that is good reason to use it in most emergency situations), nasotracheal intubation is an alternative route that may permit inserting a tube from above without much manipulation of neck and jaw and without precise visualization of the cords. With or without a stylet to maintain curvature of the tube, the angle of emergence from the nasopharynx is such that the nasotracheal tube preferentially should seek an anterior passage into the trachea (see "Tracheal Intubation," p 364).

In the presence of mechanical obstruction of the upper airway, maxillofacial injury with bony deformity and severe hemorrhage, or cervical spine injury with instability of a vertebral body that could be displaced during intubation, cricothyroidotomy is a viable alternative for direct access to the trachea (see "Cricothyroidotomy," p 366). Faster entry into the airway, less bleeding (if the incision is kept in the anterior midline), and less probability of inadvertently positioning the tube in tissue spaces outside the airway are all reasons for selecting cricothyroidotomy rather than conventional tracheostomy for direct access to the trachea in an emergency situation. Insertion of a standard cuffed endotracheal tube in an emergency cricothyroidotomy results in a very acceptable airway. In a desperate situation an intravenous catheter can be inserted as a temporary airway.

If it is decided not to intubate the airway, it is important to (1) administer supplemental oxygen by means of a loose-fitting clear-plastic face mask and (2) check the patency of the airway frequently and aspirate secretions and blood. Though oxygen saturation is normal in the majority of patients with uncomplicated hypovolemic (hemorrhagic) shock, some will be desaturated. For such patients use of increased fraction of inspired oxygen can be very important, since decrease in cardiac output and oxygen-carrying capacity accompanying hemorrhagic shock may compound the effects of acute pulmonary injury or preexisting chronic cardiopulmonary disease. A face mask allows more reliable delivery of oxygen than a nasal cannula when a nasogastric tube is in place. Frequent reevaluation of the airway and breathing is important so that the patient who was temporarily "making it on his own" doesn't later deteriorate rapidly with respiratory distress that went unnoticed in the x-ray department or while the trauma team was occupied with other details.

(*Text continues on p 368.*)

Tracheal Intubation

Indications

A. To establish or maintain an airway when obstruction is present or threatening, as in severe facial or laryngeal trauma or burns.
B. To provide adequate pulmonary toilet, prevent aspiration in comatose patients, and facilitate removal of secretions, blood, and vomitus in patients unable to clear the upper airway spontaneously.
C. To ventilate patients mechanically: with inadequate ventilation due to depressed central drive, or impaired mechanics from flail chest, open pneumothorax, ruptured diaphragm, severe lung contusion; with need for emergent open thoracotomy; with severe head injury who will benefit from lowering PCO_2 by hyperventilation.
D. To oxygenate patients with pulmonary shunting and diffusion defects related to lung contusion, aspiration, or other form of acute respiratory distress.
E. To provide adjunctive therapy in severe refractory shock.

Types of Emergency Intubation

A. Oral tracheal
Advantages: Can use a larger tube. Method of choice in cardiac arrest situations and when facial and skull fractures preclude the nasal route.
Disadvantages: Difficult in awake, uncooperative patients. Tube may be obstructed by biting. More uncomfortable if maintained for prolonged time.
B. Nasal tracheal
Advantages: Better tolerated by awake, alert patients. Can be performed more easily in uncooperative, semiconscious patients. Easier to secure tube in place and maintain for extended periods.
Disadvantages: Unless cords are visualized, cannot be used in patients without spontaneous ventilation. Must use smaller tube size (7.0–8.0 in adults). Not as fast as oral intubation in cardiac arrest scenario.

Equipment for Emergency Intubation Kit

Endotracheal tubes of various sizes (3–9) with soft, high-volume, low-pressure cuffs
Laryngoscope with adult and pediatric straight and curved blades, spare batteries, and bulbs
McGill forceps
Bag-valve-mask apparatus, with pediatric and adult masks, capable of delivering 100% oxygen
Tube of lidocaine jelly (2%) and benzocaine spray for anesthesia (Cocaine 4% solution is preferable if it can be obtained.)
10-ml syringe
2.5-cm adhesive tape or cloth tracheal tape for securing tube
Cotton applicator sticks
Stylet for endotracheal tube
Oral and nasal airways of pediatric and adult sizes
Good suction with both tonsil tip sucker and suction catheters available

Method for Nasal Intubation (Contraindicated When There Is a Possible Nasal Intracranial Fracture

PROCEDURE	COMMENTS
A. If patient is alert, counsel, explain procedure, and (to the extent possible) alleviate anxiety.	A. Patient cooperation can greatly facilitate the procedure.

B. Prepare equipment, including bag and mask apparatus adapted to deliver 100% O_2, and good suction.

B. To reduce risk one must be prepared to handle possible complications such as vomiting, laryngospasm, or inability to secure airway.

C. If patient is fully awake and has eaten, insert nasogastric tube for decompression of stomach.

C. All precautions to prevent aspiration should be utilized.

D. Unless contraindicated, place head on small pillow or rolled towel and then hyperextend head on neck (Fig. 23-1).

D. This position gives the operator the best angle for visualization of the glottis and for passage of the endotracheal tube.

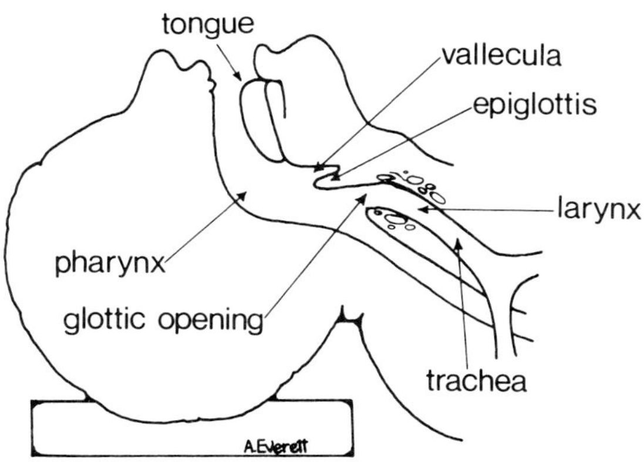

Figure 23-1. Normal anatomy of the mouth and larynx.

E. If time permits, anesthetize the nose with cocaine, using four cotton applicator sticks. Place the first into the nasopharynx and others less deeply.
After 2 to 3 minutes remove sticks and fill nasal cavity with 3 to 5 ml lidocaine jelly.

E. Good nasal anesthesia will facilitate the procedure, and cocaine will shrink the nasal mucosa and constrict vessels. This will allow passage of the tube with less difficulty and with minimal bleeding.

F. Using bag and mask that delivers 100% O_2, give the patient 10 to 15 breaths of 100% oxygen.

F. The oxygen washes out 90% of the lung nitrogen and will help prevent hypoxia during the procedure.

G. With gentle but firm pressure place the tube through the nose into the oropharynx, in which position breath sounds can be heard through the tube.
While listening to the breath sounds, advance the tube into the trachea, using rotation of the tube to adjust the tip to the right or left and extension and flexion of the neck to position the tip more anteriorly or posteriorly. If attempt is unsuccessful retract the tube into the oropharynx, place a hand over patient's mouth and using a bag, ventilate via tube with 100 O_2.
Then using a laryngoscope and McGill forceps, place the tube into the trachea by direct visualization of the glottis (Figs. 23-2, 23-3). See also oral intubation procedure.

G. With practice 80% to 90% of patients can be intubated without visualization. When breath sounds disappear the esophagus has been entered and the tube must be withdrawn slightly.
Never force the tube. If the tube does not enter easily, it is not in proper position, and force may damage glottic structures.

H. Inflate the cuff and suction the tube. Then connect tube to the resuscitation bag and ventilate the patient with 100% O_2.

H. This is to reverse hypercarbia, hypoxia, or both, which may have developed. Repeated suctioning may be necessary.

I. Listen to both hemithoraces and the upper abdomen to make sure that neither a main-stem bronchus nor the esophagus has been entered.
Secure the tube in place with 2.5-cm tape or a cloth tracheal tape tied around the patient's head above the ears.

I. Securing the tube is very important, especially in the confused patient, to prevent inadvertent extubation with potentially lethal consequences.

J. Obtain chest roentgenogram to confirm tube position.

J. The tube should be 2 cm to 3 cm above the carina of trachea.

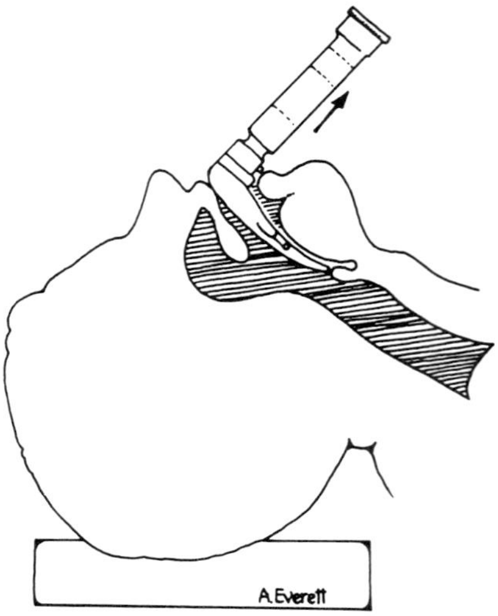

Figure 23-2. A curved-blade (McIntosh) laryngoscope is inserted to lift up the vallecula to permit insertion of the endotracheal tube. Note that the blade is behind the epiglottis.

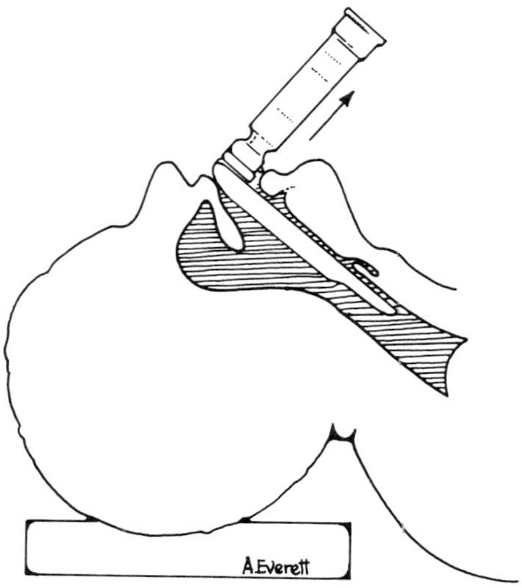

Figure 23-3. A straight-blade (Hanson) laryngoscope is inserted past the epiglottis into the trachea to permit insertion of endotracheal tube. Note that the blade is above and beyond the epiglottis.

Method for Oral Intubation

PROCEDURE	COMMENTS
A–D. Same as nasal procedure	
E. If patient is conscious and gag reflex is present, anesthetize the tongue and oropharynx with a topical anesthetic.	E. This will reduce the likelihood of gagging and vomiting during direct laryngoscopy.
F. Same as nasal procedure	
G. Open mouth with fingers and insert the laryngoscope into the mouth, sweeping the tongue to the left. Slowly advance the tip of the blade over the base of the tongue until the epiglottis comes into view. Place the tip of the blade in the vallecula if using a curved blade (see Fig. 23-1) or pick up the tip of the epiglottis if using a straight blade (see Fig. 23-2). Expose the vocal cords by lifting up on the laryngoscope, avoiding any rotation or levering action of the blade on the teeth. Place the tube through the vocal cords into the trachea under direct vision.	G. If patient is alert, cooperation is very important. Every attempt should be made to reassure the patient and obtain cooperation. If the patient is combative and fighting, some sedation may be utilized, but paralysis should be utilized only by those with experience in rapid intubation because of the dangers involved. When visualization is done properly, the laryngoscope should not touch the teeth.
H–J. Same as nasal procedure	

Cricothyroidotomy

Indication

Upper airway obstruction resulting in ventilatory insufficiency that cannot be relieved by oral or nasal intubation

Minimal Equipment Needed

1 scalpel with no. 11 blade
1 pair Mayo scissors
1 Trousseau tracheal dilator or large hemostat
1 no. 6 or 7 tracheal tube
1 pair of sterile gloves
1 bottle povidone-iodine solution
10 sterile 4 × 4-gauze pads
1 10-ml syringe with 22-gauge needle
1 bottle 1% lidocaine with epinephrine
2 sterile towels
1 self-inflating resuscitation bag adapted to deliver 100% O_2
1 suction apparatus with 14 French suction catheter

Method

PROCEDURE	COMMENTS
A. Unless contraindicated, position patient with a rolled towel under shoulders to hyperextend head on neck. Then locate cricothyroid membrane.	A. This is identified as an indentation just below the thyroid cartilage in the midline.
B. Prepare with povidone-iodine solution and drape with sterile towels.	
C. Anesthetize the skin with 1% lidocaine, then pierce the cricothyroid membrane and inject 3 ml lidocaine into the trachea. (This step may be eliminated in a comatose or severely compromised patient.)	C. By holding suction on the syringe while advancing needle through the membrane, air will be aspirated when the trachea is entered.
D. Using a no. 11 blade make a 2-cm transverse skin incision and stab through the cricothyroid membrane (Fig. 23-4).	D. The stab incision must be in the midline to avoid vascular structures.
E. Following the side of the blade, insert the curved Mayo scissors through the wound and spread firmly in the transverse direction after removing the scalpel blade (Fig. 23-5).	E. Enlarge the tracheal opening to accommodate the tracheal tube by following steps E and F.
F. Insert the Trousseau tracheal dilator and spread the opening in the longitudinal direction perpendicular to the Mayo scissors (Fig. 23-6).	
G. Using the dilator as a guide, insert the tracheal tube (see Fig. 23-6). Once the tube is in the trachea, do not let go of it until it is secured in place.	G. It is easiest to insert the tube from the side, rotating it downward as the back wall of the trachea is approached.

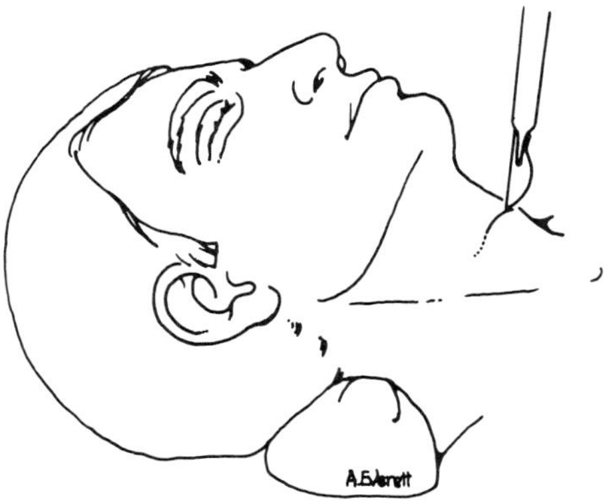

Figure 23-4. Initial incision of skin over cricothyroid membrane.

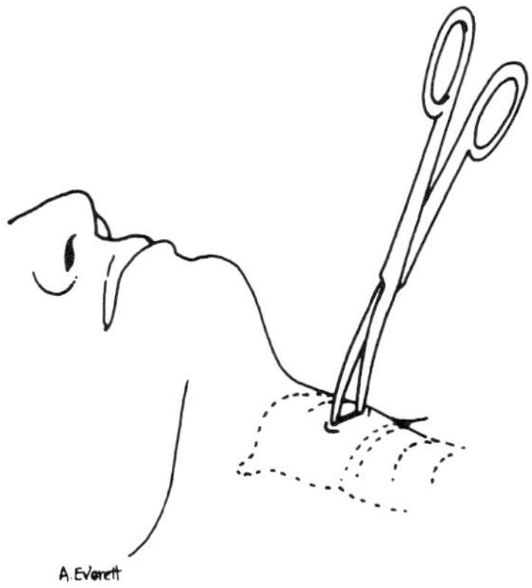

Figure 23-5. After insertion of curved Mayo scissors along side the scalpel blade, the blade is removed and the scissors firmly spread laterally.

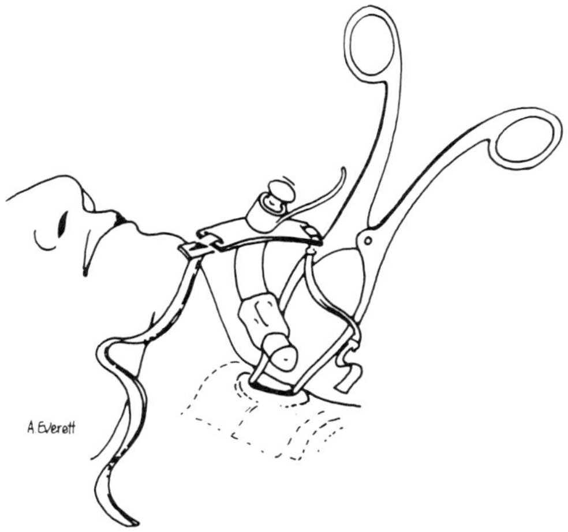

Figure 23-6. Insertion of Trousseau tracheal dilator, the scissors having been removed. The dilator is opened, spreading the wound longitudinally. The tracheal tube can then be readily inserted.

H. Inflate the cuff and suction the tube. Then connect tube to the resuscitation bag, and ventilate the patient with 100% O_2.	H. This is to reverse hypercarbia and hypoxia, which may have developed. Repeated suctioning may be necessary.
I. Listen over both hemithoraces to assure that adequate ventilation is achieved. Secure the tube by suturing it in place or tying attached strap about the patient's neck.	I. This will prevent displacement of the tube when the patient coughs.

VASCULAR ACCESS

The next priority is establishing access to the vascular space in order that intravenous (I.V.) fluid volume replacement may be accomplished as rapidly as needed. Because of the large volumes of crystalloid and blood that must sometimes be infused over a short interval if fluid resuscitation from hypovolemic shock is to be successful, it is best to have a minimum of two large-bore (at least 16-gauge, preferably 14-gauge in adults) plastic intravenous catheters. Because of the possibility of as yet undiagnosed injury to major intra-abdominal veins (particularly vena cava, renal, and hepatic) and because of risk of injury to lung, major vessels, and heart associated with (particularly emergent) percutaneous central venous catheterization, it is best to establish the initial intravenous routes in upper limbs if possible. An exception is the situation in which a crush (or blast) injury of the upper thorax is identified. In this case, potential injury to the subclavian veins and superior vena cava is a major concern, and it is appropriate to establish at least one initial intravenous line in a lower limb or in a femoral vein.

The magnitude of the deficit in vascular fluid volume and impairment of tissue perfusion is usually not defined at this point in the resuscitation effort, but there should be no delay in establishing vascular access in the trauma victim. Arm veins that may have been visible on arrival may abruptly disappear with progressive vascular collapse accompanying continuing internal hemorrhage. When two team members are available, one should work on immediately establishing an intravenous route while the other tends to initial airway evaluation and management.

USE OF MEDICAL ANTISHOCK TROUSERS AND INTRAVENOUS THERAPY IN THE FIELD

It has become common for paramedic and EMT personnel to begin intravenous therapy at the scene of the accident. It has also become common for trauma teams to employ medical antishock trousers (MAST) in the field, and even in the ED, to (1) compress bleeding sites and stabilize fractures in the lower body; (2) immediately increase effective total peripheral resistance; and (3) produce a transient "autotransfusion" of blood from the lower limbs to the upper body. These effects result, respectively, in (1) a slowing of bleeding in the lower body with preservation of valuable oxygen-carrying capacity, (2) an immediate increase in perfusion pressure at vital central organs, and (3) distention of previously collapsed veins in the upper limbs, thus permitting successful venipuncture where there would previously have been almost certain failure.

Tailored somewhat like an aviator's G suit, MAST have individual air bladder compartments that wrap around the lower abdomen, pelvis, and lower limbs. They are held in place by Velcro binders and are inflated by hand- or foot-operated pumps. MAST are conveniently applied in the field or in the ED by placing the patient on top of an open garment, prepositioned on a litter, and then wrapping the compartments anteriorly about the lower limbs, pelvis, and abdomen. Inflation pressure of the trousers is best determined in relation to the purpose for which the garment is applied. When the goal is that of restoring blood pressure (or transiently distending the veins of the upper limb), trouser pressure is increased (up to 100 mm Hg) until the desired measured systolic blood pressure of the patient is obtained. When the goal is that of hemorrhage control, a trouser pressure as low as 40 mm Hg may suffice.

It is important to note that in urban areas where transport times from scene to hospital are short, and particularly for penetrating injuries in urban areas, there is evidence suggesting that risks attendant to delay in transport related to initiation of I.V. therapy and application of MAST garments in the field may outweigh the benefits of "routine" use in prehospital care. For a severely injured patient in profound hypovolemic shock there is no question that initiation of replacement of vascular volume at the earliest moment is beneficial. However, how much time the paramedic or EMT team should invest at the scene prior to transport is not so clear-cut. If several efforts to establish vascular access fail (with the major veins in both arms being "used up") or if the shock state is due to cardiac tamponade or tension pneumothorax rather than hypovolemia, then delay at the scene in attempt to initiate I.V. therapy may well be detrimental. Emergency department physicians who regularly relate to emergency medical services personnel should establish (or become familiar with) policies regarding I.V. therapy and application of MAST in the field, for both radio contact and no-contact situations.

DECISION FOR PERCUTANEOUS CENTRAL VENIPUNCTURE VERSUS PERIPHERAL VEIN CUTDOWN

There will inevitably be those (not too common) instances where neither the transport team nor the ED team is able to start an I.V. by percutaneous venipuncture in an upper limb (even with use of MAST). In this situation, alternatives for quick vascular access are percutaneous central venous catheterization or peripheral vein cutdown. Percutaneous central venous catheterization may be performed by the subclavian or the internal jugular routes (see "Subclavian or Internal Jugular Catheter Placement," below). Cutdown may be performed, in order of decreasing convenience, to the saphenous vein 2 cm anterior and superior to the medial malleolus of the ankle, to the basilic vein 3 cm anterior and superior to the medial epicondyle of the elbow, or to the cephalic vein 2 cm below the lateralmost aspect of the prominence of the clavicle (see "Saphenous Vein Cutdown," p 371). The ease and speed with which vascular access can be established by these techniques correlate most directly with the experience of the operating physician in using the particular technique. When any of these methods are used in the emergent situation, the operator should weigh potential delay and risk involved against immediate patient need and anticipated benefit, and alternative methods.

(*Text continues on p 373.*)

Subclavian or Internal Jugular Catheter Placement

Indications

A. Peripheral vein is unavailable.
B. There is need to measure atrial filling pressure (suspected cardiac tamponade)
C. Hypertonic I.V. fluids are to be infused.

Equipment Needed

1 safety razor (disposable)
1 pair sterile gloves
2 10-ml syringes
1 22-guage needle (4 cm)
1 bottle lidocaine 1% solution
1 no. 11 (disposable) scalpel
10 4 × 4 sterile gauze pads
1 central venous catheter: preferably a no. 8 French i.d. introducer sheath with a bevel tip dilator
1 no. 18 5–7-cm thin-wall needle
1 40–45-cm-long 0.9-mm diam. floppy tip vascular guide wire
1 3-0 silk suture on a needle
1 roll 5-cm silk or adhesive tape
1 bottle Ringer's lactate
1 infusion set
1 extension tubing
1 bottle povidone-iodine solution
1 bottle tincture of benzoin
3 sterile towels

Method for Subclavian Placement

PROCEDURE	COMMENTS
A. Set up intravenous bottle and infusion line.	
B. Shave area from lower half of neck to midsternum on the side to be used.	B. This promotes sterility and helps in securing dressing.
C. Position patient with arms at sides and in a slight Trendelenburg position or with legs elevated.	C. This distends the subclavian vein and prevents air emboli in a hypovolemic patient.
D. Prepare the shaved area widely with povidone-iodine. Do not dry or blot. Drape the area with sterile towels; leave suprasternal notch visible.	D. Povidone-iodine loses some of its bactericidal action when dried. Leave enough area open to identify landmarks easily.

E. With 1% lidocaine, anesthetize the area by first making a skin wheal, then inject while advancing to the periosteum of the clavicle, particularly the posterior aspect near the vein.

F. Puncture the subclavian vein with the no. 18 thin-wall needle attached to a 10-ml syringe: Enter the skin at the midclavicular level about 2 cm to 3 cm below the clavicle. While applying suction, advance the needle under the clavicle, parallel to the horizontal plane, aiming for the suprasternal notch (Fig. 23-7). A gush of blood will return when the subclavian vein is entered.

G. When blood return is obtained, remove syringe from needle (preferably during a Valsalva maneuver if patient is cooperative), temporarily occlude the needle hub opening with thumb to prevent air embolism; then gently and smoothly advance the floppy tip guide wire through the needle into the superior vena cava.

H. Place the no. 11 scalpel blade immediately next to the guide wire at the point of skin entry; incise the skin and dermis.

I. Over the guide wire, advance the introducer sheath and bevel tip dilator, as a concentric unit, into the vein until the introducer sheath hub reaches the skin entry site.

J. Withdraw the guide wire and dilator, temporarily occluding the introducer sheath hub with thumb to prevent introduction of air; then connect syringe to introducer sheath to (re)confirm intravascular position of catheter tip by aspirating free flow of blood.

E. Not much anesthetic is needed in subcutaneous tissue because there are few nerve endings there.

F. If the vein is not entered on the first attempt, slowly withdraw the needle while applying suction—the vein may have been completely pierced. Then redirect needle and try again. (In older persons the vein frequently is more cephalad than anticipated and in obese persons deeper than anticipated.) To avoid lacerating the vein (or artery) *never change azimuth or elevation while the needle is still under the clavicle.* Always withdraw needle point to a superficial position before redirecting.

G. If, instead of the Seldinger technique thin-wall needle, an Intracath needle has been used to enter the vein, the plastic catheter is advanced through the needle into the vena cava. Never push a guide wire or catheter past an apparent obstruction: gently twist instead. If using an Intracath, never separately retract the catheter once it has been advanced past the end of the needle or it may be sheared off.

H. This will reduce resistance and avoid "fraying" the end of the catheter as the introducer sheath is advanced through the tissue.

I. Ensure that sufficient guide wire remains external to the skin so that the end of the guide wire protrudes proximal to the end of the (introducer sheath and the) bevel tip dilator before the dilator enters the skin. Then advance the introducer/dilator/wire as a unit, using gentle twisting motion. Avoid "fraying" of the distal end of the introducer sheath at the point of skin entry.

J. It usually is convenient to obtain samples for initial laboratory blood work at this time. An assistant can hand the operator a sterile 35- or 50-ml syringe for this purpose.

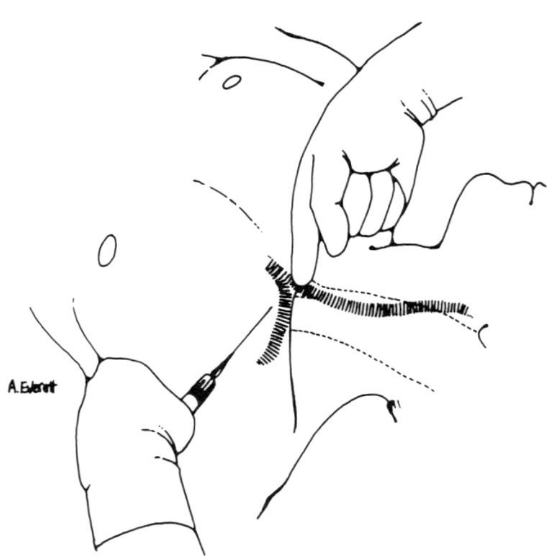

Figure 23-7. Infraclavicular approach for percutaneous subclavian vein catheterization.

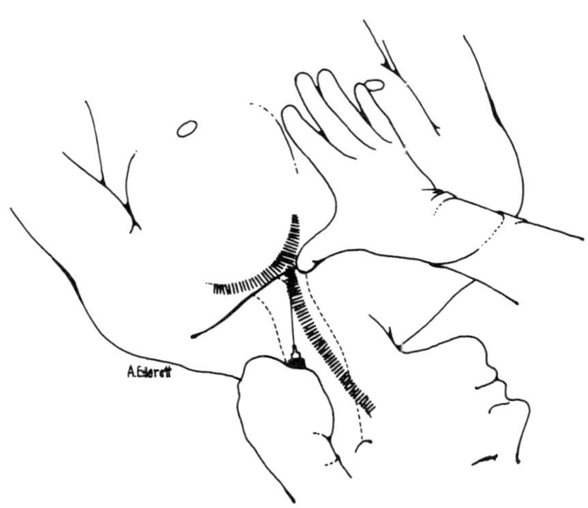

Figure 23-8. Approach for percutaneous internal jugular vein catheterization.

K. Quickly disconnect the syringe and connect the intravenous infusion line to the catheter. Begin infusion.

K. If, instead of the Seldinger technique, an Intracath has been used, then before removing the syringe from the catheter withdraw the metal needle until the tip is outside the skin. Immediately protect the catheter (from being cut by the needle) by applying the needle guard. Note that fluid runs freely when "wide open"; then adjust flow.

L. Using 3-0-silk suture, affix the catheter securely to the skin, near the skin entrance site. If items available and time permits, apply povidone-iodine ointment to skin entrance site and prep surrounding skin with tincture of benzoin.

M. Cover entrance site with 4 × 4 gauze pad held in place by tape or, preferably, if available, with flexible moisture proof clear dressing intended for maintenance of long-term vascular catheter sites. Secure a separate loop of the extension tubing to skin or dressing with a separate piece of tape.

M. This prevents traction on the intravenous tubing from dislodging the catheter.

N. Order an immediate chest roentgenogram to confirm catheter position in superior vena cava and to look for possible complications such as pneumothorax or hydro/hemothorax.

N. Total parenteral nutrition solution should not be infused into the jugular or any other small vein because administration of hypertonic fluid into a vessel without high blood flow may result in sclerosis and thrombosis.

Method for Internal Jugular Procedure

PROCEDURE

A–E. Same as subclavian procedure above

F. Puncture the internal jugular vein with the no. 18 thin-wall needle attached to a 10-ml syringe. Enter skin at the apex of the triangle formed by the clavicular and sternal heads of the steromastoid muscle and the medial third of the clavicle (Fig. 23-8). Apply suction while advancing the needle and syringe parallel to the sternum and downward at a 30-degree angle to the frontal plane. When a sudden gush of blood returns into the syringe, the vein has been entered.

G–L. Same as subclavian placement above

COMMENTS

F. If unsuccessful in entering the vein try aiming more laterally toward the ipsilateral femoral area. The vein runs from the angle of the jaw to the lateral aspect of the described triangle. If the carotid artery is inadvertently entered withdraw needle and apply pressure for 5 to 10 minutes.

Saphenous Vein Cutdown

Indication

Inability to establish intravenous access quickly by one of the standard percutaneous techniques

Equipment Needed

10 sterile 4 × 4 gauze pads
1 bottle providone-iodine solution
 sterile towels
10-ml syringe with 22-gauge needle
1 bottle lidocaine 1%
1 scalpel with no. 11 and no. 15 blades
2 small curved hemostats
2 small straight hemostats
1 suture scissors
1 small forceps
2 packs 3-0 silk sutures
2 packs 4-0 nylon or polypropylene suture on cutting needle
2 packs 4-0 polyglycolic acid or chromic gut sutures on atraumatic needles
1 14- or 16-gauge 20.5-cm plastic catheter
1 bottle intravenous solution with intravenous setup and extension

Method

PROCEDURE

A. Set up the bottle of intravenous solution and preload the infusion line.

COMMENTS

B. Prepare ankle and foot with povidone-iodine solution, drape off area, anesthetize the skin with lidocaine.
C. Make 3-cm transverse incision through the skin over the saphenous vein (Fig. 23-9).
D. Using the curved hemostats, dissect through the subcutaneous fat to locate and isolate the saphenous vein. This may sometimes be done with a single deep sweep of the hemostat through the subcutaneous tissue from one edge of the wound to the other.
E. Once the vein is isolated pass a closed curved hemostat under the vein, open the hemostat slightly, grasp two 3-0 silk sutures in the tip of the hemostat, and withdraw the hemostat to bring the sutures under the vein. Move one suture to the distalmost aspect of the isolated segment of the vein and tie a square knot in it (Fig. 23-10).
F. Grasp vein with forceps near the inferior suture and cut half way through with a no. 11 blade (Fig. 23-11).
G. Using fine-tipped forceps, lift up the anterior lip of the venotomy and insert the intravenous catheter up the vein (Figs. 23-12, 23-13). Connect to intravenous setup and start infusion.
H. Tie the vein down tightly around the catheter with the superior suture.
I. Close skin with 4-0 plastic suture on cutting needle and dress wound.

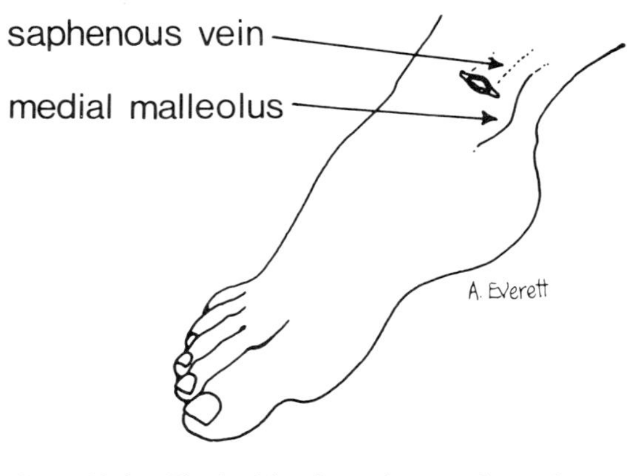

Figure 23-9. The incision is made over the saphenous vein on the medial aspect of the ankle anterior to the medial malleolus.

B. Infection in cutdown sites is a significant problem so sterility is very important, time permitting.
C. The vein is located 2 cm anteriorly and superiorly to the medial malleolus.
D. It is best to start the blunt dissection at the edges of the wound and work in to the middle. This assures that the wound remains wide enough as the dissection proceeds deeper.
E. Separate the two sutures as far as possible to the superior and inferior aspects of the wound, isolating as long a segment of vein as possible.
F. Leave forceps under vein to retract vein and control bleeding until the catheter is introduced.
G. When previous experience insures no time delay will be involved, skin closure is facilitated by bringing the intravenous catheter to the vein via a separate stab wound 2 cm inferior to skin incision.
I. The 4-0 absorbable suture on noncutting needle may be used for suture-ligature hemostasis or subcuticular tissue approximation as needed.

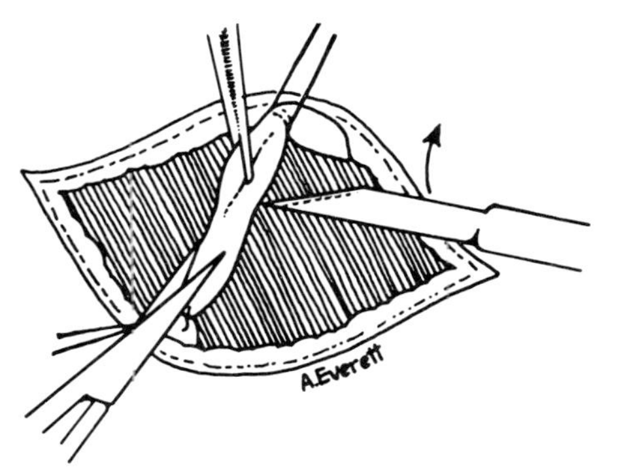

Figure 23-11. An incision is made in the isolated segment of the saphenous vein.

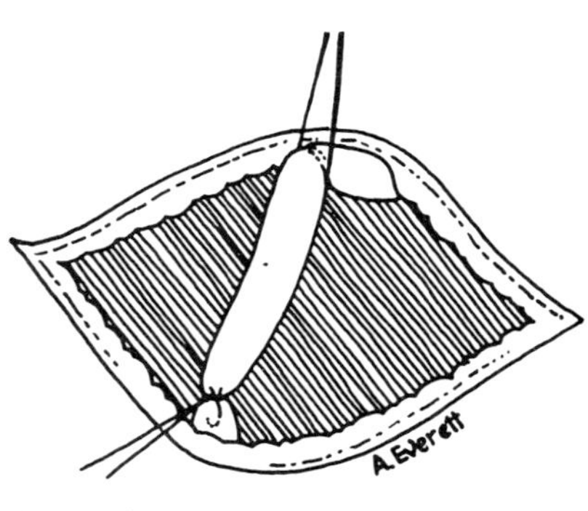

Figure 23-10. Segment of saphenous vein dissected free and tied distally, with an open loop of suture placed proximally.

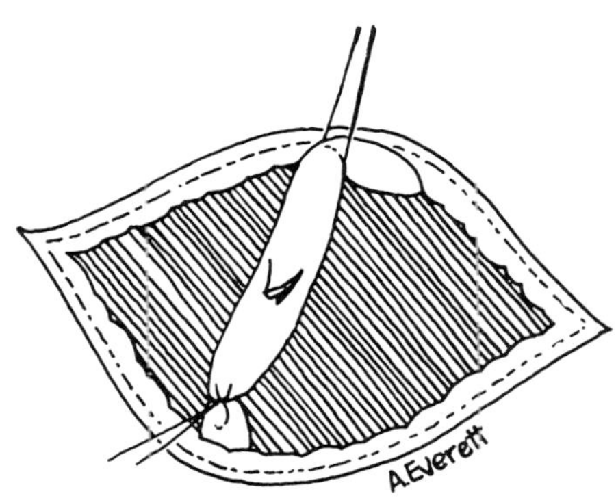

Figure 23-12. Saphenous venotomy ready for insertion of catheter.

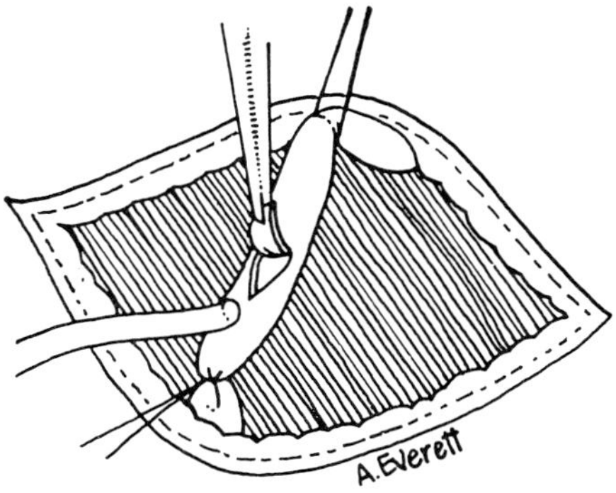

Figure 23-13. The cut edge of the vein is lifted with forceps and the catheter inserted upward for several centimeters.

In any setting it must be recognized that catheterization of the subclavian or internal jugular veins by percutaneous stick carries distinct risk of significant complications (see "Complications Associated With Percutaneous Central Venous Catheterization," below). In the already compromised multiple-system trauma patient, a pneumothorax (possibly tension pneumothorax if on positive-pressure ventilation), hemothorax, cardiac arrhythmia, or expanding hematoma next to the trachea literally represents addition of insult to injury; and in the emergent situation the probability of such complications can almost always be expected to exceed that of the "elective" situation. With severe vascular volume depletion, contracted central veins may be difficult to "stick" percutaneously, while even collapsed peripheral veins can be located by cutdown. For these reasons in some major trauma centers it is routine to place both initial intravenous lines by cutdown.

These considerations notwithstanding, it is our opinion that percutaneous central venous catheterization is the first alternative method of choice for vascular access when two large-bore upper-limb intravenous lines cannot immediately be established. (Obviously if the attempt at percutaneous central venous catheterization fails one should proceed immediately to cutdown.) In almost all cases "percutaneous stick" is significantly faster than cutdown. With hypovolemia, collapsed peripheral veins may be difficult to locate by cutdown. More soft-tissue complications at the site of entry are associated with cutdown. With increased use of introducers for elective insertion of central catheters for parenteral alimentation and monitoring of pulmonary artery pressure, physicians in training have become relatively more familiar with the percutaneous technique of catheter insertion than with the cutdown technique.

Familiarity and experience usually determine the choice of procedure: The emergent setting is not one in which to experiment with unfamiliar technique. The surgeon who most commonly uses the subclavian route for elective percutaneous insertion of catheters for administration of parenteral nutrition and for monitoring pulmonary artery pressure will do best using this route for establishing emergency vascular access. The anesthesiologist who more commonly uses the internal jugular route for establishing intravenous fluid and monitoring lines in the operating room will do best using this route in an emergent situation. The outpatient surgeon or emergency physician who does not "electively" place central catheters should learn at least one of these techniques, in accordance with the American Heart Association advanced cardiac life-support standards. It should be noted that the complications described for percutaneous central venous catheterization apply to both

COMPLICATIONS ASSOCIATED WITH PERCUTANEOUS CENTRAL VENOUS CATHETERIZATION

Related to Placement of the Catheter (Mechanical)

Arterial puncture
Malpositioned catheter
Pneumothorax
Hemothorax
Chylothorax
Perforation of vein
Perforation of atrium or ventricle (hydromediastinum with tamponade)
Intrapleural infusion
Nerve injury (brachial plexus)
Air embolus
Subcutaneous hematoma

Related to Presence of the Catheter

Mechanical
- Arrhythmia
- Venous thrombosis/thrombophlebitis
- Embolus of clot or of catheter fragment

Infectious
- Cellulitis
- Sepsis
- Endocarditis

infraclavicular and internal jugular routes of entry, pneumothorax being more common with (but not exclusively limited to) the subclavian route, and arterial and nerve injury being more common with the neck route. In the absence of previous experience or preference, we suggest that the physician first acquire familiarity with the infraclavicular subclavian route inasmuch as this location is also most favorable for longer-term aseptic maintenance of electively placed catheters for parenteral delivery of nutrition and central pressure monitoring and thus might be considered more versatile.

Two kinds of catheters are readily available and in common use for percutaneous central venipuncture: the Intracath type and the Seldinger introducer type. With the Intracath method, initial entry into the vein in an adult is made with a 5-cm 14-gauge (2.1-mm) steel needle, through which a 20.3-cm 16-gauge (1.7-mm) plastic cannula is advanced so that the catheter tip reaches the superior vena cava. With Seldinger catheter introduction, initial entry into the vein is made with a 5-cm to 7-cm 18-gauge, thin-wall steel needle, through which a 40-cm to 45-cm 0.9-mm floppy-tipped Seldinger-type vascular guide wire is advanced into the superior vena cava. (A 5-cm 16-gauge Angiocath or the 5-cm 14-gauge steel needle from an Intracath can also be used for initial venipuncture, but with somewhat more risk than with the thin-walled 18-gauge needle.) The needle is then removed, and a 12.5-cm 8 French lumen (2.7-mm) plastic introducer catheter sheath concentrically fitted over a bevel-tipped dilator sleeve 21 cm long is advanced over the guide wire into the superior vena cava. The guide wire and the inner expander sleeve are removed, leaving the 8 French plastic introducer cannula for central venous fluid administration. This conduit equals or exceeds the luminal diameter of any peripheral cutdown line it is possible to establish, yet initial percutaneous venipuncture is accomplished with only an 18-gauge needle. The complication rate of central venous catheterization by the Seldinger technique has been acceptably low, whereas the success rate in achieving small-bore needle entry into even volume-contracted central veins has been high.

During percutaneous central venous catheterization the catheter should advance with minimum resistance, and there should be free backflow of blood with the catheter in the fully inserted position. If this is not the case, placement of the catheter outside the vein, kinking of the catheter, or vessel injury must be suspected. Rapid infusion of fluid under these circumstances (if the fluid will run at all) may result in hydrothorax or superficial soft-tissue "salinoma." Instead, that catheter should be removed and another catheter inserted. In removing an Intracath it should be noted that once the plastic cannula is advanced beyond the tip of the steel needle, the needle and cannula must be withdrawn together. Pulling the catheter back with the needle still in the vein may result in the sharp bevel of the needle shearing off the catheter tip with resultant foreign body embolus to the right side of the heart or the pulmonary artery. This can be a life-threatening problem (because of arrhythmia, valvular malfunction, thrombosis, infection, or cardiac perforation) necessitating removal by thoracotomy and cardiotomy if extraction using a fluoroscopically guided intravascular angiographic catheter is unsuccessful.

Immediately after percutaneous central venous catheterization the hemithorax should be auscultated to determine whether breath sounds are the same as those before the puncture. If this is not the case, pneumothorax should be suspected and confirmed or disaffirmed by a roentgenogram. If pneumothorax is present, tube thoracostomy should be performed (see p 383). The central catheter can be left in place if free backflow of blood can be obtained and fluid can be infused freely.

Regardless of the ease with which central venous catheterization is accomplished, the final position of the catheter and integrity of the lung must be confirmed by roetgenography. Unless the patient is in imminent danger of exsanguination, when bilateral attempts at central venous catheterization are made, a chest roentgenogram should be obtained to exclude the presence of pneumothorax on the first side before proceeding with percutaneous puncture on the other side. When chest injury is suspected, percutaneous central venous catheterization should be performed (first) on the side of the injury so that pneumothorax does not compromise the patient's only good lung.

INITIAL LABORATORY BLOOD WORK

When the first (in hospital) intravenous catheter has been inserted and free backflow of blood obtained, it is convenient to attach a large (35- to 50-ml) syringe and withdraw blood for initial laboratory work. The apparently seriously injured patient is obviously going to be admitted to the hospital (if only for observation); therefore minimum indications are for a complete blood count, prothrombin time, partial thromboplastin time, determinations of platelet count, electrolytes, blood urea nitrogen, glucose, and enzymes (including amylase). In any comatose patient the blood alcohol level should be determined to aid in learning the cause of loss of consciousness and in guiding therapy. (When this value is requested for medical reasons, the physician need not be concerned about legal implications.) The hematocrit, coagulation time, and electrolyte, glucose, and amylase values should be reported *stat*.

BLOOD TYPE AND CROSSMATCH REQUEST

Because hemorrhagic shock is so often a complication of major trauma, and because cross matching of blood represents a key rate-limiting step in resuscitation of the patient with hypovolemic shock, a clot tube for typing and cross matching of blood is a first-order priority with regard to initial blood drawn. Though seemingly a mundane point in the midst of the furious activity in the emergency department, it is important that the clot tube be properly labeled and that the type and crossmatch requests be accurately completed and delivered to the laboratory promptly. Because of the probability both of specimen mix-up and of a multitude of legal constraints, most larger medical center blood banks will not process improperly labeled specimens. For a critically injured patient, delay in "doing it over again, right" may be unacceptable. Should faulty labeling actually result in a typing or crossmatching error, coagulopathy associated with a transfusion reaction may be disastrous to the patient in shock from profound hemorrhage.

When major hemorrhage is suspected or hypotension documented, the initial request should be for type and crossmatch of at least 6 units of blood, assuming the blood bank is capable of meeting this demand. (In smaller communities, lists may be kept of pretyped walk-in donors who can be recalled rapidly, or plans can be made in advance for rapid ground or air transport of blood from larger regional facilities.) Since early availability of blood may be a crucial factor in resuscitation, it is recommended there be a short interval follow-up call from the ED to the blood bank to confirm that the blood request has arrived and is being processed *stat*.

BLOOD GAS DETERMINATION

Arterial blood gas determination has become routine in major injury cases and should be included as a component of the initial *stat* laboratory studies. Early knowledge of acid–base imbalances and oxygenation–ventilation deficiencies can more precisely guide the resuscitation effort, and these data should be available within 10 minutes after a blood gas specimen is obtained. Though any laboratory value must be interpreted in relation to the clinical presentation, for the as yet minimally evaluated trauma patient, tissue perfusion should be considered inadequate if the initial blood gas values indicate:

pH < 7.3
$PCO_2 < 25$
Base excess < -8
CO_2 combining power ("bicarb") < 18
Hematocrit < 30 (reflects O_2-carrying capacity)

SHOCK AND FLUID RESUSCITATION: ASSESSMENT AND REPLACEMENT OF BLOOD LOSS

Once vascular access has been established and blood obtained for initial laboratory studies, intravenous administration of fluids must begin. Two decisions are required immediately: (1) what to infuse and (2) how fast to infuse it.

CHOICE OF RESUSCITATION FLUID

Unless imminent exsanguination demands immediate use of type O Rh-negative uncross-matched blood, initial intravenous fluid infusion should be begun with an "off the shelf" product until type-specific, and preferably crossmatched, blood is available. For a number of years shock and trauma experts have debated the relative merits of crystalloid versus colloid solutions for resuscitation from hypovolemic shock. It is our opinion that *initial* volume replacement should be with a balanced salt solution such as lactated Ringer's or Normosol R. Crystalloid solution is chosen in preference to colloid solution because larger volumes can be delivered (1) less expensively, (2) without risk of coagulation defects associated with dextran or antigen–antibody reactions associated with pooled plasma fractions, (3) with shorter-term retention in extravascular pulmonary tissue when extravasation occurs, and (4) with more certain immediate restoration of vascular volume.

Volume expansion with colloid presumes, in part, (1) that the infused colloid remains in the vascular compartment and (2) that extravascular extracellular fluid is available and able to translocate osmotically to the vascular compartment. However, there is good evidence that in a severe shock state (1) a capillary leak syndrome allows extravasation of proteins from the vascular compartment (thus increasing interstitial colloid osmotic pressure), and (2) impairment of cell membrane transport mechanisms allows interstitial water to follow sodium and chloride intracellularly where it is unavailable for immediate attraction to the vascular space. Thus it is *after* an initial (oligemic) shock state has been reversed that colloid can be used to best advantage. With capillary integrity and cell membrane function reestablished, increasing intravascular osmotic pressure by addition of a modest volume of colloid can further increase vascular volume through resorption of interstitial edema. On initial encounter with the multiple-injury patient, status of capillary integrity and cell membrane function are not immediately evident. Thus it is prudent to start fluid resuscitation with balanced salt solution.

RATE OF INTRAVENOUS INFUSION

The initial rate of fluid infusion will depend largely on the presence or absence of shock. By definition, shock is inadequate tissue perfusion, and, even more fundamentally, impaired respiration at the cellular level. It should be remembered that hemodynamics (systemic circulation) represents only one component set of parameters in a complicated sequence of events involved in the transport, delivery, and cellular utilization of oxygen. Yet in the trauma-related shock setting, hemodynamic parameters are among the first to be unfavorably altered. Thus it is useful to have a working clinical classification of shock from a hemodynamic standpoint, and an algorithm by which to assess adequacy of tissue perfusion rapidly.

HEMODYNAMIC CLASSIFICATION OF SHOCK

From a simplistic mechanical (hydraulic system) viewpoint, maintenance of normal perfusion requires a properly functioning pump, connected to a set of pipes of known size, in which is circulated a volume of fluid sufficient to fill the pipes, without obstruction to flow. Perfusion will be inadequate if (1) the pump fails, (2) the volume of the fluid contracts (but the size of the pipes does not contract correspondingly), (3) the size of the pipes expands (but the volume of fluid does not expand correspondingly), or (4) there is obstruction to inflow or outflow at the pump. These defects correspond to the classification currently accepted by the Society of Critical Care Medicine: shock due to cardiogenic, hypovolemic, distributive, and obstructive causes, respectively (Table 23-1). Many derangements are known to represent specific causes of these general categories of shock (Table 23-2).

IMMEDIATE ASSESSMENT OF TISSUE PERFUSION

Shock of all categories results in early increase in catecholamine output, both from the adrenal medulla and the sympathetic nervous system (to the extent that these systems remain intact). In general, epinephrine is a potent α- and β-adrenergic stimulant, and norepinephrine is a potent α- and a weak β-adrenergic stimulant. Excitation of α receptors

Table 23-1. Hemodynamic Classification of Shock

MECHANICAL COMPONENT	CORRESPONDING PHYSIOLOGIC DERANGEMENT
Fluid	Hypovolemic shock
Pipes	Distributive shock
Pump	Cardiogenic shock
Inflow–outflow restriction	Obstructive shock

Table 23-2. Causes of Shock Related to Hemodynamic Categories

TYPE OF SHOCK	GENERAL CAUSE	SPECIFIC CAUSE
Hypovolemic shock	External blood loss	Hemorrhage
	External plasma loss	Burn
	External dehydration	Vomiting, diarrhea, heat, forced diuresis
	Internal plasma extravasation	Inflammation, anaphylaxis
Distributive shock	High or normal resistance, increased venous capacitance	Spinal cord injury
		Reflex vagal stimuli (pain, viscus distention)
		Drugs (barbiturate intoxication)
		Anesthesia (ganglionic blockade)
		Bacillary infection
	Low resistance, vasodilation	Septicemia
		Inflammatory hyperemia (peritonitis, cellulitis)
		Reactive hyperemia (crush syndrome)
		Anaphylaxis
		Vasoactive amine release
Cardiogenic shock	Impaired contractility	Myocardial infarction
		Myocardial contusion
		Myocardopathy
		Chronic congestive failure
		Acute hypoxemic/ischemic failure
	Impaired filling, emptying	Tachyarrhythmia
		Bradyarrhythmia
		Valvular disease
Obstructive shock	Vena caval compression	Crush injury of chest
		Tension pneumothorax
		Subdiaphragmatic pressure
	Pericardial compression	Tamponade
	Cardiac chamber obstruction	Valvular dysfunction
		Thrombus
	Impaired pulmonary blood flow	Pneumothorax
		Hemothorax
		Pulmonary contusion
		Flail chest
		Pulmonary embolus
		Pulmonary hypertension
	Impaired systemic blood flow	Aortic injury (transection, laceration, intimal flap, aneurysmal dissection)
		Systemic hypertension

produces precapillary and postcapillary vasoconstriction; excitation of β receptors produces vasodilation and a positive inotropic effect on the myocardium. In decreasing order of α sensitivity and increasing order of β sensitivity are the vascular beds of the skin, kidney, abdominal viscera, and lung. With shock-induced intense α stimulation and consequent vasoconstriction, perfusion to these vascular beds is sequentially reduced in order to deliver limited remaining oxygenated blood flow to the most vital organs: heart and brain. With concurrently increased β stimulation, heart rate is increased toward the same goal. With injury-induced impairment of α-adrenergic activity, relative vasodilation occurs.

Thus the earliest effects of hypoperfusion and peripheral vasoconstriction are detectable on the skin by a cool, pale appearance, except when the shock is of the early distributive type, as with spinal cord injury, resulting in disruption of sympathetic α-adrenergic stimulation. In this latter case, the skin distal to injury may be warm and vasodilated despite relative systemic hypoperfusion. In either case, heart rate is increased. Progressive effects on the kidney are manifested by reduced urine output. Anxiety is an early central nervous system reaction to mild shock, while lethargy (progressing to coma) represents central nervous system manifestation of relatively prolonged and severe systemic hypoperfusion. Profound hypotension represents (1) hemodynamic collapse when compensatory diversion of available blood volume can no longer sustain adequate central circulation, (2) primary pump failure, or (3) a combination of both.

In otherwise uncomplicated hypovolemic shock it has been noted that organ system and vital sign manifestations seem to correlate with fraction of blood volume loss and severity of shock. Loss of less than 15% of original blood volume (designated class 1 hemorrhage by the American College of Surgeons' Advanced Trauma Life Support course) usually does not result in clinically significant shock. Loss of 15% to 30% of blood volume (class 2 hemorrhage) results in mild shock, characterized by tachycardia, tachypnea, decrease in pulse pressure width, delayed capillary refill, and anxiety. Loss of 30% to 40% blood volume (class 3 hemorrhage) results in moderate shock, characterized by marked tachycardia and tachypnea, decrease in systolic blood pressure, oliguria, and change in mental status. Loss of more than 40% blood volume (class 4 hemorrhage) results in severe shock, characterized by cool, pale skin, neglegible urine output, markedly depressed mental status, and hemodynamic collapse.

Therefore, in initial rapid assessment, skin color and temperature, urine output, and central nervous system function are simple and easily assessable parameters that reflect adequacy of tissue perfusion and organ function. Blood pressure, pulse, and respiration rate are readily obtainable vital signs that reflect perfusion pressure and hemodynamic function. The following are recommended as "limits" for vital signs in a trauma patient whose status has been only minimally evaluated:

Pulse: 50 to 120
Ventilation (spontaneous): 6 to 25
Blood pressure: >90 mm Hg systolic
Temperature: >97 degrees Farenheit

Values outside these limits, particularly if the extent of injuries is not yet known, are strongly suggestive of shock.

In interpretation of vital signs in the trauma victim, it is worth emphasizing (or reemphasizing) several points: (1) Classic changes in hypovolemic shock are toward increased pulse and ventilation rate, decreased blood pressure and central temperature (usually, but not always, in that temporal sequence). These are just *opposite* to those classically associated with increased intracranial pressure following ("isolated") head injury (see section on head injury). (2) Preexisting heart disease or coexisting head injury may limit maximum heart rate. (3) Because increased heart rate and peripheral vasoconstriction come into play as compensatory mechanisms to forestall collapse of central circulation, significant hypovolemia, particularly in young trauma victims, may be present without hypotension. Thus a weak, thready, rapid peripheral pulse and cool, pale extremities may reflect hypovolemia even in the presence of normal blood pressure. (4) Multiple trauma may result in shock of multiple causes.

HYPOTENSION: THE MOST COMMON DETERMINANT

It has been found that for each 100 ml of blood loss, most patients in hemorrhagic shock require infusion of about 300 ml of crystalloid solution to establish and maintain adequate perfusion. For patients who have sustained class 3 or 4 hemorrhage, infusion of blood (with or following crystalloid solution) will also be necessary.

It would be desirable to be able to categorize consistently, immediately, and precisely the hemodynamic cause of inadequate perfusion and to estimate the vascular volume deficit accurately in every trauma victim in shock. Unfortunately, in practice in the emergency department setting this is simply not possible. The issue is complicated by the facts that (1) multiple trauma can result in shock from a variety and combination of causes, (2) time pressures force immediate decisions, and (3) the data base is almost always incomplete at the time this initial decision must be made. Even the old standards of skin changes, urine output, and central nervous system function suffer difficulties related to reliability and time factors: Peripheral vasoconstriction (so often observed on arrival) may be due to recent cold exposure instead of hypovolemia, or changes of hypovolemia may be masked by vasodilation due to coexisting spinal cord injury. Urine output is not an "immediately" ascertainable number. (It also may be altered by preexisting renal disease.) With (so often concomitantly present) head trauma, central nervous system function obviously may be impaired independent of systemic perfusion deficit.

Thus despite the cautions in interpretation enumerated previously, the bottom line in *immediate* decision making as to rate of initial fluid infusion most often comes to rest with the vital signs. Although it would be well to avoid excessive salt load in the patient with severe head injury or cardiac or pulmonary contusion, prolonged ischemia of these same organs is the greater risk, should there be delay in replenishing vascular volume in the severely hypovolemic hemorrhagic shock patient. Because hypovolemia is such a common finding in the multiple injury patient, it is unsafe to assume hypotension does not equal hypovolemia until information is available to the contrary.

Therefore when initial systolic blood pressure is well below 100 mm Hg, initial infusion of crystalloid in an adult should be at a rate of 1 to 2 liters over 15 to 30 minutes. When blood pressure is "unobtainable," 1000 ml can be infused in *each* of two large-bore intravenous catheters during the first 10 to 15 minutes. In the presence of profound hypotension this brisk initial rate of infusion of saline fluid also applies to a trauma patient with obvious head injury or known chronic heart failure: If prolonged hypotension leads to an "irreversible-shock" state or terminal renal failure, finding nonedematous brain or lungs at autopsy will be of questionable benefit. In the absence of hypotension or tachycardia, fluid infusion can be begun at a moderate rate (125 ml/hr to 150 ml/hr in an adult) and adjusted accordingly as initial laboratory findings are received, urine output is established, and other data accumulate. The potential deleterious effects of a salt fluid load in a patient with head or cardiopulmonary injuries can be considered.

HYPOTHERMIA: A COMMON ENEMY

One of the most distressing complications in the resuscitation of a hemorrhaging trauma patient is the development of systemic coagulopathy. One of the most important variables influencing the development of coagulopathy is hypothermia. Although prehospital exposure often is a cause of hypothermia in trauma victims, the most common contributor to development of hypothermia is rapid intravenous infusion of solutions usually stored in environments well below body temperature. Crystalloid stored at room temperature can be a major offender because, although the temperature difference is favorable compared with blood stored at 4°C, large volumes of crystalloid often are infused. Therefore, when apparatus is available with which to warm I.V. fluids, its use is recommended for the resuscitation of major-trauma victims.

Warming may be accomplished before or during infusion of I.V. fluids. Microwave is an acceptable method of prewarming crystalloid solution. When fluids are warmed during infusion, it is important that the apparatus not impair rate of infusion. In this last regard, a device recently introduced on the market—the Bard Infuser 37 System—appears to combine adequate warming with adequate infusion rate.

RESPONSE TO INITIAL RESUSCITATION: USE OF BLOOD AND BLOOD PRODUCTS

In the hypotensive patient (or the patient who is normotensive on arrival at the ED but reported to have been hypotensive at the scene of the accident) vital signs (and airway status) should be reassessed at least every 15 minutes. If the hypotension is due to uncomplicated hypovolemia it can be anticipated that normal blood pressure will be reestablished with rapid infusion of less than 2 liters of lactated Ringer's. If the blood loss has been modest and hemorrhage has stopped, blood pressure should return to normal and stabilize simply with infusion of the balanced salt solution. The infusion rate can then be slowed and serial hematocrit values followed. In addition to accomplishing the necessary resuscitation, this process of crystalloid administration also (1) estimates the extent of blood loss, (2) significantly reduces the transfusion requirement should blood replacement be needed, and (3) is of benefit in reducing the deficit in functional extracellular fluid that occurs in an established shock state.

If blood loss has been severe or hemorrhage continues, then the increase in blood pressure and decrease in pulse rate that usually occur with rapid infusion of crystalloid will likely be transient. Hemorrhage from constricted or loosely clotted vessels may resume as intravascular pressure increases. If hypovolemic hypotension persists or recurs despite brisk infusion of crystalloid it will also be necessary to infuse blood and attempt to rapidly identify a site of continuing hemorrhage. In most cases the initial infusion of balanced salt solution will allow time for typing and cross matching before administration of blood becomes necessary.

Complete typing and cross matching requires about 45 minutes after a sample reaches the laboratory. The blood type can be identified very rapidly, however, and type-specific blood can be provided within 5 minutes of arrival of the sample. In the unusual event of imminent exsanguination, type O Rh-negative blood should be called for immediately.

Particularly when blood is administered because of apparent continuing hemorrhage, it is important to warm the blood during infusion when appropriate warming equipment is available. Most blood requested emergently is provided at about 4°C; several units infused rapidly at that temperature will have a distinctly negative impact on coagulation mechanisms.

When available, whole blood is useful for emergent rapid transfusion in a hemorrhaging trauma patient because (1) whole blood is what is being lost; (2) it contains useful colloid and coagulation factors; and (3) it runs in faster than packed cells through *any* delivery system. More leisurely replacement of oxygen-carrying capacity in a normotensive trauma patient whose vascular volume has been effectively reexpanded with crystalloid calls for use of packed cells (1) because red cells are the specific component needed to increase the hematocrit value and improve oxygen transport and (2) because their selective use decreases risk of antigen–antibody reactions to the unneeded components. Similarly, component therapy is also indicated in replacement of platelets and coagulation factors in a normotensive patient after volume expansion (even with concurrent elective red cell replacement).

PHYSICAL EXAMINATION AND INITIAL TREATMENT OF SPECIFIC INJURIES

When the airway is secure, vascular access established, initial laboratory work in progress, and fluid resuscitation under way, attention can be turned to identification and management of specific injuries. A combined systems–anatomic approach is useful to ensure complete evaluation. Assessment usually depends on history and physical examination, laboratory data, x-ray study, special studies, and consultation. These must be in appropriate sequence to permit diagnosis and initiation of treatment of potentially life-threatening and permanently disabling conditions before time and attention are devoted to lesser, even though perhaps more readily recognized, problems.

History and physical examination are obviously first. It is appropriate to perform physical examination of a trauma patient in two phases: On the "first pass" one looks for injuries that, if identified, would mandate immediate intervention, consultation, or confirmatory study. The appropriate actions are promptly initiated. On the "second pass," examination of each organ system or anatomic region is completed and management or further study of less critical or immediately life-threatening injuries is initiated. Recording each apparent injury or study needed, as it is identified on the second-pass examination, can help prevent omission and aid in efficient sequencing of further studies.

FIRST-PASS PHYSICAL EXAMINATION: IMMEDIATE INTERVENTIONS

On the first pass the sequence of examination should direct attention first to those systems: (1) in which injury could be aggravated by manipulations involved with subsequent physical examination, diagnostic procedures, or therapeutic maneuvers, and (2) in which even short delay in recognition and treatment of injury could adversely affect outcome. An appropriate first-pass starting point with regard to the former is spinal cord evaluation; with regard to the latter it is anterior neck, chest, and abdominal examination.

Spinal Cord Injury: Immediate Considerations

Cervical spine injury should be suspected in any patient unconscious from head trauma or with significant injuries to scalp, face, or shoulders. Likewise, thoracic or lumbar spine injury should be suspected in the patient with major thoracoabdominal injury. These suspicions should begin at the scene of the accident, and EMT and paramedic teams should protect such patients by transporting them to the hospital on rigid spine boards or orthopaedic "scoop" stretchers.

Protecting the Spinal Cord in the ED. When there is indication or suspicion of spinal cord injury, the neck should be immobilized with a cervical collar (unless direct access to the trachea is needed to maintain the airway) and the head blocked bilaterally with foam rubber wedges or sandbags until roentgenograms can be obtained of the cervical spine. A conscious but uncooperative and combative patient should be similarly protected.

The ED team may be pressured by the transport team to immediately return the backboard or stretcher on which the patient arrived. A two-piece orthopaedic scoop stretcher can be removed with safety once collar and sandbags are in place. However, a patient with a potential neck injury should not be lifted from a one-piece spine board until examined further and until adequate help is available for lifting. Having backboards available in the ED for exchange is a nice solution to this problem.

First-Pass Evaluation of Spinal Cord. A conscious and cooperative patient should be questioned directly about pain in the neck or back, sensation and strength in limbs, and ability to move about at the scene of accident. The posterior aspect of the cervical spine should be gently palpated without movement of the head or back. Peripheral sensation can be grossly assessed by light finger touch over distal aspects of each limb. In the absence of significant hand or foot injury, bilateral finger grip and ankle flexion–extension against resistance of the examiner's hand provide quick checks of motor function and symmetry of strength.

In an unconscious or uncooperative patient the presence of absence of bilateral symmetry of limb motion and ability to withdraw from noxious (pin prick or pinch) stimuli should be observed.

Acute local pain is the principal symptom of fracture of the spine. Thus pain in the midline neck or upper back, even without palpable injury or sensorimotor deficit, is sufficient indication to protect the cervical spine with a collar, even if preliminary neck films are normal. (Tomograms, computed tomography, or magnetic resonance imaging may be necessary to rule out spinal fracture unequivocally; even in the absence of fracture, neck musculature may be relaxed by cervical collar support.) A lateralizing deficit in sensation and motor strength is particular cause for concern about spinal cord injury and strong indication to provide protection until definitive studies can be accomplished.

If (portable or ceiling-mounted) roentgenography is available in the ED, then after steps 1 to 4 of the general plan of action protocol are accomplished and immediately life-threatening chest injuries have been excluded or dealt with, it is appropriate to interrupt the physical examination to obtain films of the cervical spine (and anteroposterior views of the chest and pelvis).

Anterior Neck Injury: Immediate Considerations

The anterior area of the neck contains so many major pulmonary, vascular, neurologic, and digestive system conduits within a relatively small and compact cross-sectional area that any penetrating or blunt injury must be considered potentially life threatening. Disregarding an apparently innocent superficial neck wound or allowing concomitant head or chest trauma to divert attention from the possibility of a serious neck injury may lead to morbid or fatal consequences due to delayed hemorrhage, airway obstruction, deep neck infection, or cerebral infarction.

Brisk external bleeding and airway obstruction, both discussed in earlier sections, are the most immediate considerations in neck injury in the multiple-injury patient. It must again be emphasized that external bleeding from major neck vessels should be controlled by pressure until adequate exposure can be obtained in the operating room. Attempts in the ED to apply hemostats to bleeding points deep within the neck are apt to result in permanent injury to the carotid artery, vagus nerve, laryngeal nerves, or branches of the brachial plexus.

Indication for Primary Tracheostomy. Direct injury to the posterior pharynx or larynx, avulsion of the larnyx from the trachea, or compression of the trachea by an adjacent tense hematoma may result in airway obstruction and preclude passage of an endotracheal tube from above. The immediate alternative, cricothyroidotomy, may be complicated by loss of the cricothyroid-notch landmark by traumatic shift of laryngeal structures or obliteration by surrounding hematoma, subcutaneous emphysema, or both. Such circumstances might constitute a rare indication for emergent airway entry lower in the neck, by means of third-ring tracheostomy, without an endotracheal tube already in place.

Chest Injury: Immediate Considerations

Thoracoabdominal injuries are among the most immediately lethal in multiple-injury patients. About 25% of all trauma deaths result primarily from chest injuries, with most of these occurring before the victims reach a hospital. However, for those who reach the hospital, rapid evaluation and management in the ED can result in salvage from even severe and immediately life-threatening thoracic trauma and prevent life-threatening developments from lesser chest injuries.

Evaluation of integrity and function of the cardiopulmonary system begins when the patient is first sighted, in conjunction with assessment of airway patency and adequacy of ventilation, as described in the earlier section on airway management. It continues with measurement of vital signs and determination of the presence or absence of shock. Even prior to a chest examination, with the victim's upper clothing partially opened, the examiner knows something about the symmetry of chest motion with inspiration, bilateral breath sounds, arterial pulse pressure and contour, and apparent perfusion of skin and CNS. For adequate chest examination the patient's upper body clothing must be removed as soon as possible after arrival in the ED. If upper limb or spinal cord injury is present or suspected, clothing should be cut away.

First-Pass Chest Examination. Visual inspection can immediately identify blunt contusions, penetrating wounds, asymmetry of motion, flail chest, and deviation of the trachea. Listening can immediately identify gross obstruction of the upper airway and sucking at an open chest wound. Auscultation of breath and heart sounds with a stethoscope can identify hypoventilation, upper airway fluid accumulation, rales, wheezing, pleural or pericardial rub, and diminished heart sounds. Percussion can reveal hyper-resonance, suggesting pneumothorax, or hyporesonance, suggesting hemothorax, and may elicit tenderness over a rib fracture or chest wall contusion.

Lateral cross-chest rib compression and anteroposterior compression of the sternum may elicit pain in chest wall contusion or rib fracture(s). Pain produced at a site away from where pressure is applied helps distinguish fracture from contusion or muscle strain. Palpation may demonstrate chest wall instability and pain directly over fractures of ribs or sternum and presence of air in subcutaneous soft tissues (crepitance). When x-ray equipment is available within the ED resuscitation room, a chest roentgenogram should be requested as soon as chest injury is suspected. As with the lateral cervical spine film for evaluation of neck injury, when steps 1 to 4 of the protocol are accomplished it is appropriate to interrupt the physical examination for an anteroposterior supine chest film as soon as x-ray personnel are ready.

The "Rapid Killers." There are a limited number of conditions related to blunt or penetrating thoracic trauma that may begin minutes to hours after initial injury, evolve rapidly to cause severe cardiopulmonary distress leading to early death, yet successfully respond to treatment if recognized quickly. These conditions are airway obstruction, open pneumothorax, tension (or severe) pneumothorax, massive hemothorax, flail chest with severe pulmonary contusion, and cardiac tamponade. These rapid killers should be specifically sought in every multiple-injury patient, particularly when shock is recognized *soon* after injury and hypotension does not respond rapidly to initial infusion of balanced salt solution. Identification of any of these problems in the hemodynamically unstable patient mandates immediate intervention. Airway evaluation and management, always leading the list, have already been discussed.

Pneumothorax may result from air entering the pleural space externally through a defect in the chest wall (open pneumothorax) or internally through a defect in lung, bronchus, trachea, or esophagus (closed pneumothorax). Such injury may therefore result from penetrating or blunt chest trauma. If a penetrating wound is relatively small, orientation of the tissue defect may constitute a one-way valve such that air is drawn into the pleural space from outside the chest during inspiratory effort ("sucking" chest wound), or is pushed into the pleural space during positive-pressure ventilation via tracheal intubation tube or face mask, but is unable to exit during the expiratory phase. When pressure in the pleural space exceeds that in the lung, the lung will collapse. Further increase in pressure results in shift of the mediastinum away from the side of injury. This condition constitutes tension pneumothorax. Shift of the mediastinum impairs venous return and causes the trachea to deviate away from the side of injury. Collapsed lung results in marked intrapulmonary shunting. Shock of the obstructive category is the life-threatening consequence, because of impaired cardiac filling and emptying and profound hypoxemia. If a chest wound is relatively large in a nonintubated patient, with inspiratory effort and expiratory relaxation, air will move in and out through the defect (with or without sucking, depending on size of the defect) rather than through the tracheobronchial tree. If the chest wall opening is larger than the trachea, effective ventilation of the lungs may cease.

Massive hemothorax can produce shock of both the hypovolemic and obstructive types. Bleeding may be from lung or chest wall vessels or from a penetrating heart wound whose associated pericardial wound communicates freely with the pleural space. Both loss of blood and compression of lung tissue impair cardiopulmonary function.

The most certain diagnosis of pneumothorax and hemothorax is made roentgenographically. The most definitive treatment of pneumothorax and hemothorax is tube thoracostomy. The optimal site of insertion of a chest tube is in the midaxillary line at the fifth, sixth, or seventh intercostal space. When the problem is pneumothorax without hemothorax, it is appropriate to insert a relatively small tube (22 to 28 French in an adult) at the fifth intercostal space, with the tip directed to the anterosuperior aspect of the hemithorax where intrapleural air will accumulate in the supine patient. When the problem is hemothorax with only a small associated pneumothorax, it is appropriate to insert a large tube (32 to 38 French in an adult) at the sixth or seventh intercostal space, with holes at both distal and proximal aspects of the chest tube and with the tip directed to the posterosuperior aspect of the hemithorax. When the problem is hemothorax with a large pneumothorax, insertion of both tubes may be necessary to evacuate the blood and reexpand the lung (see ''Emergency Chest Tube Placement,'' below).

Emergency Chest Tube Placement

Indications in the Trauma Victim

A. Large pneumothorax or hemothorax
B. Bilateral pneumothoraces
C. Anticipation of requirement for mechanical ventilation in the operating room, x-ray suite, or intensive care unit, even if ''only'' a small pneumothorax, several rib fractures, or pulmonary contusion has been identified.

Equipment Needed

Chest tubes of various sizes, no. 28 to 40F
Water-seal drainage apparatus or Heimlich valve
1 scalpel with blade
1 curved Mayo scissors
1 large (15 cm to 20 cm) hemostat clamp with slightly curved jaws
1 needle holder
1 0 silk suture on a cutting needle
10 sterile 4 × 4 gauze pads
1 pair sterile gloves
4 sterile towels (and preferably a ''double half sheet'' surgical drape)
1 sterile petrolatum gauze pad
1 bottle povidone-iodine solution
1 roll 5-cm adhesive or silk tape
1 10-ml syringe with 4-cm 22-gauge needle
1 bottle 1% to 2% lidocaine

Method of Placement

PROCEDURE	COMMENTS
A. Set up water-seal drainage.	A. This later may be placed to 20-cm water suction.
B. Mark the incision area over fifth, sixth, or seventh rib in midaxillary line.	B. To avoid inadvertent placement of the tube below the diaphragm, the fifth or sixth intercostal space usually is selected.
C. Don gloves and mask. Then prepare area with providone-iodine solution and drape area with sterile towels.	C. Whenever possible strict sterile technique should be used.

D. Anesthetize the area of skin incision just below the target rib with lidocaine. Then anesthetize the periosteum of the rib, moving the needle cephalad until it drops over the rib. Holding suction, advance the needle until air or blood comes back. Then slowly withdraw it until flow stops, and place 2-ml to 3-ml lidocaine between the muscle and pleura.

E. Make a transverse skin incision large enough to admit the little or index finger just over or below the target rib.

F. Using first the Mayo scissors and then the large hemostat, tunnel over the superior margin of the rib. Then with gentle spreading of the intercostal muscles and using firm pressure, pop the hemostat (or the scissors) into the pleural space. Open the clamp partially and withdraw open to create a tract (Figs. 23-14, 23-15).

G. Via the tract, place a finger into the pleural cavity and feel for adhesions or noncollapsed lung.

H. With the large clamp, grasp the chest tube near tip (Fig. 23-16) and insert into pleural space via finger tract (Fig. 23-17). Advance cephalad until proximalmost tube hole is within the pleural cavity, but avoid inserting so far that distal end of tube "kinks" against apex of thoracic cavity or mediastinum.

I. Connect to water seal.

J. Place pursestring suture around tube (Fig. 23-18) and tie with single surgeon's knot. Then wrap ends around tube several times and tie with square knot.

K. Wrap petrolatum gauze around tube, cover with sterile 4 × 4 gauze pad, and tape in place.

D. Using generous amounts of local anesthesia and infiltrating the correct location can make the procedure much more tolerable for an alert patient.

E. Making the incision large enough facilitates placement of the tube; making it too large encourages air leak at the chest wall.

F. It takes significant pressure to force the clamp into the pleural space. Therefore back pressure should be applied with the other hand to avoid going too far and lacerating the lung. A gush of air or blood will indicate that the pleural space has been entered.

G. When the lung is stiff from contusion it may not collapse away from the chest wall.

H. Trocars may puncture lung. If a trocar is used to stiffen the tube, retract sharp tip back into the tube about 0.5 cm. If blood is present use a 36 F or larger tube in adults. Once the tip of the tube is directed cephalad between the parietal and visceral pleura, it should proceed to the desired location superiorly as the tube is advanced—without wandering into a fissure or toward the mediastinum. "Fogging" of the tube indicates pleural space location.

I. This should be done quickly so as to reexpand the lung, which now may be totally collapsed.

J. The (lengthy) loose ends can be used later to seal the hole by tightening the pursestring when the tube is pulled.

K. If available and time permits, use tincture of benzoin to prepare surrounding skin.

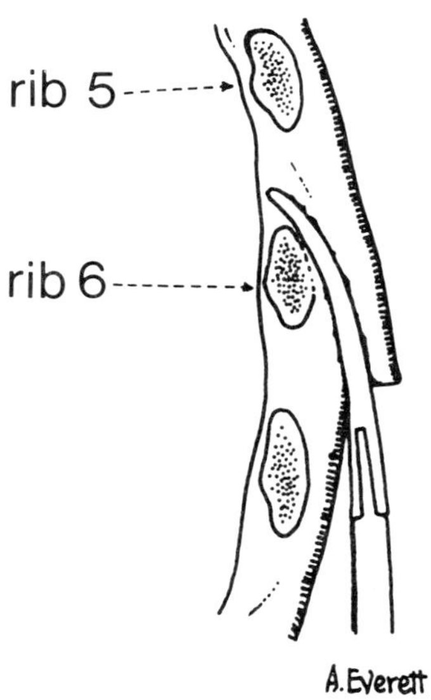

Figure 23-14. Technique for tunneling over the 6th rib into the pleural space.

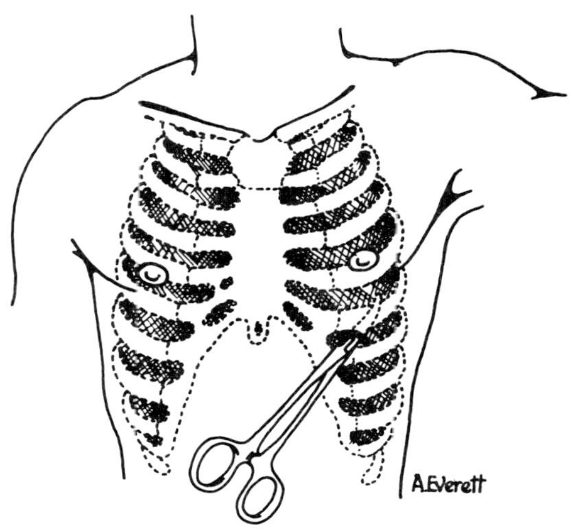

Figure 23-15. After the hemostat has been pushed gently into the pleural space, it is withdrawn partially open to create a tract.

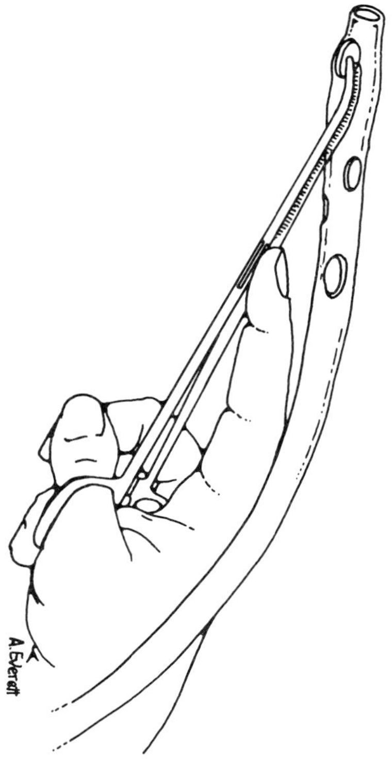

Figure 23-16. The chest tube is grasped near its tip prior to insertion into the chest cavity after a tract has been created as described in Figure 23-15.

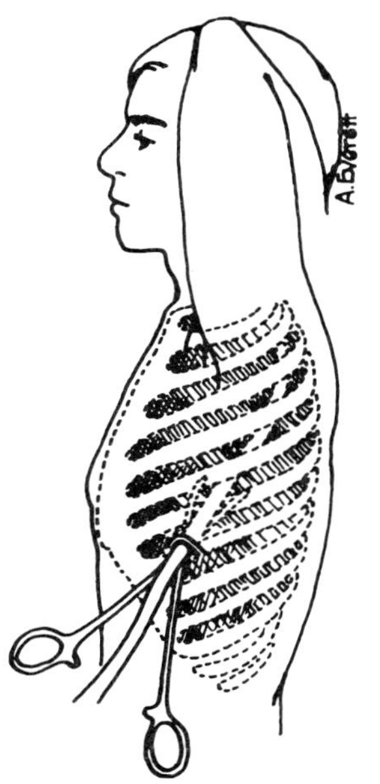

Figure 23-17. The chest tube is inserted into the pleural space by "feeding" it with a clamp and guiding the tip toward the apex of the hemithorax.

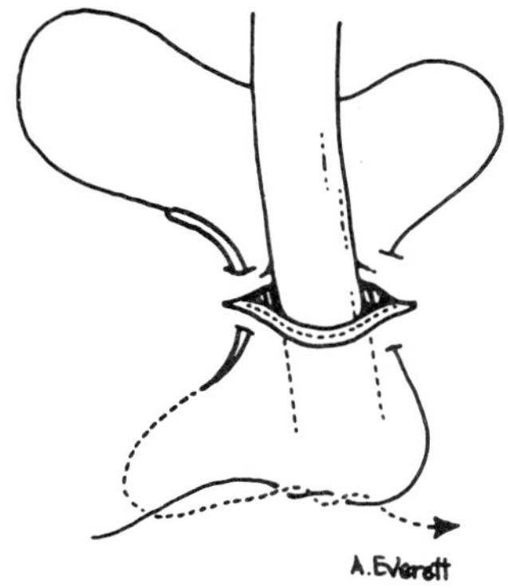

Figure 23-18. A pursestring suture is placed around the chest tube. After the suture is tied it should be wrapped around the tube several times and then tied again.

However, with major chest injury, the extreme condition of the patient may necessitate immediate intervention before there is time to obtain a roentgenogram and accomplish tube thoracostomy. Thus the ability to make a diagnosis before a roentgenogram can be obtained and to effect temporary relief before a chest tube can be inserted is life saving in certain circumstances.

Open Pneumothorax. Open or sucking wounds of the chest should be readily evident from observing and listening. If the patient is intubated (usually for other indications) and being assisted by positive-pressure ventilation, such a wound may simply constitute a temporary vent by means of which pleural space air can exit during the inspiratory cycle of lung expansion. In a nonintubated patient (a sucking wound alone is not always sufficient indication for intubation), pulmonary mechanics will be substantially improved by covering such wounds with a sterile, airtight dressing of petrolatum gauze or metal foil taped in place or by temporarily closing the skin with towel clips or a pursestring suture. Since some degree of pneumothorax invariably accompanies these wounds, and since the temporary wound cover or skin closure will convert an open pneumothorax to a closed pneumothorax with risk of developing tension, a chest tube or (temporary) Heimlich valve will be needed at short interval. In rare cases a *clean* wound itself may be a serendipitous site for insertion of a temporary tube; however, preference is for tube thoracostomy at a location away from the original wound. Intravenous administration of a good tissue-perfusing antibiotic is indicated for open or penetrating chest wounds (see "Use of Antibiotics in Multiple Trauma," p 451).

Tension Pneumothorax. Both tension pneumothorax and massive hemothorax may result in prominence of the hemithorax with poor excursions, diminished breath sounds, and a shift of the trachea to the opposite side. Diagnosis of *tension* pneumothorax on the basis of rapid physical examination is aided by apparently "contradictory" findings: On the side of injury there is absence of breath sounds to auscultation despite hyperresonance to percussion. With swing of the mediastinum, neck veins may be distended because of impaired cardiac filling; thus (potential) venous return is visible despite profound hypotension. Immediate needle aspiration can both confirm the diagnosis and relieve the acute distress of tension pneumothorax. This can be accomplished by insertion of a 16- to 20-gauge plastic (Angiocath type) intravenous catheter into the chest through the second intercostal space at the midclavicular line to allow the air accumulated under pressure to escape. (Use of a plastic catheter lessens chance of injury to the lung if it expands.) This maneuver converts the situation to that of an open pneumothorax, but with an opening so small that functionally it is little worse than a simple pneumothorax.

A convenient alternative, if the device is available, is to make the initial thoracocentesis with a Heimlich valve. The unidirectionally outward airflow characteristic of this valve will allow the lung to reexpand if it is intact. A plastic intravenous catheter can be converted to a one-way flow valve by securing the open end of a finger cut from a surgeon's rubber glove to the hub of the catheter and incising the finger distally. Air is prevented from entering the chest because the sides of the tubular glove finger collapse together as soon as the pleural cavity develops any (relatively) negative pressure. This seal can be somewhat enhanced by moistening the rubber with sterile water or saline.

Definitive treatment, however, requires placement of a chest tube. Placement of the tube in the midaxillary line is preferred over placement in the second intercostal space anteriorly, both to avoid an unsightly scar over the breast of a (young) female and to avoid bloody dissection through the thick pectoralis muscle of a (young) male. Nevertheless the anterior second intercostal space represents an alternative site for emergent tube thoracostomy to relieve life-threatening tension pneumothorax.

Massive Hemothorax. Diagnosis of massive hemothorax (with small pneumothorax) on the basis of physical examination, without (or before) the use of roentgenography and thoracocentesis, is more difficult than that of severe tension pneumothorax. With hemothorax, subcutaneous emphysema is less likely to be associated, and the neck veins are not full. A dull percussion note posteriorly is the chief diagnostic differential. (Since hemothorax will almost always have some degree of associated pneumothorax, the percussion note anteriorly may be misleading.) If roentgenography is not immediately available, small-bore needle aspiration posterolaterally can confirm the diagnosis (unless the blood is clotted) but will obviously not relieve immediate distress. In truly massive hemothorax, immediate distress is as much related to hypovolemia as to pulmonary dysfunction. In addition, abrupt drainage of hemothorax may eliminate some tamponade effect. Therefore treatment of massive hemothorax consists first of blood replacement and then of placement of a large chest tube with dependently located drainage holes. Choice of the site of entrance of a dependently placed tube for hemothorax is somewhat of a compromise requiring care and judgment: If the tube is inserted too far superiorly it may not satisfactorily evacuate the blood; if it is inserted too far inferiorly it may injure the diaphragm and underlying abdominal viscera.

Problems Associated With Emergency Tube Thoracostomy. Initial connection of chest tubes to simple water-seal drainage bottles may suffice to permit lung reexpansion and sterilely evacuate blood in the pleural space. If there is a large continuing air leak, 20 cm of water-pressure suction should be added as soon as convenient. A chest roentgenogram is needed early after thoracostomy to confirm tube position(s) and demonstrate lung reexpansion and removal of blood.

If a pneumothorax is not rapidly evacuated and the lung reexpanded, errors in tube management must be considered first: improper position, inadequate size, inadequate number, inadequate amount of suction. The underlying pathologic lung condition is considered next: occlusion of bronchi with secretions, a large tear of the lung parenchyma, a leak from one of the larger bronchi. Suspicion of major airway injury is an indication for immediate thoracic surgery consultation and for early fiberoptic bronchoscopy to clear the bronchi and identify damage to the tracheobronchial tree. If a tear of a larger bronchus is found, early operative repair is the treatment of choice. A moderate airleak from a smaller airway or peripheral air space is well tolerated: Operative control is rarely required and usually follows a relatively long trial of conservative management with tubes.

If a large hemothorax will not evacuate through well placed tubes it may be clotted. The retained blood not only may prevent immediate lung expansion but may become infected and result in a peel around the lung that can lead to entrapment and empyema. Early removal by open thoracotomy may be indicated, particularly if the hemothorax continues to enlarge. If after initial evacuation of a large hemothorax by tube thoracostomy, brisk bleeding into the chest tube bottle continues and hypotension persists despite rapid infusion of 2 to 3 liters of crystalloid and blood, immediate thoracotomy is indicated to control the bleeding. When bleeding sufficient to necessitate thoracotomy persists, injuries to major named arteries such as intercostal, internal mammary, and branches of the aortic arch or to the heart, rather than to the lower pressure vascular system of the lung, are likely to be responsible. Fortunately, a pressing need for thoracotomy is the exception rather than the rule: A stable clotted hemothorax will usually resorb spontaneously over several weeks, and post-thoracostomy bleeding at an initial rate of less than 200 ml/hour will usually subside spontaneously over several hours.

Clearly, insertion of a chest tube and even closed-chest needle throacocentesis are procedures that present a chance to harm, as well as to help, the patient. Should a sharp metal needle (such as the tip of an Angiocath type of intravenous catheter) be inserted into a hemithorax in which the lung is not collapsed, particularly when positive-pressure ventilatory assistance is being applied, there is a good possibility of lacerating the lung and generating pneumothorax. Should this occur as a result of insertion of the catheter in the wrong hemithorax (e.g., hemothorax on the right makes the relatively hyperresonant left hemithorax suspect for tension), bilateral pneumothorax may be the unfortunate consequence. Thus when the patient's condition permits and x-ray equipment is immediately available in the ED resuscitation room, confirmation of pneumo/hemothorax by chest roentgenogram, before intervention, is recommended.

Placement of a chest tube for major thoracic trauma is sufficient indication for early thoracic or general surgery consultation. Failure of tube thoracostomy to rectify rapidly one of the life-threatening conditions just described is an indication for immediate thoracic or general surgery assistance.

Flail Chest With Severe Pulmonary Contusion. Visual inspection can immediately identify the paradoxical ventilatory motion of the chest wall associated with flail chest. Fracture of two or more adjacent ribs at two or more sites on each rib often results in instability of the chest wall so that the affected segment is drawn inward rather than expanded during inspiratory effort. If a large enough segment is involved, ventilatory mechanics may be impaired.

The more critical injury, however, is likely to be the almost certain contusion of the underlying lung. Pulmonary contusion results in bleeding into alveoli, airways, and interstitial tissue. Airways and alveoli collapse or become filled with blood, and the distance separating alveoli and adjacent capillaries increases because of interposed hemorrhage and edema of injury. There is consequent decrease in lung compliance, loss of functional residual capacity, increased intrapulmonary shunting, and increased alveolar–arterial oxygen tension gradient. These are all pathologic manifestations of acute respiratory distress syndrome (ARDS or "shock lung"), and indeed the patient with massive pulmonary contusion exhibits the clinical, laboratory, and radiographic features that usually lead to initial diagnosis of ARDS: marked dyspnea (and tachypnea), profound hypoxemia on arterial blood gas determination despite administration of supplemental oxygen, and diffuse fluffy parenchymal density on the chest roentgenogram (occasionally unilateral, depending on mechanism of injury). Embarrassment of ventilatory mechanics by the paradoxical motion of the chest wall obviously compounds the oxygenation problem related to lung injury.

The most definitive ED treatment of this problem is tracheal intubation and application of positive-pressure ventilation. Intubation can be avoided only if (1) there is not significant dyspnea, (2) arterial blood gas values are (and remain) acceptable, and (3) large or multiple contusions are not evident on the chest roentgenogram. Even with intubation and mechanical ventilation using an increased fraction of inspired oxygen, repeat blood gas determinations may show persistent desaturation and low arterial oxygen tension. As with treatment of ARDS, this situation calls for application of positive end-expiratory pressure (PEEP). Mention has already been made of the risk of rapidly generating pneumothorax or tension pneumothorax in a trauma patient who is intubated and given positive-pressure ventilation before the extent of potential lung injury is evaluated. A patient with flail chest and underlying lung injury who requires PEEP represents an even greater risk for complications of pneumothorax, particularly the rapid development of tension. Therefore, when using positive-pressure ventilation to treat a large pulmonary contusion, it is wise to perform tube thoracostomy prophylactically. If prophylactic chest tube insertion is not performed when such a patient receives positive-pressure ventilation in the ED, frequent reassessment is mandatory to prevent the potentially disastrous consequence of development of tension pneumothorax while ED personnel are busy with other details.

Cardiac Tamponade. Cardiac tamponade is most often a result of penetrating rather than blunt chest trauma. Injury to the surface of the heart with the pericardium grossly intact may result in bleeding that rapidly fills the pericardial sac with blood unable to escape to the pleural space or unable to escape as fast as it enters. The resultant pericardial pressure may severely impair cardiac filling. Pulse pressure width narrows: It may close to within 10 mm Hg before blood pressure falls to shock level. Pulse rate may remain comparatively slow for the degree of hypotension.

The classic findings are known as Beck's triad: hypotension, distended neck veins, and decreased or muffled heart sounds. Pulsus paradoxus, cyanosis, and an enlarged cardiac silhouette on the chest roentgenogram may also be observed. When present, these may be helpful in making the diagnosis, but review of a large series of cases has shown the unreliability of all except hypotension: (1) Neck veins may not distend if much blood has been lost; (2) heart tones may be subjectively normal with severe tamponade; (3) pulsus paradoxus represents only a transient early stage in the development of tamponade; (4) cyanosis is difficult to appreciate in dark-skinned patients; concurrent hypovolemia may prevent accumulation of sufficient desaturated blood to allow recognition even in light-skinned patients; (5) less than 200 ml of blood in the pericardium may cause fatal tamponade, yet 300 ml or more may be present without an appreciable increase in size of the cardiac silhouette.

The invariable feature of life-threatening tamponade is hypotension. If profound hypotension persists in a multiple-trauma patient with chest injury (particularly penetrating) who has an adequate airway and who is receiving adequate ventilation and brisk vascular volume replacement, the explanation is usually exsanguinating hemorrhage or pericardial tamponade. The chest tube return and paracentesis (see "Abdominopelvic Injury," p 397) may reflect the former. If the differentiation is not readily apparent, central venous pressure should be monitored via a subclavian or internal jugular catheter already in place; if not already in place, a central venous catheter should be advanced into the superior vena cava by one of these routes (see "Subclavian or Internal Jugular Catheter Placement," p 369). If the central venous pressure is high or becomes high in response to crystalloid and blood infusion, the diagnosis of cardiac tamponade is virtually assured. If the initial central venous pressure is low, this does not exclude significant tamponade in the presence of marked volume depletion. If the central venous pressure stays low, however, cardiac tamponade is unlikely (and the central catheter can be used as an additional route for vigorous volume expansion).

Once cardiac tamponade is diagnosed, or strongly suspected in a patient in extremis, immediate treatment consists of needle pericardiocentesis with a 9-cm 18-gauge cardiac needle mounted by way of a 3-way stopcock on a large syringe, inserted just to the left of the midline at the xiphocostal angle, and directed inward and upward at a 30- to 45-degree angle to the horizontal during aspiration (see "Pericardiocentesis," below). In adults, entry from below, rather than at the left sternal border, lessens chance of injury to the anterior descending coronary artery as the ventricle expands. In smaller children peristernal entry at the fourth intercostal space, rather than subxiphoid, lessens the chance of lacerating the relatively large left lobe of the liver.

If time permits, the precordial V lead of an electrocardiograph can be attached by an alligator clip to the cardiac needle (Fig. 23-19). With penetration of the pericardium, a pop should be felt, a sharp increase in the QRS complex should be noted, and aspiration should yield nonclotting blood. If the needle goes beyond the pericardial space into the epicardium, an injury current (elevation of ST segment, premature ventricular contractions) should be apparent, and pulsations should be transmitted to the syringe.

Once the needle is in the pericardium, as much blood as possible should be aspirated. (Without detaching the syringe it can be emptied into a pan through an intravenous extension tubing attached to the three-way stopcock.) Blood that clots in the syringe or other container has probably been drawn from the heart; this will not result in hemodynamic benefit. Blood aspirated from the pericardium should not clot, having been defibrinated within the pericardial sac by motion of the heart; its removal should result in distinct hemodynamic improvement. It is surprising

Pericardiocentesis

Equipment Required

sterile gloves
1 bottle povidone-iodine solution
10 4 × 4 sterile gauze pads
2 sterile towels
1 5–10-ml syringe with 22-gauge needle
1 bottle 1% or 2% lidocaine
1 20–30-ml syringe and 3-way stopcock
1 18-gauge needle 8–10 cm long
1 intravenous extension tubing (sterile)

Equipment Desired

ECG machine with 12 lead capability and strip chart recorder
1 sterile wire with alligator clips on both ends

Method

PROCEDURE	COMMENTS
A. Connect arm and leg leads of ECG machine to the patient (if ECG machine available).	A. The chest lead later connects to the pericardiocentesis needle via the alligator clip wire.
B. Prepare epigastric area with providone-iodine solution and drape with sterile towels.	
C. If patient is conscious anesthetize skin site 3 cm to 4 cm below xiphoid just medial to the left costal margin.	C. If site is too cephalad it becomes difficult to get under the xiphoid with an angle that is shallow enough.
D. Connect 3-way stopcock and 9-cm 18-gauge needle to 20-ml syringe. Connect one end of alligator clip wire to hub of needle and other end to chest lead (V lead) of ECG machine (see Fig. 23-19).	D. This constitutes an exploring electrode to allow the operator to know when the myocardium is touched.
E. Make skin entry with needle at preselected site and advance needle under the xiphoid at a 30-degree downward angle aiming at the left midclavicular area. Apply suction to the needle; continue to advance until blood or fluid is obtained, or myocardium is touched (see Fig. 23-19).	E. Another person should continuously watch the ECG write-out with the machine set on "V". (Use the position knob to keep recording in the midposition.) When the myocardium is touched with the needle there will be a sudden elevation of the ST segment.
F. Withdraw as much pericardial fluid or blood as possible, then turn stopcock and discharge fluid via the side port into a container. Repeat until no more fluid can be obtained.	F. By connecting a sterile intravenous extension tubing to the side port, the discharged fluid can easily be placed into a container without losing needle position.
G. Withdraw needle and send fluid for appropriate studies.	G. If it is anticipated that reaspiration will be required, the metal needle may be withdrawn over a floppy tip guide wire so that a plastic catheter immediately may be returned to the pericardial sac.

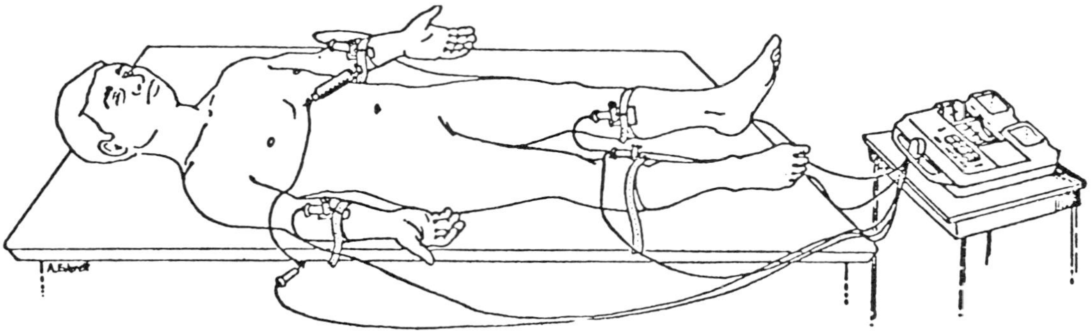

Figure 23-19. The limb leads of the electrocardiograph are attached to the patient before pericardiocentesis. The syringe and needle are advanced under the xiphoid process at a 20- to 30-degree downward angle toward the left midclavicular point. Note that one end of an alligator clip wire is connected to the hub of the needle and the other to the V lead of the machine. The needle is slowly advanced as suction is applied to the syringe and while the ECG tracing is observed for evidence of injury.

what sudden and dramatic increase in cardiac output and blood pressure can be realized with removal of as little as 30 ml to 40 ml of blood from a tensely distended pericardial sac.

Despite dramatic initial relief after aspiration of hemopericardium, it is likely that blood will reaccumulate and tamponade will occur again. Additional pericardiocentesis may be necessary to reverse recurrent hemodynamic failure. Rate of redevelopment of tamponade can be used as an index to determine whether management should consist of repeated pericardiocenteses or early thoracotomy and open pericardiorrhaphy. When there is doubt (and there usually is) it is probably wiser to lean toward early thoracotomy. The presence of a penetrating chest wound, the need to use pericardiocentesis to relieve tamponade, and probable need for early operative intervention are all strong indications for obtaining immediate thoracic surgical consultation and alerting the operating room to stand by. Priority of surgery for life-threatening cardiac tamponade equals or exceeds that for any injury in a trauma patient.

Open Thoracotomy and Cardiorrhaphy in the Emergency Department. In the "limit," discussion of early intervention for otherwise rapidly fatal chest injury usually leads to consideration of benefit versus risk of performance of thoracotomy in the ED. Some major trauma centers have reported series of dramatic "saves" as a direct result of cardiorrhaphy performed in the ED. It should be noted that most of these centers (1) receive patients at short interval following injury, rather than after long-distance transport, (2) have pump-oxygenator bypass and autotransfuser capability immediately available in the operating room or the ED, and (3) have EDs continuously staffed by surgical residents familiar with use of this equipment and with performing thoracotomy. Yet in addition to the advantages of minimal postinjury delay in transport, proper equipment, and experience, success in these centers in large part can also be attributed to careful definition of indications for ED thoracotomy and a well-defined plan for what is to be accomplished once the chest is opened. The only crucial piece of equipment not commonly present in an ED is a self-retaining chest (rib) retractor.

Among problems that warrant emergent thoracotomy are (1) cardiac tamponade that is unrelieved by pericardiocentesis or in which tamponade rapidly recurs; (2) profuse external bleeding from a penetrating chest wound; (3) profuse bleeding from a chest tube following evacuation of a massive hemothorax by means of thoracostomy; and (4) profound apparent cardiogenic shock that is unresponsive to measures described in the next section (a less absolute indication). The decision on whether to perform emergent thoracotomy in the ED or whether to await early removal of the patient to the operating room will depend on (1) the immediate status of the patient, (2) how long since injury the patient has apparently been successfully tolerating the insult, (3) response to transfusion and hemodynamic support in the ED, and (4) anticipated delay in moving the patient to the operating room. With a moribund patient a few minutes after injury, not responding to resuscitation efforts, in a setting where an operating room is not immediately available, the decision is reasonably clear-cut. With a patient who is less moribund, who has already tolerated the injury for more than a few minutes, who has shown some response, in a setting in which an operating room is immediately available, the decision is not so distinct. The very real risks and potential complications of thoracotomy performed in a nonsterile environment by a nonthoracic surgeon who has a scant data base for his decision cannot be ignored. It is particularly devastating when the extreme state prompting the intervention is discovered to be related not to one of the heart or intrathoracic major-vessel injuries just described, but to some other cause such as severe pulmonary injury. If no lesion is found that can be *benefited* by thoracotomy, then the creation of a large (contaminated) wound in the chest of an already very sick patient will almost certainly result in further deterioration. Thus the procedure should be reserved for truly desperate "what-is-there-to-lose" cases for which the specific indications have been described.

For performance of emergency thoracotomy and efficient control of bleeding, in addition to the self-retaining chest retractor it is very helpful to have available in the ED, in sterile packs, a long needle holder, long vascular (DeBakey) forceps, long dissecting scissors, a set of vascular clamps, and surgical drapes and gown. A cutdown tray, suture packs, surgeon's gloves, and suction apparatus—standard in any ED—complete the equipment list. Good variable directional overhead lighting is essential.

When immediate thoracotomy is indicated, effort at aseptic technique, consistent with the emergent necessity for the procedure, should be attempted. Rapid skin preparation with providone-iodine and hasty application of drapes are usually possible. Unless there is a unilateral right-sided penetrating wound without left hemothorax, a left anterolateral incision approximately in the fourth intercostal space is recommended. (When necessary to obtain additional exposure this incision can be extended transsternally into the right side of the chest or combined with median sternotomy. The need for temporary occlusion of venous inflow to facilitate repair of a heart injury would require such exposure.) A moribund patient requires no anesthesia. Should the intubated patient later react when resuscitation becomes effective after control of the lethal chest injury, a paralyzing agent (succinylcholine 1 mg/kg or pancuronium 0.1 mg/kg) and a narcotic (morphine 4 mg to 10 mg) can be repeatedly administered intravenously to achieve control and analgesia.

There are three major immediate objectives to be achieved by emergency thoracotomy in the ED post-trauma: (1) stop massive blood loss so that resuscitation becomes effective; (2) relieve cardiac tamponade; and (3) assist a terminally failing heart. Thus once in the chest, blood should be evacuated quickly by hand and by suction, and certain problems should be specifically sought. The most immediately obvious of these is a pulsatile or spurting bleeding point; such bleeding should be immediately occluded by hand. If bleeding is from a wound in the heart, temporarily plugging the hole by inserting a finger is often effective. If there is any evidence of cardiac tamponade or free bleeding from the heart, the pericardium should be widely incised to relieve tamponade or permit visualization of the cardiac wound or both.

Once bleeding sites are identified and controlled digitally and pericardial tension is relaxed, additional maneuvers in the chest will depend on the technical experience of the ED surgeon versus anticipated length of time it might be necessary to arrest bleeding digitally before moving to the operating room. The decision made by an emergency physician in a rural community hospital ED without surgical backup immediately available may vary considerably from that made in a major medical-center shock-trauma room with a cardiac surgery team available in an adjacent operating theater. Particularly when transport to a distant facility is contemplated, there is increased pressure (though not an absolute necessity) to attempt some measure of temporary repair so as to permit withdrawing the hand(s) and closing the chest. Immediate telephone consultation with the thoracic surgeon who will be receiving the patient is recommended in this interesting situation.

If there is a hole in an atrium, it may be possible to exclude the wound from the rest of the chamber with a vascular clamp, without occluding ventricular inflow. If there is a hole in the ventricle and bleeding can be controlled by insertion of a finger until the operating room is reached, this may be the safest temporary management. Such injuries may be sutured by passing interrupted 2-0 nonabsorbable stitches (preferably mounted on pledgets) under the occluding digit before tying them, but there is risk of catching a coronary vessel, a branch of the conduction system, or a component of a valve mechanism with this maneuver. If there is a hole in the aorta or a great vessel, the principle of proximal and distal control applies. This may necessitate incising adjacent fascia to permit application of vascular clamps. When applicable, partially occluding or "side-biting" clamps are indicated to preserve perfusion distal to a site of great-vessel injury. When hematoma and soft-tissue injury make dissection around a major vessel difficult and confusing and active bleeding can be controlled by digital pressure, then continued application of pressure until the operating room is reached may be the safest course of action. Again, the primary immediate objective of performance of thoracotomy for massive intrathoracic hemorrhage in the ED is to stop blood loss so that crystalloid and blood being infused will be retained in the vascular compartment and effective perfusion will be reestablished. If directing attention to technical details of dissecting, clamping, and suturing in the chest results in release of what was an adequately occluded major bleeding point, the effect of several minutes of vital resuscitative effort may quickly disappear through the suction line.

If a major intrathoracic bleeding site and tamponade are not discovered, or if control of identifiable bleeding sites and release of pericardial tension does not result in rapid improvement in response to fluid resuscitation, the situation is even less hopeful. The problem may be (1) preexisting vascular volume deficit so severe that it is not yet corrected by the rate of fluid infusion, (2) ongoing exsanguinating hemorrhage in the abdomen or pelvis, or (3) terminal failure of a severely injured myocardium. In this situation it is appropriate to (1) cross-clamp the descending thoracic aorta (incision of adjacent fascia may be necessary to facilitate this), (2) commence direct cardiac massage, and (3) continue vigorous fluid infusion, including by means of an intravenous line inserted directly into the atrium. This may buy enough time to do one or more of the following: (1) achieve needed volume expansion, (2) identify and surgically control an extrathoracic bleeding site, or (3) apply a mechanical cardiac-assist or bypass device to sustain circulation until a specific cardiac injury can be defined and studied. Cross-clamping of the supradiaphragmatic aorta for more than 20 minutes can be expected to lead to ischemic injury of the spinal cord, kidneys, and abdominal viscera, but then, most assuredly, so will absence of any perfusion pressure even with the aorta unclamped.

Whenever decision is made for emergent thoracotomy in the ED, it is obvious that immediate consultation with a thoracic surgeon should be obtained (if this individual is not already present), and the operating room staff should be notified to expect the patient directly. As with any penetrating chest wound, but particularly with thoracotomy in the ED, early intravenous administration of high doses of antibiotics with good tissue-perfusing characteristics is indicated. A cephalosporin is an appropriate first choice (see "Use of Antibiotics in Multiple Trauma," p 451).

Head Injury: Immediate Considerations

Although it often is not the immediate cause of death, head injury is involved in over 70% of motor vehicle accident fatalities. It is an associated injury in many nonfatal multiple-systems trauma cases, and its early management may significantly affect both short-term and long-term morbidity. Yet only a small percentage of patients require neurosurgical operations or even come under the care of a neurosurgeon. Neurologic evaluation by outpatient surgeons and emergency-care physicians is therefore a frequent and important component of trauma care.

The unconscious or semiconscious patient may have lost reflexes that protect patency of the airway, and ventilatory drive may be altered. The first considerations in evaluation and management of a head injury, therefore, are establishing an adequate airway and maintaining adequate ventilation and oxygenation of the *patient*.

Oxygenation of the *brain* may be impaired by inadequate ventilation, inadequate systemic circulation, or compromise of cerebral circulation by diffuse swelling or an expanding mass within the rigid cranial box. The importance of maintaining a patent airway, particularly in the unconscious or semiconscious patient with poor gag reflex and inability to clear secretions, and of assessing adequacy of (oxygenation and) ventilation by blood-gas measurement has already been stressed. In the hypotensive trauma patient (cause as yet not necessarily known), vigorous fluid resuscitation was initiated as the first step in improving systemic circulation.

Closed-head injury is the other cause of hypoxic impairment of CNS function. Closed-head injury can be loosely categorized as *primary,* resulting from acceleration-deceleration forces transmitted to the brain as a whole at the time of impact, and *secondary,* resulting from diffuse swelling, focal hemorrhage, or infection, which may develop in injuries that initially were not so severe. Dual goals in management of head injury are to ensure favorable circumstances for recovery from primary brain damage and to recognize any secondary problem early enough to minimize its damage. Thus it is necessary to establish a baseline as soon as possible in order to distinguish secondary events from initial injury.

A baseline neurologic examination should include assessment of the level of consciousness, vital signs, and pupillary response (brain stem reflexes). This "mini" neurologic examination is kept brief so that it can be repeated frequently and consistently. Some assessment of peripheral sensorimotor function has already been obtained with spinal cord evaluation. Deep tendon reflexes and babinski signs are often unreliable in patients with head injury and the information not immediately useful, although it may be later in lateralization of intracranial lesions. Detailed examination of scalp, skull, face, ears, and cranial nerves can be accomplished at a more convenient time after all systems have been initially evaluated.

Level of Consciousness: The Glasgow Coma Scale. In assessment of the severity of head injury, the level of consciousness is the single most important indicator of the patient's condition. A change in the level of consciousness is the most important prognostic indicator. Thus if the patient is unconscious on arrival, it is useful to know whether he or she was conscious at the scene of accident or during transport, and if conscious on arrival, whether unconscious at the scene.

It is now recognized that any interval of unconsciousness, even so-called concussion without clinical sequelae, implies some permanent structural brain damage, however slight. A history of unconsciousness is sufficient, although in a patient with an isolated head injury not always necessary, indication for hospital admission and observation.

A system for assessing impaired consciousness must be simple and based on clearly defined criteria if it is to be of maximum practical value. The Glasgow Coma Scale, introduced in 1974, is such a system and has enjoyed widespread application and acceptance (Table 23-3). The scale evaluates three separate aspects of a patient's responsiveness: the stimulus required to induce eye opening, the best verbal response, and the best motor response. Each is described according to a series of responses that indicate increasing degrees of dysfunction. Modifiers can be used to indicate inability to test eye opening when lids are closed by swelling, inability to test verbal re-

TABLE 23-3. Glasgow Coma Scale

TEST	STIMULUS	RESPONSE	SCORE
Eye opening	Spontaneous	Opens eyes on own	4
	Speech	Opens eyes when asked to in loud voice	3
	Pain	Opens eyes when pinched	2
		Does not open eyes	1
Best verbal response (talking)	Speech	Carries on a conversation correctly and tells examiner patient's name, location, month, and year	5
	Speech	Seems confused, disoriented	4
	Speech	Talks but makes no sense	3
	Speech	Makes unintelligible sounds	2
	Speech	Makes no verbal sounds	1
Best motor response	Commands	Follows simple commands	6
	Pain	Pulls tester's hand away when pinched	5
	Pain	Withdraws limb when pinched	4
	Pain	Flexes body inappropriately to pain: decorticate	3
	Pain	Body becomes rigidly extended when pinched: decerebrate	2
	Pain	No motor response to pinch	1

sponse when intubated, and concomitant influence of alcohol.

It is recommended that in every patient with multiple injuries the initial level of consciousness be described in terms of Glasgow Coma Scale responses and that in every patient suspected of having a head injury the level of consciousness be reassessed by this scale and recorded every 15 minutes (along with vital signs and pupillary size).

Vital Signs. With isolated closed-head injury and a rapid rise in intracranial pressure, decrease in pulse and respiration and increase in blood pressure and temperature may be observed. In a multiple-injury patient, however, it should be noted that coexisting injuries and blood loss may obscure these classic head trauma signs, and even in an isolated closed-head injury these manifestations are often late in developing.

A further rise to intracranial pressure may lead to a state of decompensation. Decompensation is associated with dangerously low cerebral oxygenation due to compression of cerebral circulation. In this state some of the vital signs become reversed: Pulse and respiration become rapid (pulse may fluctuate), blood pressure may or may not decrease, and temperature usually remains elevated. Early surgical intervention will usually be required to prevent death.

In patients with expanding supratentorial lesions progression of deterioration is usually orderly with impairment of consciousness and hemispheric signs preceding those of tentorial herniation and brain stem dysfunction. Changes in vital signs hardly ever presage depression of consciousness. Clearly, the issue then is to intercede when the level of consciousness deteriorates, before the appearance of foreboding late changes in vital signs. A more valuable use of monitoring of vital signs every 15 minutes in a multiple-trauma patient with head injury is to assess the adequacy of systemic perfusion, inasmuch as this so critically influences CNS function.

It is of significance to note that the initial alterations in vital signs "classically" occurring in head injury with increased intracranial pressure are the opposite of those classically associated with hypovolemic shock. Thus attributing shock to a closed-head injury or a scalp laceration alone is a pitfall to be avoided. Given the limited expandable space, it is almost impossible to sequester sufficient blood within the intact cranial vault to produce hemodynamically significant hypovolemia. (A large subdural hematoma in an infant can be an exception.) It is possible, but less probable than other possibilities in a patient with multiple injuries, that hemodynamically significant hypovolemia is due solely to hemorrhage from a scalp laceration.

Brain Stem Function: Pupillary Response. Integrity of brain stem function is reflected by the breathing pattern, size and reactivity of pupils, eye movements, and eyelid reactivity. Table 23-4 presents a scoring scheme by which brain stem function can be systematically assessed and reassessed. In a head-injury patient, pupillary size and reactivity can be conveniently reassessed at 15-minute intervals, along with level of consciousness and vital signs.

In a fully alert and oriented patient, pupillary dysfunction due to third-cranial nerve involvement generally means damage to this nerve in the orbit, in the superior orbital fissure, or in the cavernous sinus. If the level of consciousness is definitely depressed, third-nerve involvement is more likely due to a lesion in the pons or to compression from transtentorial herniation.

With an acute pontine lesion, pupils are constricted (but perhaps still reactive). With an expanding supratentorial lesion, hypothalamic dysfunction may initially produce small pupils. With herniation there is compression of one side of the midbrain and third cranial nerve, so that the pupil on the same side as the mass becomes dilated and nonreactive to light as its constrictor muscle is paralyzed (and ipsilateral lid ptosis may be observed). Shining a light in the eye with the fixed pupil should result in consensual constriction of the opposite pupil, distinguishing a third-nerve lesion from an optic nerve injury. With further herniation the midbrain may be pressed against the opposite tentorial edge, producing bilateral dilation and fixation of the pupils.

Motion of the globe is controlled by the third, fourth, and sixth cranial nerves; these traverse both midbrain and pons. Thus brain stem injury may be reflected by impairment of eye movements. A not-inviolable rule is that in brain stem injury the eyes tend to turn away from the side of the lesion, whereas in cortical injury the eyes tend to turn toward the lesion.

TABLE 23-4. Assessment of Brain Stem Function

FUNCTION	SCORE
BREATHING PATTERN*	
Normal (cerebrum and upper midbrain control breathing)	5
Cheyne-Stokes (low-midbrain and upper-pontine breathing)	4
Sustained hyperventilation (mid-pontine breathing)	3
Shallow slowing or gasping (low-pontine or medullary breathing)	2
Apnea (no CNS control of breathing)	1
EYE MOVEMENTS†	
Spontaneous conjugate movement in all directions	5
Spontaneous but dysconjugate gaze, nystagmus, or both	4
No spontaneous movement but intact doll's eyes	3
Doll's eye reflex absent but caloric reflex intact	2
Caloric reflex absent	1
EYELID RESPONSE	
Normal spontaneous blinking	5
Blinks only to bright light, loud noise, or threat	4
Blinks only to eyelash touch	3
Blinks to corneal but not eyelash touch	2
Does not blink to corneal touch	1
PUPILS‡	
Both pupils normal and reactive (may be slightly unequal)	5
Both pupils constricted but reactive (upper pons)	4
Unequal in size and one unreactive (ipsilateral third-nerve dysfunction)	3
Both dilated and unreactive (bilateral third-nerve dysfunction or terminal anoxia)	2
Both pupils midposition and fixed (brain stem death)	1

* Remove patient from ventilator for evaluation.
† Do not test doll's eye response if neck is injured.
‡ If in doubt, use the lower score.

Laceration or contusion of one hemisphere or the other may produce conjugate deviation or nystagmus. Extraocular eye motion can also be impaired by eye muscle entrapment or compression by orbital fractures. If a patient is not sufficiently alert to carry out voluntary eye movements following head trauma, then neck injury must also be suspected. In this event, testing for the doll's eye phenomenon should be deferred until spinal cord injury is ruled out.

The doll's eye phenomenon is a vestibuloocular reflex that can be used in an unconscious patient: Rapid rotation of the head induces currents in the semicircular canals that, by reflex mechanism, result in movement of the eyes away from the direction in which the head is turned. If this expected eye movement does not occur, it may be because consciousness is only slightly impaired (with reflexes suppressed) or as a manifestation of brain stem injury. The caloric response distinguishes between these two states.

Early Decision for and Timing of Surgical Intervention: The Value of Computed Tomography. Based on these serial assessments of level of consciousness, vital signs, and pupillary response, patients with head injuries can be assigned to one of three categories. The statements of witnesses and transport personnel make this possible even at the time of first examination in the ED.

1. Patients whose condition is improving: Progressive improvement in consciousness indicates recovery from primary damage, and only supportive care and continued observation are likely to be required.
2. Patients whose condition is stable: It is likely these patients also have only primary damage, but of greater severity. They are more likely to develop secondary complications, and observation needs to be particularly close. The patient who is "stable" but remains unconscious should receive early neurosurgical consultation and probably is a candidate for study by computed tomography (CT) or magnetic resonance imaging (or transfer to a facility capable of performing such studies) after all systems have been evaluated and initial ED management completed.
3. Patients whose condition is deteriorating: It is in this group that secondary brain damage due to an expanding intracranial hematoma is very likely; such a lesion may require early operative intervention. However, it is even more likely that increasing diffuse cerebral edema may be responsible; this condition does not warrant operative intervention. Special diagnostic radiographic studies, particularly CT scanning, are usually necessary to make this critical distinction. Occasionally cerebral angiography may be needed. In the multiple-injury patient it is also likely that inadequate pulmonary ventilation–oxygenation and

impaired systemic circulation may play a major role in deteriorating CNS function. Thus reassessment of vital signs, blood gas, and hemodynamic parameters is important in decision making.

In a patient with a head injury who is deteriorating, as determined by any of these criteria, rapid neurosurgical consultation is necessary even by telephone if that is the only contact immediately available. The neurosurgeon will usually request that the patient undergo CT scanning as soon as practicable on completion of physical examination and priority ED studies such as roentgenography of the chest, electrocardiography, and peritoneal lavage—provided that no life- or limb-threatening thoracic, abdominal, or peripheral vascular injuries requiring immediate attention are identified. When life- or limb-threatening thoracic, abdominal, or peripheral vascular injury is identified (i.e., cardiac tamponade, exsanguinating hemothorax, hemoperitoneum, major vascular damage in a limb), the neurosurgeon and the general surgeon (and possibly the cardiovascular-thoracic surgeon) will need to confer quickly regarding relative priorities of action. Unstable life-threatening thoracoabdominal injuries, particularly major airway damage, cardiac tamponade, or persistent major hemorrhage, take priority and mandate immediate removal to the operating room.

On the other hand, a large intracranial hematoma (particularly when located epidurally) or massive cerebral edema also represents a life-threatening condition warranting prompt treatment. Optimal intervention for a focal mass lesion requires localization on CT scan, followed by prompt surgical evacuation in the operating room with minimum use of general anesthesia. Optimum intervention for generalized edema or contusion requires use of a CT scan to distinguish the diffuse process from a focal lesion, often followed by surgical placement of an intracranial pressure (ICP) monitoring device to guide subsequent therapy in the intensive care unit directed to lowering ICP.

These surgical procedures may be accomplished by the neurosurgeon during the same anesthesia interval required for repair of thoracoabdominal injuries by the general surgeon, thoracic surgeon, or both. Thus when operable thoracoabdominal injuries are *stable* (a common example being nonexpanding hemoperitoneum with adequate perfusion established after vascular volume expansion with crystalloid), it is advantageous for a patient with a head injury who is unconscious or whose neurologic condition is deteriorating to go quickly through the CT scanner en route to the OR, with close monitoring and necessary support measures in the x-ray department being provided by an ED nurse and a physician member of the trauma team. The alternatives, that is, a potentially long delay before the head can be studied or random placement of craniotomy or multiple burr holes that may miss a clot entirely or encounter only cerebral edema, seem to be of equal or (usually) greater risk than the relatively brief delay caused by a well-coordinated preoperative CT study.

The multiple-trauma patient with head injury severe enough to warrant urgent CT study certainly could have other injuries for which no symptoms can be elicited. As just noted, this patient may proceed to the OR for an interval under anesthesia during which further examination may be limited. Therefore once a multiple-injury patient is in the CT scanner for obligatory head imaging (with members of the trauma team in attendance), it has become the practice of some centers routinely to invest only a few more minutes to obtain several widely spaced cross-sectional views of the thoracic inlet, mediastinum, and upper abdomen, to screen for otherwise occult injuries to the great vessels, aorta, liver, spleen, pancreas, and kidneys.

Like peritoneal lavage in the evaluation of abdominal trauma, one of the greatest contributions of the CT scan to management of head trauma has been a dramatic reduction in the number of unnecessary "exploratory" operations, with concomitant reduction in associated morbidity. The CT scan has proved itself so exceedingly accurate, first, in distinguishing edema from a hemorrhagic mass and, second, in precisely localizing a clot when it is present that a neurosurgeon dealing with head trauma will almost never operate without this crucial study. For these reasons the "emergency (blind) burr hole" made by a rural surgeon or family physician in a patient a long way from a neurosurgeon has practically become a thing of the past. Currently in a rural setting in a head-injury patient whose condition is deteriorating, management consists of (1) intravenous administration of a pharmacological dose of steroid (dexamethasone, 50 mg in an adult, or methylprednisolone, 30 mg/kg); (2) immediate telephone consultation with a neurosurgeon; (3) stabilization of other major injuries; (4) and transport by the fastest means available to a neurosurgeon (or his trauma team) at a facility where CT head scanning can be performed.

Abdominopelvic Injury: Immediate Considerations

In multiple-trauma patients, serious abdominal injuries are neither as frequent nor as lethal as serious chest and head injuries. Yet (1) serious abdominal injuries tend to be less obvious and more difficult to diagnose than serious injuries to head, chest, and limbs; (2) more patients with serious abdominal injuries (almost 75%) are likely to have a concomitant major head, chest, or limb injury that may divert attention from the abdomen than vice versa; and (3) more patients with serious abdominal injuries than patients with major head, chest, and limb trauma who die subsequent to reaching a hospital (about 20%) do so because of delayed, inadequate, or inappropriate treatment rather than "uncorrectable" organ damage. Thus abdominal evaluation of a multiple-injury patient presents the emergency physician and outpatient surgeon with a challenge for accuracy and speed in diagnosis, the reward for which is a high probability of being able to intercept and surgically correct what are otherwise potentially fatal injuries.

Abdominal trauma may be conveniently categorized as blunt or closed versus penetrating or open, and such classification is an immediate aid in assessment of potential organ injury. With blunt trauma the probable force and location of impact and with penetrating trauma the velocity of a bullet or size and path of entry of a knife are important factors to be considered in estimating the probable extent of damage to specific intra-abdominal structures. In any patient capable of perceiving it, abdominal pain is almost always present with contusion, hematoma, or penetration of the abdominal wall, stretching of a visceral capsule or wall by an expanding hematoma, irritation of the peritoneum by contact with free blood or upper gastrointestinal contents, or injury to adjacent skeletal structures. Thus a brief history, if obtainable from either the patient or transport personnel, is helpful in assessing potential severity of abdominal injury.

Removal of Medical Antishock Trousers. Adequate physical examination requires early removal of all clothes. (When spinal cord or lower-limb injury is probable, clothing should be cut away.) A single and very notable exception to this dictum is if medical antishock trousers (MAST) have been applied to the patient prior to arrival in the ED. Unfortunately, ill-timed removal in the ED has accounted for most of the complications related to use of these pneumatic compression devices. Should MAST be abruptly deflated on a patient who is or has recently been in shock, any of the following may occur alone or in combination: (1) Marginally adequate central vascular volume may be rapidly redirected to previously contracted peripheral vascular beds in the pelvis and lower limbs with a resultant precipitous drop in blood pressure; (2) previously compressed bleeding points in the lower abdomen, pelvis, or thighs may open up, with a precipitous drop in blood pressure; or (3) lactic acid accumulated during the period of restricted blood flow to pelvis and limbs may rapidly "wash out," with resultant profound systemic acidemia and hypotension.

Abrupt hypotension, decreased cardiac return, and increased acid load in an already critically ill patient may lead to rapid cardiac arrest. Therefore whenever a patient who is or was hypotensive arrives with MAST applied, the garment should be left in place until one of the following is true: (1) adequate perfusion pressure has been reestablished and an extra-abdominopelvic injury by which to explain the original shock has been identified and at least temporarily corrected or controlled; (2) adequate perfusion pressure has been reestablished, and, if the thoracic, abdominal, or pelvic injury probably responsible for the original shock is not well defined or controlled, a surgeon is in attendance and an operating room is ready; or (3) if adequate perfusion cannot be readily reestablished and if the thoracic, abdominal, or pelvic injury probably responsible for the persistent hypotension will require immediate surgery, the patient is first moved to the operating room.

When MAST are removed, deflation of the garment should be accomplished in stages, with vital signs being monitored repeatedly. A small amount of air is first released from the abdominopelvic compartment, the valve closed, and blood pressure checked. If blood pressure remains stable, additional trouser pressure is released in a stepwise manner. If blood pressure declines by even 5 mm Hg to 10 mm Hg, trouser deflation should be discontinued until additional vascular volume expansion with crystalloid or blood or both can be accomplished. Trouser pressure is thus reduced in a gradual manner, proceeding from proximal to distal compartments, until the garment is completely deflated. This process may require as much as 20 to 30 minutes.

Even when MAST are removed in the operating room immediately prior to emergent celiotomy or thoracotomy, the abdominopelvic compartment should be (gradually) deflated first, so as to allow prepping the chest and abdomen, with deflation of the lower limb segments being deferred until the anesthesiologist has been able to correct the deficit in blood volume.

Because of the potential of lactic acidemia on removal of MAST from poorly perfused limbs, measurement of the blood pH is helpful during the deflation process. Intravenous administration of sodium bicarbonate may be necessary to buffer the metabolic acid load. This is not likely to be required if the patient's systolic blood pressure consistently exceeded trouser pressure during most of the period of application. However, if the patient's systolic blood pressure was well below trouser pressure for a significant interval, and blood gas determination is not immediately available, an acceptable rule of thumb is to administer one or two (45 mEq) ampules of sodium bicarbonate as the trousers are deflated.

First-Pass Physical Examination. Once the victim's clothing is removed, visual inspection can immediately identify abrasions, contusions, ecchymoses, lacerations, penetrating wounds, and distention. With penetrating trauma it is particularly important that the back, buttocks, and perineum be visualized and that wounds of exit and entrance be specifically sought. Auscultation can reveal absence of bowel sounds associated with retroperitoneal or mesenteric injury or presence of bruit associated with vascular injury. Percussion can identify tympany associated with distention of the stomach with air swallowed during an accident or during pulmonary resuscitation and free intraperitoneal air from a ruptured hollow viscus; it can also identify dullness associated with hemoperitoneum or a full bladder. Palpation can reveal tenderness due to contusion of the abdominal wall or fracture of ribs, spine, or pelvis; guarding and rigidity associated with peritoneal irritation from free blood or spill of upper gastrointestinal contents; tenderness associated with an expanding hemoperitoneum; and asymmetry or absence of femoral pulse(s) associated with aortoiliac injury. Compression of the lower ribs and application of anteroposterior pressure to the region of the pubic symphysis can identify lower rib fractures, which may be associated with injury to liver or spleen, and pelvic fractures, which may be associated with injury to ureters, bladder, and rectum. Rectal examination, too often omitted in connection with an initial abdominal examination and particularly in a trauma patient, can reveal anorectal laceration, peritoneal tenderness, blood in the lower bowel, superior displacement of the prostate associated with transection of the urethra, and altered sphincter tone associated with spinal cord injury. (It also ensures observation of the buttocks and perineal area.)

Use of narcotics should be specifically avoided until results of abdominal examination have been demonstrated to be normal or until the surgeon who must decide whether or not an operation is indicated has had an opportunity to complete an examination.

Unless the patient is intubated and receiving controlled ventilation so that intravenous analgesia or muscle relaxant or both can be administered, any vicera protruding from a penetrating abdominal wound should simply be covered with sterile saline moistened dressings until their return to the peritoneal cavity can be accomplished in the operating room. Without use of general anesthetic or muscle relaxant, attempts to reduce traumatically herniated viscera are likely to be unsuccessful and may only injure intestines and result in further contamination.

Nasogastric Intubation. Except in the presence of nasopharyngeal facial injuries that would preclude its use, in every multiple-trauma patient a double-lumen sump nasogastric tube routinely should be passed and connected to constant suction (negative 60 mm Hg to 100 mm Hg). This is beneficial in several ways: (1) Removing air that was swallowed during the accident or during resuscitation with mouth-to-mouth or face mask and bag techniques relieves pressure on the diaphragm and immediately improves ventilatory mechanics. (A double-lumen sump tube effectively removes air; a single-lumen Levin tube usually does not.) (2) Emptying the stomach of liquid and particulate contents reduces the probability of vomiting and aspiration. (This is particularly important before ground or air transport to a distant facility.) (3) In penetrating trauma the presence of blood in the nasogastric aspirate provides evidence of upper gastrointestinal visceral injury. (In blunt trauma the more common source of bright red blood initially returned on nasogastric aspiration is an injury to nose, mouth, or face, but if the return does not clear rapidly, further investigation is warranted.) (4) The patient who ate or drank shortly before being injured (and this is more often than not the case) and who subsequently must go to surgery for repair of any injury will do better if the stomach is emptied prior to receiving an anesthetic. (5) Many multiple-injury patients, particularly those with injuries to abdominal viscera, the retroperitoneum, or the spine, can expect a period of ileus before the gastrointestinal tract resumes normal function, and they will need nasogastric suction.

The Question of Exsanguinating Hemorrhage. Hemorrhage is the most immediate threat to life in abdominal trauma. Identification of exsanguinating intra-abdominal hemorrhage is the most immediate consideration on first-pass abdominal examination. In the presence of obvious abdominal injury, shock should be assumed to be due to intra-abdominal hemorrhage until proved otherwise. Given the poor tamponade capability of the peritoneal cavity, resuscitation efforts may never become effective until high-flow abdominal or pelvic bleeding points are mechanically controlled. Therefore obvious penetrating or blunt abdominal injury associated with hypotension that is unresponsive to rapid upper-limb or central intravenous infusion of 2 liters of lactated Ringer's is indication for (infusion of whole blood and), and rapid removal to the operating room for emergent celiotomy. Priority of this surgery is secondary only to that for immediately life-threatening thoracic injury such as major airway damage, exsanguinating hemorrhage from the chest, or cardiac tamponade. For the patient in extremis, delay in the radiology department for head CT scanning or aortography may be impossible. If an operating room is not available immediately for such a patient, consideration should be given to application (or reapplication) of MAST in the ED in order to tamponade abdominopelvic hemorrhage and direct reduced remaining blood volume to perfusion of the heart, brain, and upper body.

For the patient with no blood pressure whose abdomen is rapidly expanding or who has a large-caliber high-velocity bullet wound or a close-range shotgun blast wound, the decision for immediate removal to the operating room is straightforward and clearly offers the best chance for survival. When the nature of abdominal injury is not so obvious and there has been (at least some) response to fluid resuscitation, immediate removal to the operating room may precipitate complications related to (1) commencing major surgery when the patient is in a suboptimal preoperative hemodynamic state and when crossmatched blood may not yet be available, and (2) neglecting yet undiagnosed associated injuries, one of which may be a greater contributor to the shock state or more life-threatening than the presumed abdominal injury. Anesthetizing a patient with contracted vascular volume may lead to further decompensation and arrest. During a prematurely commenced abdominal operation, coexistent but preoperatively undefined epidural hemorrhage, subtle cardiac tamponade, aortic arch or great-vessel injury, or peripheral vascular injury may progress to a life- or limb-threatening point of no return, unrecognized during an extended interval under anesthesia. A complicated renovascular or vena caval injury may be much more difficult to define only by extensive (even dangerous) exploration of a tense hemorrhagic retroperitoneum that it would be by preoperative pyelography, angiography, or venography followed by directed exploration and control. The probability of such complications can be markedly reduced when time is available and invested to do the following: (1) accomplish reasonably adequate fluid resuscitation; (2) complete physical examination; (3) perform crucial ED studies such as roentgenography of the chest, electrocardiography, and peritoneal lavage; (4) obtain key radiographic studies such as CT scan, angiography, and intravenous pyelography, as indicated; and (5) arrange (when appropriate) for simultaneous participation of more than one surgical specialty team before the patient goes to the operating room.

In hemorrhagic abdominal injury the factor determining whether time is available for this preoperative evaluation and preparation is whether the vascular volume can be refilled at a rate faster than the intra-abdominal leak. Fortunately for most patients with abdominal injury who require early removal to the operating room, sufficient time does exist to complete preoperative evaluation and preparation.

Urinary Tract Injury: Immediate Considerations

Diagnostic Limitations of Physical Examination. Initial ED evaluation of the urogenital system is conveniently integrated with that of the abdomen and pelvis. In an alert cooperative patient, certain aspects of history may lead to a suspicion of urinary tract injury. Deep flank pain and bloody urine suggest renal damage. Suprapubic pain, inability to void, or passage of blood per urethra suggests bladder or urethral injury or both. However, in a patient with multiple injuries history is frequently unavailable, unreliable, or nonspecific. Although inability to void is more specific than many complaints, most multiple-injury patients will not have attempted to void prior to arrival in the ED. Subsequent to arrival, pain from associated injuries and the general confusion of the ED scene may inhibit even an alert patient from attempting to void even in the absence of specific lower-tract injury.

Except for external genitalia trauma, physical examination is also unreliable and nonspecific in detecting urinary tract injury. Deep flank pain (or mass) may or may not be present with renal injury and if present may be due to associated extrarenal trauma. Deep flank eechymosis may require several days to become superficially evident after a major perirenal hemorrhage. Suprapubic tenderness may or may not be present with bladder injury, and if present may be due to abdominal wall contusion or pubic fracture without bladder injury. Generalized abdominal tenderness may or may not be present with intraperitoneal bladder rupture and extravassation of urine, and if present may be due to abdominal wall contusion or injury to other intra-abdominal organs. A rectal mass may or may not be present with perivesical hemorrhage, and if present may be related to pelvic fracture without bladder damage. Superior displacement of or inability to palpate the prostate (and inability to void) strongly suggest disruption of the urethra above the urogenital diaphragm, but normal position of the prostate (and ability to void) does not exclude incomplete laceration of the urethra. A drop of blood at the urethral meatus and perineal or penile hematoma may or may not be present with laceration of the anterior urethra.

Urinalysis and Insertion of a Bladder Catheter. With these limitations of history and physical examination to identify significant urologic injuries, an algorithm is needed for evaluation of the urinary tract, particularly in a multiple-trauma patient. Of two key principles in that algorithm, the first is that every patient with any of the foregoing symptoms or findings, and every multiple-trauma patient, deserves a urinalysis early in the course of ED evaluation. Particular attention must be given to the presence or absence of hematuria. The alert, cooperative patient without limitation of motion imposed by associated injuries should be asked to void into a urinal, shallow bedpan, or bedside commode, as appropriate; blood in a spontaneously voided specimen cannot be due to iatrogenic urethral trauma in an attempt to pass a catheter. For a patient who is unconscious, uncooperative, or unable to void, the menstruating female, or a female with associated injuries that prevent placement of even a shallow bedpan, it will be necessary to attempt to pass a urethral catheter to obtain the initial urinalysis specimen. An indwelling bladder catheter should be placed to monitor urine output continuously in any patient who is or was initially in shock.

The issue of when, post-trauma, a Foley bladder catheter should be passed is without uniform agreement. Ideally, to prevent the possibility of converting an incomplete urethral laceration to a complete disruption, it would be well to exclude the presence of urethral laceration before inserting a urethral catheter. (Transection of the posterior urethra is difficult to repair by any means, with a high incidence of stricture, incontinence, and impotence.) Identification or exclusion of this injury requires retrograde urethrography (10 ml to 30 ml of full-strength contrast material used for intravenous injection is introduced into the urethral meatus by means of a catheter-tipped syringe). To prevent the possibility of obscuring visualization of a lower ureteral injury by extravasation of contrast material from a bladder laceration, is is well to perform excretory pyelography before retrograde cystourethrography. This sequence involves relatively extended-interval contrast studies before obtaining the initial urinalysis and establishing a track on urine output. For a patient with isolated pelvic injury—particularly with inability to void, a bloody discharge from the urethra, or both—if the condition remains stable this is an acceptable, even preferred, sequence. However, this optimum sequence for ruling out the rare (but important) urologic injury that urethral laceration represents is neither realistic nor altogether safe from the standpoint of overall evaluation and management of the majority of multiple-injury patients, particularly those who are hypotensive. Therefore for trauma patients with the aforementioned indications for bladder catheterization (except in a stable, isolated pelvic injury), it would seem an acceptable compromise for the ED physician to make one gentle attempt, under sterile conditions, to pass a Foley catheter (see "Insertion of Bladder Catheter," below).

Failure to pass the catheter implies need for further study before any more attempts are made. Pelvic fracture is associated with almost every posterior urethral laceration from blunt trauma. If pelvic fracture is clinically evident or suspected and a catheter does not pass immediately, a urethrogram is definitely needed. If there is not a penetrating injury and pelvic fracture is neither clinically evident nor seen on a plain film of the pelvis, there is little probability of urethral disruption.

Insertion of Bladder Catheter

Minimal Equipment Needed

Note: The first six items usually come sterilely prepackaged in a bladder catheterization kit.

1 pair sterile gloves
2 sterile towels or drapes, preferably 1 of which is fenestrated
1 sterile package of sterile lubricant jelly
1 pack of several sterile cotton balls or gauze pads
1 sterile package of povidone-iodine solution
1 sterile urine specimen collection bottle
1 sterile 10-ml syringe with no. 20 needle
1 30-ml bottle of sterile saline or water
1 Foley catheter with 5-ml balloon (16 or 18 F is appropriate for the average adult male: 14 F for the average adult female. Where resistance due to stricture or prostatic hypertrophy is anticipated or encountered, use of a larger catheter is advised to provide more "stiffness.")
1 closed-system urine collection bag and connector tubing, preferably with integral "urinometer" cup with graduated milliliter scale for measuring urine output.
1 roll 5-cm silk or Scotch skin tape

Method

PROCEDURE	COMMENTS
A. Position male patient in supine position or female patient in a modified lithotomy position (heels drawn up toward buttocks, knees apart, unless hip or lower limb injury precludes). Position a bedside stand or equipment table near patient's leg on side corresponding to operator's dominant hand. (Right-handed operator puts table near patient's right leg.) Set up urine collection bag and preposition connector tubing near patient's thigh.	
B. Open bladder catheterization kit on bedside table. Open sterile syringe container so as to drop syringe onto sterile field of the open kit. Place Foley catheter package on table and carefully peel back top so that catheter can be picked up sterilely after gloves are on.	B. Prepositioning these items before putting on gloves will minimize the number of moves that will subsequently be required of an assistant. If sterile gloves are not included in kit, open the glove package separately.
C. Put on the sterile gloves. Place the nonfenestrated drape over the upper thighs of male patient, or caudad of the buttocks of female patient. Place the fenestrated drape over the pelvis and lower abdomen to expose the genitalia in the window.	

D. Load the 10-ml syringe with sterile saline or water.

D. An assistant will need to hold the inverted fluid bottle, and, if a needle is not already affixed to the syringe, hold the needle container to permit sterile attachment of the needle to the syringe. If everything else is prepositioned as described, these are the only moves for which an assistant is needed. The patient, if alert and cooperative, can be utilized as an assistant.

E. Carefully pick the Foley catheter out of its package. Attach the syringe, inject 5 ml to 10 ml fluid into the balloon to test its function; then withdraw fluid and leave syringe attached. Apply lubricant jelly generously to tip of the Foley catheter; then carefully position the catheter on the sterile drapes.

F. Open the package of povidone-iodine solution and pour it into the partitioned cup portion of the catheterization kit.

F. If povidone-iodine does not come prepackaged in the kit it should be poured from a separate container into a sterile cup before proceeding with step C.

G. With the nondominant hand pick up the male penis or spread the labia of the female vagina.

G. Once this move is made, the now nonsterile nondominant hand remains in this position until the catheter has been inserted.

H. With the still sterile gloved dominant hand, pick up a cotton ball or gauze pad, dip it in the povidone-iodine, and, beginning at the urethral orifice and moving outward in expanding concentric circles, prepare the periurethral portion of the genitalia. Repeat at least three times until the area is adequately cleansed.

H. When there is a limited quantity of prepackaged povidone-iodine solution, dipping each pad in the solution just before use (rather than pouring the solution over the pads before starting) will ensure maximum application of solution to the genitalia.

Care should be taken to ensure that the sterile gloved hand contacts only the prepared pads, not the genitalia.

I. With the still sterile gloved dominant hand, pick up the Foley catheter (with syringe attached) and insert it into the urethra to the maximum extent, using steady gentle pressure.

I. When the catheter is fully inserted, the now nonsterile nondominant hand may finally be released.

J. With one hand holding the catheter "hub" and the other on the syringe, inflate the Foley balloon with 5 ml to 10 ml fluid. Then detach the syringe and withdraw the catheter gently until the balloon "seats" against the bladder outlet.

J. Urine flow usually will not begin until the catheter is withdrawn a few centimeters. Should urine flow before ready for collection, simply compress the catheter between fingers and thumb.

K. Collect some urine in specimen bottle for analysis. Then connect catheter to closed-system collection-bag connector tubing and secure to patient by taping the *plastic connector tubing* (not the rubber catheter), to the midanterior thigh, using 5-cm-wide silk or Scotch skin tape, in an overlapping crisscross pattern in order to secure the "mesentery" over the tubing so that it is less likely to "lever" away from the skin. (Fig. 23-20).

K. If a single short strip of 2.5-cm adhesive tape is attached directly to the rubber catheter, it usually pulls rapidly away from the skin, allowing the urine bag to "hang" from the urethra by the Foley balloon, and leaves the rubber catheter "gummed up" with contaminated adhesive tape a few centimeters from the urethral orifice; both situations are undesirable.

Prepare the thigh by shaving and application of benzoin prior to applying the tape when time permits.

Location at which the connector tubing is secured must obviously be modified in the presence of lower-limb injury.

L. If the catheter will not readily pass and urethral laceration has not yet been ruled out, cease efforts until urethrography can be performed.

L. If the catheter will not readily pass and urethral laceration has been deemed unlikely, techniques such as using a larger-bore (hence stiffer) catheter and using a syringe to preload the urethra with a mixture of lidocaine and lubricant jelly may be tried. Particularly for a less-experienced operator, however, urology consultation should probably be sought before proceeding to use a metal catheter stylet, because use of such devices carries increased risk of serious urethral injury.

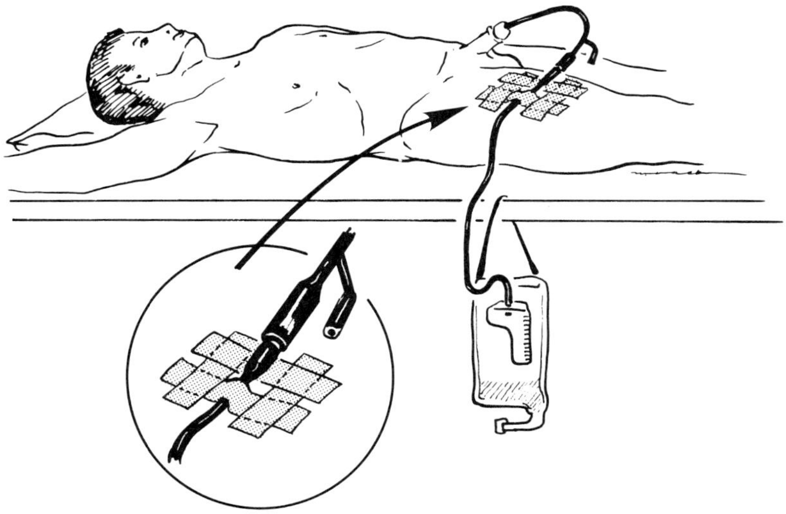

Figure 23-20. After the Foley catheter is connected to the plastic connector tubing of the urine collection bag, the tubing is secured to the anterior aspect of the thigh with a tape 5 cm wide. An overlapping crisscross pattern is used so the "mesentery" (of the tape) over the tubing will not pull away.

Fortunately, in the majority of trauma patients with indication for bladder catheterization, it is possible to insert a Foley catheter with ease on the first attempt. Success allows early determination of presence or absence of hematuria and early monitoring of urine output. Except in the presence of gross hematuria, a urine specimen should be sent to the laboratory for immediate microscopic urinalysis (or should be spun down and examined in the ED).

It should be noted that degree of hematuria does not correlate well with magnitude of urinary tract injury: Minor renal contusion may result in grossly red urine, whereas major pedicle damage with obstruction to renal artery flow may be accompanied by little or no hematuria. Gross hematuria out of proportion to the trauma apparently sustained has often been discovered to be due to preexisting renal disease (neoplasm, glomerulonephritis, hydronephrosis, congenital malformation). Distinct hematuria may result from traumatic insertion of a catheter. Urinalysis is normal in about one-third of patients with isolated ureteral injury. These qualifying observations notwithstanding, more than 90% of kidney and bladder injuries result in hematuria, and gross hematuria clearly represents significant hemorrhagic injury to the urinary tract.

The Question of Exsanguinating Hemorrhage. Exsanguinating hemorrhage may occur from an injury severe enough to fragment a kidney or disrupt the renal vascular pedicle. When associated with shock unresponsive to rapid infusion of 2 liters of crystalloid, such injury is indication for infusion of whole blood and rapid removal to the operating room for emergent celiotomy and control of the renal pedicle followed by ligature or repair. Profound shock, gross hematuria, and an expanding flank mass suggest critical renal injury, but in most cases the presenting features are not specific. The situation is more likely to be that of apparent intra-abdominal injury, specific organs unknown. Decision for immediate removal to the operating room versus delay for pyelography and arteriography must be based on the patient's condition and response to resuscitation efforts, as described under immediate considerations in the section on abdominal injuries.

Limb Injury: Immediate Considerations

A common pitfall in approaching a multiple-injury patient is to allow a striking deformity of a limb associated with a skeletal injury to attract immediate attention, with resultant diversion of that attention from other less obvious, but more serious, injuries. Yet early recognition, reduction, and splinting of fractures and dislocations can relieve pressure on and prevent further damage to major vessels, nerves, and joints; often providing the margin of protection necessary to make the difference between permanent disability and recovery of function. Thus although it is an important adage in the management of multiple trauma that (particularly skeletal) injury of the limbs is seldom the most urgent problem, it is also important to recognize that limb injuries are frequently associated with multiple trauma; the presentation of some of the more serious limb injuries may be rather subtle; and the early evaluation and management of a limb injury often determines the survival and function of the limb.

Traumatic Amputation. The most obvious and dramatic limb injury that may confront an examiner is a traumatic amputation or partial amputation of a major part. As always, control of brisk external hemorrhage is the first consideration. In accordance with Step 1 of the overall protocol, this should already have been accomplished by application of direct pressure. Selective ligation of an *exposed* vessel is often the most efficient means of gaining definitive control in order to permit more convenient and complete examination. However, for reasons previously detailed, blind application of hemostats and use of a tourniquet are to be avoided: It is always important to prevent further injury to vessels, nerves, and skin of a functional limb. With recent major advances in reconstructive surgery and limb replantation techniques, it is also important to avoid further damage to vessels, nerves, and skin of both proximal and distal components of a severed or partially severed limb: A thin bridge of intact skin and soft tissue may maintain significant perfusion to a distal part, whereas even a completely severed limb might be returned to function following replantation if precise neurovascular anastamoses can be accomplished.

It has traditionally been agreed that when there is major destruction or irreversible damage to any three of the five major limb components (skin, muscle and tendons, nerves, vessels, and bone), limb survival is in such serious doubt as to constitute sufficient criteria for immediate amputation or completion of amputation. However, with current reparative procedures, each one of these damaged systems has the potential of being restored. Thus it is recommended (1) that every detached major segment of an injured limb be initially retained and protected in a clean, cool (but not frozen) environment; and (2) that the emergency physician or outpatient surgeon not make a unilateral decision to complete a partial amputation or discard a traumatically amputated component before consultation with a plastic, orthopaedic, or hand surgeon with experience in the management of major limb injuries and knowledge of the current state of the art of limb replantation.

History and Physical Examination. In the alert and cooperative patient, history is very important in the evaluation of limb trauma. A description of the mechanism of injury, if known, can be most helpful in guiding suspicion of specific lesions: A dashboard injury of the knee, for instance, may cause a posterior dislocation of the hip in addition to the more obvious fracture of the patella and possibly of the femoral shaft. Complaint of localized pain, limitation of motion, and loss of sensation are the most common symptoms associated with limb injury. In the alert patient, specific inquiry about each of these symptoms should be made relative to each joint and segment of each limb. Whether or not the patient was able to use each limb at the scene of the accident provides an immediate index of probable severity of injury.

Thorough examination demands removal of all upper and lower limb clothing. Early removal of clothing immediately becomes more complicated when the patient arrives in the ED with a limb splint or traction device already applied. Should emergent removal to the operating room be required to manage an immediately life-threatening thoracoabdominal injury, immobilization of an injured limb should be maintained during the related transfers. If the patient's condition permits evaluation in the ED and x-ray is immediately available in the resuscitation area, it may be useful to define radiographically the skeletal injuries prior to removal of the originally applied immobilization gear. It often is necessary to remove or loosen splints and traction devices in order to cut away enough clothing to accomplish adequate first-pass limb examination. Where fractures are suspected or documented, it is important to apply (or reapply) immobilization gear before manipulation for second-pass examination or transfer to other locations within the hospital: inadequately immobilized fracture fragments may result in (additional) neurovascular injury.

On first-pass limb examination it is usually convenient to evaluate concurrently the status of skin, soft tissue, major peripheral nerves, major peripheral vessels, and skeletal members. A rapid but relatively thorough evaluation of all components is markedly facilitated by a systematic approach such as that outlined by the following steps:

1. Each limb should first be visually inspected, with specific attention directed to identification of external hemorrhage, soft-tissue avulsions, cyanosis or pallor, contusions, abrasions, swellings (with or without ecchymoses), lacerations, and deformities. Although it is unlikely that a trauma patient will arrive in the ED without significant external bleeding at least temporarily under control, it is quite possible that when a previously applied splint is removed to permit examination, a vascular injury may resume bleeding as the tamponade effect of the splint is released. Should this occur, hemostasis should be regained by application of a sterile dressing and direct pressure; for reasons previously detailed, use of a tourniquet or immediate application of hemostats is to be avoided. Open wounds should be covered with gauze pads moistened with povidone-iodine, in a manner that will not interfere with the remainder of the limb examination.

2. The alert and cooperative patient should then be asked to demonstrate active range of motion at each major joint in each limb that has not sustained a major injury as evidenced by visual inspection. In addition to evaluating joint function, these active motions demonstrate motor function of the five major nerves in each upper limb and the three major nerves in each lower limb: Abduction of the arm establishes integrity of the shoulder joint and motor function of the circumflex nerve (deltoid). Flexion (and extension) of the forearm establishes integrity of the elbow joint and motor function of the musculocutaneous nerve (biceps, brachioradialis). Flexion, extension, abduction, and adduction at the wrist establish integrity of these joints and proximal motor function of the median, ulnar, and radial nerves (radial forearm flexors, ulnar forearm flexors, and forearm extensors, respectively). The distal motor function of these three nerves is selectively tested in the patient's hand against resistance applied by the examiner's hand: ability to oppose the thumb firmly to the little finger demonstrates the median nerve, ability to spread the fingers firmly demonstrates the ulnar nerve, and ability to extend the thumb firmly, including the distal phalanx, demonstrates the radial nerve.

With the heel partially drawn up toward the buttock, ability to roll the knee alternately outward and inward and ability to cross the leg over the other lower limb establish integrity of the hip joint and motor function of the obturator nerve (adductors of the thigh). Flexion and extension of the leg establish integrity of the knee joint and motor function of the major trunk of the sciatic and the femoral nerves, respectively. Dorsiflexion and plantarflexion of the foot against resistance applied by the examiner's hand establish integrity of the ankle joint and motor function of the peroneal and tibial branches, respectively, of the sciatic nerve.

In the uncooperative or combative patient, an incomplete assessment of joint integrity and motor strength can be obtained by observation of spontaneous movements and withdrawal from noxious stimuli. In the unconscious or stuperous patient, joint integrity can be partially assessed by gentle passive range of motion with attention to detection of crepitance, in apparently uninjured limbs. However, it is best to defer passive maneuvers until Step 3 has been completed.

3. Each limb should then be gently palpated over the major joints and intervening long bones (the clavicles, scapulae, and pelvis are to be included), with specific attention given to identifying sites of deformity, tenderness, crepitance, the mass effect of an effusion or hematoma, and abnormal skin temperature. Particular attention should be devoted to the examination of any site at which pain was elicited on active range of motion maneuvers. During the course of this palpation in the alert patient, the sensory function of the five major nerves in each upper limb and the three major nerves in each lower limb can also be evaluated by inquiring about presence and symmetry of light touch sensation: The skin of the deltoid area corresponds to the sensory distribution of the circumflex nerve, the radial aspect of the forearm corresponds to the musculocutaneous nerve, the palmar surface of the first three digits of the hand corresponds to the median nerve the palmar surface of the fifth digit corresponds to the ulnar nerve, and the dorsal aspect of the web space between digits 1 and 2 corresponds to the radial nerve. The skin of the medial aspect of the thigh corresponds to the sensory distribution of the obturator nerve, the medial aspect of the leg and foot corresponds to the femoral nerve, the lateral aspect of the leg and foot corresponds to

the peroneal branch of the sciatic nerve, and the heel and sole of the foot corresponds to the tibial branch of the sciatic nerve.

In the unconscious or stuperous patient neck injury will have been suspected, and a cursory peripheral neurologic examination already will have been performed as described in the section on "first-pass spinal cord evaluation," the sensory component of which involves the ability or failure to withdraw from noxious (pinprick or pinch) stimuli. Where light touch response is in doubt during limb examination in the alert patient, sharp stimulation can be substituted.

4. In each lower limb without obvious damage to these joints, the ligamentous integrity of the knee and ankle should be briefly evaluated. With the joint in slight flexion, the knee should be stressed in valgus and varus to determine if there is opening of the joint medially or laterally. More than 15 degrees of opening either medially or laterally indicates serious damage to the corresponding collateral ligament. With the knee slightly flexed and the foot fixed, the tibia should be pulled forward and pushed posterior on the femur. Excessive displacement relative to the opposite normal knee indicates compromise of the corresponding cruciate ligament. The foot should be everted and inverted at the ankle: Excessive displacement relative to the opposite foot indicates compromise of the deltoid or lateral collateral ligaments, respectively.

5. Careful palpation for arterial pulsation should then be performed bilaterally at the brachial, radial, femoral, dorsal pedal, and posterior tibial locations. In the absence of a corresponding distal pulse or the presence of an overlying hematoma, the popliteal pulses should also be evaluated. In addition, in any limb without distal pulse where vascular injury is likely, it is important to note capillary filling and evaluate distal circulation using a Doppler ultrasound flow velocity detector. These findings not only are of interest diagnostically, but correlate fairly well with limb viability and therefore are of value in establishing priority of treatment in the multiple-injury patient.

Diagnostic Criteria. *Fracture injury* in a limb should be suspected whenever one or more of the following are present:

1. Obvious deformity
2. Persistent and localized pain
3. Swelling, effusion, ecchymosis, hematoma, or crepitance
4. Neurovascular compromise distal to any of these findings
5. Inability or unwillingness to use the part, or marked limitation of motion

Dislocation should also be suspected when any of the preceding findings are localized to a joint. Findings characteristic of the more common dislocations are as follows:

1. Acromioclavicular: prominence of the outer third of the clavicle
2. Shoulder: lateral subacromial depression or hollow, compromise of the axillary artery
3. Elbow: posterior prominence at the elbow, compromise of the brachial artery
4. Hip, posterior: internal rotation of the thigh, sciatic nerve compromise, associated patellar fracture
5. Hip, anterior: external rotation of the thigh, femoral artery and nerve compromise
6. Knee, anterior: anterior prominence of the proximal tibia, compromise of the popliteal artery and peroneal nerve
7. Patella: lateral prominence of the patella
8. Ankle, medial: prominence of the lateral malleolus
9. Ankle, lateral: prominence of the medial malleolus, compromise of the posterior tibial artery

Ligament injury should be suspected whenever there is a fracture or dislocation or when there is joint instability. Ecchymosis and swelling are very characteristic.

Tendon injury should be suspected whenever there is inability to selectively flex, extend, abduct, or adduct a part distal to a laceration over the course of the corresponding tendon.

Peripheral nerve injury should be suspected whenever one or more of the following are present:

1. Paralysis
2. Paresthesia
3. Asymmetry of strength
4. Selective loss of motor function with preservation of sensation
5. Loss of light touch sensation with preservation of pain
6. Prolonged dislocation of the elbow, hip, knee, or ankle

Brachial plexus injury should be suspected when there is (1) loss of function of all five major nerve distributions in the upper limb (complete injury), (2) selective loss of function of the shoulder and elbow with motion and sensation of the hand remaining intact (segmented upper lesion), or (3) loss of function of all three nerves in the forearm and hand with preservation of function at the shoulder and elbow (segmental lower lesion).

Arterial injury should be suspected whenever one or more of the following are present:

1. Brisk external bleeding, particularly if bright red and pulsatile
2. A rapidly expanding hematoma
3. A penetrating wound near the course of a major vessel
4. Severe soft-tissue damage (crush, avulsion, blast) near the course of a major vessel
5. A long bone fracture or prolonged joint dislocation, particularly if associated with one or more of the signs or symptoms described in the next item
6. One or more of the six "p's" classically associated with an acutely ischemic limb: pulselessness, pallor, poikilothermia, pain, paresthesia, paralysis
7. A systolic bruit or thrill over a pulsating hematoma, or a continuous bruit over a penetrating wound
8. Absence of distal flow by Doppler ultrasound study in the presence of one or more of the preceding findings

Compartment syndrome should be suspected when any of the signs of neurovascular compromise (the six "p's") develop distal to a swollen segment of a limb. Asymmetry of strength may be a subtle early indicator: Weakness of dorsiflexion of the foot, for instance, may herald increasing pressure in the anterior compartment of the leg.

First-Pass Management. Following hemostasis, the first consideration in management of limb injury is reduction of dislocated joints and severely displaced fractures with which significant neurovascular compromise might be associated. The most common of these skeletal injuries have been stated previously. The second consideration is to splint identified or suspected fractures in order to provide comfort and prevent injury to adjacent structures by motion of fracture fragments.

When an obvious dislocation or grossly displaced fracture is identified on physical examination, decision must be made on whether to attempt immediate reduction in the ED or to immobilize the limb and defer manipulation until roentgenograms have been obtained. Two imperatives impose on the emergency physician regarding this decision: In general, all dislocations should be reduced at the earliest possible time. Several sequelae related to delayed reduction have previously been stated. However it is also preferable to perform roentgenography prior to manipulation of a skeletal injury, in order to (1) document the original injury, (2) look for a fracture that might be associated with a dislocation (or vice versa), and (3) provide guidance for more accurate reduction efforts.

If the limb distal to a skeletal injury is not anesthetic or ischemic, splints should be applied and manipulation avoided until roentgenograms are obtained. Even if the limb distal to a skeletal injury is anesthetic, or ischemic as judged by the six "p's" criteria previously stated , but x-ray is immediately available, it is probably worth the brief delay involved to define the skeletal injury radiographically prior to manipulation.

However, if (1) the limb distal to a dislocated or grossly displaced skeletal injury is clearly anesthetic or ischemic or both, (2) the patient's overall condition argues against immediate removal to the x-ray suite, and (3) x-ray equipment of adequate quality is not available immediately in the resuscitation room of the ED, then attempt at immediate reduction is indicated. Specific techniques for reducing the more common dislocations and fractures are described in other chapters.

At short interval after joint dislocation (before associated muscle spasm becomes severe) or in an unconscious or stuperous patient, reduction without analgesia may be possible. More often, titrated intravenous administration of an analgesic such as morphine or meperidine, with or without supplemental injection of local anesthetic, will be needed to accomplish reduction in an alert patient. Intravenous administration of narcotic, even in carefully titrated doses, should be undertaken in the multiple-trauma patient only in the presence of adequate blood pressure and control of the airway or readiness to immediately gain control and support ventilation if necessary. In an extremely muscular patient or a complicated dislocation, use of general anesthesia may be necessary.

Where possible, it is best to have an orthopaedic surgeon present in the ED for these procedures. If reduction results in improved distal perfusion, the limb can be splinted in that position for protection during subsequent studies. If attempt at reduction fails to improve distal perfusion, then limb films (to guide more accurate attempts at reduction) and arteriography (to define the associated vascular injury) become urgent priorities, secondary only to evaluation and management of immediately life-threatening thoracoabdominal and head injuries.

SECOND-PASS PHYSICAL EXAMINATION: DECISIONS FOR TREATMENT

On the second pass, completeness is a key objective. During the second-pass examination, a head-to-toe sequence is often most convenient.

Spinal Cord Injury: Second-Pass Considerations

On the second pass, neurologic examination should be more detailed, including more refined evaluation of peripheral sensation, reaction to pain stimulus, symmetry of motion and motor strength, deep tendon reflexes, abdominal and cremasteric reflexes, and anal sphincter tone. The sensory and motor function of the hand is especially important in evaluation of brachial plexus injury: Distribution of the median, ulnar, and radial nerves must be checked individually. Since *changes* in neurologic symptoms and findings are a prime influence on management of spinal cord (and head) injuries, it is important that this initial examination in the ED, almost never done by the consulting neurosurgeon, be carefully documented. Since it is almost certain that someone else will be repeating neurologic examinations and comparing earlier findings, it is important to use straightforward *descriptions* of observations and responses to specific stimuli rather than *diagnostic* deductions or guesses.

Spinal Roentgenography. With x-ray equipment available in the ED, a lateral roentgenogram of the cervical spine (1) can be obtained quickly, with minimal interruption of other evaluation–resuscitation efforts; (2) produces a film of sufficient quality to permit definitive interpretation; and (3) provides information that influences the immediate course of action. These are sufficient reasons for obtaining this film (and anteroposterior supine views of chest and pelvis) early in the evaluation of a multiple-trauma patient. In radiographic evaluation of integrity of the cervical spine the key is alignment of the posterior aspect of the vertebral bodies. The spinal cord traverses the canal immediately posterior to the bodies. Posterior displacement of a body relative to the one adjacent can be expected to compress the cord; this is very poorly tolerated. Nondisplaced fractures of body, arch, or process of a vertebra or loss of height of body or disk space may be much more subtle findings; it is fortunate that they are also usually less of an immediate threat than are some other injuries.

Imaging of the thoracic and lumbosacral spine in the ED may be less definitive. Ceiling-mounted x-ray equipment should provide images of diagnostic quality; the same is not true of all portable units. Injury to the spine below the level of the neck should be suspected in patients (1) who have symptoms referable to levels below the neck; (2) who have cervical spine fractures; (3) who have other major thoracoabdominal injuries; or (4) who are unconscious and unable to offer any complaint. Caution should be exercised in repositioning such patients for physical examination or other procedures until the spine can be "cleared."

Contusion of the spinal cord may occur in association with major or minor fractures or in the absence of any fracture. To identify minor fractures or cord contusion, it may be necessary to perform computed tomography or magnetic resonance imaging later in the radiology department or after the patient's transfer to a larger facility.

Use of Skeletal Traction and Corticosteroids. Identification of spinal fracture with cord injury and sensorimotor deficit is an indication to treat with corticosteroid (dexamethasone 50 mg intravenously), obtain immediate neurosurgical consultation, and apply axial traction (in line with the vertebral column).

Identification of cervical spinal fracture, even without sensorimotor deficit, is usually indication to apply skeletal traction. Exceptions may be small chip fractures of the anterior margin of the bodies, small avulsions of the spinous processes, or fracture across the base of the odontoid without displacement of the vertebra. Skeletal traction (tongs-in-skull above the ears) is the most comfortable and effective means of immobilizing the cervical spine. Gardner–Wells type of tongs require little or no scalp preparation and can be relatively easily applied in the ED setting. Initial traction is established by applying (on an adult) 12 pounds to 20 pounds of weight to the end of a rope led from the tongs over a pulley projecting from the head of the bed or table. Countertraction (in the absence of continued hypotension or contraindicating injury) can be achieved by elevating the head of the bed or table. If tongs are unavailable or the emergency physician is unfamiliar with their use, immobilization of the neck can be maintained with cervical collar and bilateral head block until neurosurgical consultation can be obtained.

Decision for Surgical Intervention Versus Expectant Management. Interruption of spinal cord function may be partial or complete. When cord dysfunction is partial and there is evidence of improvement with treatment by traction, further diagnostic or operative procedures usually are not indicated. The traction should be maintained and the patient carefully observed. As long as there is continued improvement there is no rush to obtain permanent stabilization. When cord dysfunction is partial and there is evidence of progressive neurologic deficit, early operative decompression of the injured cord (and fusion stabilization of the spine) will probably be necessary to attempt to prevent what otherwise will be almost certain permanent sensorimotor deficit. A preoperative CT scan or myelogram is often of value in determining whether the anterior or posterior approach should be used. Unless there is a need for rapid removal to the operating room for immediate attention to life- or limb-threatening thoracic, abdominal, or peripheral vascular injuries, the postaccident interval needed to establish evolution of a spinal cord injury should always allow time to complete physical examination, important ED studies such as ECG and peritoneal lavage, and crucial radiographic studies such as computed tomography or magnetic resonance imaging.

Documentation of complete cord interruption on initial examination carries a grave prognosis in terms of response to any (operative or nonoperative) therapy or rehabilitation effort. Neurosurgeons note there probably has never been a documented patient with total areflexive sensorimotor paraplegia or quadraplegia who has regained sufficient neurologic function for independent ambulation.

Early Sequelae of Spinal Cord Injury. Spinal cord injury, particularly transection, may be the cause of distributive shock. Recognition is aided by apparently "contradictory" findings: moderate hypotension in the presence of warm vasodilated extremities. Initial treatment, directed to the problem of inadequate venous return, consists of intravenous volume expansion with crystalloid solution to compensate for increased venous capacitance caused by loss of vascular tone.

Spinal cord injury may result in ileus and urinary retention. In accordance with the general protocol for initial management of a patient with multiple-systems injuries, a patient with spinal cord injury should be permitted nothing by mouth, and a nasogastric tube and Foley bladder catheter should be inserted.

In a patient with complete paralysis, pressure areas leading to ischemic necrosis develop with surprising rapidity. Therefore special measures for skin care can be initiated in the ED, particularly if prolonged detention is necessary. If other injuries permit, paralyzed parts should be protected by change of position at frequent intervals. As soon as practical the patient should be placed on an alternating-pressure air mattress or, if that is not available, a foam-rubber matress. Skin care is also a consideration during transport to a distant facility.

In all cases of spinal cord (and cervical spine) injury, early neurosurgical consultation is recommended, even if only by telephone.

Head Injury: Second-Pass Considerations

More detailed evaluation of a head injury in a multiple-injury patient should continue with examination of scalp, skull, face, and ears and should include evaluation of cranial nerve function and the eyes. Thorough evaluation of peripheral sensorimotor function and deep tendon reflexes has already been described as a second-pass component in evaluation of spinal cord injury (though these components of the neurologic examination will often be better sequenced after second-pass attention to head injury evaluation). As with evaluation of spinal cord injury, it is important to document findings carefully, in terms that are unambiguous and descriptive, rather than to state what is surmised. A code such as "intact," "WNL," "benign" does not allow precise comparison with findings by a subsequent observer. Early description in terms of presumed pathologic finding ("concussion," "contusion," "laceration") is of limited value, because in most cases the pathologic condition will never be known. Since *changes* in neurologic symptoms and findings are a prime factor in the management of head injury, it is most useful to record what is observed and what stimulus produces what response so that the record may reflect differences in status at a later hour.

Scalp. The scalp should be carefully examined for laceration or contusion. Scalp injuries at either extreme of severity are associated with well-recognized pitfalls of multiple-trauma management. A small scalp injury, sometimes overlying a major skull or brain injury, or both, may go unrecognized because it is obscured by thick hair or dried blood. A large laceration of the scalp, often with persistent hemorrhage reflecting its generous blood supply, may detract attention from more immediately threatening injuries before all systems have been evaluated and more pressing diagnostic and therapeutic procedures accomplished.

Blood about the head or shoulders is an indication of possible scalp injury. A subtle laceration should be searched for, through matted or blood-clotted hair if necessary. Scalp lacerations should be briefly and gently inspected, using a sterile gloved finger, and sterile forceps if necessary, for early identification of continuing hemorrhage or presence of an obvious depressed or open skull fracture. The lacerated scalp can be a source of extensive blood loss. Although most superficial hemorrhage can easily be controlled by minimal pressure applied to an overlying sterile gauze pad, an occasional persistent brisk skin bleeder may require control by application of a small (sterile) hemostat, either directly to the vessel or to the galea so as to reflect it over the scalp, or by focal suture-ligature with a figure-of-eight stitch (preferably with polyglycolic acid absorbable suture). (Obviously, pressure should not be applied directly over an open skull fracture with brain exposed.)

Skull. Identification or strong suspicion of skull fracture is an indication to obtain skull films before closing an overlying scalp laceration. An open skull fracture or leakage of CSF from the ears or nose is an indication for intravenous administration of antibiotics (see "Use of Antibiotics in Multiple Trauma," p 451). Elevation-reduction in the operating room by a neurosurgeon is almost always indicated in a depressed skull fracture. Priority of exploration for open skull fracture is second to that for major thoracic, abdominal, and peripheral vascular injuries, unless two teams can safely operate simultaneously, without operating room personnel hindering each other and with no cross contamination of wounds. In the absence of need for rapid removal to the operating room for immediate surgical treatment of life- or limb-threatening thoracic, abdominal, or peripheral vascular injuries, elevation of a skull fracture can await completion of physical examination, important ED studies such as roentgenography of the chest, electrocardiography, and peritoneal lavage and crucial radiographic studies such as CT scanning, angiography, and spinal tomography.

Except for depressed or open fracture, it is rare for treatment of a closed head injury to be influenced by the presence or absence of a skull fracture. In addition, radiographs of the skull obtained on a portable machine in the ED may be of such poor quality that more definitive studies have to be repeated later in the radiology department. Therefore, unless appropriate x-ray equipment is available immediately in the ED, roentgenography of the skull may be deferred until removal of the patient to the x-ray suite or operating room.

Face. Face and neck lacerations are usually obvious. Identification of intraoral and intranasal lacerations will usually require specific examination. (The mouth should already have received a quick examination in conjunction with initial airway assessment.) Bleeding from an injury to face, mouth, or nose can be a source of significant blood loss and of aspiration in the patient with depressed consciousness. With exception of carotid artery laceration, hemorrhage from face and neck usually can be readily controlled by pressure applied over sterile gauze. It is both unnecessary and dangerous to attempt instrument clamping of facial vessels in the ED because it is too easy to crush adjacent branches of the facial nerve, causing paralysis.

Persistent hemorrhage from the nose or mouth necessitates repeated suctioning to keep the nonintubated airway clear, may require insertion of a pressure packing at the involved site, and may be an indication for tracheal intubation to prevent aspiration. Nasal hemorrhage usually ceases spontaneously or is temporarily controlled with anterior packing. The occasional stubborn posterior nasal hemorrhage can be temporarily controlled by passing (Foley) balloon catheters through the nares into the posterior pharynx, attaching gauze packs to the catheters, then applying traction on the catheters so as to draw the packs up behind the palate to act as a tamponade on the posterior choanae.

Positioning the patient on the side or in a face-down position to prevent aspiration usually is prohibited because of possible spinal cord injury and access needed to attend to injuries of chest, abdomen, pelvis, and limbs. Application of pressure to the face or neck or use of packs to control hemorrhage will depend on the presence or absence of associated fractures.

Common facial fractures are of mandible, maxilla, orbit, zygomatic arch, and nose. A brief but systematic second-pass examination of the facial skeleton should include inspection of teeth and palpation over alveolar ridges, over bony prominences of the cheeks, along the orbital rims, over the nose, and along the zygomatic arches. Extraocular movements have already been checked in the alert patient. The alert patient should be asked to close and open the jaw and put teeth together in a bite. Occlusion in an unconscious patient can be partially evaluated with passive motion of the mandible. The interior of the mouth is inspected with a light and a tongue blade; the interior of the nose, with nasal forceps and a light, or an otoscope.

Fractures of the mandible and maxilla are identified most readily by malocclusion of the teeth (particularly an open anterior bite), sensory loss in the mental distribution of the inferior alveolar nerve (mandibular fracture), and mobile upper incisor-gum unit (maxillary fracture). Fractures of the orbit are identified by asymmetry of the cheek prominences, discontinuity in the orbital rim, hypoesthesia in the distribution of the infraorbital nerve, and diplopia. Diplopia can occur as a result of (1) fracture high along the lateral orbital rim (trimalar fracture or Le Fort III fracture); (2) fracture of the orbital floor with entrapment of the inferior rectus muscle (blowout fracture); or (3) nerve paralysis or muscle contusion with or without fracture of the orbit. The alert patient should be questioned about double vision with eye movements to the periphery in all quadrants. Fractures of the nose are identified by asymmetry, hypermobility and crepitus at the nasal bridge, and displacement of the septum.

Identification or strong suspicion of a facial fracture indicates the need to obtain facial films later before closing overlying lacerations. Failure to identify facial skeletal injury or standard skull films does not exclude such fractures. However, along with the skull films, a single Water's view roentgenogram will provide almost all the diagnostic information needed in emergency care of fractures of facial bones. For maxillary and orbital fractures the definitive roentgenogram is the Water's projection, with particular attention to fluid "clouding" the maxillary sinus, discontinuity along the orbital rim, or both. The zygomatic arches may be demonstrated slightly better on a submentooccipital view. Tomography may be desirable when clouding of the maxillary antrum prevents definition of the orbital floor or when better definition of the temporomandibular joints is needed. For evaluating more subtle injuries or better definition of already identified injuries, a Zonarc x-ray study or facial CT scan may be indicated.

For nasal fractures the appropriate plain films are lateral, obtained with soft-tissue technique. Nasal films are of very low priority since a decision for (later) manipulation is usually based on the physical examination.

Intravenous administration of antibiotics is indicated in open fractures, fractures into the sinuses, and fractures with leakage of CSF (see "Use of Antibiotics in Multiple Trauma," p 451). Major maxillofacial skeletal injury is usually an indication for manipulation and fixation in the operating room by a plastic surgeon, otolaryngologic surgeon, oromaxillofacial surgeon, ophthalmologic surgeon, or a combined team. Timing of surgical intervention depends on several factors, the two most important of which are the patient's overall condition and extent of facial edema.

If there are no other injuries of greater priority and swelling and bruising are minimal, it is probably advantageous to achieve early realignment and fixation of displaced bones. These conditions are likely to coexist in a minority of patients with multiple injuries. Facial fractures are of much lower priority than major thoracoabdominal injuries, brain and spinal cord injuries, peripheral neurovascular injuries, major orthopaedic fractures, and major soft-tissue loss. Edema and ecchymoses in soft tissue overlying the facial skeleton usually make accurate appraisal of contour of features difficult and technically complicate surgical reduction. Fortunately, operative manipulation of most facial fractures in adults can safely be delayed up to 2 weeks following injury. (In children, facial fractures should be reduced within a few days after injury. Even in adults, the fine bone of the orbital floor if fractured and displaced may become difficult to manipulate after 7 to 10 days because of fibrous fixation.) A delay of several days before operative reduction of facial fractures in a multiple-trauma patient has the advantages of (1) allowing partial resolution of swelling, (2) avoiding (more) general anesthesia during a period of critical illness, (3) permitting attention to be directed to more immediately threatening injuries, and (4) providing an interval for transport to a larger facility if someone with maxillofacial surgical expertise is not locally available.

Cranial Nerves and Eyes. Examination for cranial nerve injury and eye damage can conveniently be accomplished simultaneously with the examination of the face and mouth just described. Assessment of cranial nerve integrity and eye function consists of both active and passive elements: those that require patient cooperation and those that the physician can complete whether the patient is conscious or unconscious. Even if intubated and unable to speak, an alert patient usually can communicate, by nod or other signal, sufficiently to provide meaningful information.

Eyes and Third, Fourth, and Sixth Cranial Nerves. Evaluation of pupillary size and reaction and interpretation of abnormalities have already been described as a first-pass component of the assessment of brain stem function (third nerve, passive). Extraocular movements are evaluated by asking the alert patient to track the examiner's finger as it is moved into all quadrants of vision, by inquiring about the presence of double vision, and by noting the presence or absence of nystagmus at extremes of gaze. Restriction in globe movement or diplopia, alone or together, may signal compression or other injury to cranial nerves III, IV, or VI anywhere along their course, fracture(s) about the orbit with ocular muscle entrapment, or both. The fourth (trochlear) nerve supplies the superior oblique ocular muscle; the sixth (abducens) nerve innervates the lateral rectus muscle. The other three recti and the inferior oblique are supplied by the third (oculomotor) nerve. The most common limitation of voluntary motion is of upward gaze, caused by entrapment of the inferior rectus muscle in a blowout fracture of the orbital floor.

As in any evaluation of the eye it is important to determine and record visual acuity early in the examination, if possible. For an alert nonintubated trauma patient still in the supine position, a convenient and reasonably accurate assessment can be made by asking the person to read, with each eye separately, an appropriate-sized label from a medical supply package. For an alert patient with more grossly impaired vision or one who cannot talk, identifying the number of fingers extended from the examiner's hand provides a crude but objective test. Unilateral blindness may be a result of laceration of the second (optic) nerve associated with a fracture involving the optic foramen. It is more likely that impaired visual acuity in an alert patient is due to injury around or within the globe. Documentation of loss of visual acuity indicates the need for early ophthalmologic consultation.

Each eye should then be examined with an ophthalmoscope from the conjunctival and epithelial surfaces anteriorly to the retina posteriorly. If facial trauma is severe this should be accomplished as soon as first-pass attention to other injuries permits, because the lids may become swollen so rapidly that the globes can be visualized in only a cursory fashion without forceful separation with lid retractors. The lids must be at least partially everted, without applying pressure to the globe, to permit adequate inspection of the conjunctival surfaces and their fornices. Initial gross inspection of the surfaces of the conjunctiva, cornea, and sclera is facilitated by oblique illumination with a bright hand-held light.

Superficially located foreign bodies that do not penetrate the globe should be removed. After insertion of a drop of topical anesthetic a light touch with a moistened cotton-tipped applicator or gentle irrigation will suffice to remove most superficial grit and contact lenses. Contact lenses are mentioned particularly because of their widespread use and the problem of corneal abrasion and edema if they are allowed to remain in place over many hours in the trauma patient who is not alert enough to suggest their removal. If a small foreign body remains stuck in the superficial corneal epithelium despite the preceding maneuvers, it may be removed under topical anesthesia, after the rest of the physical examination is complete and major injuries are under control, by flicking it out with the tip of a sterile 25-gauge needle under four-power loupe magnification. (If superficial rust particles remain they should be similarly removed to prevent permanent staining.) After removal of a foreign body from the superficial corneal epithelium or with discovery of a corneal abrasion, antibiotic solution should be instilled and the eye (semipressure) patched for 24 hours before reexamination. (The closed lid and tear milieu assured by the patch should obviate need for continued use of anesthetic or analgesics. Because of risk of aggravation of a herpetic infection of the cornea, no steroid-containing medication should be used in an eye with a corneal abrasion or ulcer.) If a superficial foreign body has not entered the corneal stroma, the corneal epithelium will rapidly regenerate 1 to 2 days after its removal and no corneal scarring will result. If a foreign body is embedded deeply enough to have penetrated Bowman's membrane into the corneal stroma, its removal should probably be left to an ophthalmologist, particularly if it is close to the visual axis, because some scarring is likely to occur.

Injury to the eyelids, particularly penetrating injury and laceration, should raise suspicion of injury to the globe and possibility of intraocular foreign body. A conjunctival laceration is an indication for careful exploration under topical anesthesia after the rest of physical examination is complete and major injuries under control, with attention directed to discovery of an occult foreign body. Pronounced acute conjunctival edema (chemosis) with or without hemorrhage may be due to a retained intraorbital foreign body, fracture of the orbit, scleral rupture, or carotid-cavernous fistula, and it may prevent adequate protection of the surface of the eye by the lids.

Discovery of a deep laceration of the cornea or sclera or of an intraorbital foreign body with or without obvious defect in the anterior surface of the eye is indication for topical application of antibiotic drops (solution), initiating intravenous antibiotic therapy (see "Use of Antibiotics in Multiple Trauma," p 451), protecting the eye with a shield, and obtaining early ophthalmologic consultation. These injuries should be managed by an ophthalmologist prepared to suture the eye in the operating room. A number of complications may ensue if such injuries are explored or extraction of a penetrating foreign body is attempted in the ED by someone without an ophthalmologist's expertise: (1) The anterior chamber of the eye may collapse and not reform. (2) The iris or lens may be extracted with a foreign body or may be indistinguishable from blood and fibrin clot and, if partially extruded through a wound, may be wiped away when the injury is inspected. (3) Inept manipulation of a foreign body may result in part or all of it being lost within the globe, making subsequent surgical removal much more complex or impossible. (4) Permanent scarring of the cornea or lens (traumatic cataract) may occur. (5) Delay in recognition and treatment of prolapse of the iris or ciliary body may increase the possibility of sympathetic ophthalmia: bilateral granulomatous uveitis originating from unilateral injury and probably resulting from autosensitivity to uveal pigment from disorganized cells in the injured eye.

Early ophthalmologic consultation is also indicated in a nonpenetrating intraocular contusion. Blood in the anterior chamber (hyphema) may signal rupture of the arterial circle of the ciliary body or traumatic disruption of the iris from the ciliary body (iridodialysis). In hyphema there is risk of (1) delayed (3 to 5 days) rehemorrhage, (2) persistent elevation of intraocular pressure, and (3) staining of the cornea with blood pigment. Administration of diuretic may be indicated to reduce intraocular pressure, as may surgical removal of a nonresorbing blood clot. Increased depth of the anterior chamber and shimmering of the iris (iridodonesis) are findings suggesting partial detachment and subluxation of the lens. Damage to a retinal vessel may cause vitreous hemorrhage, with loss of the red reflex and inability to visualize the fundus, or retinal hemorrhage. More severe force may result in rupture of the choroid with hemorrhage or retinal detachment. Almost all these injuries can be identified or suspected from examination with a hand-held ophthalmoscope, and almost all have significant implications with regard to permanent visual impairment.

When symptoms or ophthalmoscopy strongly suggests the presence of a foreign body, inability to readily identify a corneal (or scleral) epithelial defect is an indication to stain the surface of the eye with fluorescein; the palpebral conjunctiva is touched with a sterile fluorescein-impregnated strip moistened with sterile saline. When there has been obvious penetration of the surface of the globe, inability to visualize a foreign body is indication for later radiographic study of the orbits and skull in the x-ray department (or specific inspection for orbital foreign body on the skull films obtained later in connection with evaluation of concomitant head injury). Inability to characterize readily the depth or extent of a penetrating injury to the anterior surface of the globe using a hand-held ophthalmoscope is indication for a slit-lamp examination, if and when the patient's overall condition permits.

The general philosophy of surgical approach to serious eye injuries is that unless there is no light perception and almost total destruction of the eyeball, an ophthalmologist will usually make a maximal effort to repair each eye as carefully and completely as possible. Timing of surgical intervention in a multiple-trauma patient depends on the nature of injuries to the eye relative to other major organ systems. For eye injuries in which potentially serious complications are usually delayed, once the eye is protected as indicated, detailed ophthalmologic evaluation can be deferred until completion of the physical examination, other ED studies, and important radiographic studies, and until major thoracic, abdominal, peripheral vascular, and orthopaedic injuries have been operated on or stabilized. For ocular trauma involving persistent collapse of the anterior chamber, extrusion of contents with impairment of circulation, or ongoing leakage of vitreous substance, optimal management consists of early surgical repair. For these more serious injuries, surgical priority with regard to preserving sight is equal to that for major thoracic, abdominal, neurologic, and peripheral vascular injuries with regard to saving life and limb. Therefore when major eye damage coexists with need for early and lengthy thoracoabdominal, neurologic, or peripheral vascular operative procedures, it is usually best to have the ophthalmologist operate simultaneously with other surgical teams. It is highly recommended that every multiple-injury patient receive a careful eye examination and that any significant eye injury receive early ophthalmologic consultation (even if only by telephone).

Other Cranial Nerves. In the alert cooperative patient the fifth (trigeminal) nerve can be tested by subjective response to light touch over its various sensory-division distributions to the face and by determining by palpation the symmetry of masseter muscle tension on bite and observing the symmetry of jaw alignment on mouth opening. In the alert patient the seventh (facial) nerve can be tested by observing symmetry of motion on various facial expressions, and deficits can be localized to upper or lower motor neuron (UMN, LMN) lesions. Inability to raise the brow and wrinkle the forehead and inability to frown and tightly close an eyelid are associated with LMN lesion. A symmetric smile may still occur with UMN lesion, but inability to puff out cheeks or raise the mouth to show teeth occurs with injury to UMN or LMN.

In the unconscious or uncooperative patient the fifth nerve can be evaluated by testing the corneal reflex to light touch with a cotton-tipped applicator, by tickling the nose with a cotton-tipped applicator, or by applying a painful stimulus to the supraorbital ridge. As the fifth nerve is tested the response may demonstrate an intact seventh nerve: A blink response to corneal stimulation and facial grimace in response to nasal tickling and to supraorbital irritation require seventh-nerve function.

Response to verbal commands demonstrates eighth (acoustic) nerve function in the alert patient. Response to cold caloric stimulation, when this test is indicated for other reasons in the comatose patient, indicates some eighth nerve function.

In the alert nonintubated patient the ninth (glossopharyngeal) and tenth (vagus) nerves can be tested by looking for deviation of the uvula from the side of injury when the patient says "Ah" and by observing symmetry or absence of gag reflex in touching each side of the posterior pharynx with a tongue blade. In the unconscious patient, inability to swallow secretions readily without choking may indicate ninth and tenth nerve injury, and testing the gag reflex to tongue blade stimulation may be possible if the mouth can easily be opened.

In the alert cooperative patient the eleventh (spinal accessory) nerve can be tested by palpating for symmetry of strength and motion of the shoulder shrug (trapezius) and head turning (sternocleidomastoids) against resistance of the examiner's hand.

In the alert cooperative patient the twelfth (hypoglossal) nerve can be tested by looking for deviation toward the injured side on maximal effort to protrude the tongue and by palpating for symmetry or absence of strength in pushing the tongue against each cheek.

Ears. Laceration, contusion, or loss of tissue of the external ear is usually obvious. Injury to cartilage of the ear may require specific examination. The canal of the external ear and the tympanic membrane should be viewed with a clean otoscope. A foreign body should be carefully removed with the patient not struggling or moving. Hemotympanum, with or without blood or clear fluid (CSF) in the external canal, is presumptive evidence of a basilar skull fracture, even if such a fracture cannot be identified on a roentgenogram. Bleeding or leakage of CSF from within the ear and laceration or contusion of the external ear exposing underlying cartilage are indications to initiate antibiotic therapy (see "Use of Antibiotics in Multiple Trauma," p 451).

Blood in the external ear on initial examination may be from laceration of the external ear, scalp, or face. If this appears likely, reexamination, after careful removal of superficially located blood with a sterile sucker tip or sterile swab, or gentle irrigation with sterile water or saline, may be necessary to confirm or deny ongoing bleeding from within the ear. Bleeding from within the ear may be a manifestation of fracture of bones surrounding the ear; such fractures are potentially dangerous because of risk of introducing infection into the middle ear or inner ear, or, if a fracture extends through the dura, into the brain. Thus when the ear is bleeding, any manipulation in the ear canal should be performed under sterile conditions or should be avoided.

One such manipulation of concern, which may be performed during the second-pass neurologic evaluation, is caloric stimulation. Caloric stimulation is indicated when the doll's-head maneuver fails to move the globes in an unconscious patient or when neck injury precludes use of the maneuver. In a multiply-injured patient it should be appropriately sequenced after initial assessment of thoracoabdominal injuries. It is not part of the pupillary response component of the frequently repeated mini-neurologic examination. It should not be performed when there is obvious tympanic membrane injury or when blood or CSF is draining from an ear. Airway precautions should be used with this test because it is uncomfortable to the patient and can cause nausea and vomiting, which may be accompanied by aspiration. When possible, this test should be done by the neurosurgeon who may later have to interpret the results.

To test response to caloric stimulation, cold water is introduced into the external ear with a syringe. When brain stem function is not severely depressed, the cold fluid provokes eye movements after a half-minute delay. Nystagmus is observed if the reticular activating system is functioning, whereas complete absence of eye movements signals a severe degree of brain stem dysfunction. Intermediate dysfunction may be reflected by sustained ocular deviation. If sustained ocular deviation is dysconjugate (motion of only one eye toward the irrigated ear), there may be a lesion of the third nerve or of the medial longitudinal bundle within the brain stem.

Suturing of Head Injury Lacerations: Considerations Regarding Repair of Special Structures. Suturing of multiple lacerations of the scalp and face is a time-consuming process that should be deferred until (1) physical examination has been completed, (2) ED management of major thoracoabdominal, neurologic, and orthopaedic injuries has been accomplished or initiated, and (3) urgent ED and radiology department special diagnostic studies have been completed or are under way. In the interim, wounds may simply be covered with sterile gauze pads moistened with sterile saline or povidone-iodine. If early operation is necessary, lacerations can most efficiently be repaired in the operating room following, or concurrently with, the major surgical procedure. In contrast to soft-tissue wounds elsewhere on the body, clean lacerations of the face may be closed as long as 24 hours after injury with considerable benefit to final healing.

Closure of scalp lacerations requires little description. Rich blood supply, sameness of adjacent tissue (except perhaps at the hairline), and ability to undermine permit some debridement to convert ragged or stellate wounds to sharp-edged ellipses that facilitate linear closure, often with a single layer of (deep bite) cuticular sutures. Lidocaine with epinephrine can be used to aid hemostasis and duration of anesthesia. In contrast, as a general principle, facial lacerations should receive minimal debridement. This is particularly true of complex lacerations and partially avulsed soft-tissue fragments that will require plastic surgical repair in an operating room. Fragments of composite tissue from ears, nose, eyelids, and lips may be made to survive by careful reapproximation or as grafts; such tissue is almost impossible to duplicate by grafting tissue from elsewhere on the body. Face wounds should be irrigated thoroughly, and foreign particulate matter and necrotic edges should be debrided. Viable obliquely sliced edges need not be debrided to right angles, however. Any debridement must be accomplished with care to avoid injury to the relatively superficial underlying nerves and ducts abundant about the face. Lidocaine with epinephrine can be used only in locations where blood supply from more than one direction is assured, but the vasoconstriction produced by the epinephrine must be avoided at extremity locations such as the ear or tip of the nose, or partially avulsed tissue fragments. Where underlying facial muscle has been divided, the muscle should be reapproximated as an independent layer in an attempt to restore normal facial expression. In the absence of division of underlying muscle, as few interrupted subcuticular sutures as needed should be used to reduce tension on skin stitches. These subcuticular sutures should be placed as deeply as possible within the dermis, with knots buried in the subcutaneous fat, and care should be taken to align opposing dermal margins precisely; sutures of 4-0 and 5-0 polyglycolic acid are appropriate for muscle and subcuticular layers. Interrupted skin sutures should be placed within 2 mm to 4 mm of the wound margin to avoid inversion of edges, be tied loosely to avoid "crosshatch" suture scars, and be removed in 3 to 4 days (and the wound covered with sterile paper tape strips); 6-0 monofilament plastic (nylon, polypropylene) is an appropriate facial cuticular suture.

Among pitfalls in evaluation and management of facial wounds are failure to recognize injury to one or more of the special tissues or structures closely underlying a skin laceration and failure to accomplish adequate repair of such injuries. Several of these special structures and their repair deserve mention.

EYELIDS. The eyelid should be regarded as a double-layer structure: The anterior layer is composed of the skin and orbicularis muscle; the posterior layer is made up of the tarsal plate and the palpebral conjunctiva. A "gray line" at the mucocutaneous junction marks the demarcation between these layers. Each of these layers should be closed separately in any lid laceration that transects the tarsus. A lid laceration near the superior portion of the orbit may transect the levator tendon of the lid, which requires repair, or it may contain fat, signaling a penetration of the orbital septum. A vertical laceration involving the lid margin requires meticulous repair of the tarsus to prevent notching of the lid, a condition that will prevent complete coverage of the cornea during sleep (upper lid) or result in leakage of tear fluid (epiphora, lower lid).

LACRIMAL APPARATUS. Lacerations within the medial fourth of the eyelids or at the superior-lateral aspect of the nose may impair tear drainage to the nose by direct injury to the puncta, the (upper or lower) canaliculi, the lacrimal sac, or the nasolacrimal duct. A high index of suspicion can greatly increase the probability of identifying such injury. Repair requires use of a plastic tube stent and an operating microscope by an eye surgeon or plastic surgeon.

MEDIAL CANTHAL LIGAMENT. Lacerations in the region just described for the lacrimal apparatus and bony injuries of the nasoethmoid region may sever or disrupt the medial canthal ligament of the orbicularis oculi muscle. Reconstitution of this tendon with nonabsorbable suture and restoration of the normal intercanthal distance are necessary to achieve the proper cosmetic result and ensure normal function of the lid and lacrimal apparatus.

EAR AND NASAL CARTILAGE. Full-thickness lacerations of the ear or nose should be closed in three layers, independently approximating the cartilage with fine monofilament or polyglycolic acid sutures. Splinting the ear with wet cotton dressings or with petrolatum gauze packs may help prevent hematoma. With injury of cartilage or infection of a hematoma, serous perichondritis is a possible sequela of an apparently simple laceration of these structures.

PAROTID GLAND AND DUCT. Any deep laceration involving the cheek from the anterior border of the masseter muscle back toward the ear should arouse suspicion of injury to the parotid gland or duct. The duct emerges from the parotid substance, runs across the lateral surface of the masseter, turns medially at the anterior border of the masseter and opens into the mouth opposite the second upper molar. Intraoral catheterization of the parotid duct with or without sialography may be helpful in diagnosing parotid injuries. Failure to repair the capsule and a severed duct of an injured parotid gland may result in cyst formation or salivary fistula.

FACIAL NERVE. The facial nerve divides into two major branches within the parotid gland. Thus facial lacerations in the area just described may involve a potentially reparable facial nerve injury. Early repair by a plastic surgeon using an operating microscope and nerve stimulator may result in surprisingly good restoration of function.

COMPLEX FACIAL LACERATIONS. Lacerations that are stellate, that have one or more angular flaps, or that involve full-thickness loss of skin may require special suturing techniques, undermining and flap advancement, or the use of other plastic closure techniques to prevent loss of tissue at corners and angles and to achieve an optimum result. Management of complex and compound facial injury is determined by careful assessment of the extent of injury and early consultation with a plastic surgeon before burning any bridges.

Anterior Neck Injury: Second-Pass Considerations

Blunt or penetrating neck trauma can result in injury to major arteries, veins, lymphatic channels, nerves, larynx, trachea, pharynx, esophagus, and intrathoracic structures, any of which warrants early operative repair. With delay in recognition and intervention there is risk of major complications: Arterial injury may lead to delayed hemorrhage with abrupt compression of the airway at a time the patient is not under close surveillance. Cerebral infarction may be a consequence of delayed attention to arterial intimal damage. Venous injury may result in massive air embolism. Thoracic duct injury may lead to chylothorax or persistent lymph fistula. Nerve injury amenable to early repair may later be neither identifiable nor reparable. Laryngeal and tracheal injury may lead to stricture, stenosis, and fibrosis, all of which may be prevented by early repair. Pharyngeal and esophageal injuries may lead to deep neck infection with formation of abscesses, cysts, and fistulas. Associated thoracic injuries present a number of life-threatening possibilities that will be described in the next section.

Critique of Diagnostic Criteria for Surgical Intervention. Immediately evident on physical examination should be the presence or absence of a skin defect, hematoma, and subcutaneous emphysema. Less evident (particularly in the presence of hematoma or subcutaneous emphysema) are palpable fracture of larynx or trachea or displacement of the normal architecture of these structures. Uncommonly, auscultation may reveal a bruit associated with arterial injury or stridor associated with laryngeal injury. (A systolic bruit is characteristic of traumatic false aneurysm; a continuous bruit, of traumatic false aneurysm; a continuous bruit, of traumatic arteriovenous fistula.) Hoarseness may be present with injury to the larynx, laryngeal nerve, or the vagus nerve, but quality of voice is not necessarily a good indicator of severity of injury to these structures (and of course cannot be assessed in the intubated patient).

Examination for intactness of the brachial plexus and cranial nerves (IX to XII) in the neck has been described in spinal cord and cranial nerve evaluation. These assessments will always be compromised in an unconscious or uncooperative patient. Phrenic nerve injury is likely to be a late diagnosis.

The lateral cervical spine film and the anteroposterior chest roentgenogram already ordered (or obtained) at this point in the evaluation may be helpful. In addition to cervical spine alignment, the neck films should be examined for displacement of the trachea, narrowing of the airway, subcutaneous emphysema, and radiopaque penetrating foreign bodies. The chest roentgenogram may demonstrate a multitude of abnormalities (described in the next section), including intrathoracic injuries to great vessels, airway, or esophagus, from which dissecting hematomas and subcutaneous emphysema extend into the neck.

A skin defect with or without hematoma is strongly suspicious of vascular injury. Subcutaneous emphysema with or without hematoma, hemoptysis, or hematemesis is suspicious of injury to airway, posterior pharynx, or esophagus. However, hematoma and subcutaneous emphysema in the neck are not specific for a particular injury, and either could be due to intrathoracic injury, just as a penetrating wound of the neck could well extend into the thorax. Transient post-traumatic hemoptysis and hematemesis are often related to aspirated or swallowed blood from nose, mouth, or facial injuries. Given the nonspecificity of these physical and plain-film radiographic findings and the dire consequences of missing a significant injury, the following guidelines are offered to direct additional specific investigation when there is a high index of suspicion of neck injury.

Penetrating Trauma and Suspected Vascular Injury. Any penetrating injury and any significant hematoma of the neck are suspect for vascular injury. Any wound that penetrates or is suspected of penetrating the platysma muscle in the anterior region of the neck usually deserves early exploration (in the operating room) by a surgeon experienced in operating in this region and in vascular reconstruction. Probing of neck wounds in the ED is never justified, although careful superficial exploration under local anesthesia may be useful in assessing wound depth relative to the platysma.

Angiography is extremely valuable in assessment of potential vascular injuries. When a chest roentgenogram shows a widened mediastinal shadow, an aortogram is mandatory to demonstrate or exclude aortic transection. When there is a large hematoma in the lower neck without penetrating injury, an aortic arch study is mandatory to demonstrate or exclude great-vessel injury. (Disruption of the thoracic aorta or great vessels is indication for early operative repair by a thoracic surgeon; see the section entitled "Chest Injury," p 382.) When exploration is indicated for a penetrating injury in the anterior region of the neck, location of the wound of entrance may determine if preoperative arteriography is to be performed. Three "zones" are considered: lower third (base of neck), middle third (midcervical), and upper third (above the angle of the mandible).

Injuries near the base of the neck may involve not only cervical vessels but any vessels coming from the aortic arch; thus planning exploratory incisions to provide retrosternal and retroclavicular exposure when needed is facilitated by preoperative definition of the injury. Injuries above the level of the mandible (and close to the base of the skull) present problems of exposure and distal-vessel control so difficult that internal carotid artery ligation is often necessary; hence preoperative knowledge about the status of internal carotid arteries and intracerebral circulation is helpful in weighing the feasibility of repair against the consequences of ligation. Injuries confined to the midcervical zone are more easily exposed and repaired, and therefore arteriography is not always essential for their evaluation. The problem is in being sure that injury involved in a penetrating midneck wound of entrance is confined to the midcervical region. Once exploration is under way, the presence of tissue contusion and hematoma may make precise limits of the tract and damage difficult to define. Thus if stability of the patient's condition allows the time, angiography is helpful when surgery is contemplated for any major vascular injury about the neck.

Suspected Nerve Injury. Major nerve branches in the neck (brachial plexus, ninth to twelfth cranial, phrenic, laryngeal) may be injured by contusion, compression (as from hematoma), laceration, and avulsion. Contusion and compression injuries warrant conservative management. Laceration results from penetrating injury, for which exploration usually is indicated (as described earlier). Should one of the major nerve trunks be found at exploration to be severed (and such injury should specifically be sought when functional deficit has been identified preoperatively), attempt at repair is indicated, preferably with an operating microscope. Avulsion of brachial plexus roots is a complex injury warranting neurosurgical consultation and management. Spinal cord injury clearly warrants neurosurgical management, as described in a previous section.

Suspected Laryngeal and Tracheal Injuries. Post-traumatic airway obstruction, alteration of voice (dysphonia), persistent hemoptysis, and cervical subcutaneous emphysema not immediately and convincingly explained by injury of the lung or chest wall are all absolute indications for direct laryngoscopy and tracheoscopy by someone capable of interpreting the findings. Even without these findings, any suspicion of such injury is sufficient indication for these examinations. Finding of fracture, displacement, or laceration of the larynx is indication for operative repair by an ENT surgeon. Finding of a major tracheal or bronchial tear is indication for early operative repair by a thoracic, ENT, or general surgeon, depending on its location and associated injuries. A laryngeal injury is usually indication for a standard third-ring tracheostomy. Whenever possible this should be done in the operating room, over a prepositioned endotracheal tube. A laryngeal injury with airway obstruction that precludes safe passage of an endotracheal tube, and structural displacement or swelling that prevents safe identification of the cricothyroid membrane, may be one of the rare indications for early third-ring tracheostomy without a tracheal tube already in place.

Suspected Posterior Pharyngeal and Esophageal Injuries. Post-traumatic dysphagia (or inability to pass nasogastric tube), persistent hematemesis, and subcutaneous emphysema not convincingly explained by thoracic airway or pulmonary injury are absolute indications for fiberoptic esophagoscopy and contrast esophagography. Barium or a water-soluble contrast agent may be used. It is true that if extravasation occurs it would be preferable to have water-soluble material rather than barium in soft tissues. However, if extravasation is seen, the defect requires exploration as soon as the patient's overall condition permits; hence the barium will be removed within a short interval. In addition, aspiration of barium is tolerated better than aspiration of water-soluble contrast material. Observation of a full-thickness rent in the posterior pharynx or esophagus or demonstration of extravasation on an esophagogram is indication for early operative repair and drainage by a thoracic, otolaryngologic, or general surgeon (depending on its location and associated injuries).

Combined Injuries. Combinations of the preceding injuries are highly probable, particularly with penetrating trauma. Extensive tissue contusion and hematoma may make difficult precise determination of presence, extent, and depth of external injury to trachea and esophagus. While adequate exposure and debridement are essential, overly aggressive dissection to "make sure" carries some risk of iatrogenic injury to these structures, adjacent nerves, and endocrine glands. For these reasons, in a patient whose condition is stable, when a decision is made to explore the neck for penetrating injury (particularly high velocity), preoperative laryngoscopy, tracheoscopy, esophagoscopy, and arteriography are highly recommended. (If not conveniently completed in the ED, the endoscopic procedures can be accomplished in the operating room.) Finding an internal tear or hematoma in the airway or esophagus guides the surgeon to a specific point where maximum time can be invested in meticulous dissection; the absence of any such finding eliminates demand to visualize these structures totally at points distant from the apparent wound tract.

Timing of Neck Surgery. Brisk external bleeding and high-grade airway obstruction receive immediate attention in the ED, as described. Since these problems are of necessity the first to be brought under control, those neck problems that remain will usually not be of immediate threat to life or limb (although holding pressure on a major bleeding point may be inconvenient). Priority of neck exploration is secondary to that of major thoracic, abdominal, neurologic, or peripheral vascular injuries unless there is a poorly controlled carotid artery laceration or unless simultaneous operation by two teams can be accomplished safely with respect to interactions of operating room personnel and potential cross contamination of wounds. In absence of need for rapid removal to the OR for immediate attention to life- or limb-threatening thoracoabdominal, neurologic, or peripheral vascular injury, neck exploration can await completion of physical examination, important ED procedures, and crucial radiographic studies.

Potential complexity of injury and relation of outcome to precision of operative repair are factors that argue strongly for operative management of neck injuries in a setting where there are surgeons intimately familiar with the varied anatomy involved. Therefore in a hospital without immediate access to a surgeon with such expertise, if exploration is indicated, a neck injury patient whose condition is stable should be transported to a major medical center where general, thoracic, and otolaryngologic surgeons are available and where angiography and endoscopy can be performed. A transport team capable of airway management and fluid resuscitation en route should be in attendance.

Chest Injury: Second-Pass Considerations

The six potentially fatal chest injuries previously described as "immediate considerations" are usually manifested by significant early cardiopulmonary distress, and the problems can be diagnosed quickly by physical examination. Another half dozen potentially lethal chest injuries may cause the victim only modest cardiopulmonary distress at time of arrival in the ED, and the problems are usually not diagnosed readily on the basis of physical findings. These conditions are rupture or laceration of the aorta, the diaphragm, the tracheobronchial tree, and the esophagus and contusion or infarction of the lung and of the heart.

The diagnosis of the first five of these is most likely to be made by proper interpretation of a chest roentgenogram. Hypoxemia detected by arterial blood gas determination, particularly when oxygen is being administered, may reflect (but is not specific for) pulmonary contusion. ECG changes may provide the only clue to a myocardial contusion or infarction. Indeed, electrocardiography, blood gas determinations, and roentgenography of the chest represent such crucial ED studies in the evaluation of chest injury that unless one of the so-called rapid killers mandates immediate intervention in a patient in extremis, these studies should be obtained as soon as possible after airway control and vascular access have been established and while physical examination is in progress.

A myriad of potential diagnoses awaits the careful examiner of a single anteroposterior roentgenogram of the chest (Table 23-5). In addition to findings related to the "chest cavity," numerous other problems may be evident on the film, including fracture or dislocation of the clavicle and humerus; fracture of scapula, spine, or mandible; penetrating foreign bodies; and foreign bodies in the upper airway.

Rupture or Laceration of the Aorta. Rupture of the aorta is the most common fatal chest injury in traffic accident victims who do not reach the hospital alive. Aortic disruption due to nonpenetrating deceleration injury occurs most commonly at sites of vessel fixation. The sites, in order of frequency, are (1) at the ligamentum arteriosum just beyond the origin of the left subclavian artery, (2) as the ascending aorta exits the heart, and (3) at the diaphragm. It is at these points that shear forces combine with a severalfold increase in intra-aortic pressure to generate the injury. For those (10% to 20%) with such aortic injury who do arrive alive there is a spectrum of severity, from exsanguinating hemorrhage into the left chest to partial intimal disruption well contained within an aneurysmal dilatation of surrounding muscular or adventitial layers or both. Those toward the latter end of this spectrum offer the best chance for successful surgical treatment, but they may also have the fewest diagnostic signs. Indeed, pulses may be intact beyond a point of almost total discontinuity of the aortic wall, with or without an obvious pressure gradient between upper and lower limbs.

A chest roentgenogram usually provides the first suspicion of aortic rupture. A widened mediastinal shadow, representing mediastinal hematoma, is the most easily recognized finding; more subtle indications include loss of definition of the aortic "knob" and the perispinous "stripe," and a (left) pleural cap. It is not uncommon for any or all of these findings to be present on an anteroposterior supine film but be absent on an erect chest roentgenogram. Absence on an erect film equals absence of (plain) radiographic suspicion of aortic injury. Therefore when there is doubt and the patient's condition and other injuries permit,

TABLE 23-5. Thoracic Diagnoses by Chest Roentgenography

FINDING	PROBABLE OR POTENTIAL PROBLEM OR ASSOCIATED DEFECT
Malpositioned tip of endotracheal tube	Airway obstruction; hypoventilation of left lung
Altered cardiac contour (unreliable)	Hemopericardium, preexisting cardiac disease
Widened mediastinum	Aortic injury
Indistinct aortic "knob"	Aortic injury
Indistinct perispinous "stripe"	Aortic injury
Pleural "cap"	Aortic injury
Deviated mainstem bronchus	Aortic injury
Pneumomediastinum	Bronchial or esophageal tear
Deviated mediastinum, hyperlucent hemithorax	Tension pneumothorax
Fine peripheral pleural line	Small pneumothorax
Perihilar density, hyperlucent hemithorax	Large pneumothorax with lung collapse
Parenchymal lung densities	Pulmonary contusion, aspiration; lung collapse, ARDs
Fluid in pleural space	Hemothorax, hydrothorax, chylothorax, esophageal leak
Elevated diaphragm ± viscera in chest	Ruptured diaphragm
Free air under diaphragm	Ruptured abdominal viscus
Lower rib fractures	Injury to spleen or liver
Middle rib fractures	Injury to lung, heart
Upper rib (and sternal) fractures	Tracheobronchial tear, great vessel injury
Subcutaneous emphysema	Injury to airway, lung, or esophagus
Malpositioned tip of CVP catheter	Erroneous monitor data, poor infusion, perforation of vessel
Malpositioned chest tube	Poor tube function; iatrogenic injury to mediastinum, diaphragm, or abdominal viscera

findings suggestive of aortic rupture should be confirmed on an erect chest film.

Aortography is the definitive confirmatory radiographic study. History of a likely mechanism of injury, even without obvious findings on plain chest films, constitutes sufficient (although not necessary) indication for obtaining an aortogram. The appropriate management is rapid operative repair by a thoracic surgery team (with or without bypass technique to maintain spinal cord perfusion). When a laceration or contained rupture of the aorta is not diagnosed and repaired promptly after the accident, the incidence of uncontained rupture, which is often fatal, within the subsequent 48 hours is as high as 50%.

Therefore suspicion on plain chest roentgenogram of aortic injury is indication to (1) obtain immediate thoracic surgical consultation, (2) notify the operating room to stand by, (3) expedite completion of physical examination and priority ED procedures such as peritoneal lavage, and (4) obtain an aortogram (by retrograde arterial catheterization) as soon as the patient can safely be moved to the x-ray suite. If, concurrent with presence of a mediastinal hematoma, there is significant bleeding into the left side of the chest or a rapidly expanding abdomen, immediate transfer to the operating room is justified. In this situation an attempt may be made to obtain a one-shot forward "flush" aortogram, with an x-ray film cassette under the ED litter or operating table, by injecting a large bolus of contrast material into a central venous catheter.

Identification of mediastinal hematoma in a relatively stable patient received in a setting where angiography and thoracic surgery are not available is indication to obtain immediate telephone thoracic surgery consultation and arrange rapid transfer (preferably with a physician-nurse transport team in attendance en route) to a facility that has these capabilities. A thoracic vascular injury requring operative repair is indication to begin intravenous antibiotics (see "Use of Antibiotics in Multiple Trauma, p 451).

Rupture or Laceration of the Diaphragm. Most diaphragmatic injuries (90%) are on the left side. In a multiple-trauma patient who is likely to have ileus, hypoventilation due to splinting of an injured chest wall, and some degree of associated hemothorax, physical examination is unreliable in immediate diagnosis or exclusion of diaphragmatic rupture and herniation: the absence of bowel sounds over the lower hemithorax does not deny the diagnosis, nor do diminished breath sounds there affirm it. Earliest suspicion is likely to be aroused by recognition on the chest roentgenogram of elevation of the left hemidiaphragm, with or without radiolucent areas of intestinal lumen bordered by soft-tissue density above the usual level of the diaphragm. Elevation of the diaphragm by underlying air-dilated stomach or colon can be confusing. A nasogastric tube has usually been inserted prior to obtaining the initial chest roentgenogram; the position of the tube may identify the location of the stomach relative to the diaphragm. If a nasogastric tube has not been placed, radiographic discovery of distended gut under the diaphragm is indication for insertion. If it cannot be passed into the stomach, the reason may be distortion at the cardia by herniation of the stomach into the chest. Definitive confirmation of herniation of stomach or colon into the chest may require fluoroscopy with or without a water-soluble or barium-contrast study when physical examination and ED evaluation are complete and the patient's overall condition permits.

The diagnosis may well be missed at first, but when it is made, early operative reduction of the hernia and repair of the diaphragmatic rent should be undertaken. The presence of such a hernia may be threatening because of ventilatory compromise, which can be managed preoperatively by tracheal intubation and assisted ventilation, and because of strangulation of herniated gut, which is rare acutely. Priority of surgery is secondary to that for more immediately life-threatening thoracic, abdominal, neurologic, or peripheral vascular injuries, but repair can obviously be accomplished at thoracotomy or celiotomy performed for whatever indication. In the absence of apparently significant chest injury or previous upper abdominal surgery, an abdominal approach is usually used to allow evaluation of the abdominal viscera to which there is a high incidence of associated injury. In the presence of a major hemothorax or other significant intrathoracic injury, or if previous abdominal operations offer a good possibility of complicating the abdominal approach, the approach should be through the chest. Combined approaches may be needed in difficult cases. The general surgeon supervising overall care should determine the approach.

Tear in the Trachea or a Bronchus. Most tracheobronchial tears in a multiple-injury patient are the result of severe blunt trauma rather than of penetrating injury, and most occur within the first 2 cm to 3 cm of a main stem bronchus, just distal to the carina, where shear forces combine with a large increase in airway pressure against a closed glotis. When first seen the victim may be in extremis, with airway obstruction or tension pneumothorax or with lesser signs and symptoms of subcutaneous emphysema, hemoptysis, and pneumothorax. Most cases do not constitute an immediate threat to life, and the presence of the other "characteristic" findings is variable. The most constant findings are likely to be associated fractures of one or more of the upper five ribs (usually one of the top three), and mediastinal emphysema if the mediastinal pleura remains intact versus pneumothorax if the pleura is torn, with or without cervical subcutaneous emphysema. Thus the diagnosis in most cases is likely to be suggested by the chest roentgenogram. Confirmation depends on fiberoptic bronchoscopy, and early consultation with a thoracic surgeon is indicated.

Sufficient indications for early fiberoptic bronchoscopy include (1) airway obstruction or tension pneumothorax not rapidly improved by the procedures described as immediate considerations, (2) significant or persistent hemoptysis, (3) increasing mediastinal emphysema following blunt trauma, (4) failure of a collapsed lung to expand, and (5) persistence of a large air leak following tube thoracostomy for pneumothoax.

Visualization of any rent in the tracheobronchial tree is indication for administration of intravenous antibiotics (see "Use of Antibiotics in Multiple Trauma," p 451). Visualization of a large or irregular rent or one involving more than a third of the circumference of a major bronchus is indication for early operative repair. If the patient is tolerating the leak reasonably well and there are no other problems immediately threatening life or limb, surgery can await completion of physical examination, important ED procedures such as electrocardiography and peritoneal lavage, crucial radiographic studies, and stabilization of other injuries. Reliable ventilation must certainly be ensured before surgery is undertaken for coexisting injuries. If the patient is tolerating the leak poorly or if there are coexisting thoracic, abdominal, neurologic, or peripheral vascular injuries that do represent immediate threat to life and limb, rapid removal to the operating room is indicated. Along with control of exsanguinating hemorrhage and release of cardiac tamponade, operative repair of a life-threatening ineffective airway is of top priority.

Esophageal Injury. Early signs of esophageal injury may be even more subtle, but the devastating consequences of delayed recognition make rapid diagnosis even more crucial. Hematemesis is a helpful but inconsistent sign. Mediastinal emphysema or pneumothorax is usually present. Early subcutaneous emphysema is less consistent, depending on the level of injury. If mediastinal emphysema is present and fiberoptic bronchoscopy does not reveal obvious airway damage, esophageal injury should be suspected. If pneumothorax is present and chest tube drainage demonstrates return of gastric fluid, a persistent air leak, or both, esophageal injury should be suspected. As soon as physical examination is complete, important ED studies such as electrocardiography and peritoneal lavage have been accomplished, and management of more immediately life-threatening injuries is under way, any suspicion of esophageal rupture is an indication for esophagography using a water-soluble contrast medium or barium. Should removal to surgery for a more emergent life- or limb-threatening injury preclude esophagography, fiberoptic esophagoscopy may be performed in the operating room. Demonstration of an esophageal rent is an indication for intravenous administration of antibiotics (see "Use of Antibiotics in Multiple Trauma," p 451) and for early repair and drainage by a thoracic, otolaryngologic, or general surgeon, depending on location and associated injuries. Operative priority is second to control of hemorrhage and other immediately life- and limb-threatening cardiopulmonary, neurologic, and vascular injuries.

Pulmonary Contusion, Aspiration, and ARDs. Massive pulmonary contusion with cardiopulmonary decompensation was described in the discussion of immediate considerations. Pulmonary contusion without immediate symptoms is likely to be diagnosed by the characteristic appearance of fluffy densities on the chest roentgenogram. This radiographic appearance may be indistinguishable from that in other problems common to a multiple-injury patient: aspiration and ARDS. The apparent degree of dyspnea, arterial blood gas values, and size of densities on the chest film are major determinants of need for mechanical ventilatory support for these conditions. Progressively poor lung compliance and low arterial oxygen tension despite an increasing fraction of inspired oxygen are characteristic. Thus if mechanical ventilatory support is needed, the patient is also likely to benefit from use of PEEP. Less agreed on but probably also beneficial are (1) early intravenous administration of a single pharmacologic dose (30 mg/kg) of methylprednisolone sodium succinate, (2) intravenous administration of antibiotics (see "Use of Antibiotics in Multiple Trauma," p 451), and (3) when vascular volume expansion and adequate tissue perfusion are assured, judicious use of fluid restriction to reduce fluid accumulation in the lung, and diuretics (furosemide 20 mg to 40 mg intravenously) to enhance urine output.

While excessive administration of crystalloid may produce pulmonary edema in any patient, a trauma patient with pulmonary contusion is at special risk. Even minimal overloading with crystalloid can increase pulmonary capillary congestion, interstitial edema, and intra-alveolar fluid. When pulmonary contusion is identified without evidence of coexisting blood loss and systemic perfusion deficit, crystalloid fluid restriction can be instituted immediately in the ED. However, in a patient with multiple trauma in whom pulmonary contusion or ARDS coexists with other injuries, the need to expand the vascular volume sufficiently to ensure adequate tissue perfusion must initially take priority over the desire to restrict fluid infusion in order to reduce fluid accumulation in the lungs. This is because experience has shown that sacrificing renal and other systemic perfusion to dry out the lungs will usually result in *increased* morbidity and mortality. The best one can safely do in this situation in the ED is to lean toward relatively greater use of blood, in preference to crystalloid, to replace estimated blood losses, provided that adequate urine output (≥0.5 ml/kg/hr) and perfusion pressure can be maintained. Fluid and ventilatory management in this situation requires hemodynamic monitoring in an intensive care unit if critical adjustments relative to both these priorities are to be achieved. If this level of care is not available at the facility at which a patient with a major pulmonary contusion is initially received, early transfer to a critical-care facility, with a transport team in attendance capable of providing ventilatory support en route, is indicated.

The presence of a large pulmonary contusion clearly implies significant mechanical damage to lung tissue. Preoperative prophylactic insertion of a chest tube is indicated in a trauma patient with pulmonary contusion who requires surgery under general endotracheal anesthesia for other injuries.

Myocardial Contusion; Myocardial Infarction; Cardiogenic Shock. Myocardial contusion or myocardial infarction may contribute to early cardiogenic shock but more likely will be evidenced in the ED only by ECG changes characteristic for injury: elevation of ST-T segment, inversion of T wave, premature ventricular contractions, and later by enzyme changes. As with myocardial infarction, latent development of arrhythmias or heart failure represents threat to life following cardiac contusion. Thus diagnosis or suspicion of myocardial contusion is an indication to treat as for myocardial infarction: bed rest, continuous ECG monitoring, serial 12-lead ECGs and cardiac enzyme determinations, and appropriate treatment of any arrhythmias that develop. With an older patient, there is always the confusing possibility of a myocardial infarction being superimposed on other injuries. The myocardial event may be primary, the heart attack having caused the patient to fall off the ladder or drive into the power pole, or secondary, the stress of the impact triggering the myocardial infarction. Even in an alert nonamnesic patient the history may obscure the diagnosis, chest pain easily being accounted for by the impact or even superseded by discomfort from other injuries.

Myocardial infarction, severe myocardial contusion, or preexisting left ventricular disease may indeed result in shock of the cardiogenic category and is very likely to confound the trauma surgeon initially if diagnosis is not obvious on the ECG. The problem facing the trauma team may well be hypotension and oliguria that persist despite (1) apparently adequate fluid resuscitation, (2) apparently adequate effort to correct any airway or pulmonary problems that have been identified, and (3) apparent exclusion of distributive and obstructive causes of shock on the basis of physical examination. As with cardiac tamponade the explanation lies between continuing blood loss and pump failure.

Monitoring filling pressure of the right side of the heart by means of a central venous pressure (CVP) catheter may not immediately provide an accurate distinction. A high CVP (above 14 cm H_2O) should exclude hypovolemia, but it does not distinguish right-sided heart failure (due to fluid overload relative to what the pump can handle) from tamponade. A low or normal CVP should exclude tamponade and right-sided heart failure but does not distinguish hypovolemia from left-sided heart failure. (Note: In the presence of left ventricular disease or injury, left atrial pressure may be distinctly elevated although right atrial pressure is normal. Accurate assessment of left-sided filling pressure requires use of a Swan–Ganz pulmonary artery catheter.)

Since hypovolemia is the most common explanation for hypotension in the presence of a low or normal CVP in a trauma patient, and since insertion of a Swan–Ganz pulmonary artery catheter usually awaits removal to the intensive care unit, the usual course of action in the ED is to vigorously infuse more fluid and blood. In the patient with myocardial infarction or severe cardiac (or pulmonary) contusion, this may lead to further decompensation. To avoid this risk in the patient in whom the differential rests between hypovolemic and cardiogenic shock, the following alternative is applicable in the ED (or the ICU): Unless medical antishock trousers are already in place or lower body injuries preclude their use, MAST can be applied and inflated, rapidly increasing effective peripheral vascular resistance. If the cause of hypotension is persistent hypovolemia, there should be immediate improvement in circulatory dynamics. Vigorous volume expansion should be continued, and the MAST gradually deflated as described in the section on abdominal injuries. However, if the hypotension is cardiogenic in origin, the increased resistance will result in no improvement, or even deterioration, in cardiovascular performance. The MAST can then be rapidly deflated, with return to baseline before pulmonary edema can develop. (Caution must be exercised in interpreting response to fluid challenge in the trauma patient whose shock is suspected of being cardiogenic in origin. As previously noted, multiple trauma may result in shock of multiple causes.)

With or without ECG evidence of myocardial injury, persistent hypotension despite (1) apparently ensuring adequate vascular volume, (2) providing satisfactory ventilation, and (3) excluding cardiac tamponade is an indication to begin an intravenous drip of dopamine in the ED (starting at 2 μg/kg/min to 4 μg/kg/min and titrating to the desired increase in blood pressure) to support systemic circulation.

At this point a number of absolute indications for hemodynamic monitoring have accumulated: There is urgency in determining if heart failure is present, because if this is indeed the problem, excessive vascular volume expansion may lead to pulmonary edema; while at the other extreme, "flogging" an injured heart with an inotropic agent in the presence of an insufficient ventricular preload will also be detrimental. At this juncture things are sufficiently confusing so that definitive diagnosis demands measurement of pulmonary artery occlusion (wedge) pressure as an index of left ventricular filling, and preferably determination of cardiac output so that stroke work index, as an indication of left ventricular function, and systemic vascular resistance, as an index of afterload, can be calculated. If systemic vascular resistance is increased, pharmacologic measures to decrease afterload (nitroprusside) are indicated in addition to those already under way to increase contractility (dopamine). Use of nitroprusside also mandates continuously monitoring arterial pressure. To do all of the above requires (1) insertion of a Swan–Ganz pulmonary artery catheter (preferably with a thermistor tip for use in the thermodilution method of determination of cardiac output) and (2) insertion of an indwelling arterial cannula. These procedures are accomplished better in an intensive care unit or operating room than in the ED.

Thus evidence or strong suspicion of cardiogenic shock and need for pharmacologic circulatory support are indications for early removal to the intensive care unit or operating room as soon as the physical examination and crucial ED studies can be completed. If circulatory dynamics do not respond quickly to appropriate fluid balance and pharmacologic manipulations as indicated by monitored and calculated hemodynamic parameters, consultation with a critical-care specialist is indicated. Consideration may be given to support with a mechanical circulatory assistance device or transfer to a facility that has one, a transport team being in attendance en route.

Follow-up Studies. Beyond these dozen specifically described major chest injuries, what remains are less serious problems of rib fractures and lesser degrees of pneumothorax or hemothorax, pulmonary or myocardial contusion, with regard to which need for early diagnosis and treatment is less critical unless there is a sudden change or evolution. To prevent omission or sudden change from leading to catastrophe because of delayed recognition, repeat chest examination, particularly in conjunction with airway reassessment, is an important component of ED management of the multiple-injury patient. Repeat roentgenography of the chest is indicated shortly after any invasive manipulation, including tracheal intubation, placement of central venous catheters, thoracocentesis, pericardiocentesis, and insertion of chest tubes. Repeat films should also be obtained within 4 hours after identification of any thoracic abnormality that could abruptly and progressively change in a trauma patient, such as pneumothorax, hemothorax, enlarged cardiac or mediastinal shadow, pneumomediastinum, pulmonary contusion, and aspiration pneumonia. Standard roentgenography of the chest is the subsequent study of choice when rib fracture is suspected (whether or not demonstrated on the initial chest film). A common error in this situation is to send the patient to the x-ray department for a lengthy (and costly) series of rib-detail films, when potential injury to structures underlying the chest wall is of much more immediate concern.

Some problems may remain lethal sleepers, particularly vascular injuries. Although widening of the mediastinum may not be obvious with chest roentgenography, angiography should also be considered when there is a penetrating wound in proximity to great vessels; a history of blood previously spurting from a wound; an expanding hematoma in the lower neck; or severe chest wall trauma, particularly fracture of the sternum or first two ribs.

Abdominopelvic Injury: Second-Pass Considerations

The two major threats to life in abdominal trauma are hemorrhage and infection. Although hemorrhage remains the most immediate threat, intra-abdominal sepsis has become a more common cause of death in those patients who survive the initial insult and are successfully resuscitated. The source of peritoneal cavity contamination is most commonly internal, from hollow viscus injury; less commonly external, a result of direct entry from a penetrating wound (poorly cared for surgical drain sites included); and even less commonly, hematogenous seeding of devitalized injured tissues. The presence of significant intra-abdominal hemorrhage, a perforated or ruptured hollow viscus, or laceration or severe contusion of the pancreatobiliary tree structures are all absolute indications for early exploratory celiotomy. Surgical exploration per se is an almost certain means of identifying or excluding such injuries. However, although there will likely be benefit from a procedure that accomplishes something therapeutic, it is in the patient's interest to avoid an operation that is only diagnostic. Prolonged observation or extensive studies to confirm severity of injury, and unnecessary celiotomy in a patient with serious and complicated associated injuries, may be equally disastrous. The crucial question in assessment of abdominal trauma in the ED, therefore, is how to determine rapidly and accurately whether there is injury to major vessels, gut, or solid viscera that requires early celiotomy for control and repair. A survey of the usual means of assessment—history, physical examination, laboratory data, and radiographic studies—unfortunately discloses that they are not always accurate.

Critique of Diagnostic Criteria for Surgical Intervention. History is too often unavailable, as with unconscious or intubated patients, or unreliable, because of intoxication or, in certain assault cases, intent to evade. Pain remains the most significant complaint, but its perception may be significantly modified by coexisting injuries and by the effect of alcohol and drugs. Intense pain at fracture sites may divert attention from abdominal discomfort. Primary shoulder injury and abdominal injury with referred discomfort due to irritation of the diaphragm both may elicit a compliant of shoulder pain. Nausea and vomiting are common to many trauma patients and are nonspecific.

Physical examination, repeated at close intervals to detect changes, remains the cornerstone of diagnosis in abdominal trauma as in other abdominal states. Although careful physical examination may reveal a number of highly significant findings (see "Immediate Considerations," p 397), many deserve some qualifying comments. Absence of obvious abdominal wall injury does not rule out the presence of extensive intra-abdominal damage. There may be a 3- to 4-day delay before the appearance of extensive ecchymoses associated with retroperitoneal or deep abdominal wall injuries. The intrathoracoabdominal pathway of missiles cannot be predicted reliably from entrance and exit wounds because of a variety of possible positions of a patient at the time of injury and the possibility of internal skeletal deflections. In a crouching individual the diaphragm may reach the level of the fourth intercostal space; therefore any penetrating chest wound below the nipple line must be considered a potential thoracoabdominal injury. The presence or absence of bowel sounds is a poor criterion on which to base a decision in the immediate post-trauma setting, inasmuch as about 30% of patients with a significant intra-abdominal injury will have active bowel sounds, and 30% of patients with a quiet abdomen will not have operative abdominal injuries. The presence of bowel sounds in the chest is very suggestive of a diaphragmatic defect (acute or chronic), but their absence in that location does not rule out such injury. A bruit is present only in the minority of acute vascular injuries. The presence of a palpable pulse distally does not exclude the presence of major vessel injury proximally. Abdominal wall contusion or lower rib fractions may result in muscle spasm of the abdominal wall that prevents deep palpation and that can easily be confused with guarding related to chemical irritation of the peritoneum from blood or upper gastrointestinal contents. Reaction of different individuals to free blood or bile in the peritoneal cavity is quite variable, one person experiencing intense irritation from slight bleeding, while another may tolerate a large hemoperitoneum or bile leak without complaint. Leakage from the colon may exist without symptoms for hours, until a secondary inflammatory reaction is established. Alcohol and drugs in the system at the time of injury may markedly alter findings on abdominal examination.

Certain laboratory data can be quite helpful when abnormal, but otherwise are nondiagnostic. Except in chronic anemic states such as renal failure, a very low hematocrit value after injury must be interpreted as reflecting acute hemorrhage (particularly if some time has passed since injury and intravenous crystalloid has been administered). However, a normal hematocrit value after injury does not exclude significant acute hemorrhage: Initially what leaves the vascular compartment and what remains within it have the same fraction of red cells. Only when what remains within the vascular compartment becomes diluted by translocation of interstitial fluid or by intravenous crystalloid infusion will the hematocrit value decrease. As previously described in the section on shock and fluid resuscitation, when a prolonged period of profound hypotension is associated with hemorrhage, a substantial fraction of what was formerly functional extracellular fluid may become unavailable for immediate attraction to the vascular space. Thus even with acute hemorrhage to the point of shock, several hours may pass before there is a significant fall in the hematocrit value. For most multiple-trauma patients delivered to the ED shortly after injury, a significant decline in the hematocrit value is detected only after crystalloid fluid resuscitation.

Initial white blood cell counts in the range of 20,000 to 30,000 or more are associated with splenic injury, myocardial injury, and retroperitoneal bleeding, but counts in this range are so common in multiple-injury patients in general, particularly those experiencing blunt deceleration trauma, that early postinjury leukocytosis can usually be given no specific interpretation. It certainly cannot be interpreted as representing infection. A persistent increase in serum amylase is fairly diagnostic of significant pancreatoduodenal contusion or laceration or small-bowel perforation. However, even in the presence of significant pancreatoduodenal injury, the amylase level becomes elevated less than half the time, and often the elevation is not observed for 1 or 2 days after injury. Thus in the absence of readily diagnosed pancreatoduodenal damage, serial serum amylase determinations are needed after abdominal trauma, and normal values in the first 24 hours do not exclude significant injury.

Roentgenographic examination of the abdomen in the ED is not always helpful. Even high-quality anteroposterior supine plain films are notoriously unreliable in detecting small amounts of free air or even large quantities of free blood in the peritoneal cavity (because of unfavorable distribution and poor-density contrast with adjacent tissues). To increase probability of demonstrating free intraperitoneal air it is necessary to leave the patient in the left lateral decubitus (liver up) position for several minutes, or better, obtain a posterioanterior chest film after the patient has been upright for several minutes. Unfortunately, the overall condition and associated injuries of most multiple-injury patients preclude such positioning with safety.

Therefore, because of (1) the lack of specificity and difficulty in interpretation of abdominal findings on initial physical examination and laboratory and ED x-ray studies, (2) the potentially calamitous consequences of delayed recognition of and intervention for a significant vascular or visceral injury in the abdomen, and (3) the desire to minimize the number of unnecessary celiotomies performed, an algorithm is needed to determine whether the need is for early removal to the operating room or for additional study and observation of the patient with a suspected abdominal injury (Fig. 23-21). The first decision in this protocol is whether the abdominal injury is penetrating or nonpenetrating.

Penetrating Abdominal Injuries. Penetrating abdominal injuries can be further categorized as high velocity or low velocity. It is generally agreed that all gunshot wounds, other high-velocity missile injuries, and high-speed deceleration "impalement" injuries of the abdomen deserve urgent exploration. The benefit-to-

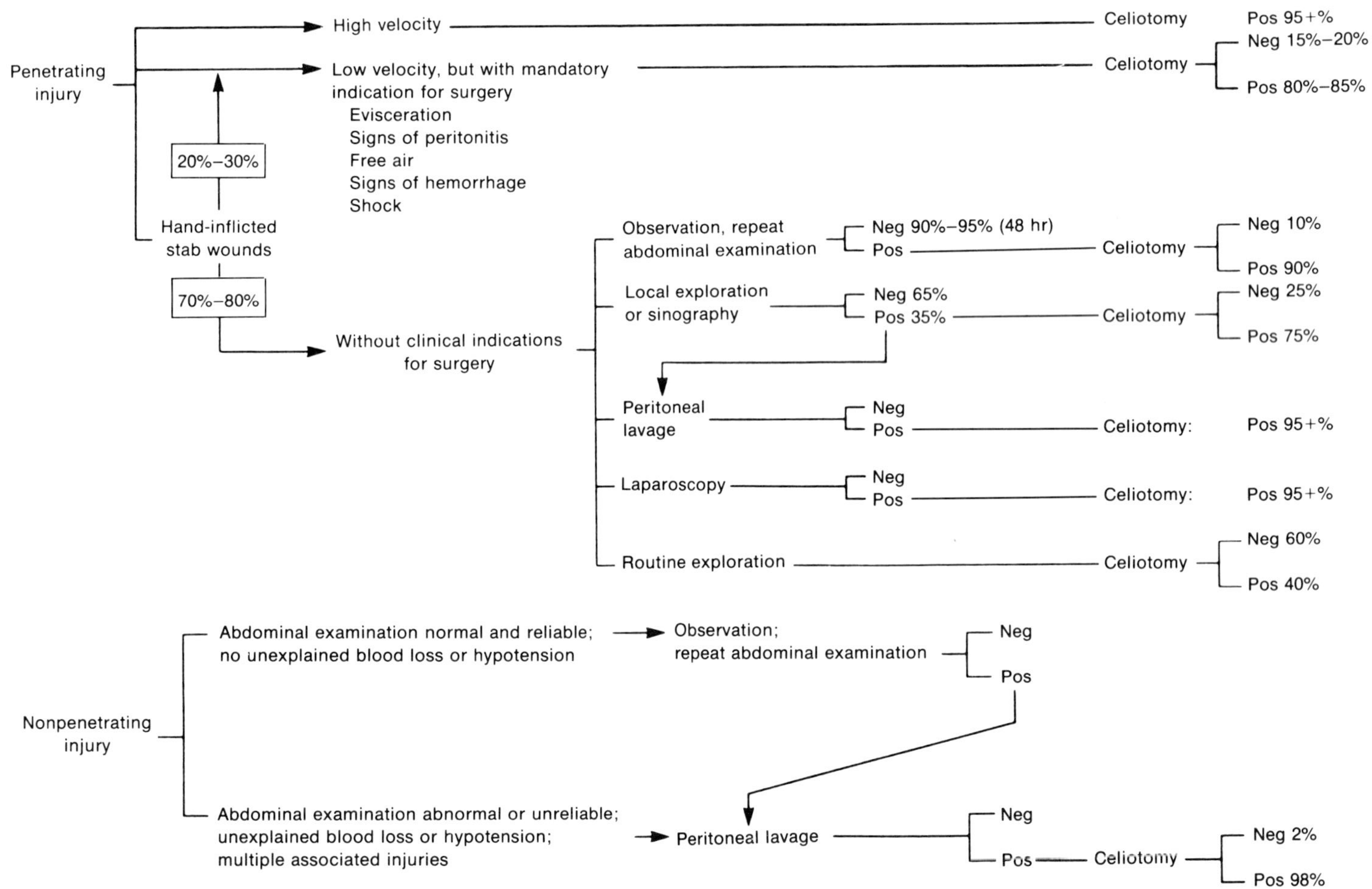

Figure 23-21. Algorithm for triage of abdominal trauma and decision for surgery.

risk ratio for routine exploration is favorable because of the high probability that a rigid object impacting the abdominal wall at high velocity will penetrate the peritoneal cavity, and that, having penetrated, it will retain sufficient energy to cause significant visceral or vascular injury or both. Even tangential bullet wounds that apparently miss the peritoneal cavity should usually be explored, as visceral disruption can result from energy absorbed. Possible exceptions to this dictum are small-caliber, relatively low-velocity bullet wounds that appear to be tangential, and wounds in which the slug is visible superficially in the abdominal wall (.22-caliber weapon and "long-range" shotgun wounds manifested by a few subcutaneous pellets embedded in a wide pattern are in this category).

Also of general agreement is urgent exploratory celiotomy for low-velocity penetrating abdominal wounds in patients who exhibit any of the following "mandatory" indications for surgical intervention: (1) evisceration, (2) signs of peritonitis (guarding, rebound tenderness, absence of bowel sounds), (3) free air, or (4) evidence of intra-abdominal hemorrhage (shock, gastrointestinal bleeding, hematuria, positive paracentesis or peritoneal lavage). These findings are present in about 20% to 30% of all stab-wound patients received in EDs.

Of less than total agreement is the philosophy that hand-inflicted stab wounds of the abdomen in patients presenting without any of the preceding mandatory indications for early exploration can be managed selectively, under close observation, with celiotomy being reserved for those who manifest specific indications rather than being performed routinely. Routine immediate exploration of stab-wound patients has generally fallen into disfavor because of a high percentage of negative explorations (well over 60%), coupled with high percentages of morbidity and mortality associated with them (reported as high as 33% and 7%, respectively, in some series). The benefit-to-risk ratio for routine exploration would be expected to be much less favorable than that for high-velocity penetrating wounds because a considerably smaller fraction of hand-inflicted wounds actually penetrate the peritoneal cavity, and, even with penetration, there is often only surgically insignificant injury (60% to 75% of cases).

Nevertheless there are definite risks for the 5% to 10% of stab-wound patients who have serious abdominal injuries but who, on admission, do not have clinical indications for surgery. Close observation implies repeated abdominal evaluation at 1- to 2-hour intervals by the same examiner, plus frequent complete blood counts and abdominal plain-film studies, a costly routine that lends itself only to an environment where full-time in-house physician coverage is available, and even then not to a trauma service so busy that personnel are unavailable to frequently reexamine the patients who are being "observed." For the multiple-injury patient, as previously described, associated extra-abdominal injuries (particularly head injury) and the effect of alcohol and drugs may invalidate abdominal findings. For these reasons, alternatives to the polar choices of routine exploration or observation have been widely used. In ascending order of probability of accurately identifying a surgically significant vascular or visceral injury these include (1) an x-ray contrast sinographic study of the stab wound, (2) local exploration of the stab wound, (3) diagnostic peritoneal lavage, and (4) laparoscopy. Although valuable adjuncts, all of these precedures have distinct drawbacks in evaluation of abdominal knife wounds.

The first two, a "stabogram" and exploration of the wound under local anesthesia, are intended to determine if the knife has penetrated the peritoneum; a positive result constitutes sufficient indication for celiotomy, and a negative result excludes intra-abdominal injury. Both of these procedures suffer from three common defects: (1) a relatively high rate of false-negative results (sinography more than exploration), (2) additional tissue irritation at the wound site that is confusing in a subsequent abdominal examination if operation is not immediately undertaken, and (3) the fact that proof of entry into the peritoneal cavity does not equal proof of surgically significant intra-abdominal injury for most hand-inflicted wounds with a small knife blade. The false-negative problem arises in part from the altered orientation of layers of the abdominal wall, one to another, at the time of stabbing, compared to orientation at the time of injection of contrast medium or of dissection while the victim is lying supine on a litter. This Z-track effect tends to obliterate the straight-in path taken by the blade.

Yet in reports of large series of abdominal

stab wounds evaluated by either of these methods, although findings are positive in only 35% of patients, of those in whom penetration of the peritoneum is demonstrated, definite intra-abdominal injuries are found at operation in three out of four. Thus despite their defects, these procedures have contributed to reduction of unnecessary celiotomies.

Peritoneal lavage (see "Diagnostic Peritoneal Lavage," p 433) is so accurate in detecting free intraperitoneal blood that a heme-negative result (in conjunction with normal findings on abdominal examination) virtually rules out significant intraperitoneal hemorrhage, whereas a heme-positive result is sufficient indication to operate. In the absence of this obvious surgical indication, laboratory examination of recovered lavage fluid for white cells and amylase content is a significant aid in extending ability of the procedure to detect hollow-viscus laceration. Failure to demonstrate elevated leukocyte or amylase levels in the lavage fluid does not exclude perforation of the gut, but (again in conjunction with normal findings on abdominal examination) it certainly reflects a low probability of an established leak with significant spill. In most instances it is surprising how insignificantly peritoneal lavage alters response on subsequent abdominal examination.

Except in posterior stab wounds, laparoscopy offers excellent opportunity to identify penetration of the peritoneum and laceration of the liver (among solid viscera the most commonly injured by penetrating trauma), of the anterior aspect of the diaphragm, and of the superior aspect of the bladder. There is also high probability of detecting a significant amount of free blood or gastrointestinal contents, although a small hemoperitoneum or gut laceration without large spill could well be missed. Laparoscopy usually requires removal of the patient to the operating room and administration of a general anesthetic and incurs the added cost of a surgical fee for two procedures if exploratory celiotomy follows, all major drawbacks that preclude convenient or frequent performance.

As assessment procedures for abdominal stab wounds, peritoneal lavage and laparoscopy offer greater opportunity to determine the presence or absence of significant vascular or visceral injury, as opposed to simply determination of penetration or nonpenetration of the peritoneum by the other two procedures. From our point of view the former determination is of distinct advantage in a multiple-injury patient because an unnecessary celiotomy may have a distinctly negative influence on management of coexisting extra-abdominal injuries. Peritoneal lavage and local wound exploration are particularly attractive from the standpoint of being inexpensive and rapidly performed procedures that provide an immediate decision-making result without need to remove the patient from the ED. This affords the ED trauma team maximum opportunity to gain and maintain control of associated injuries and to evaluate them simultaneously.

Circumstances surrounding each patient's presentation and relating to the setting of each surgeon's practice must necessarily be weighed in the decision regarding the most appropriate management for any individual abdominal stab wound. An asymptomatic person who appears many hours after a single penknife wound of the abdomen is obviously a candidate only for continued observation. An assault victim who arrives unconscious a short time after apparently being stabbed in the abdomen, shot in the chest, and kicked in the head will suffer either from delay in surgical intervention, should there be serious intra-abdominal injury, or from an unnecessary celiotomy; thus peritoneal lavage in the ED may be the best guide to immediate management in relation to associated injuries. A busy major medical center trauma service may have insufficient house staff in relation to ED volume to perform either exploratory celiotomy or hourly abdominal reexamination on each stabbed patient who does not initially have clinical indications for surgery. In this situation, exploration of wounds under local anesthesia in the ED might be the best compromise. The benefit-to-risk ratio associated with early exploratory celiotomy is increased in multiple stab wounds and stab wounds near the lower rib margin in which there is high likelihood of penetration of the diaphragm. A community hospital surgeon in private practice without house staff coverage who infrequently treats abdominal trauma and rarely sees abdominal stab wounds cannot be faulted for leaning toward exploration of abdominal stab-wound patients who appear at short interval after injury and without significant contraindication to surgery.

Identification of penetrating abdominal injury with decision for celiotomy is indication to administer intravenous antibiotics preoperatively in the ED (see "Use of Antibiotics in Multiple Trauma," p 451). When an abdominal injury is declared to be penetrating but the decision is for observation instead of operation, antibiotics should probably be withheld. Their use in this circumstance is more likely to delay recognition of peritonitis than to prevent infection. Things obviously become more complicated in a multiple-injury patient when antibiotics administered for an extra-abdominal injury may obscure a problem developing in the abdomen.

Nonpenetrating Abdominal Injury. Nonpenetrating injury is the more common form of abdominal trauma associated with multiple injuries in civilians. For purposes of assessment of potential intra-abdominal injury, patients with nonpenetrating trauma may be conveniently divided into two groups: (1) those in whom abdominal examination reveals no abnormalities (the examination being judged reliable) and who have suffered neither unexplained blood loss nor hypotension, and (2) those in whom abdominal examination shows abnormalities, whose examination is judged to be potentially invalid, or who have unexplained blood loss or hypotension, or both. In a patient who is alert and cooperative and who does not have confusing associated injuries, the presence or absence of abdominal pain and the findings on physical examination are highly accurate in identifying the presence or absence of significant blunt intra-abdominal injury.

For patients in group 1, absence of abdominal complaints or findings in the presence of normal vital signs, normal hematocrit, and active bowel sounds virtually rules out significant hemoperitoneum or visceral perforation with spill of upper gastrointestinal contents, and physical examination therefore constitutes sufficient evaluation.

For patients in group 2, abdominal pain plus guarding and rebound tenderness are very suggestive of peritoneal irritation from blood or intestinal contents. Unfortunately, these same symptoms and signs may be present (in the absence of hemoperitoneum or intestinal spill) due to associated injuries such as abdominal wall contusion or fractured ribs or pelvis, or they may be absent (in the presence of hemoperitoneum or intestinal spill) due to variable patient response, associated neurologic injury, or altered state of consciousness, any of which may make abdominal examination unreliable. When hypotension, unexplained blood loss, or both are present, the inability to distinguish quickly and accurately the presence or absence of hemorrhagic injury within the abdomen on the basis of physical examination becomes even more distressing. Unlike other locations where major hemorrhage is easily discernible by physical examination and roentgenography (thorax, long-bone fracture sites), or in which spontaneous tamponade is likely (fracture sites, retroperitoneum), the peritoneal cavity is able to sequester a significant volume of blood that is not readily evident and where tamponade does not readily occur. Thus in blunt trauma, basing decision to explore or not explore the abdomen only on physical examination (and plain x-ray study) too frequently has resulted in either unnecessary celiotomy or late surgical intervention. It is for this reason that diagnostic peritoneal lavage has become the mainstay in the evaluation of blunt abdominal trauma for patients in group 2 (see "Diagnostic Peritoneal Lavage," p 433).

Popularized by Root and associates in 1965, peritoneal lavage has assumed this key role in diagnosis of blunt abdominal trauma because it is a procedure that has demonstrated itself to be (1) extremely accurate in identifying the presence or absence of significant intraperitoneal hemorrhage (false-positive and -negative rates less than 2%), (2) very safe (associated morbidity less than 5%), and (3) inexpensive and easy to perform in the ED to produce a decision-making result early in the course of overall evaluation without need to remove the patient from immediate supervision of the trauma team. The guidance provided by peritoneal lavage, both in avoiding unnecessary celiotomy and in earlier identification of hemoperitoneum and intestinal leakage as indications for celiotomy, is so important in evaluation and management of a multiple-injury patient, and the procedure so simple, that every emergency physician and outpatient surgeon who must deal with abdominal trauma should be familiar with its use.

The majority of multiple-injury patients with blunt abdominal trauma fall into group 2. "Indications and Contraindications for Diagnostic Peritoneal Lavage" (p 432) lists indications for and relative contraindications and

INDICATIONS AND CONTRAINDICATIONS FOR DIAGNOSTIC PERITONEAL LAVAGE

Indications in Group 2 Blunt Abdominal Trauma Patients

Abdominal pain, positive abdominal examination, or both
Hypotension, unexplained blood loss, or both
Neurologic injury, altered state of consciousness, or both, rendering patient unable to complain or abdominal examination unreliable
Associated injuries (extensive abdominal wall contusion, gross hematuria, fractured lower ribs, spine, pelvis) that make intra-abdominal injury suspect and that may confuse abdominal examination
Extra-abdominal injuries requiring an interval under anesthesia for early repair

Absolute Contraindications

Decision to operate anyway (penetrating injury, rapidly expanding abdomen, and hypotension)
Gravid uterus near term

Relative Contraindications (A Seldinger Technique Entry Can Be Made at a Site Away From Scar or Hematoma)

Inability to empty the urinary bladder (unlikely)
Previous lower abdominal surgery
Abdominal wall hematoma

Alternatives

Bilateral needle paracentesis*
Repeated abdominal examination and monitoring of vital signs
Computed tomography imaging of the abdomen
Exploratory celiotomy

* Caution: up to 40% false-negative rates reported

alternatives to use of peritoneal lavage in evaluation of group 2 patients.

Diagnostic Peritoneal Lavage. Two kinds of catheters are readily available and in common use for diagnostic peritoneal lavage: the trocar type and the Seldinger technique introducer type. With the trocar method (Peridial or Trocath) initial entry of a 27-cm-long plastic dialysis catheter into the peritoneal cavity is made either by direct cutdown ("minilaparotomy") or by applying firm pressure to a 2-mm-diameter steel stylet inserted through the dialysis catheter so as to pop through the abdominal wall fascia and peritoneum. With the Seldinger catheter introducer method (Lazarus–Neson or Arrow) initial entry into the peritoneal cavity is made with 7.5-cm, 18-gauge thin-wall steel needle, through which a 36-cm, 0.9-mm-diameter floppy tip vascular-type guide wire is inserted into the peritoneal cavity. The needle is removed; a 14.5-cm, 2-mm-internal-diameter bevel tip plastic catheter with several side holes is advanced over the guide wire into the peritoneal cavity; the guide wire then is removed (see "Diagnostic Peritoneal Lavage: Seldinger Technique," p 433).

Choice of catheter should be influenced by ease of use, effectiveness in performing a diagnostically meaningful lavage, and associated complication rate. Trocar dialysis catheters provide superior return of lavage fluid because of length and rigidity, allowing dependent placement in the pelvis, and large diameter with multiple side holes, facilitating rapid flow. However, if the catheter is introduced by direct cutdown, the time required for the surgical procedure (during which other diagnostic and therapeutic procedures usually are "on hold") largely negates any advantage related to rapid fluid recovery. Significant complications associated with minilaparotomy include inadvertent enterotomy, incisional hernia, wound infection, wound hematoma, and wound separation. Associated with stylet placement have been lacerations of mesenteric vessels, lacerations of iliac artery and vein, and perforations of small bowel, colon, and uterus.

With the shorter Seldinger technique catheters, more time may be required to achieve desired recovery of lavage fluid. (Gentle "sloshing" manipulation of the lateral abdominal wall may enhance return.) However rapidity of catheter introduction and ability to resume other diagnostic and therapeutic procedures promptly while lavage is under way usually more than compensate for relatively slower fluid outflow. Seldinger technique introduction of diagnostic lavage catheters may be complicated by misplacement between tissue planes in the abdominal wall instead of entry into the peritoneal cavity, as well as by perforation of viscera and vessels. Yet in the hands of nonsurgeons, and when used to evaluate patients with relative contraindications to diagnostic lavage, the complication rate associated with use of the smaller wire-guided catheters appears to be lower than with use of the larger dialysis catheters. With the Seldinger technique, initial entry into the peritoneal cavity with an 18-gauge needle obviates need for either deep cutdown or great pres-

Diagnostic Peritoneal Lavage: Seldinger Technique

Equipment Needed

prepackaged peritoneal lavage catheter tray
1 intravenous tubing set with drip chamber
1 liter bag of normal saline (or Ringer's lactate)
sterile gloves
1 bottle 1% lidocaine with epinephrine
1 bottle povidone-iodine
10 4 × 4 sterile gauze pads
1 safety razor

Method

PROCEDURE	COMMENTS
A. Have patient void, or insert Foley catheter, then assume supine position.	A. This will ensure that the bladder is not punctured.
B. Set up fluid with tubing.	
C. Shave the abdomen, don mask and gloves, prepare site with povidone-iodine solution, and drape with (fenestrated) sterile towels.	C. The preferred site is located 2 cm to 3 cm below the umbilicus in the midline. Choose another site if there is a previous lower midline surgical scar.
D. Anesthetize the skin, fascia, and peritoneum with 1% lidocaine with epinephrine. Make a skin wheal and inject a generous amount just above the peritoneal surface.	D. Lidocaine with epinephrine will reduce the likelihood of false positive lavage from abdominal wall bleeding. Not much anesthetic need be used in the subcutaneous fat layer.
E. Make a 3-mm to 5-mm stab incision through the dermis with a no. 11 blade, down to or partially through the fascia.	E. This facilitates placement of the dialysis catheter by reducing resistance to entry.
F. The 18-gauge needle is then introduced posteriorly at a slightly inferior direction in the midsagittal plane (Fig. 23-22, *large drawing*) so that it is pointed toward the center of the pelvic hollow. When the fascia and peritoneum are penetrated, the needle should be advanced another 2 mm to 3 mm within the abdominal cavity.	F. The patient will momentarily experience pain as the needle penetrates the peritoneum. If the patient is able to cooperate, tension of the abdominal muscles during introduction of the needle aids this step.
G. The floppy end of the wire guide is introduced through the needle into the peritoneum (Fig. 23-22). If the guide wire does not fall easily into the abdomen, remove the wire and advance the needle several millimeters until the wire does fall freely into the abdominal cavity.	G. The guide should fall easily into the abdomen if the needle has in fact penetrated the fascia and the peritoneum.

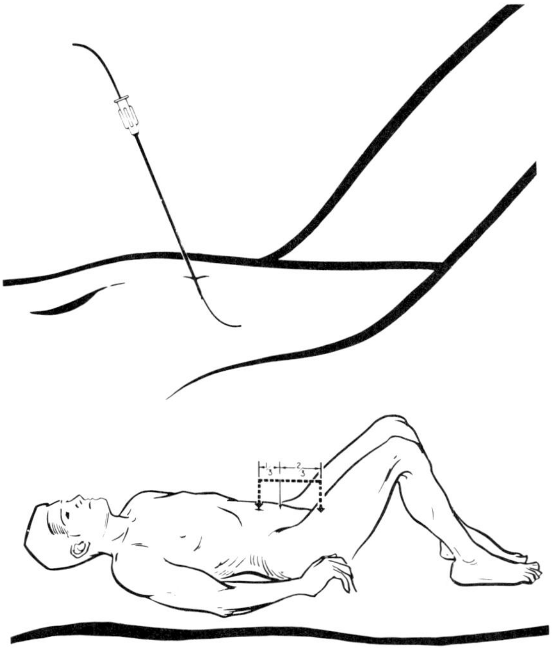

Figure 23-22. In the Seldinger technique for peritoneal lavage, an 18-gauge needle is introduced (large drawing) into the peritoneal cavity in the midline, one-third of the distance between the umbilicus and the symphysis pubis (small drawing). A floppy tip guide wire is inserted through the needle. (Lazarus HM, Nelson JA: A technique for peritoneal lavage without risk or complications. Surg Gynecol Obstet 149:889–892, 1979)

H. After approximately half the length of the wire is in the peritoneum, remove the needle.	H. Always leave sufficient wire outside the abdomen so that it can easily be grasped for withdrawal.
I. The plastic catheter is now placed over the wire and introduced into the peritoneum with a twisting, pushing motion applied to the catheter at the skin level so as to penetrate the fascia (Fig. 23-23).	I. The stiff end of the wire must be visible exiting from the end of the catheter.
J. After the catheter is introduced and advanced, the wire guide is removed.	J. The catheter is now ready for aspiration and lavage.
K. Attach connector tubing to the proximal end of dialysis catheter. Then connect a 10-ml syringe to the connector tube fitting and aspirate.	K. If at least 10 ml of gross blood is freely obtained, then the tap is positive and one need not continue.
L. If the aspiration is nondiagnostic, connect intravenous tubing to the catheter and run in 20 ml/kg or up to 1 liter of Ringer's lactate or normal saline as fast as possible.	L. The fluid should run in a steady stream with the valve wide open. If not, the position of the catheter in the peritoneal cavity should be questioned.
M. After the fluid is in the peritoneal cavity, manipulate the abdomen to help mix fluids. Then invert the solution bag and set it on the floor to siphon the fluid back out.	M. Abdominal massage and minor adjustment of catheter depth may enhance return.
N. After 100 ml have returned, the fluid may be tested by trying to read newsprint through the fluid in the tubing.	N. Inability to read the newsprint constitutes a grossly positive test.
O. If gross analysis of the lavage fluid does not result in decision for celiotomy, send an aliquot of the fluid to the laboratory for red cell count, white cell count, Gram stain, culture, and amylase.	O. Red cell count greater than 100,000 is positive. A positive stain or culture usually means an injured bowel. Increased amylase or WBC count suggests pancreatic or bowel injury (see "Criteria for Interpretation of Recovered Fluid in Diagnostic Peritoneal Lavage," p 435).
P. In cases of closed head injury or cardiopulmonary injury, it is beneficial to recover as much salt solution as possible from the peritoneal cavity.	P. In such cases, recovery of lavage fluid may be attempted after infusion of only 10 ml/kg salt solution. If there is sufficient return to permit diagnosis, no more fluid need be instilled.

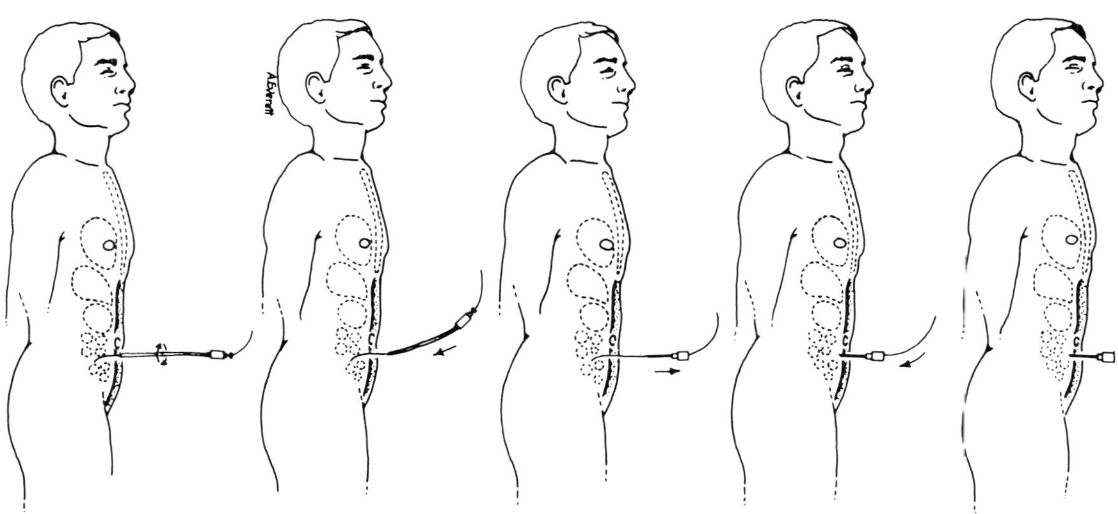

Figure 23-23. The plastic catheter is placed over the guide wire and introduced into the peritoneal cavity by means of a twisting motion at the skin level. After the catheter is advanced, the guide wire is removed. (Lazarus HM, Nelson JA: A technique for peritoneal lavage without risk or complications. Surg Gynecol Obstet 149:889–892, 1979)

sure. There is good control and sense of when the fascia and peritoneum are penetrated. (Penetration is confirmed by the ease with which the guide wire "falls" into the abdomen.) This eliminates risks associated with cutdown, or "lunging" into the peritoneal cavity with the relatively long, dull dialysis trocar. With the Seldinger technique, once the soft, floppy tip wire is in place, the only sharp object (the short 18-gauge needle) is removed. Although catheter insertion in the lower midline usually is preferred, insertion at other locations off midline can be accomplished with both ease and safety with a wire-guided catheter in contrast to a trocar catheter. (The ability to introduce a catheter elsewhere has made previous lower-abdominal surgery a "relative" contraindication to diagnostic lavage.)

Once the lavage catheter is in place, a syringe is attached for aspiration. Recovery of enteric contents or of at least 10 ml of blood is diagnostic of significant intraperitoneal injury. In this case the procedure is terminated and the catheter removed. Otherwise the catheter is connected via intravenous infusion tubing to an elevated bag of normal saline and the fluid is allowed to drain rapidly into the abdomen (a liter usually is used for lavage of adults; 15 ml/kg is used for pediatric patients). When empty, the bag is placed on the floor to recover lavage fluid by gravity and siphon effect. Recovery of all the fluid infused is desired; recovery of as little as 100 ml, particularly if "mixed," may be diagnostic.

Criteria for interpreting lavage fluid return are presented under "Criteria for Interpretation of Recovered Fluid in Diagnostic Peritoneal Lavage," above. Although accuracy of identifying laceration of a hollow viscus or of the pancreas on the basis of laboratory quantitation of white blood cell and amylase content of lavage fluid does not approach that for identifying significant hemorrhagic injury on the basis of red cell content, visceral injury is certainly suspect if these values are markedly elevated. Normal white blood cell and amylase values in lavage fluid by no means exclude such injury, particularly to retroperitoneal portions of duodenum, pancreas, or colon. However, the majority of patients with significant retroperitoneal injuries have associated peritoneal cavity injuries and, hence, heme-positive peritoneal lavage.

If lavage results are indeterminant and the patient is relatively stable and in a setting where close observation is possible, the lavage catheter may be left in place, sealed with a sterile syringe, and covered with a sterile dressing; the lavage may be repeated within 2 to 4 hours.

With closed abdominal injury, the presence of hemoperitoneum and the decision for celiotomy on that basis alone is not an absolute indication for commencing administration of antibiotics. Elevated WBC count or amylase concentration in lavage fluid, identification of free air suggesting rupture of a hollow viscus, or evidence of lower urinary tract injury (see next section) are definite indications for administration of intravenous antibiotics preoperatively in the ED (see "Use of Antibiotics in Multiple Trauma," p 451).

CRITERIA FOR INTERPRETATION OF RECOVERED FLUID IN DIAGNOSTIC PERITONEAL LAVAGE

Positive

Return of gross blood on initial syringe aspiration of catheter immediately following insertion
Lavage fluid exists via Foley catheter or chest tube
Lavage return is grossly bloody
Lavage return is bloody to extent newsprint cannot be read through fluid in the intravenous tubing
Quantitative RBC $> 100{,}000/mm^3$ ($>20{,}000/mm^3$ for penetrating injury)
Quantitative WBC $> 500/mm^3$
Quantitative amylase $> 175\ \mu/dl$

Negative

Lavage return clear
RBC $< 50{,}000/mm^3$
WBC $< 100/mm^3$
Amylase $< 75\ \mu/dl$

Equivocal

Insufficient fluid recovered to fill intravenous tubing
Lavage fluid pink, but newsprint can still be read across intravenous tubing
RBC 40,000–100,000 mm^3 (10,000–20,000/mm^3 for penetrating injury)
WBC 100–500/mm^3
Amylase 75–175 μ/dl

Abdominal Plain-Film Imaging. Along with lateral cervical spine and anteroposterior chest roentgenograms, an anteroposterior plain film of the abdomen, to include the pelvis, usually is included as a routine component of early radiographic survey of a multiple-injury patient while still in the ED. Like the C-spine and chest images, a plain film of the abdomen/pelvis can be obtained quickly and provides information that influences immediate decision making. Many injuries may be suspected from careful examination of a plain film of the abdomen (Table 23-6), although such diagnoses are made less "directly" than those gleaned from chest roentgenograms. Many of these diagnoses relate to injuries for which diagnostic peritoneal lavage would be positive; therefore decision for celiotomy would be reached independently. However, often a plain film of the abdomen provides the first indication of retroperitoneal and pelvic damage; these are injuries usually invisible to peritoneal lavage. Thus the indirect evidence of retroperitoneal or pelvic hematoma provided by an abdominal film may be very helpful in accounting for lost blood when peritoneal lavage and the chest roentgenogram are normal. Enough hemorrhage may occur in and remain confined to the retroperitoneal and pelvic spaces (several liters in an adult) to produce profound hypotension without any overt localizing sign until appearance of flank ecchymosis several days later.

As regards immediate decision making: Identification of fracture of the lumbosacral spine suggests neurologic injury that could be aggravated by injudicious repositioning during subsequent physical examination. Fracture of the pubis suggests possibility of urethral injury that could be aggravated by insertion of a bladder catheter. Of particular importance is observation of a major (class 3 or 4) pelvic fracture with marked displacement and instability. With these injuries there is almost always significant hemorrhage. While hemorrhage associated with most pelvic fractures will spontaneously tamponade, that associated with major displacement may persist at an uncomfortably brisk rate until fragments are realigned and (externally) stabilized. Therefore identification of a major pelvic fracture is indication to order at least 8 units of blood typed and cross-matched and plan to initiate blood infusion early *even in the absence of obvious signs of hypovolemic shock.*

Contrast Studies of Retroperitoneal Structures. The retroperitoneum is a difficult area to evaluate thoroughly at exploratory celiotomy. Should instability of the patient's condi-

TABLE 23-6. Diagnoses From Plain Films of the Abdomen

FINDING	PROBABLE OR POTENTIAL INJURY
Free air	Laceration or perforation of hollow viscus
Extraluminal gas (stippled or bubble appearance) in mid-upper abdomen	Retroperitoneal rupture of duodenum
Extraluminal gas in left lower quadrant	Rupture of rectosigmoid colon
Lower rib fractures	Injury to spleen or liver
Large water density mass effect in lateral upper quadrant	Injury to spleen or liver
Medial displacement of stomach with indentations along greater curvature	Splenic injury with hemorrhage into gastrosplenic ligament
Bowel-gas pattern in chest	Ruptured diaphragm
Loss of psoas shadow	Retroperitoneal hemorrhage
Enlarged renal mass shadow	Renal hemorrhage
Fracture of transverse lumbar spinous processes (particularly L1, L2)	Renal injury, pancreatic injury, retroperitoneal hematoma
Fracture of lumbosacral spine	Neurologic injury
Fracture of pubis	Bladder injury, urethral injury
Fracture of acetabulum, upper femur	Major hip injury
Fracture of iliac wing, displacement of sacroiliac joint, major acetabular disruption	Major hemorrhage
Bladder (or Foley catheter balloon) displaced upward or laterally	Pelvic hematoma, ruptured bladder
General "ground-glass" haziness, small-bowel-gas pattern "floated" to center of abdomen, separation of left or right colon-gas pattern from flank fat line	Hemoperitoneum (late signs, with large quantity of free blood)
Bullet or shrapnel fragment	Location aids in defining intra-abdominal trajectory
Nasogastric tube not in stomach	Poor tube function
Chest tube in abdomen	Iatrogenic perforation of diaphragm (± viscera)

tion deny the luxury of time to obtain this information preoperatively in the x-ray suite, intravenous pyelography, abdominal angiography, and venography can, when needed, be accomplished while the patient is on the operating table, provided that the table's configuration can accept a film cassette. An intravenous pyelogram to demonstrate the kidneys immediately before operation can be obtained by intravenous (slow, hand) injection of a bolus (100 ml to 150 ml) of diatrizoate meglumine (Renografin-60) over a 5-minute interval just prior to obtaining a supine plain film of the upper abdomen. An intraoperative aortogram or vena cavogram can be obtained by rapid upstream hand injection ("butterfly" needle-catheter attached to large syringe) of 50 ml iothalamate (Conray-60) directly into the vessel of interest. However, intraoperative roentgenography always adds anesthesia time, and the interpretation of films so obtained will always be compromised compared to that for the same studies in the x-ray suite. Thus when there is strong suspicion of retroperitoneal injury—hematuria, evidence of major arterial or venous compromise, extraluminal stippling of free air, or other question of duodenal injury—and stability of the patient's condition permits, it is very helpful to perform appropriate radiographic studies (intravenous pyelography, arteriography, venography, diatrizoate meglumine (Gastrografin) by nasogastric tube), as indicated, *before* the patient goes to the operating room.

Related to these studies in a critically ill trauma patient, three cautions are offered: (1) Rare, but significant, anaphylactic reactions have been associated with intravenous administration of these contrast agents. Positive control of the airway, or preparation for rapid intubation, and immediate availability of injectable diphenhydramine hydrochloride (50 mg in 1-ml ampule), epinephrine (1 mg in 1-ml ampule), and methylprednisolone sodium succinate (500 mg vial with dilutent) are therefore recommended. (2) Intravenously administered hyperosmolar contrast agents act as osmotic diuretics, with danger of further depleting the fluid volume of a still hypovolemic trauma patient. After an extended session of pyelography and angiography, a short interval of relative polyuria may be followed by a long interval of oliguria if continuing intravenous volume replacement is insufficient. (3) If, for special imaging studies, the patient must be transported from the ED resuscitation area to the radiology department, it is important that the patient be accompanied and constantly attended by at least one member of the trauma resuscitation team.

Synchronizing Abdominal Evaluation With CT Head Scanning. CT head scanning deserves mention again at this juncture because of the frequent association of head injury with serious abdominal injury. For a multiple-trauma patient, surgery for abdominal injury is second in priority only to that for life-threatening thoracic injury such as major airway damage, continuing hemothorax, and cardiac tamponade. Nevertheless, should a multiple-trauma patient require early removal to the operating room because of a life-threatening abdominal injury, it is best to arrange for other specialty teams to operate simultaneously on coexisting injuries that might also be threatening to life, limb, or eye. With the exception of angiography for widened mediastinum and for peripheral vascular damage, for the other major injuries (chest, limbs) commonly associated with serious abdominal injury, adequate preoperative assessment to guide emergent surgery can be made on the basis of physical examination and imaging performed in the ED. However, for assessment of intracranial bleeding, CT scanning is the ultimate means of distinguishing hemorrhage from diffuse edema and in localizing clot, and the neurosurgeon prefers not to operate without this critical information. As with unnecessary celiotomy versus unnecessary delay, the patient will not benefit from craniotomy for diffuse cerebral edema; yet in case of a rapidly expanding epidural hematoma, it may be too late on return from the operating room to obtain a CT scan. Thus when serious head injury (for which the neurosurgeon desires a CT scan) coexists with abdominal injury that mandates early celiotomy, and stability of the patient's condition permits, it is very advantageous to obtain a CT head scan before commencing a potentially lengthy abdominal operation.

Angiography. Except in aortic and renal injuries (discussed in the next section), angiography is usually not considered among the crucial studies in the initial evaluation of abdominal trauma. The information provided adds little to the initial operative approach in the vast majority of hemorrhagic injuries within the peritoneal cavity. We have found *pre*operative angiograms most helpful in connection with (1) decision for *re*operation in a complicated injury to liver, pancreas, or root of mesentery; (2) *re*evaluation (and occasionally therapeutic clot injection) of persistent bleeding from around pelvic fractures; (3) *re*-evaluation of the condition of a high-risk patient for whom unnecessary celiotomy is highly undesirable and for whom the decision for or against surgery still cannot safely be made on the basis of physical examination, vital signs, and diagnostic peritoneal lavage. With the possible exception of a patient transferred to a major medical center ED from a rural community hospital, these situations usually arise hours after initial ED evaluation. Obviously, if a patient is undergoing angiography for other reasons (evaluation of aortic arch, great vessels), access has been established via a femoral artery, and excessive contrast has not yet been injected, valuable information relative to the incremental time invested may be added by imaging vasculature of the liver, spleen, and kidneys "on the way out." Excretion of contrast provides a nephroureterogram of quality comparable to an intravenous pyleogram (IVP); therefore decision to obtain an angiogram obviates the need to order a separate IVP to image the urinary tract.

Abdominal Cross-sectional Imaging. Recently, CT scanning has been described by some trauma centers as an alternative to diagnostic peritoneal lavage for guiding the decision to perform or withhold celiotomy for nonpenetrating abdominal injury. Previously, radionuclide scanning had been suggested to fill a similar role. We suspect that in the near future, trials comparing magnetic resonance imaging (MRI) to diagnostic lavage will be reported. At present, these special imaging techniques remain subordinate to diagnostic peritoneal lavage in guiding the decision to perform exploratory celiotomy for the majority of multiple-trauma patients, for the following reasons: (1) Diagnostic lavage can be performed relatively quickly and early in the course of evaluation in the ED with the entire resuscitation team in immediate attendance and without need for transport equipment, whereas cross-sectional imaging usually must await removal from the resuscitation area to a special radiology suite for a more lengthy procedure and it involves a transport team and often "special" life support equipment. (For critically ill patients, even "elective" MRI scanning may have to await development of life support equipment compatible with the powerful magnetic forces involved.) (2) The findings related to diagnostic lavage are easily interpretable by the ED and trauma team personnel in attendance at any hour, whereas "definitive" interpretation of cross-sectional images usually requires a "special studies" radiologist, who often is not immediately available at the hours trauma patients are most likely to arrive. (3) The likelihood of the most undesirable error—a false negative result—is anticipated to be higher when a decision is based on images of organs rather than the presence or absence of free blood and intestinal content: A "small" crack in liver or spleen seen on scan may induce a false sense of security as regards severity of (present or future) hemorrhage; a visceral perforation may be missed altogether on a scan. Without contrast enhancement, scan sensitivity may be reduced markedly; yet administration of intravenous and intraluminal contrast may involve significant risk in the multiple-injury patient. (4) In an era of cost containment pressures, the diagnostic lavage procedure wins hands down over special imaging as regards cost effectiveness.

The foregoing arguments notwithstanding, abdominal cross-sectional imaging can be an important component in the evaluation of a stable patient with abdominal injury suspected (or even confirmed by diagnostic lavage) for whom an abdominal operation would be dangerous or difficult. Examples in this category include a massively obese patient with multiple rib fractures (hence anticipated ventilatory difficulty) or a patient whose positive lavage probably relates to a severe pelvic fracture and in whom the risks of disturbing the pelvic hematoma and failing to be able to close the incision exceed the (small) chance of presence of visceral perforation (which would not be identified on cross-sectional imaging). Cross-sectional imaging also makes sense in the evaluation (or reevaluation) of a stable and relatively asymptomatic patient received at a medical center in transfer from a smaller hospital a number of hours after injury. This patient already has demonstrated ability to survive an acute hemorrhagic injury; therefore presence or absence of blood in the peritoneal cavity is not a *necessary* indication for celiotomy. However, radiographic "visualization" of extent of organ damage is useful for prognostication and management planning. As above, cross-sectional imaging may fail to identify an enteric perforation in such a patient, but this is an injury having a low probability of occurrence in blunt trauma, and, if present, there is low probability of the abdomen remaining asymptomatic over many hours.

As just noted, identification or suspicion of hemoperitoneum is not always an absolute indication for celiotomy. This is particularly true in young children. Further, increased emphasis is being given to preservation of injured splenic and hepatic tissue. Nevertheless, for the majority of trauma patients presenting without significant contraindication to exploration and for the majority of surgeons practicing outside a major medical center pediatric surgical environment, celiotomy remains the safest management of hemoperitoneum. If splenic or hepatic injury is repaired rather than resected, cross-sectional imaging and scintigraphy offer excellent means of following healing and assessing function in the postoperative period.

The Rural Community Hospital: Decision for Immediate Surgery Versus Transfer. For the abdominal trauma patient with indication for celiotomy, received in a rural community hospital at which a general surgeon is unavailable, the question of whether to perform the operation at the local facility or to transfer the patient to a major medical center will sometimes arise. The answer will depend on the stability of the patient's condition and the nature of associated injuries, anticipated delay in effecting a transfer, care available during transport, expertise of surgeons available in the community hospital, and ability of the local facility to support a major surgical effort. Fortunately, with most potentially life- and limb-threatening injuries (cerebral, thoracic, peripheral vascular, skeletal) the level of specialty expertise needed to repair the probable lesion successfully can be fairly well estimated preoperatively. The issue is less clear-cut with abdominal trauma, in which the precise nature of the injury is usually unknown before celiotomy.

Hemorrhagic injury, the most immediate threat to life in abdominal trauma, is also the most immediately evident. If hypotension persists in a trauma patient in whom hemoperitoneum was identified by peritoneal lavage, a family practitioner who does limited abdominal surgery in a remote setting may serve that patient well by removing a ruptured spleen. But if on opening the abdomen a major liver laceration, pancreatoduodenal injury, or renovascular-caval disruption is encountered, the outcome may be less satisfactory. Use of thoracoabdominal exposure, caval bypass shunts, hepatic artery occlusion, and laser-knife resection for major hepatic injuries; resection with or without Roux-en-Y pancreatojejunostomy for complicated pancreaticoduodenal injuries; repair of renal vessels; and partial resection of kidneys for complicated renal injuries are procedures that challenge the expertise even of surgical teams in major trauma centers, yet often provide the patient the best chance for recovery. Even the experienced trauma surgeon would find hepatic lobectomy or renovascular repair a formidable problem in a rural community hospital without assistants and without liberal blood bank support.

Injury to a hollow viscus, less immediately threatening to life, is also less immediately evident. Nevertheless, when overlooked or mismanaged operatively, the resultant intestinal leak can kill just as surely as hemorrhagic injury, although it does so more slowly. Decisions regarding repair versus resection of a perforated gut, primary anastomosis versus temporary ostomy, and repair and drainage of complicated rectoperineal injuries challenge the trauma surgeon to provide the correct solution during the first operative intervention, since failure to do so may preclude opportunity for successful revision several days later.

Therefore when an abdominal-injury patient in whom celiotomy is indicated is received in a community hospital but a general surgeon is not available, if rapid transfer to a major medical center with care during transport can be arranged, the ED physician in the community hospital should confer by telephone with the trauma surgeon in the medical center to select the optimum location for the operation according to the specific circumstances surrounding the individual case. When emergent surgery for abdominal trauma is undertaken in a community hospital and complicated viscerovascular injuries are encountered whose definitive repair is beyond the capability of the local surgeon, straightforward methods should be employed to gain control of continuing hemorrhage (packing, ligatures as appropriate) and irrevocable procedures avoided. Early transfer to a major medical center for reoperation should then be arranged.

Urinary Tract Injury: Second-Pass Considerations

Injuries to the urogenital system can be conveniently classified in several ways: Anatomically it is useful to localize the site of injury to kidney (parenchyma, collecting system, pedicle), ureter (upper, middle, lower), bladder (intraperitoneal, extraperitoneal), urethra (posterior, anterior), or external male genitalia. Etiologically, it is helpful to categorize the injury as penetrating or nonpenetrating. Clinically, it is meaningful to identify renal injuries as minor, major, and critical.

The kidney is frequently injured, being second only to the spleen as the viscus most commonly injured by blunt abdominal trauma. Contusion of the renal parenchyma without rupture of the capsule or tear into the collecting system is a minor injury to the kidney. Hematuria may or may not be gross initially but usually abates rapidly. Any signs and symptoms related to the contusion should steadily improve; observation only is indicated. Over 80% of all renal injuries fall into this group. Major injury to the kidney consists of parenchymal laceration with extension through the capsule and into the collecting system but without disruption of the renal pedicle. Shock and hematuria may or may not be present initially, but signs and symptoms are likely to intensify rather than abate with time. Less than 15% of all renal injuries fall into this group. Fragmentation of the kidney or extension of a laceration into the vascular pedicle is a critical injury. Blood loss is likely to be severe within a short interval. Less than 5% of renal injuries fall into this group.

Most ureteral injuries are a result of penetrating trauma.

Lacerations of the bladder from penetrating injuries vary in location according to the pathways of the missile. Ruptures of the bladder from blunt trauma are almost equally distributed between extraperitoneal (usually associated with pelvic fracture) and intraperitoneal locations (usually associated with disruption of a full bladder at its weakest point, the dome), with less than 10% being combined intraperitoneal and extraperitoneal injuries.

Injuries to the urethra are usually classified according to their location in relation to the urogenital diaphragm: Those below (anterior) are more frequent, whereas those above (posterior) pose more difficult management problems. Injuries confined to the membranous urethra, which traverses the urogenital diaphragm, are extremely rare. Posterior injuries result from blunt trauma that causes the prostate to be sheared from its connection to the urogenital diaphragm and puboprostatic ligaments and the urethra to be disrupted. Posterior urethral tears are about equally divided between complete and incomplete. Even when the urethra is severed, the sphincteric activity of the bladder outlet remains intact. Thus the bladder is likely to remain full and there may be only minimal or no extravasation of urine.

External Genitalia. It is useful to classify the injuries as penetrating or nonpenetrating. A wound that has probably penetrated the tunica albuginea of a testis or a corpus cavernosum of the penis, or a blunt injury that has resulted in a large scrotal hematoma, is indication for early exploration in the operating room, preferably by a urologist. Similarly, loss of significant skin covering of the penis or scrotum is indication for early repair by a urologist or plastic surgeon. This surgery is clearly second in priority to that for major thoracic, abdominal, neurologic, peripheral vascular, and even many orthopaedic injuries, but often it can conveniently be accomplished simultaneously with or immediately following other operations in a multiple-injury patient. Thus early urologic consultation should be sought. While the patient is awaiting surgery, it is helpful to elevate and apply an ice bag to the scrotum if there is a hematoma and to place sterile-saline or povidone-iodine–moistened gauze dressings on scrotal and penile wounds denuded of skin. Fragments of partially avulsed scrotal skin should not be debrided in the ED, as they may be invaluable in reconstituting an intact scrotum.

Blunt injury to the scrotum that has resulted in only minimal swelling, ecchymosis, and tenderness may be treated conservatively. Whenever there is doubt, early urologic consultation is recommended. Since rupture of the testis may occur secondary to blunt trauma and salvage can be accomplished only by prompt exploration and repair, many urologists are taking a relatively aggressive approach with regard to early exploration of scrotal hematoma.

Identification of a penetrating wound of the genitalia or of a scrotal hematoma which is to undergo exploration is indication to initiate intravenous antibiotic therapy (see "Use of Antibiotics in Multiple Trauma," p 451).

Intravenous Pyelography. The remainder of the initial evaluation of urinary tract injury is radiographic. The second key principle in the algorithm for urinary tract evaluation is that the finding of gross or microscopic hematuria is *sufficient* indication for intravenous pyelography (IVP). In patients stable enough to undergo the study, the finding of any hematuria is an absolute indication for IVP in the presence of (1) shock (or history of preresuscitation shock), (2) other major multiple injuries, (3) other abdominopelvic (or flank) symptoms or findings, (4) obtundation with absence of any symptoms. If none of these four conditions exist, there is less agreement about the indication for IVP in a patient with only microscopic hematuria ($\geq$10 RBCs/HPF). Some authorities now advocate omitting the emergency IVP and following these patients with serial abdominal exam and urinalysis.

A history of an allergic reaction to previous intravenous iodinated contrast studies is a relative contraindication to intravenous pyelography. As observed in the section on abdominal injury, anaphylactic reaction to a contrast agent is a risk associated with intravenous pyelography. When there is vague history of an allergic reaction to iodine compounds, a 1-ml test dose of the contrast agent may be slowly injected into an intravenous line and the patient observed carefully for at least 10 minutes before intravenous delivery of a 100-ml to 150-ml bolus of 60% solution over 5 minutes. Positive control of the airway, or preparation for rapid intubation, and immediate availability of injectable diphenhydramine, epinephrine, and methylprednisolone sodium succinate (which must be reconstituted from powder) are recommended. When there is both serious question of iodine sensitivity and urgent need to obtain the contrast study, potential reactions can usually be blocked by infusing 250 mg methylprednisolone sodium succinate intravenously, followed by intravenous injection of diphenhydramine, 1 mg/kg up to 50 mg prior to the study. (Diphenhydramine itself, in rare cases, has associated side-effects, including respiratory depression.)

Performance of pyelography usually awaits completion of physical examination and other key ED studies (roentgenography of the chest, electrocardiography, peritoneal lavage) but precedes removal to the operating room or intensive care unit. Particularly when exploratory celiotomy is indicated, it is most helpful to have a preoperative IVP. This relates both to the difficulty in thoroughly evaluating the retroperitoneal area at surgery and the need to confirm the presence and function of the contralateral kidney prior to nephrectomy should a badly damaged kidney be judged not salvageable. However, if the patient's extreme condition and failure to respond to resuscitation efforts mandate immediate removal to the operating room or intensive care unit, an abbreviated (renal phase) intravenous pyelogram (IVP) can be obtained on the operating table (or in a bed in the intensive care unit) as described in the section on abdominal injury.

Interpretation of the IVP is outlined in Table 23-7. Radiographic demonstration of extravasation of contrast medium is the most convincing diagnostic feature on excretory urography. False-negative rates for extravasation on the initial IVP are as high as $\frac{1}{3}$ in large series of major injuries to kidney and ureter, and higher in injuries to the bladder in which a tamponade effect of perivesical hematoma may prevent extravasation or concentration of contrast agent may be inadequate to visualize small rents. (When a Foley catheter is in place, it should be clamped during the initial phases of excretory urography to permit visualization of the bladder.)

Although not all the potential findings are specific, many of them represent indications for additional x-ray studies or surgical intervention. An accounting of these indications follows.

Kidneys. Bilateral poor visualization or nonvisualization (most often due to low flow state) is an indication for nephrotomography if available.

Unilateral nonvisualization or other strong suspicion of renal vascular pedicle damage is indication for selective renal angiography by the retrograde femoral route. Identification of renal artery thrombosis or other vascular pedicle injury is indication for early operative intervention by a vascular surgeon, urologist, or

TABLE 23-7. Urinary Tract Diagnoses by Intravenous Pyelography

FINDING	PROBABLE OR POTENTIAL PROBLEM
Fracture of transverse processes of L1, L2	Renal injury, possibly severe enough to involve vascular pedicle
Bilateral nonvisualization of kidneys	Low flow state (hypovolemia, hypotension) vs bilateral injury, or preexisting disease
Small kidneys or marked disparity in size	Preexisting renal disease
Bilateral delayed or poor visualization	Low flow state vs bilateral contusion or renal artery spasm
Unilateral nonvisualization	Renal contusion, renal artery spasm, renal artery occlusion by intimal tear flap, congenital (or surgical) absence
Nonvisualization or poor visualization of a segment and its calyx	Renal laceration or rupture
Extravasation of contrast from a kidney	Renal parenchymal laceration extending into collecting system
Dilated (hydronephrotic) ureter	Distal ureteral injury with obstruction, obstruction of ureter by hematoma
Extravasation of contrast from ureter	Ureteral laceration
Fracture of pelvis	Bladder injury
Distorted shape (tear drop, crescentic) or displacement (upward, lateral) of bladder or both	Perivesical hematoma; bladder injury
Extravasation of contrast agent from bladder:*	Bladder rupture or laceration:
into peritoneal cavity	at dome
into retroperitoneum	at extraperitoneal site

* May need postdrainage film to detect.

general surgeon. By repair of a defect as simple as an intimal flap tear, a kidney may be salvaged that would otherwise be lost to ischemic necrosis. Priority of this surgery is equal to that for other abdominal injuries.

Extravasation of contrast material from a kidney is evidence of major renal injury and indication to obtain early urologic consultation, even if initially by telephone and while in the operating room. Treatment of major renal injury depends on whether the trauma is penetrating or nonpenetrating, the extent of damage to parenchyma and collecting system, and presence or absence of continuing hemorrhage. Thus once major renal injury is identified or strongly suspected from the IVP, selective renal arteriography is extremely useful to assess more precisely the extent of both damage and hemorrhage, which in turn guides the decision concerning operative intervention and whether to attempt repair or to remove the kidney. When IVP obtained on the operating table shows major renal injury, an intraoperative arteriogram can be obtained, as described in the section on abdominal injury.

Penetrating renal injuries and those with evidence of continuing hemorrhage deserve early exploration by way of an anterior transperitoneal approach, preferably by a urologist. Priority of this surgery is equal to that for other penetrating and hemorrhagic abdominal injuries. When other penetrating or hemorrhagic abdominal injuries are coexistent, it is best to have the urologist operate with the general surgeon. Although the general surgeon should seldom need assistance with total nephrectomy, advances in ability to salvage kidney function by partial nephrectomy and renoplasty represent a changing state of the art with which the urologist should always be better versed than the general surgeon.

Despite extravasation, major renal injury resulting from blunt trauma that is not complicated by continuing hemorrhage or evidence of infection is often best managed expectantly. For such injuries, surgical intervention in the early post-trauma period too often results in nephrectomy for otherwise viable kidneys; bleeding that had been checked by compression resumes when Gerota's fascia is opened, making it difficult to assess damage precisely. Conservative management should be pursued with urologic consultation.

Ureters. Evidence of ureteral injury (extravasation, hydronephrosis) is indication to obtain early urologic consultation. Any ureteral injury requires operative repair, preferably by a urologist. Priority of this surgery is equal to that for other penetrating abdominal injury (without massive hemorrhage). When other penetrating abdominal injury coexists, it is best to have the urologist, who is well versed in the multiple options related to ureteroplasty, stenting, nephrostomy, cystostomy, reimplantation-vesicoplasty, and ureteroureterostomy, operate with the general surgeon. When stability of the patient's condition and operative priority of associated injuries permits, the urologist will usually wish to perform preoperative retrograde pyelography to define precisely the location and (in combination with the excretory pyelogram) extent of the ureteral defect.

Bladder. Extravasation of contrast medium from the bladder is evidence of laceration or rupture. Except perhaps for small extraperitoneal perforations, all bladder defects should be surgically closed by way of a suprapubic or intra-abdominal approach as appropriate, using three layers of running absorbable suture and establishing postclosure drainage via suprapubic cystostomy (a Foley urethral catheter may suffice in a female in the absence of associated urethral or pelvic injury). Priority of this surgery follows that for other abdominal injuries (without massive hemorrhage).

Whether or not extravasation from the bladder is noted during the excretory phase of intravenous pyelography, after the bladder collection phase the patient should be asked to void, or if a Foley catheter is in place it should be unclamped, to drain the contrast material accumulated in the bladder. Another film should then be obtained: Minimum extravasation of contrast material from a small defect in the bladder or lower ureter, previously obscured by density of contrast agent in the bladder, may then become evident.

When extravasation is not detected but there is strong suspicion of bladder injury (suprapubic pain, inability to void, pelvic fracture, distortion of bladder contour) and a Foley catheter is in place, 200 ml to 400 ml of contrast material should be introduced into the bladder by gravity drainage from the barrel of a large syringe attached to the Foley catheter. Anteroposterior and lateral oblique films are obtained before and after subsequent bladder drainage.

Urethra. For a patient in whom there is strong suspicion of urethral laceration (pelvic fracture, inability to void, bloody urethral discharge, displacement of the prostate) or a patient in whom an attempt to pass a Foley catheter has failed, a retrograde urethrogram is indicated. Demonstration of a partial or complete urethral disruption (or if there is continued inability to pass a Foley catheter after inability to demonstrate a laceration) is indication for early urologic consultation. Whether or not the urologist elects to manipulate the urethra in the immediate post-trauma period, suprapubic drainage of the bladder must be established. There is obviously some urgency in accomplishing this for a patient who can neither void nor have a Foley catheter inserted. The most definitive and certain technique is placement via surgical incision in the operating room. However, when instability of the patient's condition or priority of ED management of associated injuries precludes early removal to the operating room, percutaneous placement of a suprapubic bladder drainage catheter may be necessary.

When percutaneous suprapubic bladder catheterization is contemplated after trauma, it should be remembered that the same pelvic injury and associated hematoma that may be preventing catheter insertion per urethra may distort and displace the bladder so as to complicate a percutaneous approach from above. As with introduction of a peritoneal lavage catheter, complications of suprapubic bladder catheterization in the ED can be minimized by use of the Seldinger technique instead of a trocar or a deep cutdown. In fact, a peritoneal lavage tray contains appropriate components for safely establishing the desired drainage: An 18-gauge needle is the sharpest object that must locate the bladder through a hematoma; certainty of approach to the lumen of the vesicle is assured before advancing the larger plastic catheter (see "Diagnostic Peritoneal Lavage," p 433).

Identification of penetrating injury to the urinary tract (as in other penetrating abdominal injuries) and identification of urinary tract injury with extravasation are indications to administer intravenous antibiotics (see "Use of Antibiotics in Multiple Trauma," p 451).

Limb Injury: Second-Pass Considerations

Classification and Description of Limb Injuries. It is useful to consider limb injury in terms of five components: skin, underlying soft tissue (muscle and tendon), nerves, vessels, and bone. However, in the multiple-trauma patient it is important to note that injuries to these systems seldom are isolated phenomena. Coexistence of damage to arteries, veins, and nerves, and destruction and contamination of adjacent muscle and soft tissue, in addition to fractures and dislocations, are factors that bear heavily on overall management and outcome of limb injury.

It is also useful to categorize limb injuries according to mechanism of injury: those which are a result of penetrating trauma versus those which are a result of blunt trauma. Knowledge of mechanism of limb injury immediately provides a great deal of insight into which components may be injured, in what manner, and to what extent.

SKELETAL INJURY. The major skeletal injuries of the limbs are fractures, dislocations, and traumatic amputations. It is not uncommon for such injuries to exist in combination in the multiple-injury patient.

It is convenient to classify fractures according to whether they are open (in communication with a defect in the skin) or closed. This distinction is not always obvious: A significant defect in the skin may not necessarily communicate with an immediately underlying fracture, whereas a minimal skin defect may communicate with a fracture some distance away. A closed fracture is almost certain to be a result of blunt trauma, whereas an open fracture may be caused by blunt or penetrating trauma: The skin defect communicating with a fracture may be a result of laceration by a fragment of broken bone from within, in blunt trauma, or of entry by a missile from without, in penetrating trauma.

It is convenient to describe dislocations in terms of direction of displacement of the distal skeletal member relative to the proximal joint surface. Anterior or posterior is the distinction usually appropriate in specifying a dislocation at the shoulder, elbow, hip, or knee.

Specification of whether a dislocation is anterior or posterior or whether a fracture is open or closed represents much more than an exercise in nomenclature: It immediately suggests what adjacent neurovascular structures might be compromised or injured and determines the nature of manipulation or surgical intervention that might be urgently required, as will be described.

It is important to recognize that significant blood loss may be associated with major fractures: It is not uncommon that 4 to 5 units may be sequestered in the thigh of an adult with a femur fracture, and 1 to 2 units may be present in the upper arm of an adult surrounding a fracture of the humerus. Even larger quantities of blood may accumulate in extraperitoneal soft tissues adjacent to fractures of the lower back or pelvis. Fortunately, in most cases of closed fractures, this bleeding will tamponade spontaneously.

NEUROVASCULAR INJURY. Peripheral neurovascular injuries can also be categorized according to type of injury: those injuries that result in perforation or laceration of a vessel or nerve versus those that result in compression, contusion, or stretching. A laceration may be partial, or may sever a vessel or nerve completely. Lacerations and perforations are most commonly associated with penetrating trauma but may occur from contact with sharp fracture fragments created by blunt trauma. Laceration by a fracture fragment may occur during the original accident or may result from motion of fracture fragments during subsequent transport and manipulation of the patient.

Stretching, compression, or contusion of a major peripheral nerve may result in complete loss of function, affecting motor, sensory, and autonomic components, or may result in partial loss of function. The larger, more rapidly conducting nerve fibers are more easily damaged by stretching or compression; thus with a partial lesion there is likely to be motor deficit with sparing of sensation and loss of light touch sensation with preservation of pain sensation. Neurologic deficits associated with nonlacerating injury to peripheral nerves are often at least partially reversible.

Compression of a vessel to the point of cessation of flow over a prolonged interval is likely to result in thrombosis. Contusion may result in hemorrhage into a vessel wall with resultant high-grade narrowing of the lumen, damage to the intima, or both. An injured intima predisposes to primary thrombosis, or to formation of an intimal "flap" with occlusion of flow and subsequent thrombosis.

Injury to vessels and nerves must be suspected whenever there is a penetrating wound near the course of major neurovascular bundles. With high-velocity (>1500 ft/sec) missile injury, the effects of energy absorption and cavitation of the surrounding tissue may result in significant damage to a vessel or nerve at points several centimeters from the path of the missile. In addition, the wound may be contaminated with bits of clothing and dirt or bacteria from the skin that have been "sucked in."

Blunt neurovascular injury is most often associated with fracture of a long bone or a severe dislocation. Vessels and nerves may be contused or compressed by a displaced bone or may be lacerated by the sharp, ragged end of a fractured bone. Common sites for blunt injury to vessels and nerves are (1) subclavian artery and vein and brachial plexus in association with fractured clavicle, (2) axillary artery and nerve in association with dislocated shoulder, (3) radial nerve in association with midshaft fracture of the humerus, (4) brachial artery and radial or median nerve in association with supracondylar fracture of the humerus or posterior dislocation of the elbow, (5) femoral artery and nerve in association with anterior dislocation of the hip or femur fracture, (6) sciatic nerve in association with posterior dislocation of the hip, (7) popliteal artery in association with dislocated knee or high tibial fracture, (8) peroneal nerve in association with fracture of the proximal fibula, and (9) posterior tibial artery in association with fracture/dislocation of the ankle.

SOFT-TISSUE INJURY. The major soft-tissue injuries of the limbs are lacerations of tendons, contusions and crush of muscle, and avulsion of segments of muscle and overlying skin. Tendon lacerations may be partial or complete. Associated with severe muscle crush injury may be (1) profound reactive hyperemia, (2) significant blood loss, (3) release of large quantities of myoglobin, and (4) a great deal of pain and prolonged limb dysfunction.

Critique of Diagnostic Criteria and Indications for Subsequent Studies. SKELETAL INJURY. The signs and symptoms by which a fracture or dislocation is suspected are not specific: Deformity and pain may be due to soft-tissue damage instead of skeletal injury. Distal neurovascular compromise may be due to primary nerve and vessel injury without fracture or dislocation. Limitation of motion may relate entirely to pain or proximal impairment of innervation. In the unconscious or stuperous patient a large amount of information is unavailable because local pain, distal light touch sensation, and active range of motion cannot be assessed. However, in the multiple-trauma victim, any of the complaints or findings by which fracture or dislocation should be suspected constitutes sufficient indication for x-ray study of the appropriate components of the affected limb.

The appropriate components include the joints proximal and distal to a potential long bone fracture and the supporting bones proximal and distal to a suspected joint injury. With doubt concerning epiphyseal injury in a child, a picture of the contralateral uninjured limb may need to be obtained for comparison. Two views are almost always desirable and occasionally a third view, special angle, or stress film is needed. The ED physician should be as specific as possible in describing the suspected injuries on the x-ray requisition. If a radiologist is not immediately available and the x-ray technician is not familiar with the standard views or the ED physician is not familiar with the pertinent x-ray findings relative to the injuries suspected, then the ED physician should consult an orthopaedic surgeon or refer to a textbook of trauma roentgenography. Poor-quality films should be repeated rather than accepted. Adherence to these principles should lead to roentgenographic definition of even those fractures and dislocations whose presentations are relatively subtle.

An all too common error in trauma management in the emergency department is to send an unaccompanied and unstable multiple-injury patient to the x-ray department early in the course of overall evaluation to roentgenographically confirm an already obvious fracture. With possible exception of a dislocation that cannot be readily reduced and with which is associated obvious neurovascular compromise, removal to the radiology department for skeletal films that cannot be obtained in the ED should await completion of physical examination and all crucial ED studies. If removal to the radiology department is necessary in order to obtain *any* or *all* x-ray studies, then, for a multiple-injury patient, films of the cervical spine, chest, and pelvis should be obtained and reviewed *prior* to investing time imaging limb injuries. Knowledge of injuries to the spine, chest, or pelvis leads to immediate action in the ED that otherwise might not be taken; once splinted to provide comfort and protect adjacent structures, most limb skeletal injuries do not require immediate attention.

When moved to the radiology department, the multiple-trauma patient should be accompanied by a member of the ED trauma team. With the exception of presence of an associated limb-threatening vascular injury, priority of skeletal roentgenography follows that for studies related to major thoracoabdominal and head injuries.

TENDON AND PERIPHERAL NERVE INJURY. In the alert and cooperative patient, the functional assessment of active limb motion and sensation represents a straightforward and accurate means by which to diagnose significant injuries to tendons and nerves. In the unconscious or stuperous patient this initial data base will be incomplete, since assessment will be limited to observation of spontaneous motion and withdrawal from noxious stimuli. Operable tendon or nerve injury is extremely unlikely in the absence of a laceration or penetrating wound. Possible exceptions include (1) joint dislocation (which may mechanically block motion, avulse an adjacent tendon insertion, or impinge on an adjacent nerve) and (2) closed displaced fracture (which may lacerate an adjacent nerve or tendon from within). A functional deficit in the presence of an open wound over the corresponding tendon or nerve is sufficient indication for surgical exploration, at which definitive diagnosis will be made. In the presence of a deep laceration, absence of a functional deficit does not exclude the possibility of a partial transection of a tendon or nerve.

VASCULAR INJURY. With trauma to bones and joints, nerves, and soft tissue of the limbs, significant injuries are usually readily determined by physical examination, or suggestive findings lead to immediately available noninvasive roentgenographic study by which a definitive diagnosis is established. Unfortunately, the same does not pertain as frequently to significant vascular injuries.

Bleeding may be relatively minimal or absent in the presence of a significant penetrating or blunt vascular injury. With complete transection of an artery, constriction and retraction of the muscular vessel ends may markedly restrict or stop bleeding. With thrombosis and intimal flap formation associated with compression/contusion injuries, a limb may quickly be jeopardized with no evidence of bleeding or hematoma.

Conversely, the presence of (nonpulsatile) bleeding with a penetrating wound or soft-tissue injury, or of a hematoma, is not specific for major vascular injury: The external bleeding or hematoma formation may be due only to smaller vessel injury associated with extensive soft-tissue damage. Similarly, a major fracture or dislocation may be present without any injury to vessels or compromise of perfusion.

Even the six ''p's'' are not infallible: Pulses distal to significant arterial injury have been present in up to 27%, and normal in 10% to 15%, of patients in various series. Pallor does not always develop with arterial insufficiency and is difficult to appreciate in dark-skinned patients. If there is a concomitant venous injury, the limb is likely to appear cyanotic rather than pale. Skin temperature may be maintained if there is sufficient collateral flow and superficial vessels are dilated or if the ambient temperature is high enough. Pain may rapidly subside and a limb become anesthetic when ischemia is severe. Paralysis and paresthesia are *late* signs of severe ischemia to distal muscles and motor nerves, and to peripheral sensory nerves, respectively, and therefore are not very helpful in early diagnosis. Paralysis and paresthesia may also result from direct injury to motor and peripheral sensory nerves. In addition to these specific limitations, many of the foregoing signs and symptoms may appear as a result of hypovolemic shock and/or severe cold exposure, in the absence of arterial injury.

As previously mentioned, a bruit is a rare early finding, present only in the minority of acute vascular injuries.

A confusing factor is the question of spasm: as a relatively *rare* event, *temporary* segmented narrowing of an artery may be observed as a result of sustained local constriction of vascular smooth muscle without definable damage to the vessel. In the trauma setting when such ''spasm'' persists, it is dangerous not to suspect underlying injury.

Thus given (1) the nonreliability and nonspecificity of the symptoms and findings on which diagnosis of peripheral vascular injury is classically based, (2) the potential of limb loss as a consequence of delayed recognition and delayed surgical correction of a significant arterial injury, and (3) the desire to avoid unnecessary exploratory surgery; an ancillary study is needed by which to assess accurately the status of limb circulation in patients with suspected vascular trauma. Arteriography, preferably by the percutaneous Seldinger method, has become clearly established as the single most accurate diagnostic modality for evaluation of vascular trauma. It is of particular value in identifying or excluding operable injuries in cases where the clinical evidence is not conclusive. Arteriography can (1) precisely locate a site of contrast extravasation from a laceration, (2) identify a level of occlusion, (3) define an intimal flap obstruction, (4) demonstrate a false aneurysm or arteriovenous fistula, (5) evaluate the status of collateral circulation, and (6) help differentiate segmental spasm from true occlusion (although it may be difficult to be sure whether segmental narrowing is due to spasm rather than intimal injury).

For the reasons just given, an arteriogram is usually of great value as a preoperative "road map." Therefore in general, in a patient with suspected vascular trauma, a preoperative arteriogram should be routinely omitted only when the presence and location of an arterial injury are essentially certain, as in a penetrating wound with brisk bleeding or expanding hematoma. Preoperative arteriography in the radiology department should be selectively omitted only when it is determined that anticipated delay in obtaining the study may jeopardize limb survival, or when coexistence of life-threatening thoracoabdominal or head injuries mandates immediate removal to the operating room. In these instances, consideration should be given to obtaining a preoperative or intraoperative arteriogram on the operating table. (The operating table should always be configured for x-ray during peripheral vascular surgery because a postrepair arteriogram is often helpful in confirming a successful result.)

On completion of physical examination and urgent ED studies such as chest x-ray, ECG, and peritoneal lavage, priority of peripheral arteriography is secondary only to that for radiographic studies related to rapidly life-threatening thoracoabdominal and head injuries. Absence of angiographic capability in a community hospital is sufficient indication to transfer a suspected vascular injury patient rapidly to a larger facility that has, immediately available, both angiography and vascular surgical expertise.

Indications for Consultation and Surgery for Limb Injuries. FRACTURES. All open fractures, open-joint injuries, and fractures for which operative reduction and fixation are indicated should undergo early exploration, debridement, and repair in the operating room by an orthopaedic, plastic, or hand surgeon. Selection of the surgeon should obviously be influenced by the site of injury and the experience and interests of the available specialists.

Simple reduction and initial immobilization of nondisplaced or minimally displaced closed limb fractures that do not involve joint surfaces or growth centers and debridement and subsequent care of peripheral soft-tissue injuries that do not involve tendons are procedures with which most general surgeons are familiar. Many of these procedures are described in Chapters 32 and 33. The trauma surgeon will usually undertake initial management of this nature, with subsequent consultation as necessary at the convenience of the orthopaedic or plastic surgeon.

However, even with closed fractures (1) that are displaced such that complicated maneuvers or traction may be required to achieve functional anatomic reduction, (2) that involve joints or growth centers, or (3) in which the need for open reduction and fixation is controversial or in doubt, it is best to get an orthopaedic surgeon (or plastic or hand surgeon) involved in the *initial* management. In the presence of one or more of these injuries and the absence of an orthopaedic surgeon, reference to an orthopaedic text and early telephone consultation are recommended. Failure to recognize the potential severity of certain injuries or to take the proper action within an appropriate time frame or both may preclude an orthopaedic or plastic surgeon from achieving an optimal functional result when repair or reconstruction must be undertaken as a delayed procedure.

TENDON LACERATIONS. All tendon lacerations should be repaired in the operating room by an orthopaedic, plastic, or hand surgeon. Even in the absence of an obvious functional deficit, presence of a deep laceration directly over the course of tendons may be sufficient indication for exploration. (Failure to diagnose and repair a partial tendon laceration may result in delayed rupture of the tendon or in scarring of the tendon in its sheath.) By tradition, tendon lacerations associated with lower limb, and proximal upper limb and joint injuries usually are repaired by orthopaedic surgeons, whereas lacerations affecting function of the hands (and sometimes the feet) are usually repaired by plastic or hand surgeons. Selection of the appropriate surgeon again depends on the experience and interests of the available specialists.

PERIPHERAL NERVE INJURY. Peripheral neurologic deficit in a limb without a penetrating wound or fracture probably represents nerve contusion, for which only expectant initial treatment is indicated. In open or penetrating limb injury, it is unusual for a major peripheral nerve to be lacerated without concomitant injury to adjacent soft tissues, vessels, and bones. The usual indication for early surgery will therefore be other than suspected nerve transection. Should a sharply transected major nerve be identified in a clean wound without associated major injuries, primary anastamosis may be undertaken by a plastic or neurologic surgeon using an operating microscope. Should a lacerated nerve be identified by a general or orthopaedic surgeon in a contaminated wound or in association with complicated injuries of higher operative priority, the wound ends may be tagged with nonabsorbable monofilament suture to facilitate identification for delayed repair by a plastic or neurologic surgeon.

PERIPHERAL VASCULAR INJURY. In general, a penetrating wound near the course of a major artery should undergo early exploration in the operating room by a surgeon experienced in peripheral vascular reconstruction. An acceptable exception is a wound resulting from low-velocity penetration in a patient whose neurovascular physical examination and angiogram are normal. A closed limb injury in a patient whose physical examination and angiogram are even suspicious for arterial injury usually also warrants early exploration.

SOFT-TISSUE INJURY. Presence of a large soft-tissue defect, major skin loss, a grossly contaminated wound, or a significant mass of devitalized muscle are all indications for early debridement in the operating room. Strong suspicion of developing compartment syndrome is sufficient indication to perform fasciotomies in the operating room.

WOUNDS. In many cases exploration of a wound may be the only certain means by which to establish or exclude the presence of operable injury to vessels, nerves, or musculoskeletal structures of a limb. However, exploration and debridement or suturing of a limb wound in the ED should be limited to the combination of circumstances in which there is (1) only a modest skin and soft-tissue defect with minimal contamination; (2) low index of suspicion about presence of and communication with an underlying fracture, laceration of joint capsule or tendon, or major arterial injury; (3) ability to provide a sterile field and appropriate anesthesia; (4) availability of adequate lighting, instruments, and assistance; (5) readiness to achieve hemostasis rapidly, including by inflation of a proximally placed circumferential pressure cuff if appropriate; and (6) no other injury identified or diagnostic study remaining that commands higher priority of action. In all other circumstances, exploration, debridement, and repair should be carried out in the operating room. In the multiple-trauma patient who will require early removal to the OR for attention to other injuries, even superficial limb wounds should await exploration and repair at that time and in that setting.

USE OF ANTIBIOTICS. Antibiotics should be administered preoperatively by the intravenous route in the ED whenever one or more of the following problems have been identified: (1) open fracture or joint injury, (2) tendon laceration, (3) operable vascular injury, and (4) major soft-tissue or crush injury (see "Use of Antibiotics in Multiple Trauma").

Timing and Priority of Surgery for Limb Injury. **FRACTURES AND DISLOCATIONS.** Once major joint dislocations (with which might be associated neurovascular compromise) are reduced and fractures are splinted, skeletal injuries rank relatively low on the list of operative priorities for the multiple-trauma patient, following surgery for life-threatening thoracoabdominal and head injuries, limb-threatening vascular injuries, and sight-threatening eye injuries. However, a sense of complacency regarding the need for early and vigorous debridement and irrigation of open fractures and joint injuries is not to be encouraged. Although with early administration of antibiotics, delay up to 6 hours is probably without significant difference in outcome, delay in debridement of such wounds beyond 12 hours is unquestionably fraught with a distinctly higher incidence of long-term infection despite use of antibiotics. Fortunately, the anatomic site of many skeletal injuries permits the orthopaedic or plastic surgery team to operate simultaneously with another surgical team dealing with an injury of higher priority.

By use of skeletal traction or cast support easily established in the ED, ICU, or OR, definitive repair of many closed fractures can be deferred safely for days. When such a fracture is the only indication for surgery identified in an unstable multiple-trauma patient, use of these orthopaedic techniques to defer removal to the OR allows the trauma surgeon uninterrupted attendance to resuscitation and monitoring during the crucial early postinjury hours.

TENDON LACERATIONS. Tendon repair is also of low operative priority for the multiple-trauma patient. However, within 6 hours of injury it is highly desirable to (1) complete necessary debridement and irrigation of the associated wound and (2) be under way with an anastamosis if it is intended to accomplish a primary repair. The time imperative for the first issue relates to the incidence of subsequent long-term infection; the time imperative for the second issue relates to poor suitability (due to edema and softening) of the tissue for anastamosis between 12 and 48 hours postinjury. As with skeletal injury, the anatomic site of many tendon lacerations permits the orthopaedic or plastic surgeon to repair a tendon while another surgical team deals with an injury of higher priority.

Severed tendons related to powerful muscles in the proximal aspects of the limbs should be reapproximated as soon as possible in order to prevent permanent shortening due to muscle contraction. The smaller muscles and tendons related to hand function offer more latitude. Except in the case of immediate anastamosis in a clean, sharply incised wound, it remains controversial whether primary repair of these smaller tendons is superior to that which is delayed by 2 to 6 days. In wounds with gross contamination and crushing injuries, tendon repair should be deferred until infection has cleared and tissues are soft and pliable. Thus in the multiple-trauma patient, once the associated wound is cleansed and debrided as necessary, delayed repair of a tendon laceration may be preferable.

PERIPHERAL NERVE INJURY. Peripheral nerve laceration itself poses no immediate threat to limb survival. Provided the cut ends can later be identified, success of nerve repair delayed by 6 or more weeks is comparable to that of primary anastamosis. Thus when laceration of a peripheral nerve is suspected or identified at surgery for other trauma, operative priority is low, following that for peripheral vascular and musculoskeletal injuries. Arguments in favor of delayed repair in the multiple-trauma patient include (1) better definition of the extent of nerve injury when scar tissue has developed and (2) technically easier anastamosis to perform when the perineurium has thickened.

PERIPHERAL VASCULAR INJURY. As with life-threatening injuries to head, neck, and trunk, time is a factor in dealing successfully with limb-threatening arterial injuries. It has been demonstrated that when vascular repair is undertaken within 6 hours of acute arterial occlusion, the incidence of subsequent gangrene and amputation approaches zero, whereas when delay in repair exceeds 12 hours, the incidence approaches 30% or more. When arterial injury is associated with a fracture or dislocation, delay in repair results in a severalfold increase in late amputation rate. Thus priority of surgery for limb-threatening vascular injury is secondary only to that for immediately life-threatening thoracoabdominal and head injuries. Where such injuries coexist and the life-threatening injury mandates immediate removal to the OR, it may be best to have the peripheral vascular team operate simultaneously if this can be accomplished safely with respect to interactions of OR personnel and potential cross contamination of wounds.

On the other hand, once the potential of exsanguinating hemorrhage has been controlled, a vascular injury might present no immediate threat to life *or* limb. This may be true even in the absence of distal pulse, as long as (1) capillary refill is good, (2) distal flow can be verified by Doppler ultrasound, and (3) paresthesia and paralysis are absent. (It should be noted that apparent skin viability does not necessarily correlate with viability of more perfusion-sensitive underlying muscles and nerves.) In the multiple-injury setting, trauma to other systems may deserve more immediate attention. In this event it is important to verify, by repeated close interval reexamination, that the vascular injury indeed continues to remain non-limb-threatening.

A setting in which it is common to have to establish operative priorities is the coexistence of an arterial injury and an associated fracture or dislocation. The question of which injury to correct first frequently arises.

If it is the decision of the orthopaedic surgeon to use *external* fixation to stabilize the fracture (a common choice with contaminated open wounds), the sequence easily is determined: the vascular repair should be accomplished first, while the entire limb is accessible.

When it is the choice of the orthopaedic surgeon to use internal fixation or distal skeletal traction, it is in theory desirable to reduce and stabilize a fracture before repairing an associated vascular injury. This prevents application of force to an arterial repair during manipulation of the skeletal injury and prevents tension on or kinking of the arterial repair should reduction of the fracture result in lengthening or shortening of the associated limb segment in comparison to the prereduction skeletal configuration.

However, the most important determinant of operative sequence is the ischemic time factor. It is not uncommon that (1) a prolonged prior interval of arterial insufficiency is judged by the vascular surgeon to constitute an immediate threat to limb survival or that (2) the orthopedic surgeon estimates that reduction and fixation of the skeletal injury are likely to require an extended period of time (with intraoperative x-ray confirmation of alignment, etc.). In either or both of these situations the most immediate priority is reestablishment of limb perfusion. One option by which to accomplish this rapidly is the temporary use of a nonthrombogenic arterial shunt, a technique that permits early restoration of distal flow *and* allows reduction and fixation of the skeletal injury prior to definitive arterial repair. A shunt also provides a convenient means by which to perfuse the distal vascular bed selectively with heparin and allows time to repair major venous injuries before arterial repair.

In any event, when there is an operable arterial injury and an associated operable fracture or dislocation, it is important to have the vascular and the orthopaedic surgeons present simultaneously at the time the patient goes to the operating room. Presence of both surgical teams (1) facilitates the most meaningful exchange of opinions regarding relative operative priorities and potential complications related to sequencing one procedure after the other, (2) allows the vascular surgeon to achieve proximal and distal vessel control before the orthopaedic surgeon manipulates a skeletal injury with which is associated a yet-to-be-repaired arterial laceration or perforation, and (3) allows the vascular surgeon to continue to observe and thus "protect" an arterial repair that has been accomplished prior to manipulation and fixation of an associated skeletal injury.

Success of vascular trauma surgery has been shown to correlate well with the peripheral vascular reconstructive experience of the surgeon. Therefore with a stable patient in a setting without availability of vascular surgical expertise, identification of a major vascular injury is strong indication to arrange rapid transfer of the patient, with a transport team in attendance en route, to a larger facility where a vascular surgeon and angiographic capability are immediately available.

SOFT-TISSUE INJURY. Compartment syndrome and ischemic muscle necrosis due to progressive infection both represent complications of soft-tissue trauma that are truly limb threatening secondary to progressive ischemia. Since the perfusion deficit is usually an evolving one rather than one of abrupt onset, the threat to limb survival is usually less immediate than that of an acute arterial occlusion. However, once well under way, there is no reconstructive surgical procedure by which these processes may be effectively reversed; there is only ablative surgery by which to attempt to remove diseased tissue. Therefore when fasciotomy or wide debridement of devitalized muscle are indicated, early removal to the operating room should be effected. Priority for these procedures follows that for repair of major vascular injury.

Sequelae of Limb Injuries. SKELETAL INJURY. The earliest sequelae of skeletal injuries of the limbs are usually related to delay in relieving associated vascular compromise. Some of the more common examples are (1) Volkmann's ischemic contracture of the forearm due to prolonged arterial compression associated with delayed reduction of a displaced supracondylar fracture or a posterior dislocation of the elbow, (2) gangrene of the leg and foot due to prolonged compression and contusion of the popliteal artery associated with delayed reduction of dislocation of the knee, and (3) necrosis and sloughing of overlying skin due to prolonged pressure associated with delayed reduction of a fracture/dislocation of the ankle. Among later sequelae of skeletal limb injuries are those related to inability of bones, joint surfaces, and surrounding ligaments to heal. Some of the more common examples are (1) nonunion at a fracture site, a phenomenon profoundly influenced by the presence or absence of infection, which is in turn greatly influenced by whether an open fracture was adequately debrided; (2) aseptic necrosis of the femoral head due to damage to capsular vessels occurring with prolonged dislocation of the hip; and (3) chronic instability of the knee or shoulder joint subsequent to serious disruption of supporting ligaments, with delayed recognition or inadequate repair.

Fat emboli, phlebothrombosis, and pulmonary emboli are problems associated with skeletal injury whose occurrence is relatively independent of technique of management.

PERIPHERAL NERVE INJURY. The sequelae of peripheral nerve injuries are sensorimotor defects and muscle atrophy, which most often can be predicted on the basis of deficits identifiable immediately post-trauma. Occasionally a neurologic deficit will develop de novo during the healing process when a peripheral nerve becomes entrapped in the formation of scar tissue or bone callus.

PERIPHERAL VASCULAR INJURY. The most common late sequelae of vascular lacerations are formation of false aneurysms and arteriovenous fistulas. If a partially severed artery is not repaired, the associated hematoma may develop a cavity in a continuity with the vessel lumen. Since such a cavity does not contain the layers of the vessel wall, it constitutes a "false" aneurysm. Potential complications include pressure on adjacent structures and "blow out." When concomitant lacerations of an artery and an adjacent vein are not repaired, arterial blood may be persistently shunted through the associated hematoma into the injured vein. As the hematoma resolves and retracts, the defects in artery and vein may be brought into direct continuity. Potential complications include increased cardiac output, even to the point of high-output cardiac failure.

SOFT-TISSUE INJURY. Serious sequelae of soft-tissue injury include renal failure, ischemic necrosis, and necrotizing fasciitis and gas gangrene. Muscle crush plus hypovolemia can result in marked myoglobinemia. Inadequate fluid resuscitation in the presence of myoglobinemia can result in concentration of myoglobin in the urine, with subsequent renal tubular failure. Where adjacent fascial planes and bone limit ability of contused soft tissue to swell, the pressure of contained edema and hemorrhage may increase to the point that first venous outflow and then arterial inflow are compromised ("compartment syndrome"). Crush injury may result in primary compromise of vascular supply to muscle. When a significant mass of soft tissue becomes devitalized, particularly in the presence of a penetrating wound and in the absence of adequate debridement, conditions are optimum for the development of the relatively rare but always devastating complications of necrotizing fasciitis or clostridial myositis with gas gangrene.

USE OF ANTIBIOTICS IN MULTIPLE TRAUMA

As ability to treat specific organ system injuries has improved, more seriously injured trauma patients survive the initial insult but later succumb to simultaneous failure of multiple-organ systems. The factor most commonly responsible for this multiple-organ failure, or that itself leads to death, is infection. In fact, infection is the second most common cause of death of major-trauma patients. Once resuscitation and control of major hemorrhage have been accomplished, infection becomes the leading cause of mortality and morbidity and markedly increases the cost of hospitalization of trauma victims. Therefore prevention of infection and early and proper treatment of established infection are crucial considerations in management of trauma.

Host Defenses and Resistance to Infection. Susceptibility of the trauma patient to infection appears to be related to a relative immunosuppressed state, which in turn results from a combination of factors. These relate to magnitude of tissue injury, nature of bacterial inoculation, adequacy of tissue perfusion, and nutritional status of the patient.

The following parameters have been shown to influence host defenses in trauma patients:

- Duration and severity of shock
- Impairment of local circulation
- Devitalization of contused or partially avulsed tissue
- Dead spaces (hematomas and seromas)
- Extent and nature of any contamination
- Location of soft-tissue injury
- Association of orthopaedic injury
- Association of bowel injury
- Severity and multiplicity of associated injuries
- Time elapsed from injury until surgical or medical therapy was instituted
- Status of the host
  - Age
  - Associated diseases (preexisting cardiopulmonary decompensation, diabetes, uremia, etc.)
  - Obesity
  - Nutritional status
  - Immune state (steroids, antimetabolites)
  - Preexisting infections
- Iatrogenic factors
  - Vascular catheters
  - Urinary catheters
  - Tracheal intubation
  - Chest tubes and other drains
  - Improper use of antibiotics

These factors must be considered in decisions concerning extent of debridement, timing of wound closure, whether or not to leave a drain in place, when to use antibiotics, and which antibiotics to choose. The decision-making capabilities of the best physicians are tested because of the complexities of multiple injuries, the patient's diminished host defenses, and the numerous varieties of pathogenic bacteria. Because of these complexities, every physician who treats trauma victims should have a well-thought-out plan to handle infections or potential infections as they arise in these patients.

Timing of Antibiotic Administration. Timing of administration is important if antibiotics are to be of maximum benefit. When used prophylactically because contamination at surgery is anticipated, antibiotics are most effective when given preoperatively, less effective when given intraoperatively, and of minimum or no value when given postoperatively. It obviously is impossible to administer antibiotics before or during most injuries. However, the interval from injury until initiation of antibiotic therapy is important: The earlier antibiotics are given, the greater their efficacy. Beyond 3 hours after injury, antibiotics are of minimum value in prevention of infection.

Indications for Early Use of Antibiotics in Trauma. In the following situations, the patient should receive antibiotics as soon as possible:

- Open head injury (open skull fractures, fracture into sinuses, CSF rhinorrhea or otorrhea)
- Open or penetrating injury to airway or esophagus
- Open or penetrating chest wound (including thoracotomy in the ED)
- Severe pulmonary contusion, aspiration
- Penetrating abdominal injury with indications for celiotomy, or
  - Suspected perforation or laceration of gastrointestinal tract
  - Suspected injury of biliary tract
  - Suspected perforation or laceration of urinary tract
- Vascular injury that may require repair with a prosthetic graft
- Wounds entering a joint space or associated with an open fracture.
- Penetrating injury to tendons and tendon sheaths
- When adequate debridement is not feasible or will be delayed
- When the wound is heavily contaminated
- When the injury is prone to develop clostridial infection as in
  - Extensive devitalization of muscle
  - Compromised arterial blood supply
  - Deep gross contamination with dirt or fecal material
- Whenever an infection is present at the time of the injury, including infection of
  - Skin
  - Sinus
  - Urinary tract
  - Biliary tract
  - Respiratory tract

Choice of Antibiotics. Use of antibiotics subjects a trauma patient to the dangers of (1) potential allergic and idiosyncratic reactions inherent in administration of any drug; (2) toxicity to various organs related to high dose and extended use of certain agents, particularly in the presence of already compromised function of kidneys or liver; (3) selection of resistant strains of less desirable organisms that may establish a septic state worse than that associated with the original infection. These risks associated with use of any antibiotic in a trauma patient must be weighed against the probable efficacy of a particular antibiotic in preventing clinical infection or dissemination of an established infection. The ideal, of course, would be to cover the specific organisms that are present in contaminated tissue with a highly selective antibiotic. Unfortunately, specific organisms are unknown at the time of injury. Since cultures are obtained infrequently in the ED or operating room, there is difficulty in rationally stopping or modifying the antibiotic regimen after 24 to 48 hours.

Despite these drawbacks there are several studies showing efficacy of early use of antibiotics in trauma patients, and enough bacteriologic data to estimate accurately the most common and prominent organisms associated with various injuries. On the basis of these data, the following suggestions are offered as guides to initial selection of antibiotics in the indicated situations. These choices should be modified by Gram stains, cultures, and good clinical judgment.

Open Head Injury. For open head injuries manifest by obvious open fractures, rhinorrhea, otorrhea, pneumoencephalus, or large, deep lacerations through the galea, it is best to (1) cover the most common organisms tending to cause meningitis (2) with an antibiotic that penetrates well into the CSF but (3) that has minimal toxicity. Since there is a predominance of *Streptococcus* in post-traumatic meningitis and penicillin is a good CNS perfuser with low toxicity, a penicillin such as ampicillin is an acceptable choice. To provide broader-spectrum coverage of potential external contaminants such as *Staphylococcus* while retaining the desirable characteristic of CNS penetration, a second-generation cephalosporin such as cefuroxime is also an obvious choice.

Major Soft-Tissue Injury, Penetrating Chest Wounds, Vascular Injuries, and Open Fractures and Joint-Space Injuries. In major soft-tissue injuries, penetrating chest wounds, vascular injuries, and orthopaedic injuries that are not ischemic or severely contaminated with dirt, feces, or both, the predominant organisms are *Staphylococcus* and *Streptococcus,* along with some common aerobic gram-negative rods. *Bacteroides* or *Pseudomonas* is rarely involved. The immediate issue is prevention of wound infection, not treatment of septicemia. Therefore the choice of antibiotic is a fairly narrow-spectrum agent with low toxicity that is active against the anticipated organisms and has good tissue-perfusing characteristics. A first-generation cephalosporin fits this description, with clindamycin a reasonable substitute.

When there is severe crush injury or much devitalized tissue, or when there is extensive contamination by soil or fecal matter, a clostridial infection must be considered along with infection due to other anaerobes and gram-negative bacteria. Clostridia may be covered, in descending order of preference, by high doses of penicillin, of clindamycin, or of a first-generation cephalosporin. Because other gram-negative aerobic infections are common in this situation, an aminoglycoside is usually added. When *Bacteroides* contamination is suspected or possible, clindamycin is added (as a third antibiotic, if penicillin is also used).

Because of relatively high incidence of gram-negative organisms recovered from open fracture sites, many orthopaedic surgeons add an aminoglycoside to their first-generation cephalosporin coverage.

The combination of extensive tissue damage and contamination demands early and aggressive surgical debridement, followed by frequent reexamination and additional debridement as indicated. Antibiotics represent only an adjunct to the primary therapy: adequate surgical debridement. Nevertheless, use of antibiotics to prevent gas gangrene is well worth the risk involved, since once such an infection is well established, treatment is difficult at best.

Penetrating Abdominal Injury or Suspected Gastrointestinal Injury. Identification of penetrating abdominal injury with decision for celiotomy is indication for early administration of antibiotics. Blunt abdominal injury with suspicion of injury to bowel, biliary tract, or urinary tract also warrants preoperative antibiotic treatment. Only when an abdominal injury is declared potentially penetrating but decision is made to observe instead of operate should antibiotics be withheld, since their use in this circumstance is more likely to delay recognition of peritonitis than to prevent infection.

Violation of bowel integrity exposes to infection with a wide spectrum of organisms. Appropriate culturing techniques demonstrate massive counts of anaerobes, particularly *Bacteroides fragilis,* along with numerous species of gram-negative aerobes. Therefore most authorities recommend double coverage with an aminoglycoside to prevent development of early overwhelming septicemia plus clindamycin or another agent that has strong activity against *Bacteroides,* to prevent abscess formation.

Because this combination is not very active against enterococci, ampicillin often is added as a third antibiotic; however, this is not a critical issue as regards immediate postinjury coverage. It must be reemphasized that it is impossible to cover every possibility; therefore most authorities advise covering the more common organisms with relatively nontoxic antibiotics.

When injury is limited to the liver or biliary tract but there is a significant amount of necrotic tissue, drains are used, or organisms are seen on Gram stain, then antibiotics may be continued in the postoperative period. In this situation it makes sense to select an antibiotic that (1) has low toxicity, (2) is concentrated in the bile, (3) is fairly specific for the more common organisms that may appear in the biliary tract (note: *Pseudomonas* and *Bacteroides* are rarely found in unobstructed bile), and (4) also covers the common skin contaminants (*Staphylococcus* and *Streptococcus*) so often responsible for drain tract infections. In this regard, a first- or second-generation cephalosporin is a good choice.

In isolated splenic injury antibiotic administration may be discontinued unless drains are left in place because of iatrogenic injury to the tail of the pancreas during splenectomy. When drains are placed in the left upper quadrant, the incidence of subphrenic abscess due to introduction of staphylococci through the drain tract is high enough to warrant continuation of staphylococcus antibiosis postoperatively.

Treatment of Preexisting Infections in a Trauma Victim. Patients who already have an established infection, such as an infected wound, skin abscess, sinusitis, or urinary tract infection, or in whom there are positive findings on Gram stain of the bile, should be treated with an appropriate antibiotic on the basis of the Gram stain and good clinical judgment. Following trauma the immune system is impaired, and these preexisting "slowly smoldering" infections tend to disseminate rapidly if not treated promptly.

Summary of Initial Antibiotic Usage. The suggested guidelines for the early use of antibiotics in major trauma are:

Open head injury
- Ampicillin, 1 g intravenously (I.V.) every 4 hr
- *or*
- Cefuroxime, 1.5 g I.V. every 8 hr

Massive soft-tissue or open fracture injury:
- First- or second-generation cephalosporin (cefazolin or cefamandole, respectively), 1 g I.V. every 6 hr
- *plus (often added)*
- Aminoglycoside (gentamicin or tobramycin), 1.5 mg/kg I.V. every 8 hr

Massive soft-tissue injury with heavy dirt or fecal contamination
- Penicillin, 5 million units I.V. every 4 hr
- *or*
- Clindamycin, 900 mg IV, every 8 hr
- *plus*
- Gentamicin or tobramycin, 1.5 mg/kg I.V. every 8 hr
- *with or without addition of*
- Cefazolin, 1 g I.V. every 6 hr, to cover *Staphylococcus* (note: clindamycin or tobramycin provides reasonably good coverage of non-hospital-acquired staphylococcal infection).

Penetrating chest wound or peripheral vascular injury that may require use of graft
- First- or second-generation cephalosporin, 1 g I.V. every 6 hr

Abdominal injury with suspected bowel involvement
- Gentamicin or tobramycin, 1.5 mg/kg I.V. every 8 hr
- *plus*
- Clindamycin, 900 mg I.V. every 8 hr

These suggestions (doses applicable to adults) must be modified according to cultures, Gram stains, allergies, renal dysfunction, and other clinical data that may be available.

BIBLIOGRAPHY

Background

Baker SP, O'Neill B, Karpf RS: The Injury Fact Book. Lexington MA, Lexington Books, 1984

Committee on Trauma Research, Commission on Life Sciences, National Research Council: Injury in America. Washington, DC, National Academy Press, 1985

Nahum AM, Melvin J (ed): The Biomechanics of Trauma. East Norwalk CT, Appleton-Century-Crofts, 1985

Pekkanen J: Our no. 1 medical need. Readers' Digest pp 100–07, July 1985

General

Baxt WG (ed): Trauma: The First Hour. East Norwalk CT, Appleton-Century-Crofts, 1985

Committee on Trauma, American College of Surgeons: Advanced Trauma Life Support Course. Chicago, The American College of Surgeons, 1985

Maull KI (ed): Advances in Trauma, Vol. 1. Chicago, Year Book Medical Publishers, 1986

Moore EE, Eisman B, Van Way CW II (ed): Critical Decisions in Trauma. St Louis, CV Mosby, 1984

National Conference on Cardiopulmonary Resuscitation and Emergency Cardiac Care: Standards and guidelines for cardiopulmonary resuscitation and emergency cardiac care. JAMA 255(21):2905–2989, 1986

Salvatore JA, Sclafeni MD, Panetta T et al: The management of arterial injuries caused by penetration of zone III of the neck. J Trauma 25(9):871–884, 1985

Shires GT (ed): Principles of Trauma Care, 3rd ed. New York, McGraw-Hill, 1985

Trunkey DD, Lewis FR (ed): Current Therapy of Trauma, Vol 2. Philadelphia, BC Decker, 1986

Wiener SL, Barrett J: Trauma Management for Civilian and Military Physicians. Philadelphia, WB Saunders, 1986

Zuidema GD, Rutherford RB, Ballinger WF: The Management of Trauma, 4th ed. Philadelphia, WB Saunders, 1985

Prehospital Care

Lewis FR: Prehospital intravenous fluid therapy: Physiologic computer modelling. J. Trauma 26(9):804–811, 1986

Mattox KL, Bickell MD, Pepe PE, Mangelsdorff AD: Prospective randomized evaluation of antishock MAST in posttraumatic hypotension. J Trauma 26(9):779–786, 1986

Smith JP, Bodai BI, Hill AS, Frey CF: Prehospital stabilization of critically injured patients: A failed concept. J Trauma 25(1):65–70, 1985

Trauma Scoring System

Baker SP, O'Neill B, Haddon W, Long WB: The injury severity score: A method for describing patients with multiple injuries and evaluating emergency care. J Trauma 14(3):187–196, 1974

Champion HR, Sacco WJ, Carnazzo AJ et al: Trauma score. Crit Care Med 9(9):672–676, 1981

Champion HR, Gaines PS, Yackee E: A progress report on the trauma score in predicting a fatal outcome. J Trauma 26(10):927–931, 1986

Fischer RP, Flynn TC, Miller PW, Rowlands BJ: The economics of fatal injury: Dollars and sense. J Trauma 25(8):746–750, 1985

Vascular Access

American Heart Association: Intravenous techniques. In Textbook of Advanced Cardiac Life Support. Dallas, American Heart Association, 1986

Bernard RW, Stahl WM: Subclavian vein catheterizations: A prospective study. I. Non-infectious complications. Ann Surg 173:184, 1973

Brinkman AJ, Costley DO: Internal jugular venipuncture. JAMA 223:182–183, 1973

Daily PO, Griepp RB, Shumway NE: Percutaneous internal jugular vein cannulation. Arch Surg 101:534–536, 1970

Defalque RJ: Percutaneous catheterization of the internal jugular vein. Anesth Analg 53:116–121, 1974

Moosman DA: The anatomy of infraclavicular subclavian vein catheterization and its complications. Surg Gynecol Obstet 136:71–74, 1973

Mostert JW, Kenny GM, Murphy GP: Safe placement of central venous catheter into internal jugular veins. Arch Surg 101:431–432, 1970

Williamsen J: Prevention and early recognition of complications of central venous catheterization. Am Heart J 92:667–679, 1976

Fluid Resuscitation

Holcroft JW, Trunkey DD: Extravascular lung water following hemorrhagic shock in the baboon: Comparison between resuscitation with Ringer's lactate and Plasmanate. Ann Surg 180:408–417, 1974

Schwab CW, Shayne JP, Turner J: Immediate trauma resuscitation with type-O uncrossmatched blood: A two-year prospective experience. J Trauma 26(10):897–902, 1986

Shires GT, Carrico CJ, Canizaro PC: Shock. Major problems in clinical surgery. Surg Clin North Am 53:1341–1366, 1973

Trunkey DD, Holcroft JW, Carpenter MA: Monitoring resuscitation of primates from hemorrhagic and septic shock. JACEP 5:249–252, 1976

Head and Neurologic Injuries

Bakay L, Glauser FE: Head Injury. Boston, Little, Brown & Co 1980

Cooper PR (ed): Head Injury. Baltimore, Williams & Wilkins, 1982

Gurdjian ES, Gurdjian ES: Acute head injuries. Surg Gynecol Obstet 146:805–820, 1978

Miner ME, Wagner KA: Neurotrauma. Boston, Butterworths, 1986

Javid M: Head injuries. N Engl J Med 291:890–892, 1974

Jennett B: Assessment of the severity of head injury. J Neurol Neurosurg Psychiatry 39:647–655, 1976

Teasdale G: Assessment of head injuries. Br J Anaesth 48:761–766, 1976

Teasdale G, Jennett B: Assessment of coma and impaired consciousness: A practical scale. Lancet 2:81–84, 1974

Cornell SH, Chiu LC, Christie JH: Diagnosis of extracerebral fluid collections by computed tomography. Am J Roentgenol 131:107–110, 1978

Dublin AB, French BN, Rennick JM: Computed tomography in head trauma. Radiology 122:365–369, 1977

Forbes GS, Sheedy PF, Piepgras DG, Houser OW: Computed tomography in evaluation of subdural hematoma. Radiology 126:143–148, 1978

Koo AH, LaRogue RL: Evaluation of head trauma by computed tomography. Radiology 123:345–350, 1977

Merino-De Villasante J, Taveras JM: Computed tomography in acute head trauma. Am J Roentgenol 126:765–778, 1976

Zimmerman RA, Bilaniuk, LT, Gennarelli T et al: Cranial computed tomography in diagnosis and management of acute head trauma. Am J Roentgenol, 131:27–34, 1978

Chest

Blaisdell FW, Trunkey DD (ed): Trauma Management, Vol III: Cervicothoracic Trauma. New York, Thieme Stratton, 1986

Feliciano DV, Mattox KL: Indications, techniques, and pitfalls of emergency center thoracotomy. Surg Rounds 4:32, 1981

Mattox KL, Beall AC Jr, Jordan GL Jr, DeBakey ME: Cardiorrhaphy in the emergency center. J Thorac Cardiovasc Surg 68:886–895, 1974

Abdominal Injury: Peritoneal Lavage

Blaisdel FW, Trunkey DD (ed): Trauma Management, Vol I: Abdominal Trauma. New York, Thieme Stratton, 1982

Fischer RP, Bevelin BC, Engrav LH et al: Diagnostic peritoneal lavage, 14 years and 2586 patients later. Am J Surg 136:701–704, 1978

Jergens ME: Peritoneal lavage. Am J Surg 133:365–369, 1977

Lazarus HM, Nelson JA: A technique for peritoneal lavage without risk or complications. Surg Gynecol Obstet 149:889–892, 1979

Lazarus HM, Nelson JA: Peritoneal lavage with low morbidity. JACEP 8:316–319, 1979

Merlotti GJ, Marcet E, Sheaff CM, et al: use of peritoneal lavage to evaluate abdominal penetration. J Trauma 25(3):228–231, 1985

Parvin S, Smith DE, Asher M, Virgilio RW: Effectiveness of peritoneal lavage in blunt abdominal trauma. Ann Surg 181:255–261, 1975

Root HD, Hauser CW, McKinley CR et al: Diagnostic peritoneal lavage. Surgery 57:633–637, 1965

Ryan JJ, Kyes FN, Horner WR et al: Critical analysis of open peritoneal lavage in blunt abdominal trauma. Am J Surg 151(2):221–223, 1986

Urinary Tract

Blaisel FW, Trunkey DD (ed): Trauma Management, Vol II: Urogenital Trauma. New York, Thieme Stratton, 1985

Demetriades D, Rabinowitz B, Sofianos C, Landau A: Haematuria after blunt trauma: The role of pyelography. Br J Surg 72(9):745–747, 1985

Fortune JB, Brahme J, Milligan M, Wachtel TL: Emergency intravenous pyelography in the trauma patient: A reexamination of the indications. Arch Surg 120(9):1056–1059, 1985

Lang EK, Sullivan J, Frentz G: Renal trauma: Radiologic studies. Comparison of urography, computed tomography, angiography, and radionuclide studies. Radiology 154(1):1–6, 1985

Nicolaisen GS, McAninch JW, Marshall GA et al: Renal trauma: Re-evaluation of the indications for radiographic assessment. J Urol 133(2):183–187, 1985

Peters PC, Bright TC III: Management of trauma to the urinary tract. Adv Surg 10:197–244, 1976

Uehara DT, Eisner RF: Indications for intravenous pyelography in trauma. Ann Emerg Med 15(13):266–269, 1986

Vascular

Kerstein MD (ed): Management of Vascular Trauma. Baltimore, University Park Press, 1984

Rich NM, Spencer FC: Vascular Trauma. Philadelphia, WB Saunders, 1978

Imaging, General

Federle MP, Brant-Zawadzki M (ed): Computed Tomography in the Evaluation of Trauma, 2nd ed. Baltimore, Williams & Wilkins, 1986

Greenbaum EI: Radiology of the Emergency Patient. New York, John Wiley & Sons, 1982

Heller M, Holgerjend H, Genaut HK (ed): Computed Tomography in Trauma. New York, Thieme Stratton, 1986

Jurkovich GJ, Zingarelli W, Wallace J, Curreri PW: Penetrating neck trauma: Diagnostic studies in the asymptomatic patient. J Trauma 25(9):819–822, 1985

Schwartz SS (ed): Trauma. Radiol Clin North Am 11 (Dec), 1973

Computed Tomography Versus Diagnostic Peritoneal Lavage

Davis RA, Shayne JP, Max MH et al: The use of computerized axial tomography versus peritoneal lavage in the evaluation of blunt abdominal trauma: A prospective study. Surgery 98(4):845–850, 1985

Fabian TC, Mangiante EC, White TJ et al: A prospective study of 91 patients undergoing both computed tomography and peritoneal lavage following blunt abdominal trauma. J Trauma 26(7):602–608, 1986

Goldstein AS, Salvatore JA, Kupferstein NH et al: The diagnostic superiority of computerized tomography. J Trauma 25(10):938–946, 1985

Marx JA, Moore EE, Jordan RC, Eule J Jr: Limitations of computed tomography in the evaluation of acute abdominal trauma: A prospective comparison with diagnostic peritoneal lavage. J Trauma 25(10):933–937, 1985

Peitzman AB, Makaroun MS, Slasky BS, Ritter P: Prospective study of computed tomography in initial management of blunt abdominal trauma. J Trauma 26(7):585–592, 1986

Trunky DD, Federle MP: Computed tomography in perspective. J Trauma 26(7):660–661, 1986

Pediatric Management

Brooks BF (ed): The Injured Child. Austin, University of Texas press, 1985

Eichelberger MR, Randolph JG: Pediatric trauma: An algorithm for diagnosis and therapy. J Trauma 23(1):91–97, 1983

Hoelzer DJ, Brian MB, Balsara VJ et al: Selection and nonoperative management of pediatric blunt trauma patients. The role of quantitative crystalloid resuscitation and abdominal ultrasonography. J Trauma 26(1):57–62, 1986

Antibiotics in Multiple Trauma

Atherton ST, Wright DM, White DJ, Jones ES: An antibiotic policy for bacterial infections after thoracic and other injuries. Thorax 32:596–600, 1977

Burke JF: The effective period of preventive antibiotic action in experimental incision and dermal lesions. Surgery 50:161–168, 1961

Cerise EJ, Pierce WA, Diamond DL: Abdominal drains: Their role as a source of infection following splenectomy. Ann Surg 171:764–767, 1970

Fuller WD, Hunt J, Altemeier WA: Prophylactic antibiotics in penetrating wounds of the abdomen. J Trauma 12:282, 1972

Grover FL, Richardson JD, Fewel JG et al: Prophylactic antibiotics in the treatment of penetrating chest wounds. J Thorac Cardiovasc Surg 74:528–536, 1977

Jones RC: Antibiotics in trauma. J Surg Pract Sept–Oct: 26–31, 1977

Karl RC, Mertz JJ, Veith FJ et al: Prophylactic antimicrobial drugs in surgery. N Engl J Med 275:305, 1966

Pankey GA: Posttraumatic antibiotic management. Bull NY Acad Med 55:272–283, 1979

Patzakis MJ, Dorr LD, Hammond W, Ivler D: The effects of antibiotics, primary and secondary closure on clostridial contaminated open fracture wounds in rats. J Trauma 18:34–37, 1978

Patzakis MJ, Harvey JP, Ivler D: The role of antibiotics in the management of open fractures. Bone Joint Surg 56-A:532–541, 1974

Quintilian R: Antibiotic combination therapy in posttraumatic infection. Bull NY Acad Med 55:257–265, 1979

Romanoff H: Prevention of infection in wall chest injuries. Ann Surg 182:144, 1975

Schimpff SG, Miller RM, Polakavefz S et al: Infection in the severely traumatized patient. Ann Surg 179:352–357, 1974

Thadepalli H, Borback SL, Broido P et al: A prospective study of infections in penetrating abdominal trauma. Am J Clin Nutr 25:1405–1408, 1972

Weinstein WM, Onderdonk AB, Bartlett JC et al: Antimicrobial therapy of experimental intraabdominal sepsis. J Infect Dis 132:282, 1975

Patient Transfer Criteria

Committee on Trauma, American College of Surgeons: Field categorization of trauma patients. ACS Bulletin, October 1986, pp 17–21

24 The ABCs of Pediatric Trauma

MICHAEL E. MATLAK

CHILDREN'S TRAUMA IN PERSPECTIVE

Trauma has been the number-one killer of children in the United States for many years. Nevertheless, this complex disease process is still poorly understood, frequently mismanaged, and largely ignored. Management strategies in every community need improvement so that children receive expert care at the scene of an accident, during transport, and in the emergency room. This chapter focuses on the field management and emergency room resuscitation of seriously injured children, because outcome, favorable or otherwise, depends strongly on the care given during the first critical hour following injury. Delays in obtaining expert management are costly.

MAGNITUDE OF THE PROBLEM

Trauma is responsible for over half of the deaths in people between the ages of 1 and 35 years and causes nearly one third of all deaths in children less than 1 year of age. Annually, about 25,000 children die because of accidents. For every death from trauma there are four children permanently disabled and 100 temporarily disabled. In our area half of all injured children are preschool age; nationwide almost 40% of all injuries occur in this age group. Two thirds of these injuries occur in boys.

NATURE OF INJURY

Understanding the mechanism of injury helps with management planning. The motor vehicle is the major cause of serious injury in the pediatric age group. Almost one third of these injuries involve automobile occupants. Few children ever sustain life-threatening or disabling trauma if they are properly restrained while riding in a car. Despite this well-known fact, few parents regularly "buckle up" their offspring. Two thirds of the injuries occur in children riding bicycles or crossing or playing in the street. Motorcycle injuries account for less than 1% of vehicular accidents, but these children are always seriously maimed. Recently, the all-terrain vehicle has become another frequent cause of serious injury. In Utah six children died in one recent spring while riding these new vehicles.

Falls from heights or against objects account for a great number of injuries in childhood. Most serious injuries involve a fall from a substantial height (20 feet), but not all. For example, infants falling from a high chair may sustain life-threatening neurologic damage. Also, the impact of a bicycle handlebar is concentrated in one narrow area, which can result in a splenic or hepatic laceration, small-bowel perforation, or pancreatic transection. Major trauma also occurs with physical abuse and during sports or recreational activities.

In most pediatric centers blunt trauma accounts for 90% of all injuries. As a rule, multiple organs are injured. These patients are difficult to evaluate, and physical findings may be subtle or masked despite serious injury. This is especially true with the head-injured child. The solid organs are injured most frequently; in decreasing order of frequency these organs include the brain, lung, liver–spleen, pancreas, and kidney. Injuries to hollow organs also occur and should not be overlooked. These include perforations of the proximal jejunum, duodenum, or bladder. Fractures of the long bones occur in 20% to 25% of these children.

Penetrating injuries are encountered infrequently, except in some centers located near large inner-city populations. Gunshot wounds and stabbings are usually easy to diagnose. Both hollow and solid organs are frequently involved. The immediate concern with this type of injury is the risk of life-threatening hemorrhage from a major vascular injury.

FOCUS OF INITIAL DIAGNOSIS AND MANAGEMENT

Trauma deaths may be grouped into three distinct subsets. The first group is composed of children who die immediately at the scene from irreparable central nervous system injury or from lacerations of the heart, aorta, or major vessels. The only effective treatment for this category of children is prevention. The second group of deaths occurs within 1 to 3 hours, usually from ventilatory impairment, bleeding, or neurologic damage. The major focus of this chapter is on the recognition and management of this group of children. In the third group death results from sepsis, irreversible brain damage, or multiple organ failure, usually 3 to 4 weeks postinjury. Many of these children would not die if they had initially received prompt and expert treatment.

Head injury is the major cause of morbidity and mortality in the pediatric age group. In the Intermountain West, three fourths of the injured children have a neurologic injury. Sixty percent of the time this is the most severe injury. Half the children have isolated head injuries; the other half have the devastating combination of a head injury and an injury to another body region. In this latter group death or a vegetative state occurred three times more frequently than in the group that had only a head injury.

The thorax is the second most commonly injured body area, with a frequency of injury of 40%. The extremities and bony pelvis, face and neck, and abdomen and pelvic contents were each injured in one fourth of the children. Less than 10% of the deaths resulted from chest injuries; fewer than 5% came from abdominal injuries.

Over 85% of the deaths were categorized as due to head trauma. Yet approximately half of these children seemed to die or be disabled for the wrong reason: they suffered from untreated or prolonged hypoxia and shock. Frequently, the brain and spinal cord did not appear to be damaged by the impact that occurred during the accident; rather, the brain had sustained global ischemia and hypoxia. Are many of these deaths avoidable?

It is not unusual for three or four people to be injured simultaneously in an auto accident. Usually the child, often the youngest child, receives care last because few paramedical personnel feel comfortable or have the necessary training to deal with this situation in an expert fashion. Sometimes the same uncomfortable feeling permeates the emergency room. This treatise focuses on the specifics of the emergency management of the critically injured child, emphasizing brain resuscitation. It is hoped that the application of these principles will save many lives and prevent permanent disability.

APPROACH TO THE CHILD WITH POLYTRAUMA

One of the most important principles of trauma triage is to establish priorities. Evaluation must proceed in an orderly sequence from the most to the least life-threatening conditions. The diagnosis of a life-endangering problem is suspected or proved almost exclusively by careful and repeated physical examination. Diagnosis and management occur simultaneously.

Airway patency and ventilatory support must be securely established before transportation to the hospital. This is especially true for air transport where the pathophysiologic derangement of ventilation will be aggravated during high-altitude transport in an unpressurized aircraft. Furthermore, it is extremely difficult to insert an endotracheal tube or a chest tube during air transport, making it mandatory to establish a secure airway on the ground. At the scene, a determination must also be made if exsanguinating bleeding is likely. If it is, the shortest possible transport time is extremely important. A secure airway is established with immobilization of the neck, pneumatic antishock trousers are inflated, and immediate transport to the trauma center is undertaken. Most children, however, do not fall into this category. Thus, although transport should be expeditious, time can be given to ensure that proper resuscitation is initiated at the scene and continued during transport. Therapy always includes control of the airway, but it may also involve establishment of vascular access, a thoracentesis or chest tube insertion, splinting fractures, and other treatments.

In the emergency room each member of the trauma team is assigned specific areas of responsibility. The anesthesiologist is responsible for airway management. Another physician checks for lethal injuries of the chest and performs a tube thoracostomy if necessary. A nurse or physician ensures that good venous access is established. Another nurse records the patient's status, medications, laboratory results, and other useful information. An organized team of four to six people should efficiently complete 1 hour's work in 20 minutes. The resuscitative skills required to deliver this type of care can be mastered by all primary care givers.

Management priorities based on body systems are:

1. Airway
2. Cardiovascular
3. Central nervous system
4. Gastrointestinal and genitourinary
5. Orthopaedic and plastic surgery

Initially, attention should not be focused on establishing a specific diagnosis; rather, the goal should be to identify lethal or potentially lethal conditions by physical examination and the prompt restoration of vital functions. This is the key to trauma and brain resuscitation. For example, an unconscious child may have a ruptured spleen (usually a level 4 priority). It takes considerable time in the radiology department to establish this diagnosis. The real question, however, is whether the child has any evidence whatsoever of shock (a level 2 priority). If this is the case, time is better spent restoring blood volume, as normovolemia is best for cerebral perfusion. This principle may seem obvious, but in practice too many patients undergo radiologic evaluation before they are properly resuscitated.

WHAT ARE THE ABCs?

The ABCs for cardiopulmonary resuscitation (CPR) help us remember treatment priorities. The same is true for pediatric trauma. The important differences between the ABCs in adults and children are presented in the next section.

*A*irway and cervical spine protection
*B*reathing
*C*irculation with hemorrhage control
*D*isability: Brief neurologic evaluation
*D*iagnose shock.
*E*xpose: Completely undress the child.
*E*nvironment: Temperature control

AIRWAY, BREATHING, AND CERVICAL SPINE PROTECTION

The first key to successful resuscitation is airway management. The goal is to optimize oxygenation and ventilation while protecting the cervical spine.

ANATOMY OF THE PEDIATRIC AIRWAY

The anatomy of the airway in children less than 8 years of age is very different from that of the adult. The consequences of these differences are described later. At age 8 or 9 years the anatomic configuration of the airway becomes similar to that of the adult. Thus in preadolescents or older children the principles of airway management are the same as those for adults except for the size of the equipment employed.

Young children have big heads and weak neck muscles. In the unconscious state it is difficult for them to maintain a patent airway. Also, if the child is riding unrestrained in a car, his head serves as a heavy lead point that smashes against the dashboard or windshield.

The oral cavity in children is small, filled with a large tongue, and the glottis is partially obscured by a floppy epiglottis. These features make intubation difficult and help explain the airway obstruction that easily occurs with unconsciousness. The nasal cavity is narrow, the mucosa bleeds easily, and the nasopharynx is partially blocked by adenoidal tissue after 6 months of age. This partially explains why nasal intubation is avoided in youngsters. More important, the larynx is displaced in an anterior and cephalic direction, making blind nasotracheal intubation impractical in children under 8 years of age. The endotracheal tube must negotiate too acute an angle to allow easy access into the glottis. These anatomic features also explain why oral intubation can be challenging in infants and toddlers.

The vocal cords are delicate and easily injured. The narrowest part of the airway is the cricoid ring in children and the vocal cords in adults. The diameter of the cricoid approximates the size of the little finger or anterior nares. Because of the cricoid narrowing, cuffed endotracheal tubes are not recommended in children less than 8 years of age, although there are exceptions to this guideline, namely, children with severe pulmonary contusion or hemorrhage. The usual site for tracheal stenosis in children is the subglottic area; in adults the narrowing occurs at the distal trachea.

One last anatomic difference deserves mention. The trachea of the child is narrow and short. During intubation there is constant danger of right mainstem intubation or accidental dislodgment of the tube into the esophagus.

RESPIRATORY PATTERNS

The first item to check in an injured child is the respiratory pattern. It may be normal, apneic, or obstructed.

Apnea

Apnea following injury is bad news. It implies a severe neurologic deficit secondary to prolonged hypoxia, major brain damage, or spinal cord transection. The child must be given 100% oxygen immediately. The best method to accomplish this is oral intubation with assisted ventilation. Mouth-to-mouth breathing delivers only 16% to 18% oxygen, and bag and mask ventilation delivers only 40% to 60%. This is too little oxygen for the hypoxic brain.

Airway Obstruction

The obstructed airway is the most common preventable cause of death in pediatric trauma. The signs of airway obstruction are air hunger, nasal flaring, cyanosis, stridor, noisy breathing, coughing, a hoarse cry, retractions, tachypnea, harsh rhonchi, wheezing, and diminished breath sounds.

There are two common and two uncommon causes of airway obstruction. The common causes include unconsciousness with posterior displacement of the tongue against the hypopharynx, and the accumulation of foreign matter, such as blood or vomitus, at the glottis. An automobile accident in which the child hits the windshield is typical of accidents that result in airway occlusion. The youngster has a head injury with unconsciousness, maxillofacial trauma with bleeding, and a suspected cervical spine injury. Occasionally, confusion arises concerning the best method of handling the airway. Surprisingly, the simple things—proper positioning and frequent suctioning—usually correct this problem.

The uncommon causes of airway obstruction are direct trauma to the cervical airway and glottic edema resulting from smoke inhalation. Inhalation injuries are best treated by early intubation before obstruction becomes complete. Direct trauma to the larynx or trachea is unusual in the pediatric age group, probably because of the elasticity and pliability of the cartilaginous support. Occasionally, the larynx is fractured or the trachea is lacerated when an older child encounters a clothesline or wire fence while riding a bicycle, snowmobile, or all-terrain vehicle. Although uncommon, these injuries and the accompanying spinal cord trauma may prove fatal. Manifestations include hoarseness, hemoptysis, crepitus, and subcutaneous emphysema. Most of these children can be transported to a hospital without sophisticated airway management. Bronchoscopy is necessary to determine the nature and extent of the injury, thus guiding subsequent treatment.

AIRWAY PATENCY

Initial Therapy

The first step in the establishment of a patent airway is proper positioning. The optimum position for ventilation is the "sniffing position," with the neck flexed forward, the head extended on the neck, and the jaw held forward as shown in Figure 24-1. The mandible can be advanced forward to help open the airway by either pushing on the angle of the jaw (jaw thrust) or pulling on the chin (chin lift). The neck must be maintained in the neutral position to avoid spinal cord injury. Often positioning is the only treatment required to maintain an open airway.

The mouth should be opened and inspected for foreign matter. Any foreign debris, such as blood, vomitus, food, broken teeth, and so forth, should be removed manually or preferably with a large sucker or suction catheter. Suctioning must be repeated regularly to remove secretions. If the child vomits do not turn his head to the side. This may damage the spinal cord. Rather, the head, neck, and torso should be turned as a unit, preferably with the youngster taped to a backboard, so that a rotational injury to the neck does not occur.

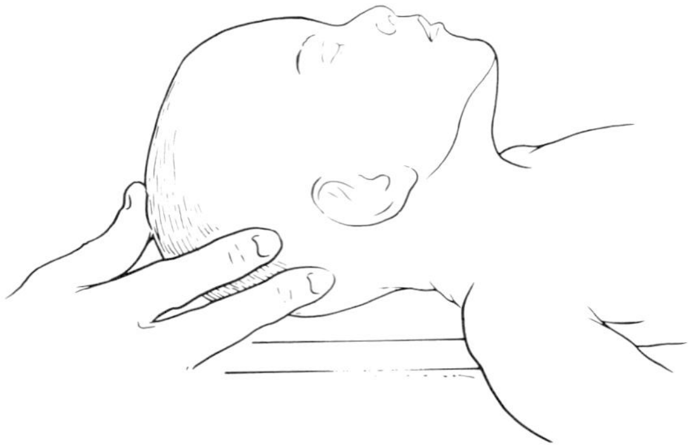

Figure 24-1. In the "sniffing position" the neck is flexed forward, the head extended on the neck, and the jaw held forward for effective ventilation.

High-flow oxygen is very beneficial and should be given as soon as possible.

Mechanical Devices

If proper positioning, suctioning, and oxygen do not relieve the signs of respiratory insufficiency, then mechanical means of improving ventilation must be employed. This is particularly true in the unconscious child. The mechanical methods include an oral-pharyngeal airway, nasopharyngeal airway, endotracheal intubation, and cricothyroidotomy.

Oral Airway. If properly used, a simple plastic oral airway may be quite beneficial in maintaining airway patency. It should only be employed in the unconscious child. Insertion must be done gently so that bleeding from the palate or tongue does not develop. This airway might be poorly tolerated and result in coughing, gagging, and vomiting. If this occurs, remove the device and consider inserting a nasopharyngeal tube. The correct size is not always available. Placement of the wrong-sized tube may totally obstruct the airway. Once the tube is inserted make certain that breathing is improved. If bag and mask ventilation is necessary, the oral airway is a very helpful means of keeping the airway patent.

Nasopharyngeal Airway. The nasopharyngeal airway is better tolerated than the oral airway and can be used in a semiconscious or unconscious child. These devices are not readily available in pediatric sizes, but a suitable nasal airway can be fashioned by trimming an appropriately sized endotracheal tube. Nasal tubes of any kind (nasopharyngeal airway, nasogastric tube, or nasal endotracheal tube) should not be inserted if there is a chance of cannulating the brain: anterior basal skull fracture, midfacial fracture, or cerebrospinal fluid rhinorrhea.

Endotracheal Intubation. If airway patency is still difficult to maintain or ventilation is insufficient with the preceding maneuvers, then endotracheal intubation is necessary. Guidelines for selection of laryngoscope blades are as follows: prematures, No. 0 straight; newborns to 3 years, No. 1 straight; 3 years to adolescents, No. 2 straight or curved; and adolescents, No. 3 straight or curved. The properly sized tube may be selected from Table 24-1. In the field the tube size should approximate the nares or little finger. Before intubation is attempted, the child should be preoxygenated. Also, it saves time to select a tube one size larger and smaller in case the tube size chosen for intubation is wrong. Try to avoid inserting an endotracheal tube that is too large. The single passage of a big tube may strip off the tracheal mucosa, resulting in irreparable airway damage. Uncuffed tubes are used in children less than 8 years old for reasons mentioned in the anatomy section. Inflation of a cuffed tube in a young child may result in a laceration of the membranous portion of the trachea with subsequent pneumomediastinum, pneumopericardium, and even bilateral tension pneumothoraces, as shown in Figure 24-2. This can be a disastrous complication and is best avoided by following the guidelines already mentioned. A properly fitted tube should develop an air leak at 15 cm to 20 cm H_2O inspiratory pressure. If it does not, the tube is too

TABLE 24-1. Guidelines for Selection of Endotracheal Tubes

AGE	TUBE SIZE (MM)
Newborn	
<1000 g	2.5
1000–2000 g	3
2000–3000 g	3.5
6 mo	3.5
18 mo	4
3 yr	4.5
5 yr	5
6 yr	5.5
8 yr	6
12 yr	6.5
16 yr	7

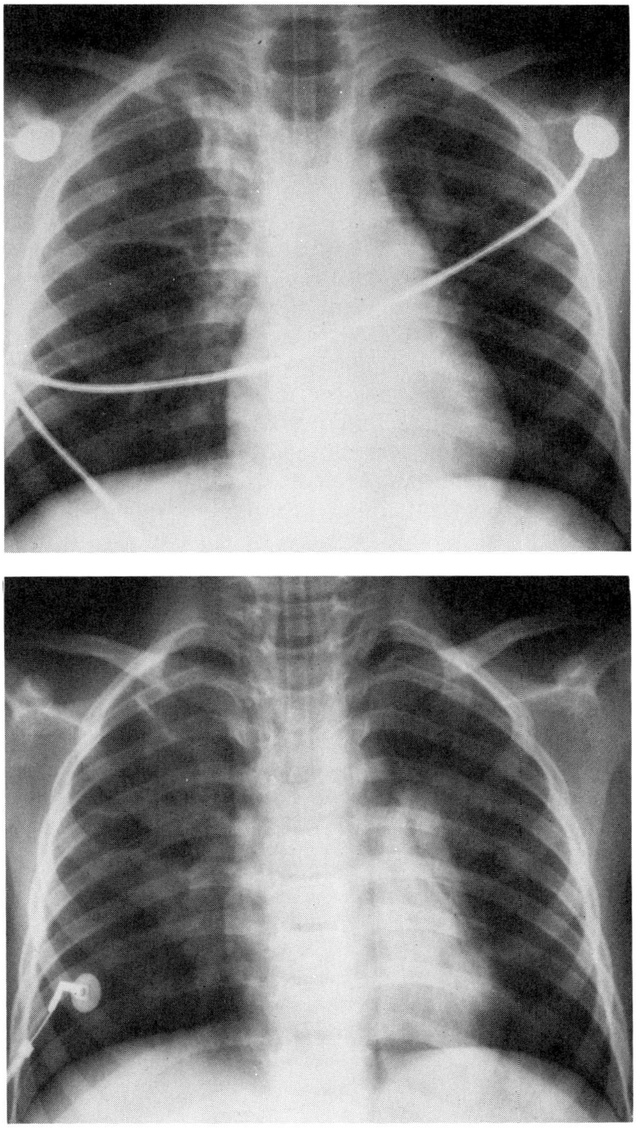

Figure 24-2. (*Top*) Cuffed endotracheal tubes in young children can overdistend the airway and perforate the membranous portion of the trachea. (*Bottom*) When the balloon is deflated, it uncovers the injury and a pneumomediastinum and pneumopericardium develop.

big. If air leaks at 5 cm to 10 cm H_2O pressure, the tube is too small.

Oral intubation is preferred when the child is less than 8 years old, has an unobstructed airway, is apneic, and has normal cervical spine films. Blind nasal intubation is preferred when the child is preadolescent or older, has partial airway obstruction, has spontaneous breathing, and may have a cervical spine injury. The nasal tube may be secured better during transport, and it cannot be occluded by the teeth. The nasal route should be avoided if there is danger of the tube entering the brain. The child is then ventilated according to his age: infants, 30 breaths/min; pre-school-aged children, 20 breaths/min; and school-aged children, 15 breaths/min.

Errors With Intubation

The following are six common errors with intubation.

Oropharyngeal trauma
Hypoxia
Right main stem intubation
Esophageal intubation
Accidental dislodgment
Bronchopleural fistula

The structures of the mouth and pharynx may be injured, especially in the combative, agitated child. This can result in further bleeding or aspiration.

Probably the most common avoidable problem is hypoxia. This occurs because the intubation takes too long. It can be avoided by following the practice of holding your breath when you start the intubation process and continuing to do so until the child is successfully tubed. If you run out of breath before the intubation is completed, it is best to resume bag and mask ventilation.

As stated previously, the trachea in children is short. Right mainstem intubation occurs frequently, and the physiologic consequences may be substantial. Atelectasis of the entire left lung and right upper lobe results in profound and prolonged cyanosis because of arteriovenous shunting. This has deleterious effects on brain resuscitation until corrected. Another major complication may develop if the inexperienced physician misinterprets the chest radiograph as representing a left-sided hemothorax as shown in Figure 24-3. Since the child is doing poorly, a chest tube may be inserted; frequently the tube is advanced into the lung parenchyma. Needless to say, this delays proper resuscitative efforts. During the past year this iatrogenic complication has occurred three times in outlying hospitals in our area. We can now suspect this diagnosis on the telephone and help the referring physician avoid this messy situation.

A fourth error is esophageal intubation. This occurs because of the anterocephalic location of the glottis and the short length of the trachea. Intubation may be difficult, and the tip of the endotracheal tube may bounce off of the posterior rim of the glottis instead of passing through the vocal cords. Also, with coughing, gagging, or movement of the neck, the tube may slip out of the airway into the esophagus. The diagnosis may escape detection and may be masked by spontaneous breathing. With esophageal intubation there is danger of hypoxia, gastric dilation, and aspiration. Be certain that breath sound and chest expansion are clearly augumented by large tidal volumes delivered through the endotracheal tube. Listen for noise over the stomach. If there is any question about the tube's location, perform laryngoscopy again or attempt reintubation.

A fifth error, accidental dislodgment of the endotracheal tube, may occur if the tube is not taped carefully or if it is bumped when the child is moved. Secretions accumulate under the tape, and retaping may be required to prevent this problem.

Finally, an iatrogenic bronchopleural fistula

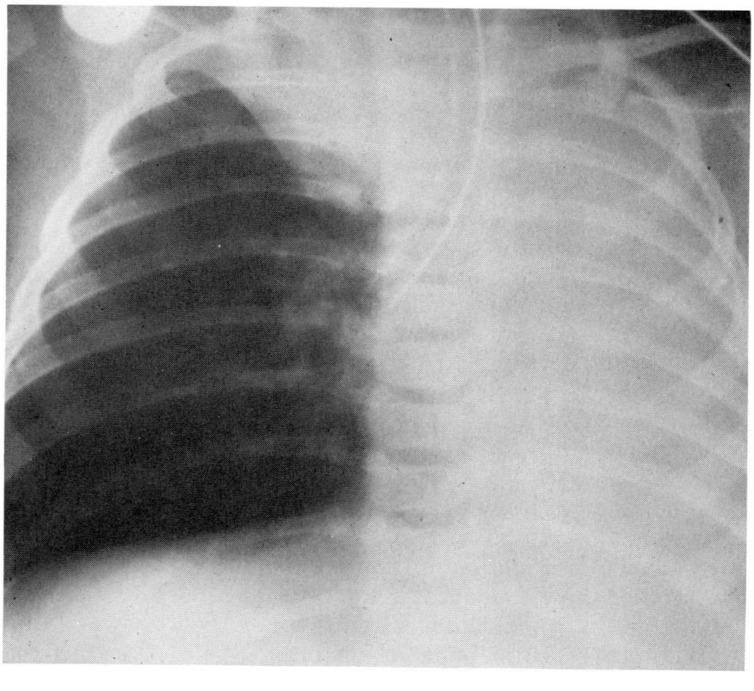

Figure 24-3. Right main stem intubation results in atelectasis of the left lung and right upper lobe. Do not misinterpret this film as demonstrating a left hemothorax.

and pneumothorax may develop in infants and young children with deep suctioning or deep insertion of the endotracheal tube. The usual scenario is the sudden onset of respiratory distress following suctioning. The secretions are blood-tinged, and the pneumothroax is almost always right sided. A chest tube is required, and an air leak may persist for several days. This problem can be avoided if the suction catheter is not advanced more than 2 cm to 3 cm beyond the tip of the endotracheal tube.

Cricothyroidotomy

The indications for a cricothyroidotomy are high-grade or complete upper-airway obstruction associated with ineffective assisted ventilation or an ability to intubate the trachea. The usual setting is severe maxillofacial trauma, a fractured larynx, laryngeal foreign body, or epiglottitis. In a life-threatening situation a standard tracheostomy is not recommended, because it cannot be performed quickly enough to prevent hypoxia, and it is a difficult procedure in a struggling, agitated child.

A needle criothyroidotomy is performed by inserting a 14- or 16-gauge angiocatheter through the cricothyroid membrane as shown in Figure 24-4. Because this membrane is soft, care must be taken to avoid cannulation of the esophagus. The needle is placed directly in the midline and advanced at a 45-degree angle until air is aspirated. After the plastic catheter is advanced, the steel stylet is removed. An intermittent jet of oxygen is delivered to the catheter Luer-lok hub through either oxygen tubing attached to a Y-connector or a 3-mm pediatric endotracheal tube adapter attached to a ventilating bag. Oxygen must be given at high flow rates (10 liters). The chest should rise when oxygen is delivered, but exhalation occurs passively. Manual compression of the chest wall may assist the exhalation process. A needle cricothyroidotomy is only a temporary airway, as hypoxemia and hypercarbia develop in 30 to 45 minutes. This allows enough time for the physician to perform a standard tracheostomy with added safety.

A surgical cricothyroidotomy is performed by incising the cricothyroid membrane in the midline. Use a No. 10 or 15 scalpel blade and avoid using a pointed No. 11 blade, which may perforate the esophagus. Use the knife handle or a hemostat to spread the cartilages apart and insert a small endotracheal tube (3.5 mm to 4 mm). Avoid deep intubation by listening for breath sounds bilaterally and by checking the location of the tube tip with a radiograph. The surgical procedure allows rapid access to

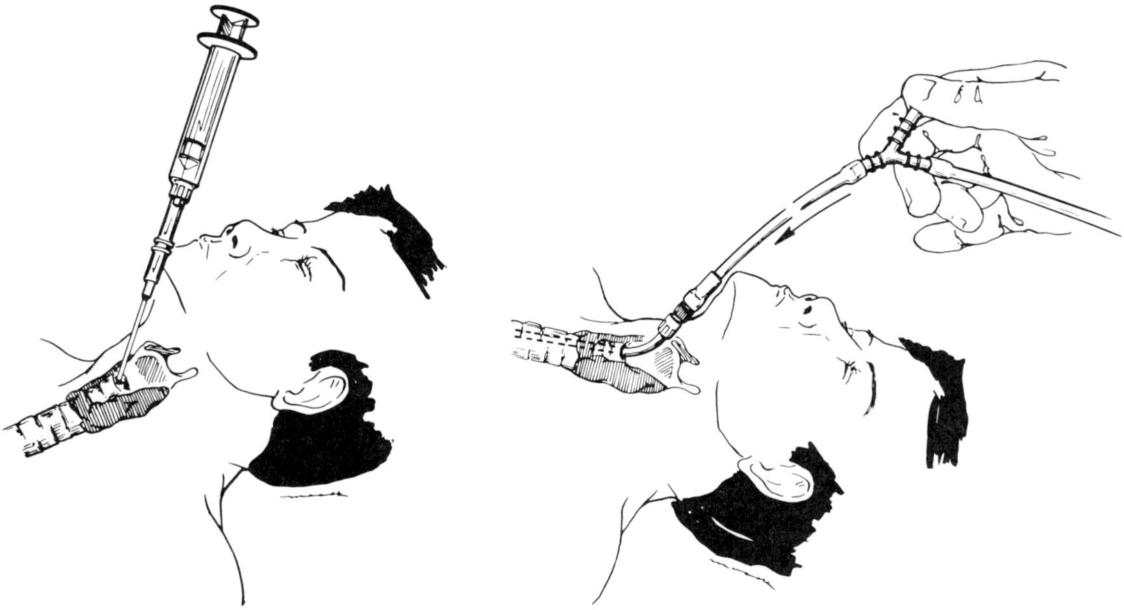

Figure 24-4. (*Left*) A needle cricothyroidotomy can be performed quickly by advancing a 14- or 16-gauge angiocatheter through the cricothyroid membrane. High-flow oxygen is delivered as shown in photo on right.

the airway and improved oxygenation–ventilation, but it has a higher complication rate than that of the needle technique.

SIGNS OF APPROPRIATE VENTILATION

As soon as any one of these maneuvers is completed and the cervical spine is immobilized, check for clinical signs of improved ventilation. The steps in this evaluation are as follows: expose the chest, assess the rate and depth of respiration, inspect and palpate the neck and chest wall, and auscultate the lungs and heart. Signs of appropriate ventilation are bilateral chest expansion, bilateral breath sounds, an increase in heart rate to normal, and an improvement in color. Normal physiologic parameters for infants and children are presented in Table 24-2.

CERVICAL SPINE PROTECTION

Cervical spine injury should be suspected in all head injuries, in unconscious children, and with injuries above the clavicles. The cervical spine is stabilized by one of the following: sandbags–tape–backboard, rigid cervical collar, gentle manual axial traction, or Gardner–Wells tongs. Neck protection is maintained until a cross-table lateral radiograph shows seven normal cervical vertebrae. If a cervical spine injury is suspected or proved, the neck should never be hyperextended to establish an airway. Remember, it is crucial to maintain a patent airway, and this must be done even if one is fearful of a cord injury. Also remember that the head should not be turned to the side if vomiting occurs.

TABLE 24-2. Physiologic Parameters for Infants and Children

	VITAL SIGNS		URINE OUTPUT
	Breaths/min	Pulse	(ml/kg/hr)
Infants	30	140	2
Preschool-aged	20	120	1
School-aged	15	100	1

BLOOD PRESSURE

Systolic B.P. = 80 + 2 times age (years)
Diastolic B.P. = $\frac{2}{3}$ systolic B.P.

ESTIMATED BLOOD VOLUME

80–85 ml/kg

LETHAL INJURIES OF THE THORAX

Injuries of the thorax may affect ventilation and circulation; thus they are of prime importance in the injured child. In adults thoracic trauma accounts for one of four deaths secondary to accidental injury. In our experience with children, one of 10 deaths was directly attributed to thoracic trauma, but in 25% to 50% of the instances thoracic trauma contributed significantly to neurologic deterioration or brain death. Surprisingly, most deaths resulting from chest injuries occur after hospitalization. Ninety percent of these problems can be handled with simple measures, including intubation, assisted ventilation, thoracentesis, chest tube insertion, volume replacement, and pericardiocentesis. Only 10% require an open thoracotomy.

Blunt trauma, especially resulting from motor vehicle accidents and falls, is the predominant mechanism of injury. Iatrogenic injuries are also common. These problems may develop while the child is on the ventilator or during deep endotracheal suctioning, during insertion of a chest tube or nasogastric tube, or with endoscopy. Penetrating trauma from a missile or weapon is relatively uncommon but often lethal.

Two of the lethal injuries of the chest have already been discussed in detail: apnea and airway obstruction. The other causes are tension pneumothroax, open pneumothorax, massive hemothorax, flail chest with pulmonary contusion, and cardiac tamponade.

PHYSICAL DIAGNOSIS

All the lethal injuries of the chest can be diagnosed or suspected by careful physical examination of the airway, neck, chest, and heart. Time delays may prove fatal. Do not delay treatment if sudden deterioration develops. Refer to Table 24-3 for physical signs helpful with the differential diagnosis. Remember, a chest radiograph is an essential diagnostic study in all seriously injured children.

After securing the airway, immobilizing the neck, and establishing effective ventilation, the next step in management is careful examination of the neck, chest, and heart. The neck veins are assessed and the location of the trachea is carefully checked. Collapsed neck veins suggest hypovolemia, whereas distended veins suggest a tension pneumothorax,

TABLE 24-3. Differentiation of Common Respiratory Emergencies Occurring With Polytrauma

SIGNS	RIGHT MAIN STEM INTUBATION	ESOPHAGEAL INTUBATION	RIGHT TENSION PNEUMOTHROAX	CARDIAC TAMPONADE	MASSIVE RIGHT HEMOTHORAX
Neck veins	Flat	Flat	Distended	Distended	Usually flat
Tracheal position	Midline or to left	Midline	Left	Midline	Midline
Chest Expansion or Breath Sounds					
Right	Normal	Absent	Absent	Normal	Decreased
Left	Absent	Absent	Normal	Normal	Normal
Percussion					
Right	Tympanitic	Tympanitic	Tympanitic	Tympanitic	Dull
Left	Tympanitic	Tympanitic	Tympanitic	Tympanitic	Tympanitic
Heart sounds	Normal	Normal	Slightly decreased	Muffled	Normal
Shock	No	No	Yes	Yes	Yes

cardiac tamponade, or cardiac failure from a myocardial or endocardial injury. The mediastinum and trachea are very mobile structures in children. For this reason deviation of the trachea may occur with tension pneumothorax or significant atelectasis such as that related to a right main stem intubation. The relationship of the trachea to the suprasternal notch and the status of the neck veins should be checked early in the clinical course, since they may suggest the etiology of a thoracic emergency.

Crepitus or subcutaneous emphysema of the neck or chest occurs with a penetrating wound, tracheobronchial tear, esophageal perforation, or pneumothorax. The neck is also checked for masses, and carotid pulses are palpated.

The entire chest wall is then examined for signs of blunt or penetrating trauma. Compression of the sternum may elicit pain, suggesting a serious injury to the chest wall, ribs, or sternum. Percussion of the chest is performed to check for fluid in the pleural cavity. Unilateral dullness suggests a hemothorax. Auscultation of the heart may reveal tachycardia and muffled heart sounds indicating a shocklike state, tamponade, or a tension pneumothorax. Unilateral diminished breath sounds may indicate a tension pneumothorax or hemothorax. The breath sounds will be absent on the left side with a right main stem intubation.

CHEST TUBE INSERTION

Insertion of a chest tube adequately treats approximately 90% of serious chest injuries in children. The function of a chest tube is to drain blood, monitor the rate of bleeding, and evacuate air. The tube is inserted in the midaxillary line at the level of the nipple or slightly higher. This space is devoid of thick musculature and allows for easier access through the chest wall. We do not recommend insertion of a chest tube over a trocar. This device is too dangerous for routine use. The technical details for tube thoracostomy are described in Figure 24-5. During transport the chest tube is attached to a one-way Heimlich valve, which allows the exit of blood and air and is less cumbersome than an underwater seal system. Occasionally, the Heimlich valve sticks together and needs to be changed during transport. After the tube is inserted, a chest radiograph is taken and the vital signs are reevaluated.

TENSION PNEUMOTHORAX

A tension pneumothorax is a common cause of impaired ventilation and low cardiac output in the injured child. These injuries may occur with or without rib fractures. The pathophysiology of the combined cardiorespiratory failure is due to elevated pleural pressure, collapse of the ipsilateral lung, shift of the mediastinum, compression of the contralateral lung, kinking of the vena cava, and decreased venous return. The clinical signs are summarized in Table 24-3.

If a tension pneumothorax is suspected on clinical grounds, the immediate treatment is a diagnostic and therapeutic thoracentesis. The objective is to quickly convert a life-threatening condition, a tension pneumothorax, into a less threatening condition, a simple pneumo-

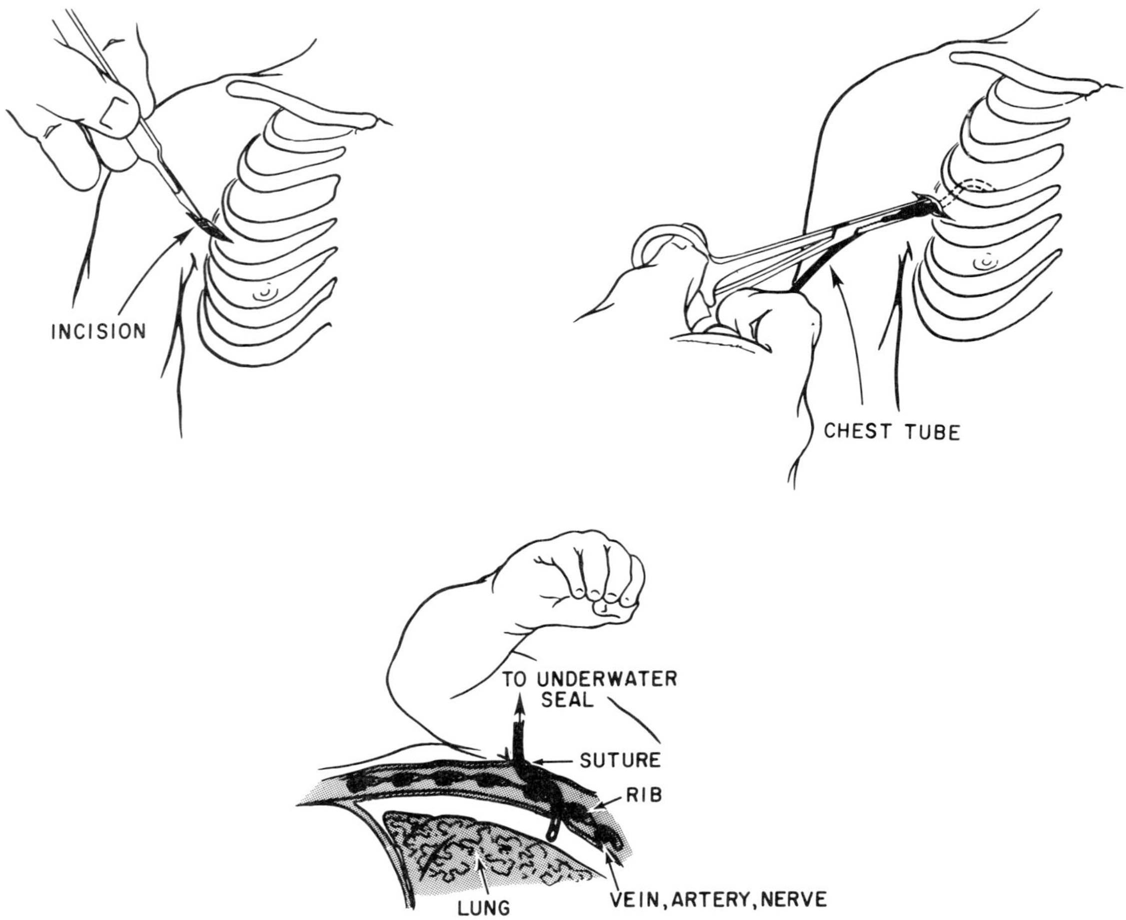

Figure 24-5. Chest tube insertion. The upper arm is elevated to expose the axilla. The skin is prepped, and a local anesthetic is injected intradermally, subcutaneously, and into the chest wall muscles. A 1–1.5-cm transverse skin incision is made in the midaxillary line just above the level of the nipple (4th or 5th intercostal space). A curved hemostat is used to dissect an oblique tract from the skin site to the next higher intercostal space. The clamp is bluntly passed through the intercostal space just above the rib to avoid injury to the nerurovascular bundle. The tip of the chest tube is grasped with a clamp, and the tube is inserted into the pleural cavity in a superior and posterior direction. The most proximal hole in the chest tube must be well inside the chest wall. The incision is closed snugly around the chest tube. The chest tube is securely anchored to the skin with sutures and tape. Petroleum jelly gauze and a small dressing are placed around the tube to ensure an airtight seal. The chest tube is attached to an underwater seal with 20 cm to 25 cm H_2O suction or to a one-way Heimlich valve.

thorax. The thoracentesis gives one additional time to insert a chest tube more safely. The equipment for a needle aspiration is a 14- or 16-gauge angiocatheter attached to a three-way stopcock and a 60-ml syringe. The needle is inserted in the midaxillary line at the level of the nipple. Removal of as little as 50 cc of air may be life-saving. Keep the angiocatheter in the pleural cavity until a chest tube is inserted.

Remember, a tension pneumothorax develops more frequently after the child arrives in the hospital than during transport. This is especially true if the child is intubated and receiving assisted ventilation. Sudden clinical deterioration might require an immediate thoracentesis for diagnosis and temporary therapy.

A simple pneumothorax or a combined hemopneumothorax are the most common type of chest injuries in the pediatric age group.

Quite often management simply involves bed rest, oxygen, and chest physiotherapy. A chest tube is required for a pneumothorax of 15% or greater, respiratory symptoms, air transport, prolonged transport, general anesthesia, or ventilator support. Persistent air leaks may be due to disruption of pulmonary parenchyma, a tracheobronchial tear, or an esophageal perforation.

OPEN PNEUMOTHORAX

The diagnosis of a sucking chest wound is obvious on inspection. Although an open pneumothorax occurs less frequently than a closed pneumothorax, the pathophysiology is basically the same. There is an inability to generate negative intrathoracic pressure, a collapsed lung, and often a tension pneumothorax. The most acceptable therapy is application of an occlusive dressing and a tube thoracostomy at a site some distance from the injury. Generally, it is not wise to insert the chest tube through the sucking wound, since this may aggravate bleeding. When a chest tube cannot be inserted by transport personnel, a lightly fitting occlusive dressing can be applied to the wound but taped on only three sides. This allows for exit of air and blood, but the dressing seals the wound during inspiration. Alternately, the wrist of the sterile surgical glove can be taped circumferentially around the wound. One of the fingertips of the glove is cut off, making a simple one-way flutter valve.

HEMOTHORAX

A small to moderate amount of blood in the pleural cavity frequently accompanies blunt thoracic trauma. A supine chest radiograph may miss significant amounts of blood in the pleural space, and for this reason an upright or semiupright film is desirable. A chest tube is used to monitor the amount of bleeding, which is usually from intercostal vessels and will stop spontaneously.

Occasionally, large quantities of blood fill the thorax from a major crush injury to the chest wall or from injury to the great vessels or lung parenchyma. This can occur with severe blunt trauma, but it happens more often from gunshot wounds or stabbings. The physical findings are tabulated in Table 24-3.

When a massive hemothorax is suspected, hypovolemia must be treated aggressively. Several large intravenous lines must be started and blood must be given freely. A chest tube is essential. Open thoracotomy is indicated for continued bleeding, persistent shock, or an acute blood loss of one third or more of the estimated blood volume. Sometimes the bleeding is so massive that autotransfusion is required to salvage the situation.

FLAIL CHEST

A flail chest develops when multiple ribs are fractured on both sides of a zone of impact. The involved segment is unstable and not in continuity with the rest of the chest wall. The condition may be suspected on chest radiograph, but the diagnosis is established by physical examination. The hallmark is paradoxical chest movement: the chest wall moves inward on inspiration and outward on expiration. This results in an inability to generate negative intrathoracic pressure, and air cannot move in and out of the trachea. Furthermore, all these children have a severe pulmonary contusion.

The emergency treatment attempts to immobilize the flail segment. This can be done by gentle manual compression or by placing the injured side down. If severe respiratory distress persists, intubation and ventilatory assistance are mandatory. Once the patient is intubated the risk of pneumothorax is about 25%. Factors that predispose to early intubation include continued ventilatory insufficiency, preexisting lung disease, neurologic or abdominal injury, immobilization from skeletal injuries, or renal failure. Currently, many of these children are managed without ventilator support. This requires vigorous monitoring of respiratory care and careful titration with narcotics, preferably by continuous infusion of morphine. Intercostal nerve blocks are generally not done in children because they hate shots.

CARDIAC TAMPONADE

Cardiac tamponade is an unusual cause of circulatory collapse in the injured child. It results from accumulation of blood in the pericardial sac. The heart cannot fill with blood during diastole, and low cardiac output develops. The most common cause is penetrating trauma. The physical findings reveal profound shock, distended neck veins, marked hepatomegaly, and muffled heart sounds. The trachea is not deviated, and breath sounds are normal bilaterally.

The emergency treatment consists of the rapid infusion of the large bolus of intravenous fluids (20 ml/kg) to help increase the diastolic filling pressure. This is followed immediately by a pericardiocentesis, as shown in Figure 24-6. Evacuation of a small volume of blood may be life-saving. Blood in the pericardial sac becomes defibrinated and does not clot. Blood aspirated from the heart chamber clots in a few minutes. The angiocatheter is left in the pericardial sac in case further aspiration of blood is required. In very urgent cases an emergency department thoractomy, with pericardiotomy and release of the cardiac tamponade, is preferred. Cardiac repair can often be done without cardiac bypass.

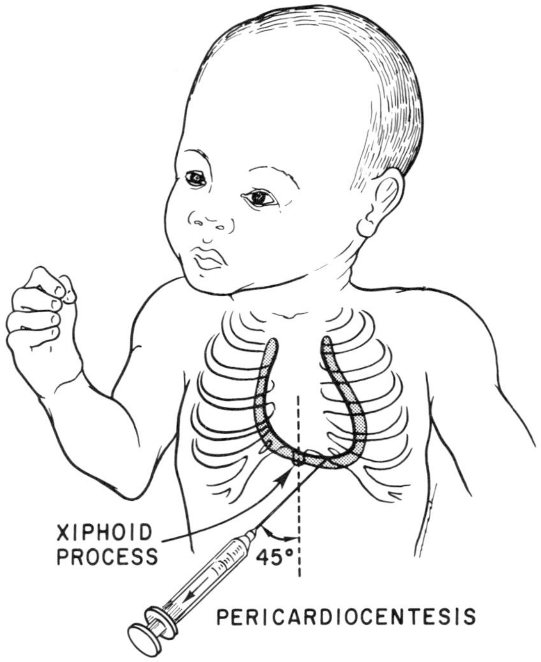

Figure 24-6. Pericardiocentesis. Cardiac tamponade can be relieved by aspiration of a small volume of fluid from the pericardial space. An 18-gauge angiocatheter is inserted into the subxiphoid area just to the left of the midline. The needle tip is aimed at the tip of the left scapula, 45 degrees laterally and 45 degrees superiorly. The syringe is aspirated during advancement of the needle. Aspirated blood from the pericardial cavity will not clot, but blood from the heart chamber will. The plastic catheter can be left in situ in case further aspiration is required.

RIB FRACTURES

Rib fractures in children less than 8 to 10 years of age are quite uncommon. The rib cage is quite compliant and elastic. It is not unusual to have the thorax run over by a car without any fracture developing. On the other hand, the pliability of the chest wall does not afford great protection to the thoracic viscera.

The lesson to emphasize is that young children with rib fractures have sustained major chest wall trauma. They require admission to the hospital for 24 to 48 hours. Serious consideration should be given to associated injuries to the head, neck, spine, lung, great vessels, and brachial plexus. Also consider nonaccidental trauma as a possible etiology. Remember that rib fractures are frequently missed or not seen on routine chest radiographs. Repeated studies or oblique films may be helpful in establishing the diagnosis.

CIRCULATION AND CONTROL OF BLEEDING

Shock is a dynamic process defined as inadequate tissue perfusion causing impaired cellular respiration. In the injured child it is usually caused by hypoxia or blood loss. Signs and symptoms of shock reflect the compensatory mechanisms that come into play to restore effective circulation. The degree of shock, as mirrored by progressive physical findings, is proportionate to the amount of blood loss. Classification of shock depends on an understanding of normal physiologic variables as well as the components of normal homeostasis. The keys to successful management are early recognition, prompt fluid replacement, and arrest of further bleeding. Remember to ventilate and oxygenate the child while concurrently initiating shock therapy.

RECOGNITION OF SHOCK

Vital signs and other physiologic parameters vary with a child's age and size. Normal physiologic variables are listed in Table 24-2 and a chart to estimate a child's weight is presented in Table 24-4. These charts will be of assistance in recognition and treatment of shock. The principles described in this section pertain to hemorrhagic shock, the most common type seen in an injured child.

TABLE 24-4. Weight According to Age

AGE	WEIGHT (KG)
Newborn	4
6 mo	8
12 mo	10
18 mo	12
2–3 yr	14
5–6 yr	20
8 yr	25
10 yr	30
14 yr	50
18 yr	65

A blood loss of 15% or less of the estimated blood volume (E.B.V.) is well tolerated in most children. There will be local findings of bleeding and tachycardia, but the other vital signs are normal. Most traumatized children have tachycardia, which is usually attributed to fear, pain, or crying. It is better to assume that the rapid pulse is secondary to volume loss until proved otherwise. While the veins are still full, an intravenous line (I.V.) can be started and a fluid challenge given.

Mild shock develops with a blood loss of 15% to 25% of the E.B.V. Specific physical signs must be carefully checked so that shock is diagnosed early and not overlooked. Again tachycardia is present, but now the diastolic blood pressure is elevated and the pulse pressure is narrowed. In most emergency rooms the diastolic blood pressure is not checked in children and narrow pulse pressures are not appreciated. Special automatic blood pressure monitoring equipment that utilizes air pressure transducers or a doppler probe is required to detect accurately the low pressures in young children. Generally, the diastolic pressure is two thirds of the systolic. Thus a blood pressure of 90/60 in a 5-year-old is normal, but 90/70 suggests hypovolemia. The other physical findings are slight prolongation of capillary refill (longer than 2 seconds); slight cooling, pallor, or mottling of the skin; tachypnea; anxiety; and thirst. These physical findings may not seem very impressive or worrisome. Children initially compensate well for mild to moderate amounts of blood loss. They masquerade the disaster that lurks ahead. For example, it is not unusual for a child to look "good" clinically one minute and the next minute have the "bottom drop out" as the youngster develops circulatory collapse. This problem can be avoided if meticulous care is given to the early recognition of shock as stated earlier.

A blood loss of 25% to 50% of the E.B.V. results in moderate shock. Most children can transiently compensate for losses approaching 40% of the blood volume, but then they decompensate rapidly. For the first time the blood pressure falls and the child is hypotensive, the skin is cool and mottled, capillary refill is prolonged, the urine output is decreased, and the child is confused. Laboratory studies reveal acidosis: *p*H less than 7.3, base excess less than 8, bicarbonate less than 18 mEq/liter, and a lactate over 2.5 mg/dl. Aggressive resuscitation is required.

Blood losses over 50% of the blood volume are potentially life-threatening, and surgical control of bleeding may be indicated. Clinical manifestations are profound hypotension and marked metabolic acidosis. Treatment requires rapid blood replacement.

TREATMENT OF SHOCK

Hemorrhagic shock must be recognized early and treated promptly. Fluids are given in a bolus fashion with large volumes administered over a period of minutes. Comparison of preinfusion and postinfusion physiologic parameters is crucial in detecting hemodynamic instability. If the vital signs do not improve, more volume is required and surgery may be necessary.

Vascular Access

Establishing vascular access in the pediatric age group may be a challenging ordeal, especially if the child is chubby or has impending shock. The following information should help with establishing a strategy toward approaching this sometimes frustrating but always important aspect of shock management.

Percutaneous Peripheral Intravenous Line. The preferred initial sites for venous access in the injured child are the peripheral veins. These sites are the simplest, safest, and usually the quickest way to start. The preferred veins are the saphenous, cephalic, or basilic at the elbow; the interdigitals of the hand (especially the vein between the fourth and fifth finger); the cephalic at the wrist; the external jugular; and the scalp veins in infants.

The following guidelines are helpful in starting a peripheral I.V.:

1. Restrain the extremity on a padded board.
2. Apply a warm compress to dilate the vein.
3. Properly apply a tourniquet proximal to the site.
4. Flush the needle with heparinized saline prior to cannulation.
5. Puncture the skin first with a larger needle than the angiocatheter.
6. Attach a T-connector to help prevent catheter dislodgment.
7. Tape securely.

Transillumination with a high-intensity light may help to locate veins in the hands or feet of chubby toddlers.

Avoid starting an intravenous line in injured extremities, as the fluid may not reach the central circulation and additional swelling may produce a compartment syndrome. An I.V. should be started in the lower extremity if there is trauma to the base of the neck or upper thorax. Reliable venous access usually requires two lines that are working well.

Saphenous Vein Cutdown. The saphenous vein at the ankle is the best place to perform a cutdown in a child. The vein is usually quite large, and even a newborn will accept a 20-gauge angiocatheter. The technical details of the procedure are illustrated in Figure 24-7. If during the dissection a small vein is identified, this is probably just a tributary. Look deeper for the larger vein located against the tibial periosteum. During shock the saphenous vein may develop marked venospasm. This makes cannulation difficult, and fluid may not flow into the vein by gravity drip. Fluid may have to be pushed in with a syringe.

A cutdown can also be performed on the external jugular or basilic vein. During shock it may be difficult to differentiate between the brachial artery and basilic vein. A doppler can be placed on the radial artery at the wrist to help avoid accidental arterial cannulation.

Pneumatic Counterpressure Device. The pneumatic counterpressure device can be a useful adjunct to the treatment of shock in the critically injured child. Scientific studies documenting their efficacy are lacking, but there are still valid reasons for their continued use in children. Inflation of the garment results in an autotransfuion of 5% to 10% of the E.B.V. Equally important, application of the trousers transiently bulges the veins in the upper extremities. This phenomenon lasts for only a few minutes, but it usually allows enough time to establish several good percutaneous I.V. lines. The garment is very helpful in stablizing pelvic fractures and fractures of the lower extremities. Soft-tissue bleeding is tamponaded, pain is relieved, and the body temperature is maintained—all helpful adjuncts to shock management.

There are some disadvantages to the trousers. Inflation of the abdominal component interferes with ventilation, and endotracheal intubation is required in most patients. The device interferes with examination of the abdomen and does nothing to slow intra-abdominal bleeding. As stated previously, the garment may prove very helpful in diminishing the blood loss from pelvic fractures, but bleeding into the peritoneal cavity is not affected. One of the major disadvantages of the device is that few people know how to use it properly. The details of management will not be presented here, but they need to be mastered if the trousers are employed in your area.

The trousers now come in two sizes. There is a pediatric size for children from 4 to 10 years of age and a toddler size for ages 18 months to 4 years. Elastic wraps can be used in children younger than 2 years of age.

Intraosseous Infusion. In a critically ill or injured child, valuable time may be wasted trying to start a peripheral I.V. line or venous cutdown. In a life-threatening situation a rapid and effective method for delivering fluids, medications, and blood products is the intraosseous route. This procedure is recommended for children 5 years of age or younger. Between the ages of 3 and 5 years the bone marrow starts to be replaced with fat, which can nullify the usefulness of this approach. Nevertheless this method should be attempted in this age range, but occasionally it will not be successful. We suggest this technique be used if venous access cannot be established in 2 minutes following a cardiorespiratory arrest or in 5 minutes following trauma resuscitation. The intraosseous site should be considered a temporary route, and as soon as a good I.V. line is started it should be discontinued.

The equipment required is a bone marrow needle or 16- to 20-gauge spinal needle, a syringe, and a T-connector. The insertion site is the anteromedial surface of the tibia 1 cm to 2 cm below the tibial tuberosity. The needle is

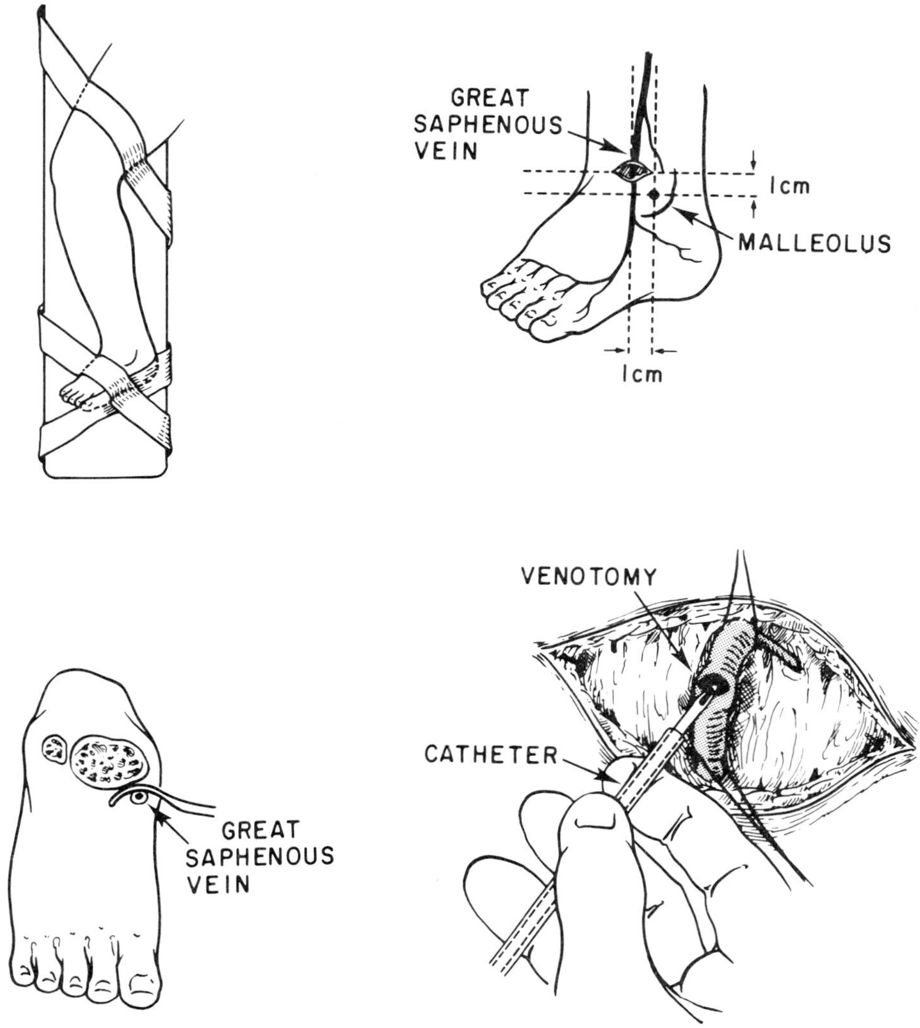

Figure 24-7. Saphenous vein cutdown. The leg and foot are taped to a padded board with the medial side up. The skin is prepped and a local anesthetic is injected intradermally. A 3–5-mm transverse incision is made superior and anterior to the tip of the medial malleolus. A fine, curved hemostat is inserted into the posterior aspect of the incision until the tibia is encountered. The tip of the hemostat is scraped forward against the bone, and all the tissue is scooped up and brought out through the incision. The hemostat is gently opened and the vein isolated from the fatty tissue and nerve. The vein is tied distally with an absorbable suture. The vein may be directly cannulated with an angiocatheter, but frequently the posterior wall of the vessel is perforated. A safer technique is a transverse venotomy made with a No. 11 scalpel blade, with insertion of the catheter facilitated by use of a vein introducer. The catheter is anchored to the vein with another absorbable suture. Careful skin closure completes the procedure.

inserted perpendicular to the tibial surface aiming slightly in an inferior direction to avoid damage to the epiphysis. The needle is advanced in a screwing or boring fashion. Proper placement is verified when blood and bone marrow are aspirated and a gentle infusion does not cause subcutaneous infiltration. Blood may clot quickly in the needle. The obstruction can be relieved by reinsertion of the stylet. Medications should be diluted to lessen the chance of bone marrow damage.

The technique is quick, safe, and effective. Large quantities of fluid can be administered in a short time. Paramedical personnel can be trained to use this procedure in the field. It will help save lives.

Limitations of Central Venous Access. Central venous access, even under ideal circumstances, is difficult to establish in children less than 8 years of age. The procedure requires a great deal of experience and skill to be done safely. In a seriously injured child the chance for successful cannulation is low, and valuable time will be wasted trying to insert this line. Furthermore, the procedure is associated with a long list of significant complications. For these reasons this is not recommended as a primary route for vascular access during the resuscitative phase of management.

Volume Replacement

Ringer's lactate (RL) is the fluid of choice for resuscitation of the pediatric trauma victim. Fluid replacement is divided into two phases: initial therapy and total replacement. Initial therapy is based on an estimation of the severity of shock. Fluids are administered rapidly via a push of RL with a 60 ml syringe. Vital signs are carefully checked before and after bolus therapy. If vital signs are not improved immediately, more volume is given. Total fluid replacement approximates 3 ml of RL for every 1 ml of estimated blood loss. Remember, these are guidelines for initiation of therapy. If a child does not respond appropriately, suspect continued bleeding, check for causes of refractory shock, or consider operative intervention.

Mild shock (15% to 25% blood loss) is initially treated with a bolus of RL at 20 ml/kg. If the vital signs do not move toward normal, a second bolus of 20 ml/kg is given. If the vital signs improve, the maintenance I.V. rate is 5 ml/kg/hr. Total volume replacement is 3 ml of RL for every 1 ml of blood loss.

Moderate shock (25% to 50% blood loss) is initially treated with a bolus of RL at 40 ml/kg. If there is no improvement, 10 ml/kg to 20 ml/kg of packed red blood cells or 20 ml/kg to 40 ml/kg of RL is rapidly infused. Lack of improvement suggests the need for operative control of bleeding unless there is a clear-cut explanation for the lack of response, such as multiple fractures with continued bleeding. If the child improves after the first bolus of fluids, the maintenance I.V. rate is 5 ml/kg/hr. One-half of the total blood loss should be replaced with packed red blood cells and the other half with RL at a ratio of 3 ml RL to 1 ml of blood loss.

Severe shock (greater than 50% blood loss) is treated by continuous boluses of RL and type-specific blood until the child's vital signs improve. If there is evidence of continued bleeding into the thorax or abdomen and the child is not responding to rapid fluid replacement, then life-saving surgery is required.

Control of Bleeding

The control of bleeding from trauma depends on many variables. The hemorrhage may be acute, with large quantities of blood loss in a short time. Obviously, aggressive fluid replacement and/or surgical control of bleeding may be required if bleeding continues or if hemodynamic instability persists.

On the other hand, there are injuries associated with sizable blood losses but that are best treated by nonoperative therapy. For example, one can anticipate a blood loss approaching or exceeding the total blood volume in a child with a closed head injury, scalp laceration, and fractured femur and pelvis. The bleeding occurs over several hours. Treatment includes volume replacement, splinting or traction of fractures, and repair of the scalp laceration. Most pelvic fractures require simple bed rest, but occasionally the pneumatic antishock garment or interventional angiography is required to stop pelvic bleeding.

Recognition of occult blood loss may require a long period of observation. Significant occult bleeding is usually intra-abdominal or retroperitoneal, but occasionally it is within the thoracic cavity. The CT scan is very helpful in assessing occult bleeding. Remember that children can lose life-threatening quantities of blood from scalp lacerations or intracranial injuries.

External bleeding should be arrested by direct pressure over the bleeding point. Elevation may greatly reduce blood loss, and this is particularly true with brisk bleeding from scalp wounds or dural sinus lacerations. On occasion, spurting vessels may be clamped with hemostats, but only if the bleeding points are clearly visible. Remember that nerves are generally adjacent to vessels, especially in the extremities and the face. The only blood vessels that may be clamped without significant risk of permanent nerve injury are those of the hair-bearing portion of the scalp.

Bleeding from the extremities may be controlled temporarily by tourniquets. Blood pressure cuffs serve as useful tourniquets under these conditions. The tourniquet must be tight enough to obliterate the distal pulses or else blood loss will be promoted. Ischemic pain usually becomes unbearable within 15 to 20 minutes after application of the tourniquet, and ischemic damage may be present within 30 to 45 minutes of application. Within a few minutes the tourniquet should be replaced by a sterile pressure dressing. Pneumatic splints or the pneumatic antishock garment are also useful in splinting extremity fractures and decreasing blood loss.

Refractory Shock

If the child does not respond as expected to fluid replacement, there may be other causes for continued shock. Airway patency, oxygenation, and ventilation should be checked again. Has the child developed a lethal chest injury? Is there an unrecognized source of bleeding? Also consider whether the child has gastric dilation, diabetic ketoacidosis, hypoadrenalism, or neurogenic shock.

DISABILITY AND DIAGNOSIS OF SHOCK

Since head injuries occur so frequently in children, the triage should include a brief neurologic evaluation. The objectives of this evaluation are to detect deterioration in the level of consciousness and to note the appearance of a lateralizing nuerologic deficit that may require operation or intensification of nonoperative management.

Initially, the neurologic examination means assessment of the level of consciousness, detection of motor weakness, and pupillary size and reactivity. There are four levels of consciousness: alert, responsive to verbal stimuli, responsive to painful stimuli, and unresponsive. This brief neurologic assessment should be rechecked serially. A more detailed evaluation is done after the child is stable from a hemodynamic and respiratory standpoint.

The symptoms of increased intracranial pressure are headache, nausea and vomiting, diplopia, transient obscurations, lethargy, and drowsiness. The signs are papilledema, sixth nerve palsy, decreased awareness, a bulging fontanel in infants, palpable suture spread, progressive head enlargement, and signs of internal herniation.

The keys to the emergency management of the head-injured child include adequate oxygenation (PaO_2 80 torr to 100 torr), hyperventilation ($PaCO_2$ 25 torr to 30 torr), restoration of normovolemia, and elevation of the head. More intensive therapy includes diuretics, muscle paralysis, control of seizures, short-activity barbiturates, hypothermia, and a host of newer investigational therapies. A neurosurgeon should direct this management. If a diuretic is given for neurologic deterioration, the bladder must be effectively drained. Failure to do so may result in a bladder perforation.

Remember, shock may be difficult to diagnose in a child, and sudden deterioration can occur if it is not treated properly. Serially reassess the child for the subtle, early signs of circulatory insufficiency.

EXPOSURE AND ENVIRONMENT

All clothing is removed from an injured child so that he can be inspected from head to toe and front to back. The body wall is examined for the presence of contusions, abrasions, lacerations, and penetrating wounds that suggest underlying injury. Several hours may be required for some of the injuries to become apparent.

Because of the relatively large body surface area of children and an immature thermoregulatory mechanism, body heat can be easily lost, resulting in acidosis and hemodynamic instability. Rectal temperature is carefully monitored. Keep the child warm. This can be done by surface rewarming with blankets, warm compresses, or heat lamps or by turning up the room temperature. In infants the head has a large body surface area. Cover it and keep it warm. Core rewarming is done by infusing warm fluids that have been heated by a blood warmer or microwave oven. Heat can also be given by warming the air given through the endotracheal tube. In a near-drowning setting, rewarming is done by lavage into the stomach, rectum, or peritoneum, and consideration is given to partial cardiac bypass.

NASOGASTRIC TUBE AND URINARY CATHETER

The final steps in the initial management of the injured child are insertion of a nasogastric tube and bladder catheter. A properly functioning nasogastric tube prevents aspiration, removes swallowed air, and checks for blood. A nasally inserted tube is contraindicated if there is danger of intubating the brain: CSF rhinorrhea, midfacial fractures, and an anterior basal skull fracture. Suspect an anterior basal skull fracture in the presence of "black and blue" eyes and lateral scleral hemorrhages. Under these circumstances the gastric tube should be inserted orally, and a bite block may also be necessary. Insertion of a nasogastric tube is very painful. Make certain that the neck is immobilized while this procedure is being done. If the child is gagging, retching, or struggling during the insertion, do not force the tube down. The tube can accidentally perforate the hypopharynx and be advanced into the mediastinum and right pleural cavity. Fortunately, most of these lesions heal without operation.

Acute gastric dilatation frequently accompanies childhood trauma, even minor trauma. It develops from swallowed air or esophageal intubation. This condition may fool the unwary physician. Not only is the abdomen distended, but in many cases respiration is compromised and the child appears to be in shock. The diagnosis is established and definitive treatment rendered by inserting a nasogastric tube. Gas comes out the tube under pressure, and the physical findings quickly return to normal.

A urinary catheter is inserted to monitor urine output and to check for hematuria. Urine output is of little value in the initial phases of shock evaluation, but it is an excellent index of circulatory perfusion in the ongoing management of the injured child. The catheter is inserted unless contraindicated: pelvic fracture, resistance to passage, or suspect urethral injury. If the bladder is distended and the urethra cannot or should not be cannulated, an angiocatheter can be inserted suprapubically for temporary bladder decompression.

CONCLUSIONS

Outcome, favorable or otherwise, depends on the care the child receives during the first critical hour following injury. The resuscitative skills, the ABCs, can be mastered by all primary care givers. If a dent in the pediatric trauma epidemic is to be made in our lifetime, we will have to create a team of people who regularly and expertly perform these skills at the scene, during transport, and on arrival to the hospital emergency department. I trust this information will help in this worthwhile endeavor.

BIBLIOGRAPHY

Committee on Trauma, American College of Surgeons: Advanced Trauma Life Support Course. Chicago, American College of Surgeons, 1984.

Eichelberger MD, Randolph JG: Thoracic trauma in children. Surg. Clin North Am 61:1181, 1981

Mayer TA, Matlak ME, Nixon GW, Walker ML: Emergency Management of Pediatric Trauma. Philadelphia, WB Saunders, 1985

Standards and Guidelines for Cardiopulmonary Resuscitation (CPR) and Emergency Cardiac Care (ECC). JAMA 255:2954

25 Thoracic Trauma, Other Common Cardiothoracic Problems, and Diagnostic Procedures

WILLIAM A. GAY, JR., AND S. V. KARWANDE

THORACIC TRAUMA

Although many thoracic surgical diagnostic procedures can be accomplished on an ambulatory basis, for the most part thoracic surgery is a hospital-based specialty. However, recognition and early treatment of thoracic trauma should certainly be part of the skills of every physician providing ambulatory surgical care. This chapter is structured so as to deal first with the recognition and early management of thoracic injuries, then with the diagnostic and minor therapeutic procedures suitable for ambulatory management.

Major advances in transporting injured patients and providing on-site and in-transit care by highly skilled paramedical personnel have resulted in many seriously injured patients surviving long enough to reach a medical facility. Major thoracic trauma is present, either alone or in combination with other injuries, in 75% of fatally injured patients. The medical staff responsible for the patient's evaluation and early treatment must therefore act quickly and correctly. Delay in diagnosis or treatment may be a major factor contributing to morbidity and mortality in victims of chest trauma.

Trauma to the thorax includes injury to the thoracic cage, pleura, lung, esophagus, diaphragm, heart, and great vessels. In many instances there is a combination of injuries, and the trauma may be unilateral or bilateral. It often is associated with injury to other parts of the body.

Early treatment of patients with chest injuries is based on two principles: (1) assurance of adequate ventilatory function and (2) control of bleeding and restoration of intravascular volume. Injuries to the thorax are characteristically classified according to etiology as either blunt or penetrating.

THORACIC STRUCTURES AND TYPES OF INJURIES

It is helpful to recall the structures that may be injured in trauma to the chest. From such an orderly approach, one is less likely to miss recognizing injuries:

1. Chest wall—rib fractures, lacerations, stab wounds, and the like
2. Lung—tears and contusions
3. Bronchus—disruption, partial or total
4. Trachea—tears and contusions
5. Mediastinum—contusions, lacerations
6. Esophagus—perforation
7. Great vessels—perforation, tears, or disruptions
8. Diaphragm—tears and perforations

MANIFESTATIONS OF INJURIES TO THESE STRUCTURES

1. Chest wall—flail chest, open pneumothorax with a sucking wound, localized pain
2. Lung—closed pneumothorax or tension pneumothorax, tears with bleeding, respiratory insufficiency
3. Bronchus—total or partial disruption with massive air leak and moderate bleeding
4. Trachea—mediastinal or subcutaneous emphysema, injury to larnyx

5. Mediastinum and contents—mediastinal emphysema, mediastinal widening, pericardial tamponade, cardiac contusion
6. Esophagus—severe pain, pleural effusion, pneumothorax
7. Great vessels—bleeding, often severe, usually associated with rapid deceleration injury
8. Diaphragm—rupture with bowel in chest (usually left side) with symptoms referable to obstruction

GENERAL TREATMENT

When a patient is felt to have had major thoracic trauma, he or she should be sent to the hospital as quickly as possible. Transportation in the erect or semierect position is advisable with the injured side *dependent,* as this aids respiration and lessens the chance of flooding the opposite side with blood and secretions. Tension pneumothorax is an extreme emergency and timely insertion of a chest tube may be life-saving. Sucking wounds of the chest require immediate sealing with dressing. The general treatment of such injuries is similar to the treatment of trauma in general, with special emphasis on the treatment of failing respiration and circulation. In treatment of hypovolemic shock, adequate fluids must be administered, but it is important to avoid overloading the circulation and causing pulmonary edema. Blood should be used in adequate quantities. Pain must be relieved to minimize shock, but narcotics should be used sparingly because they depress respiration. Meperidine (Demerol) is recommended by intravenous route. Local intercostal nerve blocks are helpful. Sometimes better pain control can be obtained by using an epidural catheter and injecting preservative-free morphine into the epidural space. Using this technique, significant and long-lasting analgesia may be obtained with small narcotic doses that do not affect hemodynamics. The patient, however, needs monitoring for respiratory depression, apnea, and urinary retention, preferably in an intensive care unit. Respiration and cough are encouraged, and oxygen, when indicated, is best administered by nasal catheter or through an endotracheal tube.

Maintenance of a patent airway is basic to the treatment of chest trauma. Retention of bronchial secretions is caused by severe chest wall pain, which results in involuntary immobilization of the chest wall, making cough ineffectual because of abnormal mobility of the chest wall and depression of the cough reflex. Treatment is therefore directed toward relieving chest wall pain and clearing the airway of secretions. This may be accomplished by encouraging deep breathing and coughing. When this is not feasible, intratracheal aspiration may be employed.

Aspiration is performed by inserting a fairly stiff 16 to 18 French catheter through the nose. The patient is placed in a semisitting position with the back supported and the head and neck extended. The lubricated catheter is passed through the nose and pharynx without suction apparatus attached. The patient is instructed to take a deep breath, and during inspiration the catheter is passed into the trachea. If the patient gags, the catheter is in the esophagus and not the trachea. Suction is applied intermittently when the catheter is passed into the tracheobronchial tree.

An endotracheal tube should be placed in serious chest injuries because it makes removal of secretions much easier and lessens the work of breathing. A tube with a high-volume, low-pressure balloon should be used because it decreases the possibility of pressure necrosis of the trachea. *The importance of maintaining a patent airway cannot be overemphasized.*

Reexpansion of the lung should be effected as early as possible, so it is important to diagnose accurately the presence of air, blood, chyle, or abdominal viscera in the pleural space. Pneumothorax or hemothorax requires prompt insertion of an adequate-sized chest tube (30 to 36 French) in the fifth to seventh intercostal space in the midaxillary line (Fig. 25-1). In a patient known to have rib fractures it is wise to insert a chest tube concomitantly with endotracheal intubation and institution of positive pressure ventilation to prevent tension pneumothorax. In a supine patient great care must be exercised if the chest tube is placed below the fifth intercostal space to prevent intra-abdominal insertion of the tube and injury to the liver or spleen. If the diaphragm is elevated by dilated stomach or bowel, nasogastric decompression will allow an increase in pulmonary reserve.

Prophylactic use of antibiotics is controversial and depends on the type of wound, contamination, and so forth. In grossly contami-

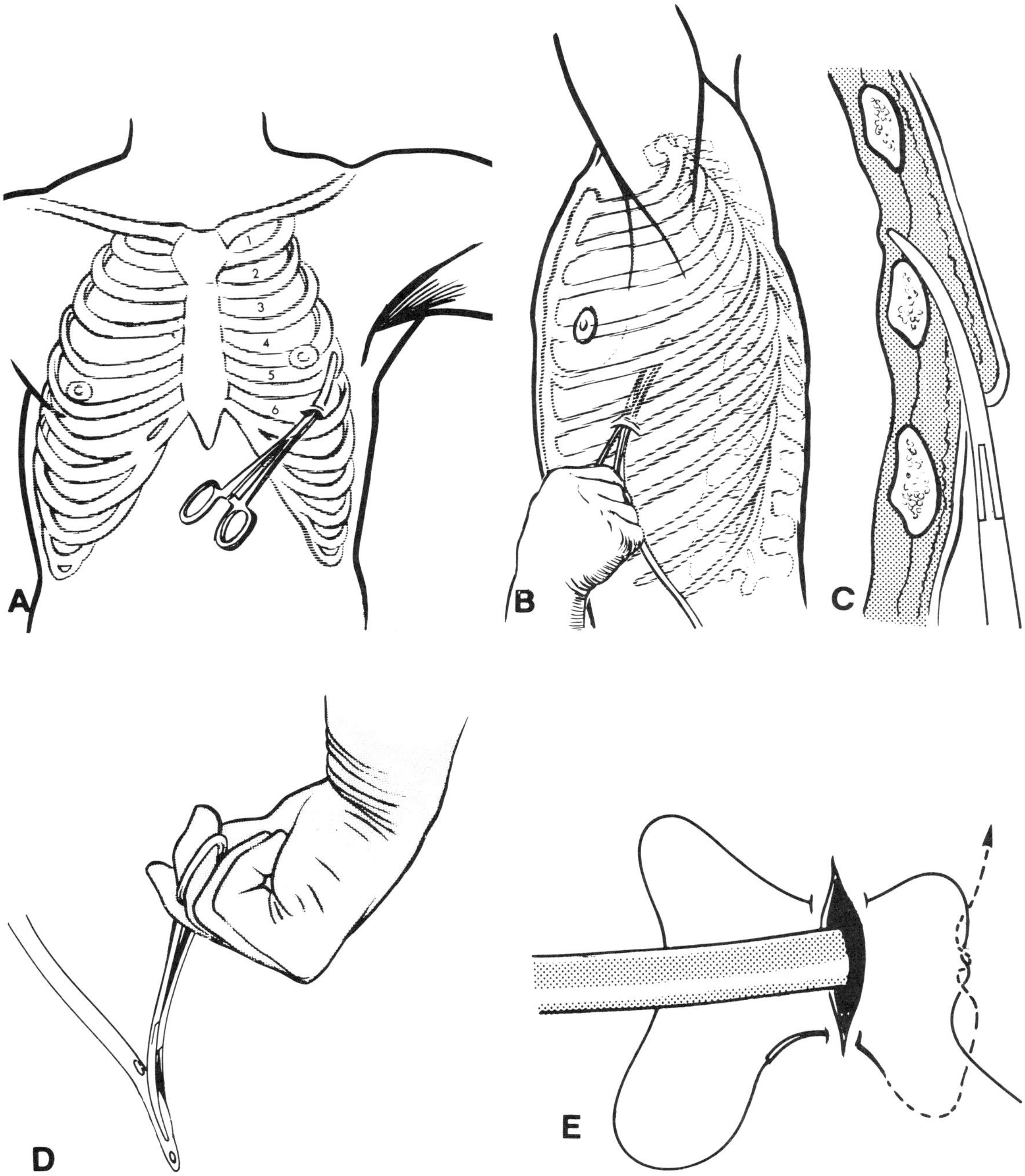

Figure 25-1. Placement of an intercostal tube. (*A*) Anterior approach in the nipple line into the sixth intercostal space. A Kelly hemostat is used after the area is first infiltrated with local anesthetic and a 2-cm incision is made with a scalpel just through the skin. (*B*) Lateral approach in the midaxillary line in the sixth interspace. (*C*) Blunt dissection over the top of the rib to avoid nerve and vascular structures. (*D*) Grasping the catheter in the hemostat. (Sometimes grasping is easier if about 1 cm of hemostat extends beyond the end of the catheter.) (*E*) Placement of stitch to hold the tube in place.

nated wounds it is justified to start with a broad-spectrum antibiotic and then to change to a more specific antibiotic once a culture is obtained. In severe lung contusion or hemothorax it is probably wise to administer a first-generation cephalosporin immediately and switch, if appropriate, after cultures are obtained and reported.

It is important to have a routine to follow in resuscitating a patient with penetrating or closed-chest injury and in evaluating the injury.

1. Examine the entirely exposed neck and chest for evidence of injury requiring immediate respiratory assistance.
2. Start intravenous administration of fluids and infuse rapidly up to 2000 ml of lactated Ringer's solution if the patient has been known to have had significant blood loss.
3. Obtain blood specimens for:
   - Type and crossmatch
   - Complete blood count
   - BUN, glucose, serum electrolytes, and blood gases when appropriate.
4. Insert nasogastric tube
5. Insert Foley catheter to:
   - Obtain specimen for urinalysis
   - Determine hourly urinary output
6. If the patient is hypotensive, be suspicious of cardiac tamponade or mediastinal shift due to tension pneumothorax. Obtain portable chest roentgenogram if condition is stable and ECG as soon as feasible.
7. Obtain a complete history.
8. When condition permits, obtain additional roentgenograms:
   - Stab wounds—upright posteroanterior projection of chest; upright, supine, and left lateral decubitus projection of abdomen
   - Gunshot wounds-upright posteroanterior and laterial projection of chest; supine and lateral projections of other body regions suspected of containing a missile
   - Hematuria—infusion pyelography or cystography (or both)
9. When pneumothorax or hemothorax is confirmed, insert a thoracostomy tube. Often aspiration with syringe and needle indicates need for insertion of a thoracostomy tube if air or blood is obtained and the patient is too ill for roentgenography.
10. Administer tetanus prophylaxis.
11. Transport patient to operating room or observation unit as indicated by condition.

SPECIFIC TREATMENT

Blunt Thoracic Trauma

INJURY	TREATMENT
Rib fracture	Analgesics; intercostal nerve block
Flail chest	Endotracheal tube and volume-cycled respirator
Pneumothorax	Chest tube to underwater seal and suction
Pulmonary contusion	Observation; respirator support as needed
Tracheobronchial	Surgical repair as soon as possible
Spinal	Neurosurgical or orthopaedic care
Cardiac	Observation; supportive treatment; surgery as indicated
Aortic disruption	Surgical repair immediately
Diaphragmatic rupture	Surgical repair as soon as possible

Penetrating Thoracic Injuries

In a penetrating thoracic injury if the vital signs are stable and chest film is normal, only observation is necessary.

INJURY	TREATMENT
Pneumothorax or hemopneumothorax	Chest tube to underwater seal and suction
Sucking chest wound	Occlusive dressing; chest tube
Cardiac	Pericardiocentesis if suspicion of tamponade; may need surgical repair, usually immediately

INJURY	TREATMENT
Aortic	Surgical repair immediately
Pulmonary vascular	Chest tube; may need surgical repair, depending on amount of bleeding
Tracheobronchial	Surgical repair as soon as possible
Esophageal	Surgical repair and drainage immediately
Transdiaphragmatic to abdomen	Abdominal signs usually present and exploration needed promptly
Spinal	Neurosurgical or orthopaedic care

THORACIC CAGE

Rib Fractures. After the general measures of treatment are carried out, injuries to various parts of the chest must be treated. In the thoracic cage nonpenetrating injuries sometimes result in fractures. In rib fractures intercostal nerve block and narcotics in small amounts are usually adequate (Fig. 25-2). One or two ribs above and below as well as the involved rib must be blocked because of overlapping nerve supply. The complications of these, pneumothorax or hemothorax, must be kept in mind. Elderly patients with poor cardiopulmonary reserve, underlying chronic lung disease, arterial hypoxia, and associated pleural effusion may require hospitalization.

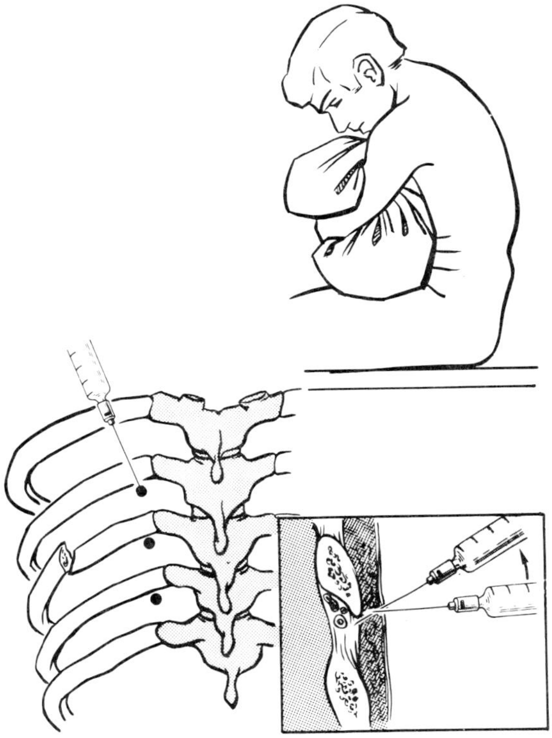

Figure 25-2. Intercostal nerve block in rib fracture. This position of the patient opens the intercostal spaces somewhat. Note that the site of the block is well posterior, just lateral to the transverse processes and the undersurface of the rib, and that one rib above and one below the fractured rib are blocked. The inset shows the technique of going down to the rib and then "walking the needle downward until it just drops off the edge of the rib." By advancing the needle about 1 cm at this point the nerve bundle is reached. Before injection of local anesthetic, aspiration is mandatory to avoid intravenous injection.

Sternal Fractures. Sternal fractures are usually incomplete or undisplaced. Such an injury may be effectively treated by injection of local anesthetics. There is no loss of stability of the chest wall, and the chief concern is the possibility of injury to the heart or great vessels (Fig. 25-3). Complete fractures with displacement can cause instability of the chest wall; open reduction and fixation with wire may be required.

Flail Chest. Severe crushing injuries to the chest may result in flail chest, a paradoxical motion of the chest wall due to multiple rib fractures (Fig. 25-4A and B). In addition, there is usually associated contusion of the lung beneath. The paradoxical motion of the chest wall causes a decrease in breathing capacity and a total ventilatory deficit proportional to the volume of the paradoxical segment.

It was believed for many years that the main component of pulmonary insufficiency and the morbidity and mortality associated with crush injuries of the chest were due to this instability of the chest wall. It is now recognized that the pulmonary contusion usually associated with crushing injury contributes to the defect and is of considerable importance.

Management of the patient with a flail chest consists of endotracheal intubation, mechanical ventilation, and initiation of positive end-expiratory pressure (PEEP) only if the arterial PO_2 cannot be maintained above 60 torr. It is also important to restrict fluids and to provide pain relief by narcotics, nerve blocks, or prolonged epidural analgesia. Extubation is done when satisfactory blood gas levels are ob-

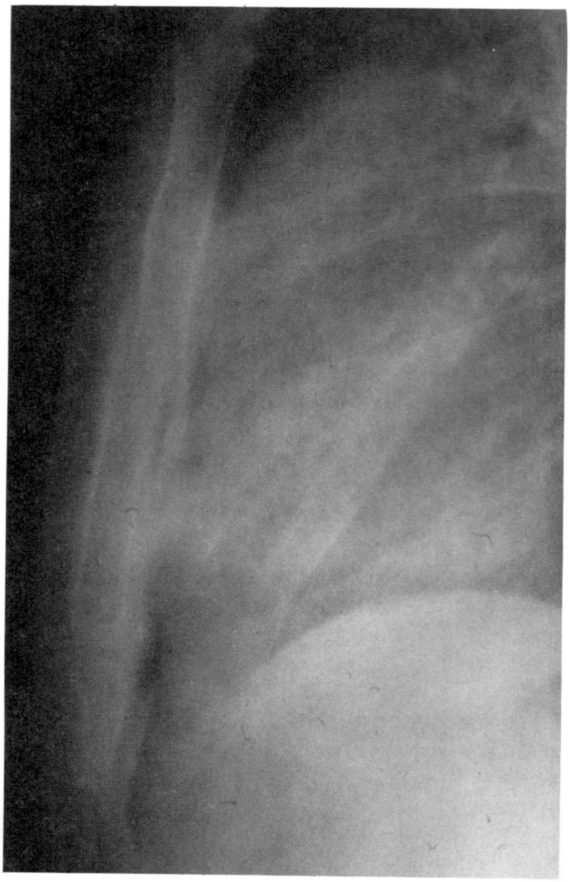

Figure 25-3. Fracture of the body of the sternum. Surgery is usually not needed.

tained. Stabilization of the chest by operative insertion of Steinmann pins, Kirschner wires, or Judet's struts has been reported, but this is probably rarely necessary. It is important to realize that although the value of endotracheal intubation is well known, many such patients can be managed without intubation.

General guidelines for early intubation are as follows:

Initial respiratory rate >25/min
Pulse rate greater than 100/min
Systolic blood pressure <100 torr
Poor initial arterial blood gas (PaO_2 <60 torr)
The presence of multisystem trauma

First Rib Fracture. Because the first rib is short, broad, and well protected by musculoskeletal structures, it can be fractured only by a significant force. The significance of fractures of the first rib has been debated. From recent reviews one may conclude that upper rib fractures including the first rib are "a hallmark" of severe trauma. This should raise the index of suspicion for major vessel injury.

LUNG

Pneumothorax–Hemothorax. Penetrating injuries produce trauma to deeper structures. However, nonpenetrating injuries causing rib fractures may result in lacerations of lung parenchyma. Occasionally, blunt trauma will lacerate a lung. Hemorrhage is a serious com-

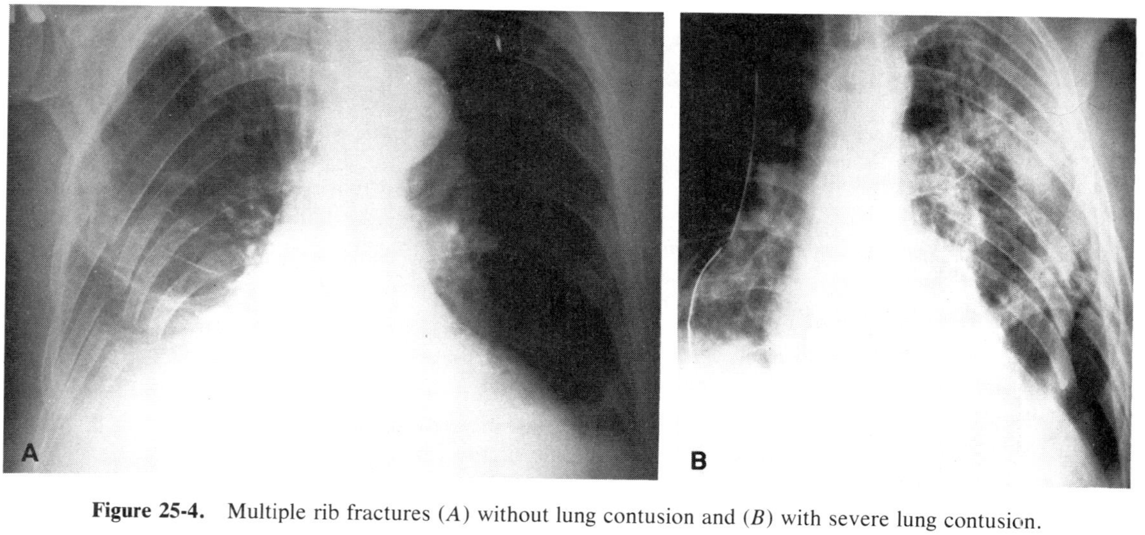

Figure 25-4. Multiple rib fractures (*A*) without lung contusion and (*B*) with severe lung contusion.

plication if it is not recognized or readily controlled. This may result from intercostal, internal mammary, or great vessel bleeding. Uncontrollable bleeding is one of the indications for immediate surgical intervention. After initial removal of accumulated blood, loss of over 200 ml/hr for 4 to 5 hours is indication for open thoracotomy to locate and control bleeding.

Penetration of the pleura must be suspected in all cases of laceration of the chest wall or epigastrium. If the pleura is opened, pneumothorax and possibly hemothorax may occur. With simple thoracic injuries in which only a small pneumothorax is present, the lung may reexpand without further interference. If pneumothorax is more massive, insertion of an intercostal tube is necessary. Hemothorax, if the amount of blood is significant, is not difficult to diagnose (Fig. 25-5). The patient is dyspneic and cyanotic, and the percussion note is flat. Breath and voice sounds are usually distant over the greater part of the chest. Free return of blood on thoracentesis confirms the diagnosis, and a large-bore (32 to 36 French) catheter should be placed in the fifth to seventh intercostal space. Simple aspiration with a plastic catheter and syringe in the second or third intercostal space in the midclavicular line will confirm the presence or absence of pneumothorax. The needle should be inserted carefully on the upside of the rib and just through the parietal pleura. Catheter aspiration of a simple traumatic pneumothorax may be performed safely but is not recommended for the multiply injured patient.

Tension Pneumothorax. Tension pneumothorax, or pressure pneumothorax, indicates accumulation of air under pressure in the pleural cavity, compressing the lung and thereby seriously interfering with ventilation. Dyspnea and cyanosis are common findings, and there is a shift of the trachea (Fig. 25-6) and heart to the uninjured side with loss of breath sounds over the involved side. The combination of hypoxia and interference with cardiac filling may lead to circulatory collapse. Treatment is immediate decompression, which is best accomplished by introducing a catheter into the second or third interspace anteriorly 4 cm lateral to the sternum and connecting it to water-seal drainage.

Open Pneumothorax. Open injuries of the chest wall present another problem. Because of the opening intrapleural pressure is atmospheric. If the wound allows air to enter the pleural space but not to escape (sucking type of wound), the patient's condition deteriorates rapidly. These wounds must be treated as soon as possible. A simple occlusive dressing of petrolatum gauze and a large dressing and

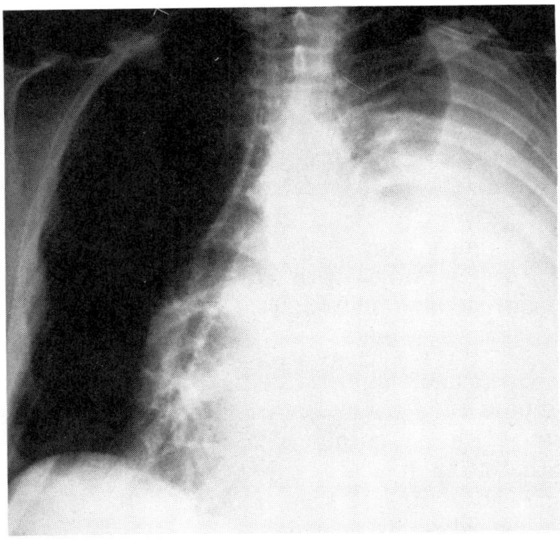

Figure 25-5. Massive hemothorax on the left.

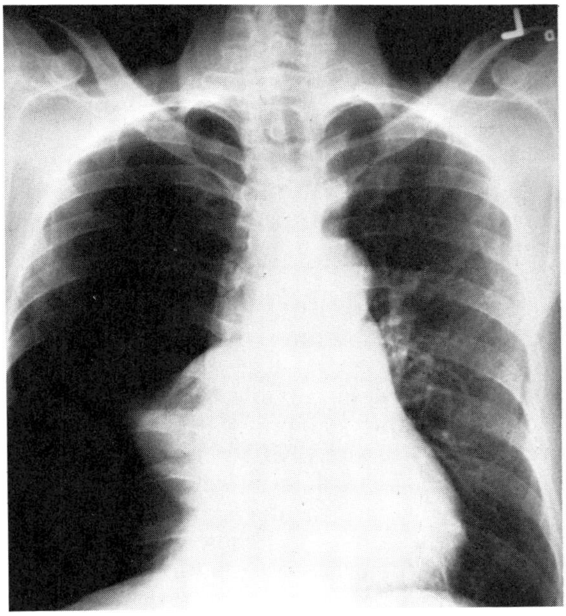

Figure 25-6. Pneumothorax with some tension on the right as demonstrated by tracheal shift to the left.

adhesive tape are adequate as an emergency measure. (Initial surgery requires adequate wound debridement and airtight closure. Water-seal drainage is used in the pleural space to evacuate air and fluid.)

Subcutaneous Emphysema. Air in the subcutaneous tissue usually indicates a tear in the lung or bronchus, trachea, or esophagus. Such injury may be due to penetrating or blunt trauma or occasionally may occur spontaneously or with very heavy exertion when a Valsalva maneuver is prolonged and excessive. Subcutaneous emphysema may occur anywhere over the thorax but is often greatest at point of penetration and may rapidly spread to involve face, arms, and abdomen, depending on continued air leak.

Mediastinal Emphysema. Mediastinal emphysema is much more subtle and noted only on closely inspecting the roentgenogram. Air dissects upward into the suprasternal notch, where it should always be sought. It may dissect out along the bronchial tree and lead to pneumothorax. Air in the mediastinum denotes injury to esophagus, trachea, or bronchus. Occasionally, it can occur spontaneously, usually as a result of severe straining or violent coughing. Treatment is directed toward the primary cause of the air leak.

Contusion. Associated with blunt trauma or blast, pulmonary contusion can vary from minimal to profound. Manifestations may take several hours to appear and are caused by edema and bleeding into the interstitial space and alveoli, often producing severe ventilation-perfusion abnormalities. Roentgenographic evidence is a patchy pulmonary infiltrate under the site of maximal trauma (Fig. 25-4B).

Management consists of treatment of hypovolemia, pain control, and respiratory toilet. Antibiotics are indicated, since contused lungs are more susceptible to bacterial invasion. Respiratory support with positive end-expiratory pressure (PEEP) is indicated if arterial blood gases deteriorate. The extent of contusion on chest roentgenogram or the presence of concomitant flail chest are not predictive of need for assisted ventilation. The initial PO_2/FIO_2 is a better indicator of the extent of pulmonary injury, with an initial ratio of more than 300 predictive of the need for mechanical ventilation and indicative of the likelihood of serious complications. Steroids are not indicated. Associated injuries are important determinants of mortality and morbidity.

Laceration of Parenchyma. Laceration of the lung parenchyma is usually due to a penetrating wound but can result from blunt trauma. Such injury may cause tension pneumothorax or hemothorax. Bleeding from the lung usually stops spontaneously when the lung collapses. Minor lacerations seal off readily; the larger ones may require suture or occasionally lobectomy. Insertion of a 30- to 36-French intercostal tube in the fifth to seventh interspaces in the midaxillary line is the first treatment. The tube is connected to an underwater-seal bottle and suction. Decision for or against exploration then rests on observation. Excessive air leak or continued bleeding indicates early exploration.

Tracheal or Bronchial Tears. Tracheal or bronchial tears should be suspected, especially in severe blunt chest trauma, occasionally in penetrating injuries in which air leak is massive, and especially if there is associated mediastinal emphysema. Diagnosis is by bronchoscopy, and treatment consists of prompt repair. Delay in repair may result in loss of excessive lung parenchyma.

ESOPHAGUS

Esophageal injury
- Gunshot or stab wounds
- Blunt external trauma
- Operative accidents

Intraluminal causes
- Intrinsic (pressure from within body)—vomiting
- Extrinsic (pressure from without)—severe compression
- Foreign body—with or without perforation
- Iatrogenic—instrumental or ingestion of caustics, acid

Esophageal injuries are uncommon in chest trauma and, if they occur, are usually associated with lacerations of the great vessels or penetrating injuries of the thorax. There is leakage of air and fluid into the mediastinum or pleural cavity. Diagnostic measures may include administration of iodized oil (lipidol) or

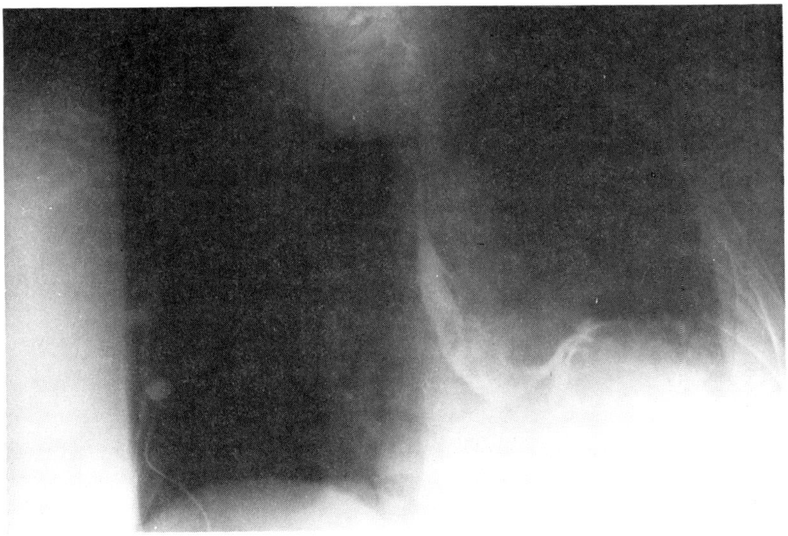

Figure 25-7. Esophageal rupture from severe compression injury. Note iodized oil (lipidol) smear and effusion of the left.

a similar substance by mouth with roentgenographic confirmation of the leak (Fig. 25-7). The treatment of choice is early operative repair before severe mediastinitis occurs. Drainage of the pleural cavity after early repair is usually adequate.

DIAPHRAGM

Severe compression of the lower part of the chest and upper abdominal area can cause acute rupture of the diaphragm, usually on the left. Laceration can occur from penetrating trauma. Diaphragmatic rupture should be kept in mind in dealing with crush injuries in which there is increasing dyspnea along with abdominal symptoms. Diagnosis may occasionally be made by chest roentgenography. The presence of the stomach in the left chest may be documented in some instances by passing a nasogastric tube and taking a chest roentgenogram. A study with diatrizoate meglumine (Gastrografin) may also show the stomach in the pleural cavity; a barium enema study should be used if herniation of the colon is suspected. Treatment is operative repair either by thoracotomy or abdominal approach. A hernia may occur at the time of injury, but if it is small it may not be noticed, with symptoms not occurring until years later (Fig. 25-8).

HEART AND GREAT VESSELS

The heart may be injured in penetrating and nonpenetrating thoracic injuries. After chest trauma, cardiac contusions may be the most common unsuspected visceral injury leading to death. Contusions result from violent compression of the chest. The diagnosis of cardiac contusion is based on serial ECGs and cardiac isoenzyme studies and may be further confirmed by a two-dimensional echocardiography demonstrating localized contraction abnormalities. Patients with two-dimensional echocardiographic abnormalities may manifest cardiac arrhythmias and should be observed and managed in an intensive care unit under myocardial infarction precautions.

Causes of Blunt Cardiac Trauma

Automobile accidents
Compression of chest between two large objects
Direct blows from a fist, baseball bat, golf ball, helmeted head, hoof, or during cardiac resuscitation
Falls
Blasts

Types of Cardiac Injury From Blunt Trauma

Myocardium
- Contusion
- Laceration
- Rupture
- Septal perforation
- Aneurysm, pseudoaneurysm
- Hemopericardium, tamponade
- Thrombosis, systemic embolism
- Foreign body in either heart or ventricle

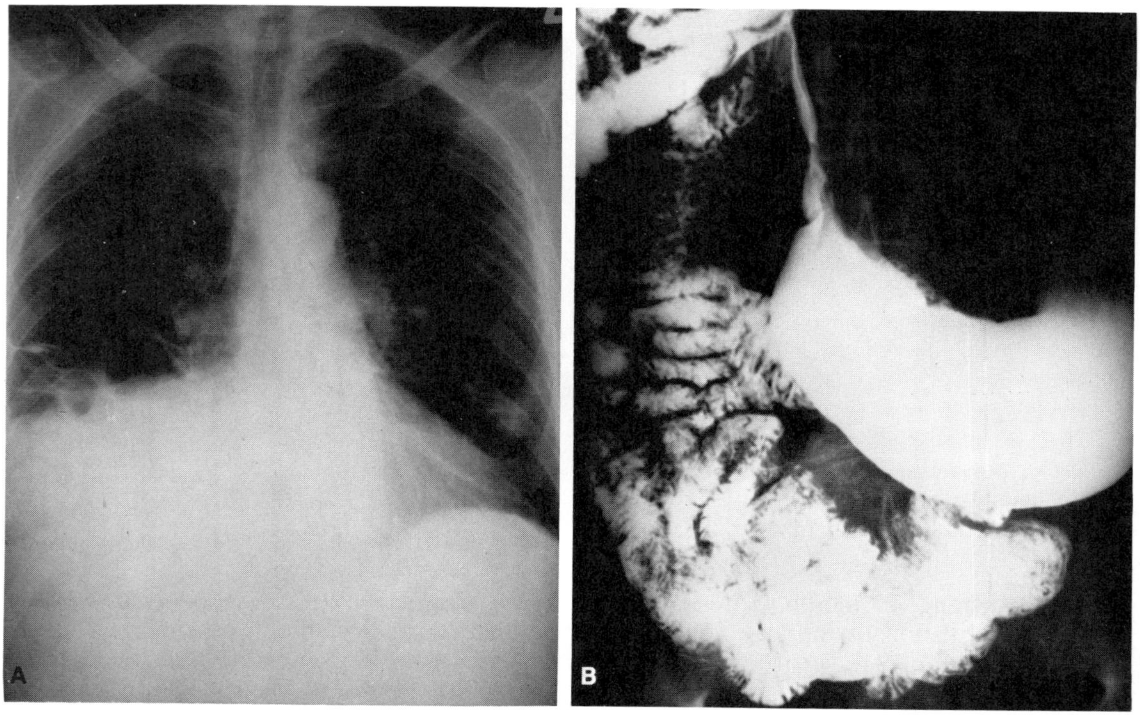

Figure 25-8. (*A*) Rupture of the right hemidiaphragm with air–fluid levels suggesting small bowel in the right hemithorax. (*B*) Demonstration of small bowel after a barium swallow.

- Pericardium
  - Pericarditis
  - Postpericardiotomy syndrome
  - Constrictive pericarditis
  - Pericardial laceration
  - Cardiac herniation
- Endocardial structures
  - Rupture of papillary muscle
  - Rupture of chorda tendineae
  - Rupture of atrioventricular and semilunar valves
- Coronary artery
  - Thrombosis
  - Laceration
  - Fistula

Perforating wounds of the heart usually result in massive bleeding into one of the pleural cavities, and occasionally to the outside, but in perforating wounds of one of the ventricles, blood may escape from the heart more rapidly than from the pericardial sac, resulting in tamponade. Cardiac tamponade usually results from wounds that penetrate the chest wall in the area in which the pericardium is not covered by pleura. Blood rapidly fills the pericardial sac, and as it becomes distended, the opening is displaced away from the chest wall opening with little bleeding to the outside. The typical picture of cardiac tamponade is dusky cyanosis, distention of neck veins, a markedly narrow pulse pressure—as low as 10 torr even before the blood pressure falls to shock level—distant heart sounds, and a pulse that is not as rapid as would be expected from the degree of shock. Of these classic signs, distention of neck veins, even when the head and shoulders are elevated, distinguishes this condition from others in shock. If the wound is small the picture may be less striking. The classic picture will eventually develop, but in the meantime, permanent damage to brain and kidneys may have occurred. Chest roentgenography is worthless. Fluoroscopy may show reduction in pulsation of the cardiac shadow.

If foreign intrapericardial bodies are present they may be removed when lacerations are repaired, but they are not an emergency if there is no tamponade. However, foreign bodies in the chambers of the heart or great vessels are a potential danger and should be removed as soon as the patient is stable. Metallic bodies in the ventricular muscle need not be removed.

The clinical presentation of serious acute cardiac trauma falls into two distinct groups: cardiac tamponade and hemorrhagic shock. When there are signs of hemorrhagic shock with brisk chest tube drainage, thoracotomy should be done immediately. Cardiac injuries, both penetrating and blunt, can be approached via either median sternotomy or thoracotomy. We prefer the former, because it is a more utilitarian incision that gives more options. If tamponade is suspected because of hypofusion and elevated central venous pressure, the patient is positioned on a surgical table and a subxiphoid pericardial window is performed under light general or local anesthesia. If blood is encountered in the pericardium, the incision can be extended into a median sternotomy and the cardiac wound repaired. Needle pericardiocentesis has a high incidence of false positives and negatives and is not recommended for diagnosis or treatment except as a temporizing measure in a monitored patient with tamponade during transport to the operating room.

Blunt Injuries to Branches of the Aortic Arch (Clinical)

Manifestations include the following findings:

Widened mediastinum or mass
Decreased distal pulse and blood pressure
Ischemic extremity
Superior vena cava syndrome
Bruit
Palpable pulsatile mass
Dysphagia
Recurrent nerve palsy
Symptomatic subclavian steal

The usual injury is to the thoracic aorta at the level of the ductus arteriosus (Fig. 25-9). The tear may be complete or partial.

The first step in management is to suspect the possibility of injury in all severe trauma. A widened mediastinum is indication for an arch aortogram. Treatment is prompt surgery with repair.

THORACOABDOMINAL INJURIES

Trauma to chest and abdomen are discussed as separate entities. However, they frequently occur simultaneously, and a knowledge of correct handling of such injuries is necessary for good results.

Thoracoabdominal injuries are greater emergencies than trauma to chest or abdomen alone. Delay before surgical intervention is limited to the time needed for resuscitation and complete evaluation of the existing injuries. Thoracoabdominal injury, particularly perforation of a hollow viscus, is an indication for immediate surgical intervention. Preoperative correction of altered intrathoracic physiology is necessary and should be accomplished first. When surgery is required in the chest, it takes precedence.

Operation should be confined to the abdomen if possible. Only a few thoracoabdominal injuries need be submitted to combined exploration: Upper abdominal and lower thoracic injuries that are not accessible through laparotomy wounds alone include liver wounds located at the dome of the right lobe near the inferior vena cava, injuries of the lower end of the esophagus, and trauma to the cardiac end of the stomach. Perforation of the diaphragm or the anatomic likelihood of such is an indication for laparotomy rather than thoracotomy. In case of massive hemothorax the pleural space is aspirated, and, if present, a sucking wound is handled prior to the laparotomy. If a hollow viscus of the abdomen is perforated, the pleural space is irrigated with saline prior to closure of the tear in the diaphragm.

Independent chest and abdominal injuries present no particular problems. Usually the chest injury is taken care of first, followed by laparotomy. Restoration of cardiorespiratory physiology to as near normal as possible enables the patient to endure abdominal exploration with greater safety.

With the increasing number of injuries produced by high-speed transportation in civilian life, general knowledge of evaluation, of logical sequence of treatment, and of emergency measures is necessary to reduce the high mortality that exists.

EMERGENCY ROOM THORACOTOMY

The value of emergency room thoracotomy is questionable except under selected circumstances. Patients who are without vital signs at the scene rarely survive and, except in cases of hypothermia, should not be resuscitated. Patients who have suffered penetrating car-

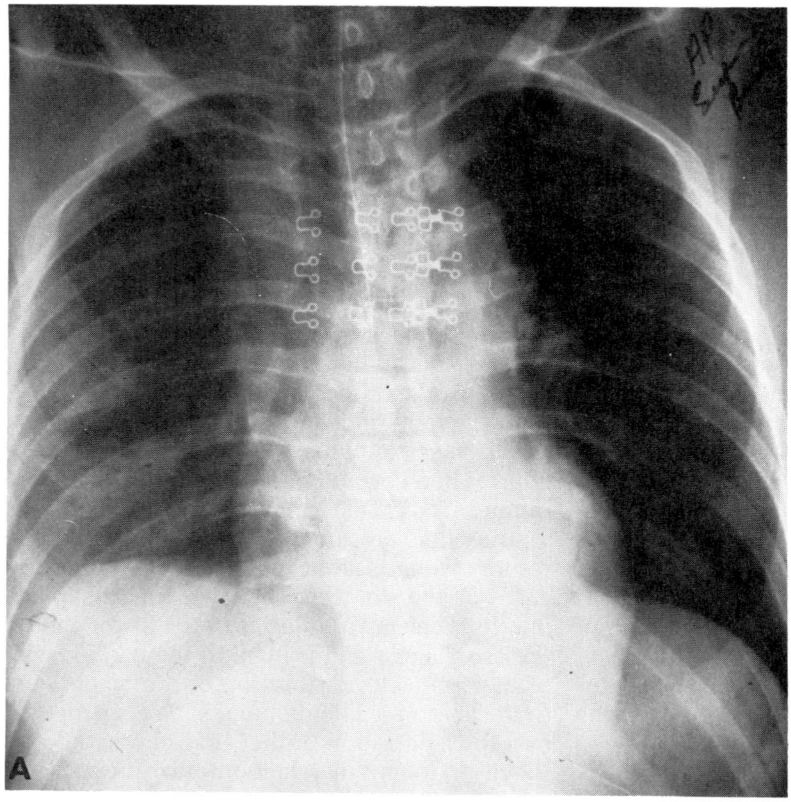

Figure 25-9. (*A*) Mediastinal widening in patient with a tear of the thoracic aorta due to blunt trauma. (*B*) AP and lateral arch aortograms, demonstrating a tear in the thoracic aorta at the level of the ductus arteriosus, the usual site.

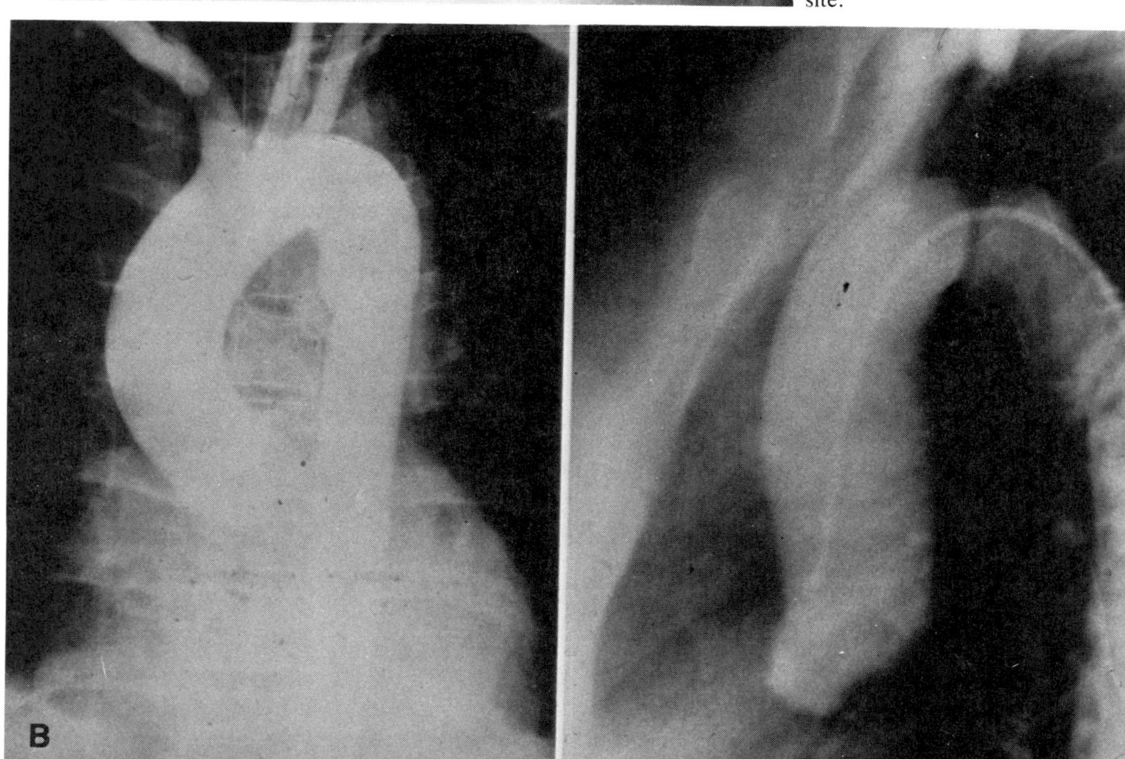

INDICATIONS FOR EMERGENCY SURGICAL INTERVENTION IN THORACIC TRAUMA

Urgent Thoracotomy

Uncontrollable hemorrhage
Cardiac injury with shock
Abnormal thoracic aortogram (showing aortic tear)
Bullet embolus in heart

Semiurgent Thoracotomy

Continued hemorrhage
High-volume air leak
Abnormal bronchogram or tracheogram
Abnormal esophagogram
Bowel or stomach above diaphragm

diac trauma and arrest in the emergency room or shortly before arrival have the best survival and are candidates for emergency room thoracotomy. Indications for emergency room thoracotomy include unmanageable hemorrhage with cardiac laceration suspected or pericardial tamponade that cannot be relieved in other ways. Rarely, a suspected laceration of the aorta or vena cava may be controlled or a major bronchial rupture contained by emergency room thoracotomy and swift appropriate action.

AUTOTRANFUSION AND CARDIOPULMONARY BYPASS

Patients who have extensive blood loss may benefit from autotransfusion. A number of these systems are commercially available and are able to quickly provide large amounts of compatible blood and reduce demands on the blood bank.

Femoral vein to femoral artery bypass may be rapidly initiated in the emergency room; its use is indicated in patients who cannot be adequately ventilated, patients with cardiac injury and exsanguination, and patients with hypothermia.

CAUSES OF ALVEOLAR HYPOVENTILATION

It is good to keep in mind the multiplicity of causes of hypoventilation other than the obvious thoracic trauma:

- Depression of respiratory center
  - Drugs
  - Acid-base imbalance
  - Head trauma
- Inadequate chest wall expansion
  - Chest pains
  - Tight strapping of chest
  - Injury of chest wall
- Inadequate lung expansion
  - Pneumothorax
  - Hemothorax
  - Diaphragmatic hernia
- Airway obstruction
  - Oral airway block
  - Tongue, foreign bodies
  - Secretions, blood in lower airway, bronchostenosis
- Emergency traumatic chest situations
  - Respiratory obstruction
  - Flail chest
  - Open pneumothorax

COMMON CARDIOTHORACIC PROBLEMS OTHER THAN TRAUMA

The purpose of this section is to acquaint the physician briefly with some common thoracic conditions that may be encountered in the office or emergency room to improve his or her ability to recognize and occasionally carry out some simple or even life-saving procedures.

CHEST WALL

PAIN

Etiology. Pain may be due to a recent thoracotomy incision, contusion, rib fracture, metastatic disease or direct invasion by a primary tumor of the lung, costochondral injury, or occasionally no apparent cause.

Diagnosis. The diagnosis rests on a history of operation, trauma, cancer in the thorax or elsewhere. During physical examination, moving the thoracic cage by compression other than at the site of pain may suggest a fracture. A roentgenogram is usually diagnostic of fracture and malignant invasions, either local or metastatic. A bone scan may be helpful.

Treatment. Pain relief can be gained by intercostal block with a long-acting local anesthetic (see Fig. 25-2). Strapping is ineffectual and usually results in greater discomfort as a result of skin excoriation.

Malignant involvement, either metastatic or local, requires in-depth evaluation and possibly chest wall resection.

Costochondral injuries are slow to heal and occasionally necessitate resection of a piece of cartilage if nonunion occurs; pain may persist for several months.

Idiopathic chest wall pain is usually transient and can be treated with mild oral analgesics and reassurance, since such pain is often misinterpreted by the patient as being of cardiac origin.

ABSCESS

Etiology. An abscess may be a local infection of skin and subcutaneous tissue, or it may be empyema that has penetrated through to the skin (empyema necessitatis).

Diagnosis. Empyema must be excluded, and this can best be done by roentgenography of the chest.

Treatment. Incision and drainage are the treatment of choice in a superficial chest wall infection. In the case of empyema a large tube, 36 to 40 French, should be placed in the most dependent position possible and connected to a closed drainage system. (This is usually a hospital procedure.)

TRACHEA AND BRONCHUS

OBSTRUCTION

Etiology. Obstruction may be due to extrinsic pressure from a tumor or hematoma but more commonly is due to tumor or foreign body in the trachea or bronchus.

Diagnosis. Symptoms of bronchial obstruction consist of cough and dyspnea. Tracheal obstruction is an emergent and life-threatening episode characterized by choking, gasping attempts at respiration, cyanosis, and loss of consciousness.

A chest roentgenogram may show only atelectasis of a segment or lobe or may show a foreign body if radiopaque. It is rarely necessary or desirable to use a contrast medium to delineate an obstruction.

Treatment. TRACHEAL OBSTRUCTION. Removal of the foreign body with a laryngoscope and grasping forceps may be necessary. However, many times such equipment is not immediately available and use of the Heimlich maneuver may be life-saving. A condition often referred to as a "cafe coronary" occurs when a foreign body, often a bolus of food too large to swallow, gets stuck in the hypopharynx and obstructs the laryngeal orifice, with strangulation resulting. In such a situation the Heimlich maneuver should be promptly instituted (Fig. 25-10). It consists of upward compression into the upper abdomen (Fig. 25-10A and B). Done suddenly, this elevates the diaphragm, which in turn compresses the lungs, suddenly increasing the intrabronchial air pressure and popping the foreign body out of the hypopharynx and often completely out of the mouth.

The Heimlich maneuver is performed two different ways, depending on whether the victim is standing or lying.

Rescuer standing: If both rescuer and victim are standing proceed as follows:

1. The rescuer stands behind the victim with both arms wrapped around the victim's waist (Fig. 25-10A).
2. The rescuer grasps one fist with the other hand and places the thumb side of the fist against the victim's abdomen, slightly above the naval and below the rib cage (Fig. 25-10B).
3. The rescuer presses this fist into the victim's abdomen with a *quick* upward thrust, repeating several times if necessary.

The action consists of sharp flexion movement at the elbows rather than a "hug." This emphasis on the hands rather than on the hug prevents possible rib fractures. If the victim is sitting, the rescuer stands behind the victim's chair and performs the maneuver in a similar manner.

Rescuer kneeling: If the victim is supine, the maneuver is performed as follows:

1. With the victim supine on his or her back, the rescuer faces the victim and kneels astride the victim's hips (Fig. 25-10C).
2. The rescuer places one hand on top of the other, then places the heel of the bottom

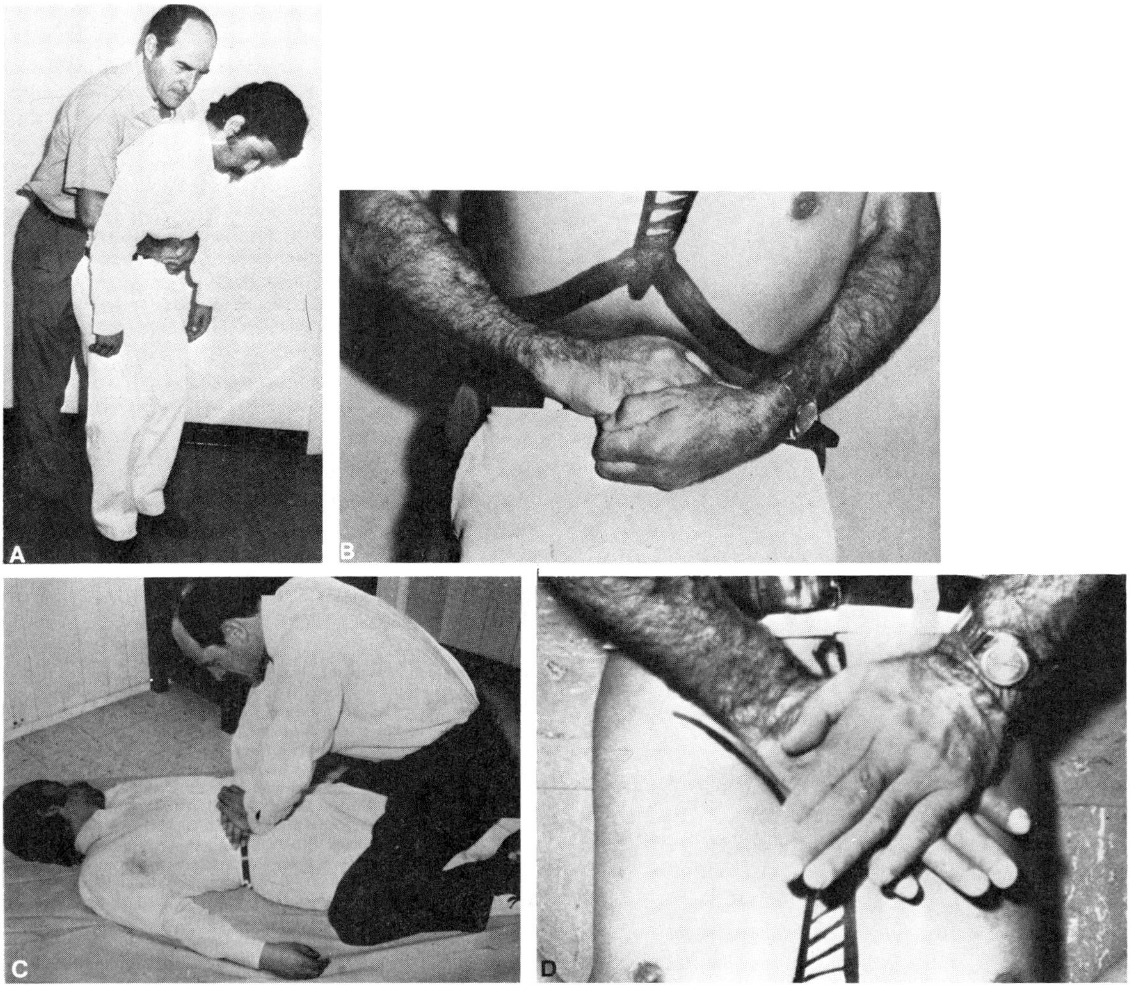

Figure 25-10. The Hemlich maneuver. (*A*) If the victim is standing, the procedure is performed with the resuscitator behind. (*B*) The resuscitator's grasped hands are placed below the rib margin against the upper abdomen. (*C*) If the victim is supine the resuscitator straddles him. (*D*) The resuscitator's hands are one on top of the other. (The head of the victim is toward the bottom of the photograph.)

hand on the abdomen slightly above the navel and below the rib cage (Fig. 25-10D).

3. The rescuer presses into the victim's abdomen with a *quick* upward thrust, repeating several times if necessary.

A child often cannot reach around an adult; therefore if a child is rescuing an adult, the maneuver should be performed in the supine position as just described. If the victim is alone, the Heimlich maneuver may be carried out in one of two other ways. Grasping one's own fist and placing it on the abdomen just below the naval and below the rib cage, the victim presses quickly upward, repeating if necessary several times. An alternate technique when alone is to position oneself over the edge of a chair back, railing, or table edge and press the abdomen into the edge with quick movements.

If the victim is an infant, he or she should be placed on a hard surface. Only the index and middle finger of both hands are placed on the infant's abdomen, just above the navel and below the rib cage, and pressed into the abdomen with quick upward thrusts.

Hughes in 1976 reported on 563 attempts and observed that most rescuers were untrained (70%) in cardiopulmonary resuscitation techniques. The Heimlich maneuver is usually performed on the victim of a choking attack. Between 94% and 96% of such attacks occur in the presence of a second person. Usually no more than four to six thrusts are necessary to expel the obstruction.

The Heimlich maneuver can be quickly tried with drowning victims who may have aspirated water. However, if it is not immediately successful, cardiopulmonary resuscitation by the usual mouth-to-mouth technique and external cardiac massage should be immediately started.

BRONCHIAL OBSTRUCTION. Removal of a bronchial obstruction is best accomplished under light general anesthesia using a rigid bronchoscope and appropriate instruments for grasping and removing a foreign body. (See the technique in the section entitled "Endoscopy" at the end of this chapter.)

LUNG AND PLEURA

SPONTANEOUS PNEUMOTHORAX

Etiology. Rupture of a bleb or bulla may cause spontaneous pneumothorax. It can occur at any age but is found most often in those under 45 years of age.

Diagnosis. Onset is usually sudden, with sharp chest pain followed by shortness of breath. Often there is a history of a similar episode. Physical examination usually reveals increased resonance on percussion and breath sounds that are distant to absent. A simple way to confirm the diagnosis is to carefully insert a 20-gauge needle attached to a 10-ml syringe into the second intercostal space anteriorly, being careful to go just through the pleura. Aspiration of air confirms the diagnosis. Roentgenography is helpful and should be done prior to needle aspiration or definitive treatment unless the patient is in serious condition from respiratory distress.

Treatment. Insertion of a 20- to 28-French catheter under local anesthesia (see Fig. 25-1 for technique) that is connected to an underwater-seal bottle connected to a low-suction apparatus is the treatment of choice. In the usual pneumothorax, the second anterior interspace in the midclavicular line permits easy and quick access to the pleural space. If fluid is present, the fifth to seventh interspaces in the midaxillary line are best, since drainage of the fluid as well as evaculation of air is necessary. Ambulatory management of spontaneous pneumothorax has been described. Repeated spontaneous pneumothoraces on the same side or an air leak persisting for more than 3 or 4 days is indication for open thoracotomy with pleural abrasion or stripping and closure of the air leak.

EMPYEMA

Etiology. Empyema is most commonly associated with a pulmonary infection such as pneumonia or lung abscess, but it may be associated with fungal disease, tuberculosis, or infected hemothorax, or it may occur after pneumonectomy.

Diagnosis. The patient is usually febrile, appears ill, and may have a cough and some chest pain and dyspnea, especially in large empyema or when empyema is associated with significant lung disease.

Roentgenography confirms the physical findings of dullness to percussion and distant to absent breath sounds over the area of the thorax involved. Differential diagnosis includes pleural effusion, thickened pleura, mesothelioma, or hemothorax. Needle aspiration should make the diagnosis definite.

Treatment. Except for diagnostic aspiration, treatment should be in the hospital—either tube thoracostomy if it is early nonpurulent empyema or limited open thoracotomy at the lowest level possible with placement of one or two large 40 to 50 French soft chest tubes.

HEMOPTYSIS

Etiology. Hemoptysis has many causes. Most common are bronchiectasis, tumors of the bronchus, chronic pulmonary infections such as tuberculosis or fungus diseases, pulmonary embolism, and mitral stenosis.

Diagnosis. Diagnosis requires hospitalization with careful observation, roentgenography of the chest, and early bronchoscopy to ascertain the site of bleeding.

Treatment. Treatment is usually a hospital procedure. (Conservative measures of support, modest cough suppression, and correction of any coagulation defect are often all that is needed.) Urgent operation is occasionally required and can be life-saving. Prior localization of the bleeding site is mandatory. Resection of tubercular or fungal infected lung tissue frequently is necessary, since usually those cases represent treatment failures.

ESOPHAGUS

OBSTRUCTION

Etiology. Esophageal obstruction may be due to tumors, both benign and malignant, foreign bodies, achalasia, stenosis from esophagitis, or chemical burns.

Diagnosis. A history of increasing dysphagia suggests any of the preceding causes except foreign bodies. Sudden obstruction suggests ingestion of a foreign body. Roentgenography after a swallow of contrast medium should define the level of obstruction, and esophagoscopy with biopsy of suspicious lesions should make a definite diagnosis.

Treatment. Except for removal of a foreign body, which can be done on an ambulatory basis (see "Endoscopy" at the end of this chapter), treatment of esophageal obstruction should be carried out in the hospital. Dilatation of chronic strictures with various dilators (Hurst, Maloney, or Tucker) can be accomplished in an ambulatory setting (Fig. 25-11). In achalasia dilatation is accomplished with hydrostatic bag dialators. This is a safe procedure in the hands of an experienced physician and may be all that is needed. However, most patients require myotomy.

INJURY

Etiology. Rupture may occur as a result of either blunt trauma or vomiting. Perforation may be from without, such as a gunshot or knife wound, or from within as a result of ingestion of sharp material or iatrogenically at time of esophagoscopy.

Diagnosis. In case of rupture or perforation, prompt appearance of pain in the neck area or posteriorly in the chest is common. Fever follows within a matter of a few hours. Subcutaneous air in the suprasternal notch is common and appears promptly within an hour or so.

Treatment. Prompt surgical intervention is of the utmost importance.

DISSECTING ANEURYSM

Etiology. Caused by a tear in the intima, 70% of dissecting aneurysms occur in the ascending aorta and 30% in the arch or descending aorta with subsequent dissection of blood downward between the layers of the aorta. This may either reenter lower down or rupture to the outside.

Diagnosis. Diagnosis is suggested by acute chest or back pain, widening of the mediastinum, a history of hypertensions, and diminished or absent pulses in the arch vessels. There may be stigmata of Marfan's syndrome

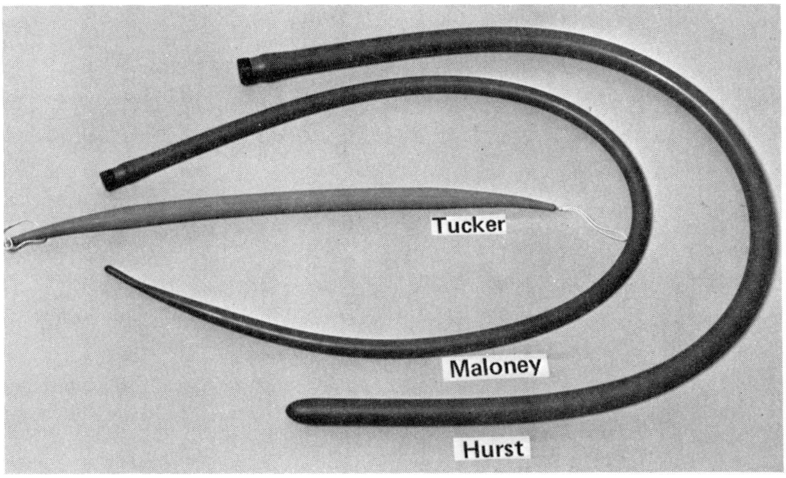

Figure 25-11. The esophageal dilators usually employed are the Tucker, Maloney, and Hurst. A number of other types are occasionally used.

or there may be aortic valve insufficiency. An aortogram is diagnostic.

Treatment. This is always a hospital-treated condition. If aortic insufficiency is a complication, treatment includes immediate surgery with resection of the diseased segment and replacement with a prosthetic graft and aortic valve. Immediate operation is indicated if the aneurysm involves the ascending aorta, if there is obstruction of a major aortic branch, or if bleeding from the aneurysm occurs.

Pharmacologic management consists of reduction of the blood pressure with nitroprusside and reduction of cardiac impulse with beta blockers. This must be maintained for several days with appropriate monitoring of blood pressure, as well as regular checking with ECGs and periodic checks with posteroanterior and lateral chest roentgenograms.

DIAGNOSTIC PROCEDURES

ENDOSCOPY

Bronchoscopy, esophagoscopy, thoracoscopy, and mediastinoscopy may often be done in an ambulatory setting. Usually these are best done with short-acting general anesthesia; however, local or topical anesthesia can be used in some cases. De Meester uses local block of the glossopharyngeal and superior laryngeal with excellent results to perform bronchoscopy and/or esophagoscopy.

BRONCHOSCOPY

Figures 25-12 and 25-13 show the most commonly used bronchoscopes, rigid and flexible. They range from the 5-mm infant size to the standard 8-mm adult size.

Accessory equipment is shown in Figure 25-14. Included are a suction trap for collecting bronchial secretions and brushes, slides, and fixative for collection of cytologic samples. Grasping forceps for removal of foreign bodies are shown in Figure 25-15.

INDICATIONS

Diagnostic. Bronchoscopy is used to obtain samples of cells by brush, from secretions, or by biopsy for diagnosis of tumors of the lung or bronchus and to obtain secretions for culture. Transbronchial biopsy with or without

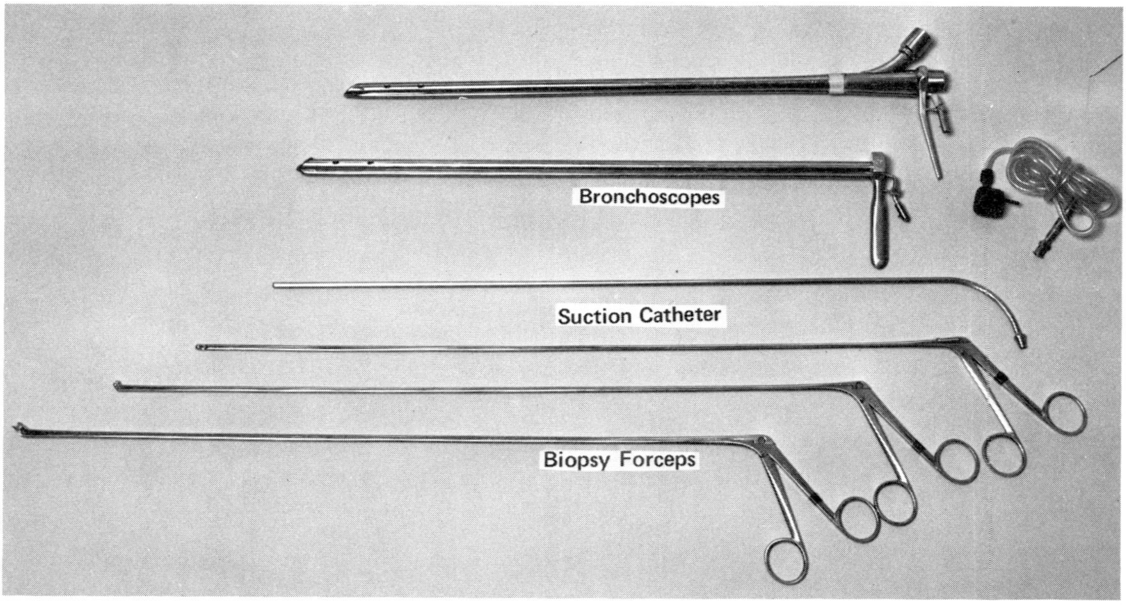

Figure 25-12. Two types of rigid bronchoscopes: suction catheter and biopsy forceps, and at upper right, a Venturi apparatus that, when connected to an oxygen source and with a flush valve attached, permits adequate oxygenation bronchoscopy.

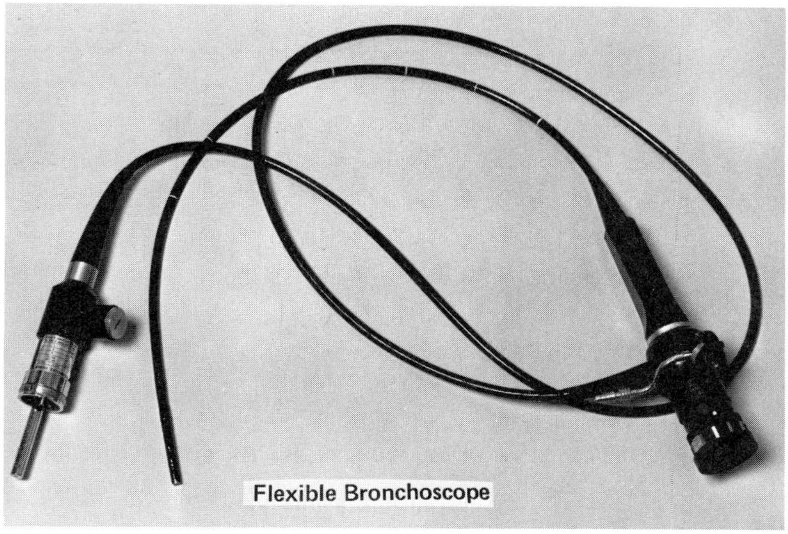

Figure 25-13. This flexible bronchocsope can be passed through the nose or by means of a special endotracheal tube with an attachment that provides a tight seal while ventilation is provided through a side part.

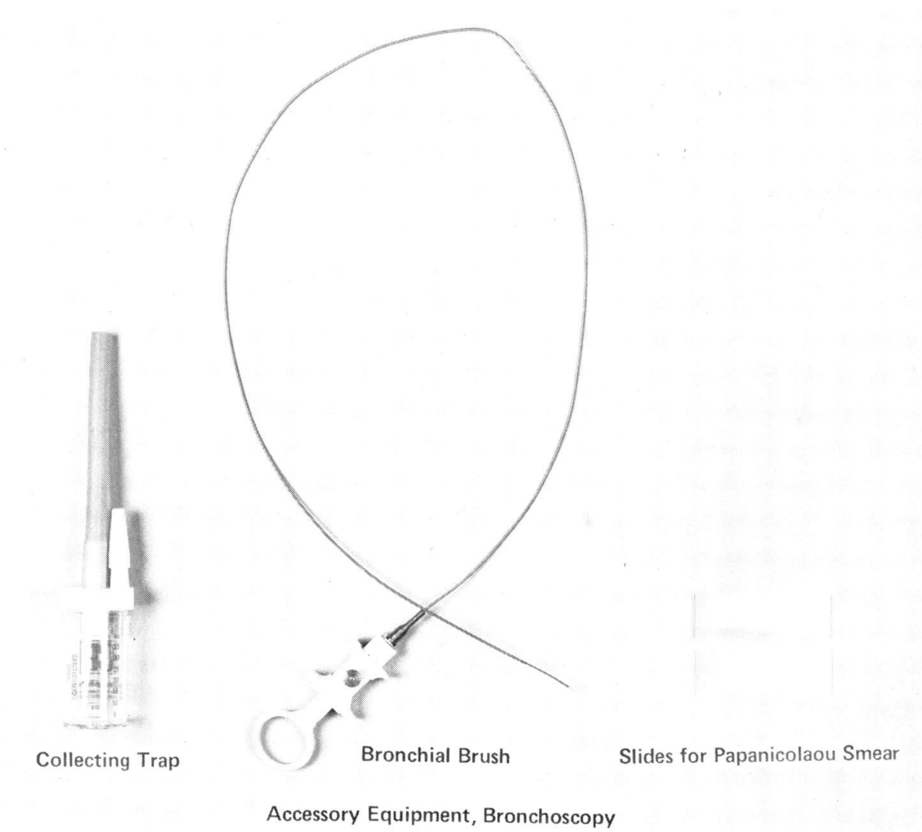

Figure 25-14. Accessory equipment for bronchoscopy: suction tubing, suction trap for collecting secretions for culture or cytology, bronchial brush for collecting cells for study, and glass slides and fixative for preserving specimens collected with the brush.

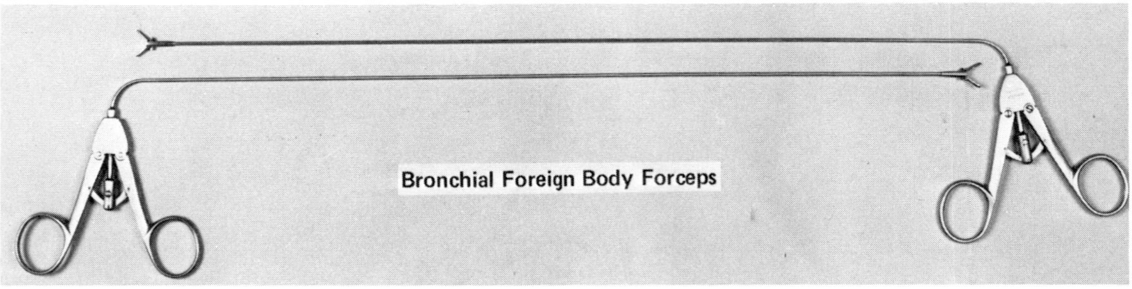

Figure 25-15. Two types of forceps for grasping a bronchial foreign body. There are many types.

fluoroscopic guidance is often done on an ambulatory basis.

Therapeutic. Bronchoscopy is used therapeutically in removal of aspirated matter, foreign bodies, or retained secretions.

TECHNIQUE

The most satisfactory technique is that with the patient supine, with the head slightly extended or with a small pillow under the shoulders, and in a slight 10-degree Trendelenburg position.

Insertion of the bronchoscope is simple once the technique is learned. Care should be exercised to protect the teeth and gums. The safest means of maintaining ventilation is with the Venturi apparatus in combination with the ventilating bronchoscope.

An unhurried and orderly approach should be taken with careful inspection of all orifices and observation of the size and fixation of the carina, of mucosal lesions, and of types of secretion.

The advent of the fiberoptic brochoscope has further increased the ease, safety, and applicability of ambulatory bronchoscopy. The straight bronchoscope is probably best for removal of foreign bodies since the size of the grasping forceps for use in the fiberoptic bronchoscope limits somewhat the size and type of foreign body that can be removed.

ESOPHAGOSCOPY

The usual types of esophagoscopes are shown in Figure 25-16 along with accessory equipment, including suction tube, biopsy forceps, and foreign-body forceps.

INDICATIONS

Diagnostic. Esophagoscopy is indicated for observing the esophageal mucosa for tumors, ulcerations, or inflammation.

Therapeutic. Dilatation of benign strictures, removal of foreign bodies, and occasionally hydrostatic dilatations in achalasia are all readily done in an ambulatory setting. Injection of bleeding esophageal varices is an inhospital procedure in most situations.

TECHNIQUE

Having the patient supine with the head slightly elevated and in a 10-degree Trendelenburg position is quite satisfactory. Either local or general anesthesia can be used. If general anesthesia is selected, an endotracheal tube should be used to assure proper ventilation.

Insertion of the esophagoscope is simple if one has had some training. It is highly important to control the instrument well and to use great care on insertion, being especially careful not to put pressure on the posterior area of the esophagus where it passes over the cervical spine. Occasionally in arthritic patients there may be spurs on the cervical vertebrae that can lead to tearing of the esophagus on insertion of the esophagoscope.

Use of a small bougie is very helpful in locating the esophageal opening. The esophagoscope can then readily be passed over the bougie and into the esophagus. One must never try to pass a narrowed area by use of force.

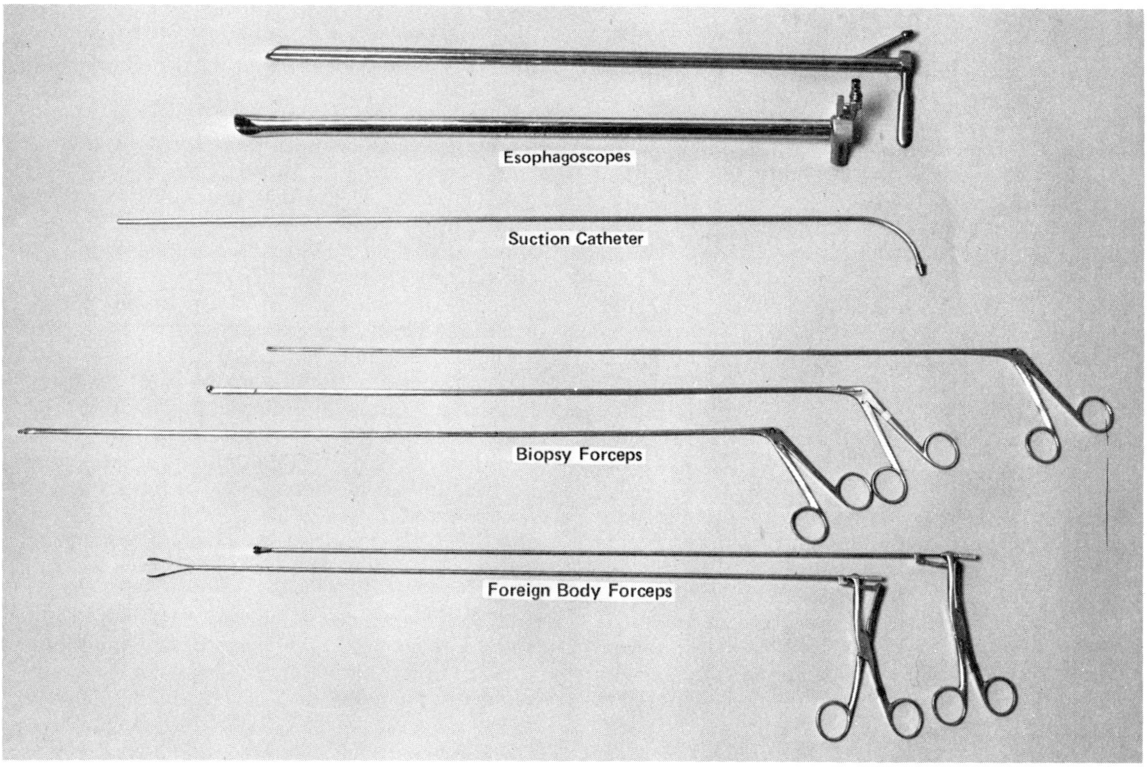

Figure 25-16. Two types of esophagoscopes: suction catheter and biopsy forceps, including two types of forceps for removing a foreign body. There are a number of other types of forceps that may be used for removal of certain types of foreign bodies.

THORACOSCOPY

INDICATIONS

Thoracoscopy is primarily of value in determining the causes of pleural disease, effusions, or tumors in which knowing the tissue specificity helps in future management. It is also valuable in diagnosis of pleuropulmonary disease, biopsy of pulmonary lesions, preoperative screening, and spontaneous pneumothorax to define the cause and help determine need for thoracotomy.

TECHNIQUE

The procedure can be done on an ambulatory basis under local anesthesia. The technique is not difficult but should be undertaken only after some experience with the instruments and knowledge of precautions have been achieved.

MEDIASTINOSCOPY

Although some advocate the use of mediastinoscopy in an ambulatory setting, it is our opinion that it should usually be reserved for a hospitalized patient as a means of determining operability of a proved carcinoma of the lung or as an aid in diagnosing certain other mediastinal tumors.

BIBLIOGRAPHY

Thoracic Trauma: Books

American College of Surgeons Committee on Trauma: Early Care of the Injured Patient. Philadelphia, WB Saunders, 1976

Naclerio EA: Chest Injuries: Physiologic Principles and Emergency Management. New York, Grune & Stratton, 1971

Skillman JJ: Intensive Care. Boston, Little, Brown & Co., 1975

Thoracic Trauma: Articles

Appelbaum A, Karp RP, Kirklin JW: Surgical treatment for closed thoracic trauma. J. Thorac Cardiovasc Surg 71:458, 1976

Barone JE, Pizzi WF, Nealon TF, Richman H: Indications for intubation in blunt chest trauma. J Trauma 26:334–338, 1986

Beall AC, Crosthwait RW, Crawford ES, DeBakey ME: Gunshot wounds of the chest. J Trauma 4:328, 1976

Brooks JW: Blunt traumatic rupture of the diaphragm. Thorac Surg 26:199–207, 1978

Braun RA et al: Cervical tracheal transection with esophageal fistula. Arch Otolaryngol 96:67–72, 1972

Bryan PM et al: Operative stabilization of nonpenetrating chest injuries. J. Thorac Cardiovasc Surg. 70:619–630, 1975

Bryan-Brown CW, Shoemaker WC: Acute respiratory failure after trauma and surgery. Semin Drug Treat 3:269–288, 1973

Castagna J et al: Blunt injuries to branches of the aortic arch. J Thorac Cardiovasc Surg 69:521, 1975

Comer PG: Airway maintenance in patients with long term endotracheal intubation. Crit Care Med 4:211, 1976

Cowie RL: Flail chest. S Afr Med J 46:1724–1725, 1972

Cullen P et al: Treatment of flail chest. Arch Surg 110:1099, 1975

Ellis R: Traumatic lung cysts. JAMA 236:1976–1977, 1976

Esteban A et al: Ten cases of acute unilateral pulmonary edema following rapid reexpansion of pneumothorax. Bull Am Coll Chest Physicians, 14:28–30, 1975

Franz JL et al: Effect of methylprednisoline sodium on experimental pulmonary contusion. J Thorac Cardiovasc Surg 68:842, 1974

Frazee RC, Mucha P, Farwell MB, Miller FA: Objective evaluation of blunt cardiac trauma. J Trauma 26:510–520, 1986

Hancock EW: Constrictive pericarditis. JAMA 232:176, 1975

Herung DP, Meir I: Cardiac and vascular sequelae of sternal fractures. J Trauma 26:553–555, 1986

Hughes RK: Thoracic trauma. Ann Thorac Surg 1:778–804, 1965

Huller T et al: Blast injuries of the chest and abdomen. Arch Surg 100:24–30, 1970

Humphreys RL et al: Rapid reexpansion of pneumothorax: A cause of unilateral pulmonary edema. Radiology 96:509, 1970

Jackson DH et al: Nonpenetrating cardiac trauma. Mod Concepts Cardiovasc Dis 45:123–128, 1976

Johnson JA, Cogbill TH, Winger ER: Determinants of outcome after pulmonary contusion. J Trauma 26:695–697, 1986

Jones RJ et al: Current management of civilian thoracic trauma. Am J Surg 114:289–296, 1967

Jones RJ et al: Esophageal injury. Ann Thorac Surg 19:216, 1975

Kirsh M et al: Management of tracheal-bronchial disruption secondary to nonpenetrating trauma. Ann Thorac Surg 22:93–101, 1976

Lajos TZ et al: Pericardial decompression. Ann Thorac Surg 19:47, 1975

Lewis F et al: Control of respiratory therapy in flail chest. Ann Thorac Surg 20:170–176, 1975

Lindskog GE: Some historical aspects of thoracic trauma. J Thorac Cardiovasc Surg 42:1–11, 1961

Love JW: Chest injuries. JAMA 232:385–387, 1975

Maurer ER et al: Modern methods of managing traumatic rupture and amputation of the bronchus. Dis Chest 48:587–594, 1965

Modig J et al: Early recognition and treatment of post traumatic pulmonary microembolism. Crit Care Med 40:180–185, 1976

Moore BP et al: Operative stabilization of nonpenetrating chest injuries. J Thorac Cardiovasc Surg 70:619, 1975

Obeid FN, Shapiro MJ, Richardson HH et al: Catheter management for simple pneumothorax (CASP) in the outpatient management of simple traumatic pneumothorax. J Trauma 25:882–886, 1986

Parham AM, Yarbrough DR, Redding JS: Flail chest syndrome and pulmonary contusion. Arch Surg 113:900–903, 1978

Poole GV, Myers RT: Morbidity and mortality rates in major blunt trauma to the upper chest. Ann Surg 193:70–75, 1986

Reul GJ et al: Recent advances in the operative management of massive chest trauma. Ann Thorac Surg 16:52–66, 1973

Sawyers JL et al: Esophageal perforation. Ann Thorac Surg 19:233, 1975

Schmidt GB et al: Continuous positive pressure in the prophylaxis of the adult respiratory distress syndrome. Surg Gynecol Obstet 143:613–618, 1976

Sherman RT et al: The role of intrapleural blood in fibrothorax. Am Surg 31:1, 1965

Sturm JT: Hemopneumothorax following blunt trauma of the thorax. Surg Gynecol Obstet 141:539, 1975

Shoemaker WC: Pathophysiologic basis of therapy for shock and trauma syndromes. Semin Drug Treat 3:211–229, 1973

Shoemaker WC, Bryan-Brown CW: Resuscitation and immediate care of the critically ill and injured patient. Semin Drug Treat 3:249–267, 1973

Stallone RJ et al: Management of major acute thoracic vascular injuries. Am J Surg 128:249–254, 1974

Stein L et al: Recognition and management of pericardial tamponade. JAMA 225:503–506, 1973

Symbas PN et al: Acute penetrating tracheal trauma. Ann Thorac Surg 22:473–477, 1976
Taryle DA, Chandler JE, Good JT et al: Emergency room intubations—complications and survival. Chest 75:541–543, 1979
Trinkle JK: Management of flail chest without mechanical ventilation. Ann Thorac Surg 19:355, 1975
Trinkle JK et al: Management of the wounded heart. Ann Thorac Surg 17:230–236, 1974
Turney SZ et al: Traumatic rupture of the aorta. J Thorac Cardiovasc Surg 72:727–734, 1976
Williams JR: Pulmonary hematomas secondary to nonpenetrating injury. South Med J 55:622–625, 1962
Wiot JF: The radiologic manifestations of blunt chest trauma. JAMA 231:500, 1975
Wilson JM, Boren CH, Peterson SR, Thomas AN: Traumatic hemothorax: Is decortication necessary? J Thorac Cardiovasc Surg 77:489–495, 1979
Wilson JM, Thomas AN, Goodman PC, Lewis MD: Severe chest trauma. Arch Surg 113:846–849, 1978
Wilson RS: Acute respiratory failure diagnostic and therapeutic criteria. Crit Care Med 2:293–304, 1974

Heimlich Maneuver

Heimlich J, Hoffman KA, Canestri FR: Food choking and drowning deaths prevented by external subdiaphragmatic compression. Ann Thorac Surg 20:88–195, 1975
Hughes T: Computerized analysis of Dr. Henry J. Heimlich's data for 530 case reports of the application of the Heimlich maneuver. Submitted to National Research Council/Committee on Emergency Medical Services, Washington, 1976

Bronchoscopy

DeMeester TR, Skinner DB, Evans RH, Benson DW: Local nerve block anesthesia for peroral endoscopy. Ann Thorac Surg 24:278–283, 1977
Landa JF: Diagnostic and therapeutic applications of the bronchoscope. Chest 73:685–778, 1978
Zanda DC: Diagnostic fiberoptic bronchoscopy: Techniques and results of biopsy in 600 patients. Chest 68:12–19, 1975

Esophagoscopy

Burke EI, Sturm J, Williamson D: The diagnosis of microscopic carcinoma of the esophagus. Dig Dis Sci 23:148–151, 1978
Eastman MC, Gear MWL, Nicol A: An assessment of the accuracy of modern endoscopic diagnosis of esophageal stricture. Br J Surg 65:182–185, 1978
Halter F, Witzel L, Gretillat PA et al: Diagnostic value of biopsy, guided lavage, and brush cytology in esophagogastroscopy. Dig Dis Sci 22:129–131, 1977
Lanza FL, Graham DY: Bougienage is effective therapy for most benign esophageal strictures. JAMA 240:844–847, 1978
Pearson FG, Henderson RC: Long-term follow-up of peptic stricture managed by dilatation, modified Collis gastroplasty and Belsey hiatal hernia repair. Surgery 80:396–404, 1976

Thoracoscopy

Bloomberg AE: Thoracoscopy in perspective. Surg Gynecol Obstet 147:433–443, 1978
Oldenburg FA Jr, Newhouse MT: Thoracoscopy: A safe, accurate diagnostic procedure using the rigid thoracoscope and local anesthesia. Chest 75:45–50, 1979

26 The Unconscious Patient—Differential Diagnostic Work-up

CLARK A. MILLIKAN AND NANCY FUTRELL

What does one do when confronted with an unconscious patient (Fig. 26-1)?

Priority one: Examine respiratory action.

1. Remove foreign objects, vomitus, or blood (may need forceps or endotrachael suctioning).
2. Supply oxygen—2 to 3 liters/min until arterial blood gas parameters are available.
3. Employ a bag and mask or endotracheal tube with mechanical ventilation if spontaneous respiration is inadequate.

Priority two: Examine cardiac action.

1. Pulse. Do closed chest massage if a pulse is not present. Because the circulation of poorly oxygenated blood is detrimental to recovery, this maneuver should not be done until respiration is established.
2. IV access—volume expansion.
3. Take a blood pressure.
4. Electrocardiogram (ECG).

Priority three: Examine and treat the metabolic status.

1. Bicarbonate—pressor agents per advanced cardiac life support (ACLS) guidelines.
2. Give 50 ml 50% glucose and check with a Dextrostix.
3. Give 100 mg thiamine.
4. Give naloxone (Narcan) 0.4 mg IV or IM.
5. Draw blood for glucose, blood urea nitrogen (BUN), creatinine, sodium, white blood cells (WBCs), red blood cells (RBCs), hemoglobin (Hb), hematocrit, phosphorus, serum glutamic–oxaloacetic transaminase (SGOT), gases, serum *p*H, $PaCO_2$, HCO_3, drug screen, and cardiac enzymes in nontrauma cases.

Priority four: Simultaneously with priorities one, two, and three, get a history and begin thinking through the differential diagnosis, based on initial observations.

Priority five: Examine the patient fully to establish the anatomical diagnosis; an etiologic diagnosis may also be possible.

1. Assess and define the patient's "state of consciousness" and record it for short-range and long-range comparison.
2. Evidence of injury (scalp, face, ears, nose, tongue, elsewhere)
3. Evidence of blood loss
4. Cranial nerves, retina, and neck
5. Motor system examination, including respiration
6. Reflexes

Now make an anatomical and, if possible, an etiologic diagnosis.

Priority six: Select additional procedures.

1. Computed tomography (CT) scan of the head: Primary brain tumors, metastatic tumors, abscesses, freshly extravasated intracerebral blood, most subarachnoid hemorrhages, and acute epidural and acute and subacute subdural hematomas are detected by CT of the head. Brain swelling, either focal or generalized, is also displayed. This ability to demonstrate many abnormalities has made CT the best neuroradiologic procedure in the diagnosis of coma. A negative scan may be almost as helpful as a positive one because such a scan may rule out intracranial bleeding. Rarely, subarachnoid hemorrhage of limited quantity may not be detected by CT, and cerebrospinal fluid ex-

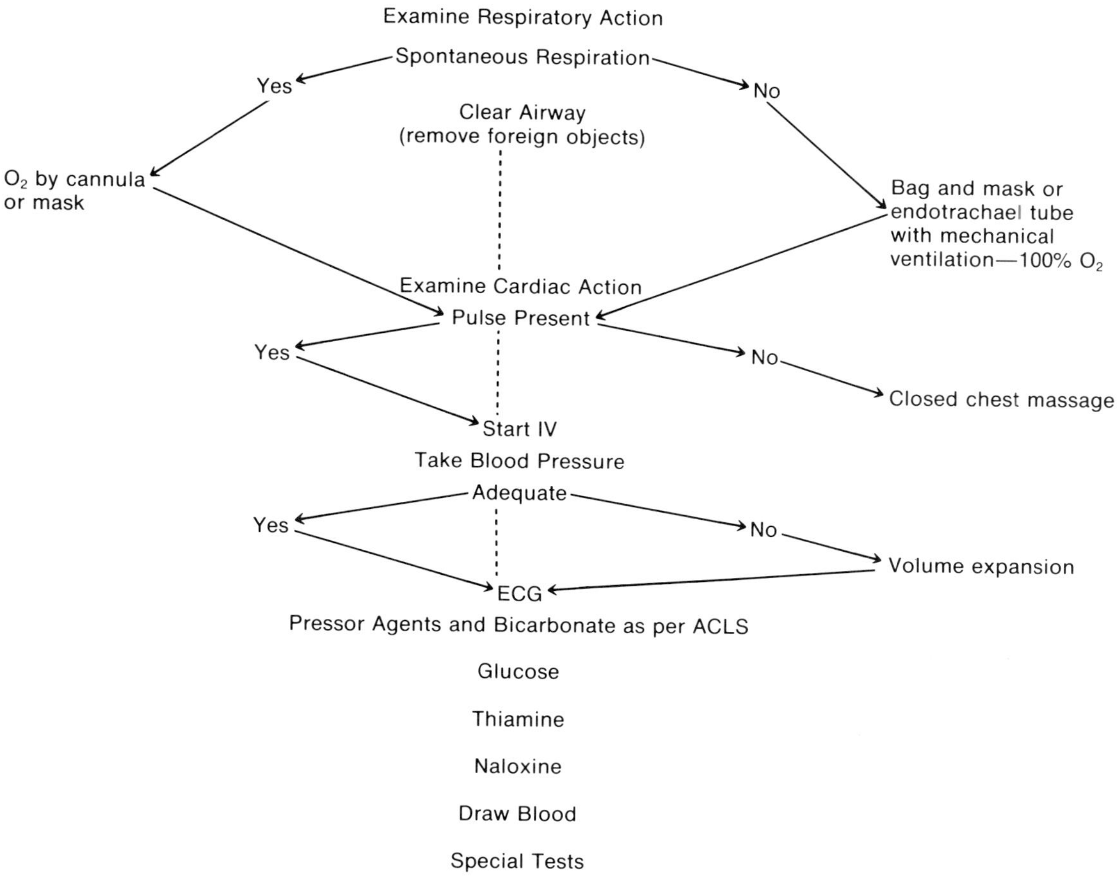

Figure 26-1. Schematic for evaluation of the unconscious patient.

amination may be necessary. Contrast enhancement may be necessary, but injection of 40 g of iodine creates a large osmotic load that may be dangerous in patients with impaired cardiac reserve or with impaired renal function.

2. X-rays of the cervical spine if evidence of trauma is present
3. X-rays of the head if a CT scan of the head is not available
4. Urinalysis
5. Electroencephalography (EEG)? Some examples of stupor or coma caused by inflammatory processes such as herpes simplex encephalitis, subacute sclerosing panencephalitis, or Creutzfeldt–Jakob disease may have the diagnosis suggested by EEG.

Metabolic and toxic encephalopathies, if severe, may cause coma and change the EEG. Patients in coma with uremia, hypoglycemia, hepatic insufficiency, or combinations of these may have EEG changes, but the diagnosis is usually established by doing the basic chemical tests.

In coma caused by focal cerebral vascular occlusion, EEG is generally not necessary. In rare instances in which infarction or bleeding involves the central core of the brain stem near the pontomesencephalic junction, EEG may contain predominant alpha activity that resembles the EEG pattern of normal wakefulness. This has been called "alpha-coma." In contrast to focal cerebral ischemia (hypoxia), diffuse cerebral hypoxia often causes diffuse nonspecific slow wave abnormalities. If the hypoxia is moderate, this change may be reversible, but more severe hypoxia may cause residual EEG abnormalties that may become paroxysmal. Very severe prolonged diffuse hypoxia causes generalized electrocerebral inactivity associated with irreversible coma or death.

In acute focal or diffuse traumatic encephalopathy, EEG is not necessary for the primary diagnosis of coma. Sequential recordings may be helpful in assessing the recovery process, or its absence, after severe brain trauma.

6. Cerebrospinal fluid examination. Usually the above work-up will lead to the diagnosis of the cause of the coma. Very seldom is infection the single cause unless something in the history is suggestive of infection. The purpose of a cerebrospinal fluid examination in this setting is to rule out infection.

DEFINITIONS OF CONSCIOUSNESS

To establish an orderly approach to a diagnostic–treatment problem and to make accurate records for immediate and future use, it is important to have precise definitions of *consciousness*.

The term *normal consciousness* indicates, by the person's behavior (including speech), that there is a generally accepted "awareness" of self and surroundings. This awareness is measured and assessed in terms of the patient's response to verbal, visual, and tactile stimuli. This awareness or normal consciousness has two fundamental components: (1) alertness (arousal, waking state [eyes open], including the capability of responding to some stimuli) and (2) cognitive power (thinking: effective processing of verbal and visual stimuli to produce accepted verbal and motor responses).

As one seeks words to describe abnormal states of consciousness, one reads about lethargy, obtundation, somnolence, confusion, delirium, drowsiness, semi-stupor, stupor, semi-coma, coma, deep coma, and so forth. There is no standard classification for changes in normal consciousness. In acute-care hospitals, intensive care units, and emergency rooms it is important that words be selected, then defined and used in a standard fashion. (The examination methodology must also be standardized.) The following definitions are suggested but can be changed for local use.

Sleep. Sleep, in a way, is normal unconsciousness. It is a cyclic physiologic absence of alertness and cognition that reverses spontaneously or is reversed by a variety of auditory, visual, or tactile stimuli. The sleeping person shows no evidence of awareness (unless the process is reversing), has his eyelids closed (no blinking), has his eyes in an abnormal position, and often has decreased muscle tone. However, he may dream and be able to recall the contents of the dream. But let a fly light on the face—sleep is reversed.

TERMS DESCRIBING ABNORMAL COGNITIVE POWER OR CONTENT OF CONSCIOUSNESS

Confusion. Confusion is a state in which a person cannot think and make appropriate responses (verbal and visual stimuli) with usual coherence and accuracy. There may be relevant answers to some simple questions (name, age, etc.) but disorientation for time and place. Attention span is short and memory faulty, but the patient is alert. In this sense confusion is not decreased consciousness; rather, cognitive functions are faulty, while arousal response is intact. Confusion should be considered a different phenomenon than drowsiness. It is also important to distinguish confused responses from those of an aphasic person (one with a focal brain lesion). Aphasic responses include the use of wrong words, distorted words, or new words and the repetition of the same word or phrase. Aphasic patients tend to have a poverty of speech production, but confused patients usually have normal or increased quantity of speech.

Delirium. Delirium is a state characterized by confusion with agitation and hyperactivity. These are usually concurrent with vivid visual or auditory hallucinations (false sensory perceptions), illusions (false interpretations of a sensory perception; *e.g.,* seeing a cane and believing it is a snake), or delusions (false ideas). There is often tremulousness and sweating. The person is overalert and may respond with a startle reaction to a mild unexpected sound or tactile stimulus.

TERMS DESCRIBING PATHOLOGICALLY DECREASED ALERTNESS (DECREASED RESPONSE TO EXTERNAL STIMULI AND INABILITY TO SATISFY INNER NEEDS)

This arousal capability is a spectrum; at one end is semi-stupor, somnolence, and so forth, where the person drifts off to sleep but is roused by a normal voice stimulus; at the other is deep coma, where there is no response to any stimulus.

Semi-stupor (Somnolence, Drowsiness, Light Stupor). Semi-stupor is a state in which the person goes to sleep (eyes closed) but is easily aroused by various stimuli, including the normal level of a voice. When aroused, questions are answered and commands followed accurately. When stimuli are stopped, the person drifts off to sleep. Spontaneous movements are common.

Stupor. Stupor is a state in which the person appears to be asleep and will respond only to painful tactile, loud auditory, or bright visual stimuli. Repeated stimuli may arouse the person to a point at which the person will try to answer the simplest questions in monosyllables or will follow simple commands. Arousal capability is so defective that processing of material for cognitive action is not possible.

Semi-coma. Semi-coma is a state in which there is only a nonspecific, ineffective response to painful stimuli. There may be occasional spontaneous movements, aimless picking at bedclothes (carphologia) or variable restlessness.

Coma. Coma is a state in which there is no significant response to painful stimuli. Stretch reflexes, pupillary reactions, and corneal reflexes are generally intact.

Deep Coma. Deep coma is a state in which there is no response to painful stimuli. Stretch reflexes, pulpillary reactions, and corneal reflexes are absent; respirations may begin to fail.

CROSSOVER TERMS

Much of the uncertainty concerning descriptive terms describing abnormal consciousness is caused by using a word that refers to cognition when the patient's state is impaired alertness or arousal. In some instances there is a defect in both; a person is confused and semi-stuporous. In such an instance both terms should be used. When alterness is decreased to the state of "semi-coma," cognition cannot be tested; only the one term is used.

SPECIAL TERMS

Aphasia of Various Types. In aphasia the person is alert, but cognition is faulty because of a focal brain lesion that produces a defect in the comprehension and/or production of spoken or written language. This is quite different from the traditional terms concerning consciousness.

Akinetic Mutism (Rare). In akinetic mutism the patient has his eyes open and appears alert but is mute and makes no movements except ocular rotation, swallowing, and breathing.

Locked-in Syndrome (Rare). Locked-in syndrome is much the same as akinetic mutism, but the patient signals by moving the eyes.

Vegetative State. The natural course of prolonged coma is either death or a chronic vegetable state. The latter is characterized by the return of the sleeping-waking cycle. There may be purposeless movements. This state can occur after severe brain damage whether due to trauma, surgery, hypoxia, or whatever.

Examples of Grading Coma

PHENOMENA TO BE OBSERVED	GRADE
Eye Opening	
Spontaneous	4
To voice	3
To pain	2
None	1
Speech	
Oriented (normal)	5
Confused	4
Dysphasia	3
Incomprehensible	2
None	1
Motor	
Correctly follows instructions	6
Localizes painful stimulus	5
Withdraws	4
Flexion, upper (decorticate)	3
Extension, upper (decerebrate)	2
None	1

STATE OF CONSCIOUSNESS

1. Normal
2. Semi-stupor (lethargy—response slowed)
3. Stupor (appropriate response to verbal stimulus)
4. Deep stupor (purposeful response to noxious stimulus)
5. Semi-coma (nonspecific response to pain)
6. Coma (above reflexes present—no response to pain)
7. Deep coma (absent deep tendon reflexes, pupillary reactions, and corneal reflexes; no response to pain)

EXAMINATION AND MEANING OF FINDINGS

In the section on definitions appears the term *painful stimuli*. How does one produce a painful stimulus? We have watched a variety of techniques: pressure over the styloid process of the temporal bone, pressure over the supraorbital ridge of the frontal bone, thumping the sternum, rubbing up and down on the sternum, and pinching the skin on the medial superior surface of the arm or thigh. Forceful rubbing up and down on the sternum, or pinsticking should not be done (see the discussion of psychogenic coma under Examination of Reflexes). All are obvious but may appear to be unusual to some observers in the patient's room. We prefer exerting heavy pressure on a fingernail bed by pressing an object (tuning fork base) into the nail bed. Observers are often unaware that a very painful stimulus is being exerted. The examiner can then make some estimation of the degree of alertness; obviously, the stimulus is ineffective if the sensory pathway from the site being stimulated is interrupted. This method has the important advantage of being applicable to each extremity.

CRANIAL NERVES OF IMPORTANCE

Pupils

The size of each pupil depends on the relative contraction–relaxation of the sphincter muscle (parasympathetic system) and the dilator fibers (sympathetic system). Parasympathetic system fibers arise in the oculomotor nucleus, travel in the oculomotor nerve, and synapse in the ciliary ganglion. The sympathetic fibers arise in the hypothalamus; descend through midbrain, pons, medulla, and spinal cord to exit at C7–8 and T1; ascend in the cervical sympathetic chain; pass along the internal carotid artery; and travel with the nasociliary branch of the ophthalmic division of the trigeminal nerve into the orbit, then in the long ciliary nerve to the dilator fibers of the pupil. Areas of the brain stem important to consciousness and control of the pupils are close together. Since these brain stem loci for control of pupils are relatively resistant to metabolic abnormalities, the presence or absence of the pupillary light reflex and the size of the pupils are of importance in determining the anatomical substrate of coma and even the cause of the coma (a supratentorial bilateral metabolic cause rather than morphologic focal destruction of infratentorial tissue).

The size of the pupils is recorded, and the direct light reflex is tested by flashing a bright light into the eye (dimly lighted or dark room). If an abnormality is present, consensual reflexes are also tested.

Oculomotor Phenomena in Coma

Ocular movements are directly controlled by impulses traveling along the oculomotor, trochlear, and abducens (the 3rd, 4th, and 6th cranial) nerves, which originate in the midbrain and rostral pons. The control of conjugate gaze (eyes moving in unison) begins in supranuclear centers in the frontal and occipital lobes, then travels into the brain stem, where there are complex interrelationships between fibers carrying vestibular phenomena and the medial longitudinal fasciculus, which connects the 3rd, 4th, and 6th cranial nerve

LOCALIZING VALUE OF PUPILLARY ABNORMALITIES IN COMA

Ciliospinal reflex: seldom performed (homolateral dilatation following pinching of the neck); disappears with brain stem damage
Horner's syndrome: ipsilateral pupillary constriction and slight ptosis. The lesions may be anywhere in the sympathetic nervous system from the hypothalamus through the brain stem, in the spinal cord to the level of T2, sympathetic cervical chain, or intracranially to the eye.
Midbrain damage (tectal or pretectal): pupils in midposition (5–6 mm) light-fixed; the ciliospinal reflex may be present.
Third nerve involvement (unilateral): pupil dilated, eye abducted, ptosis
Pontine damage: bilateral small pupils (sympathetic pathway damage)
Lateral medullary damage: small pupil, slight ptosis (Horner's)

PHARMACOLOGIC AND METABOLIC EFFECTS ON THE PUPIL

Atropine and scopolamine: dilated and fixed
Doriden (glutethimide): midposition or mild dilatation, often fixed
Barbiturate, meprobamate, phenothiozine, bromide, alcohol: small, reactive; ciliospinal reflex intact
Opiates: pinpoint pupils
Anoxia: fixed, dilated pupils
Metabolic encephalopathy: small but reactive pupils

nuclei. These anatomical pathways are adjacent to the brain stem (hypothalamus, midbrain), the anatomical area controlling consciousness; observation of the position of the eyes and their movements is important to the anatomical diagnosis of coma.

Open the patient's eyelids. If extraocular muscles are not working, the eyes are often equally slightly divergent; each eye is centered in the axis of its orbit. If the oculocephalic (Doll's eyes) reflex is absent, it means brain stem damage until proven otherwise. If the eyes are open as well as divergent, the prognosis is grave. Roving eye movements: generally the brain stem is intact.

Abnormal Conjugate Gaze (Eyes Deviated in Unison to the Functioning Side of the Body; Opposite Side Hemiplegic). Abnormal conjugate gaze is commonly caused by a destructive lesion (infarct) on the side of the brain toward which the eyes are rotated; the eyes "look at the lesion." Rarely, in so-called irritative or convulsive phenomena, conjugate deviation may be away from the pathophysiology, such as early in the course of an intracerebral bleed. In some brain stem lesions there may be conjugate deviation away from the lesion.

Skew Deviation. Skew deviation, malalignment of the eyes with one eye down and the other up, is produced by a brain stem lesion.

Oculocephalic Reflex (Doll's Eyes). Holding the eyelids open, turn the patient's head to the right; the eyes move in unison to the left. Then turn the head to the left; the eyes move in unison (conjugate gaze) to the right. In the comatose patient this reflex is intact in bilateral hemispheric dysfunction, intact in metabolic coma unless it is very deep, and impaired or lost in brain stem lesions. *Do not do this test if there is a chance of traumatic damage to cervical spine.*

Oculovestibular (Caloric) Reflex. With the patient supine, the head is raised about 30° (check the ear drum and external auditory canal) and the ear irrigated with up to 100 ml of cold water. In normally alert people, nystagmus develops, slow component to the irrigated side. In comatose patients the eyes deviate to the irrigated side (hemisphere pathology). If the pathology is in the brain stem, this reflex is lost.

Partial Internuclear Ophthalmoplegia (Comatose Patient). Test the oculocephalic reflex (Doll's eyes). If one eye does not adduct when the other abducts, it is a sign of a brain stem lesion until proven otherwise (on the same side as the adducting eye).

Retina

Important information can be obtained by using the ophthalmoscope for a few seconds on each eye. *Papilledema* means increased intracranial pressure, until proven otherwise. This may be associated with trauma, an expanding intracranial mass, malignant hypertension, or infection (meningitis or encephalitis). Rarely, it is caused by drugs or metabolic encephalopathy. *Hemorrhage* into the retina may occur within many minutes or a few hours after intracranial bleeding, whether subarachnoid or intracerebral. *Retinal emboli (cholesterol or platelet–fibrin)* are evidence of atheromatous arterial disease, usually at the carotid bifurcation. *Cotton-wool* patches are commonly caused by occlusion of arterioles and capillaries; diabetes and hypertension are causes. Papilledema, hemorrhages, and cotton-wool patches may appear together in malignant hypertension.

OTHER CRANIAL NERVES

Trigeminal Nerve (V)

Corneal Reflex. Hold the eyelids open, touch the cornea with a moistened compact cylinder of cotton or tissue paper. Normally, there is an immediate attempt to close the eye. This may quantitatively diminish as coma deepens.

The intranasal sensory reaction may be tested by inserting the same sort of cylinder into each nostril. The normal response is for the person to wrinkle the nose slightly. There may be a protective hand motion.

Facial Nerve (VII)

Observation of the position of the buccal angles may reveal a blowing out or relaxing of one angle, commonly caused by a contralateral supratentorial lesion. A painful stimulus (see earlier under Examination and Meaning of Findings) may cause wincing or retraction of the buccal angles. If one buccal angle "lags" or does not retract, suspect a contralateral supranuclear lesion.

Glossopharyngeal Nerve (IX)

The glossopharyngeal nerve can be tested by touching the posterior wall of the pharynx with a wooden tongue depressor or applicator stick. Normally, there is contraction of the pharyngeal muscles. However, we have not found this test to be of much importance in the comatose patient.

Neck

With any evidence of trauma, it is prudent to be very cautious in moving the patient's neck until x-rays of the cervical spine have been done. Irritation of the meninges (whether due to blood or infection) commonly causes stiffness of forward flexion of the neck but not of rotation to either side.

MOTOR EXAMINATION INCLUDING RESPIRATION

Motor activity is not necessarily directly related to the depth of coma. Patients with bilateral subdural hematomas, exogenous poisons (sedatives), or diffuse brain hypoxia (cardiac arrest) are often hypokinetic. Those with trauma, brain abscess, metablic encephalopathy, and brain tumors are more likely to have motor activity, which may include asterixis, tremors, shivering, and decerebrate posturing.

Observation of the patient may reveal:

An abnormal position

- Decorticate rigidity: flexion of elbow, wrist, and fingers and extension and internal rotation with plantar flexion in the lower extremity. When unilateral, this indicates pathology in the opposite hemisphere and/or internal capsule. Bilaterality of this posture means bilateral lesions.
- Decerebrate rigidity: straight-line torso or opisthotonos, upper extremities extended, internally rotated (hyperpronated) and adducted, while the lower extremities are extended with the feet plantar flexed and often internally rotated. This state is usually caused by bilateral pathology in the diencephalon (thalamus, hypothalamus), pretectal region, and midbrain.
- Poverty of spontaneous movements: simple observation may reveal that there is no protective or other movement of one side of the body (or one extremity as compared to the other side). Such a finding may be a valuable clue pointing to a focal motor system lesion.

Involuntary movements: particularly noteworthy are asterixis, tremors, and myoclonic jerks. Asterixis (sudden relaxation of the wrist extensors when the wrists are extended or hyperextended) is most commonly elicitable when the patient is in an early stage of decreased consciousness. Various irregular coarse tremors, often interspersed with myoclonic jerks or twitches, frequently occur in metabolic encephalopathy; these are rare in focal supratentorial lesions. Aimless, almost purposeful, movements (seeming to pick at the bedcovers, etc.) are also often present in metabolic encephalopathy.

Vomiting may occur (in which case the airway must be protected), but rarely is vomiting a clue to localizing the nervous system abnormality.

Yawning that occurs frequently as alertness fails usually means brain stem pathophysiology. The primary pathology may be supratentorial, and central herniation may be the cause of yawning.

Hiccup (singultus) associated with decreased consciousness may be produced by a central lesion, usually in the medulla or nearby. One must recall that an expanding lesion (as in the cerebellum) may produce an effect on a nearby structure (any portion of the brain stem).

Muscle tone is tested after observing the patient's behavior. Commonly, tone in an upper extremity is tested by rather swiftly flexing and extending the elbow, moving the part through the full range of the joint's action, then alternately flexing and extending the wrists. It is particularly important to compare the tone on the two sides of the body. Abnormalities include:

Hypertonicity

- Spasticity: with the rapid movement the resistance of the muscle increases and then subsides or relaxes (clasp-knife phenomenon) with the continuing stretching of the muscles. This is usually seen when there is focal structural damage to the corticospinal tract(s). It is generally associated with hyperactive stretch reflexes and a Babinski sign.
- Rigidity: there is steady (plastic) resistance to muscle stretch throughout the range of joint action. One type of rigidity is sometimes called paratonia or gegenhalten. There is probably extrapyramidal patho-

physiology when rigidity is present, as it is in certain frontal lobe or hemisphere lesions. When it is definitely more severe unilaterally, it may assist in determining which hemisphere is involved.

Hypotonicity (loss of normal tone): the muscles offer less than normal resistance to the passive movements. Again, compare the two sides of the body. Absence of observed movement and ipsilateral hypotonia are often due to a contralateral acute hemisphere or internal capsule lesion (infarct or hemorrhage). Hypotonia may change to hypertonia with such a lesion. As coma deepens, hypertonia subsides, and generalized hypotonia appears.

Now a noxious stimulus is applied to the upper and lower extremities on each side (see earlier under Examination and Meaning of Findings). The quality and quantity of the response are noted and recorded for comparison with future serial testing. As mentioned, it is incorrect to absolutely equate motor response with depth of coma; however, there is often a significant relationship, which may be very helpful as one reexamines the patient.

Quality of response includes purposeful protective movements (indicating effective sensory function, motor response, and modest depression of consciousness), decorticate rigidity (see earlier in this section), decerebrate rigidity, or fragments of these abnormal responses. There may also be nondescript defensive-reflex withdrawal movements that do not have a direct protective quality.

The quantity of response often decreases and disappears as coma deepens. Compare the quantity (as well as quality) on the two sides of the body. Definite unilateral decrease or absence of response usually indicates contralateral damage to the corticospinal system (cortex, internal capsule, peduncles, etc.).

RESPIRATION

Great emphasis has been placed on the anatomical–etiologic meaning of certain patterns of abnormal respiration (Cheyne-Stokes, central neurogenic hyperventilation, etc.). We have not found an individual pattern of respiration to be of great specificity in the anatomical–etiologic diagnosis of coma. If one stays at the bedside of a patient in coma (whether due to trauma, poison, tentorial herniation, or infection) for several minutes, two or three different respiratory patterns may be seen. In addition, the central nervous system pathophysiology is often accompanied by pulmonary changes, which make the problem much more complex than taking a quick look at a patient with "mild central neurogenic hyperventilation" and assuming that the primary trouble is in the upper pontine tegmentum.

It is much more important to know that change in respiration is the immediate mechanism for correcting systemic acid–base imbalance. *Hyperventilation* is caused by metabolic acidosis or respiratory alkalosis, while hypoventilation is due to respiratory acidosis or metabolic alkalosis. These states are determined by emergency laboratory tests: serum *p*H, $PaCO_2$ and HCO_3.

Common causes of metabolic acidosis (hyperventilation) are diabetic coma and uremia. Respiratory alkalosis (hyperventilation) is due to pulmonary disease, hepatic coma, systemic infection, and, rarely, salicylism or hysteria. Hypoventilation associated with respiratory acidosis is due to neuromuscular disease (decreased respiratory excursions) or to pulmonary disease, while hypoventilation due to metabolic alkalosis (much less common) is a result of loss of acid from gastrointestinal or renal routes or ingestion of an excessive amount of alkali.

Slow, regular, shallow respiration (often ineffective) frequently occurs with decreased consciousness due to ingestion of sedatives.

Rapid, regular, somewhat shallow breathing occurs with pneumonia, diabetic acidosis, or uremic acidosis.

Cheyne-Stokes respiration (CSR) is a pattern in which waxing and waning hyperpnea (increasing rate than decreasing rate) alternates with shorter periods of apnea, which suggest bilateral dysfunction of cerebral structures deep in the hemispheres or diencephalon, although CSR may occur during sleep in elderly people without other evidence of central nervous system pathology.

Central neurogenic hyperventilation (CNH) is a pattern of increased rate (often 25/min or more), regular and often somewhat deep. We have found it to be of very little localizing value, although it may be present with caudal midbrain or upper pontine tegmental lesions. This may continue despite low arterial CO_2 tension and elevated *p*H.

In apneustic respiration there is a prolonged inspiratory phase followed by expiratory apnea. This occurs at a rate of $1\frac{1}{2}$ to 2 cycles/

minute. It is a rare, ominous abnormality, occasionally associated with infarction of the pons.

Irregular irregularity (Biot's or ataxic breathing) of breathing is a pattern in which deep, medium, and shallow breaths occur at randomly irregular intervals. It is associated with medullary pathophysiology and is an ominous sign.

In certain instances in which focal hemisphere lesions cause central or temporal lobe herniation, one may observe a sequence of patterns of respiration from Cheyne-Stokes respiration to central neurogenic hyperventilation to Biot's respiration to apnea.

EXAMINATION OF REFLEXES

Muscle-stretch reflexes are of limited value in the differential diagnosis of coma. Some normal persons have absent stretch reflexes, while others have maximal hyperactivity of reflexes, including clonus, without any evidence of dysfunction or disorder of the nervous system (such persons have equal reflexes on the two sides of the body). In examining the patient with abnormal consciousness, a definite difference in stretch reflexes on the two sides of the body may assist in ruling out hysteria or in determining which side is more involved.

Superficial reflexes such as the corneal reflex (see Trigeminal Nerve [V]) have been mentioned. The superficial abdominal, cremasteric, and anal reflexes are of little value in this context.

A pathologic reflex (Babinski sign, etc.) has little specificity other than to indicate the presence of pathophysiology somewhere along the corticospinal pathway. A unilateral Babinski sign is more helpful than bilateral signs. In severe hypoglycemia a Babinski sign may be present, only to disappear in minutes after the hypoglycemia is corrected. Following a grand mal attack the sign may last only a few seconds. The Babinski sign may disappear as coma deepens. This sign may aid in ruling out a diagnosis of psychogenic coma.

The evaluation of the comatose patient to this point has taken less than 10 minutes. The accompanying list summarizes the physical signs associated with the anatomical sites of the primary processes causing coma. This representation is dogmatic and is accurate when the process is precisely located. However, the trouble may be multifocal, or there may be worsening (edema, etc.) of supratentorial pathology causing supratentorial brain shift, which produces uncal or central (transtentorial) herniation. Herniation can produce direct brain stem compression, vascular occlusion in the stem, or a combination of both.

PHYSICAL SIGNS SUGGESTING THE ANATOMICAL SITE OF A PRIMARY PROCESS CAUSING COMA

Supratentorial

Focal
- Pupils: normal
- Ocular rotations: abnormal conjugate gaze—the eyes deviate toward the lesion; oculocephalic and oculovestibular reflexes are intact.
- Motor: hemiparesis or hemiplegia are apparent by observation of the patient or the patient's response to pain stimulus or unilateral decorticate phenomena; unilateral Babinski sign.

Diffuse
- Pupils: normal (see text for special pharmacologic actions on the pupils)
- Ocular rotations: roving eye movements or eyes in the midorbital position; oculocephalic and oculovestibular reflexes are intact.
- Motor: responses to painful stimuli are equal on the two sides; muscle tone, stretch reflexes, and Babinski responses are about the same on the two sides.

Infratentorial

Focal
- Pupils
  - Midbrain: ipsilateral pupil dilated, absent light reaction, eye abducted, ptosis (3rd cranial nerve palsy)
  - Pons: ipsilateral miosis and slight ptosis, light reaction present (Horner's)
  - Medulla: ipsilateral miosis and slight ptosis (Horner's), light reaction present
- Ocular rotations: dysconjugate position of eyes including skew deviation, partial internuclear ophthalmoplegia, and so forth; uncertain oculocephalic and oculovestibular reflexes
- Motor: "crossed hemiplegia"—on painful stimulation, absent retraction of the buccal angle with hemiparesis (upper and lower extremity) on the opposite side

Diffuse
- Pupils
  - Midbrain: normal size, absent light reaction
  - Pons: very small, light reaction gone or minimal
  - Medulla: small, light reaction present
- Ocular rotations: eyes in midorbital position, skew, etc.; absent oculocephalic and oculovestibular reflexes
- Motor: decerebrate position, posturing, or response to painful stimuli

Listed under Basic Mechanisms Causing Coma are the ten causes of this state. Convulsions, shock, chemical causes, bacterial infections, epidural and subdural hematomas, and deficiency states are commonly causes of coma, curable with specific treatment. These basic categories must receive specific diagnostic attention if the history and examination do not make the cause evident.

Listed under Etiologic Basic Differential Diagnosis Related to Supratentorial or Infratentorial Sites are the basic etiologic diagnoses as they relate to basic anatomical sites. With abnormal signs from the patient's examination and information from these three lists, diagnostic priorities are established and a laboratory work-up designed. CT scans of the head are now performed in most medical centers in the United States, and they aid greatly in the emergency diagnosis of expanding intracranial masses, destructive and/or bleeding lesions, and any situation in which there is a shift of the brain. Unless meningeal infection is suspected, the CT head scan has largely eliminated the need for cerebrospinal fluid examination. By the time the CT scan is completed (presuming that it is needed), the results of the blood tests listed at the beginning of this chapter under Priority three, step 5 are available.

Although an uncommon cause of decreased responsiveness, psychogenic disease including catatonia is occasionally part of the differential diagnosis in patients with altered consciousness. When present, it can be difficult to distinguish from metabolic or structural brain disease. Severely ill psychiatric patients may be resistant to painful stimuli. The technique of delivering a stimulus such as sticking the patient with a large-bore needle is sometimes used to rule out psychiatric disease. Not only is this unreliable, but it is not acceptable to inflict a puncture wound unless it is a part of a necessary phlebotomy or insertion of an arterial or venous line. Other parts of the examination (Babinski sign, pupillary size, light reaction, position of the eyes in the orbit, and caloric reflexes) are more reliable.

Listed under Differential Diagnosis of Coma (Pathological and Physiological Basis) are additional pathologic and pathophysiologic causes of coma, amplifying by subcategories the list of basic mechanisms given previously. In a sense, all causes of dysfunction of the nervous system (as in coma) are metabolically or chemically determined in that there is a defect in each and in the sum of all the physical and chemical processes by which the living neural tissue functions normally. It has be-

BASIC MECHANISMS CAUSING COMA

- Trauma (concussion, contusion, hemorrhage, etc.)
- *Convulsions* (particularly status epilepticus)
- Vascular (occlusion, hemmorhage, impaired cardiac output, *shock*)
- *Chemical (metabolic, toxic, electrolyte imbalance)*
- Expanding masses (neoplasm, *abscess, subdural hematoma, etc.*)
- *Infections (meningitis,* encephalitis)
- *Deficiency states (thiamine, cyanocobalamin)*
- Physical agents (heat, cold, electroshock)
- Psychogenic
- Other (demyelinating, Alzheimer's disease, Huntington's chorea, etc.)

ETIOLOGIC BASIC DIFFERENTIAL DIAGNOSIS RELATED TO SUPRATENTORIAL OR INFRATENTORIAL SITES

Supratentorial

- Focal
  - Trauma
  - Vascular
    - Infarction
    - Hemorrhage
  - *Expanding masses*
    - *Subdural hematoma*
    - *Epidural hematoma*
  - *Infection*
    - Abscess
- Diffuse
  - Trauma
  - Convulsive disorder
  - Vascular: ischemia (*shock, anemia, cardiac arrest*)
- Infection
  - Chemical
    - *Drugs–toxins*
    - *Metabolic encephalopathy*
    - *Deficiency states*

Infratentorial

- Focal
  - Vascular
    - Infarction
    - Hemorrhage
  - Neoplasm
  - *Infection–abscess*
  - Hypoglycemia
- Diffuse
  - Herniation (variable loci)
  - *Chemical*
    - Metabolic

come popular to use the term *metabolic encephalopathy* for any systemic process that distorts brain metabolism by producing a deficiency of nutrients, a chemical that is toxic to brain cells, or an electrolyte imbalance.

DIFFERENTIAL DIAGNOSIS OF COMA (PATHOLOGIC AND PHYSIOLOGIC BASIS)

- Trauma
  - Concussion
  - Contusion, laceration, subarchnoid bleeding
  - *Subdural hematoma*
  - *Epidural hematoma*
  - Depressed fracture
  - High spinal cord lesion
- *Convulsions (particularly grand mal, as in status epilepticus)*
- Vascular disease
  - Decreased diffuse cerebral perfusion pressure
    - Cardiac arrest—pulmonary embolism
    - Cardiac arrhythmias
    - Myocardial infarction with "pump failure"
    - Congestive failure
    - *Low blood volume (shock)*
    - Vasovagal syncope—orthostatism
    - *Hypertensive encephalopathy*
    - Polycythemia
    - Small vessel occlusions (lupus erythematosis, collagen disease, multiple fat emboli)
  - Decreased focal cerebral perfusion pressure
    - Occlusive vascular disease
      - Thrombus
      - Embolus
        - Intraluminal source
        - Cardiac source
      - *Arteritis*
    - Hemorrhage
      - Intracerebral
      - Subarachnoid
- Chemical
  - Toxins
    - *Sedative–narcotic*
    - Other (methyl alcohol, cyanide, carbon monoxide)
  - Metabolic encephalopathy
    - *Pancreas (hyperglycemia, hypoglycemia)*
    - Liver (hepatic coma)
    - Kidney (uremic coma)
    - *Lung (CO_2 narcosis)*
    - Neoplasm (remote effects)
    - Thyroid or parathyroid or adrenal states
- *Electrolyte abnormalities*
    - Metabolic and respiratory acidosis
    - Metabolic and respiratory alkalosis
    - Hypernatremia and hyponatremia
    - Potassium or magnesium or calcium abnormalities
- Expanding mass
  - Neoplasms
    - Primary
    - Secondary
  - *Abscess*
  - *Subdural hematoma*
  - *Extradural hematoma*
- Infections
  - Encephalitis
  - *Meningitis*
  - *Abscess*
  - Remote effects (typhoid, diphtheria, pneumonia)

27 Trauma of the Central Nervous System

M. PETER HEILBRUN

A recent report from the University of Pennsylvania Head Injury Research Center notes that trauma kills 140,000 persons annually in the United States, more than all other diseases combined for the population under age 35.[1] Approximately one half of all trauma deaths are due to head injury, for which the mortality rate is 40%. Generally, those head injury patients who do survive face greater costs of care and longer treatment than other trauma patients. This high morbidity and mortality in head injury is related not only to the initial brain damage produced by impact, but also to the secondary complications of hypoxia and diffuse cerebral swelling.

This chapter outlines a scheme for clinical evaluation of the head-injured patient based on analysis of:

1. The pathophysiologic state of brain function, level of consciousness, and absence or presence of focal deficit
2. The morphologic integrity of the brain, cervical spinal cord, and coverings
3. The cardiovascular and respiratory function
4. The presence of multiple organ injury
5. The time profile of the pathophysiologic state, serially observed from the time of impact to the triage point in the ambulatory care setting or the emergency room

Using this analysis, the treating physician can immediately institute measures to prevent secondary complications while he or she defines the severity of injury with appropriate radiographic imaging and laboratory studies and determines whether specialized neurosurgical consultation is indicated.

PATHOPHYSIOLOGIC STATE OF BRAIN FUNCTION

DIFFUSE AXONAL INJURY

Most head injuries result from motor vehicle accidents. A smaller number are related to direct blows to the head with a blunt instrument, and a smaller proportion is related to direct penetration of the cranial vault by objects such as bullets, knives, or picks. Since the most common cause is motor vehicle accidents in which the victim is moving at the time of impact, much of the effect of trauma is related to rapid differential rates of acceleration and deceleration of the highly dense cranial vault compared with the lower-density contents of the cranial vault, namely, the brain, spinal fluid, and cerebral vasculature. The differential rate of acceleration and deceleration, at its most severe state, results in a condition defined by the University of Pennsylvania Head Injury Research Center as diffuse axonal injury.[1] These researchers have demonstrated that a particular set of acceleration conditions, namely, the degree of angular acceleration with the head moving in a coronal side-to-side plane, correlates closely with the severity of diffuse axonal injury and thus with the duration of coma and neurologic outcome. Experimental results in a primate model are quite similar to the pathologic material of human fatalities studies by Strich and Adams many years ago.[2–4] This type of injury is usually associated with prolonged coma.

By contrast, these researchers have also noted that acceleration–deceleration mechanisms confined to the anterior–posterior sagittal direction generally are associated not with severe axonal disruption but with vascular disruptions that lead to polar and extra-axial hematomas. This type of injury may have a better prognosis than diffuse axonal injury associated with angular acceleration–deceleration measurements.[5] The definition of possible different outcomes from two types of acceleration–deceleration injuries has implications for motor vehicle design considerations for head injury prevention.

CEREBRAL VASOMOTOR PARALYSIS

A second pathologic condition that occurs with impact followed by bleeding and severe brain compression is cerebral vasomotor paralysis. The initial event in vasomotor paralysis is the loss of cerebral autoregulation, a condition in which the cerebral vascular resistance normally adjusts to changes in brain perfusion pressure to maintain a relatively constant blood flow and volume. With brain compression vasomotor paralysis ensues such that at the extremes of the intracranial pressure and volume curve, small increases in cranial vault volume specifically related to both brain water and cerebral blood volume can lead to further increases in intracranial pressure to the point that cerebral perfusion pressure (defined as the difference between the systemic mean arterial blood pressure and the mean intracranial pressure) can be reduced to critical levels of brain perfusion.[6]

A basic understanding of the mechanisms of angular acceleration–deceleration forces leading to diffuse axonal injury and of the potential for secondary complications of increased intracranial pressure (often related to the associated development of intracranial hematomas and eventually leading to vasomotor paralysis) allows the clinician to devise treatment protocols comfortably.

ASSESSMENT OF LEVEL OF CONSCIOUSNESS

The Glasgow Coma Scale. In the past, descriptive terms of level of consciousness were often related to extremely nondescriptive terms such as *sleep, wakefulness, comatose, semicomatose, confused,* and *loss of speech.* When physicians attempted to communicate to each other the state of the patient's level of consciousness based on the nondescriptive terms, the interpretation of the patient's actual level of consciousness often depended on the physician's personal conceptualization of the meaning of those terms. In the early 1960s Professor Bryan Jennett and his staff, particularly Graham Teasdale, at the Institute of Neurological Sciences in Glasgow, Scotland, addressed the confusion of terms describing levels of consciousness and devised a more quantitative evaluation titled the Glasgow Coma Scale (Table 27-1).[7–9] The Glasgow Coma Scale has now become accepted worldwide as a standard for communicating not only level of consciousness but specific severity of head injury.

The Glasgow Coma Scale is defined by combined scores for opening of the eyes, termed *eye opening*; speech, termed *verbal response*; and movement of the extremities, termed *motor response*. Table 27-1 outlines the grading system. This scoring can be applied efficiently in the majority of head injury problems, and its criteria are commonly understood and accepted. Patients with the most severe injury present with a Glasgow Coma Scale of 0 to 4; with moderately severe injuries, 4 to 9; and with milder injuries, 10 to 15. It has become a common observation that the break point between quality survival is often related to a Glasgow Coma Scale above 6 to 8.

TABLE 27-1. Glasgow Coma Scale

RESPONSE	SCORE
EYES OPEN	
Never	1
To pain	2
To verbal stimuli	3
Spontaneously	4
BEST VERBAL RESPONSE	
None	1
Incomprehensible sounds	2
Inappropriate words	3
Disoriented and converses	4
Oriented and converses	5
BEST MOTOR RESPONSE	
None	1
Extension (decerebrate rigidity)	2
Abnormal flexion (decorticate rigidity)	3
Flexion withdrawal	4
Localizes pain	5
Obeys commands	6
Total	3–15

If one listens to emergency room physicians and neurosurgeons communicating about the severity of an injury or the temporal course of an injury, one might hear the following conversation: "When the patient came in the emergency room, he had a GCS score of 13 and rapidly improved to 15. On the basis of this improvement, we feel that it is reasonable to observe the patient here in the emergency room for a few hours and, if there is no deterioration in Glasgow Coma Score, then send the patient home."

Focal Neurologic Deficits. Because of its qualitative and quantitative accuracy, the Glasgow Coma Scale has contributed significantly to the management of head-injured patients. However, these scores by themselves are *not* a full measure of the state of the brain injury. Thus the physician must also efficiently analyze the central nervous system for the absence or presence of focal neurologic deficit. The presence of a focal neurologic deficit can usually be related to one of two mechanisms. The first and most common mechanism is loss of neurologic function due to focal injury to a specific region of the brain at impact. For example, a blow to the temporal vault may result in loss of memory, change in speech, and commonly a pupillary abnormality; a blow or penetration of the cerebral cortex in the parietal region can lead to loss of motor or sensory function in the opposite extremity; a blow to the vertex area with disruption of blood supply to the parasagittal motor cortices can lead to unilateral or bilateral lower-extremity paresis; impact to the occipital region can lead to blindness considered cortical in nature. These deficits, which reflect severe focal injury, are often noted in patients with high Glasgow Coma Scale scores.

The second mechanism of focal injury derives from the associated swelling and shift of brain structures, which in turn cause herniation of the cerebral peduncles through or against the tentorial notch leading to focal paresis of the third nerve and corticospinal tracks manifest by abnormal pupil reactions, coma, and, again, contralateral hemiparesis.[10–12] Such hemiparesis usually denotes life-threatening compromise of brain function, but in many cases this compromise can be relieved by surgical removal of intracranial hematomas to reduce intracranial pressure and impaction. In other cases, aggressive pharmacologic regimens may be attempted to treat cerebral vasomotor paralysis and/or to lessen cerebral brain edema and thereby decrease intracranial pressure.[13,14]

MORPHOLOGIC INTEGRITY

The baseline analysis of the Glasgow Coma Scale level and the absence, presence, and types of focal neurologic deficit at both the scene of the accident and in the initial facility where physician evaluation is performed are critical.[15] However, periorbital swelling often forces eyelid closure, thus preventing analysis of the eye-opening response. Also, traumatic injuries often require endotracheal intubation, sedation, and muscle relaxation, which further compromise the observer's ability to ascertain a valid Glasgow Coma Scale and focal neurologic index.

In addition, because of the decompressive effect of open injuries down to the brain structure, particularly in silent areas such as a unilateral frontal lobe, the presence of severe anatomic disruption of these structures may not be apparent with either Glasgow Coma Scale or focal neurologic deficit indices. Therefore the integrity of the anatomic structures of the head, face, and neck must be analyzed by direct visual observation and by radiographic studies.

CARDIOVASCULAR AND RESPIRATORY FUNCTION

Severe brain dysfunction noted on examination is often associated with either primary or secondary impairment of cardiovascular tone. Sometimes this results through a simple mechanism such as blood loss secondary to extensive scalp lacerations or extremity or internal organ hemorrhage. More complex mechanisms relate to loss of systemic vasomotor tone and changes in vasomotor tone propagated from compromised brain stem structures. These mechanisms lead to states of low blood pressure, high blood pressure, cardiac arrhythmia, abnormal respirations, and abnormal oxygen uptake due to increased pulmonary fluid. All these mechanisms combine to states of hypoxia, then to combined hypoxia and hypoxemia, and eventually ischemia to the brain and associated secondary complications. Thus the physician must analyze cardiovascular status by blood pressure and pulse measurements, and he or she must also analyze respiratory patterns and oxygen saturation by blood gases or peripheral saturation meters.

MULTIPLE ORGAN INJURY

The observing physician must keep in mind that injuries to other organ systems, particularly major trauma to the chest and abdomen and proximal lower extremities, can lead to severe compromise with other ischemic effects. The management of multiple organ system failure is addressed in other chapters and will not be addressed at this point except for the reminder that oxygen and glucose requirements of the central nervous system are immediate and high; thus any compromise, particularly in body oxygenation, will quickly lead to increased brain damage.

TIME PROFILE

The natural history of recovery from brain injury in the absence of secondary complications is generally one of a state of loss of consciousness to gradual but steady return to normal consciousness and brain function. Thus the hallmark of treatment of the brain-injured patient and of decisions as to whether specific diagnostic studies or therapeutic intervention are indicated is based on serial observation of the state of the brain. This profile of the injury provides data from which one can determine whether the patient is in a state of steady but rapid or gradual improvement, fluctuating but gradual improvement, improvement followed by lack of improvement, or plateauing of neurologic status, progressive deterioration, or improvement followed by deterioration of neurologic status. If improvement is slower than should be expected, is fluctuating, or has plateaued or if deterioration is occurring, the physician must rule out secondary complications of the injury. Studies should be performed to determine brain conditions that may require either surgical intervention or medical therapeutic measures.

In summary, the physician's analysis and treatment protocols for individual patients require an evaluation of head injury based on level of consciousness analyzed by the Glasgow Coma Scale, findings of focal neurologic abnormality based on the classical neurologic examination, determination of morphologic integrity of anatomic structures, measurement of cardiorespiratory function, consideration of multiple system injury, and a time profile.[16]

Further evaluation and treatment of the head injury includes the rapid total patient assessment. If it is determined that life-threatening injuries are present, these must be treated first. Specifically, airway problems must be corrected, generally by institution of endotracheal intubation. (In the presence of associated spinal cord injury, nasotracheal intubation by a skilled practitioner may be required.) Also cardiovascular tone must be maintained by controlling hemorrhage.

It should be kept in mind that associated cervical spinal cord injury is often associated with loss of sympathetic tone. Thus decreased vasomotor tone in this situation is often associated with both hypothermia and bradycardia rather than tachycardia and should be treated with sympathomimetic drugs rather than volume replacement.

Hypotension should be treated with appropriate blood replacement and ringer's lactate. Overhydration with intravenous solutions should be avoided.

The diagnostic procedures are relatively straightforward. In the patient who has been comatose, chest and lateral cervical spine films to the T1 level as well as a CT scan should be obtained. It was once considered that CT need be performed only in patients with a Glasgow Coma Scale of 8 or less. Today, however, CT scanning is routine in most institutions, as it is helpful not only in evaluation of the brain state but also in the management of major scalp wounds, suspected fractures, and penetrating injury. In addition, Dacey has shown that combined observation and skull films and/or CT scan in patients with Glasgow Coma Scores in the range of 13 to 15 demonstrate a small but significant number of treatable intracranial hematomas, which not only is cost effective but may significantly contribute to preventing catastrophic deterioration in the patient with relatively minor head injuries.[17]

With this outline in mind, several typical head-injured patient management problems will be described. These descriptions will cover a spectrum of cranial vault and cerebral trauma, from which the physician in the ambulatory care setting may develop his or her own evaluation and treatment protocols.

CASE 1: MINOR HEAD INJURY WITH SCALP LACERATION

This 8-year-old boy was riding a bicycle at a slow speed, turned into a gravel-lined driveway, and fell off his bike, landing in the gravel. When he was found by his family, they noted that he had moderate abrasions of the face and scalp. There was a 5-cm irregular laceration in the left frontal area behind the hairline. They noted that he was alert and awake. He did not complain of headache or neck stiffness and remembered all of the events of the accident, including slipping from the bike and striking the gravel. There was no loss of consciousness. He was taken to the emergency room, where it was noted that he opened his eyes spontaneously, was oriented, and conversed and obeyed all commands. He was judged to have a Glasgow Coma Scale of 15. Neurologic examination revealed no focal neurologic deficit and there was no loss of consciousness. The anatomic evaluation showed evidence of the abrasions and scalp laceration.

MANAGEMENT

Based on the analysis scheme, this patient's management requires brief observation and debridement and cleansing of the abrasions and debridement and layered suture of the scalp laceration.

Rule Out Fracture. Visual inspection and gloved palpation of the periosteum and skull underlying the laceration are performed. If there is no disruption or swelling of the periosteum, there is probably no bony fracture; nonetheless the possibility needs to be ruled out by plain skull films or CT scan and cervical spine films. If radiographs are negative for a fracture, debridement of the wound and layered suture of the laceration, as noted, are required.

If during the period of observation and treatment, which generally would last at least $1\frac{1}{2}$ hours, there has been no change in the Glasgow Coma Scale or neurologic status, the child can be discharged under the care of a responsible adult with instructions to observe hourly for development of headache, nausea, and vomiting followed by lethargy or seizures. If any of these events occur, he should return immediately to the ambulatory care facility for reevaluation. Otherwise return for inspection of the wound and suture removal in several days is all that is necessary.

Fracture. However, if radiographs show an underlying fracture, the physician must determine whether it is linear and whether it crosses the meningeal vascular structures, particularly the middle meningeal arteries in the temporal bone, and whether it is complex and depressed. If the fracture is linear and nondisplaced, management is the same as that in which no fracture is involved, although a longer observation period is necessary and hospitalization should be considered. This type of patient should be either hospitalized or reevaluated in the ambulatory care facility at 24 hours following the injury.

If the patient is released, instructions should also advise the responsible party to watch for the development of symptoms of intracranial pressure and brain shift, which in this type of patient generally start with complaint of severe headache followed by decreasing consciousness.

If plain skull films are the only radiographic study performed and the fracture is nondisplaced but overlies vascular structure such as middle meningeal artery over the temporal bone or the sagittal sinus at the vertex or the occipital bone from the lambdoid suture to the foramen magnum, a baseline CT scan should be performed to look for early development of an extradural hematoma. (See cases 4 and 6 for management of complicated fractures.)

CASE 2: CLOSED DEPRESSED SKULL FRACTURE IN AN INFANT

This 3-month-old infant was seen in the emergency room and was noted to be awake, alert, and crying. On examination of the scalp, there was a large left subgaleal hematoma with a slight indentation in the midportion of the hematoma. There was no evidence of focal neurologic deficit. No scalp lacerations were present.

Radiographs were obtained; they showed evidence of a closed, depressed fracture in the parietal posterior region. A CT scan was obtained; it showed no evidence of cortical contusion or laceration and no evidence of chronic subdural hematoma, acute cortical contusion, or laceration in the region of the skull depression. The hematocrit was at 22.

MANAGEMENT

Management of this type of closed depressed fracture requires surgical intervention (see Fig. 27-1).

CT Scan to Rule Out Brain Parenchyma Damage. A CT scan should be taken both to rule out brain tissue damage and to provide precise data so that surgical elevation can be made through a small opening.

Surgical Elevation. This greenstick or Ping-Pong ball–type depression can be elevated by a small incision overlying the depressed fracture and a small bony opening at the edge of the depression. An appropriate instrument can then be placed between the dura and the bone, generally resulting in rapid elevation of the depressed bone to its normal position. In the absence of a CT scan a small dural incision to rule out an associated subdural hematoma must be considered.

Hematocrit Measurements. It should be noted that in a small infant significant blood loss in both the subperiosteal and subgaleal space can occur to reduce the hematocrit to critical levels. Adding even a small operative procedure can compromise hemoglobin oxygen-carrying capacity. Therefore even though there does not appear to be significant blood loss, careful evaluation of the hematocrit is essential.

In addition, careful observation for other injuries that might alert the physician to child abuse definitely must be considered when this type of fracture is noted in an infant.

CASE 3: OPEN DEPRESSED SKULL FRACTURE IN AN ADULT

This 40-year-old woman was involved in a marital dispute and was struck in the left parietal region with a baseball bat. She was initially unconscious and when brought to the emergency room was noted to be awake but seemingly confused. She opened her eyes to command and moved her left side to command but had no verbal response and could not move her right arm. Neurologic examination showed evidence of expressive aphasia and moderate right hemiparesis. Examination of the head revealed a stellate ragged 5-cm laceration in the left parietal area with exposed underlying bone and dura. No brain substance was noted.

No CT scanner or neurosurgeon was available. The wound was dressed and the patient was transported to an appropriate facility where there was noted to be no change in her Glasgow Coma Score of 11 or her focal neuro-

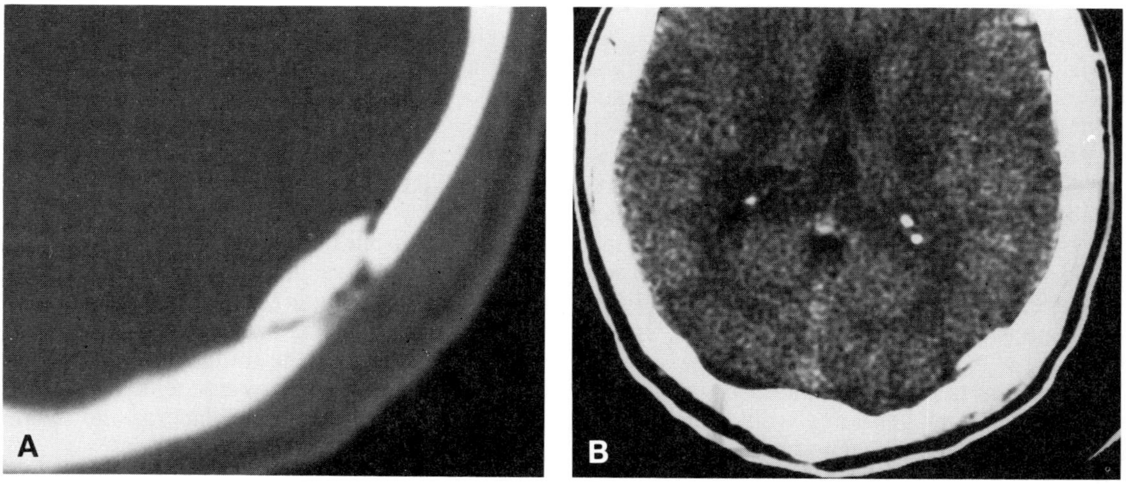

Figure 27-1. Example of depressed skull fracture requiring surgical elevation. (*A*) CT scan—bone window to define extent of fracture. (*B*) CT scan—tissue window that shows no evidence of cortical contusion or laceration.

logic deficit. A CT scan was performed that showed evidence of a bone fragment embedded in the cerebral cortex with a small surrounding zone of hemorrhagic brain.

MANAGEMENT

CT Scan for Bony Fragment and Tissue Damage. CT scan should be taken as indicated in the preceding history.

Surgery. The patient was taken immediately to the operating room, where the wound was cleansed with copious irrigation fluid, following which the scalp was prepared in the usual fashion. The stellate laceration was extended on each end and the fractured bone fragments were carefully removed by placement of multiple perforator openings at the bony edges and careful removal of all the bone fragments with the exception of the one that had pierced the dura and was embedded in the brain. When all other bone fragments were removed, the bony margin was smoothed and bleeding was controlled with bone wax; epidural bleeding was controlled with bipolar coagulation. Following this, the dural laceration was opened to the bony margin and the cortex was noted to be lacerated by the embedded bone fragment, which was carefully removed. Following removal of the embedded fragment, the surrounding cortical brain was carefully debrided of necrotic and hemorrhagic cortex. Minimal bleeding occurred; this was controlled with gentle irrigation. Next, the dura was repaired primarily. The scalp laceration and incision were repaired with a layered closure.

Postoperative Prophylactic Anticonvulsant. The patient was placed on phenytoin (Dilantin).

Result, Follow-Up, and Repair of Bony Defect. The patient quickly regained use of her right arm and leg, and over a period of several weeks her speech deficit disappeared. A postoperative CT scan showed that the hemorrhagic area was gone and no residual bone fragments were present. The patient was discharged with minimal neurologic deficit, was followed on a regular basis, and was readmitted in 6 months, at which time the bony defect was repaired with an acrylic plate fixed to the bone.

CASE 4: MODERATELY SEVERE HEAD INJURY WITH BASILAR SKULL FRACTURE AND CSF LEAK

This 20-year-old man was involved in a motor vehicle–bicycle injury. He was brought to the emergency room, where he was noted to have a decreased level of consciousness. His best eye-opening response was to painful stimulation only. He moved all extremities spontaneously. His best verbal response was inappropriate words and his best motor response was flexion withdrawal for a Glasgow Coma Scale of 8. There were no pupillary or reflex abnormalities. Examination of the head showed evidence of left periorbital ecchymoses, left postauricular ecchymoses, and blood and CSF draining from the left ear canal.

Vital signs were normal. Respiratory rate and pattern were normal. Skull and cervical spine showed no evidence of a fracture. A CT scan revealed a vertical fracture passing through the ear canal and traversing the vertical portion of the facial nerve canal. No intracranial hematoma was noted.

MANAGEMENT

CT Scan. CT scan was given as indicated (see Fig. 27-2).

Intensive Care, Antibiotics. The patient was hospitalized in the intensive care unit and placed on antibiotics. By the first postinjury day the patient was alert, opened his eyes spontaneously, had a verbal response in which he was oriented and conversed, and obeyed all commands with no evidence of a motor deficit.

Observation for Facial Nerve Damage. Over several days the patient showed no development of a facial nerve paralysis.

Drain for Continued CSF Leak. At 6 days he continued to have significant cerebrospinal fluid drainage from the left ear canal. Therefore a lumbar subarachnoid drain was placed with drainage to an external bag. Over a period of 48 hours his CSF otorrhea stopped. The drainage was continued for an additional 24 hours, following which the drainage tube was clamped for 24 hours. No further CSF drainage occurred and the lumbar subarachnoid drain was removed.

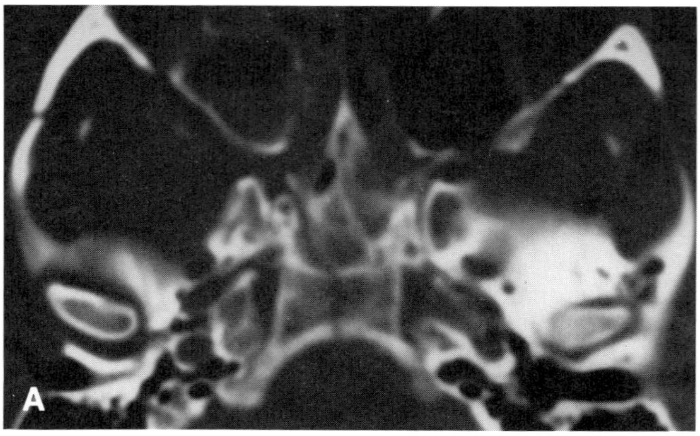

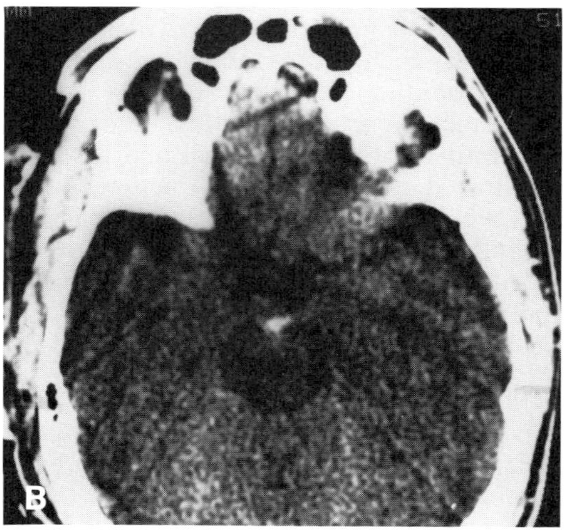

Figure 27-2. Example of basilar skull fracture. (*A*) CT scan—bone window that defines fracture line through sella and clivus. (*B*) CT scan—tissue window that shows small extraaxial hemorrhage adjacent to fracture in interpeduncular cistern.

Result. The patient was gradually ambulated over a period of 4 days and was discharged.

CASE 5: PENETRATING BRAIN INJURY

This 24-year-old man under inpatient psychiatric treatment was found in his room with a decreased level of consciousness with a No. 2 pencil penetrating the intracranial cavity through the left nostril. The patient was transported to the emergency room, where his Glasgow Coma Scale score was 8. He had localized pain, no verbal response, but opened his eyes to pain. No focal neurologic deficit was noted.

MANAGEMENT

See Figure 27-3.

CT Scan. The patient was taken to the CT scanner, where a plain scan showed the tip of the pencil to be just adjacent to the midline within the anterior portion of the third ventricle. This was followed by a contrast-enhanced scan, which suggested that the pencil abutted the A1 segment of the left anterior cerebral artery. An *angiogram* was performed, which showed occlusion of the A1 segment of the anterior cerebral artery but good filling of both anterior cerebral arteries from the right with the left filling through a patent anterior communicating artery.

Surgery. The patient was taken to the operating room, where a bifrontal craniotomy was performed and the optic nerves, chiasm, and anterior cerebral complex were identified. Under direct vision the pencil was slowly re-

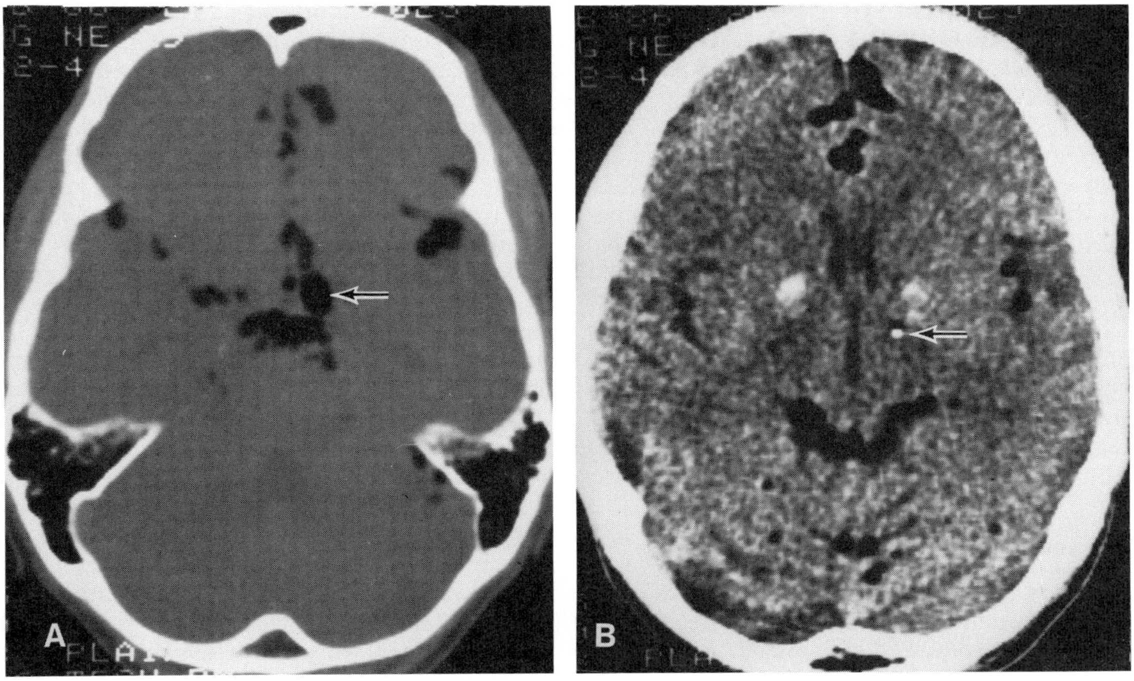

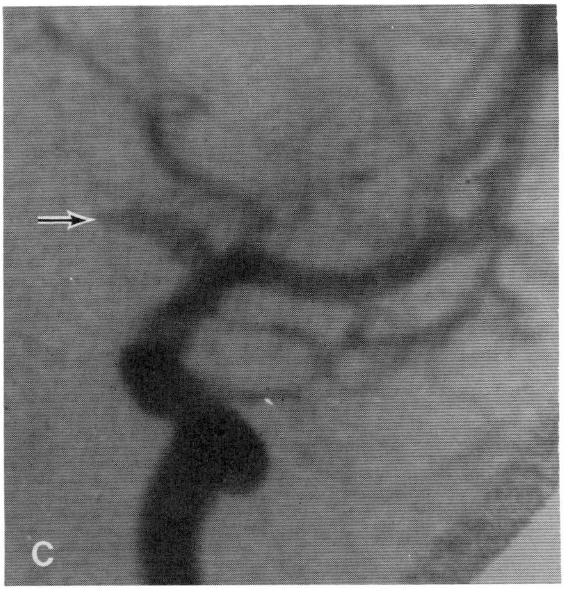

Figure 27-3. Example of penetrating injury. (*A*) CT scan—bone window showing air in cisterns and pencil tract (*arrow*). (*B*) CT scan—tissue window showing air, small zone of hemorrhage, and pencil tip in subthalamus (*arrow*). (*C*) Angiogram—occlusion of A1 segment of anterior cerebral artery by penetrating pencil.

moved from the cranial vault. There was bleeding from the A1 segment by penetration of the artery from the pencil tip. Temporary clips were placed on the anterior cerebral artery, following which it was repaired with microsurgical technique and 10-0 monofilament nylon suture.

Result. Postoperatively the patient was placed on antibiotics and gradually improved over a period of several weeks. Whereas prior to the suicide attempt he had been agitated, postoperatively his affect was calm. He was returned to the psychiatric ward for further rehabilitation.

CASE 6: LINEAR NONDISPLACED FRACTURE OVERLYING MIDDLE MENINGEAL ARTERY, EPIDURAL HEMATOMA

This 10-year-old boy was struck in the left temporal region by a hardball, following which he was unconscious. He awoke and paramedics noted that he spontaneously opened his eyes, was disoriented but conversed, and obeyed commands, resulting in a Glasgow Coma Score of 14. He was transported to an emergency room facility where a CT scan showed evidence of a linear nondisplaced fracture overlying the middle meningeal artery. No epidural hematoma or intracranial lesion was noted.

MANAGEMENT

CT Scan. CT scan was performed as indicated. On determination of a fracture, the patient was hospitalized.

Intensive Care. The patient was admitted to the intensive care unit. At 3 hours he had no change in his Glasgow Coma Scale but was complaining of left temporal headache. One hour later he was noted to open his eyes spontaneously but used inappropriate words; he obeyed commands but was noted on neurologic exam to have slight enlargement of the pupils.

Repeat Scan on Deterioration. He was returned to the CT scanner, where repeat scans showed evidence of a 2-cm epidural hematoma underlying the fracture.

Surgery. The patient was taken to the operating room, where, through a temporal craniectomy, the epidural hematoma was evacuated. The patient's subsequent course was one of resolution of the headache, return of the Glasgow Coma Scale to 15, and resolution of the pupillary abnormality.

CASE 7: SEVERE CLOSED HEAD INJURY WITH BILATERAL BALANCED INTRACEREBRAL HEMATOMAS

This 38-year-old man was involved in a motor vehicle accident and was thrown through the windshield. When found by the paramedics, he could not open his eyes. His sounds were incomprehensible and he had extension posturing of all four extremities. He was noted to have a rapid respiratory rate with some chest retraction. Both the blood pressure and pulse were evaluated. There were no pupillary asymmetries. The pupils were small and reactive to light. There was no evidence of focal hemiparesis. Examination of the scalp revealed abrasion and contusion with facial and forehead swelling but no laceration. The abdomen was distended with absent bowel sounds and the extremities showed swelling of the right hand with deformity of the wrist.

The patient was transported to the emergency room, where these observations were unchanged. The patient was placed on oxygen by mask; blood gases and oxygen saturation were normal. CBC and electrolytes were normal. Serum amylase was elevated. Peritoneal lavage was negative. The patient's cardiorespiratory status was stable and he was taken to the CT scanner, where both head and abdominal CT scans were performed. The abdominal CT scan was negative. The head CT showed evidence of a 2-cm right frontal intracerebral hematoma and a 2.5-cm left temporal lobe hematoma. The ventricular system was small. There was no shift of the midline structures.

MANAGEMENT

See Figure 27-4.

CT Scan. CT scan was accomplished as indicated for diagnosis of possible fracture, hematoma, and tissue damage. The decision was made that the balanced intracerebral hematomas did not require surgical evacuation at that time.

Intensive Care. The patient was admitted to the neurosurgical intensive care unit. At that point he opened his eyes to pain and spoke inappropriate words. The motor response of extension had improved to flexion withdrawal. However, he was agitated and thrashing about. With such agitation the patient was at risk from complications of increased intracranial pressure and brain shift.

Pharmalogic Treatment, Intubation, Pressure Monitor. It was elected to manage the patient by sedation with intermittently administered intravenous morphine, placement of en-

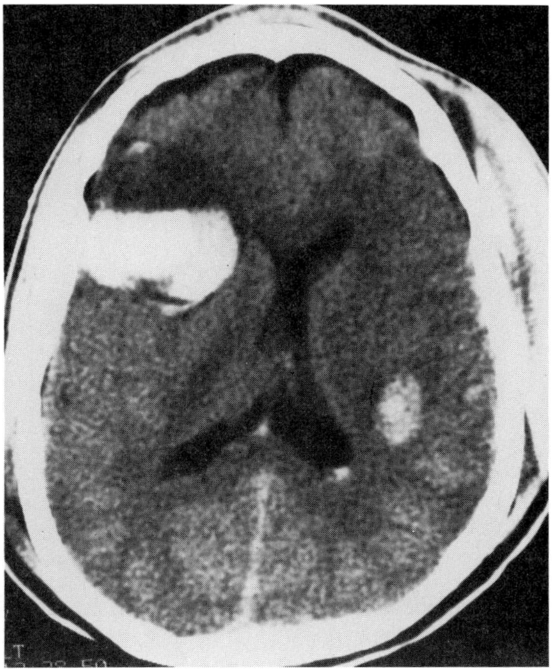

Figure 27-4. Example of balanced bilateral frontal and temporal hematoma. The large frontal hematoma required evacuation when patient showed slow improvement.

dotracheal intubation, and placement of an intracranial pressure monitoring device with a subdural screw placed in the right frontal region. On placement of the intracranial pressure monitor, the initial resting pressure was 17 torr to 20 torr, but with agitation it was increased to 30 torr to 35 torr. The opiate sedation was increased and the patient remained quiet; the intracranial pressure remained below 20. The following day the opiate sedation was decreased. The patient was now opening his eyes to verbal stimuli and again became agitated, at which time the pressure rose to 30 torr. The CT scan was repeated. There was no change in the size of the hematoma. The sedation was again increased but the patient's intracranial pressure remained elevated. The patient was started on mannitol, given every 6 hours, and the pressure fell to 5 torr to 10 torr. This was continued for 2 days and the pressure remained normal, following which the mannitol was discontinued. The pressure remained normal for 1 day. The sedation was discontinued. The patient was now awake and opened his eyes spontaneously. He spoke inappropriate words and no verbal response could be noted, but he now obeyed commands. Controlled ventilation was replaced with a T'd tube when it was clear that he could maintain adequate oxygen saturation with 20% O_2. The endotracheal tube was removed, following which he was disoriented but conversed. No dysphasia was noted.

Result. A CT scan was performed. The frontal hematoma resolved. The temporal lobe hematoma was less. The following day the intracranial pressure monitor was removed. The patient progressed to a normal level of consciousness but was noted to have marked memory deficit. He was referred to the rehabilitation service.

CASE 8: SEVERE HEAD INJURY WITH UNILATERAL EPIDURAL AND ACUTE SUBDURAL HEMATOMAS

This 40-year-old man fell from an oil rig and had evidence of severe decreased level of consciousness. He had no eye-opening response, no verbal response, and decerebrate rigidity. He was seen by the paramedics and intubated at the scene and transported directly to the tertiary care facility, where he was noted to have, in addition, a femur fracture. Cardiorespiratory signs were well controlled. Neurologic exam showed an enlarged right pupil with sluggish reaction to light. Left pupil response was normal. A CT scan showed evidence of a large, acute subdural hematoma with marked shift of the intracranial structures from right to left.

MANAGEMENT

CT Scan. CT scan showed hematoma and shift as indicated (see Fig. 27-5).

Surgery. The patient was taken immediately to the operating room, where a large frontotemporal curved horseshoe scalp incision was fashioned. A large bone flap was removed with evacuation of acute subdural hematoma and exploration of the subdural space, which showed bleeding cortical veins that were coagulated. At the termination of the procedure, the cerebral hemisphere was noted to be swollen and contused. Both a ventricular catheter and a subdural intracranial pressure monitor were placed.

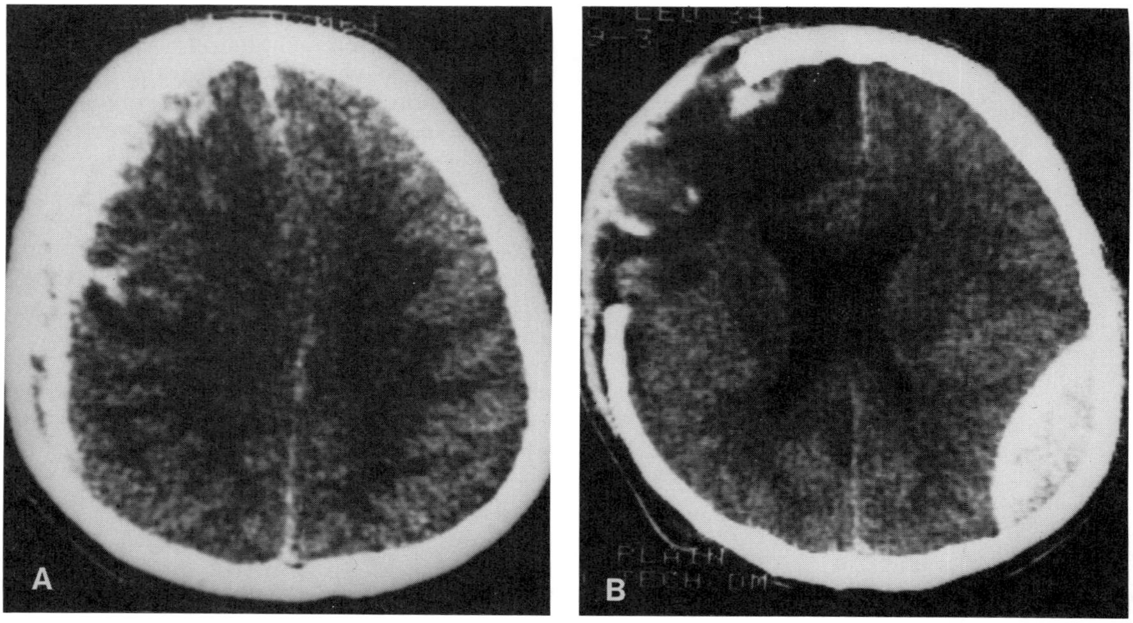

Figure 27-5. Example of acute subdural hematoma and epidural hematoma. (*A*) CT scan—large acute subdural hematoma over convexity. (*B*) CT scan—following evacuation of subdural hematoma brain herniation was noted and the patient was returned to the CT scanner, which showed interval development of a contralateral epidural hematoma requiring a second operative procedure.

Pharmalogic Treatment. After closure the patient was taken to the intensive care unit, intubated, where he was sedated and paralyzed with pancuronium bromide (Pavulon) and where intracranial pressure was monitored. However, in spite of the evacuation of the hematoma, the intracranial pressure remained over 40. Controlled ventilation to reduce the PCO_2 to 25 did not reduce the intracranial pressure. Mannitol was given every 4 hours, which only reduced the pressure to 30. There was no improvement. The repeat CT scan showed satisfactory evacuation of the hematoma but severe brain swelling with continued right to left shift. Barbiturate coma was considered, but the patient's family, when apprised of the poor outlook for quality survival, requested that barbiturate coma not be instituted.

Result. On the fifth postoperative day the patient was noted to have a sudden increase in intracranial pressure to 60. A repeat CT scan showed slit ventricles, continued shift, and no hematoma. There was no response to mannitol. The pupils were fixed and dilated. No spontaneous respirations were present and there was no motor response. An EEG showed no brain wave activity and a perfusion scan showed no intracranial circulation. On determination of absence of brain function, the family requested that the patient's organs be donated.

INSTITUTIONAL REQUIREMENTS FOR HEAD INJURY CARE—AANS GUIDELINES

At its annual meeting in 1983, the American Association of Neurological Surgeons (AANS), which is the major organization of board-certified American neurosurgeons, proposed draft recommendations for providing optimal care to the head-injured patient. These recommendations provide that treatment should be performed in medical facilities that include as a minimum a 24-hour emergency room staffed by physicians competent in endotracheal intubation and initial resuscitation, a well-equipped and staffed intensive care unit; in-house CT scanning capability, available promptly on a 24-hour basis; and ready availability of an operating room, anesthesia, and neurosurgical service. (If CT scanning or neurosurgical capabilities are not available, the facility must be able to transport the patient to the closest appropriate facility.)

The following statements outline acceptable procedures to be applied to the care of severe head injury and acceptable outcomes of care as discussed by the AANS.[18]

The majority of surgical procedures for head injury are not controversial. Intubation and maintenance of ventilation is accepted in the therapy of patients with severe head injury which is usually defined as a Glasgow Coma Score of 8 or less. Maintenance of adequate systemic arterial pressures is essential. CT scanning is an important diagnostic tool for the care of the head injured. . . . Repeat scans have become an important part of head injury management, and patients in traumatic coma or who have severely altered mental status should be cared for in facilities with CT scanners.

Treatment of Specific Lesions

a. Extracerebral (Extradural and Subdural) Hematomas
   Early evacuation of extracerebral hematomas by craniotomy is uniformly practiced. One recent report (Seelig et al. NEJM 304:1511–1518, 1981)[19] strongly supports the belief that rapid evacuation of subdural hematomas is influential in ultimate outcome. In general, mortality rates in patients with extradural hematomas admitted with varying degrees of impairment of consciousness should not exceed 25%. For those patients already in coma a mortality of 35% or less is commonly reported. Most patients with acute subdural hematomas are comatose when they reach the hospital, and mortality rates of 60% to 80% commonly are reported despite aggressive treatment including emergency craniotomy.
b. Intracerebral Hematomas
   The treatment of intracerebral hematomas is somewhat less clearly defined. In general, in patients with significant displacements of midline structures (greater than 5 mm), and in whom the hematoma is surgically accessible, evacuation may be indicated. In addition, hematomas should be considered for removal when they contribute to intracranial hypertension or are associated with significant generalized or focal neurologic deficits. Preliminary data from the National Traumatic Coma Data Bank suggests that patients with large shifts of midline structures, and relatively good initial neurologic examinations, often deteriorate if intracerebral hematomas are not removed surgically.
c. Open Fractures
   Modern military and civilian practice dictates that compound depressed skull fractures be explored. While minimal injuries sometimes are found, operative evaluation and debridement of necrotic brain and indriven fragments of bone, hair, skin and other contaminants must be done to prevent CNS infection. In awake patients with open depressed fractures, mortality rates should not exceed 3%.
d. Intensive Care
   Patients with Glasgow Coma Scores of 8 or less should be managed in an intensive care unit during the acute phase of their injury. This requires the combined skills of a number of specialists, notably neurosurgeons, trauma surgeons, anesthesiologists, internists, inhalation therapists and intensive care nurses. Intracranial pressure (ICP) monitoring is useful in both detecting and guiding rational management of intracranial hypertension although ICP monitoring has not been shown definitely to improve outcome from head injury. In comatose patients and head injury patients who have suffered multiple injuries resulting in hypoxia or shock, there is substantial risk of intracranial hypertension and ICP monitoring is warranted. The accepted medical management of intracranial hypertension includes hyperventilation, CSF drainage, sedation and paralysis with muscle relaxants when needed, hyperosmolar therapy and the maintenance of normothermia. The use of high dose barbiturates, while not considered investigational because of relatively widespread use, has not been shown to improve outcome from head injury. Despite widespread use, corticosteroids also have not been shown to improve head injury morbidity or mortality.
e. Other Lesions
   Chronic subdural hematomas generally are seen in elderly patients and mortality rates of between 1% and 8% have been reported in the literature. Mortality after concussion is minimal and patients generally require only brief hospitalization. However, recent evidence strongly suggests that mild head injury often is associated with a considerable degree of intellectual impairment which can persist for several months.

Penetrating injuries of the skull and brain require immediate and careful neurosurgical management. Picks, knives, rods or splinters penetrating the skull should be left in place during careful transport. Following patient stabilization, skull x-rays and CT scans are indicated. Under control in the operating room, foreign bodies are removed surgically. Missile or fragment wounds require expedient management. Adequate debridement of necrotic brain, bone fragments and blood clots followed by dural closure to prevent CSF fistula is advised to prevent infection and additional brain damage.

SUMMARY

The management of the head-injured patient in the ambulatory care setting requires a knowledge of evaluation schema, including use of the Glasgow Coma Scale for analysis of the level of consciousness, knowledge of classical neurologic examination, and understanding of the natural history of the brain-injured patient. What initially appear to be minor injuries must be observed carefully for development of secondary complications, which may or may not be easily treated, depending not only on the severity of the initial impact but also on the time that treatment begins following the onset of the secondary complication.

Thus the assessment of the patient with the head injury—whether by the trained layman observer immediately at the scene of the accident, by the emergency room physician in either an ambulatory or emergency room setting, or by the neurosurgeon in the intensive care unit—is based on the combined analysis of neurologic function utilizing the Glasgow Coma Scale, the neurologic examination, and the description of anatomic structures.

REFERENCES

1. The University of Pennsylvania Head Injury Research Center: Contributions to More Effective Diagnosis and Treatment of Head Injured Patients. Philadelphia, University of Pennsylvania, 1985
2. Strich SJ: The pathology of brain damage due to blunt head injuries. In Walker AE, Caveness WF, Critchley M (eds): The Late Effects of Head Injury, pp 501–524. Springfield, IL, Charles C Thomas, 1969
3. Adams JH, Graham DI, Gennarelli TA: Acceleration induced head injury in the monkey. II. Neuropathology. Acta Neuropathol (Suppl) VII:26–28, 1981
4. Gennarelli TT, Thibault LE, Adams JH et al: Diffuse axonal injury in the primate. In Dacey R (ed): Trauma of the Central Nervous System, pp 169–194. New York, Raven Press, 1985
5. Gennarelli TA, Spielman GM, Langfitt TW, et al: Influence of the type of intracranial lesion on outcome from severe head injury: A multicenter study using a new classification system. J Neurosurg 56:26–32, 1982
6. Langfitt TW, Weinstein JD, Kassell NF: Cerebral vasomotor paralysis produced by intracranial hypertension. Neurology 15:622–641, 1965
7. Jennett B, Teasdale G, Braakman R et al: Prognosis in series of patients with severe head injury. Neurosurgery 4:283, 1979
8. Jennett B, Teasdale G: Management of Head Injuries. Philadelphia: FA Davis, 1981
9. Teasdale G, Jennett B: Assessment of coma and impaired consciousness: A practical scale. Lancet i:480–484, 1975
10. Langfitt, TW: Increased intracranial pressure. Clin Neurosurg 16:436, 1969
11. Marmarou A, Poll W, Shapiro K et al: The influence of brain tissue pressure upon local cerebral blood flow in vasogenic oedema. In Beks JW, Bosch DA, and Brock M (eds): Intracranial Pressure, Vol. III, pp 10–12. Berlin, Springer-Verlag, 1976
12. Miller JD, Becker DP, Ward JD et al: Significance of intracranial hypertension in severe head injury. J Neurosurg 47:503–516, 1977
13. Miller JD, Becker DP et al: The physiological basis of intracranial pressure change with progressive epidural brain compression. J Neurosurg 47:532–550, 1977
14. Jamieson KG: Extradural and subdural haematomas: Changing patterns and requirements of treatment in Australia. J Neurosurg 33:632–635, 1970
15. Becker DP, Miller JD, Ward JD et al: The outcome from severe head injury with early diagnosis and intensive management. J Neurosurg 47:491–502, 1977
16. Becker DP, Povlishock JT: Central Nervous System Trauma Status Report, 1984. Bethesda, National Institute of Neurological and Communicative Disorders and Stroke, National Institutes of Health, 1984
17. Dacey RG, Alves WM et al: Neurosurgical complications after apparently minor head injury: Assessment of risk in a series of 610 patients. J Neurosurg 65:203–210, 1986
18. Long Range Planning Committee, Joint Committee on Trauma: Resources for Optimal Care of Nervous System Trauma. Chicago, The American Association of Neurological Surgeons, 1983 (draft report)
19. Seelig JM, Becker DP, Miller JD et al: Traumatic acute subdural hematoma: Major mortality reduction in comatose patients treated within four hours. N Engl J Med 304:1511–1518, 1981

28 Ophthalmic Accidents, Emergencies, and Surgery

HUNTER R. STOKES

Ophthalmic accidents are not common, but the potential for permanent loss of vision is almost always there and must be a consideration in the management of all cases. The ophthalmologist (a medical doctor especially trained in managing eye conditions) may not always be available, and it is essential that other physicians be knowledgeable in the evaluation and initial management of all ophthalmic accidents and in the appropriate and timely referral of those accidents that require ophthalmologic attention. True ophthalmic emergencies are rare. There are only three conditions considered absolute emergencies: alkali burn to the eye, perforation of the eye, and central retinal artery occlusion. Two of the three are accidental; therefore it is critical that the physician providing initial care to the patient be aware of appropriate management criteria.

Ophthalmic surgery has become almost entirely outpatient surgery since late 1984, and the issue will be addressed from the standpoint of the role of the general physician in evaluating patients who may be undergoing ophthalmic surgery on an outpatient basis.

OPHTHALMIC ACCIDENTS

CONJUNCTIVAL FOREIGN BODIES

Foreign bodies embedded in the conjunctiva or trapped in the conjunctival cul-de-sacs are usually quite painful and can cause permanent loss of vision if not properly managed. If transport of the patient is necessary to evaluate or manage any of these foreign bodies, the primary consideration is protection of the eye (especially the cornea) from further damage by preventing any movement (e.g., rubbing of the foreign body). A paper cup, either flat-bottomed or pointed, can be taped over the eye, which allows the foreign body to remain in place and puts no pressure on the eyeball. This management is also proper for preparation for transport of patients with corneal foreign bodies (see "Corneal Foreign Bodies," below) and with perforations of the globe (see "Perforations of the Globe").

Incidental trauma, such as an airborn foreign body in a gust of wind, can cause foreign bodies in the cul-de-sacs and under the upper lid. The typical symptom is a foreign body sensation, and often the patient describes the foreign body "moving around in the eye." The foreign body is usually embedded in the conjunctiva under the upper lid and is not moving, but with each blink, a different area of the cornea is irritated, giving the impression that the foreign body is moving.

If the foreign body is in the inferior cul-de-sac, it can be visualized by pulling the lower lid down and having the patient look up. It can then almost always be removed by simple sweeping of the inferior cul-de-sac after topical anesthesia is instilled. Foreign bodies in the superior cul-de-sac are often trapped in the substance of the conjunctiva and are not readily visible unless the upper lid is everted. This must be done in a proper fashion. With the patient looking down, the lashes of the upper lid are grasped and pressure is placed on the midportion of the upper lid with a blunt instrument, which allows the upper lid to "flip," exposing the undersurface or the superior palpebral conjunctiva. The foreign body is usually visualized and can be easily swept away using a cotton-tipped applicator impregnated with a topical anesthetic. Prior to eversion of the upper lid, a foreign body in that region can be strongly suspected if fluorescein stain is instilled into the inferior cul-de-sac and allowed to cover the entire corneal surface.

Very often the superior cornea will show a quadrant of stain, often in a vertical linear pattern in an area corresponding to where the foreign body is trapped under the upper lid. Sometimes a foreign body may be trapped under the upper lid, and with irrigation and/or tearing, the foreign body washes out. Subsequently, when definitive care is provided, no foreign body is noted. When this occurs the superior conjunctival surface should be swept with a cotton-tipped applicator impregnated with topical anesthetic. This often allows the removal of a transparent foreign body such as a small insect wing or a grain of sand. Failing to do this may lead to continued abrasion of the cornea and to a deeper injury that can cause a permanent scar.

Glass foreign bodies represent a particular problem. Often in accidents where broken glass is involved the patient may have a foreign body sensation and no foreign body may be found. In such circumstances a fine sliver of glass may have penetrated the conjunctival tissue and may be invisible to the naked eye and even with magnification. If discomfort persists, or if a corneal stain fails to heal in a reasonable length of time (24 to 48 hours), then the patient should be referred to an ophthalmologist for careful examination with the slit-lamp biomicroscope.

Occasionally, a bulbar conjunctival foreign body (the bulbar conjunctiva covers the surface of the eyeball) will be encountered that is sufficiently large (such as a sliver of wood) or sufficiently deep (an iron fragment from hammering steel on steel) that irrigation or sweeping of the area does not remove it. Under this circumstance a small toothless forceps can usually remove the foreign body. If this proves to be impossible or if grasping the foreign body creates significant pain in the patient's eye or the appearance of blood or, more important, a clear liquid coming from around the foreign body, then all manipulation should cease and the patient should be referred to an ophthalmologist. These foreign bodies may well have penetrated the globe, which is a major problem.

Conjunctival irritation by itself clears rapidly and requires no treatment other than broad-spectrum antibiotic coverage for 24 to 48 hours. However, there is often related corneal abrasion, and this requires more careful management (discussed under "Corneal Abrasions," below).

CORNEAL FOREIGN BODIES

Corneal foreign bodies create significant pain almost immediately; consequently, the patient seeks medical attention without undue delay. These foreign bodies are easily embedded in the corneal tissue and therefore are not easily irrigated, though that should be the first effort for removal once the eye is anesthetized with topical anesthetic (tetracaine HCl [Pontocaine]). The next effort should be with a sterile cotton-tipped applicator moistened with topical anesthetic. This often removes the foreign body, but if it is metallic and has been present for more than 3 to 4 hours, there may be a ring of rust in the corneal tissue that does not come out with the foreign body. It is important for rapid wound healing that this area of rust also be removed. This requires the use of either a sharp instrument or a miniature drill. This is best done using the magnification of a slit-lamp biomicroscope and should be done by an ophthalmologist. As with conjunctival foreign bodies, if an effort to remove a corneal foreign body is associated with significant pain or with the apparent leakage of fluid from the inside of the eye, then immediate referral to an ophthalmologist is indicated, because the depth of penetration of the foreign body into the cornea is obviously extensive, with entrance into the anterior chamber.

The location of a corneal foreign body is also critical in determining management. Mid-peripheral corneal foreign bodies are the easiest to remove because the threat of permanent vision loss is less, since there is little or no significant vision from the peripheral cornea and this area is usually anesthetized well with instillation of topical anesthetic drops. Foreign bodies located at the periphery of the cornea (the limbus, where the cornea and conjunctiva meet) are more difficult to remove because topical anesthetic does not give the same amount of anesthesia. In addition, there may be some bleeding from conjunctival vessels at the limbus during the effort to remove the foreign body, which makes visualization of the foreign body more difficult. Central corneal foreign bodies should always be referred for removal by the ophthalmologist. There is always the danger of scarring with corneal foreign bodies, and a central scar, even a rather faint one, can lead to a permanent loss of vision that may be disabling to the patient. The patient deserves every opportunity for this scar to be minimized and not associated with any additional trauma related to the removal of the foreign body. The ophthalmologist can best do this with the slit-lamp biomicroscope. This is a particular consideration in young children, in whom a small scar may reduce the vision enough to lead to amblyopia (lazy eye), and a scar that would reduce vision from 20/20 to 20/40 in an adult can ultimately lead to a level of legal blindness in a child under the age of 5 or 6. In addition, many of these youngsters may require general anesthesia merely to remove the corneal foreign body. Immediate referral is indicated in such cases.

Most corneal abrasions associated with conjunctival foreign bodies and most corneal foreign bodies create only a disturbance of the superficial layer of the cornea—the epithelial surface. In the absence of infection the corneal epithelium can be expected to heal without any scarring; within 1 week there will be no evidence, even under the slit lamp, of any previous injury. If, however, the abrasion and/or foreign body penetrates through the epithelial surface and into Bowman's membrane or the stroma of the cornea, permanent scarring will occur. This can be minimized by immediate treatment to reduce the incidence of infection and by careful removal.

CORNEAL ABRASIONS

Corneal abrasions are caused not only by corneal or conjunctival foreign bodies, but by other events in which a foreign body strikes the front surface of the eye and immediately falls away or is washed out by tearing or blinking. In addition, misdirected eyelashes and inappropriate wearing of contact lenses, especially the older type of hard lenses, will scratch the corneal surface. This is a painful event; management includes not only carefully searching for a foreign body and making every effort to see that the cornea heals without scarring, but also seeing that the patient is comfortable in the healing process. A broad-spectrum antibiotic solution is the preferred method of protecting against infection. Typical solutions that are effective include gentamicin, chloramphenicol, sulfacetamide and neomycin, polymyxin, and bacitracin solutions. These antibiotic drops should be used four times a day until there is no evidence of any corneal stain. Unless the area of corneal stain is very small, a topical cycloplegic, moderately long-acting, should be utilized to put the ciliary body at rest, stop ciliary spasm, and reduce pain. I prefer 0.25% scopolamine (Isopto Hyoscine), which generally begins to act approximately one-half hour after instillation and lasts for 72 hours. This usually coincides with the healing of the epithelial defect. In addition, a mild pressure dressing over the eye is indicated for 24 hours in all but the smallest abrasions. This reduces the blinking over the cornea and allows the epithelium to heal faster. The use of a patch is contraindicated when the abrasion has been present for several days at the time of initial examination or where a foreign body has created not only an epithelial disturbance but also an early area of infiltration suggesting infection. Here the critical issue is delivery of the antibiotic to the area, and the patch should be disregarded in favor of instillation of drops. In addition, if a patient has had a chemical burn to the eye, especially an alkaline burn, then it is appropriate to leave the eye open for frequent instillation of drops instead of using a patch. A patch is rarely indicated for more than 24 hours. It is more important after that time to use the antibiotic drops. A proper pressure dressing should have one or two sterile pads placed over the closed lid and then three or four strips of adhesive tape measuring 3 or 4 inches and placed over the eye pads with one end of the tape in the center of the forehead and the other end of the tape on the lateral cheek. All of the tape strips should be approximately parallel so as to give pressure to the eyelid, keeping the lid closed over the eyeball. The patient should be discouraged from attempting to repatch the eye if the patch comes off, as it is virtually impossible for a patient to reposition the patch effectively for continued pressure. Additional relief for pain is indicated for all but the smallest of corneal abrasions using analgesics or narcotics for a period of 24 to 48 hours. The patient should be warned about the pain and should be provided with a prescription for pain medication or, in the case of a late evening visit to an emergency room, should be given sufficient medication to give relief of pain for the night.

Small, uncomplicated corneal abrasions, with proper care, usually heal in 24 hours and certainly in 48 hours. Larger abrasions and those associated with foreign body removal may take an additional 24 hours to heal. Any patient whose corneal epithelial defect is still present after 3 days should be referred to an ophthalmologist for further care, as the risk of additional problems (retained transparent foreign body causing continued abrasion, early infection or defect in epithelial healing) is a consideration after this period of time.

CHEMICAL BURNS TO THE CORNEA AND CONJUNCTIVA

Alkaline burns to the external surface of the eye represent one of the true ocular emergencies, and first aid is critical in the management of these cases. Concentrated alkaline burns such as those resulting from an industrial accident or a household accident with such items as Easy Off or Drāno, can lead to immediate, total, permanent opacification of the cornea, and perhaps even result in "melting of the cornea" with perforation and loss of the eye. Even a dilute concentration of a household cleanser such as Clorox can lead to a very slow healing, painful corneal epithelial defect with a high incidence of infection and permanent scarring of the cornea. Irrigation of the eye with tap water, even immersion of the face in a bucket of water, is very important in alkaline burns, and any call to an emergency department for advice after such an accident should be handled with the encouragement for first aid at the site rather than trying to make a fast trip to the emergency area for care. Once the patient does arrive in the medical facility, copious irrigation should be carried out, with particular care to the inferior and superior cul-de-sacs, where trapped alkaline particles may continue to create burns. A topical anesthetic greatly facilitates this process of irrigation, and it is not inappropriate to irrigate 20 minutes or longer using 2 or more liters of solution. Because of the potential for long-term vision loss and slow wound healing, all cases of alkali burn should be referred to an ophthalmologist for care.

Acid burns are less serious from a long-term prognosis but are equally painful at the time of injury. With an acid agent, irrigation is again critical. Irritation to the lids and conjunctival surface as well as to the cornea may be extensive. Healing, however, occurs much more rapidly, but again, because it is a chemical injury it is best handled by an ophthalmologist.

LID LACERATIONS

Lid lacerations can be simple and managed expeditiously by emergency room personnel and other physicians not especially trained in eye care, or they may be extensive and require meticulous microsurgical plastic repair by an ophthalmologist. The lacerations will be subdivided into categories related to the unique problems that may arise and the specific types of management indicated.

Simple horizontal lacerations, upper or lower lid, no involvement of medial lid area or lid margin. These injuries are common and are often associated with blunt trauma, such as a fist or some object striking the face or the region of the eye. Pressure over the superior and inferior orbital rims creates horizontal linear lacerations that are often superficial and can be repaired with the traditional methods of closure. These wounds must be examined carefully to determine the extent of injury, to determine that no major functional parts of the lids, such as tear drainage system or levator muscle, have been involved. Closure can be with silk or nylon suture; the sutures should be removed in 5 to 7 days to allow appropriate healing with minimal scar formation.

Deep lacerations of the upper lid. Here one must be concerned with damage to the levator palpebrae superioris muscle, which elevates the lid. If the evaluation of the laceration reveals that it is deep and that muscle areas are involved, then the patient should be referred for repair by an ophthalmologist.

Deep lacerations of the lower lid. The danger with lower lid lacerations is that if the laceration is sufficiently deep, then the orbicularis muscle fibers are involved, and there is the possibility of an actual tear of the periosteal lining over the inferior orbital rim or laceration of the anterior portion of the orbital septum. With these more extensive deep injuries there is a great chance for significant tension on the scar, pulling the lash margin of the lower lid away from the globe and creating the condition of cicatricial ectropion, and this leads to a variety of problems, with tearing and exposure of the eye later. If these injuries are extensive and particularly if there is any avulsion of the tissue, then a definitive skin grafting or at least undermining of the skin may be indicated at the time of primary closure.

Lacerations of the lid margins. Lacerations of the lid margins may lead to notching, with an irregular lid surface as well as lashes turning in against the cornea. The notching of the upper lid is cosmetically unacceptable, and notching of the lower lid is functionally a problem because it prohibits the tear film from staying against the eye, which may cause a chronic epiphora. The proper repair of these lacerations along the margins requires careful closure with absorbable and nonabsorbable suture in several layers and is best reserved for the ophthalmologist.

Medial lacerations possibly involving the lacrimal drainage system. Any injury to the margin of the upper or lower lid in the region of the medial canthus or in the last 3 mm to 5 mm of the medial portion itself may involve the upper or lower lacrimal drainage system. These injuries are often difficult to repair, especially if there is any avulsion of tissue, thus making the identification of the ends of the lacerated drainage system more difficult. Appreciation of this danger by the physician providing initial emergency care and consequent timely referral to an ophthalmologist are important.

BLUNT TRAUMA

There are several significant problems that may occur related to blunt trauma to the region of the eye.

Hyphema

Traumatic hyphema occurs when a blow to the eye ruptures a blood vessel inside the eye, resulting in red blood cells in the anterior chamber. Generally this is due to a tear in the iris at its base or root causing a rupture through an area where a major artery circle is present and leading to hemorrhage in the anterior chamber. This tear in the iris root may also cause a visible dialysis of the iris, which may be evident once the blood has cleared. Smaller hemorrhages may occur with tearing of the iris in other areas such as the sphincter. The presence of a traumatic hyphema suggests sufficient trauma to the eye that the patient should immediately be referred to an ophthalmologist. The hyphema itself is potentially a major problem in management, but there may be other related injuries to the eye (dislocation of the lens, damage to the retina, etc.). The patient should immediately be placed in the hands of an ophthalmologist. The requirement for hospitalization and bilateral patching of the patients with traumatic hyphema, which was considered essential in the past, is no longer the universal method of management. Many hyphemas are treated on an outpatient basis when there is a stable home situation that allows the patient total rest. The management is still best left to the ophthalmologist. Elevated intraocular pressure, rebleeding, and blood staining of the cornea (where a persistent elevated pressure actually forces blood into the stroma of the cornea, leading to a long-term cloudy cornea) are among the problems that create the need for immediate ophthalmological care. Surgical evacuation of blood from the anterior chamber is not often necessary but one situation with which all emergency care physicians should be familiar is the 24/24 rule in sickle cell patients. If a patient with sickle cell disease has blood in the anterior chamber and an elevated intraocular pressure of 24 mm Hg or more for more than 24 hours, then the resultant ischemia to the circulation in the posterior portion of the eye can lead to a permanent major loss of vision.

Orbital Rim and Floor Fracture

The blunt trauma situations leading to orbital rim and floor fracture include sports injuries, blows from a fist, and automobile accidents. The patient has a "black eye" and the eyeball may appear to be deep in the orbit. There may be pain on motion of the eye and, significantly, there may be double vision, especially on upgaze. There may be a reduction in the sensation over the upper cheek on the involved side, and crepitus may actually be noted in the lower lid or conjunctiva. In addition, a defect may be palpable along the lower rim. A fracture of the rim itself is uncommon and is usually reserved for genuinely strong blows to the region of the orbit. However, a much less significant blow may create a fracture in the floor, causing two clinical situations. One is the "trapdoor" fracture, in which the concussive effect against the closed lids creates pressure against all the contents of the eye, popping a small fracture site in the floor. The floor is depressed immediately, during which time some tissue from the orbit, including fat and extraocular muscle, are trapped in the defect, which then pops back into position with tissue trapped in the fracture site. This leads to pain and limitation of motion with diplopia. With a more extensive injury, the second type or "blow-out" fracture may be seen, in which the floor not only is depressed but stays down owing to a displacement of some of the fragment of the floor itself. Here radiographic evidence of fracture is much more likely to be seen, and the best views for evaluating this are the stereo Waters view or the Feugers view. In these cases, however, pain on motion of the eye and diplopia may not be present, since there may not be any entrapment of eye muscles. All these patients should be evaluated immediately by an ophthalmologist. Ophthalmologists are trained to repair these injuries definitively; moreover, these patients have a significant incidence of related damage to the structure of the eyeball and therefore should be immediately evaluated to determine the status of the eye itself. Many ENT specialists, maxillofacial plastic surgeons, and oral surgeons are well trained and quite competent to operate on these patients, but ophthalmologic consultation is essential to determine the status of the eye.

Iritis and Mydriasis

Less severe blunt trauma may lead a patient to complain of blurred vision and pain, although the signs of eye injury may seem minimal to an emergency physician. The problem here is traumatic iritis with or without traumatic mydriasis. In traumatic iritis inflammatory cells are released in the anterior chamber with irritation of the iris, leading to blurring of vision with significant sensitivity to light. Usually in this situation the pupil is small and some injection of the conjunctival vessels at the limbus (perilimbal injection) may be present.

The pupil may, however, be dilated in the absence of any drugs. This condition, known as traumatic mydriasis, may persist for weeks or months, or rarely, it may even be permanent, because of damage to the pupillary sphincter muscles that constrict the pupil. A slit-lamp biomicroscopic evaluation of these patients often reveals small tears or rupture in the sphincter at the pupillary margin. Again, these patients complain of blurred vision, especially at close distances, and of sensitivity to light.

PERFORATIONS OF THE GLOBE

It is rare for blunt trauma to actually rupture the globe. However, sharp objects may penetrate the eye, leading to a rupture of the globe and loss of intraocular contents. This is another true ocular emergency and must be immediately referred to an ophthalmologist. Several points are of concern to an emergency physician. First, if perforation of the globe is suspected, then no further effort should be made to evaluate the eye; rather, the patient should be immediately referred. For the travel he or she should be patched so that there is no pressure on the eye itself. (This has previously been described under "Conjunctival Foreign Bodies.") No medication should be placed in the eye that may cause the patient to squeeze, resulting in further loss of contents of the globe or allowing medication to go inside the eye, causing damage. Patients who have extensive injuries to the face and are noted to have blood coming from an eyelid may be suspected of having a perforation of the globe. If examination reveals that the upper lid on the side of the injury is roughly flat compared with the normal convex contour of the upper lid caused by the presence of an intact eyeball behind the lid on the other side, then further evaluation should not be carried out by the emergency physician, especially if met by any resistance by the patient.

A final emergency consideration is that if a patient is seen in an emergency area and has life-threatening injuries requiring immediate surgery where an ophthalmologist will not be present and where the evaluation of the globe must be delayed until other conditions can be cared for, then the anesthesia department should be discouraged from using succinylcholine in the medication used for intubation. Succinylcholine (Anectine) can cause cocontracture of the extraocular muscles and in the presence of rupture can cause further loss of the contents of the eyeball.

Perforating injuries to the eye are seen with gunshot wounds, BB gun accidents, throwing of darts, inappropriate use of a knife for whittling or carving, automobile accidents, and a variety of other events where a sharp object comes in contact with the eyeball. These patients require immediate surgery if there is any hope of recovery of the eye. Small perforations may be suspected if examination of the eye reveals a deep abrasion or laceration of the cornea associated with an irregular pupil that seems to be peaked in the area of the corneal damage. This peaking may actually represent iris that has come in contact with or become incarcerated into a perforation of the cornea. Whenever a foreign body is expected in the conjunctiva or cornea and grasping the foreign body causes immediate pain, it is possible that this foreign body represents contents of the globe that are protruding through a small perforation. Again, this requires immediate ophthalmologic evaluation. The prognosis with perforations of the eye has improved significantly because of the greater availability of skilled ophthalmologic care in many community hospitals, excellent microscopic surgical repair with fine sutures, availability of effective antibiotics for subconjunctival injection, the ability to definitively manage such things as related traumatic cataract at the time of the initial repair, high incidence of suspicion or care for evaluation by emergency personnel, and availability of better vision support equipment, such as newer types of contact lenses, to restore vision.

OPHTHALMIC EMERGENCIES

As previously mentioned, there are generally considered to be three ophthalmic emergencies. Two of them, alkaline burns of the cornea and globe perforations, have been mentioned in the discussion of accidents. The third is the central retinal artery occlusion, and it will be mentioned only briefly, as it is not of particular concern in this section. Central retinal artery occlusions occur in older patients with the complaint of sudden, permanent loss of vision in one eye. When the patient is seen, the pupil is usually dilated, the vision is at the level of counting fingers or less and the fundus examination reveals edema of the retina with a cherry red spot in the macula and sludging of the blood in the arteries and sometimes even the veins described as "boxcarring." In addition, an embolus, white or more often golden, glistening "Hollenhorst plaque" may be seen in the retinal arterial circulation. This does represent a true ocular emergency. It is associated with significant systemic vascular disease, especially disease in the carotid artery. These patients should be immediately referred to an ophthalmologist for further evaluation.

OPHTHALMIC OUTPATIENT SURGERY

BACKGROUND

In the 1970s several ophthalmologists in the United States began to perform surgery on an outpatient basis. Most of these procedures were done through the hospital outpatient units. Douglas Williamson, of Venice, Florida, was the first to build a surgery center solely to provide outpatient eye care. In 1977 the federal government received a report to evaluate the cost, quality, and system impact of surgery in an alternative setting to inpatient hospitalization. This report showed that surgery performed in a free-standing ambulatory surgery center was 55.3% less costly than hospital inpatient surgery and 11% less costly than hospital outpatient surgery. With this as documentary evidence the Congress included, as a part of the 1980 Omnibus Reconciliation Act, authorization for Medicare to reimburse free-standing ambultory surgery centers for some procedures. This was the first time Medicare would reimburse a facility other than a Medicare-approved hospital. Over the next several years as the regulations were written for the ambulatory surgery center Medicare reimbursement and as surgery centers were developed, ophthalmic surgery began to be done on an outpatient basis. Ophthalmologists were encouraged to go to outpatient surgery with the development of the diagnosis-related group (DRG) system for hospital reimbursement in 1983, because the DRG reimbursement for cataract extraction was the same whether the procedure was done with the less expensive equipment for intracapsular extraction or by the newer technique of extracapsular extraction using expensive machines with packs as well as the implantation of intraocular lens. The final shift toward outpatient eye surgery came in 1984 with the implementation of the PRO (Peer Review Organization) process, in which each state was challenged to develop guidelines for shifting surgery to an outpatient basis for Medicare patients whenever possible. By 1985 over 90% of cataracts were done on an outpatient basis as compared with less than 10% as early as 1980.

IMPLICATIONS FOR REFERRING AND CONSULTATIVE PHYSICIANS

The traditional method of evaluating cataract surgery patients was to admit the patient to the hospital 1 or 2 days prior to surgery. During this time appropriate and sometimes excessive diagnostic tests were performed and consultations were obtained with staff internists or the patient's family physician. Then after everyone was comfortable that the patient could tolerate the procedure, the surgery was performed. The patient traditionally stayed in the hospital as much as a week after surgery, during which time the follow-up care was shared between the operating surgeon and the physician who was caring for the general medical condition of the patient. With the advent of outpatient surgery, all preoperative evaluation had to be done outside of the facility because the patient arrives at the hospital outpatient unit or the free-standing ambulatory surgery center approximately 1 hour prior to scheduled surgery. To evaluate patients properly for surgery, the history, physical, and appropriate laboratory studies must be performed prior to the arrival of the patient at the facility.

Initially, many family physicians and internists were concerned that surgery might be performed on patients whose general health would not permit it or that certain medical conditions would preclude outpatient surgery. Experience in the several years since outpatient surgery for cataract extraction has become routine shows that there are very few contraindications to outpatient intraocular surgery under local anesthesia. Physicians who are responsible for making this decision should be aware of this positive situation.

Hypertensive patients whose condition is not under control should have their hypertension brought under control prior to surgery, since cataract surgery is always elective and can be delayed until the blood pressure is satisfactory. The main complication of uncontrolled hypertension is hemorrhage occurring during surgery. This can be in the form of retrobulbar hemorrhage, which may force the surgery to be canceled after the retrobulbar block is given, or it may even take the form of an intraocular hemorrhage during surgery, which can lead to the disastrous results of an expulsive hemorrhage. Once a patient's blood pressure is controlled, surgery can be performed with minimal risk. One consideration that should be made is the deletion of a strong diuretic on the morning of surgery, because it may lead to an uncomfortably full bladder while the patient is in the operating room.

Diabetes mellitus is also a condition that, if it is under good control, does not contraindicate outpatient intraocular surgery. There is a slightly higher incidence of hemorrhage in diabetics, but this generally does not alter the prognosis. Slightly different surgical procedures may be utilized on certain diabetic patients, with a major consideration being the need for subsequent management of significant retinopathy, but this is not a concern for the physician who is evaluating the patient preoperatively. Generally, ophthalmologists are reluctant to do intraocular surgery on patients whose blood sugar is significantly out of control, but diabetic patients whose condition is under control, whether the patients are insulin dependent or not, can be safely operated on as outpatients. Different physicians use different methods of managing the diabetic's medication needs on the day of surgery. Almost universally, the patients who are on oral medication do not receive medication on the day of surgery. Patients who are on insulin may receive their insulin only after the surgery has been performed and it is determined that the patient is not having a problem with nausea and vomiting. Others prefer that half the insulin dosage be given routinely in the early morning; the patient is then operated on early in the surgery schedule. The intravenous fluids utilized during surgery will preclude any major hypoglycemic episode that might occur. Diabetics are almost always able to go back on their regular medication and diet schedule on the first day after surgery. Generally speaking, patients who are on oral anticoagulants discontinue medication 3 to 5 days prior to surgery; it is restarted 1 to 2 days after surgery. This is not absolutely essential, since the ophthalmologist may carefully do intraocular surgery on patients who are anticoagulated. Generally, the site of incision may be slightly altered in order to enter the eye in an area where there are fewer blood vessels.

There are certain medical conditions in which the potential for a life-threatening cardiac arrhythmia exists (e.g., idiopathic hypertrophic subaortic stenosis [IHSS]). Here the physician caring for the general needs of the patient feels that surgery should be performed in a hospital. Outpatient surgery is still perfectly acceptable but the family physician or cardiologist feels more comfortable if the patient is already in the hospital so that if a major problem arises the patient is near a coronary care unit. Outpatient surgery in a free-standing surgery center, on the other hand, may require a time-consuming transfer to a hospital when a patient's cardiac status may be rapidly deteriorating.

Most ophthalmologists insist that anesthesia personnel be in attendance for intraocular surgery. When regulations were being developed for ambulatory surgery centers, the American Academy of Ophthalmology sent a letter to Health Care Finance Administration in 1981, stating, "in as much as less sedation is used in ambulatory surgery, anesthesia personnel shall monitor all patients undergoing intraocular surgery under local anesthesia in order to immediately respond to an emergency or need for intravenous medications." Routinely, in both hospital outpatient centers and free-standing surgery centers, anesthesia personnel, either anesthesiologists or anesthetists, evaluate the patient preoperatively, review allergies and medications, review the information received from the physical exam done by the referring medical doctor and medical laboratory data, and then carefully monitor the patient during surgery. Intravenous fluids are started, oxygen cannulas are put into place, and a cardiac monitor is attached to the patient. In many cases, some form of intravenous medication is given to the patient before the retrobulbar block in order to reduce the discomfort often associated with that procedure. Medication is often administered during the procedure in order to have the patient relaxed or to offset any change in the patient's vital signs. Medications are sometimes necessary to keep blood pressure at a reasonable level as well as to offset any arrhythmias that may develop. It is important for the physician in charge of the patient's general health to be aware of the fact that anesthesia personnel will be available throughout the patient's surgery and to insist on a certain level of anesthesia availability for patients where the risk of some intraoperative medical problem may be greater than normal.

Ophthalmic surgery, especially cataract extraction, allows restoration of vision to more senior citizens in the United States than ever before. In 1986 more than 1 million cataract operations were performed, and in 95% of the cases, vision was restored to a level of significant improvement over the preoperative vision level. This is the number-one surgical procedure performed in the Medicare-age population, and by the end of next year, 95% of these procedures will be performed on an outpatient basis. It is important for referring physicians to be aware of the exceptionally high success rate of the operation and of the precautions and care taken to support the general condition of the patient during this operation. It is also critical that the physician be very careful in evaluating these patients preoperatively, realizing that there will be no further extensive evaluation by other medical doctors prior to surgery. The physician should be encouraged to be cautious and to communicate directly with the ophthalmologist if there is any concern that might indicate that the patient's general health would be served better by having the procedure done on an inpatient basis or by having the procedure delayed or canceled.

There are two other medical conditions that are not uncommon in elderly patients who may be undergoing cataract surgery and that must be considered by the family physician. The first of these is systemic steroids. Many elderly patients, for a variety of conditions, especially respiratory disorders and some connective tissue disorders and arthritis, may be on systemic steroids at the time that cataract surgery is performed. There is no contraindication to operating on these patients and the stress associated with the operation generally does not require any additional steroid on the day of the operation. The surgeon should be aware, however, of the patient's use of this medication, because it may alter the decision as to the site of the incision as well as the type of suture material utilized.

The other consideration has to do with patients who have chronic obstructive pulmonary disease. This is becoming progressively more of a problem in the elderly population. These patients may need to be hospitalized for several days of intensive respiratory therapy treatment so that they breathe easily and have minimal potential for coughing at the time of the operation. If the pulmonary condition is not quite so severe, the patients may be instructed to use some particular extra medication the day before and the day of surgery. It is certainly appropriate to determine, from the referring physician and from the patient, what time of day the patient seems to breathe best because this is the time that one would like to have the operation scheduled. Patients with respiratory problems may be a problem during surgery because they may be unable to lie flat on the operating table. This is a logistics problem for the surgeon, not for the referring physician, but again, communication between these two doctors is essential in planning a successful operation.

The bottom line in outpatient eye surgery is that there must be careful preoperative medical evaluation of the often elderly patient who will undergo surgery. Further, clear communication must be established between the physician who has responsibility for the general medical care of the patient and the physician who performs the surgery. Outpatient eye surgery is almost always elective and should never be performed if there is a sizable threat to the patient's general condition by an ill-timed or inappropriately located (e.g., outpatient) operation. Even with strict PRO guidelines regarding eye surgery, especially cataract extraction, inpatient surgery may be indicated, and the family physician must inform the ophthalmologist of this.

29 Hand—Soft-Tissue Injuries and Infections

RONALD J. MANN

GENERAL PRINCIPLES OF MANAGEMENT

The majority of hand and finger injuries, exclusive of fractures, which require emergency treatment, are open wounds. Brief initial evaluation of the injury determines the necessary preoperative regimen. Severe hand or multiple digital injuries should be treated in the operating room, whereas the majority of single acute fingertip injuries can be managed adequately in the emergency room or office. The first priority is to establish hemostasis. The sterile, bulky, compressive dressing (Fig. 29-1) should be supplemented by elevation and volar splint immobilization of the forearm, wrist, and hand. This treatment controls most active bleeding. Blind instrument probing of a wound to clamp a bleeder is contraindicated, since additional contamination may be introduced to the wound and since an adjacent nerve is often crushed. Soaking the injured digit or hand in a basin of soapy water or bactericidal solution is not indicated, because edema of the soft tissues is increased by the hypotonicity of the water. Such soaking has no cleansing effect. If contamination is unavoidable during this initial, cursory examination, the wound should be explored.

Appropriate laboratory and roentgenographic determinations are performed prior to the patient's transfer either to the operating suite or back to the emergency room. Roentgenographic studies are necessary for a suspected fracture, fracture dislocation, any near amputation or amputations, high-pressure injection injuries, and suspected foreign bodies. All jewelry should be removed prior to roentgenography. Comparison of roentgenographs of the injured area to the contralateral normal extremity may be helpful in a skeletally immature person to differentiate epiphyseal growth plates and the long bones and ossification centers of the carpal bones from trauma.

An inclusive history of the injury, including the mechanism of injury and environment, helps determine the type and extent of trauma and the degree of contamination. The specific type of injury should be noted. The wound should be considered contaminated if it has remained open for 10 to 12 hours since the injury, if the environment of injury was grossly contaminated, and particularly if it is a human or animal bite.

The principal areas to be examined and tested in the physical examination of a hand injury are

- Status of vascularity distal to the site of injury
- Condition of the skin in and about the wound
- Function of tendons distal to the site of injury
- Function of nerves distal to the site of injury
- Concurrent soft-tissue injury involving deep destruction, such as the intrinsic muscles of the hand
- Injuries to the skeletal system
- Degree of contamination or possible infection within or about the wound
- Mental or emotional status and any evidence of alcohol or drug abuse

If there is a problem with patient cooperation, then a more complete examination could be done directly during the exploration in the operating room with adequate anesthesia and tourniquet control.

Appropriate tetanus prophylaxis is mandatory. If a patient has received a tetanus toxoid booster within 5 years of the current open injury, no treatment is necessary. If the time interval was longer than 5 years, 0.5 ml of tetanus toxoid and usually 250 ml. of tetanus immune globulin should be given. If there is any doubt about whether proper immunization was originally received, then both toxoid and

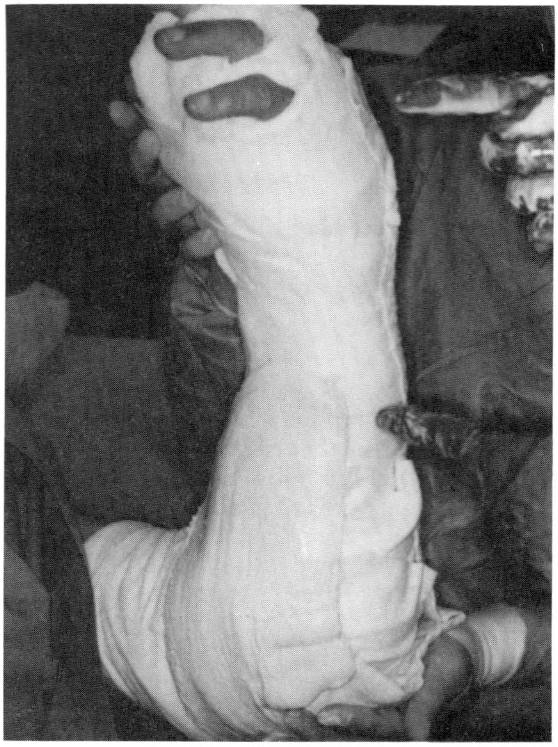

Figure 29-1. Bulky hand dressing.

antitoxin should be given. It is imperative to guarantee tetanus prophylaxis in the following injuries: human or animal bite injuries, full-thickness thermal and electrical burns, high-pressure-injection injuries, high-velocity-projection through-and-through injuries, and massive crush injuries.

FINGERTIP INJURIES

Fingertip injuries are the most common injuries to the hand. Controversy exists about how best to treat them. Improper treatment can result in persistent pain, restriction of motion, and deplorable appearance. The fingertips serve as a perceptive sensory organ of touch and discrimination, and their proper function depends on the integrity of all component parts, including skin, pulp, soft tissue, bone, and fingernails (Fig. 29-2). Because of their vulnerable, exposed position and constant physical use, it is not surprising to see fingertip injuries as a frequent medical problem. Fingertip injuries are usually defined as those that occur distal to the distal interphalangeal joint. The complexity of injury to the fingertip requires a careful assessment of the extent of loss and a critical evaluation of the viability of remaining tissues. The level and plane of injury, the location and configuration of the tissue defect, and the involvement of the component parts of the fingertip help in selecting the appropriate method of treatment (Fig. 29-3).

The basic aim of treatment should be to achieve rapid healing while retaining maximum function and mobility with minimum loss of time from work. This is generally consistent with the preservation of digital length while ensuring adequate skin and soft-tissue coverage, good sensibility, and acceptable cosmetic appearance.

The various methods of repair include open treatment, skin grafting, primary repair, digital shortening, local or adjacent flap closure, regional pedicle flaps, and distal pedicle flaps.

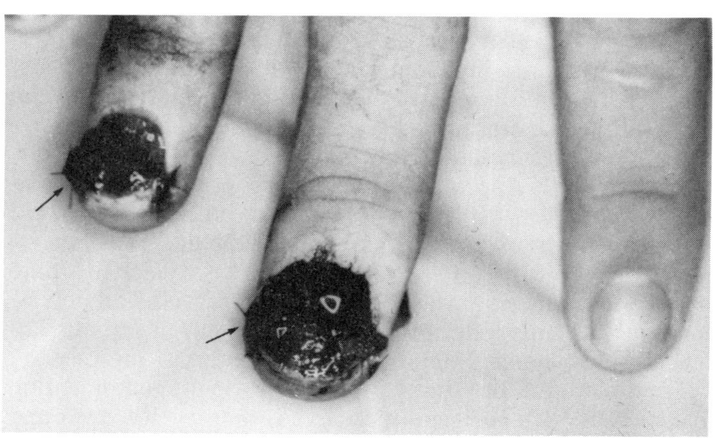

Figure 29-2. Crushed fingertips with suture repair (*arrows*) of nailbeds.

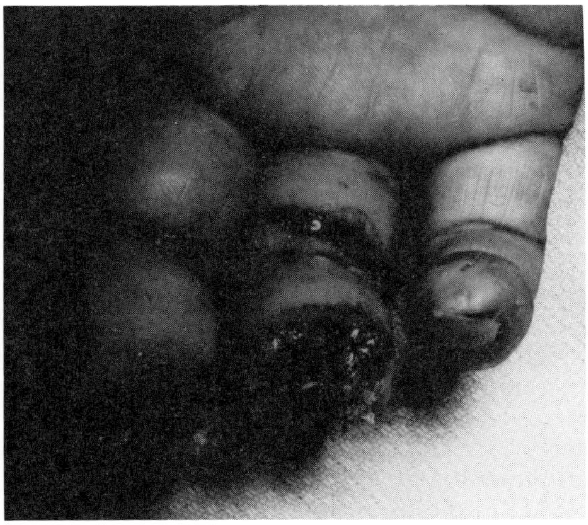

Figure 29-3. Fingertip amputations.

The open treatment consists of meticulous debridement, cleansing, and wound care. Debridement should eliminate all obviously devitalized and contaminated tissue. This may be accomplished by frequent dressing changes or the use of plaster finger casts (Fig. 29-4). Epithelialization of small skin defects usually takes 2 to 3 weeks. Wound contraction by secondary intention decreases the eventual area that may require closure by epithelialization (Fig. 29-5). With time the area obtains a normal texture, durability, and sensibility. This method may be used in all children under the age of 3 and in over 80% of adults.

NAIL BED INJURIES

Injury to the nail bed results from closing doors, fingertip compression between two objects followed by machines, saws, lawnmowers, and many others. The most commonly injured nail bed is that of the long finger (Fig. 29-6) followed by the ring, index, and small fingers and thumb. The usual injury of the nail bed is not isolated to the nail bed but involves the surrounding skin of the tip. Injury to the nail bed is caused by a blow or other deforming force that buckles the nail and compresses the nail bed between the bent portion of the nail and distal phalanx. This force may or may not cause a fracture of the distal phalanx but causes a crushing split in the nail bed. A blow from a relatively sharp object usually causes a single laceration of the nail bed, whereas a blow from a large object, such as a hammer, causes a wider area of pressure and an explosion type of injury that leaves the nail bed in many fragments. Between these two examples are many forces that cause stellate lacerations of the nail bed. It is relatively rare for a sharp object to lacerate the nail plate and the nail bed, because most sharp objects that strike the nail plate with enough force to perforate it usually sever the tip of the finger. Therefore almost all nail bed injuries are of a crushing nature, rather than sharp lacerations.

The most common injury to the nail bed is a simple laceration. This may be oriented in any direction, depending on the force applied, but

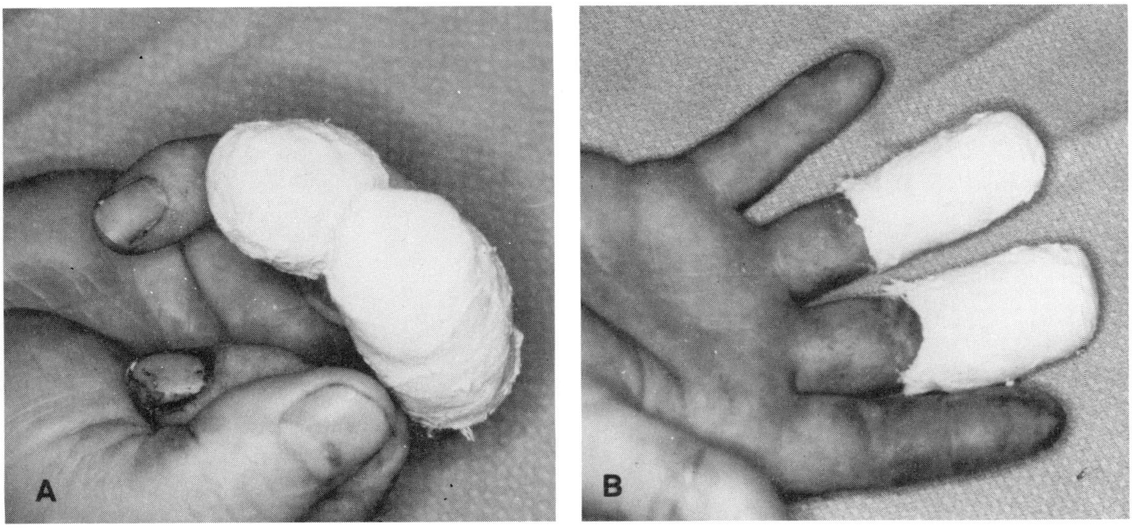

Figure 29-4. (*A*) Finger casts in flexion at PIP and MP joints. (*B*) Finger casts in extension.

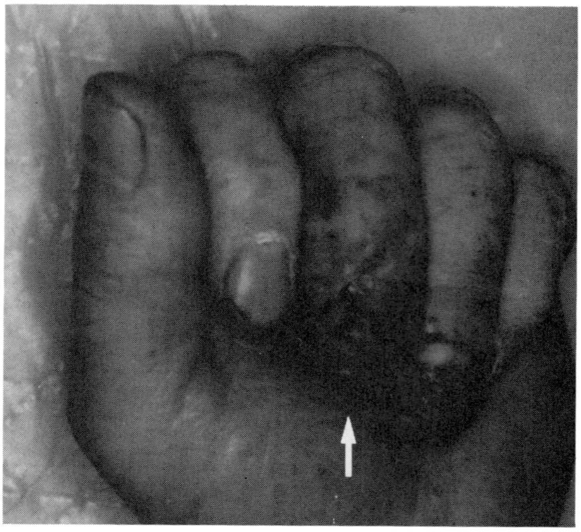

Figure 29-5. Fingertip healing (*arrow*) by secondary intention.

it is most commonly transverse. Next most common is the stellate laceration, followed by crushes and avulsions of nail bed. The most common site on a nail bed for injury is the middle third, with the distal third being a close second. Tuft fractures are associated with 50% of nail bed injuries and make roentgenographs of all nail bed injuries advisable.

Subungual hematoma can occur only with disruption of the nail bed vessels or from bending of the nail with compression of the nail bed between the bent nail and the bone. The more blood vessel injured, the larger the hematoma becomes (Fig. 29-7). The question is whether the injury to the nail bed is sufficient to warrant removal of the nail and repair if necessary. If 25% or more of the visible nail is undermined with hematoma, the nail should be removed and the nail bed explored. The removed nail should be cleaned and its undersurface scraped; it should then be replaced on the nail bed and maintained with a suture placed in the tip to hold it in the nail fold. If less than 25% of the nail is undermined with hematoma, drainage of the hematoma is indicated if the patient is having significant throbbing pain. The author's preferred method of drainage is either to use a heated paper clip or an ophthalmologic cautery. When either the cautery or the paper clip is red hot, the tip is pressed downward on the dorsum of the nail. As soon as the nail is perforated, the heated tip will be cooled by the hematoma beneath it. With extreme care, a nail bed injury should not result. One of the most devastating complications of a nail bed injury is infection and subsequent scarring.

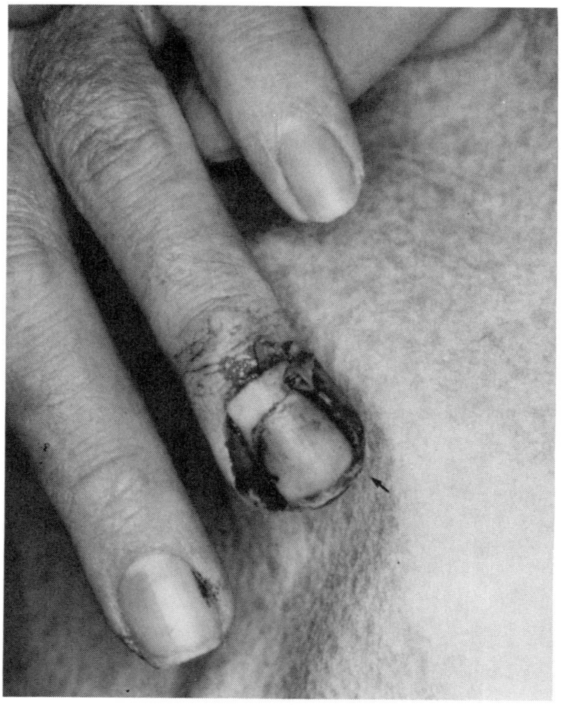

Figure 29-6. Nailbed injury to ring finger. Arrow shows separation of nail from bed.

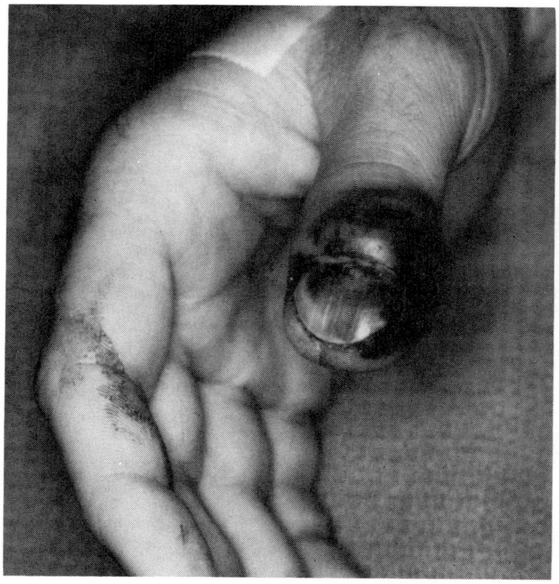

Figure 29-7. Crushed thumb in hemophiliac. Note severe hemorrhage.

Lacerations of the nail bed should be repaired by anatomic approximation. The author prefers to use a 6-0 absorbable suture using loop magnification. If the nail is removed, it can be placed back as a splint. It is important that no tension be placed on the repair. If the edges of the wound are very irregular, they can be trimmed. If the nail is not available to replace, then a piece of silastic sheeting or nonadhering gauze can be cut to resemble the shape of the nail. The nonadhering gauze I prefer is either Xeroform or Adaptic.

If there is a tuft fracture of the distal phalanx that is nondisplaced associated with a nail bed laceration, then replacement of the nail on its bed should maintain the position of the bone until healing occurs. If the fracture is unstable, then reduction should be accomplished and a Kirschner wire should be placed longitudinally through the tuft end of the proximal portion of the phalanx. This wire should be in the medullary cavity rather than beneath the nail bed. If the fracture is comminuted, then manual molding and compression of the fracture usually will allow it to be rounded into a reasonable position and maintained with nail replacement.

TENDON INJURIES

History and findings of a lacerating, penetrating, or through-and-through injury resulting in loss of, or diminished, wrist or digital motion distal to the site of injury, with or without sensory abnormalities, indicate definite tendon damage. Tendons are not usually severed in crushing injuries, but are bound down in dense scar involving soft tissue during healing and abundant callus formation in the case of a fracture. It is important to know whether the digit was flexed or extended at the time of injury to help diagnose the level of flexor tendon laceration. If the digit was extended, then the tendon laceration should be found beneath the skin laceration. If, however, the digit was flexed, then the tendon laceration will be found distal to the site of skin laceration at a variable distance relative to the extent of flexion.

The configuration of the wrist and digits at rest helps determine what tendons are lacerated. If the digit lies in complete extension, then complete laceration of both superficial and deep flexors is strongly suspected (Fig. 29-8). If the DIP joint is in complete extension (Fig. 29-9) but the PIP joint is flexed, then complete laceration of the profundus tendon and possibly partial laceration of the superficialis tendon may be found. The patient should be urged to attempt active flexion of all joints distal to the site of injury. If this is impossible because of other injuries, or if the patient is uncooperative, then the determination of the extent of the injury could be discovered during exploration in the operating room. This should be performed under adequate anesthesia and tourniquet hemostasis.

FLEXOR TENDON INJURIES

Flexor tendon injuries are categorized according to the location of injury, comprising

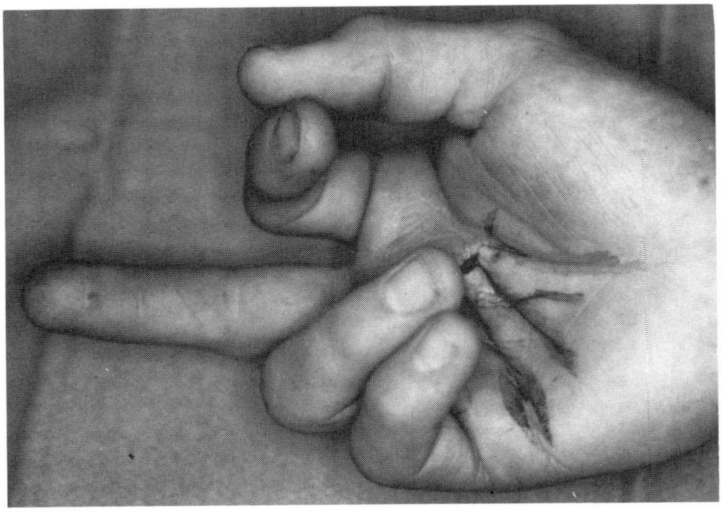

Figure 29-8. Both flexor tendons to middle finger lacerated. Note inability to flex middle finger.

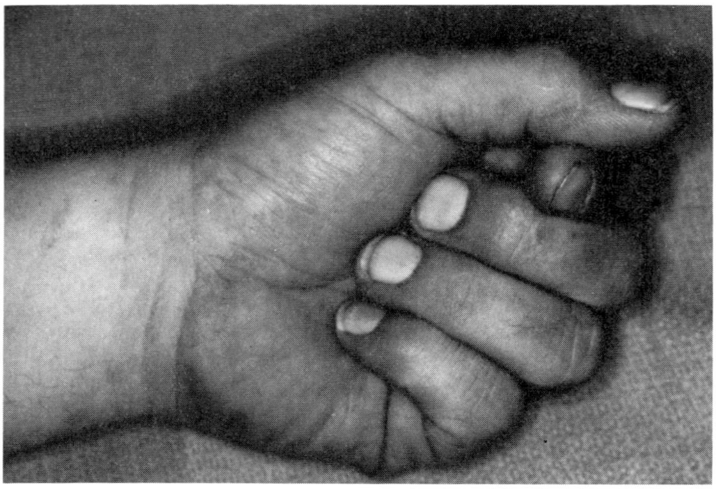

Figure 29-9. Isolated profundus laceration to index finger. Note inability to flex DIP joint.

five distinct areas in digits index through little fingers.

Zone 1 includes that area of the flexor sheath that extends distally from the distal-most determination of the superficialis tendon of insertion on the middle third of the middle phalanx past the insertion of the flexor digitorum profundus tendon on the distal phalanx.

Zone 2 includes the area commonly referred to as "no man's land," which extends from the beginning of the fibrous flexor sheath in the area of the distal palmar flexion crease distally to the distal-most determination of the superficialis tendon on the middle third of the middle phalanx.

Zone 3 includes the palm from the distal end of the transverse carpal ligament distally to the commencement of the flexor sheath at the distal palmar flexion crease.

Zone 4 encompasses the area of the wrist beneath the transverse carpal ligament contained within the carpal tunnel.

Zone 5 includes the distal forearm from the musculotendinous junctions of the forearm flexors distally to the proximal boundary of the transverse carpal ligament.

A tendon injury occurring in zone 2 presents the biggest problem with flexor tendon repairs. In this area the flexor digitorum profundus and superficialis tendons enter the flexor sheath and remain together up to the termination of the superficialis insertion at the junction of the middle and distal thirds of the middle phalanx. The profundus tendon is in intimate association with the superficialis through the decussation. One may say that there are three flexor tendons in this area between the superficialis decussation and profundus tendon.

One has several options in dealing with flexor tendon injuries. One may offer immediate primary repair of the tendons or close the skin and perform a delayed primary repair. It is also acceptable to close the wound to allow healing and later return to a secondary tendon graft. A lot depends on the appearance of the wound, the delay after the injury, and the experience of the surgeon. The concept of delayed primary repair for the questionably contaminated wound has allowed extension of early tendon repair to cases only slightly less favorable. The results of delayed flexor tendon repair are comparable to those of primary repair. Delayed tendon grafting with or without induction of a sheath using silastic rods remains appropriate for cases that are less favorable.

Incisions that have been used have been the midlateral incision or the volar zigzag incision. I prefer the volar zigzag approach (Fig. 29-10).

Whether to repair the flexor tendon sheath is controversial. It has recently been shown that the tendon sheath, which contains synovial fluid, is important to the healing of the tendon. Some authors feel that the damaged tendon sheath synovium should be repaired, even if it is repaired with free grafts of autogenous synovium. It is my feeling that this is not necessary.

Various methods of suturing have been de-

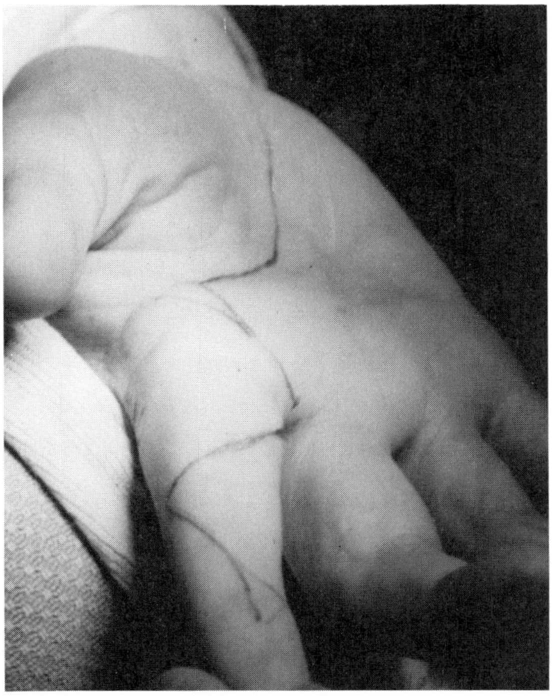

Figure 29-10. Bruner volar zigzag incision.

scribed: the classic crisscross suture, the classic crisscross suture described by Bunnell, the Kessler, and modified Kessler. My preference is to use modified Kessler with a 4-0 nonabsorbable Dacron-coated suture and then use a running 6-0 nylon around the rough edges. Some surgeons still use the classic pull-out sutures (Fig. 29-11), but I have not used this in many years.

It is important to maintain the pulley system of the tendon sheaths (Fig. 29-12). The necessity of the pulleys to prevent bow stringing was recognized early in hand surgery. The most important pulleys to maintain are the A-2 and A-4. If it is necessary to trim the pulleys, then one can start distally and trim no more than a centimeter.

At one time it was felt that repairs of the flexor pollicis longus gave better results than those of the other flexor tendons of the remaining digits. This was based on the belief that there was only one tendon in the fibroosseous tunnel. In later studies it was found that the results of repair of this tendon were not any better than the results of the repair of the other flexor tendons of the remaining digits. There are two annular pulleys, one at the MP joint and another at the IP joint; between them is an oblique pulley. It is generally agreed that the oblique pully is the most important to save or reconstruct for maintenance of flexor pollicis longus action (Fig. 29-13).

PARTIALLY SEVERED TENDONS

It is recommended that partial flexor tendon lacerations (Fig. 29-14) without beveling should not be repaired but instead should be treated with early active motion. Beveled partial tendon lacerations of less than 25% of the cross-sectional area can be either excised or

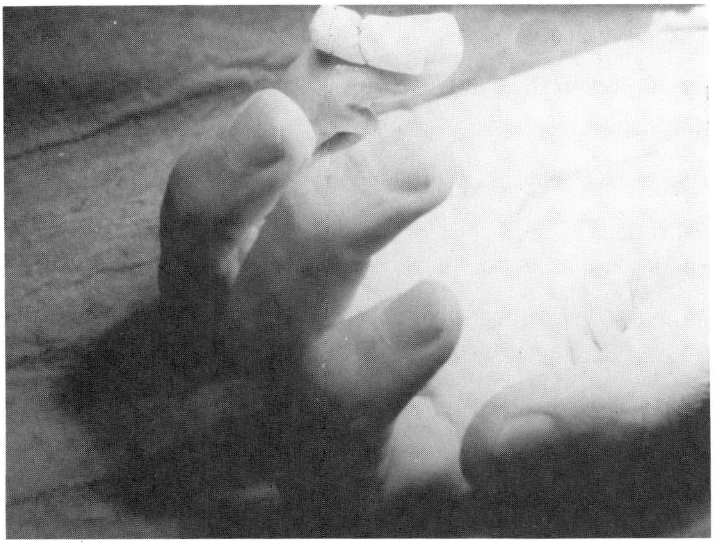

Figure 29-11. Pull-out suture tied over dental roll in little finger.

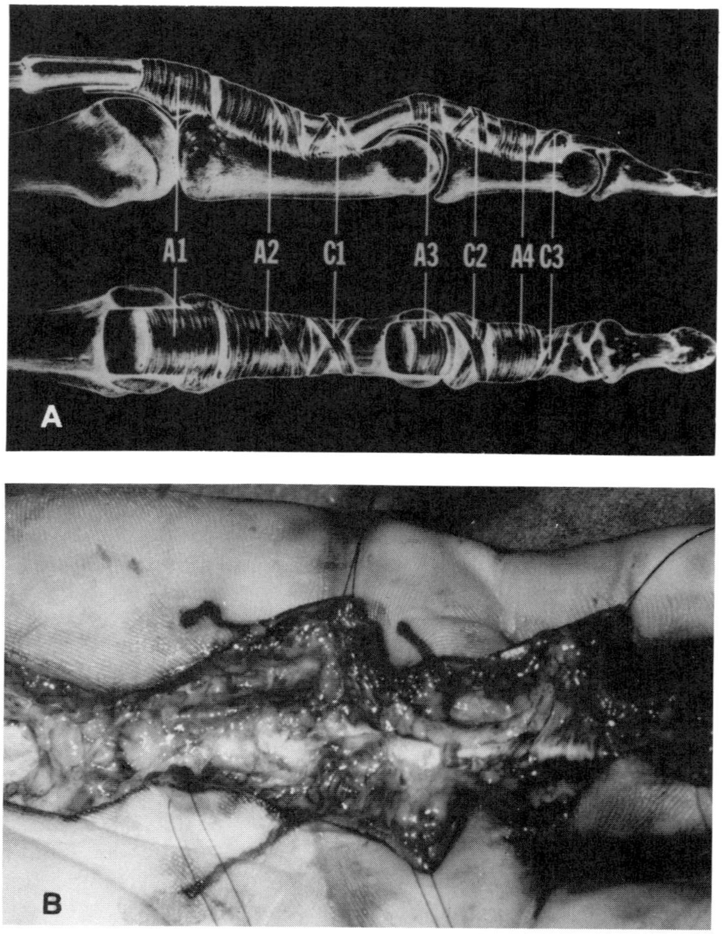

Figure 29-12. (*A*) Diagram of pulley system. (*B*) Dissection showing pulley system in ring finger.

repaired with a single stitch, whereas a larger beveled laceration should be repaired with a few simple stitches. Some surgeons believe that tendon entrapment, rupture, and triggering can result from not repairing partial tendon lacerations.

TENDON INJURIES IN CHILDREN

Primary tendon repair in children generally yields better results than those in adults, presumably because of an increased capacity for remodeling. Although the principles of tendon repair in children remain basically the same, the inability of children to cooperate, both during examination at the time of the acute injury and during mobilization of the tendon following injury, makes them worthy of separate consideration. If one suspects a tendon injury in a child, then one might expect poor cooperation in the examination, so that it is my recommendation that a dry sterile dressing be applied and the examination and exploration be done in the operating room under suitable anesthesia with tourniquet control.

Because of the ability of children to free themselves of any dressing, immobilization must be more extensive. Children are unable to participate in early guarded movement and have the capacity for more extensive remodeling. Immobilization is typically more prolonged in children, but it should not be longer than 4 weeks. Most authors recommend a plaster cast that is above the elbow; occasionally, it is recommended that with children under 6 years of age the cast be attached to the trunk by either soft bandages or a plaster Velpeau. Not only the injured finger, but all the fingers should be covered with dressing and plaster.

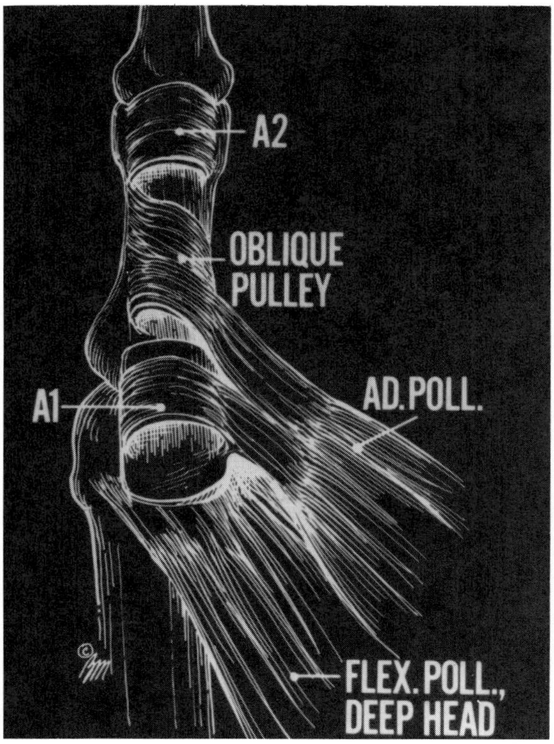

Figure 29-13. Pulley system of thumb.

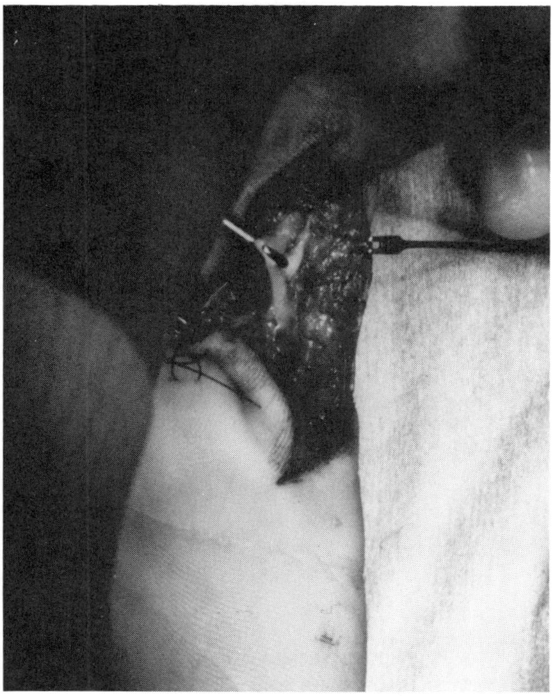

Figure 29-14. Partial laceration of profundus tendon.

EXTENSOR TENDON INJURIES

Most extensor tendon injuries of the fingers can be treated successfully by splinting alone. Only on the dorsum of the hand, where the extensor tendons are free to retract, is suturing necessary. Early treatment is preferable because it is almost impossible to restore the delicate balance of the complex extensor–flexor mechanism at late reconstruction.

Mallet Finger

The mallet finger is an interruption of the extensor tendon at the distal IP joint that results in a deformity; it is also called baseball or drop finger (Fig. 29-15). It is important to diagnose the cause of the deformity accu-

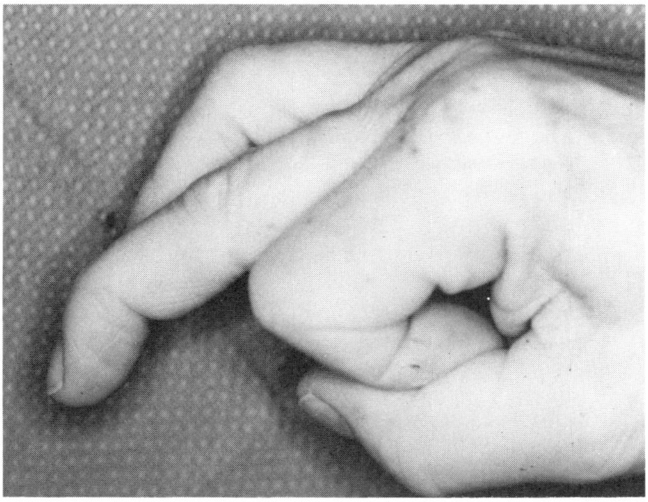

Figure 29-15. Mallet or baseball finger. Note inability to extend DIP joint.

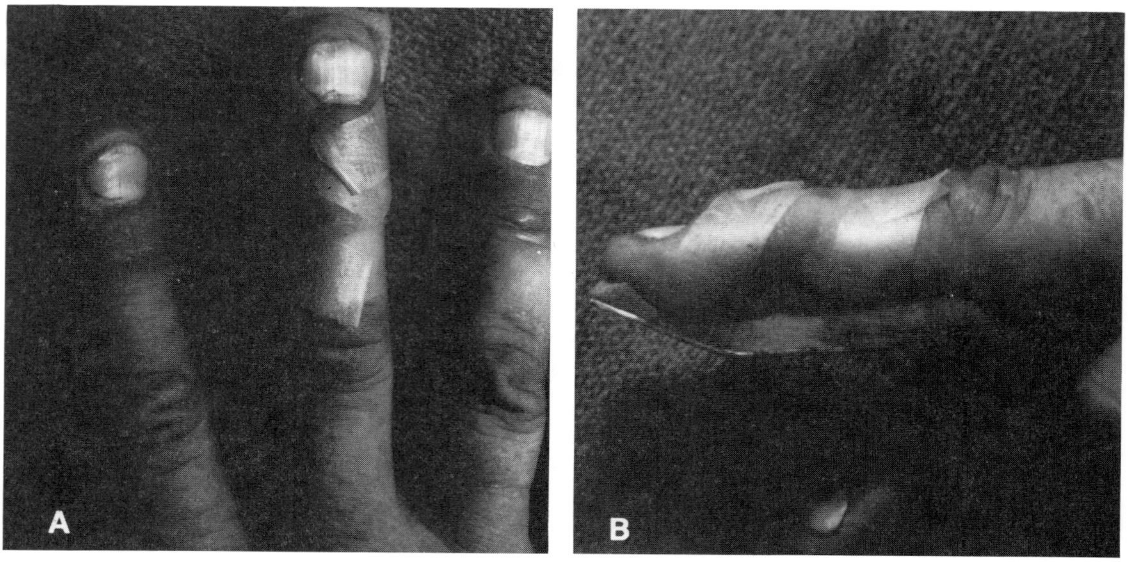

Figure 29-16. (*A*) Splint for mallet finger, dorsal view. (*B*) Splint for mallet finger, lateral view.

rately, whether a laceration, closed rupture, avulsion fracture, or fracture dislocation, because treatment and prognosis vary. In most cases conservative splinting of the distal phalanx in extension (Fig. 29-16) to very slight hyperextension for 6 weeks after injury corrects the deformity. This may be in a plaster finger cast or a splint, with the PIP joint left free.

If no treatment has been given, many patients will tolerate the deformity, as disability is slight. There may be some loss of voluntary extension of the distal joint, but flexion of the joint and hand grip will be essentially normal. To some, however, the deformity may cause the fingertip to hook on objects or be cosmetically unacceptable. The mallet finger may progress to a noticeable hyperextension of the proximal IP joint or the secondary swan-neck deformity. Many procedures have evolved to repair the acute injuries, including plastered finger casts, various splints, external sutures, Kirschner wire and immobilization, and primary tendon suture. The true fracture dislocations are discussed in the chapter on fractures. The uncertain results from direct operative reconstructions have led some authors to suggest nonintervention in the chronic mallet finger.

Boutonnière Deformity

A boutonnière deformity (Fig. 29-17) is caused by acute laceration of the central slip of the extensor tendon insertion that terminates on the dorsal aspect of the middle phalangeal base, or more commonly by blunt trauma that avulses that insertion. The central slip retracts proximally, and the adjacent lateral band on each side acutely or progressively separates and eventually migrates volar to the axis of flexion and extension of the PIP joint. The lateral bands normally are situated dorsal to the axis of flexion and extension of the PIP joint that aid in extending that joint, eventually migrating volar to the axis. Therefore any active attempt to extend the PIP joint proximally retracts the central slip further and volarly subluxes the lateral bands more severely. The result is increased PIP joint flexion by the subluxed lateral bands, which also hyperextend the DIP joint because of increased tension on their insertions on the distal phalanx base. The initial treatment of this injury must be aggressive, regardless of the etiology, to prevent sequelae of the PIP joint flexion contracture and DIP joint hyperextension contracture. The main disability of a chronic severe boutonnière deformity is fixed DIP joint hyperextension and the inability to flex that joint actively. Closed injuries should be treated by a splint with the PIP joint in complete extension for 6 weeks. The MP joint and DIP joint should be free to allow exercises while the PIP joint is splinted in full extension. Flexion contracture of the PIP joint must be passively stretched to achieve complete extension prior to immobilization; otherwise the lateral bands will remain volar to the axis of

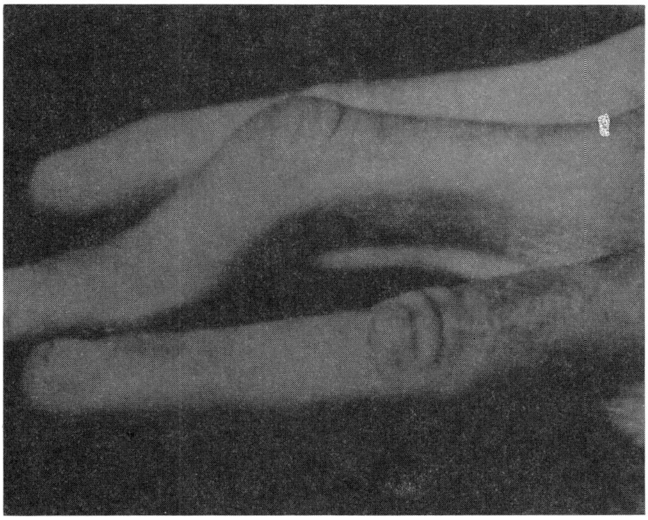

Figure 29-17. Boutonnière deformity.

flexion and extension. Only after lateral bands are anatomically relocated and the PIP joint is completely extended can conservative immobilization be successful.

Complete laceration of the central slip with or without one or both lateral bands involved should be surgically repaired. Temporary, oblique Kirschner wire fixation across the PIP joint in complete extension offers excellent protection augmented by protective external splint to immobilization or plaster finger casts.

Extensor Tendon Injuries Proximal to the PIP Joint

Extensor tendon lacerations over the MP joint should be repaired surgically. Following repair with nonabsorbable suture, the hand should be immobilized for 4 weeks with the wrist in extension and the MP joint blocked at 0 degrees and not allowed to flex.

The same treatment is advocated for extensor tendon lacerations on the dorsum of the hand and wrist and forearm (Fig. 29-18). A primary suture is indicated with immobilization for 4 weeks with the wrist in 30 degrees of dorsiflexion and the MP joints blocked at 0 degrees of extension. Four weeks of immobilization should be sufficient followed by a period of rehabilitation.

PERIPHERAL NERVE INJURIES

Following the initial clinical examination of a patient with peripheral nerve injury, decisions must be made regarding indications for exploration and/or indications for electrophysiologic studies such as electromyograms and nerve conduction velocities. A patient management plan must be instituted. For the purposes of clinically defining a level of nerve injury or evaluating the rate of recovery, muscle testing must be performed. The most commonly used electrical studies to assess neuromuscular function are the electromyogram and nerve conduction velocity studies.

A transected nerve is repaired as soon as wound conditions and other factors permit. With a closed nerve injury, a waiting period of 6 weeks or more may be appropriate for ordering EMGs or nerve conduction velocities.

Traction injuries, high-velocity missile wounds, and shotgun wounds, as well as any other type of severe traumatic injury, adversely affect the outcome of nerve repair. The degree of trauma directly relates to intraneural damage, contusion, hematoma, devitalized tissue, and infection and scarring, all of which are detrimental to functional recovery. Retrograde changes at the neuron cell body level are pronounced with this type of injury, with more proximal degneration and less potential for regeneration. In contrast, injuries caused by sharp lacerations are considerably better for prognosis.

The techniques of nerve repair are still in dispute. Epineural or perineural repairs or nerve grafting have been described by various authors. The clinical decision on which type of repair to use must be made with reference to each case, with the goals being the most accurate alignment possible with the smallest num-

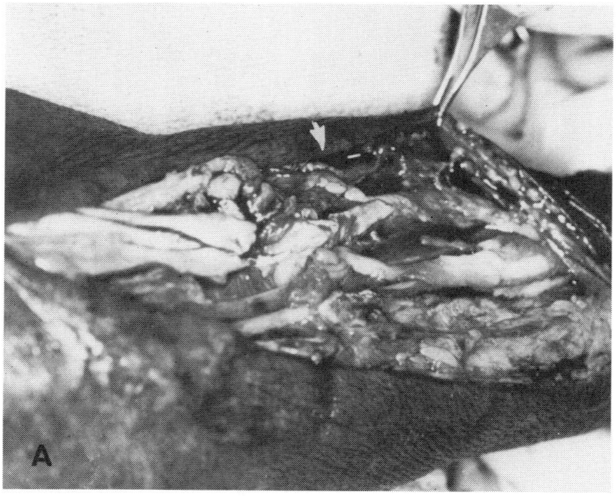

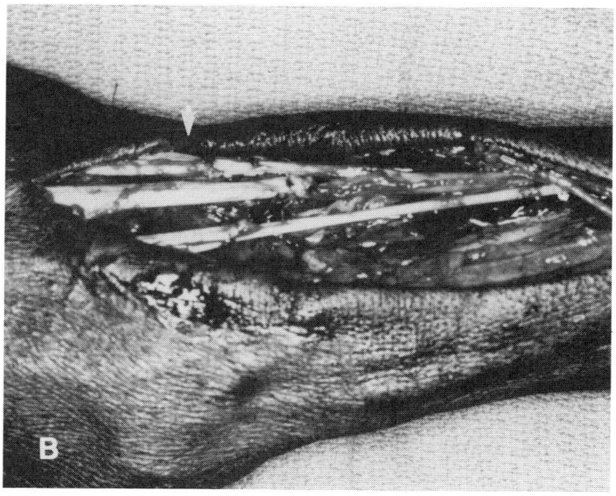

Figure 29-18. (*A*) Laceration (*arrow*) of extensor tendons at wrist. (*B*) Repair (*arrow*) of extensor tendons at wrist.

ber of sutures and dissection of nerve ends only to the extent necessary to achieve proper alignment. No matter which type of repair is used, it should be done in the operating room under tourniquet control with the use of magnification (Fig. 29-19) and adequate anesthesia.

ARTERIAL INJURIES

Sharp or blunt trauma that does not break the skin or a small puncture wound may cause a false aneurysm or thrombosis of the radial or ulnar artery. Of the two vessels, the ulnar is involved much more frequently. A false aneurysm of the ulnar artery results in a tender mass located at the hypothenar eminence and accompanied by a bruit and a positive Allen test. Secondary spasms of the more distal vessel may cause suspicion of Raynaud's disease. Treatment consists of resecting the lesion. A false aneurysm of the radial artery may cause few symptoms early and may be confused with a ganglion, so often located over this artery on the volar surface of the wrist. In this instance considerable trouble may be encountered during surgery, especially if it is carried out in a less than ideal environment. Again treatment consists of resecting the lesion. Thrombosis of the ulnar artery may be caused by a single injury or by a repeated occupational injury such as those that may occur when a heavy hammer is used frequently. It

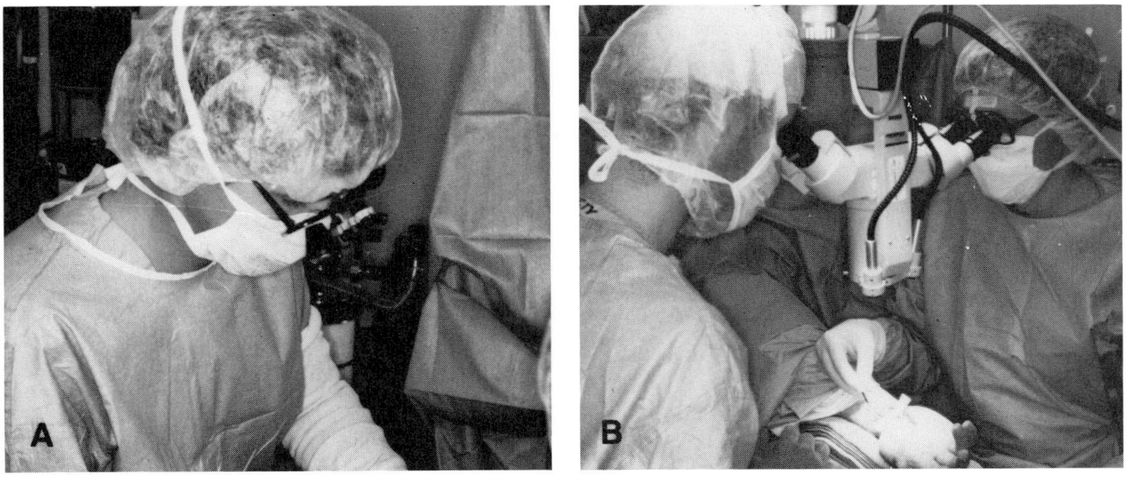
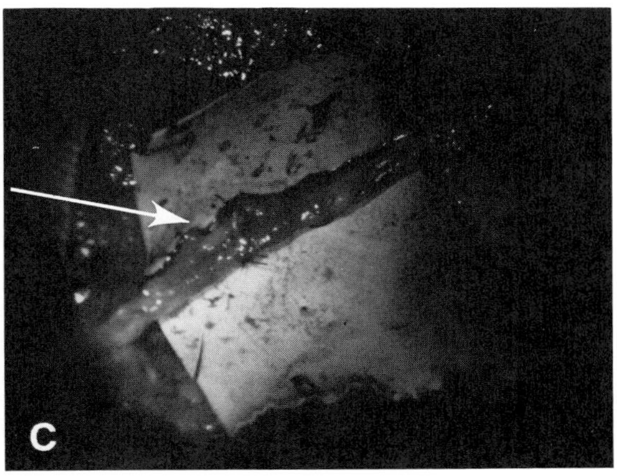

Figure 29-19. (*A*) Surgeon using loupe magnification. (*B*) Surgeon and assistant using operating microscope. (*C*) Photo through microscope showing nerve repair (*arrow*).

causes persistent secondary spasm of the more distal vessels, resulting in blanching of and pain in the ulna three digits. It may be confused with Raynaud's disease, especially since exposure to cold increases the blanching. Sometimes pain is severe and sensibility is lost over the distribution of the ulnar nerve in the hand. There is tenderness over the artery and occasionally a feeling of fullness in the wrist and hand. The Allen test is helpful in diagnosing this, but arteriography of course is diagnostic. Treatment consists of exploration of the artery and resection of the entire thrombotic mass.

The Allen test was described in 1929 as a new way to test the patency of the ulnar and radial arteries. First the patient elevates his hand and makes a fist while the examiner occludes both radial and ulnar arteries (Fig. 29-20). Then the patient extends his fingers and blanching of the hand is seen. This is usually repeated three times. Next the hand is observed while the radial artery alone is released; the color of the hand should return to normal immediately. The same maneuvers are repeated to test the ulnar artery. The test is positive when the color fails to return to normal after release of either artery alone. In thrombosis of the ulnar artery the test is positive when this artery alone is released. The patency of the digital arteries can be tested in a similar manner. This test should be a part of a complete physical examination of the hand in a patient. It should be performed prior to invading either radial or ulnar arteries diagnostically or by the use of A-lines or arterial sticks. The Allen test should be performed on both hands, since there are anomalies in which either radial or ulnar arteries are the main supply of blood to the hand.

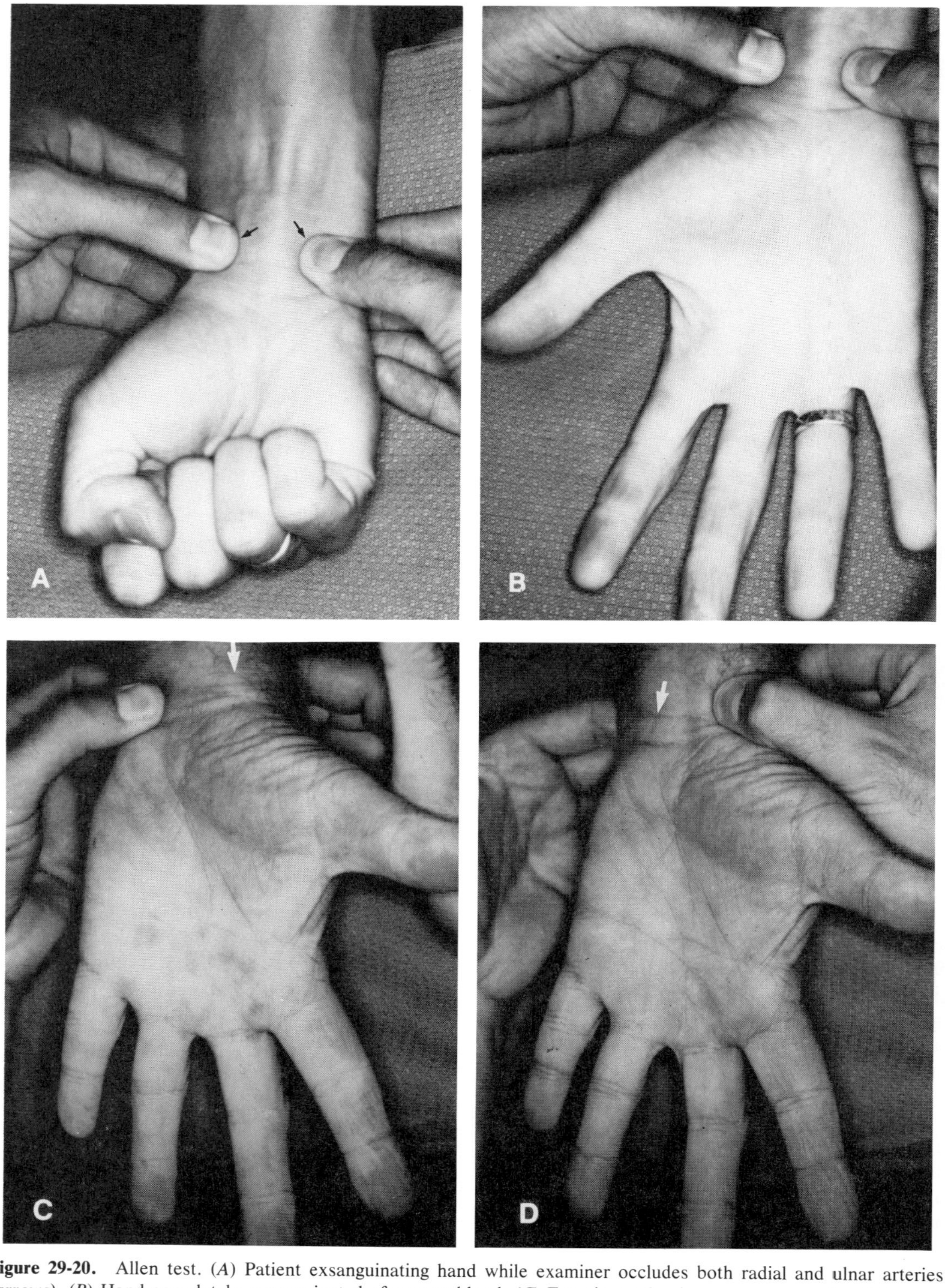

Figure 29-20. Allen test. (*A*) Patient exsanguinating hand while examiner occludes both radial and ulnar arteries (*arrows*). (*B*) Hand completely exsanguinated of venous blood. (*C*) Examiner releasing compression of radial artery (*arrow*). (*D*) Examiner releasing compression of ulnar artery (*arrow*).

REPLANTATIONS

The first successful replantation of an amputated human limb was in 1962. The success of this case encouraged many other surgeons to attempt replantation. The excellent experimental and clinical work by microvascular surgeons in this country, in Asia, and in Europe demonstrated that digits could be successfully replanted. At present, success and survival rates are approximately 90%. Success of a replantation is measured not by survival alone but by the degree of useful function. Final functional return may not be evident for many months because of slow regeneration of peripheral nerves. A lengthy recovery period may result in extreme limitation of function.

The function expected after replantation must be better than that of a prosthesis or an amputation, and the difference must be worth the risk, time, and expense. Indications for replantation are stronger for children, (Fig. 29-21) for multiple-digit amputations, for thumb amputations proximal to the interphalangeal joint (Fig. 29-22), for amputations with minimal contamination. Replantation is less strongly indicated in age groups over 50 years, with single digit amputations other than the thumb, in severe crush or avulsion injuries, and in the presence of other life-endangering injuries.

The time interval from the accident to arrival at the replantation center is critical. By cooling, not freezing, the amputated part during transport, this interval is made less critical and may be prolonged. The amputated part should be wrapped in gauze and placed in a plastic bag within an iced container. There should be no attempt to wash, irrigate, or profuse the amputated part prior to transportation. All necessary primary care must be given to the patient, crushing of exposed vessels by clamp should be avoided if at all possible because excision of the crushed ends will shorten the vessels even more.

There is no uniform agreement on preoperative, intraoperative and postoperative aspects of replantation surgery. Most agree on certain basic principles. The general physical condition of the patient should be carefully assessed. This is because the surgical procedure may last 10 or more hours. The patient and the family should thoroughly understand the possibility of complications and the possibility of loss of the amputated part. Probable necessity for multiple future procedures should also be discussed.

For preparation of the amputated part and preparation at the site of detachment, two teams are essential or highly desirable with one team in charge of each of the wounds. On each team there must be at least one member with experience in microsurgery. As with multiple procedures and surgery of the hand, adequate anesthesia and tourniquet control is necessary. All devitalized tissue must be excised first; then the bone should be reduced and fixed rigidly. One may do either the venous or arterial repair first; then the extensor tendons are repaired, followed by the transected

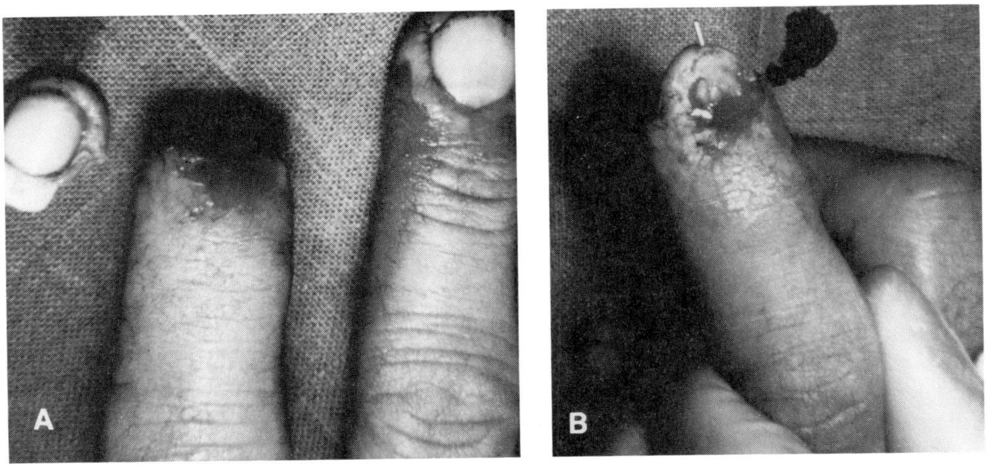

Figure 29-21. (*A*) Traumatic amputation at DIP joint. (*B*) Immediately after artery, nerve and tendon repair with K-wire fixation.

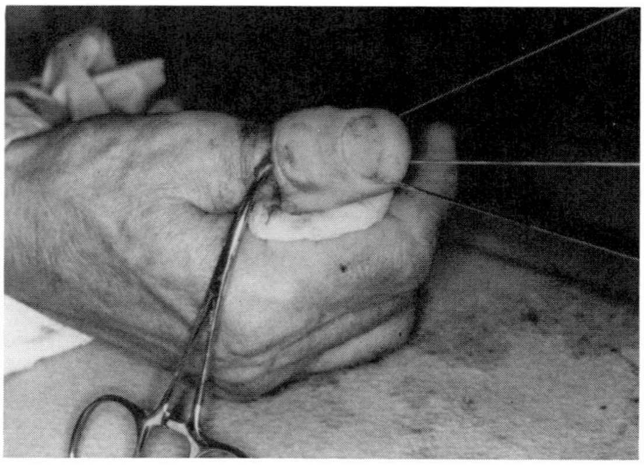

Figure 29-22. Fixation of amputated thumb with K-wires prior to vessel, nerve, and tendon repair.

nerves and the flexor tendons. A uniform hand dressing is then applied with splints. Frequent evaluations of the circulation of the part are carried out. Should vascular occlusion occur, reexploration may be necessary. Smoking should be prohibited in the room, especially by the patient. Anticoagulants, low-molecular-weight dextran, aspirin, and stellate ganglion blocks have been advocated postoperatively. The first dressing change is usually delayed for approximately 7 days.

SOFT-TISSUE INJURIES

COMPARTMENTAL SYNDROMES

Compartmental syndromes are less frequently the cause of nerve compression but are still extremely important in differential diagnosis. Increased pressure within a limiting envelope containing neuromuscular tissue may result in circulatory compromise, which may progress to muscle or nerve necrosis. Following severe trauma, clinical differentiation between direct nerve injuries or neuromuscular dysfunction secondary to compartmental syndromes may be difficult. If suspicion of increased compartmental pressure exists, direct measurement of compartmental pressures may be necessary.

Ischemic myositis ranks with impending gangrene as one of the most potentially devastating emergencies of the upper extremity. Its development may be subtle, but its sequelae are severe. Although the peripheral nerves are involved as a result of hypoxia and later entrapment, the primary pathologic finding in ischemic myositis is progressive degeneration of muscle tissue to necrosis. This is caused by a loss of circulation. The degenerated necrotic muscle tissue is gradually replaced by fibrous tissue that engulfs and strangles the remainder of viable muscles and nerves. This results in characteristic paralysis and deformity. Local factors include external compression, muscle contusion and swelling, crush and wringer injuries, fractures, infection, gas gangrene, excessive hemorrhage, chemical trauma, and direct trauma to muscle. Proximal arterial obstruction may be caused by an arterial injury, tourniquet, vasculitis, thrombosis, or medication. Each of these factors may initiate a number of events that will increase intercompartmental pressure and loss of blood flow directly or indirectly.

Frequently implicated in Volkmann's ischemia are crush injuries to the forearm, which are most common in adults, and supracondylar fractures of the humerus, most common in children. The muscles most frequently involved are the deep volar forearm muscles. Other muscles, such as the intrinsic muscles of the hand, may be directly involved with the ischemic process or may be secondarily involved by the imbalance created between extrinsic and intrinsic musculature and nerve palsies.

Compartmental syndrome can be diagnosed only when there is a high index of suspicion. The diagnosis must be made promptly, because irreversible muscle changes have been noted within 6 to 8 hours of an ischemic event. This diagnosis must be immediately suspected in a high-risk clinical setting, especially if there is excessive pain, tightness in the compartment, pain on passive stretching of muscles involved (Fig. 29-23), and peripheral nerve deficit. *Persistent and unrelenting pain of increasing severity is the most important diagnostic sign.* A loss of pulse may be a very late finding in compartment syndrome. In a comatose patient it may be helpful to measure intercompartmental pressures.

The best treatment of ischemia, obviously, is prevention. Measures include admission to the hospital and partial elevation for at-risk injuries, splinting, frequent assessment, and the removal of circular dressings or casts. Specific measure of fracture care, such as proper technique of fracture reduction, the leaving open of fascial forearm incisions and

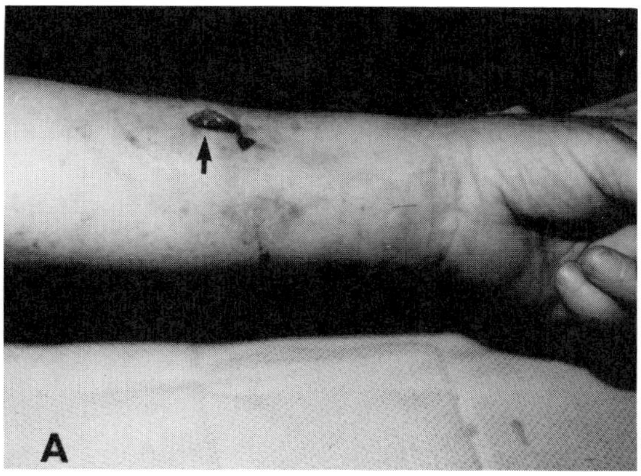

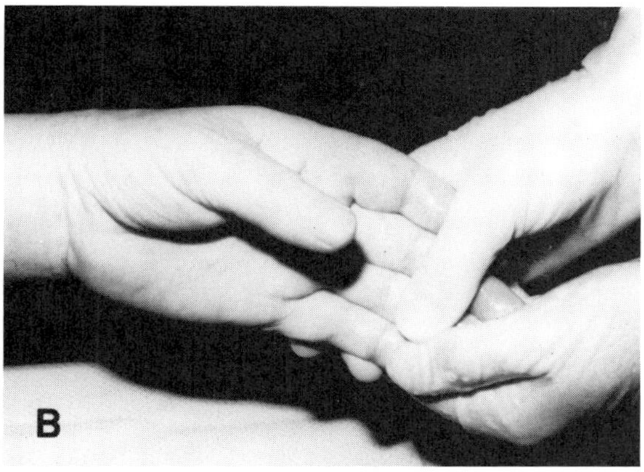

Figure 29-23. (*A*) Stab wound (*arrow*) in forearm with compartment swelling. (*B*) Limitation of passive extension of fingers.

wounds, and judicious use of the tourniquet must be performed. Once ischemia is diagnosed, the cause should be eliminated. Fasciotomy should probably be performed (Fig. 29-24). It is much preferred to release deep fascia too early than too late.

Ischemia may be caused by either crush injury to the hand or more proximal ischemia (Fig. 29-25). Both the volar and dorsal interossei are tightly confined between the metacarpals, the unyielding deep dorsal fascia, and the fascia overlying the volar surface of the ad-

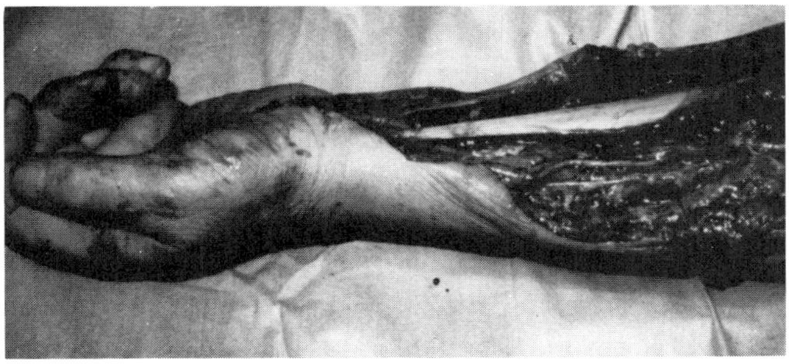

Figure 29-24. Fasciotomy performed from carpal tunnel to elbow.

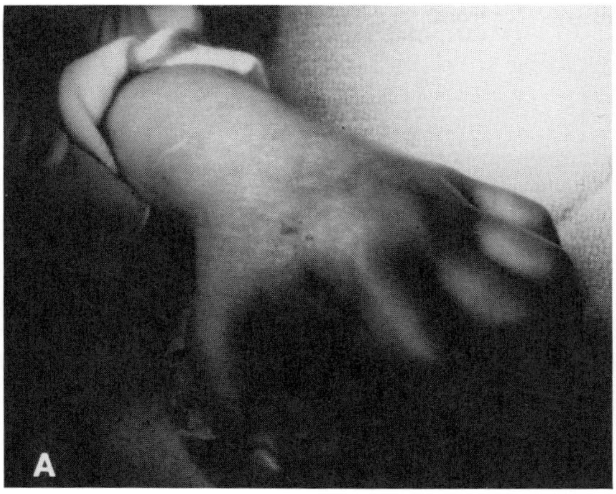

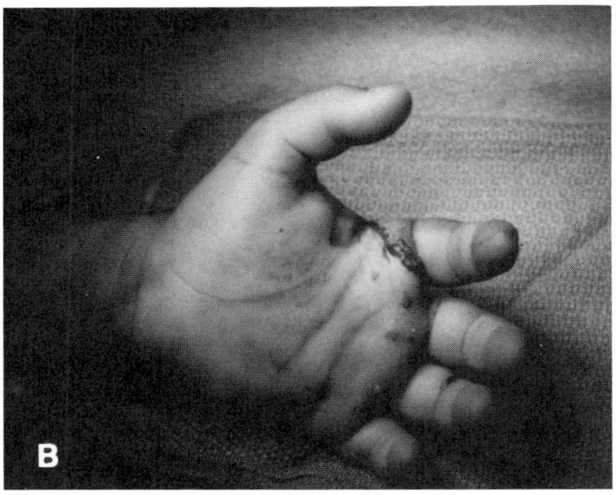

Figure 29-25. (*A*) Dorsal view of hand with intrinsic compartments tight. (*B*) Palmar view of hand with intrinsic compartments tight.

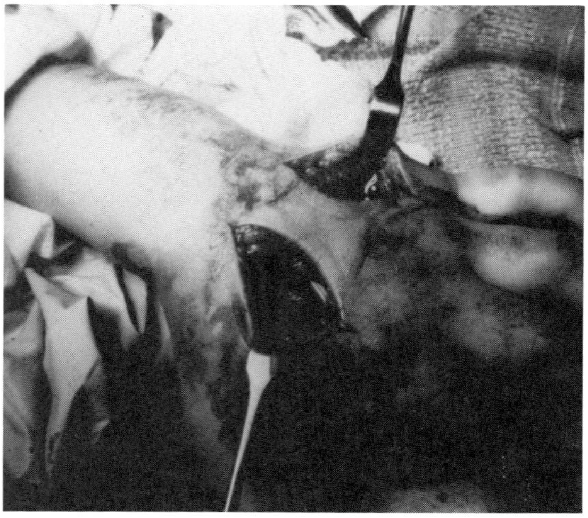

Figure 29-26. Decompression of intrinsic compartments through two longitudinal incisions on dorsum of hand.

ductor pollicis and volar interossei. The hand appears grossly edematous, but circulation and sensation of the fingertips are usually intact. The posture of the hand is generally one of varying degrees of intrinsic minus deformity with or without thumb adduction and thumb web space bulging. As with all compartment syndromes, passive stretching of the involved muscles is painful and the muscles are weak. Passive stretch is best accomplished by separate abduction and adduction of each digit. If numbness is present, decompression of the ulnar and median nerves should seriously be considered at the time of fasciotomy.

Decompression of the tight interosseous spaces is usually done dorsally with longitudinal incisions through the interosseous investing fascia and the intermetacarpal spaces (Fig. 29-26). Wounds are left open with delayed primary or secondary closure or grafting as necessary.

VOLKMANN'S ISCHEMIC CONTRACTURE

Volkmann's ischemic contracture is a late result of several different types of tissue injury; however, the earliest changes usually involve the flexor digitorum profundi muscles in the middle third of the forearm. The mild type includes ischemia of the flexor digitorum profundus muscles, frequently the result of a crush injury, and may be treated by dynamic splinting to maintain finger extension, by an exercise program, and by observation for further contracture. Muscle slide operations to lengthen the muscle mass may be indicated when the contracture involves three or four fingers. The moderate type involves not only the deep finger flexors, but the superficial finger flexors, flexors of the wrist, and the thumb flexor, all of which may be benefited by lengthening if their muscles are still functioning. In this type the median nerve should be freed by neurolysis and placed in a more vascular bed, if one is available. The severe type (Fig. 29-27) usually results from a supracondylar fracture or occasionally a fracture dislocation of the elbow; therefore it is more frequent in younger age groups. Primary reconstruction procedures should be done to position the hand and wrist in a position of function, excise scar tissue from the necrotic areas, and perform neurolysis on the nerves to enable sensory return if possible. Later tendon transfers may be indicated.

PERIPHERAL NERVE COMPRESSION SYNDROMES

In certain areas nerves pass through unyielding surroundings, as in the carpal tunnel

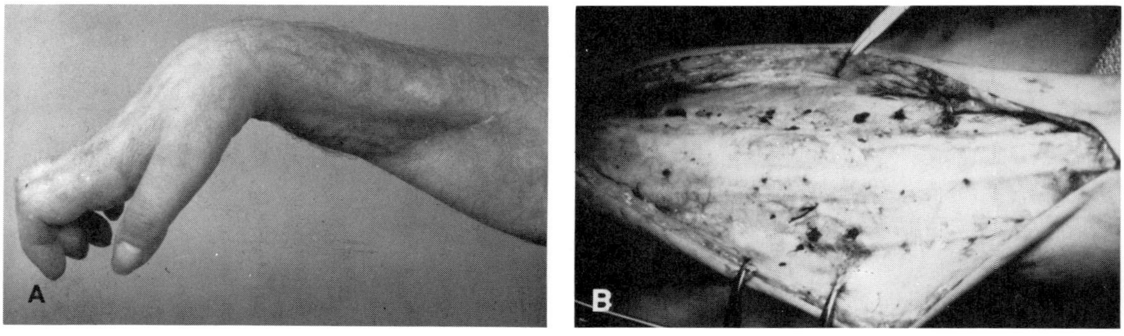

Figure 29-27. (*A*) Volkmann's ischemic contracture. (*B*) Fibrosis of muscle in forearm.

and beneath the arcade of Frohse. Many occupations or recreations require repetitive motions. If these are made in a posture that increases peripheral nerve compression, symptoms may develop. For example, the flexed wrist that increases carpal tunnel compression occurs if weight is lifted in this posture. Pronation of the forearm with an extended elbow and flexed wrist compresses the radial nerve in its tunnel at the elbow. Anomalous structures may overfill a tight compartment or may place a nerve on a stretch, as occurs in the presence of a cervical rib or a fibrous anlage. Synovitis is the most common cause of nerve compression in the carpal tunnel (Fig. 29-28). Usually nonspecific, the increased bulk of inflamed synovium cannot be accommodated by the unexpandable tunnel and compression of the median nerve results. Acute peripheral nerve syndromes require urgent release and may complicate any hand injury in which significant edema occurs. Delayed nerve compression may result from trauma, as in the tardy ulnar nerve palsy following supracondylar fractures of the humerus. Alterations in fluid distribution may well participate or exacerbate nerve compression. This is especially common carpal tunnel syndrome, in which the characteristic night numbness is due to the increased peripheral circulation that occurs during sleep, largely as a means of temperature regulation. The syndrome is more prevalent in women and is often more troublesome in the premenstrual phase and during pregnancy, when water retention occurs. Certain endocrine disorders, by disturbing fluid balance, show increased incidence of nerve compression syndromes. Thus carpal tunnel syndrome is more common in hypothyroidism and diabetes. Acute compression may occur on nerves during surgical procedures. Such injury occurs most commonly to the radial nerve, traveling as its does close to bone. It is therefore very vulnerable during internal fixation of fractures of the humerus and radius. Compression of peripheral nerves may also occur through poor positioning of the anesthetized patient. The radial nerve and the spiral groove of the humerus are most at risk, although the axillary nerve and ulnar nerve above the elbow have been injured by positioning the patient during anesthesia.

MEDIAN NERVE COMPRESSION

CARPAL TUNNEL SYNDROME

Carpal tunnel syndrome results from compression of the median nerve within the carpal tunnel. It is most common in patients between 30 and 60 years old and is five to six times more frequent in women than men. Any condition that crowds or reduces the capacity of the carpal tunnel may initiate symptoms; complex fractures around the wrist, edema from infection or trauma, tumors or tumorous conditions such as ganglion (Fig. 29-29), and lipoma are among the more frequent. In fractures around the wrist if the wrist is immobilized in marked flexion and ulnar deviation, which has been the case in Colles fractures, this has caused acute compression of the median nerve immediately after reduction.

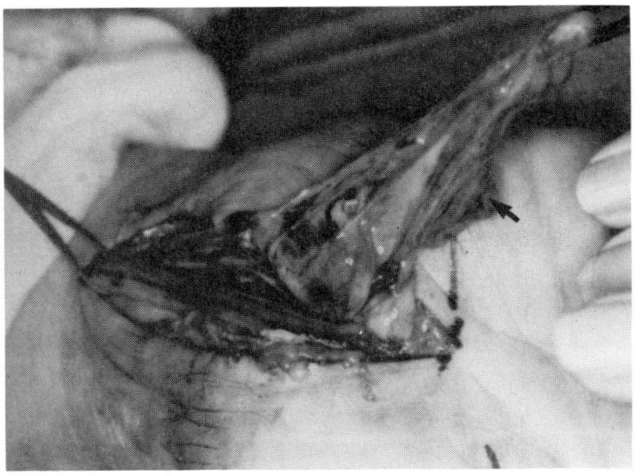

Figure 29-28. Chronic tenosynovitis (*arrow*) in carpal tunnel, vessel loop around median nerve.

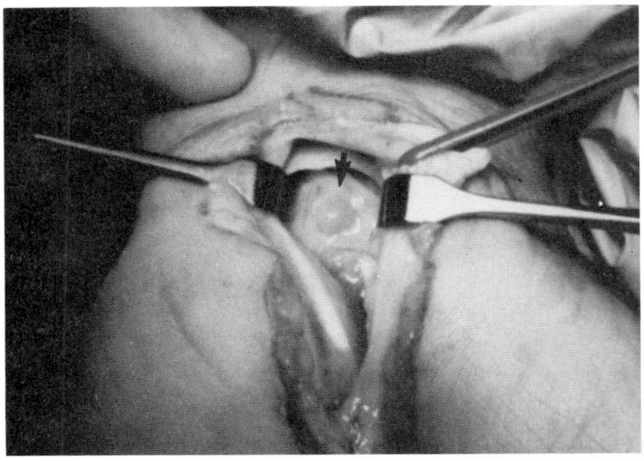

Figure 29-29. Ganglion (*arrow*) in carpal tunnel, vessel loop around median nerve.

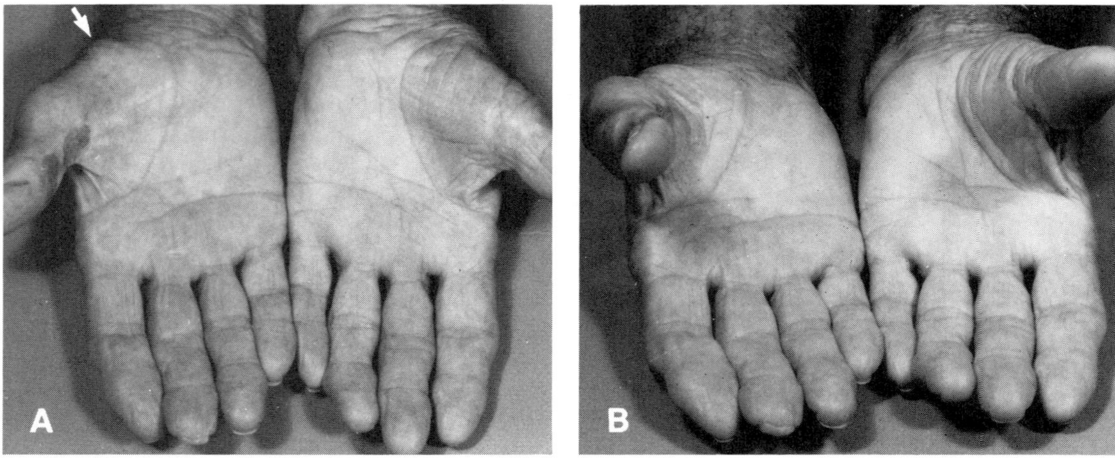

Figure 29-30. (*A*) Atrophy of thenar muscles (*arrow*) in right hand of patient with long-standing carpal tunnel syndrome. (*B*) Inability of patient in (*A*) to abduct and oppose thumb.

Paresthesias over the sensory distribution of the median nerve—that is, the radial three and a half digits with thenar atrophy—is the most common finding. It frequently awakens the patient at night with burning and numbness in the hand that is relieved by shaking the hand. A positive Tinel's sign may be demonstrated by percussing the median nerve at the wrist. Atrophy of the thenar muscles is common in half of the patients (Fig. 29-30). A positive Phalen test with acute flexion of the wrist within 30 seconds increases the paresthesias and pain. One may apply a blood pressure cuff on the upper arm sufficient to produce venous distention and initiate the symptoms. Carpal tunnel syndrome is common during pregnancy due to edema but usually disappears by the sixth week after delivery. EMG studies may show decrease in the nerve conduction velocity of the median nerve.

Early treatment may use a wrist control splint, mainly at night. Some authors suggest an injection of steroids within the carpal tunnel (Fig. 29-31). Anti-inflammatories and antidiuretics have been used. In the acute syndrome following trauma, surgical decompression is probably indicated. If there is no response to conservative measures of rest and medication, then surgical decompression may be performed.

PRONATOR SYNDROME

Pronator syndrome occurs where the median nerve passes deep to both heads of the pronator teres muscle, at the thickening of the lacertus fibrosis, or at the flexor superficial fibrous arch within the muscle belly. The significance of the pronator syndrome is that it may easily be mistaken for carpal tunnel compression. One can reproduce the proximal forearm pain on having the patient pronate the forearm and flex the wrist against resistance. The Phalen test is negative, and there is no Tinel's sign at the wrist. On the EMG studies, nerve conduction may be delayed but not at the wrist. There may be a positive Tinel's sign at the juncture of the two heads of the pronator muscle. Treatment may consist initially of splinting the forearm in pronation with or without elbow flexion. If this does not relieve the symptoms, then surgical decompression is indicated.

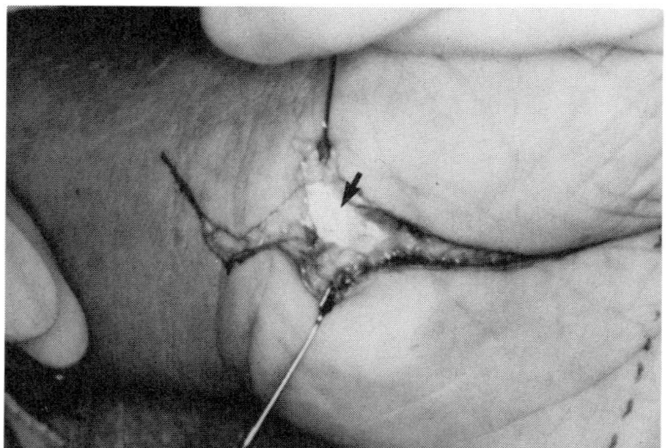

Figure 29-31. Nonabsorption of steroids (*arrow*) after injection into carpal tunnel.

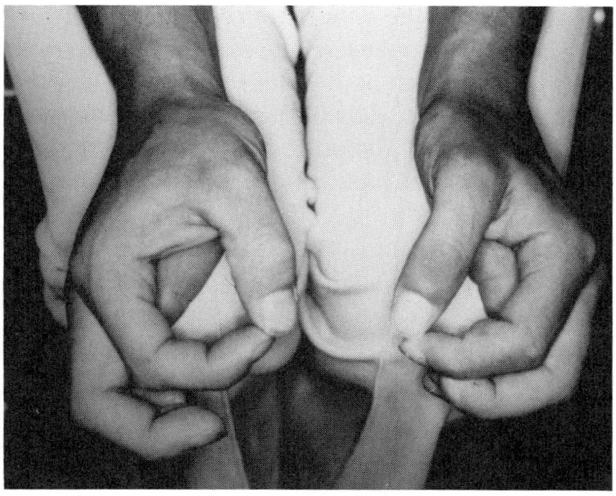

Figure 29-32. Patient with anterior interosseous nerve syndrome, left hand. Unable to make a circle. Normal on right hand.

ANTERIOR INTEROSSEOUS SYNDROME

The anterior interosseous nerve may be compressed where it crosses the tendinous origin of the deep head of the pronator teres muscle. It may also be compressed at the origin of the flexor digitorum superficialis muscle to the middle finger and the origin of a profundus muscle. There may be accessory muscles from the superficialis to the profundus muscle and a muscle known as Gantzer's muscle, which is an accessory head to the flexor pollicis longus. Pain in the forearm is very commonly the presenting symptom. The pinch attitude of the hand due to paralysis of the flexor pollicis longus and the flexor digitorum profundus at the index and long fingers is pathognomonic. When the patient is asked to pinch with a circle this is impossible (Fig. 29-32). So the pinch looks more elliptical rather than circular. Treatment usually consists of rest; if there is no improvement, surgical decompression should be done.

RADIAL NERVE COMPRESSION SYNDROMES

POSTERIOR INTEROSSEOUS SYNDROME

The posterior interosseous nerve can be compressed at the arcade of Frohse, where the nerve pierces the two heads of the supinator muscle. If the nerve is compressed partially, the extensor digitorum communis at one or more of the fingers is paralyzed. Dislocation of the elbow or a fractured dislocation such as in a Monteggia's fracture of the forearm can cause this syndrome. Synovitis associated with rheumatoid arthritis can also compress the posterior interosseous nerve. The common mistake is to consider the diagnosis of rupture of the extensor tendons at the wrist instead of the posterior interosseous nerve syndrome. Pain is frequently the first complaint and is later accompanied or replaced by weakness and paralysis. When it is fully developed, the patient complains of the inability to extend the fingers and weakness in extension of the wrist (Fig. 29-33). On attempted extension of the wrist, the wrist goes into radial deviation. Attempted extension of the fingers produces a characteristic posture in which the interphalangeal joints are fully extended but the metacarpal phalangeal joints cannot be extended beyond 45 degrees.

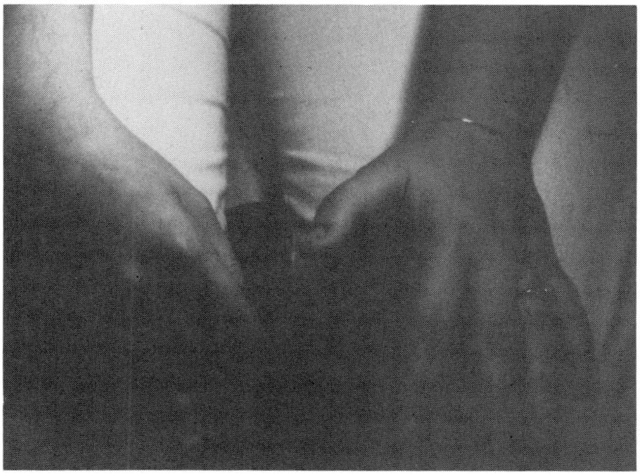

Figure 29-33. Patient with posterior interosseous nerve syndrome, right hand. Unable to extend fingers. When the patient attempts to extend her wrist, only radial deviation is accomplished. Left hand normal.

RADIAL TUNNEL SYNDROME

The fibrous bands tethering the nerve to the radial humeral joint, the extensor carpi radialis brevis, and the arcade of Frohse have been implicated in this syndrome. These anatomic structures compress the nerve when the wrist is passively flexed and pronated or when the wrist is extended or supinated against resistance. Men and women appear to be affected equally, and the dominant hand is involved. Pain is often the only presenting symptom. The patient has very frequently been diagnosed as having tennis elbow and may have had several injections in the lateral epicondylar region for this. In the pure radial tunnel syndrome, there is no sensory disturbance or motor loss. Tenderness is located along the line of the radial nerve over the radial head anteriorly and over the lateral epicondyle. Unlike tennis elbow, however, it is less severe than over the course of the nerve. Resisted supination of the extended arm may also produce pain over the radial tunnel. Conservative measures should be proposed initially, with rest from repetitive motion and injection of anti-inflammatories with steroids. If no improvement results from this treatment, then surgical exploration is indicated.

ULNAR NERVE COMPRESSION SYNDROMES

ULNAR TUNNEL SYNDROME (GUYON'S CANAL)

The volar carpal ligament, called the pisohamate ligament, that roofs over the canal of Guyon covers the ulnar nerve and artery. Ulnar nerve compression can commonly be caused here. When it does occur, it is most frequently associated with trauma or the presence of an abnormal structure. Repetitive trauma over the base of the hypothenar eminence can commonly cause this syndrome. Thrombosis of the ulnar artery can also occur in this situation. A ganglion is by far the most common cause of ulnar nerve palsy in Guyon's canal. Aberrant muscles, such as an accessory palmaris longus, duplication of hypothenar muscles, or abnormal origin of the hypothenar muscles can be the cause. Deep motor branch compression is common, and patients complain of progressive weakness of the hand, especially in pinch (Fig. 29-34). There may also be loss of sensation and paresthesias in the ulnar nerve distribution of the ulnar one and a half fingers. Electromyography shows that the nerve conduction velocity is decreased from the wrist to the first dorsal interosseous muscle. Treatment may be rest and splinting; if there is no improvement, then surgical exploration is indicated.

CUBITAL TUNNEL SYNDROME

Traumatic ulnar neuritis, tardy ulnar palsy or cubital tunnel syndrome at the elbow, was one of the first peripheral nerve compressions to be described. There may be several causes (Fig. 29-35), such as tightness of the aponeurosis between the two heads of the flexor carpi ulnaris or direct blow to the flexed elbow. Injuries to the bones of the elbow joint, especially in childhood (Fig. 29-36), may result in a tardy ulnar palsy.

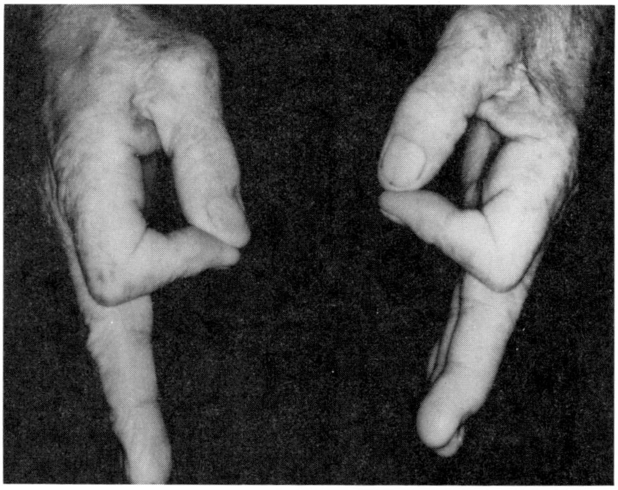

Figure 29-34. Weakness of pinch of left hand with atrophy of first dorsal interosseous and adductor pollicus muscles secondary to ulnar nerve compression.

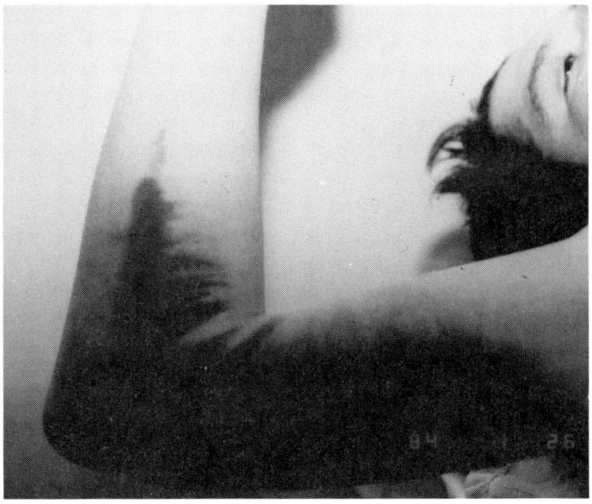

Figure 29-35. Ulnar compression at elbow secondary to hemorrhage from a fall.

Fractures of the lateral condyle and dislocation of the radial head in children can lead to a cubitus valgus with stretching of the ulnar nerve at the elbow. If the ulnar nerve is not anatomically situated in the groove or cubital tunnel, it will dislocate (Fig. 29-37), and recurrent dislocation by motion of the elbow can cause the syndrome. Symptoms are pain in the upper extremity and paresthesias and numbness involving the ulnar innervated one and a half digits. Weakness in the ulnar innervated muscles is common. There is usually a positive Tinel's sign at the elbow over the ulnar nerve. The ulnar nerve supplies the flexor digitorum profundus to the ulnar two fingers and the flexor carpi ulnaris muscles. These have been demonstrated to be weak or absent secondary to ulnar nerve compression (Fig. 29-38). With electromyographic studies, slowing of the nerve conduction velocity across the elbow is suggestive of the diagnosis. Once the diagnosis is established, surgical intervention is usually required. In early stages one may use a long arm plastic splint to rest the elbow. This may help as far as pain and paresthesias are concerned. Surgical approaches have been many and varied. All the procedures have one thing in common: transposition of the nerve away from its exposed area. I prefer submuscular anterior transposition of the ulnar nerve over the other methods.

It is imperative that the previously described peripheral nerve compression syndromes be differently diagnosed from thoracic outlet syndrome and cervical root syndromes. This requires accurate history taking and physical examination. Electromyographic studies are certainly helpful to separate central lesions, such as cervical root radiculopathy, from peripheral lesions.

STENOSING TENOSYNOVITIS

Stenosing tenosynovitis occurs more often in the hand and wrist than anywhere else in the body. When the first dorsal compartment consisting of the extensor pollicis brevis and the

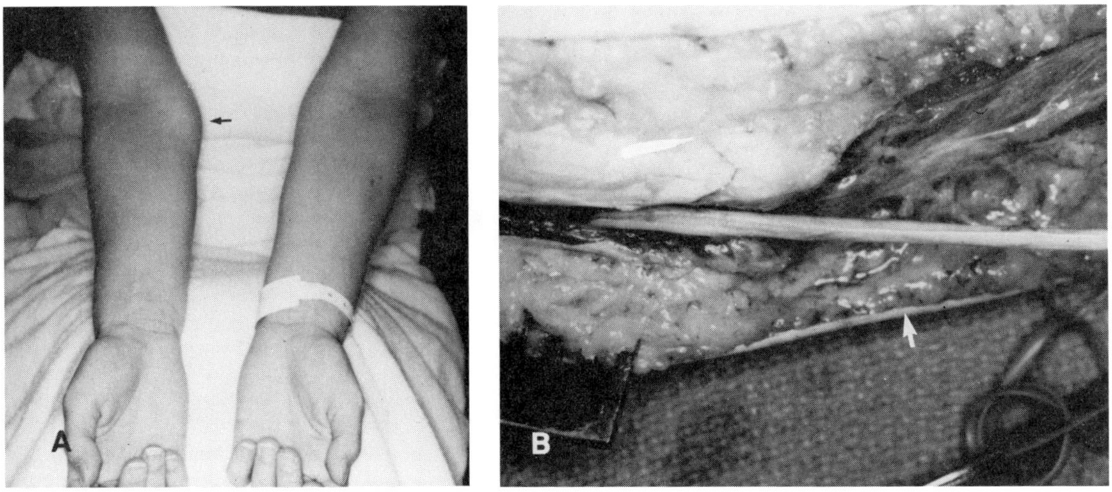

Figure 29-36. (*A*) Ulnar nerve compression at elbow secondary to cubitus valgus deformity (*arrow*) on right arm from old malunited supracondylar humerus fracture. (*B*) Tight hyperemic ulnar nerve (*arrow*) at surgery for patient in *A*.

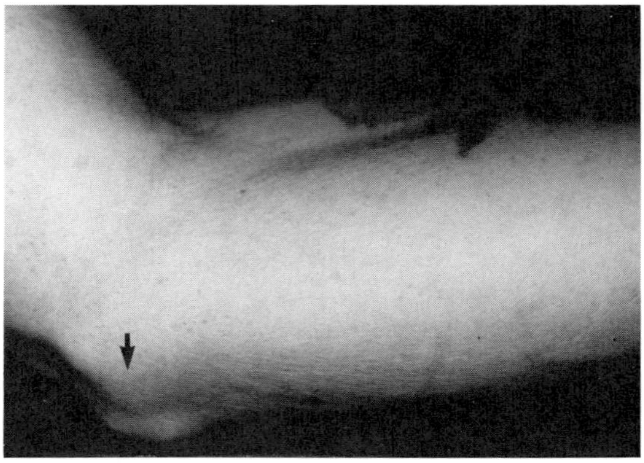

Figure 29-37. Painful "snapping" subluxing ulnar nerve (*arrow*) at elbow.

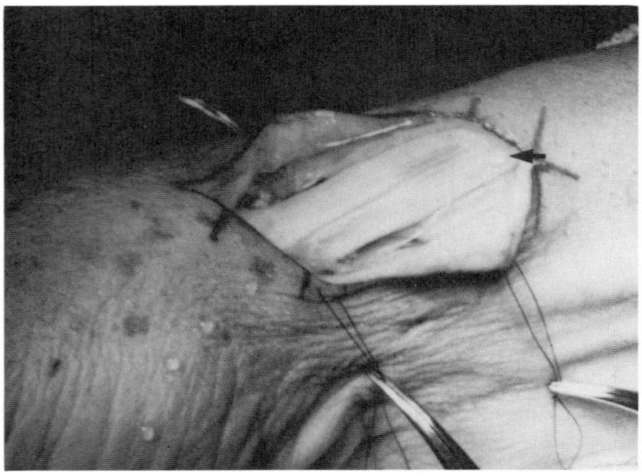

Figure 29-39. Surgical release of de Quervain's disease. Arrow indicates 1st dorsal extensor compartment.

abductor pollicis longus tendons are affected, the condition is sometimes called de Quervain's disease. When the long flexor tendons are involved, trigger thumb, trigger finger, or snapping finger occur. Less often, the extensor pollicis longus may be affected at the level of Lister's tubercle. Any of the other tendons that pass beneath the dorsal wrist retinaculum may also be involved. The tenosynovitis that precedes the stenosis may result from an otherwise dormant or subclinical collagen disease. Recurrent mild trauma, such as that experienced by carpenters, waitresses, or elevator operators, may be the cause. The case histories indicate that acute trauma may initiate the pathologic condition. The stenosis occurs at a point where the direction of the tendon changes, for here a sheath or a fibrous theca acts as a pulley and friction is maximum. Although the synovium lubricates the sheath, friction may cause a reaction when the repetition of a particular pattern of movement is necessary, as in winding a fine coil of wire or stacking laundry.

DE QUERVAIN'S DISEASE

Stenosing tenosynovitis (Fig. 29-39) of the first dorsal compartment occurs typically in women between the ages of 30 and 50 years. The cause is almost always occupational or may be associated with rheumatoid arthritis. The presenting symptoms are usually pain and tenderness at the radial styloid or the anatomic snuff box. Sometimes a thickening of the sheath is palpable. A Finkelstein's test is usually positive. This test is performed when the patient acutely flexes the wrist and places

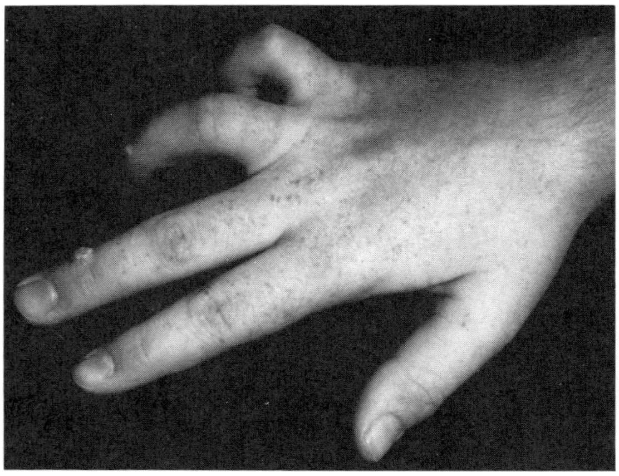

Figure 29-38. Typical clawhand deformity secondary to ulnar nerve palsy.

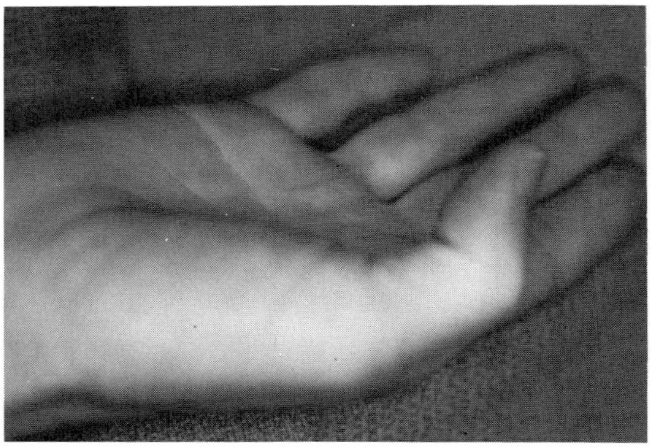

Figure 29-40. Trigger thumb in adult.

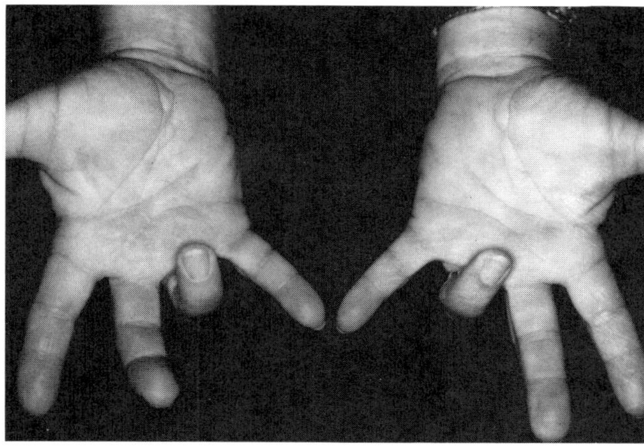

Figure 29-41. Bilateral trigger ring fingers.

it in ulnar deviation and flexes the thumb to the base of the little finger. Cases have been described in which the test is performed passively, with the examiner doing the maneuvers. The author prefers to have the patient perform the test actively. Conservative treatment consists of rest in a thumb spica splint or cast and the use of anti-inflammatories, which usually results in relief of symptoms. Local injections of steroids may be used. If a conservative regime is unsuccessful, then surgical exploration is indicated. The most common findings are aberrant tendons at the insertion of the abductor pollicis longus tendon. A common complication during surgery is injury of the superficial sensory branch of the radial nerve.

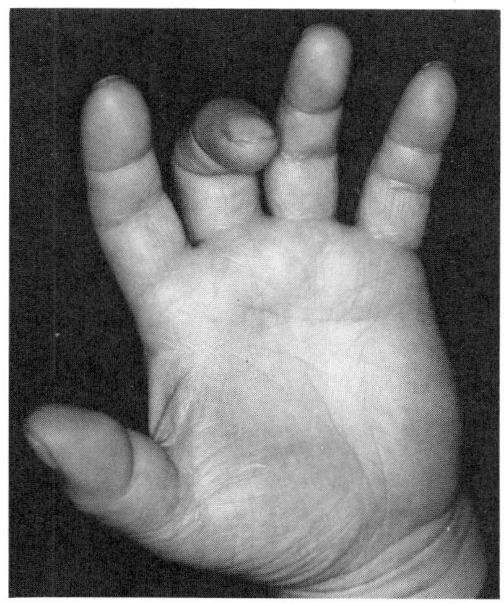

Figure 29-42. Trigger middle finger.

TRIGGER FINGERS AND THUMB

A trigger thumb may be congenital in the infant but is usually associated with a collagen disease in middle-aged adults (Fig. 29-40). Several fingers may be involved, but the ring (Fig. 29-41) and middle fingers (Fig. 29-42) are most commonly involved. A nodule on the flexor tendon may be palpated just proximal to the A-1 pulley at the distal palmar crease. As the patient flexes the finger, this nodule is forced under the A-1 pulley and locks in that position and the finger has to be passively extended with considerable pain. This can also be present in rheumatoid arthritis with flexor tenosynovitis, or occasionally a partial lacerated flexor tendon may heal with a nodule sufficiently large to cause triggering. One of the misdiagnoses is that although the constriction is opposite the metacarpal phalangeal joint, the interphalangeal joint is the one that locks or snaps. This is particularly noted in the thumb but can occur in the PIP joints of the other fingers. Treatment may be local injection of steroids or anti-inflammatory drugs with or without splinting. I feel that this is a mechanical problem and that surgical release of the A-1 pulley is indicated.

Stenosing tenosynovitis may occur with the extrinsic extensor tendon or with both flexors and extensors. This usually occurs at their bony insertions. They usually respond to conservative measures of rest, anti-inflammatories, and a local injection of steroids. If not, then surgical intervention may be necessary.

HIGH-PRESSURE INJECTION INJURIES

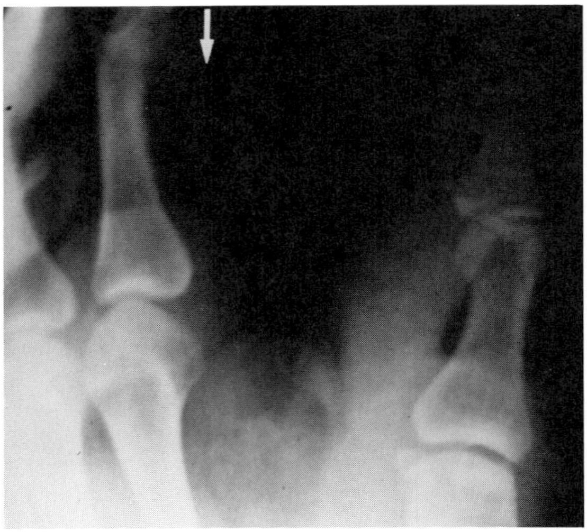

Figure 29-43. Paint gun injection injury to thumb. Radiograph showing radiopaque material (*arrow*) in soft tissue.

Accidental, inadvertent, or careless triggering of a high-pressure injection gun most commonly causes injury to the fingers. The culprit can be a high-pressure airless paint spray gun, the fuel injection mechanism of a diesel engine, a break in a faulty hydraulic line of a high-pressure system, a high-pressure grease gun, or occasionally a tear gas gun or even guns that are being used for nails and rivets.

A thin stream of fluid is ejected from the nozzle of a high-pressure system at a velocity of usually 4000 lb/sq. in. This velocity is usually as high as that of a .22 long bullet. The high-velocity jet hits the skin at a very small point of contact, which may be several inches from the nozzle of the gun. This tremendous kinetic energy is released and absorbed in the soft tissue after skin penetration. The severity of the injury depends on the velocity of the fluid, the amount of material, the type of material, and the anatomic location and penetration. From the tip of the finger proximal spread takes basically three routes: subcutaneous, through the flexor synovial sheath, and along fascial planes and neurovascular bundles. I have seen extension well into the forearm passing through Parona's space in as far as the elbow. It is important to obtain radiographs (Fig. 29-43), since most of the material is radiopaque and can be seen on the radiograph. The presenting symptoms are usually benign initially and misleading. At the time of injury usually a mild stinging sensation is noted with some digital swelling, depending on the amount of material injected. Sometimes the person does not seek immediate medical attention. Within 2 to 4 hours of injury, pain, paresthesia, and swelling increase rapidly. Paint thinners or paint solvents that contain turpentine, toluene, or naphtha cause more severe symptoms and symptoms that progress more rapidly. Because of the benign appearance of the entrance wound the first physician who sees the patient places him or her on an antibiotic and advises that the involved hand be elevated; usually the patient is also given a prescription for analgesics. Although the prognosis of a high-pressure injection injury, particularly if paint thinner or solvent is involved, is generaly poor, the only hope for reasonable salvage of function is *immediate surgery*, not conservative treatment. Immediate surgery

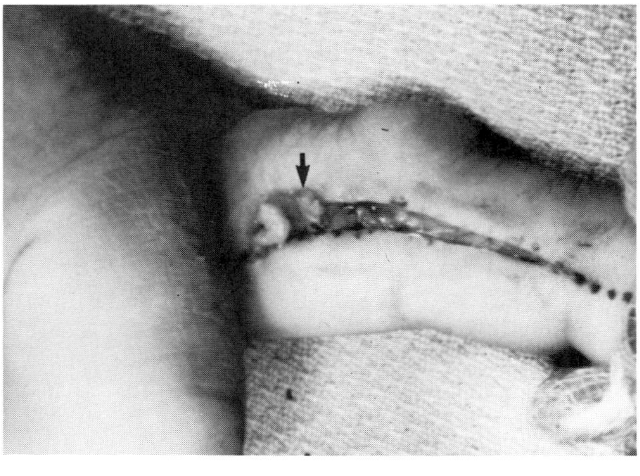

Figure 29-44. Grease gun injection injury to finger. Midlateral incision with grease (*arrow*) at base of finger.

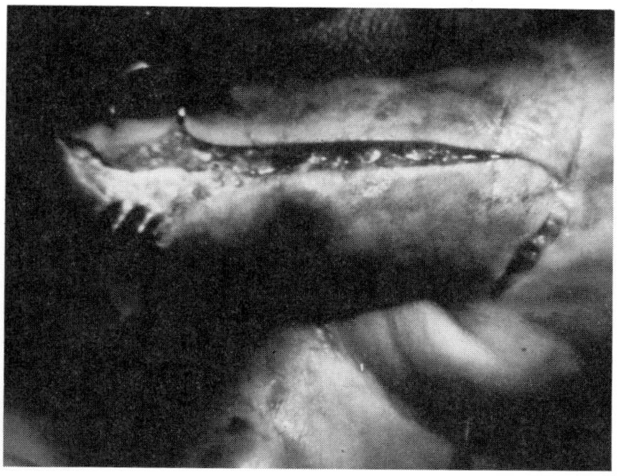

Figure 29-45. Paint gun injection injury to thumb. Midlateral incision continuing into palm.

with wide exposure to decompress and adequately debride, to eliminate chemical irritants as much as possible, to decrease pressure in a closed space, and, it is hoped, to decrease the possibility of secondary infection. The paint or grease should be carefully dissected from the fibrous tendon sheath or neurovascular bundle. The approach is midlateral (Fig. 29-44), since direct exposure by Bruner zigzag incisions may cause necrosis of the tendon sheath early on. The incisions are carried into the palm (Fig. 29-45), across the wrist, and even into the forearm as far as the elbow if necessary. The wounds are left open and the patient may have to be brought to the operating room within 48 hours for another look. The patient is treated with intravenous antibiotics. Wounds are usually healed by secondary intention and may be grafted at a later date. Only early recognition of this type of injury and immediate effective surgical intervention can prevent needless tissue destruction.

HAND INFECTIONS

CELLULITIS

Cellulitus represents the initial phase of bacterial infections. Depending on local factors, the type of infectious agent, and the method of occurrence, an infection may manifest itself as only cellulitis, abscess formation, or tenosynovitis. Because of free access to various tissue planes, the dorsum of the fingers, hand, and forearm is most commonly involved with cellulitis. An overwhelming majority of these infections are caused by gram-positive cocci. Clinically, cellulitis is manifested by erythema, swelling, mild to moderate pain, and occasionally lymphangitis (Fig. 29-46). Elevation, rest, and antibiotics are recommended. Streptococci are still the most common organisms causing cellulitis, and antibiotics appropriate for this organism are indicated. Usually high doses of penicillin are required if the patient is not allergic. The second most common organism causing cellulitis is *Staphylococcus aureus*.

PARONYCHIA

Subcuticular abscesses involving the nail fold are termed *paronychia* and constitute approximately 30% of all infectious processes presenting for treatment. Paronychia may originate as a hangnail or similar minor injury. Clinically, it is characterized by erythema, swelling, and tenderness at the nail fold. The process may involve the nail and result in an apical or subungual abscess (Fig. 29-47). Early treatment may consist of merely lifting the eponychial fold to permit drainage. If the area of involvement is large, anesthesia may be necessary for adequate drainage. Chronic paronychias are treated more aggressively by removal of the underlying nail. Causes of chronic paronychia may be a retained foreign body, necrotic nail, or possibly fungus infection. These must be eliminated for adequate treatment. Vascular insufficiency conditions such as Raynaud's phenomenon and scleroderma may occasionally be associated with chronic paronychia.

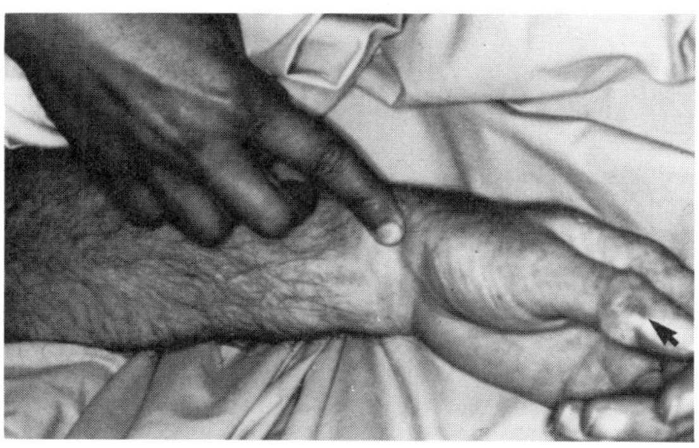

Figure 29-46. Bee sting (*arrow*) to thumb with secondary cellulitis and lymphangitis of forearm.

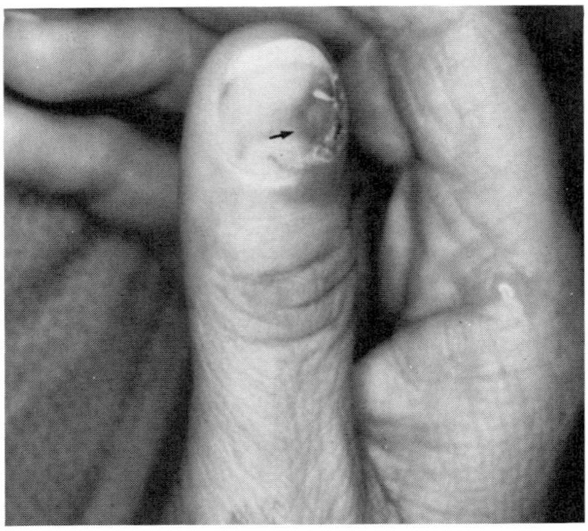

Figure 29-47. Subungual abscess (*arrow*) in thumb of physician's wife.

FELON

A felon is an abscess formation in the distal pulp involving multiple septa. This term should not be used for minor infections of the pulp, primarily because of the recommended method of treating felons. Clinically, there is extreme tenderness, with swelling, erythema, and throbbing of the fingertip (Fig. 29-48). Because of the fibrous septa in the pulp, significant destruction of tissue may quickly ensue, as well as osteomyelitis. Treatment with antibiotic therapy alone is not enough because of the rapid destruction possible with undrained felons. Surgical drainage may require separation of all septa of the pulp from the periosteum by means of incision just under the nail bed and distal phalanx. Fortunately, patients seek treatment relatively early in the disease process and through-and-through incisions are usually not necessary. To allow adequate drainage, however, the incision must still be extensive enough to separate the pulp septa from the phalanx in the area involved.

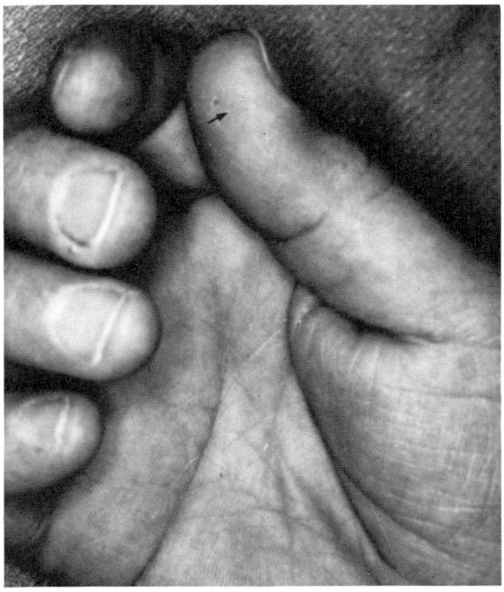

Figure 29-48. Felon (*arrow*) of thumb in heart transplant patient.

SUBUNGUAL ABSCESS

Occurring beneath the nail and above the nail bed, or matrix, subungual abscess may result from the spread of a paronychia or apical abscess or from penetrating trauma. The pus beneath the nail may be visible, and a small incision or unroofing at the site may be curative. If the abscess is not visible, the maximum point of tenderness will serve as a guide to it. Removal of the entire nail plate and clearing of the cul-de-sac are curative.

APICAL ABSCESS

Occuring at the apex of the nail and the subeponychial tissues, an apical abscess generally presents with a swollen and tender fingertip and a history of minor penetrating trauma to the area. Subsequent infection of a hyponychium leads to the apical abscess. Removal of a wedge of this pulp abscess and associated nail plate is the optimal treatment.

HERPES SIMPLEX

The presentation of herpes simplex on the hands varies from a single pale elevated vesicle to multiple vesicles within an erythematous area. Often the lesions occur simultaneously, with similar lesions around the lips and oral mucosa. Human saliva will transmit the disease, and physicians, nurses, dentists, and anesthesia personnel are at increased risk. Lesions, which may be painful, will increase in size, merge, and then dry up and heal over a 2-week period. Frequent dressing changes aid in the prevention of secondary bacterial infection of the vesicles. Elevation, immobilization, the new antiviral agent acyclovir (Zovirax), and analgesics may be helpful. Herpetic infections may progress to devastating systemic disease in the immunosuppressed patient.

PYOGENIC GRANULOMA

Pyogenic granuloma is a vascular lesion that is red, projects above the skin's surface, and is a nidus of subacute or chronic infection. It is often termed "bleeding wart" and actually represents hypertrophic granulation tissue usually caused by retained foreign material at the base of the trauma-related lesion. Treatment of the small lesion includes complete excision of the granulation tissue with excision of a narrow margin of circumferential skin and meticulous debridement of the base of the lesion to remove any foreign material. Rapid healing by reepithelization occurs. After debridement of a larger lesion occasionally a split thickness skin graft or a local transposition flap is necessary. It is important to submit the excised lesion for microscopic examination. One may see premalignant or malignant lesions that commonly occur in this area.

PALMAR AND COLLAR BUTTON ABSCESSES

The palmar space exclusive of the flexor tendon sheaths anatomically allow for free spread of infectious processes. A superficial palmar abscess may extend through the palmar fascia to deeper areas, which must be detected at the time of drainage. The spread of an abscess from palmar to dorsal surface, or vice versa, is known as a collar button abscess and should be suspected with infections in this area. Only adequate surgical drainage of both abscess cavities will effect a cure.

WEB SPACE INFECTIONS

Although infections in the web space may occur after traumatic or nontraumatic interruption of the skin, they more likely represent an infection moving proximally from digital involvement, distally from the palmar or thenar eminence, or via the lumbrical canals and fascial spaces. The anatomy of the web space area, including the MP joints, flexor and extensor tendons and their sheaths, and the neurovascular bundles to the digits, must be considered in order to avoid damage to these structures during treatment. Examination of the hand reveals a painful tender web space, with swollen tissues, the edema being most pronounced dorsally, where loose tissue planes allow for the greatest expansion. The hand is held stiffly, since movement of the MP joints is painful. The fingers are angled outward, away from the involved web space. One must drain these abscesses by longitudinal incisions on either the dorsal or palmar aspects of the web space. A transverse incision along the ridge of the web space will accomplish drainage but usually at the expense of a contracted web space after healing.

FLEXOR TENOSYNOVITIS

The flexor tendon sheaths are characterized anatomically by restrictive retinacular fibers on the palmar and lateral sides and the rigid phalanx dorsally. This is in contrast to the extensor tendon sheaths that lie in loose areolar tissue. This anatomic fact is primarily responsible for the severity of infections involving the flexor tendon sheaths. Because of the closed compartment type of process involved in tenosynovitis, rapid destruction of the gliding mechanism ensues. Kanavel's four signs of tenosynovitis (Fig. 29-49) remain the most appropriate way to make the diagnosis clinically. These four signs are generalized swelling circumferentially, including the palmar and dorsal aspect of the finger; tenderness over the flexor tendon sheath; the flexed position of the finger; and pain on attempted extension of the finger actively. Tenosynovitis involving the small finger and the thumb may result in extension to either and is called a horseshoe abscess. This is due to the anatomic proximity of the radial and ulnar bursa at the wrist. The flexor tendons of the small finger end in the ulnar bursa at the wrist and the flexor tendon of the thumb ends in the radial bursa at the wrist; therefore an infection from one may extend to the other. The surgical treatment is through a midlateral incision with an incision also made at the base of the A-1 pulley, which is the end of the bursa for each finger. The sheath must be opened in at least two locations and through-and-through irrigation must be performed. I prefer through-and-through irrigation at surgery, followed by early motion and soap-and-water wound washes within 24 to 36 hours. Other authors advise placing a catheter in the sheath for subsequent irrigation. Intravenous antibiotics and elevation are appropriate until hand washings are started.

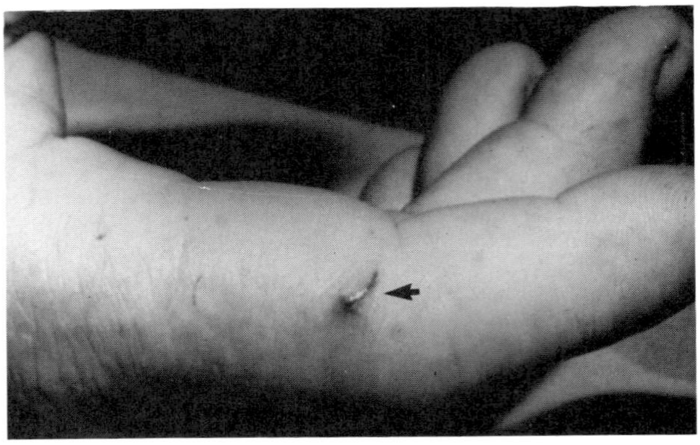

Figure 29-49. Flexor tenosynovitis of index finger. Arrow indicates entrance wound.

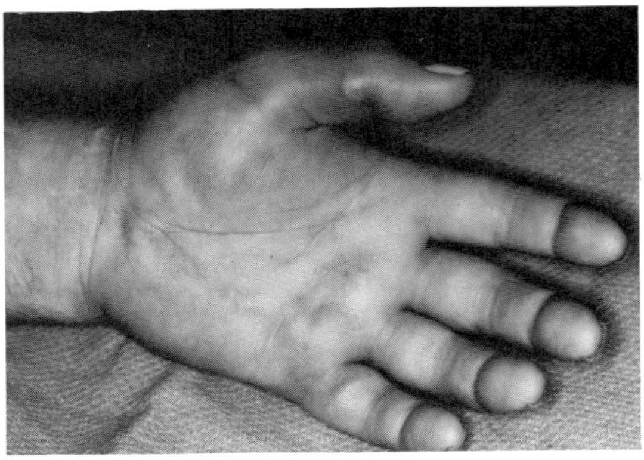

Figure 29-50. Radial bursa, thenar, and midpalmar space infection.

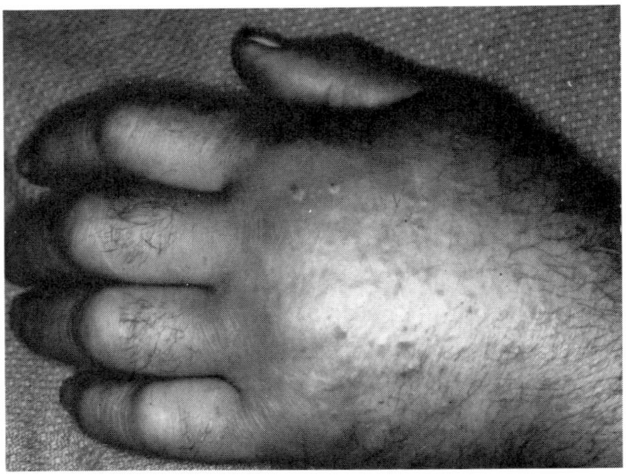

Figure 29-51. Dorsal edema secondary to lymphangitis.

DEEP SPACE INFECTIONS

Infection of a deep fascial space of the palm (Fig. 29-50) is usually caused by a direct penetrating injury or rupture of a flexor tenosynovitis or web space infections through the lumbrical canal. The chief symptom is marked tenderness over the palm. Involvement of the midpalmer space causes generalized swelling and loss of normal palmar anatomy. Involvement of the thenar space causes ballooning of the entire thenar area and the thumb index web area. Associated dorsal edema (Fig. 29-51) is remarkable and is usually secondary to lymphatic lymphangitis. Infection may spread from the thenar space into the synovial flexor sheath of the index finger and sometimes the long finger. Infection of the midpalmar space may extend into the sheath of the ring finger or the long finger. Therefore surgical drainage depends on where the abscess points. Drainage of the midpalmar space is necessary in a distal palm or on the ulnar border of the midpalm radial to the hypothenar compartment.

Drainage of the thenar space may be dorsal or palmar and incision should avoid injury to the recurrent motor branch of the median nerve and not violate the thumb index web to prevent a later web space contracture.

HUMAN AND ANIMAL BITES

One must constantly be aware of the possibility of human bites in evaluating hand injuries. The history is often misleading; therefore the seriousness of potential infections must be stressed to the patient. The mechanism of wounding, which involves a puncture wound inoculating pathogenic organisms, results in a superficial closure and deep bacterial growth. Only aggressive treatment will prevent disastrous sequelae, including digital amputation. Although these wounds appear trivial (Fig. 29-52) or may be overlooked in the treatment of more serious injuries, they are potentially disastrous, and aggressive treatment with hospitalization—including surgical debridement with open treatment, intravenous antibiotic coverage, and adequate tetanus prophylaxis—is strongly recommended. Often the history may be deceptive because the patient is embarrassed and does not wish to reveal that the cause of injury was a fight. A human bite injury should be suspected in any jagged open wound on a dorsal aspect of the MP joint area, and hospitalization is recommended if the injury extends into the bone or joint. Again, as mentioned previously, early motion and soap and water washes of wounds are performed.

Animal bites, particularly cat and dog bites, usually contain *Pasteurella multocida*, a gram-negative rod that is sensitive to penicillin alone. These rather innocuous injuries may cause prolonged morbidity if adequate treatment is not rapidly initiated.

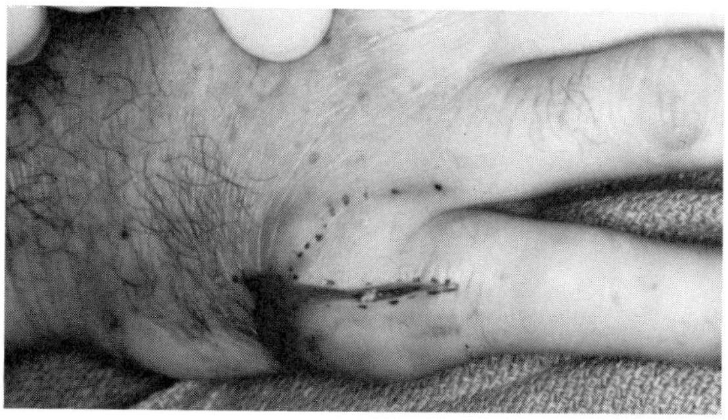

Figure 29-52. Human bite infection secondary to fight. Beginning incision showing pus culturing anerobes and staphylococci.

SPECIAL INFECTIONS

INFECTIONS ASSOCIATED WITH DRUG ADDICTS

The more common pathogens associated with hand infections in addicts (Fig. 29-53) are *Staphylococcus aureus* and *E. coli*. The increased scar tissue in the hands from the result of previous extravasation of drugs into the subcutaneous tissue often mask local signs of infection until irreparable damage is done. This coupled with the tendency of addicts to postpone early treatment results in extensive infectious involvement of the hands in these individuals. Gas gangrene and tetanus are commonly found in drug addicts because of the use of contaminated needles.

Clostridial and other gas-forming infections usually spread rapidly through muscle planes; however, gas may not be noticed until some time later. When gas is detected, either by physical examination of crepitus on palpation or roentgenographs, the diagnosis is obvious. Treatment involves adequate debridement, open treatment of the wounds, and massive doses of penicillin. Some authors have reported on the use of hyperbaric oxygenation.

MYCOBACTERIAL INFECTIONS

A high index of suspicion is necessary in mycobacterial infections. These usually involve the flexor or extensor tenosynovium of the wrist, the carpal bones, and the digital flexor tenosynovium. These may be typical tuberculosis-type infections or atypical infections secondary to atypical mycobacterium. Symptoms are variable, commonly worsening and then becoming quiescent. Swelling is constant with discomfort or pain in the wrist and

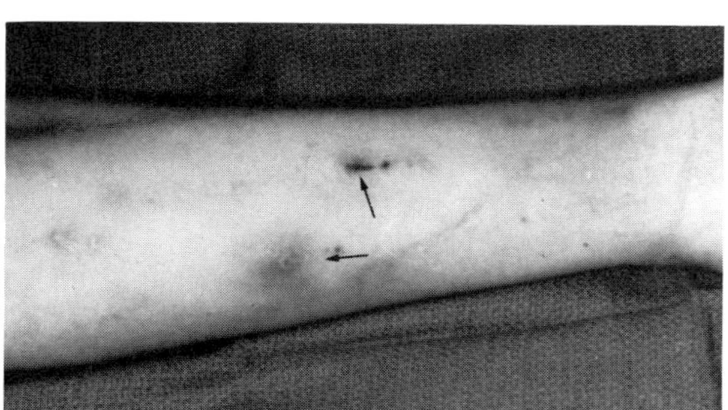

Figure 29-53. Drug addict showing intravenous injection tracks (*arrows*).

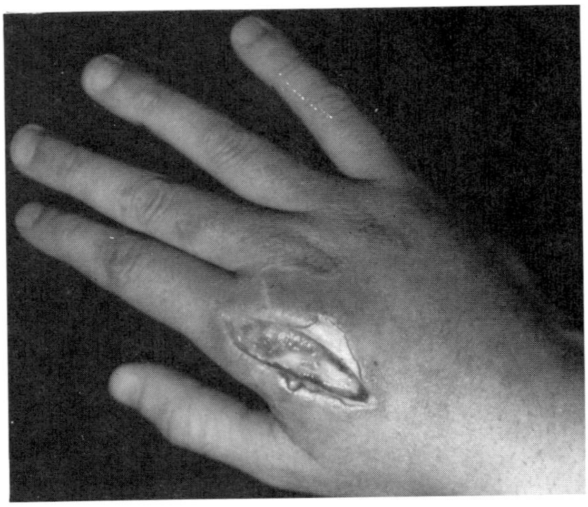

Figure 29-54. Chronic draining skin ulceration after scraping boat bottom. Finally cultured *M. Marinum*.

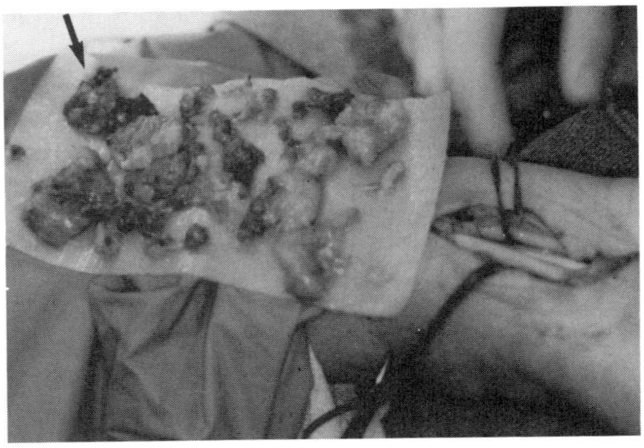

Figure 29-55. Synovectomy dorsal and palmar wrist. Finally cultured *S. Schenkii*. Arrow indicates synovium.

is often diagnosed as median nerve compression caused by tenosynovitis of the flexor tendons. In chronic cases a draining sinus may be present. The differential diagnosis suggests rheumatoid arthritis but usually only one digit is involved, whereas in rheumatoid arthritis multiple digits are involved. The diagnosis is usually decided by an open procedure with histologic granulomas and acid-fast bacilli on smear. Granulomatous changes in the synovium may be caused by foreign bodies or fungus infections. Atypical mycobacterial infections require culturing at temperatures below 37 degrees centigrade. Skin ulceration (Fig. 29-54) secondary to cleaning boats or coral injuries along the gulf coast of the United States is common. Treatment involves surgical synovectomy and chemotherapy. Chemotherapy may consist of streptomycin or rifampin and ethambutol. These treatments usually last for 18 to 24 months.

FUNGUS INFECTIONS

Fungus infections of the hand are rare, they include actinomycosis, blastomycosis, coccidioidomycosis, cryptococcosis, histoplasmosis, and sporotrichosis (Fig. 29-55). These infections are acquired through contact with soil or soil products. Fungus diseases are like tuberculosis in that they are great imitators, and the diagnosis is difficult to make. Roentgenographic findings of marked destruction or osteolysis of the bone with relatively little or no new bone formation is common (Fig. 29-56). This again must be differentiated from mycobacterial infections, neoplasm, and bacterial

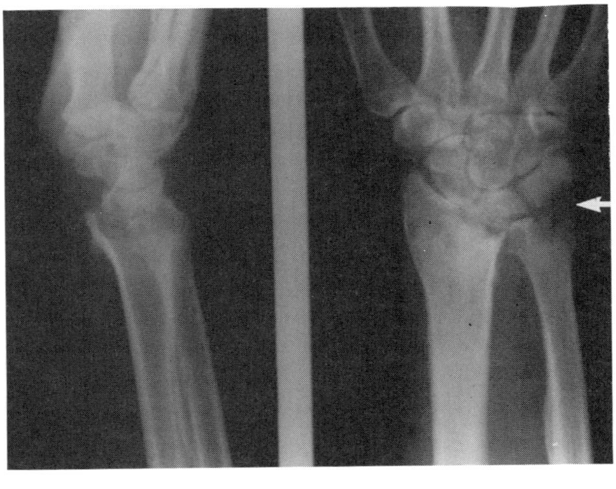

Figure 29-56. Roentgenogram of wrist of patient with positive sporotrichosis culture. Arrow indicates destroyed wrist joint.

infections. A presumptive diagnosis may be provided by skin and serological tests, but true verification comes from direct examination of the fungus or by culture.

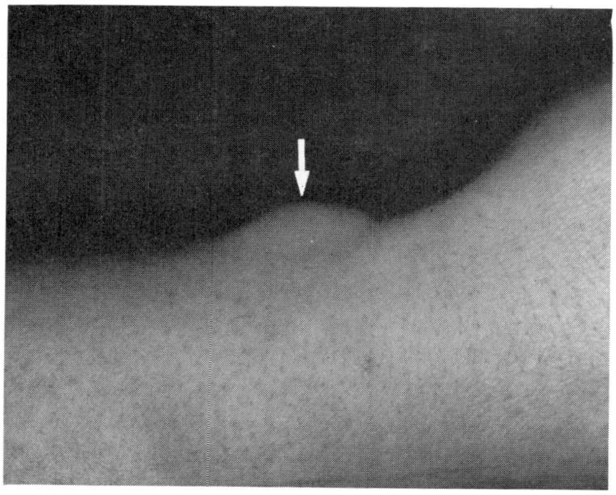

Figure 29-58. Volar ganglion of wrist.

MISCELLANEOUS LESIONS

GANGLIA

Simple ganglia of the hand and wrist are the most frequent soft-tissue tumors of the hand common during the third, fourth, and fifth decades of life. Females are affected more often than males. The etiology of the ganglion remains controversial and unknown. Trauma in the form of degenerative arthritis, however, may play an important role in other variants of the disease, such as mucous cyst and carpal boss ganglia. Common dorsal ganglia (Fig. 29-57) of the wrist usually originate from the capsule overlying the scapholunate articulation. These occur in 60% to 70% of all ganglia. Common volar ganglia of the wrist (Fig. 29-58) occurring in 15% to 20% of all ganglia commonly arise from the same joints and are in close association with the radial artery. Dorsal ganglia of the distal interphalangeal joints or mucous cysts may originate from the extensor tendon itself or more commonly from the joint capsule. Mucous cysts tend to occur more frequently in women past middle age who have osteoarthritic changes. Volar ganglia of the flexor tendon sheaths arise opposite the metacarpal neck or middle shaft of the proximal phalanx. Dorsal ganglia at the base of the second and third metacarpals (carpal bosses) (Fig. 29-59) are associated with highly localized degenerative bony lipping of the capitate and metacarpal. These lesions are rare and occasionally present with pain. The treatment of these lesions is usually nonsurgical. They are surgically excised only when they cause pain or limitation of motion. Some authors will aspirate the cyst with or without injection of steroids. Complete excision presents the best chance for cure but also results in longer time off work and may often be associated with postoperative complications such as hypertrophic scar and keloid formation, joint stiffness, nerve damage, and wound infection.

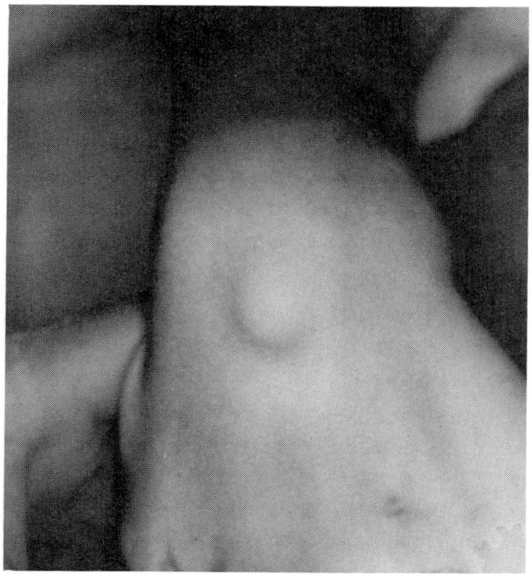

Figure 29-57. Dorsal ganglion of wrist.

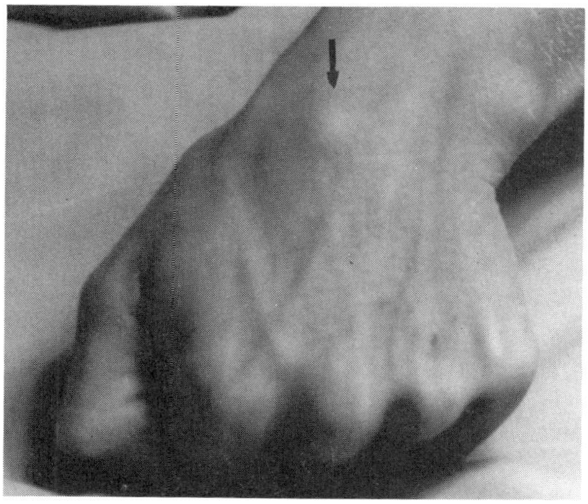

Figure 29-59. Carpal boss (*arrow*) on wrist of champion gymnast.

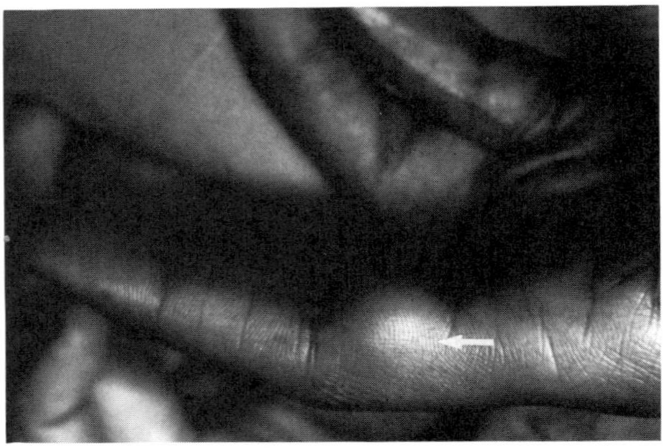

Figure 29-60. Mass (*arrow*) on removal proved to be giant cell tumor of tendon sheath.

GIANT CELL TUMOR

Giant cell tumor of the tendon sheath (Fig. 29-60) is the second most frequent subcutaneous hand tumor and comes to women during their fourth to sixth decades of life. Most tumors involve the fingers more often than any other part of the body, affecting more often the distal interphalangeal joint of the index and middle fingers. The ability of giant cell tumors to erode bone by pressure and to involve overlying dermis is well known. But its benign nature is established. Digital nerve and vessels are often in close approximation to the tumor. Treatment consists of complete local excision of the tumor.

EPIDERMOID INCLUSION CYSTS

Epidermoid inclusion cysts occur (Fig. 29-61) almost always in the palmar surface of the hand or fingers. The development of these lesions is clearly related to injury, but the trauma need not be of perforating character. Frequently, a scar overlying the cyst can be found. The latent period between injury and development of a cyst may vary from a few months to years. They are usually firm, spherical, and nontender. Local complications include infections and bone erosion or a lytic lesion of the terminal phalanx. Treatment consists of removing all the cyst lining and contents and overlying puckered skin. Curettage with a bone graft may be necessary. Also, local flap coverage or skin grafts may be necessary.

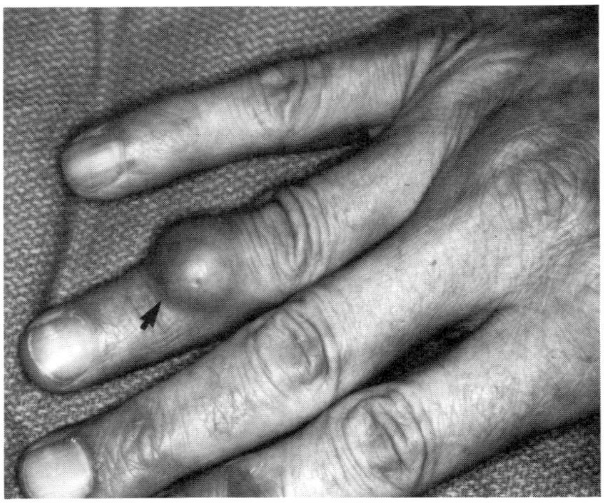

Figure 29-61. Mass (*arrow*) on ring finger proved to be epidermoid inclusion cyst.

MALIGNANT TUMORS

Basal cell carcinoma is rare on the hand but squamous cell carcinoma is not. Squamous cell carcinoma (Fig. 29-62) usually arises in the dorsum of the hand in a male who has been exposed to the sun. The axillary and epitrochlearnodes should be checked at the time of initial examination. Excision of the lesion with at least a centimeter margin is indicated.

Keratoacanthoma is a benign lesion that closely resembles squamous cell carcinoma, both grossly and histologically. It has a circular raised area with a central keratin plug that looks like a central ulceration. A history of extremely rapid growth over a 3- to 4- week period is characteristic.

Malignant melanoma is uncommon on the hands, but several insignificant-appearing lesions require excision to rule out melanoma. All nevi in the palm should be excised. Biopsies should be done of any pigmented area beneath the nail. This may present as only a brown streak of the nail bed.

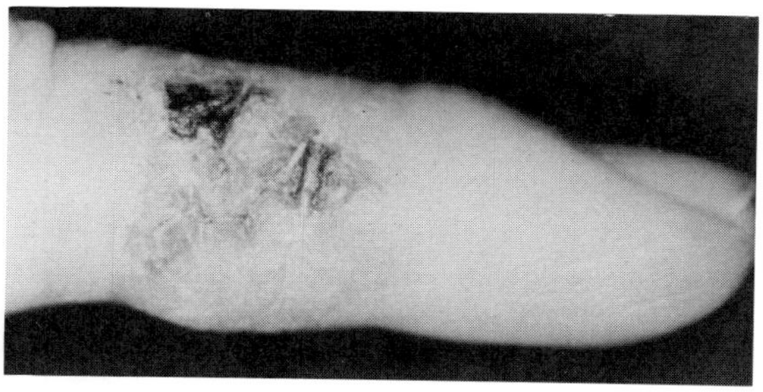

Figure 29-62. Lesion proved to be squamous cell carcinoma in situ (Bowen's disease).

BIBLIOGRAPHY

Boyes JH: Bunnell's Surgery of the Hand, 5th ed, pp 613–638. Philadelphia, JB Lippincott, 1970

Flatt AE: The Care of Minor Hand Injuries, 3rd ed. St Louis, CV Mosby, 1972

Kanavel AB: Infections of the Hand. Philadelphia, Lea & Febiger, 1925

Linscheid RL, Dobyns JH: Common and Uncommon Infections of the Hand. Orthop Clin North Am 6:1063–1104, 1975

Lister: The Hand: Diagnosis and Indications. New York, Churchill Livingstone, 1977

Mann RJ et al: Human Bites of the Hand: Twenty Years of Experience. J Hand Surg 2:97–104, 1977

Milford L: The Hand, 2nd ed. St Louis, CV Mosby, 1982

Omer GE: Injuries to nerves of the upper extremity. J Bone Joint Surg 56A:1615–1624, 1974

Sandzen SC: Atlas of Acute Hand Injuries. New York, McGraw-Hill, 1980

30 Fractures of the Metacarpals and Phalanges

RONALD J. MANN

Fractures of the hand are among the most common injuries treated by the practicing clinician. They may constitute 10% to 30% of injuries seen in an average emergency room and physician's office. There are few other fractures so commonly seen in which treatment outcome can so drastically alter the ultimate function of the patient. The treatment of these fractures has gradually evolved from nontreatment to an incredible variety of external immobilization devices to limited internal fixation and more recently, aggressive operative intervention to provide the patient with rigid internal fixation and early motion. The outcome of no treatment or various methods of external immobilization is well documented, and in certain fractures external immobilization is the treatment of choice. However, in more complicated fractures—in particular, unstable fractures, intra-articular fractures, and multiple fractures—prolonged immobilization can lead to severe loss of motion and ultimately impaired function of the hand. These are the principal factors that have generated an increasing interest in internal fixation and early motion in certain hand fractures.

Some fractures of the phalanges and metacarpals of the hand represent relatively minor injuries whose mechanism of injury is simple, recognition is obvious, treatment is easy, and end results are quite satisfactory. Others cause great difficulty for both patients and physicians. Hand fractures that are unrecognized or ignored by either patient or physician or those in which improper treatment has been given may result in hands whose total function is impaired and whose appearance is altered and, as a result, patient dissatisfaction. These exceptions are common enough to make it necessary for the physician who treats injured hands to be fully familiar with all types of hand fractures and to recognize those that respond well to simple treatment and those in which more elaborate measures are necessary.

It is also important that the physician be able to inform his patient early in the course of treatment what the probable outcome will be to avoid disillusion and disappointment with the final result. Too often patient and physician may consider the injury a minor one because of the small size of the bone involved, but a poor result will not appear so minor to the patient, whose hand will be constantly before his eyes and who will always be aware of any deformity or functional impairment. Expectations regarding the end result must be realistic; otherwise, seemingly minor complications will later assume major proportions in the patient's appraisal of the result.

METACARPAL FRACTURES

The management of metacarpal fractures regarding the indications and types of internal fixation is controversial and generally evokes many opinions from treating physicians. The treatment of these fractures depends on the location of the fracture and requires an understanding of the pertinent anatomy.

Metacarpals may be considered miniature long bones, the weakest point being just proximal to the neck. The index and middle metacarpals are relatively immobile, whereas the ring and little finger metacarpals are mobile, with 25 degrees to 45 degrees of motion in the anteroposterior plane. The metacarpophalangeal joint has an asymmetric configuration that produces a cam effect with motion. Owing to this cam effect, the collateral ligaments are tight in flexion and loose in extension. The principal deforming force on metacarpal fractures is exerted by the interossei muscles,

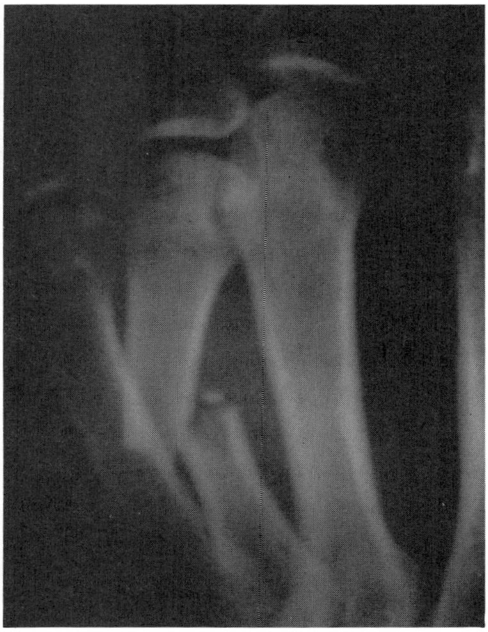

Figure 30-1. Fracture, metacarpal midshaft.

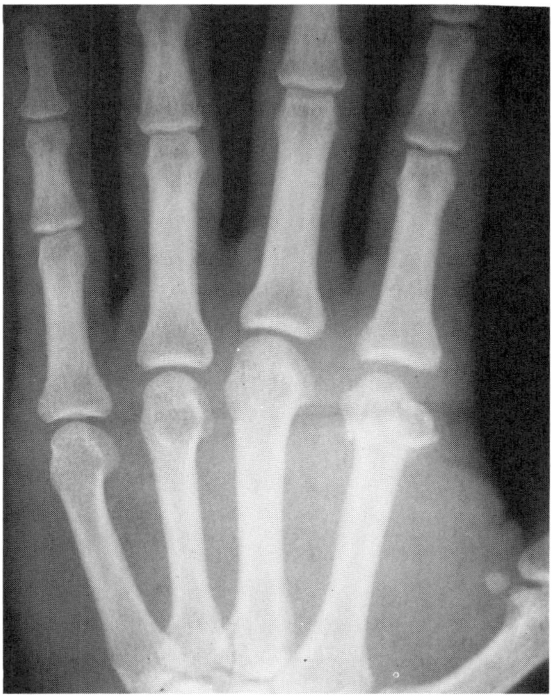

Figure 30-2. Comminuted fracture, index metacarpal head.

which account for the apex dorsal angulation in neck and shaft (Fig. 30-1) fractures. The metacarpal fractures are generally classified by location, that is, those affecting the head, neck, shaft, and base.

METACARPAL HEAD FRACTURES

Metacarpal head fractures (Fig. 30-2) frequently result from a crush injury or a high-velocity missile injury. These fractures are often intra-articular and involve the metacarpal phalangeal joint. If the fracture is grossly comminuted, the treatment would generally involve splinting and early motion. Buddy taping (Fig. 30-3) can be used by taping the affected fingers to the next finger, which acts as a splint and also enables early active motion. A large intra-articular fragment can occasionally be fixed with a Kirschner wire or a small screw.

METACARPAL NECK FRACTURES

Metacarpal neck fractures are common injuries that frequently involve the fifth metacar-

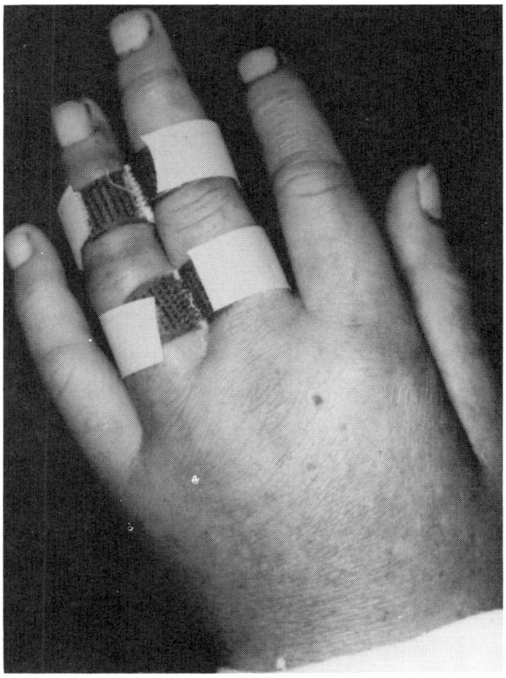

Figure 30-3. Buddy taping with Velcro straps, middle and ring fingers.

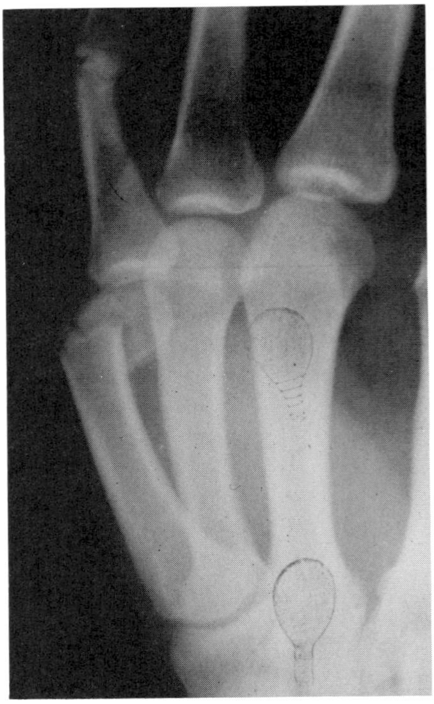

Figure 30-4. Boxer's fracture.

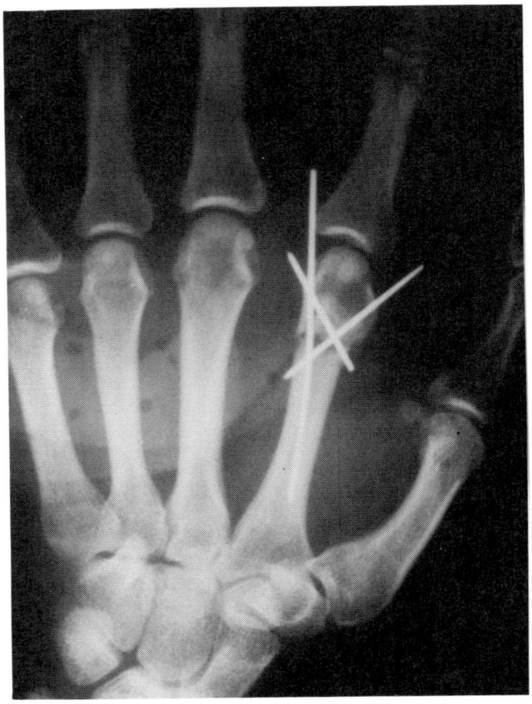

Figure 30-5. Open reduction, metacarpal neck index finger, with fixation with four K-wires.

pal or little finger metacarpal. These are generally called *Boxer's* fractures (Fig. 30-4). These are generally unstable fractures because of volar comminution. The treatment depends on the metacarpal involved. In the inner metacarpals involving the index and middle fingers, the distal fragment needs to be held near anatomic position with less than 10 degrees of angulation. Splinting and active motion are usually indicated. When there is more than 10 degrees of angulation on these fingers, then anatomic reduction and fixation (Fig. 30-5) are necessary to avoid malrotation, malunion, and a painful grip. The Boxer's fractures involving the mobile ring and little digits allow acceptance of more angulation at the fracture site. The nonoperative treatment of these fractures is controversial. I feel that one can accept up to 60 degrees of angulation as long as the patient has full active motion and no pain. The patient is told that he or she would probably have a bump in the palm of the hand because of the metacarpal head, but as long as it is not painful and does not affect the patients grip, that will be accepted. The treatment for these patients is a wrist control splint with or without buddy taping, and the patient is encouraged to move the fingers actively. These fractures are usually asymptomatic by the third or fourth week, and the patient can then return to normal activities. I have not seen any problems with malunion or painful grip in patients treated in this manner.

If the angulation exceeds 60 degrees in the ring and little finger metacarpal necks, a closed reduction is desired. With a closed reduction, one can use percutaneous Kirschner wires to immobilize the fracture. We have not used the 90/90 method of treatment because of severe joint contractures seen secondary to this method of treatment. One can also use a Kirschner wire to cross over to an adjacent metacarpal to hold the reduction anatomic.

METACARPAL SHAFT FRACTURES

The treatment of metacarpal shaft fractures depends on whether the fracture is stable or unstable. Transverse and certain spiral oblique fractures are stable and successfully treated by closed methods using a radial or ulnar gutter plaster splint or a plastic wrist control splint leaving free motion at the metacarpal phalangeal joint. Comminuted or long

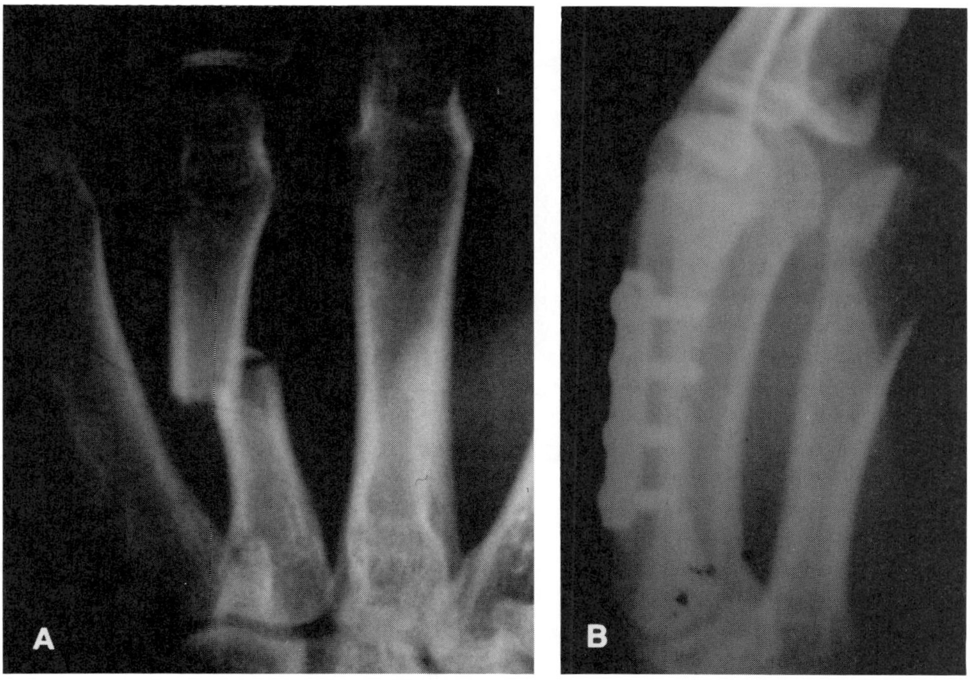

Figure 30-6. (*A*) Displaced fracture, midshaft ring finger metacarpal. (*B*) Open reduction and internal fixation with A-O plate and four screws.

spiral fractures are often unstable and tend to shorten and angulate dorsally. With these types of fractures, internal fixation is indicated (Fig. 30-6). Numerous studies have been done to test the biomechanical stability of various types of internal fixation. I tested six modes of internal fixation in a three-point bending test with cadaver metacarpals and found that dorsal plates with an interfragmentary compression screw (Fig. 30-7) were superior to other methods of fixation.

METACARPAL BASE FRACTURES

Metacarpal base fractures occur as a result of a direct blow or crush injury. These are often intra-articular, involving the metacarpal carpal joints (Fig. 30-8). They are also comminuted and can heal with rotational deformity (Fig. 30-9) and result in painful arthritis at the joint. These fractures should be reduced anatomically and may be fixed with Kirschner wires that would require an external fixation

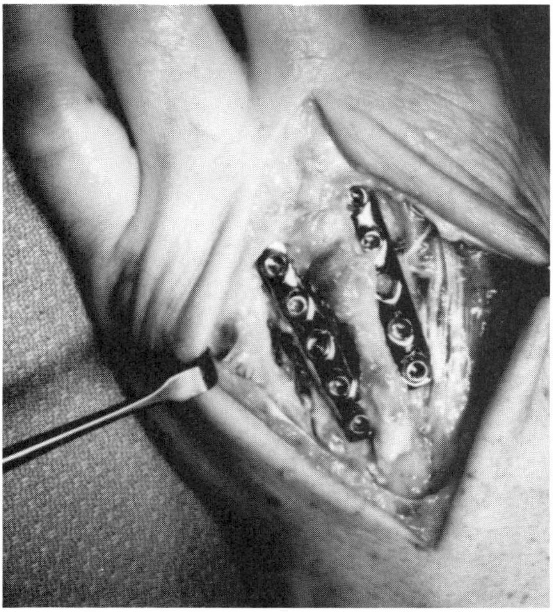

Figure 30-7. At surgery, two plates used for fixation for middle and ring finger metacarpal shafts.

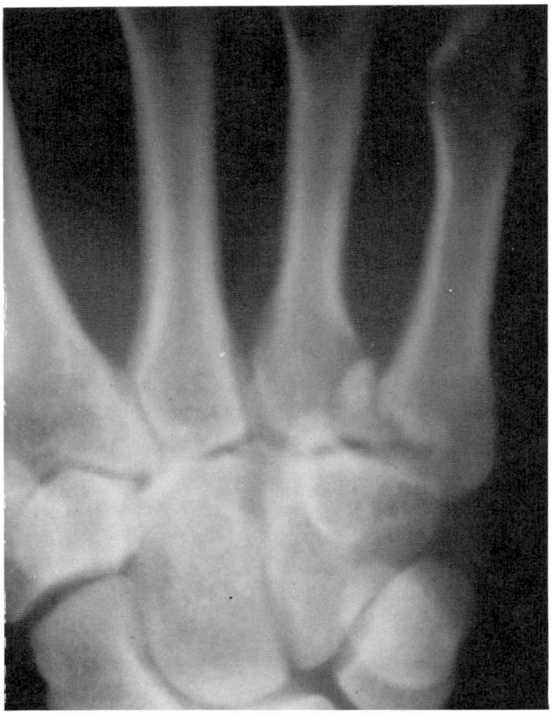

Figure 30-8. Intra-articular fracture, base of little finger metacarpal.

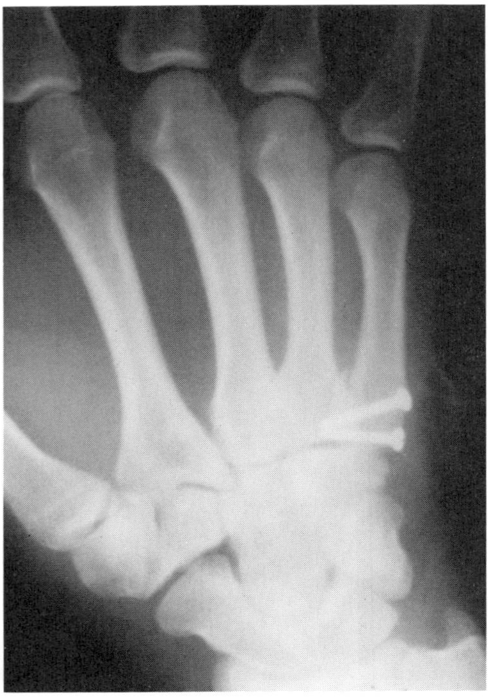

Figure 30-10. Open reduction and fixation, base of little finger metacarpal, with two A-O screws. Early motion possible.

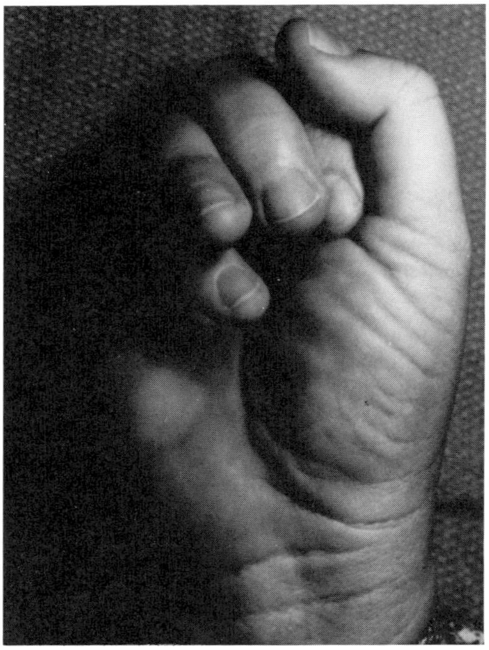

Figure 30-9. Malunited fracture with rotational deformity seen during flexion.

such as a cast or splint. If early motion is desirable, then rigid internal fixation with AO screws (Fig. 30-10) and mini plates can be done.

THUMB METACARPAL FRACTURES

The carpometacarpal joint of the thumb is far more important than any other in the function of the thumb and thus of the whole hand. Unless accurately reduced, metacarpal fractures involving this joint may cause limitation of motion, pain, and weakness of pinch and grip. The thumb metacarpal moves through a wide arc, stands apart from the other four metacarpals, and acts independently of them. It can tolerate greater deformity or distortion without significant impairment of function. Fractures of the shaft of the thumb metacarpal are more commonly transverse and tend to angulate dorsally with the distal fragment flexing toward the palm. These fractures are usually easily reduced by traction and adequately immobilized in a plaster thumb spica.

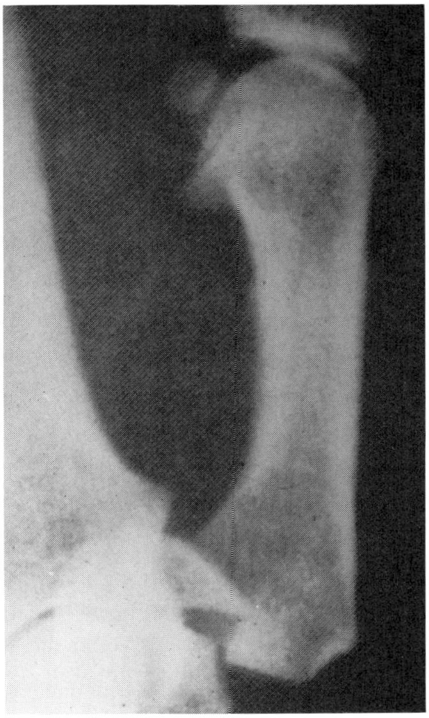

Figure 30-11. Bennett's fracture of thumb.

BENNETT'S FRACTURE

Edward H. Bennett, an Irish surgeon, described a Bennett's fracture in 1881. It is an intra-articular fracture through the base of the first metacarpal (Fig. 30-11). The shaft is laterally dislocated by the unopposed pull of the abductor pollicis longus muscle. The medial projection, or "hook," remains in place or is slightly rotated because of its capsular attachment. It is really a fracture dislocation at the base of the thumb metacarpal. If recognized early, it can generally be reduced by manual traction on the thumb and percutaneous pinning with a Kirschner wire. If reduction by traction and manipulation is not possible, the fracture should be opened and fixed internally either by Kirschner wires or by interfragmentary compression screws (Fig. 30-12). With rigid internal fixation, one can start early motion and function. If the fixation is less than desirable, then a thumb spica cast for about 4 weeks is necessary.

ROLANDO'S FRACTURE

Rolando's fracture is a comminuted fracture of the base of the thumb metacarpal. This can be treated occasionally by traction and percutaneous pinning, but an open reduction may be necessary to reassemble the fragments. The patient should be told that traumatic arthritic changes can occur and may require future reconstructive surgery, either arthroplasty or arthrodesis.

PHALANGEAL FRACTURES

DISTAL PHALANX

Fractures of the phalanges are usually incurred by smashing the fingertip with a heavy

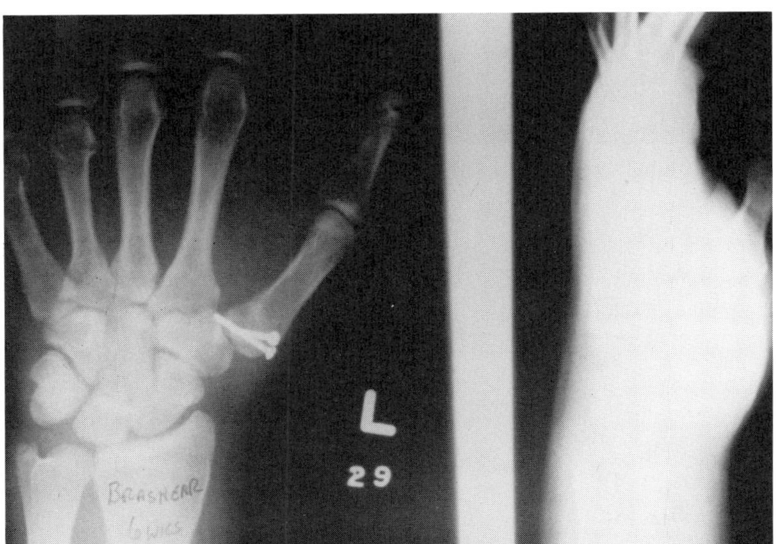

Figure 30-12. Radiographic appearance 6 weeks after operative fixation of Bennett's fracture with two A-O screws.

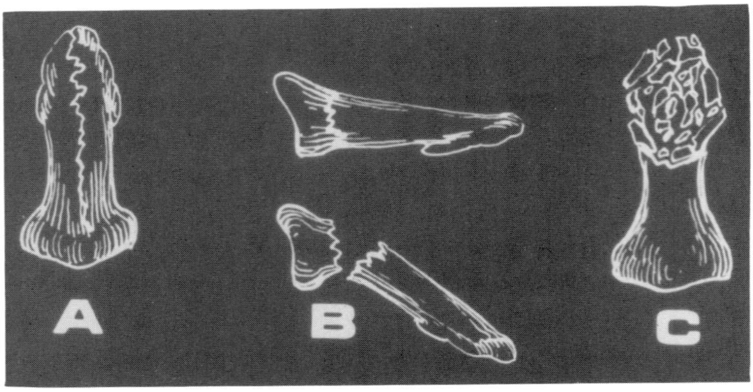

Figure 30-13. (*A*) Longitudinal nondisplaced fracture, distal phalanx. (*B*) Transverse fracture, distal phalanx, nondisplaced (*above*) and displaced (*below*). (*C*) Comminuted tuft fracture, distal phalanx.

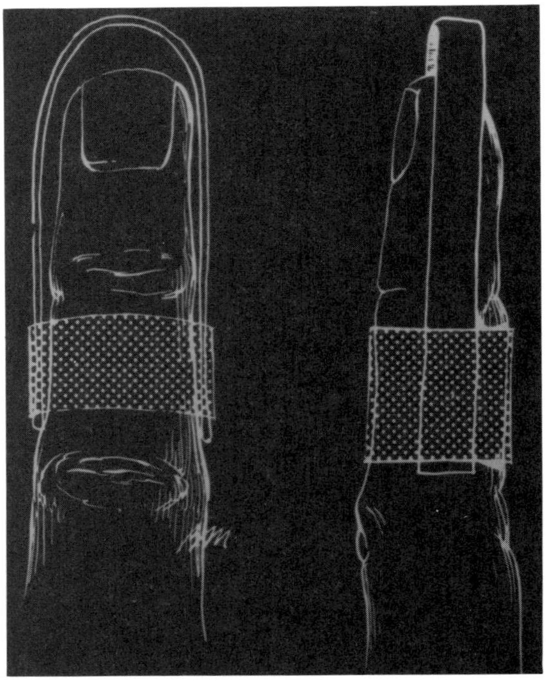

Figure 30-14. Protective aluminum splint with tape.

object or crushing it in a door. They are usually comminuted and accompanied by considerable bleeding into the distal finger pulp (Fig. 30-13). If a subungual hematoma is present, release of the blood from under the fingernail is accomplished by burning a hole in the nail with the end of a hot paperclip. This would give considerable relief of pain. Splinting is the method of treatment, and a protective aluminum splint or a plastic splint with a Velcro strap (Fig. 30-14) can be used over the tip of the finger without immobilizing the proximal interphalangeal joint.

Avulsion fractures of the extensor tendon insertion (Fig. 30-15) result in a mallet or baseball finger deformity and if one-third or more of the joint surface of the distal interphalangeal joint is involved, it is accompanied by subluxation. These common injuries result from force applied against the tip of the extended finger. A small bony fragment involving less than one-third of the articular surface can be treated by splinting (Fig. 30-16) or a finger cast. If more than one-third of the joint surface is involved, then it would usually re-

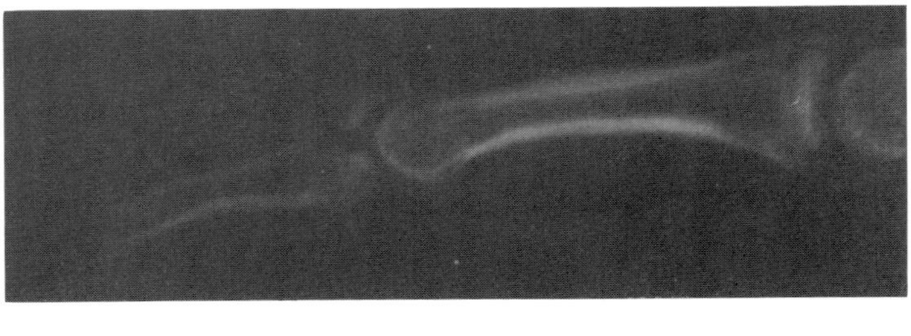

Figure 30-15. Lateral roentgenogram of finger showing mallet fracture.

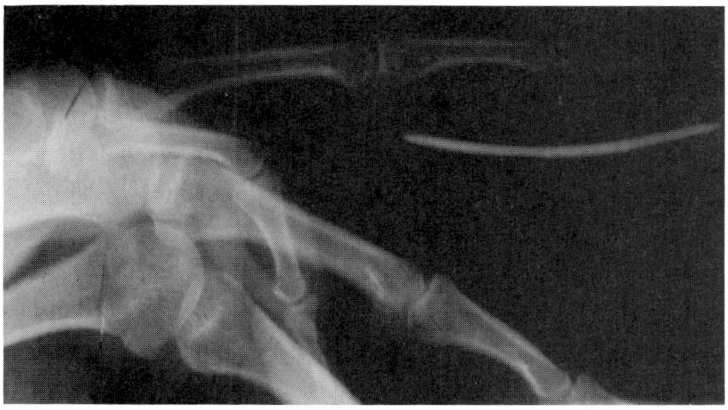

Figure 30-16. Lateral roentgenogram of finger after closed reduction and splinting. Unacceptable position of fracture fragment.

quire open reduction using internal fixation with a pull-out wire, Kirschner wire, or an interfragmentary compression screw (Fig. 30-17).

PROXIMAL AND MIDDLE PHALANX

Fractures of the proximal phalanx are much more common that those in the middle phalanx. To understand methods of treatment it is essential to review the anatomy and think about the deforming forces present on the fracture fragments. The anatomy will predict the deformity. In the proximal phalanx the proximal fragment is flexed by the insertion of the interosseous muscle. The distal fragment

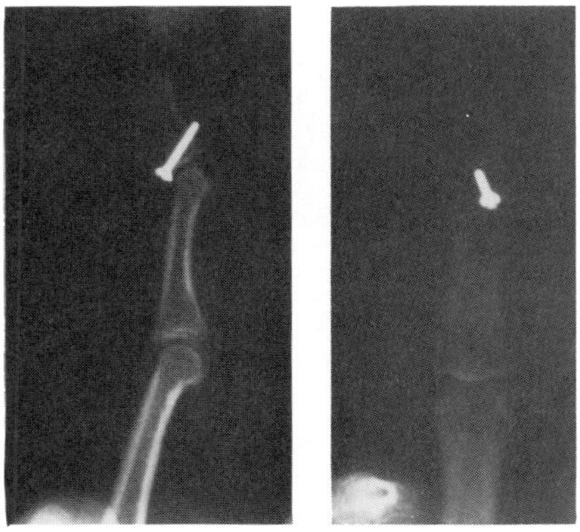

Figure 30-17. Open reduction of mallet fracture with A-O screw fixation. Acceptable position of fragment.

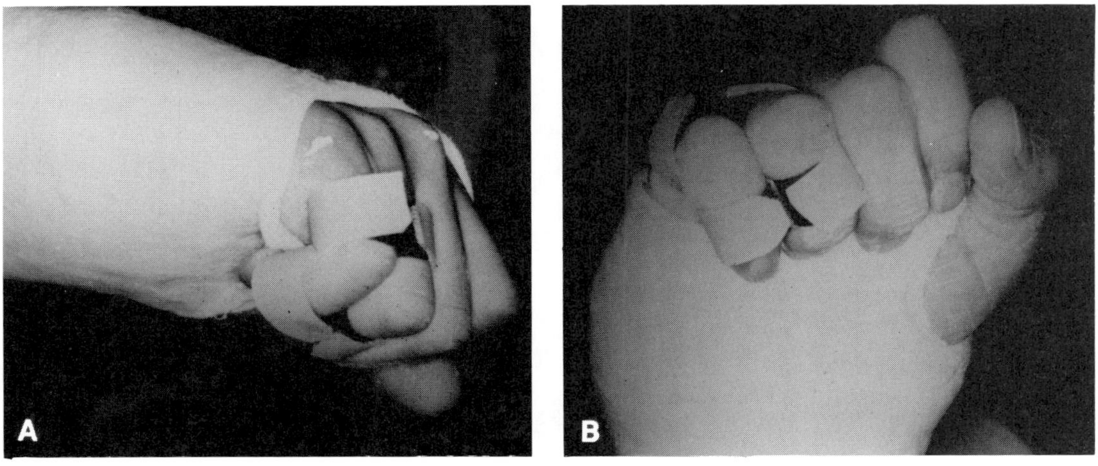

Figure 30-18. Stable fracture treated with plaster cast and buddy taping.

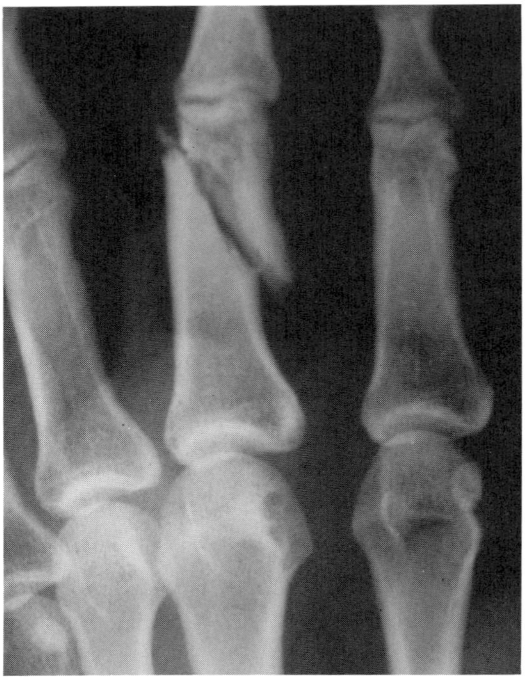

Figure 30-19. Oblique fracture of proximal phalanx with shortening.

is extended by the insertion of the central slip of the extensor tendon. In the middle phalanx the principal deforming force is the flexor digitorum superficialis muscle. Malrotation is probably the most frequent complication in treating these fractures. The treatment of phalangeal fractures is determined by whether the fractures are stable or unstable. Stable fractures can be treated with buddy taping and early active motion (Fig. 30-18). Buddy taping requires a truly stable fracture with no angulation and careful follow-up.

A variety of closed and open methods have been described to treat unstable phalangeal fractures. These fractures are frequently oblique (Fig. 30-19) or comminuted and are prone to angulation, shortening, and malrotation. Closed methods of external immobilization can certainly achieve accurate union, but the prolonged immobilization can frequently result in residual loss of motion. This is especially true at the proximal interphalangeal joint. In an attempt to overcome the problem of joint stiffness with rigid splinting, more dynamic methods have been used, including pulp and nail traction devices. By exerting pull on the collateral ligaments, further stiffness of joints will occur, with limitation of motion.

There is an increasing preference for internal fixation in these unstable phalangeal fractures with the goal of rigid immobilization and, more important, early functional motion. Kirschner wires have traditionally been used and are useful in holding small fragments (Fig. 30-20) or small intra-articular fragments. Although accurate reduction can be obtained, Kirschner wires are often not sufficiently rigid to allow unrestricted early motion. I have also done laboratory studies of the cadaver proximal phalanx in determining the best method of fixation. Interfragmentary screws (Fig. 30-21) were as good as mini plates with screws.

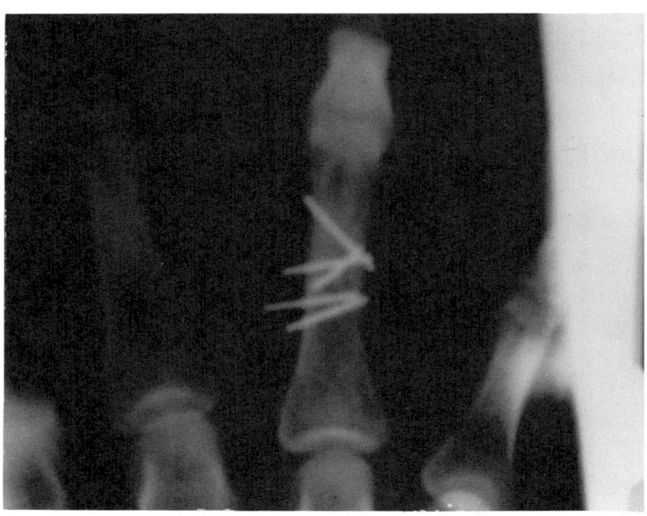

Figure 30-20. Open reduction and internal fixation with five K-wires.

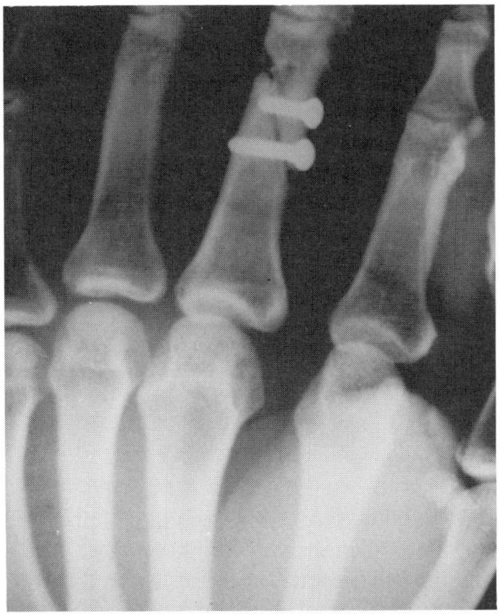

Figure 30-21. Open reduction and internal fixation with two A-O screws.

SPECIAL FRACTURES AND DISLOCATIONS

FRACTURE DISLOCATION OF THE PROXIMAL INTERPHALANGEAL JOINT

Fracture dislocations of the proximal interphalangeal joint, as a rule, result in an unstable volar displacement of the middle phalanx (Fig. 30-22) caused by disruption of the attachment of the volar plate. When there is a large single volar fragment involving at least 50% of the joint surface, open reduction and internal fixation can be carried out using a Kirschner wire, a wire pull-out suture, or even a interfragmentary screw. When the fragments, which can be comminuted, measure less than 50% of the articular surface, an extension block splint (Fig. 30-23) can be used, allowing active motion of the proximal interphalangeal joint, which gives satisfactory results, especially in those without gross displacement. The proximal interphalangeal joint is blocked in 30 degrees in flexion, allowing full flexion but blocking full extension. This can be in either a plaster cast or a plastic splint.

CARPOMETACARPAL DISLOCATION OF THE THUMB

Carpometacarpal dislocation of the thumb is usually accompanied by a fracture and this is discussed in the discussion of Bennett's fracture. When it occurs without fracture, it can be reduced closed, and if it is stable, early motion can be started but probably should be protected either with a thumb spica splint or a bivalve cast.

DISLOCATION OF THE METACARPOPHALANGEAL JOINT OF THE THUMB

Dislocation of any of the metacarpophalangeal joints is possible from hyperextension in-

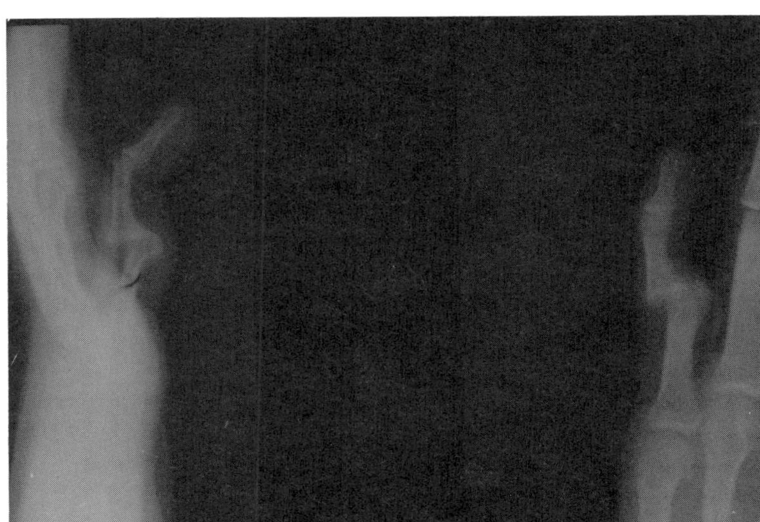

Figure 30-22. Fracture dislocation of PIP joint, little finger.

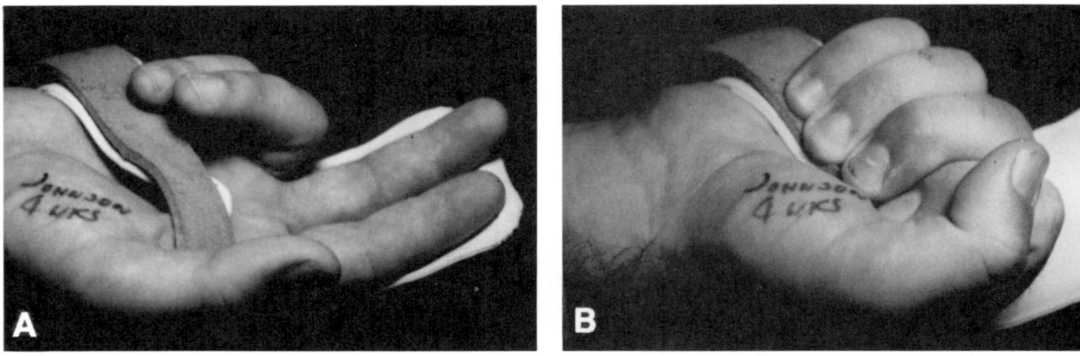

Figure 30-23. (*A*) Extension block splint blocking full finger extension. (*B*) Extension block splint allowing full finger flexion.

juries, but dorsal dislocation in the metacarpophalangeal joint of the thumb is the most common. Early closed reduction may be tried but usually this injury has to be treated by open surgery. There is a buttonhole effect on the metacarpal neck that will be accentuated by traction. If closed treatment is not successful, repeated attempts are contraindicated. Open reduction should be done to disengage the head of the metacarpal from a button-hole slit in the anterior capsule and from the flexor pollicis brevis muscle. This has been described by Kaplan and has sometimes been called the Kaplan lesion.

RUPTURE OF THE ULNAR COLLATERAL LIGAMENT OF THE METACARPOPHALANGEAL JOINT OF THE THUMB

An incomplete rupture of the ulnar collateral ligament of the thumb is common. It is frequently secondary to a ski injury and has also been known as a Gamekeeper's thumb. The treatment includes a thumb spica cast or a splint.

Complete rupture of the ulnar collateral ligament is more common in the radial, but both have been described secondary to ski injuries. It is more disabling because it renders pinch unstable. On examination, it may be suspected clinically by comparing the stability of the affected joint with that of the unaffected joint. This can be also demonstrated by stressing the metacarpophalangeal (Fig. 30-24) joint on radiographs (Fig. 30-25). This may also be compared with the normal side.

The ligament may avulse a bony fragment from the phalanx. If this is displaced over 3 mm, it would require internal fixation. This can be determined by radiographs. If it is not displaced or rotated, then it may be treated by applying a plaster thumb spica or splint for 4 to 6 weeks.

DISLOCATION OF THE METACARPOPHALANGEAL JOINTS OF THE FINGERS

Dislocation of the metacarpophalangeal joint is less common than interphalangeal dislocations. It is seen most often in the index finger and has been described by Kaplan. It usually is irreducible by closed methods because the dislocated metacarpal head is displaced volarward, and the base of the proximal phalanx is displaced dorsalward. The major obstruction preventing this reduction is the displaced volar plate, which lies dorsal to the metacarpal head.

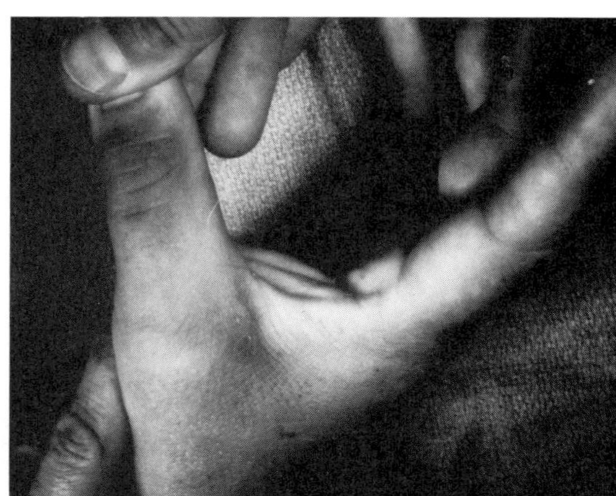

Figure 30-24. Stressing ulnar side of MP joint of thumb.

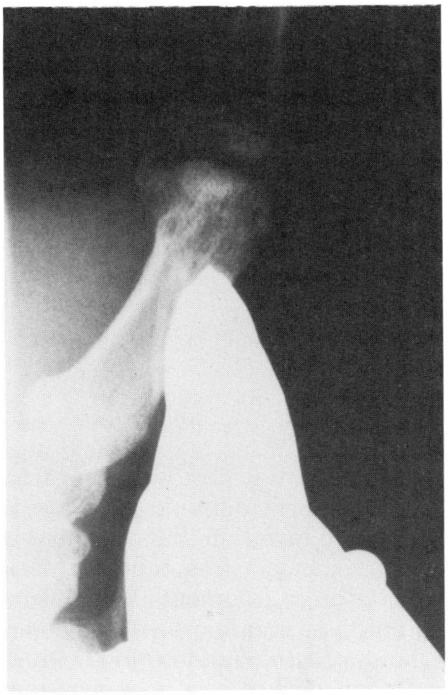

Figure 30-25. Roentgenogram showing stressing of ulnar side of MP joint of thumb. Examiner wearing lead gloves.

INTERPHALANGEAL DISLOCATIONS

Most interphalangeal dislocations are reduced immediately by the patient or by a bystander such as a trainer or a coach. If the reduction is stable, then joint motion can be started immediately when pain and swelling subsides. If both collateral ligaments are completely ruptured, they should be repaired. The most important collateral ligament is probably on the radial side of the index finger.

CHILDREN'S HAND FRACTURES

Injuries to the hand in children present challanges both diagnostically and therapeutically. Although metacarpal and phalangeal fractures are common in this age group, most can be easily treated by closed reduction, usually healing without difficulty in 3 to 4 weeks. Those fractures near the epiphyseal plate remodel nicely if displacement is in the plane of motion of the adjacent joints. Fractures near the opposite end demonstrate little remodeling but still heal rapidly.

Regardless of the proximity of a rotational deformity to an epiphyseal plate, no degree of rotation will be remodeled. At the time of reduction of a metacarpal or a phalangeal fracture, care must be taken to assure proper clinical alignment of the fingers. This is best evaluated by comparing the alignment of the fingernails of both hands following closed reduction and with the fingers in flexion.

If fractures are stable and require no reduction, immobilization can be by a simple bulky compression dressing that gently controls swelling and maintains position. Minimal displacement can be buddy taped to an adjacent finger, which protects against angulatory forces and facilitates early active motion. Young children have an enormous free disposition to either destroy or wiggle out of their immobilization. When plaster of paris is used to maintain a bony reduction of the hand, application of an above-elbow cast with the elbow flexed at 90 degrees helps retard the child's ability to maneuver out of rigid immobilization.

BIBLIOGRAPHY

Black D, Mann RJ, Constine R, Daniels AU: Comparison of internal fixation in metacarpal fractures. Hand Surg 10A:466, 1985

Black D, Mann RJ, Constine R, Daniels AU: The stability of internal fixation in the proximal phalanx. Hand Surg 11A: 1986

Edmondson, Crenshaw: Campbell's Operative Orthopaedics, 5th ed, Vol I. St Louis, CV Mosby, 1971

Heim V et al: Small Fragment Set Manual, 2nd ed. New York, Springer-Verlag, 1982

Segmuller G: Operative Stabilization in the Hand. Bern, Hans Huber AG, 1973

31 Carpal Fractures and Instability

RONALD J. MANN

FRACTURES OF THE SCAPHOID

Fractures of the scaphoid are the most common carpal fracture and constitute 50% of all wrist injuries; they take on particular significance because of their tendency for nonunion and subsequent development of a painful unstable wrist. These injuries are most common in the younger, active patient population.

History is of an injury to the wrist in extreme dorsiflexion, typically from a fall on an outstretched hand (Fig. 31-1). There is wrist pain with tenderness within the anatomic snuff box. The pain is accentuated by supination and pronation against resistance.

With a history of a fall on an outstretched right hand, multiple radiographic views should be taken. The minimum should be AP lateral oblique and a special scaphoid view (Fig. 31-2). With a suggested history and physical examination and even with negative films, the wrist should be immobilized either in a plaster cast or a splint for 10 days to 2 weeks. Then repeat radiographs should be taken with the hand out of the splint and cast. If repeat films fail to demonstrate fracture, the external support may be discontinued. It has been shown that bone scans within 72 hours of injury can be used to learn the need for continued immobilization.

Treatment for acute scaphoid fractures is immobilization. Some consider a thumb spica cast, either below the elbow or above the elbow, to be satisfactory. I prefer the three-fingered or baseball cast above the elbow. This includes immobilizing the thumb to the interphalangeal joint and the index and middle fingers to the PIP joints. This is then removed after 6 weeks and recheck radiographs are taken. If trabeculations are seen across the fracture site, a thumb spica cast is used for another 6 weeks. With good patient compliance the fracture should be healed by 12 weeks.

Many factors predispose scaphoid fractures to delayed union or nonunion. Delayed diagnosis, failure to maintain uninterrupted immobilization, displaced fragments, and inadequate reduction of fragments all contribute to delayed union or nonunion. If the diagnosis is made, then operative innervation is indicated; the treatment of choice is bone grafting. The most important factor in nonunion is lack of a sufficiently long immobilization period. The same is true for failure of union after bone grafting.

FRACTURES OF THE TRIQUETRUM

Fractures of the triquetrum are commonly associated with other carpal injuries. Isolated fractures are much less frequent, although they are reported to represent the second or third most common group of carpal bone fractures. The mechanism of injury may be a rotation or twisting motion, such as occurs when lifting heavy weights, or a sheer force during falls with the wrist in dorsiflexion and ulnar deviation. The treatment consists of a period of 2 to 4 weeks of either splinting or casting. Nonunion may occur, but this is exceedingly rare.

FRACTURES OF THE PISIFORM

The pisiform is generally injured during a fall on a dorsiflexed outstretched hand. The most frequent mechanism of injury seems to be direct trauma on the pisiform. Avulsion injuries may occur by the muscle pull of the flexor carpi ulnaris. Fresh fractures are treated by protective splinting or casting. If after con-

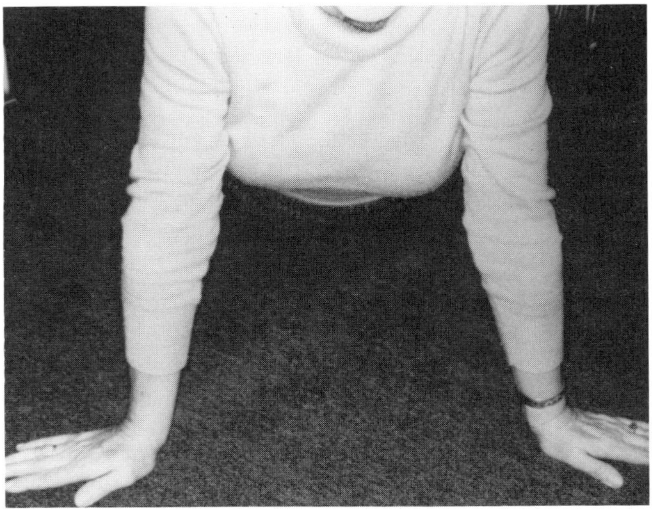

Figure 31-1. Demonstration fall on both outstretched hands.

servative therapy persistent and localized tenderness continues, excision of the pisiform is indicated.

FRACTURES OF THE TRAPEZIUM

Fractures of the trapezium constitute approximately 5% of all carpal fractures. Isolated fractures are rare, and the most frequently associated bony injury is fracture of the thumb metacarpal. Dislocation of the trapezium is rare. Treatment of these fractures is in a thumb spica cast for 4 to 6 weeks. Displaced fractures or dislocations are best managed by open reduction and internal fixation.

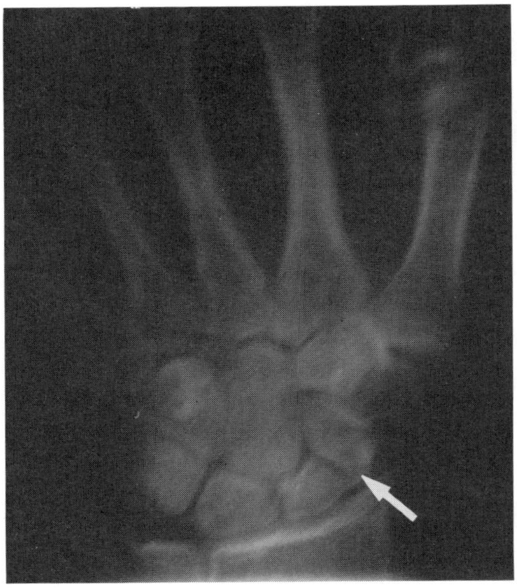

Figure 31-2. Roentgenogram showing fracture (*arrow*) through waist of scaphoid.

FRACTURES OF THE TRAPEZOID

Fractures of the trapezoid are rare because of its well-protected position unless the fracture occurs with other fractures. These fractures are managed by immobilization in plaster for 3 to 4 weeks. In cases of dislocations, closed manipulation may be attempted. If closed reduction is unsuccessful, open reduction should be done with internal fixation and plaster immobilization.

FRACTURES OF THE CAPITATE

Most capitate fractures produce pain and swelling and limitation of motion without clear localization of the injury to the capitate. The diagnosis is entirely based on careful radiographic evaluations. Nondisplaced isolated fractures should be immobilized in plaster for 4 to 6 weeks.

FRACTURES OF THE HAMATE

Isolated fractures of the hamate are rare. Fractures of the body can occur from forced

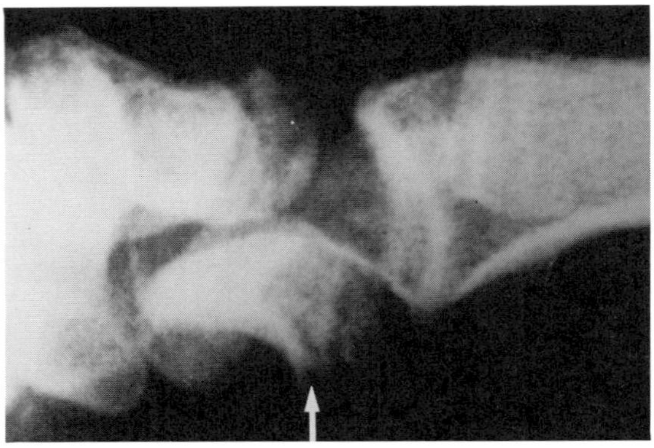

Figure 31-3. Lateral roentgenogram showing anterior (volar or palmar) dislocation (*arrow*) of lunate.

LUNATE DISLOCATIONS

The most common carpal dislocation is anterior dislocation of the lunate (Fig. 31-3). On the lateral roentgenographic view of the wrist, the half-moon-shaped profile of the lunate articulates with the cup of the distal radius proximally and with the rounded proximal capitate distally. An anterior dislocated lunate may cause acute compression of the median nerve in the carpal tunnel. When the injury is treated early, manipulative reduction is usually easy, and immobilization for 3 weeks in plaster is required. If after reduction the median nerve continues to show evidence of compression, then a carpal tunnel exploration may be necessary.

dorsiflexion and ulnar deviation. A fracture of the hook of the hamate is most likely secondary to a direct blow produced by the butt end of a golf club, baseball bat, or tennis racquet. Special radiographic examination, including oblique views and carpal tunnel views, may be necessary to make the diagnosis. Usually immobilization in a plaster cast for 4 to 6 weeks is all that is necessary. Occasionally, for fractures of the hook of the hamate with nonunion, excision of the hook surgically may be necessary.

TRANSSCAPHOID PERILUNATE DISLOCATIONS

Volar transscaphoid perilunate dislocations are extremely rare. Dorsal volar transscaphoid dislocations are more common and may be associated with other injuries of the upper extremity (Fig. 31-4). Early reduction by closed manipulation is best. When accurate reduction of the scaphoid fracture is not possible, open reduction may be necessary with internal fixation such as Kirschner wiring.

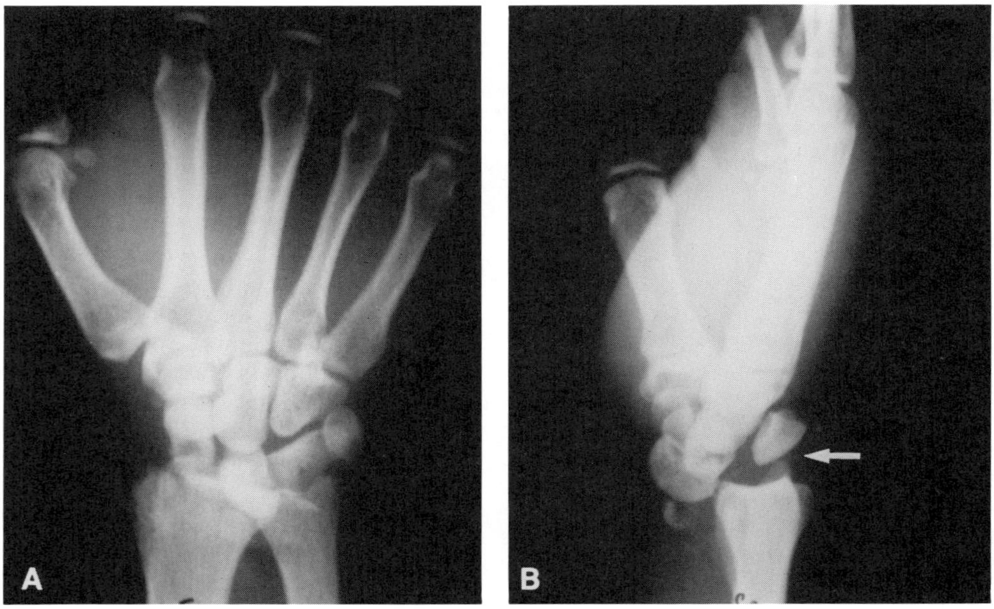

Figure 31-4. AP (*A*) and lateral (*B*) roentgenograms showing transscaphoid perilunar dislocation (*B*, *arrow*).

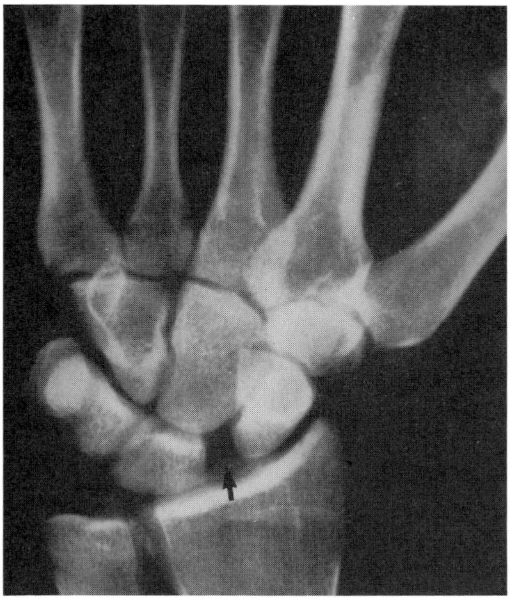

Figure 31-5. AP roentgenogram showing gap (*arrow*) between scaphoid and lunate. ("Terry Thomas sign").

ROTARY SUBLUXATION OF THE SCAPHOID

Rotary subluxation of the scaphoid may be misdiagnosed as a wrist sprain following acute dorsiflexion of the wrist after a fall. A tear of the scapholunate interosseous ligament permits a subluxation. The condition is also known as scapholunate dissociation. The scapholunate ligament is not a strong ligament and cannot withstand acute dorsiflexion injuries. The proximal pole of the scaphoid rotates dorsally and becomes more vertical in the position and permits separation of the scaphoid from the lunate. The diagnosis is made on anteroposterior roentgenograms (Fig. 31-5) by noting a gap between the scaphoid and lunate of more than 3 mm. On the lateral view measuring the scapholunate angle of more than 60 degrees helps to make the diagnosis (Fig. 31-6). The rotation of the scaphoid causes it to appear to be shortened and produces a so-called ring sign on the anteroposterior view. Occasionally, the capitate migrates proximally into the gap created by a separation of the scaphoid and the lunate. To diagnose the scapholunate dissociation patterns further, one can get special roentgenographic views with a clenched fist (Fig. 31-7), and again radial and ulnar deviation, pronation and supination, in the AP and lateral projection. Other means of diagnosis are wrist arthrography and, more recently, wrist arthroscopy.

Closed reduction may be attempted, but the preferred treatment is open reduction. The various methods of treatment may be repair of the ligament, pinning of the scaphoid lunate after reduction of the scaphoid, reconstruction of the scapholunate ligament, or limited carpal arthrodesis.

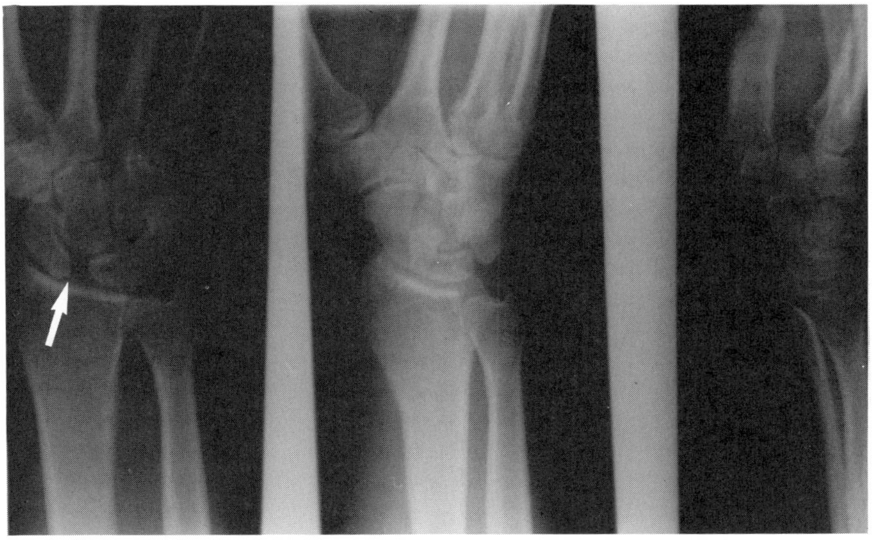

Figure 31-6. AP, oblique, and lateral roentgenograms showing gap (*arrow, left*) between scaphoid and lunate with scapholunate angle greater than 60 degrees.

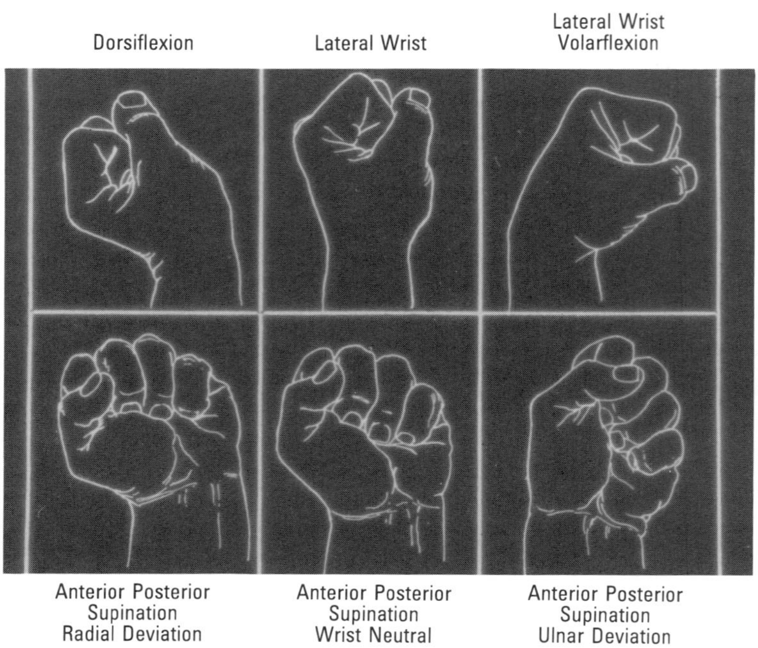

Figure 31-7. Diagram showing position of hand and wrist for special roentgenograms.

TRIQUETRAL LUNATE DISSOCIATION

Dissociation or disruption between the triquetrum and lunate may occur. The result is a fixed palmar flexion of the lunate. This may be common in the rheumatoid wrist. The diagnosis is again made most commonly by wrist arthrography or arthroscopy.

TRIQUETRAL HAMATE DISSOCIATION

Triquetral hamate dissociation is a midcarpal instability and the distal carpal row shifts dorsal or palmar to the axis of the radius. This may be painful and disabling.

KIENBÖCK'S DISEASE

Kienböck's disease is also known as lunatomalacia. The cause is elusive, and many theories have been attempted to explain the structural changes that have allowed the lunate to collapse. More frequently, Kienböck's disease is believed to be the sequel to single or multiple microscopic fractures resulting in secondary vascular impairment. The actual diagnosis is strictly made on radiographic studies (Fig. 31-8). The pain may initially be deceptively mild, and patients have poor recollection of the precipitating injury. There may be symptoms suggestive of involvement of the median nerve within the carpal tunnel. Early on, radiographs may show no abnormalities except for the presence of an ulnar-minus variant. Trispiral tomography may be helpful in early situations. Bone scans may show an abnormal lunate uptake. Many forms of

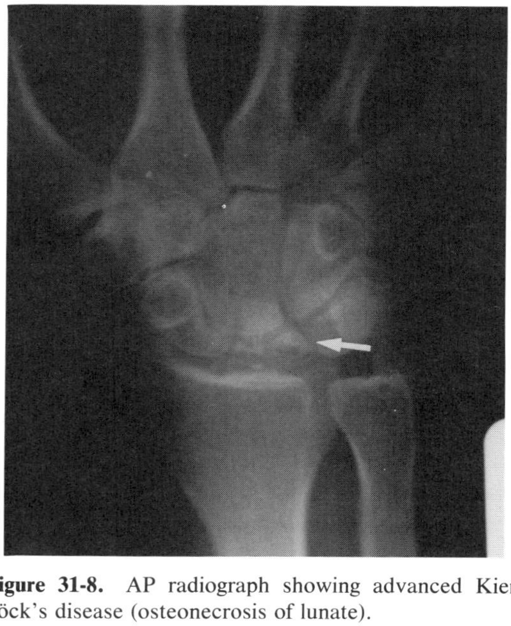

Figure 31-8. AP radiograph showing advanced Kienböck's disease (osteonecrosis of lunate).

treatment have been described, ranging from immobilization to casting or splinting to revascularization, prosthetic replacement, and arthrodesis.

BIBLIOGRAPHY

Dobyns J et al: Traumatic instability of the wrist. Instr Course Lect 24:182, 1975

Linscheid R et al: Traumatic instability of the wrist: Diagnosis, classification and pathomechanics. J Bone Joint Surg 54:1612, 1972

Palmer AK et al: Management of post-traumatic instability of the wrist secondary to ligament rupture. J Hand Surg 3:507, 1978

Taleisnik J: The Wrist. New York, Churchill-Livingstone, 1985

Watson, HK et al: Limited wrist arthrodesis. I. The triscaphoid joint. J Hand Surg 5:320, 1980

32 Upper Extremity

JAMES B. MANNING AND AARON A. HOFMANN

The upper extremity is the prehensile organ of the body. This function frequently makes it susceptible to injury. Obviously, intact neurologic and vascular function of the upper extremity is critical to normal function. Lesions of any of the major nerves or vessels in the upper extremity can cause profound dysfunction. Such injuries are not always easily suspected from the nature of the associated trauma. An example would be neurapraxia of the radial nerve with a fracture of the distal humerus. Because of the association of neurologic and vascular injuries with bone and joint injuries of the upper extremity, any evaluation of a significant upper-extremity injury should include a screening examination of the major upper-extremity neurovascular structures.

Most significant upper-extremity injuries are properly treated definitively by orthopaedic surgeons. A large percentage of upper-extremity fractures and dislocations, however, can be successfully managed in the emergency room environment and therefore are sometimes treated by primary care physicians. This chapter describes in detail the management of injuries treated in the outpatient setting. Injuries that are described briefly or not at all, such as intra-articular fractures of the distal humerus, require orthopaedic consultation.

PRINCIPLES OF MANAGEMENT

The principles of management of injuries to the upper extremity are similar to those that apply to injuries of the lower extremity. If they are followed, major errors in management can be avoided.

1. The first step in evaluating any significant upper-extremity injury is an examination of the neurologic and vascular status. This should even precede reduction of a dislocation and radiographic examination.
2. Upper-extremity dislocations should be reduced as soon as possible.
3. All upper-extremity fractures and dislocations should be effectively immobilized after the initial evaluation is complete.
4. Any upper-extremity fracture or dislocation should be imaged radiographically in two orthogonal planes (at a 90-degree angle to each other). The radiographic evaluation of shaft fractures should include the joint above and below the fracture.
5. Intra-articular fractures with significant displacement (step-off) are most effectively treated by open anatomic reduction and internal fixation, if possible, which usually means orthopaedic consultation.

NEUROVASCULAR EXAMINATION

The screening neurovascular examination of the upper extremity is performed quickly and simply. The basic presumption is that if the distal-most structure supplied by a given nerve or vessel is innervated or perfused, the nerve or vessel is intact and functioning along its entire course. The sensory innervation of the upper extremity is shown in Figure 32-1. Although this figure shows a sharp demarcation between the area supplied by the median ulnar and radial nerves in the hand, there is, in fact, significant overlap. However, certain localized areas on the hand have been identified as receiving sensory innervation from only one nerve. Intact sensation in the first dorsal web space between the thumb and index finger indicates intact radial nerve sensory function (Fig. 32-2A). The same can be said for the palmar aspect of the index fingertip and the little fingertip regarding the median and ulnar nerves, respectively (Fig. 32-2B,C). The modalities tested include light touch and sharp–dull discrimination. If the opposite hand is uninjured it can be used for comparison. More subtle deficits can be detected using two-point

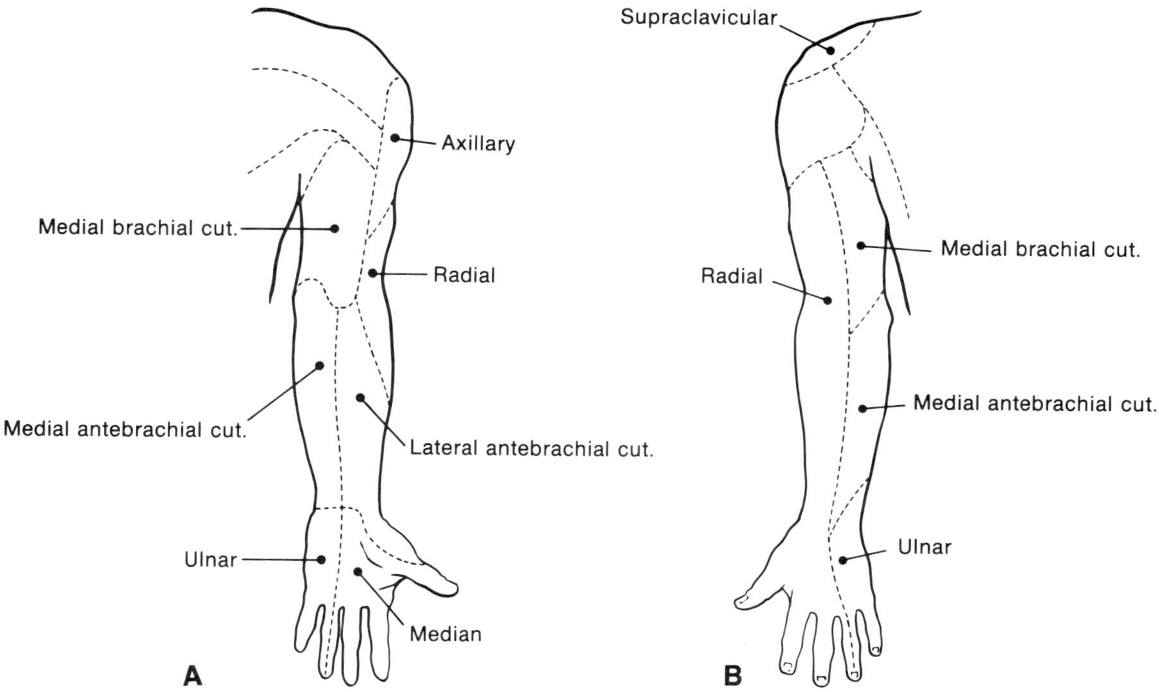

Figure 32-1. Sensory innervation of the upper extremity.

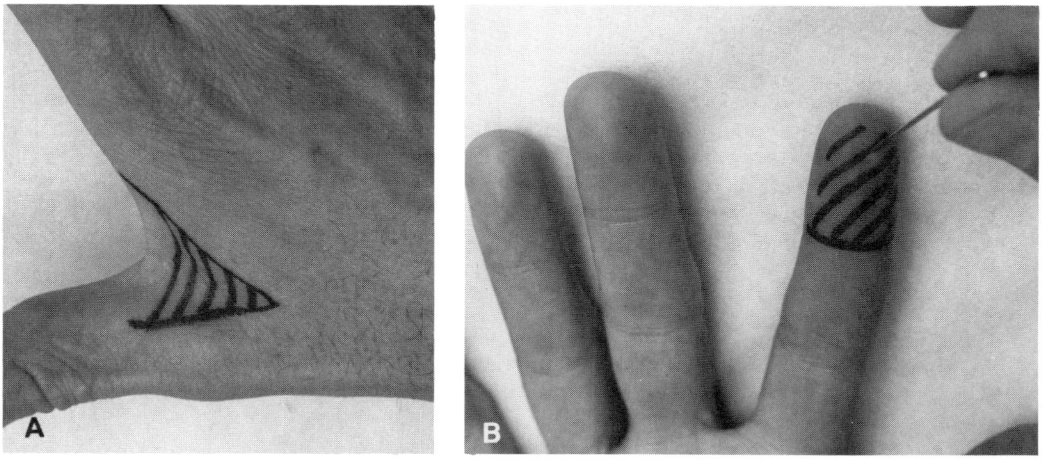

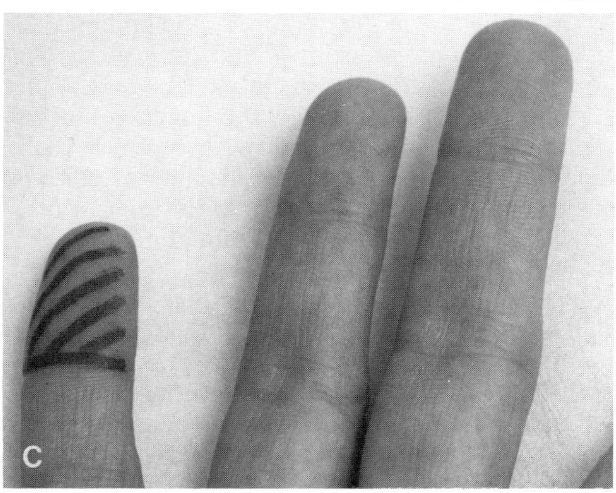

Figure 32-2. (*A*) Area indicating radial nerve innervation that has no overlap. (*B*) Area where there is no overlap for the median nerve. (*C*) Area where there is no overlap for the ulnar nerve.

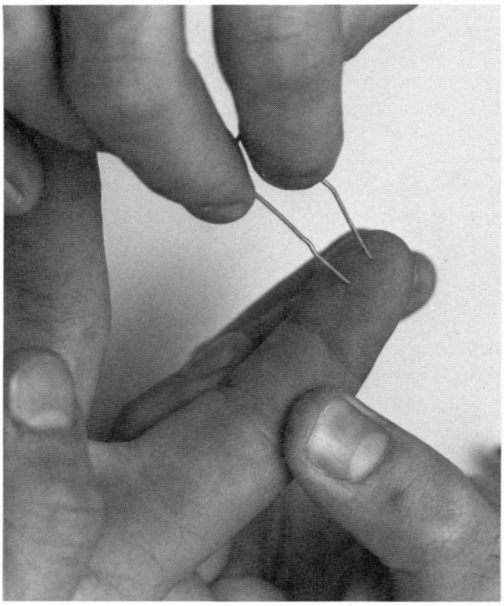

Figure 32-3. Two-point discrimination testing with a bent paperclip.

discrimination, as shown in Figure 32-3. A good test for intact motor function of the median nerve innervated muscles is the motor strength of the abductor pollicis brevis muscle (Fig. 32-4A). The interossei, which are uniquely innervated by the ulnar nerve, can be tested by measuring the strength of the abduction of the index finger (Fig. 32-4B). Innervation for index finger extension is uniquely supplied by the radial nerve and can be tested by resisting extension of the index finger (Fig. 32-4C). The other major nerves at risk in upper-extremity injuries, especially shoulder dislocations, are the axillary and musculocutaneous nerves. Their sensory distribution is illustrated in Figure 32-1.

The vascularity of the upper extremity can be assessed by palpating the radial and ulnar arterial pulses and examining the capillary refill of the fingertips. If the soft tissues are swollen from injury, a Doppler ultrasonic device may be helpful in detecting the peripheral pulses. Again, the opposite extremity, if it is uninjured, is examined for comparison. If the patient has normal pulses and capillary refill, it can be presumed, at least temporarily, that there has been no significant injury to the major vascular structures. However, it should always be remembered that injuries to the arterial intima may produce delayed arterial thrombosis.

IMMOBILIZATION OF UPPER-EXTREMITY INJURIES

It is difficult to immobilize the shoulder completely with anything less than a splint or cast that incorporates the trunk of the body. Fortunately, this usually is neither necessary nor advantageous. Most shoulder injuries can be effectively immobilized either in a standard sling (Fig. 32-5) or with a more elaborate shoulder immobilizer. Both devices hold the shoulder in the position in which it is generally most comfortable, which is adduction and internal rotation. Most other upper-extremity injuries can be effectively immobilized using some variation of the bulky dressing. These dressings have in common a thick layer of cast padding applied to the skin to provide even compression and to control swelling. A plaster splint is then applied, followed by a thin layer of padding, which facilitates the removal of the dressing. An elastic bandage or bias cut stockinette is applied as the outside layer.

Coaptation splints provide the bulky dressing used to acutely immobilize closed humeral shaft fractures. With the arm held at the patient's side and the shoulder inwardly rotated, the splints are applied to the medial and lateral surfaces of the arm as shown in Fig. 32-6.

Injuries in the elbow region are effectively immobilized with a simple posterior molded splint extending from the level of the axilla to the ends of the metacarpals (Fig. 32-7). This type of splint should not be used for humeral shaft fractures, because if the proximal end of the splint is near the level of the fracture site, it can merely act as a long lever arm on the distal fragment and actually increase the motion at the fracture. Forearm and wrist injuries can be effectively immobilized in a "sugar tongs" splint (Fig. 32-8A). This splint is applied by running a plaster slab from the metacarpal heads on the dorsum of the hand proximally around the elbow and then along the volar side of the arm distally to the end of the palm (Fig. 32-8B,C,D). If the fingers are uninjured, they should be allowed to move freely (Fig. 32-9). If there are concomitant serious hand injuries, a bulky hand dressing can provide adequate temporary immobilization for both forearm and hand injuries.

Each of the preceding dressings begins with five to ten layers of cast padding applied to the injured parts. The plaster slabs should be 10 to 20 layers thick. The plaster should be thoroughly wet before it is wrung out and applied

(*Text continues on p 596.*)

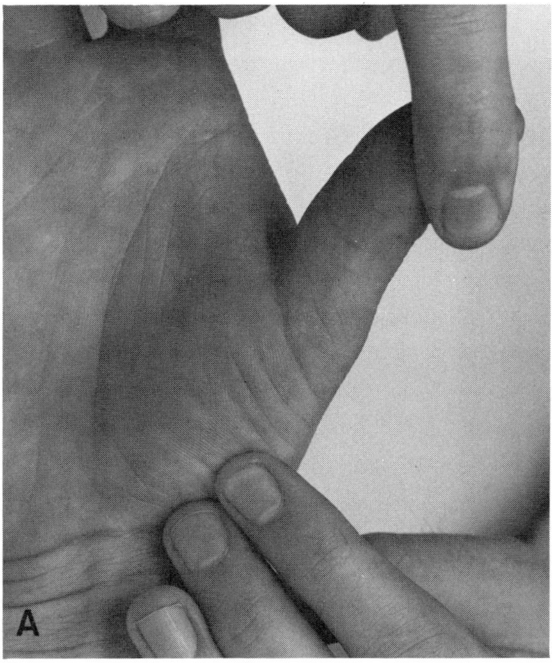

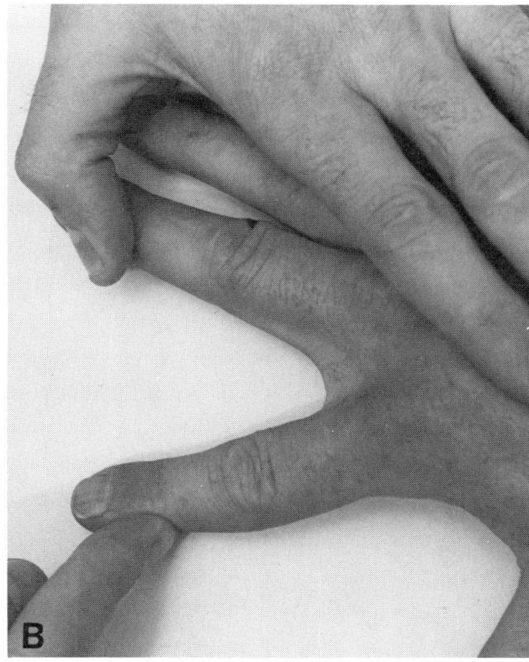

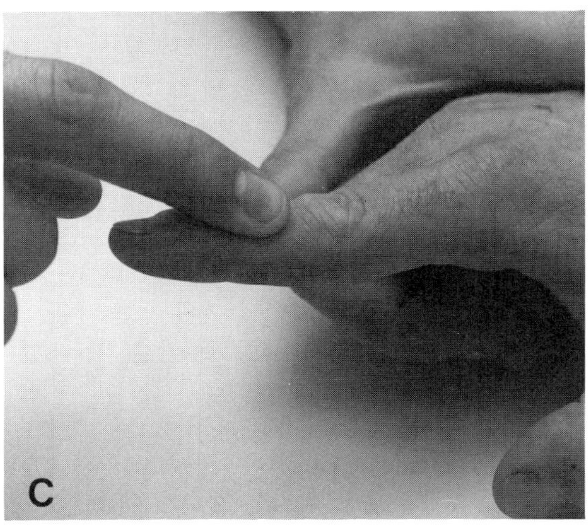

Figure 32-4. (*A*) Testing for weakness in the pollicis brevis—median nerve injury. (*B*) Testing for abduction weakness in the index finger—ulnar nerve injury. (*C*) Testing extension of the index finger—radial nerve injury.

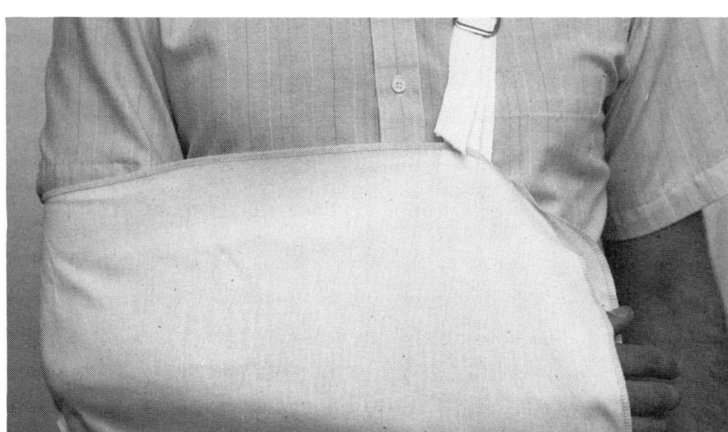

Figure 32-5. The simplest form of immobilization is demonstrated with the standard sling.

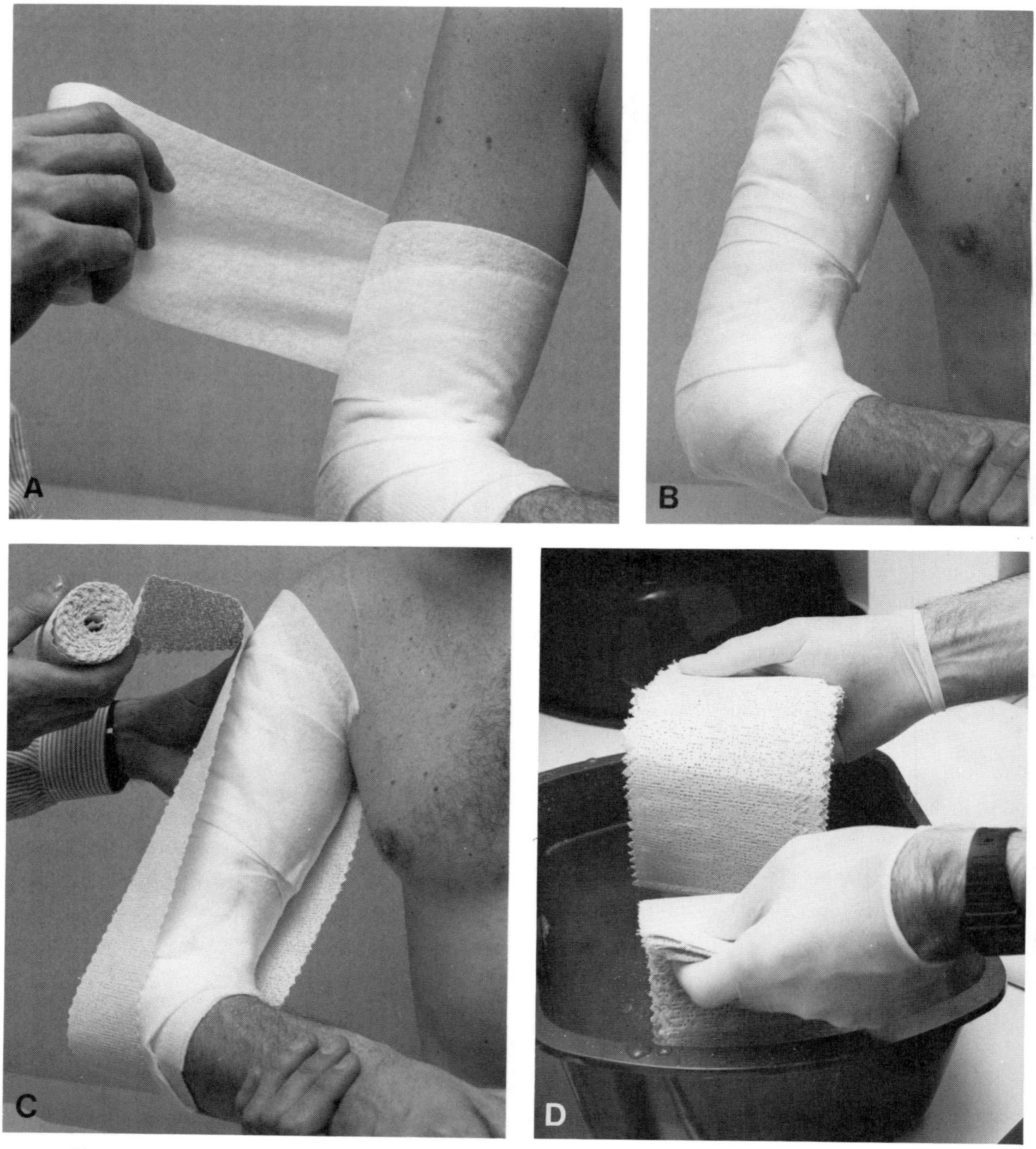

Figure 32-6. (*A,B*) Application of coaptation splints. A thick layer of cast padding is applied. (*C*) The length of the splint is measured. (*D,E*) The splint is held on either end while it is dipped and squeezed.

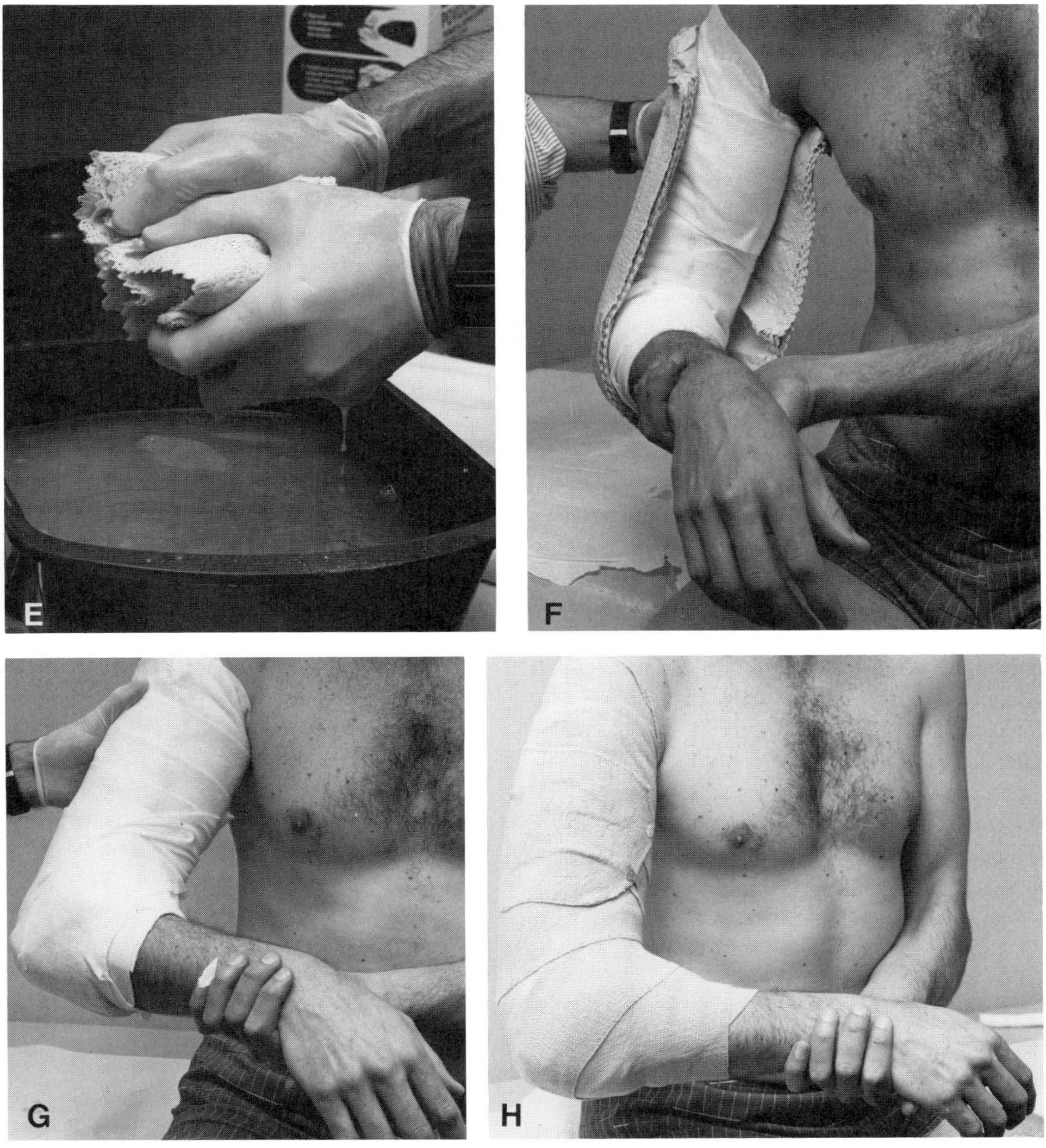

Figure 32-6 (*continued*). (*F*) The splint is applied. (*G*) A thin layer of cast padding. (*H*) An elastic bandage for the outside layer.

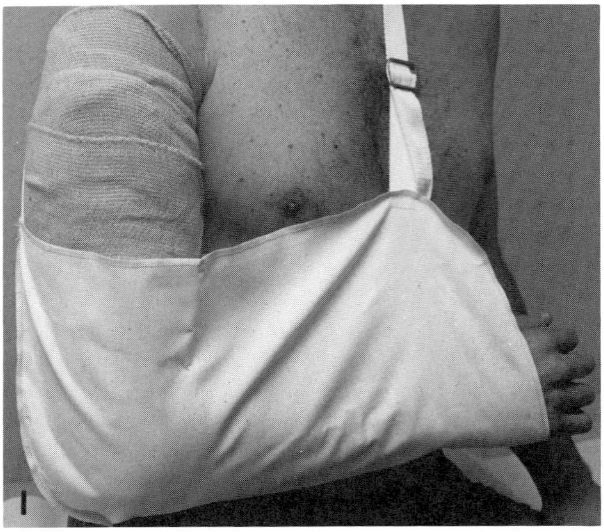

Figure 32-6 (*continued*). (*I*) A sling completes the dressing.

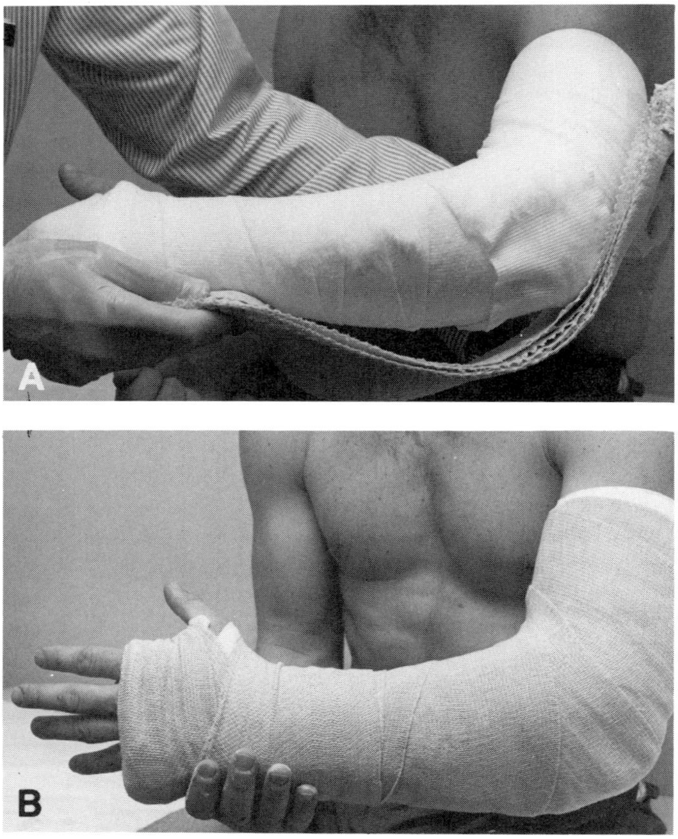

Figure 32-7. Posterior splint for distal arm and elbow injuries. The elbow is immobilized in 90 degrees of flexion, and the wrist is held in neutral position.

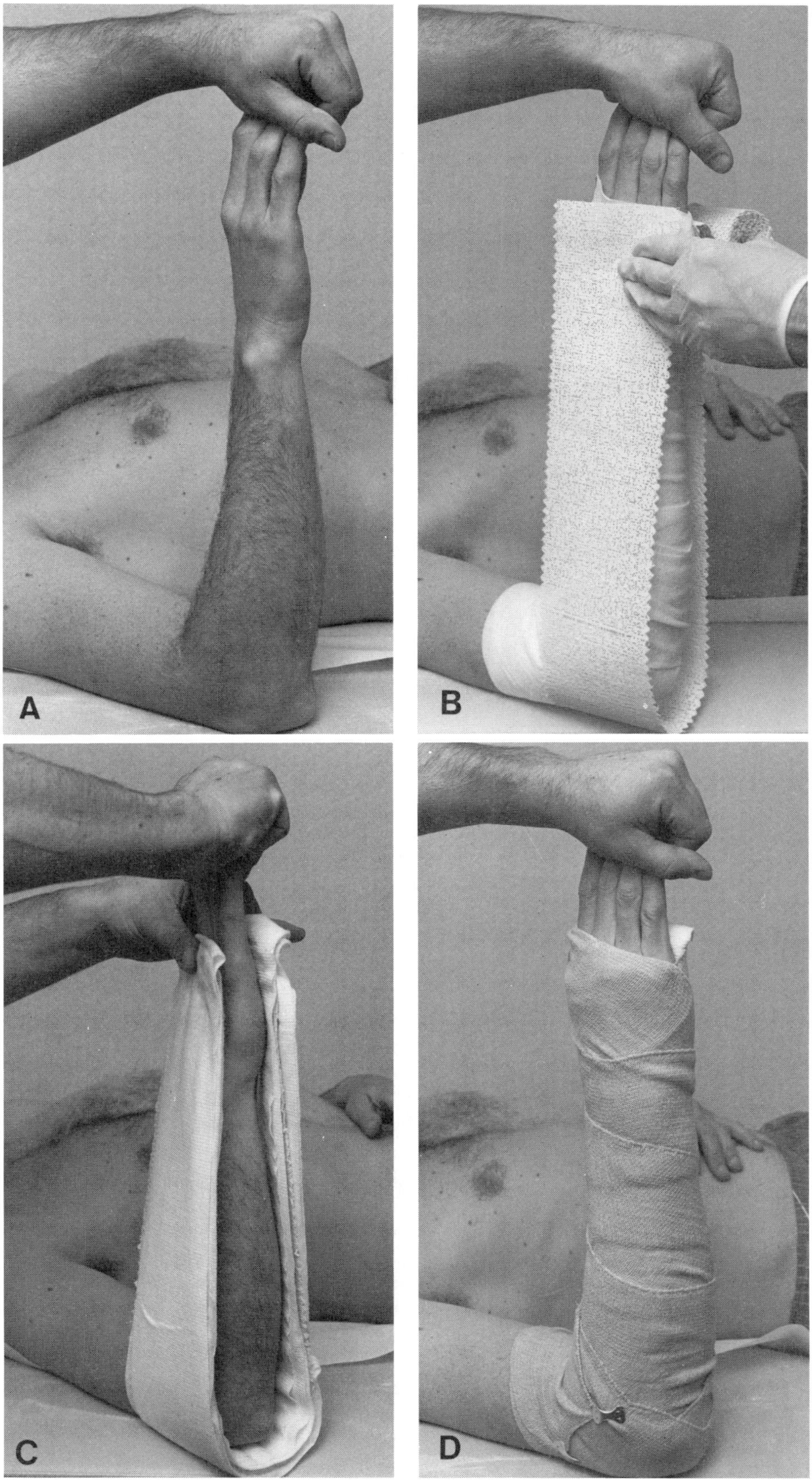

Figure 32-8. (*A*) "Sugar tongs" splint application, The forearm is supported by an assistant. (*B*) Measuring the length of the splint. (*C*) An alternative method of splint application using plaster sandwiched between layers of padding. (*D*) An elastic bandage applied as the outside layer.

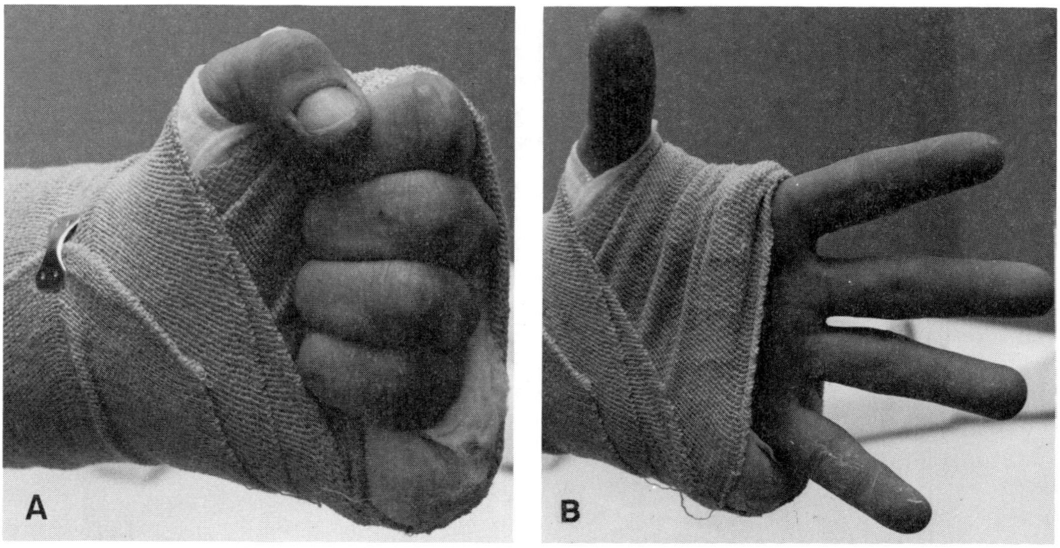

Figure 32-9. The wrist and elbow can be immobilized without immobilizing the fingers.

to prevent excessive heat dissipation during hardening, which can cause burns. Also, the plaster should not be allowed to touch the skin, because serious burns can result. The splint should not be rested directly on a plastic-covered pillow while it is setting, because this also prevents heat dissipation.

OPEN FRACTURES

Open fractures of the upper extremity are surgical emergencies. The same implications and treatment principles apply as for lower-extremity open fractures (see Chap. 33).

COMPARTMENT SYNDROMES

In the upper extremity, compartment syndromes occur most commonly in the forearm. The forearm contains two compartments, volar and dorsal. The dorsal compartment contains the extensor muscles. The volar compartment contains the flexor muscles, along with the median and ulnar nerves. The pathophysiology and treatment principles of compartment syndrome are described in detail in Chapter 33.

SHOULDER

ANATOMY

The shoulder girdle is the most mobile articulation in the body. It contains three synovial joints—the glenohumeral, the acromioclavicular, and the sternoclavicular—and two false joints—the subacromial and the scapulothoracic. In abduction, shoulder motion occurs simultaneously at the glenohumeral joint and the scapulothoracic articulation, with about two third of the motion occurring in the glenohumeral joint.

The anatomy of the clinically important bony and ligamentous structures of the shoulder is illustrated in Figure 32-10. The sternoclavicular joint is an articulation between the medial clavicle and the manubrium. It is stabilized both by the sternoclavicular ligaments and by the joint capsule. The capsule is stronger posteriorly than anteriorly, which may explain the higher incidence of anterior dislocation.

The line of the acromioclavicular joint tilts upward and outward 30 degrees and backward and inward about 20 degrees to 30 degrees. The joint is stabilized superiorly by the acromioclavicular ligament, but the major stabilizing structures are the coracoclavicular ligaments: the conoid and trapezoid. Articulation at the acromioclavicular joint allows the scapula to follow the asymmetric contour of the chest wall during shoulder motion.

The configuration of the glenohumeral joint allows remarkable motion but at the expense of bony stability. The articular cartilage of the humeral head covers an area approximately four times that of the glenoid. The glenoid labrum is a fibrocartilaginous structure around

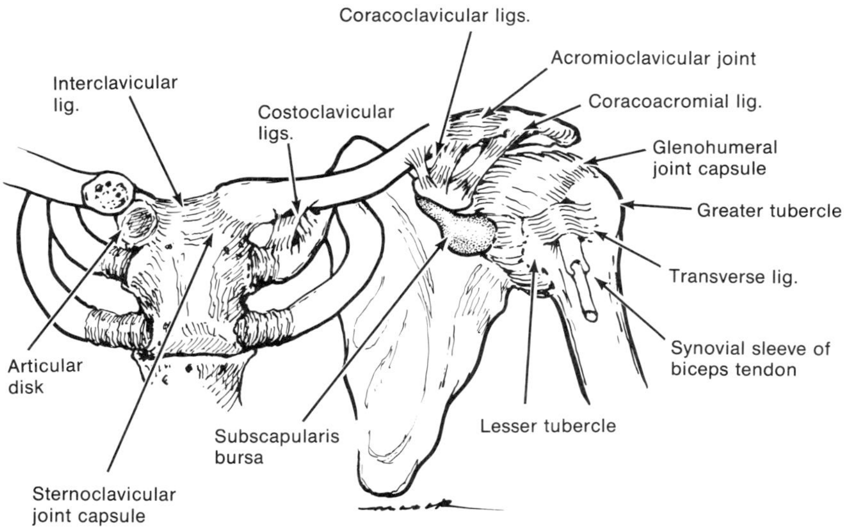

Figure 32-10. Bony and ligamentous anatomy of the shoulder.

the rim of the glenoid, which increases its concavity and hence stability. The shoulder capsule is redundant inferiorly to allow shoulder motion.

The muscles of the shoulder girdle are arranged in two layers (Fig. 32-11). The outer layer is the deltoid muscle, which provides most of the power for shoulder elevation and abduction. The deep layer is called the rotator cuff and is comprised of the supraspinatus, infraspinatus, subscapularis, and teres minor muscles. These muscles are rotators of the humerus and act to depress the humeral head within the glenoid, providing a stable fulcrum

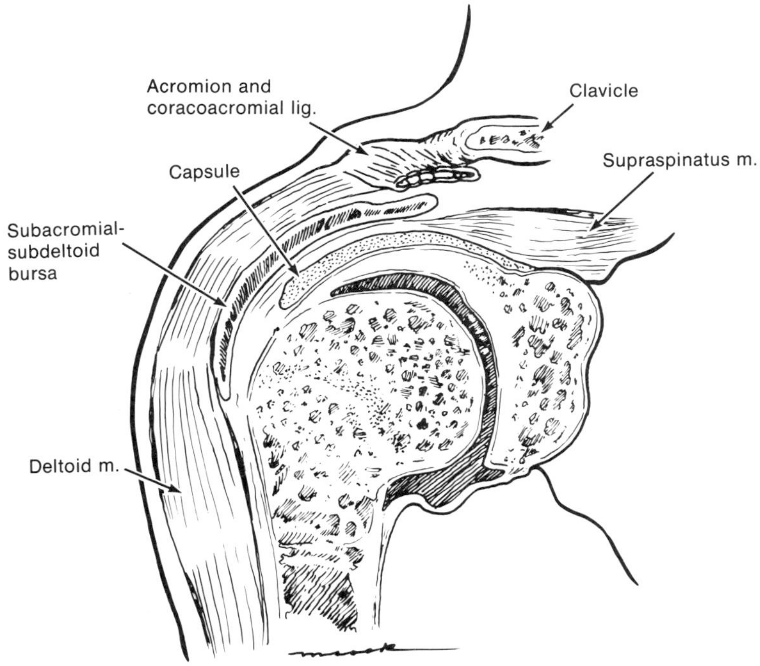

Figure 32-11. Acromial section of the shoulder joint illustrating the position of the deltoid and supraspinatus muscles in relation to the subacromial bursa and the shoulder joint.

for glenohumeral motion. The tendon of the long head of the biceps brachii muscle enters the shoulder joint through the bicipital groove and attaches to the supraglenoid tubercle. Through this attachment it also acts presumably as a dynamic stabilizer of the glenohumeral joint.

HISTORY AND PHYSICAL EXAMINATION

A thorough history is essential in the evaluation of the patient with shoulder complaints. Common shoulder symptoms include pain, giving way, and stiffness. The age of the patient and the duration and nature of the symptoms can strongly indicate a diagnosis. The patient's sex and occupation are also important.

The physical examination of the shoulder begins when the patient enters the room. It may be evident initially that a generalized disorder such as rheumatoid arthritis is present. The presence or absence of normal movement or rhythm of the shoulder during gait and any difficulty with disrobing should also be noted. To perform an adequate shoulder examination, the shoulder and upper extremity should be exposed at least down to the axilla. An appropriate gown arrangement for female patients is shown in Figure 32-12. The shoulder should be inspected closely for any asymmetry or prominence of bony structures indicating muscular atrophy. The opposite side is used for comparison. For example, the patient with a chronic rotator cuff tear can have atrophy of the supraspinatus and infraspinatus muscles, which is manifested by the soft-tissue depressions over the scapula and prominence of the scapular spine.

Palpation of the shoulder should proceed in a systematic fashion. Initially, the sternoclavicular joint is palpated for any tenderness. Palpation continues along the clavicle to the acromioclavicular joint. The anterior and lateral margins of the acromion and the bicipital groove are then palpated for any tenderness that might indicate rotator cuff pathology or biceps tendonitis. Localized areas of tenderness, called trigger points, may be found overlying the muscles of the shoulder girdle. The surface anatomy of the shoulder is illustrated in Figure 32-13.

The true motion of the shoulder is global and an infinite number of planes of motion could be identified. By convention, only a few

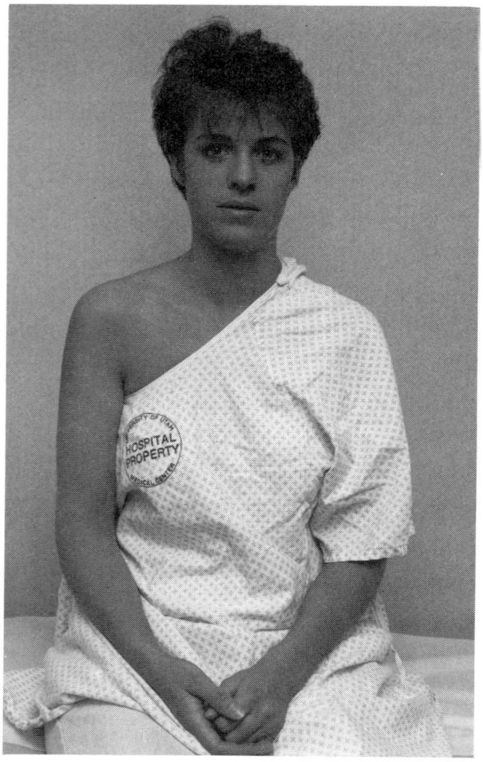

Figure 32-12. An appropriate gown arrangement for a female patient.

motions are documented. These include forward elevation, flexion, abduction and external rotation with the arm at the side and abducted 90 degrees, and internal rotation. The patient is examined in the standing, supine, or sitting positions, depending on the motion that is measured. In the standing position, the patient can compensate for a lack of shoulder motion with the movement of the spine and pelvis (Fig. 32-14). The supine or upright positions are good for measuring forward elevation, flexion, and external rotation. Abduction and internal rotation can best be evaluated with the patient upright. Forward elevation is performed with the arm abducted 15 degrees to 20 degrees, whereas flexion is performed in the sagittal plane (Fig. 32-15A). Abduction is performed in the frontal plane and begins with the extremity at the patient's side (Fig. 32-15B). The normal ranges of both these motions should be near 180 degrees. It will be necessary for the patient to rotate the shoulder externally at 90 degrees of abduction to avoid impingement of the greater tuberosity against the lateral margin of the acromion with the

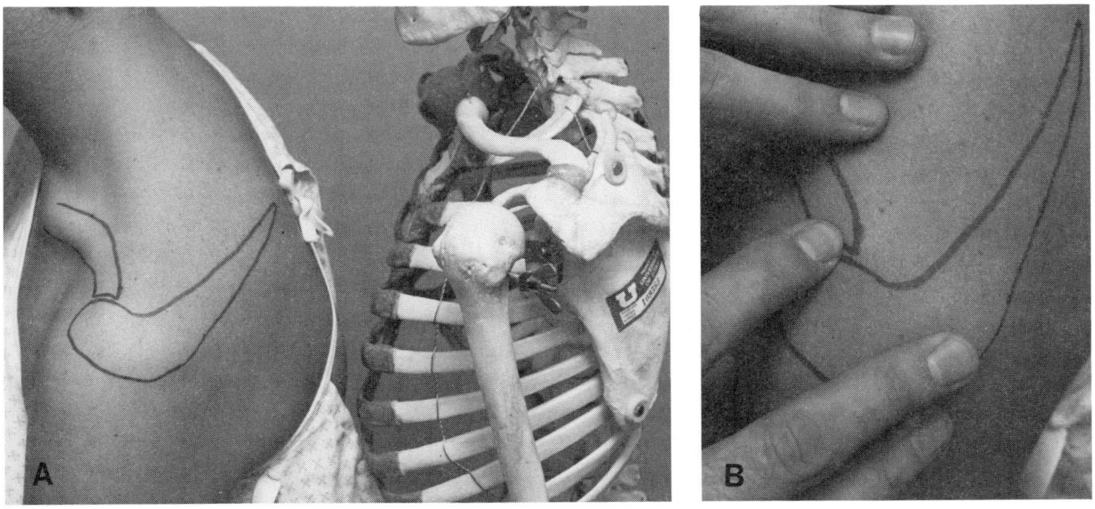

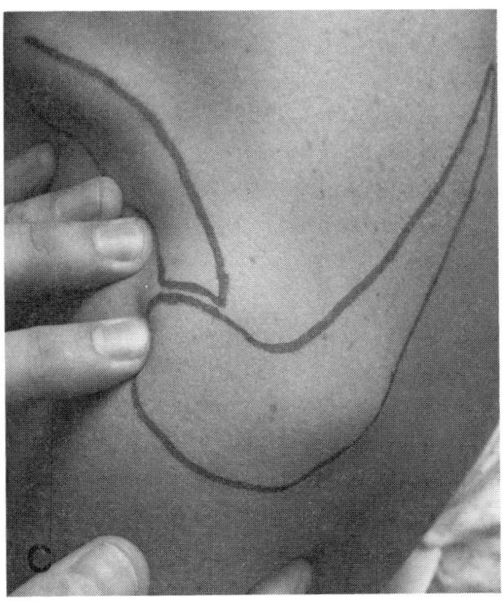

Figure 32-13. (*A*) Surface anatomy of the shoulder. (*B*) Acromioclavicular joint. (*C*) Anterior acromial margin.

further motion. External rotation begins with the arm abducted 90 degrees to the side and the elbow flexed 90 degrees (Fig. 32-15C). There is considerable individual variation in this motion and the two sides should be compared. Internal rotation is measured not in degrees but by the anatomical landmarks reached by the thumb. With progressive internal rotation the thumb will pass the greater trochanter and superior gluteal fold and the spinous processes of the lumbar and thoracic vertebrae (Fig. 32-15D). The lower border of the scapula is at about the level of the tenth thoracic vertebra. Shoulder extension is not necessarily measured, because it is incorporated into internal rotation. If full active range of motion is present, there is no need to test passive motion except to stress the shoulder at extremes to elicit a pain response. Any crepitation on shoulder motion should also be noted.

Motor examination involves testing shoulder strength while performing the motions just described. It is especially important to document strength in abduction and rotation, because weakness of these motions is a common finding in rotator cuff tears (Fig. 32-16).

Stability testing is performed with patients who have a history of frequent dislocations. It should be done with the patient lying relaxed and supine. An apprehension test for anterior shoulder instability is performed by forcefully externally rotating the shoulder with the arm abducted 90 degrees (Fig. 32-17). Discomfort

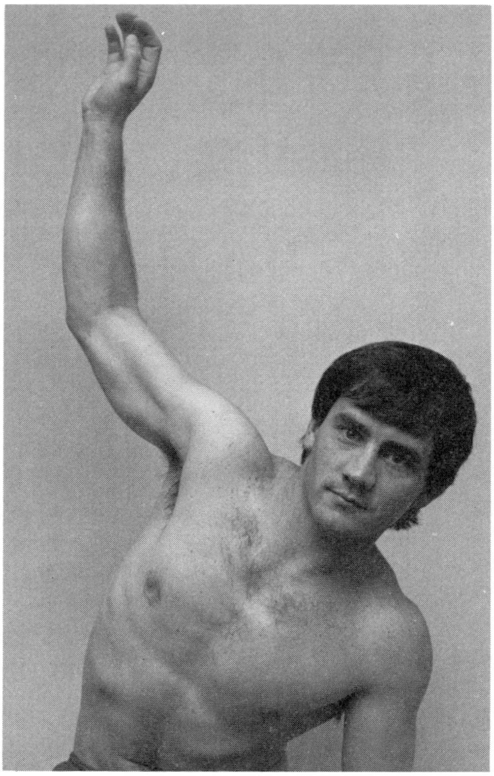

Figure 32-14. Compensating for lack of shoulder motion by bending the back.

and fear of impending dislocation on the part of the patient constitute a positive test.

DISLOCATIONS OF THE STERNOCLAVICULAR JOINT

Etiology

Dislocation of the sternoclavicular joint is a relatively uncommon injury. Usually a large amount of force is involved. Typical settings are a motor vehicle accident or a contact sport such as football.

Sternoclavicular dislocations can occur as a result of direct or indirect force applied to the joint. Direct force can be applied only from anterior to posterior and therefore produces only posterior dislocations. A blow to the lateral aspect of the shoulder can produce an indirect force that results in sternoclavicular joint dislocation. The direction in which the joint dislocates depends on the position of the shoulder at the time the force is applied. If the shoulder is held anteriorly, the medial end of the clavicle is most likely to dislocate posteriorly. However, if the shoulder is retracted at the time of the injury, an anterior dislocation is more common. In general, anterior dislocations are thought to be more common than posterior dislocations, partly because the anatomic restraints to anterior dislocation are weaker than those to posterior dislocation. In posterior dislocations the medial end of the clavicle can be displaced into the mediastinum and injure, or compress, important structures such as the great vessels, esophagus, and trachea.

Diagnosis

Although the sternoclavicular joint is a subcutaneous structure, in the setting of dislocations, soft-tissue swelling may be severe enough to make diagnosis by palpation difficult. This is usually the case if the patient is examined more than 6 hours after injury. Frequently, patients with this injury have other severe associated trauma, such as a head injury, and cannot complain of pain. The alert patient with a sternoclavicular joint dislocation will complain of localized pain in the area of the joint and of pain with shoulder motion. The history usually reveals a direct or indirect mechanism consistent with the injury. The neck of the patient is typically flexed and tilted toward the side of the injury. Shoulder motion produces pain in the localized area of the joint. The shoulder is held forward if the dislocation is posterior and is retracted if the dislocation is anterior. The patient with a posterior dislocation may complain of dysphagia and dyspnea due to compression of the esophagus and trachea by the medial end of the clavicle. If the patient presents acutely, the nature and direction of the dislocation can be detected by palpation. With an anterior dislocation a bony prominence may also be visible; a posterior dislocation, on the other hand, leaves a depression.

The diagnosis is confirmed with radiographs. Routine anterior–posterior views of the sternoclavicular joint, however, may not be diagnostic. A true lateral view is very difficult to obtain. If the x-ray tube is angled about 40 degrees cephalad with the cassette placed under the cervical spine and shoulders, enough asymmetry between the two sternoclavicular joints can sometimes be detected to make a precise diagnosis. Positioning for this view is difficult; it may be simpler and more advantageous to perform AP tomograms or a CT scan of the sternoclavicular joint, which if

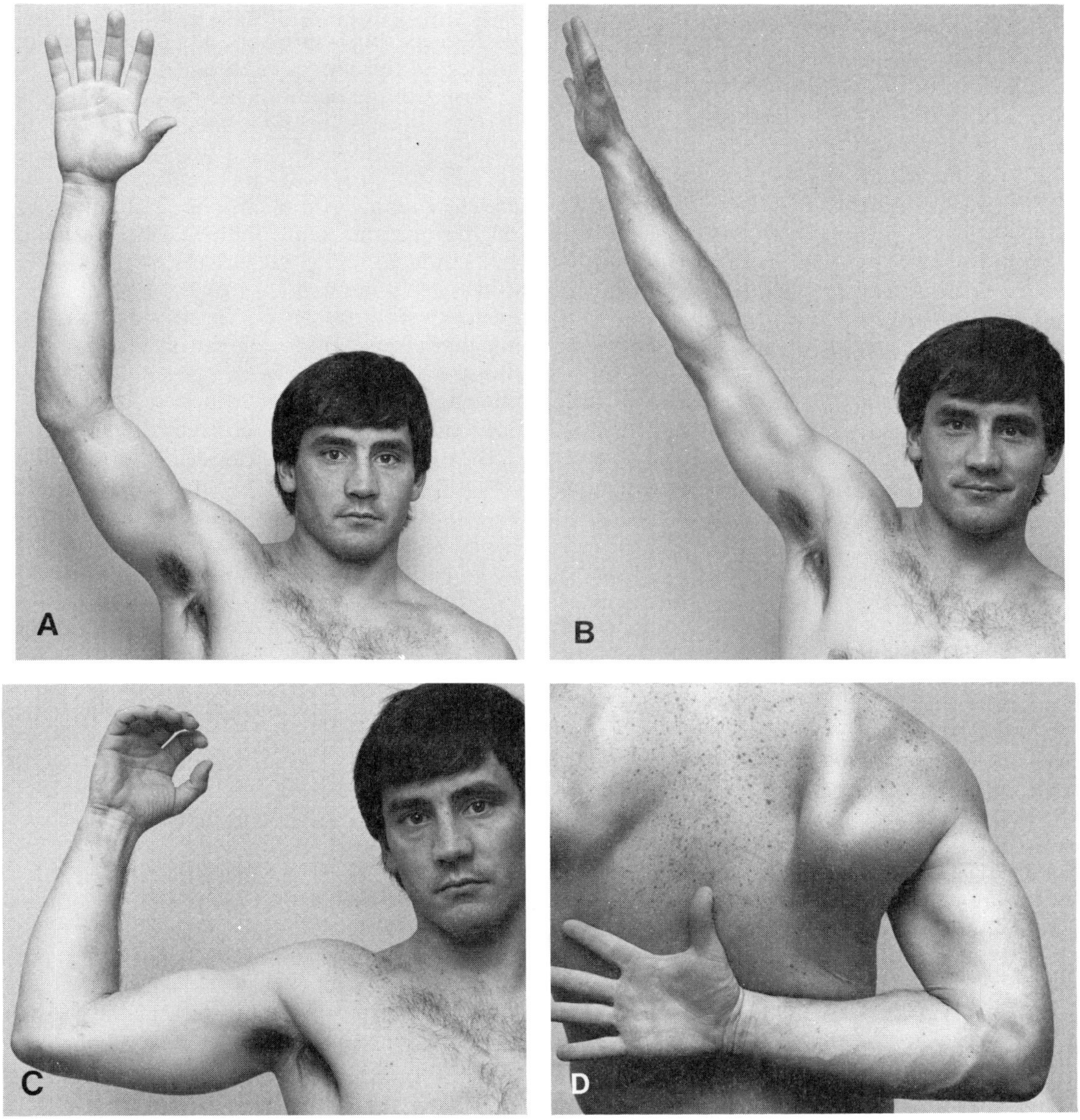

Figure 32-15. (*A*) Forward elevation. (*B*) Abduction. (*C*) External rotation. (*D*) Internal rotation.

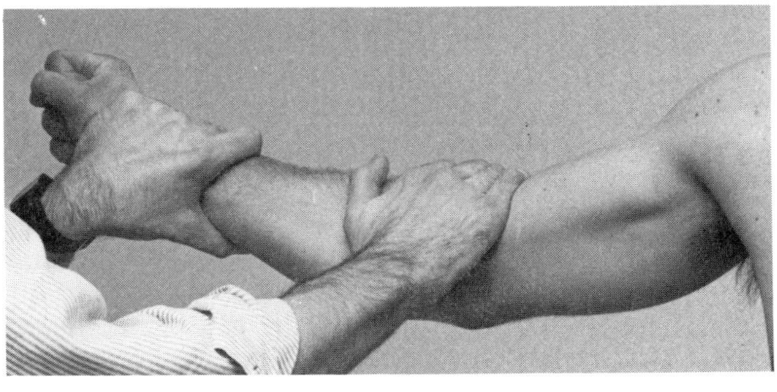

Figure 32-16. Testing for strength of shoulder abduction.

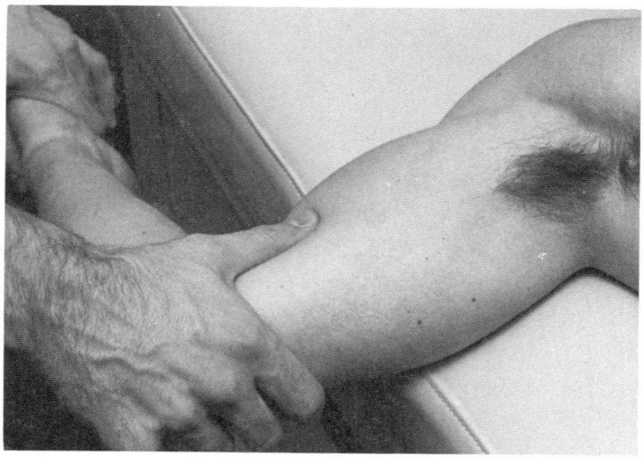

Figure 32-17. Apprehension test.

properly done can provide excellent imaging of the joint.

Treatment

The vast majority of sternoclavicular dislocations are anterior and pose no threat to the mediastinal structures. If these injuries are untreated, they are not usually associated with long-term disability. If chronic pain develops, the medial third of the clavicle can be excised without fear of compromising shoulder function.

If the diagnosis is made acutely, however, it is reasonable to attempt a closed reduction of the joint. This is done with the aid of muscle relaxants and a general or local anesthesia as appropriate. A prerequisite to performing a reduction is that a sandbag or folded towels be placed under the patient's spine to allow retraction of the injured shoulder. Traction is then applied to the upper extremity with the shoulder abducted and in line with the clavicle. A sheet placed through the patient's axilla can be used by an assistant to apply countertraction. A second assistant then applies direct anterior pressure over the medial end of the clavicle. After the reduction, the patient is immobilized in a figure-of-eight splint. The total time of immobilization in the splint should be at least 6 weeks, to allow adequate healing. The patient's activities should be limited for a total of 3 months. If the reduction is unstable, a figure-of-eight splint is unnecessary. The patient is then placed in a sling and treated symptomatically. Surgery to reduce the joint involves open reduction with some sort of internal fixation. Traditionally, this has been performed using smooth transfixing pins. However, this technique has been fraught with disastrous complications because of migration of the pins into the mediastinum.

Posterior dislocations are reduced using the identical maneuvers described for anterior dislocations. The evaluating physician must be aware that posterior dislocations can cause life-threatening complications, including pleural rupture and acute injuries to the esophagus, trachea, and great vessels. If the dislocation is left unreduced, chronic compression of these structures can occur with corresponding symptoms. The degree of symptoms is thought to correlate with the amount of the posterior displacement. Since reduction of a posterior dislocation is considered necessary, it is usually best performed in the operating room under general anesthesia. Frequently, these patients are under general anesthesia already for treatment of other injuries. Appropriate surgical backup should be available if vascular injury is suspected. If closed reduction cannot be achieved, then open reduction should be performed without delay. A posterior dislocation usually does not reduce spontaneously with traction applied to the upper extremity. Usually it is necessary to apply anterior traction to the medial clavicle using the fingertips or a towel clip to grasp the bone percutaneously. Closed reduction is most easily accomplished in the acute postinjury period. After 48 hours, the likelihood of a successful closed reduction is significantly diminished. Unlike anterior dislocations, postreduction stability is frequently good with posterior dislocations.

It is important to be aware that the growth plate at the medial end of the clavicle does not close until about the age of 18. Patients with an open growthplate tend to fracture through the plate instead of dislocating the medial end of the clavicle. Displacement can be accepted, however, since with continued growth the bone will remodel. Treatment consists of closed reduction and immobilization in a figure-of-eight splint for about 4 weeks.

CLAVICLE FRACTURES

Fractures of the clavicle are common, accounting for over 40% of all shoulder injuries and about 5% of all fractures. The clavicle is frequently divided anatomically into thirds, and the classification of clavicle fractures follows this division. Fractures of the medial

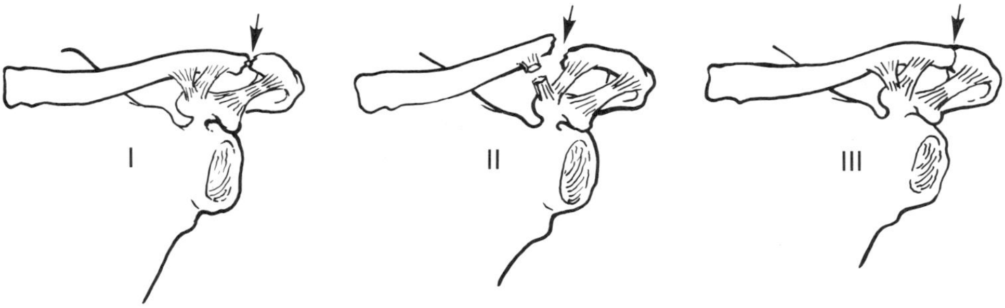

Figure 32-18. Classification of fractures of the distal clavicle. (*Left*) A type I, nondisplaced fracture with intact ligaments. (*Center*) A type II, displaced interligamentous fracture in which the coracoclavicular ligaments are detached from the proximal segment, rendering the lesion unstable. (*Right*) A type III, articular surface fracture, which is easily overlooked and may lead to post-traumatic arthritis.

third of the clavicle are the least common and are usually due to a direct blow. Unless displacement is severe, their course is usually benign. The vast majority of clavicle fractures occurs in the middle third, resulting from direct trauma or a blow to the lateral aspect of the shoulder. If the force is severe enough, significant displacement can occur. Displacement is exacerbated by the pull of the sternocleidomastoid muscle on the medial fragment and the weight of the upper extremity on the lateral fragment. Fractures of the lateral third of the clavicle are also relatively rare but account for a large percentage of the complications of clavicle fractures, including arthritis of the acromioclavicular joint, nonunion, and residual shoulder pain. They usually occur from blunt trauma to the lateral aspect of the shoulder. A useful classification of lateral third fractures places them in three groups (Fig. 32-18). A Type I distal clavicle fracture is extra-articular and does not involve disruption of the acromioclavicular ligament. In Type II fractures the coracoclavicular ligament attachment to the proximal fragment is disrupted. The result is that the proximal fragment is displaced superiorly away from the scapula by the pull of the trapezius muscle. The resulting displacement predisposes the patient to nonunion. Type III fractures involve the acromioclavicular joint and are associated with early degenerative arthritis.

Diagnosis

The patient with a clavicle fracture usually cannot localize the pain accurately and give a typical history. On exam, the shoulder has fallen downward and the elbow is supported by the opposite hand for comfort. Tenderness, swelling, and deformity at the fracture site are easily detected. Although injuries to the underlying neurovascular bundle are rare in clavicle fractures, they have been reported. Any evaluation of a clavicle fracture should include a neurovascular examination of the upper extremity as the first step. The physician should also be alert to the possibility of a pneumothorax in a patient with respiratory distress and a displaced clavicle fracture. Clavicle fractures can be associated with injuries to the sternoclavicular and acromioclavicular joints. Any associated tenderness over these joints is an indication for a thorough radiographic evaluation.

Clavicle fractures can usually be well delineated radiographically on an AP view of the shoulder. A second view with the tube angled 45 degrees cephalad more accurately demonstrates the fracture displacement. In the case of a Type I or Type II fracture of the distal clavicle with suspected disruption of the coracoclavicular ligaments, a stress AP view can be obtained, including both shoulders with 10-pound weights strapped to each wrist. A patient with a Type II fracture has significant upward displacement of the medial fragment on the stress film.

Treatment

After neurovascular injury has been ruled out, an attempt is made to achieve a satisfactory reduction of the fracture. In the vast majority of cases the fracture is in acceptable position or can be reduced by applying a figure-of-eight splint (Fig. 32-19). Occasionally, a reduction is necessary and can be per-

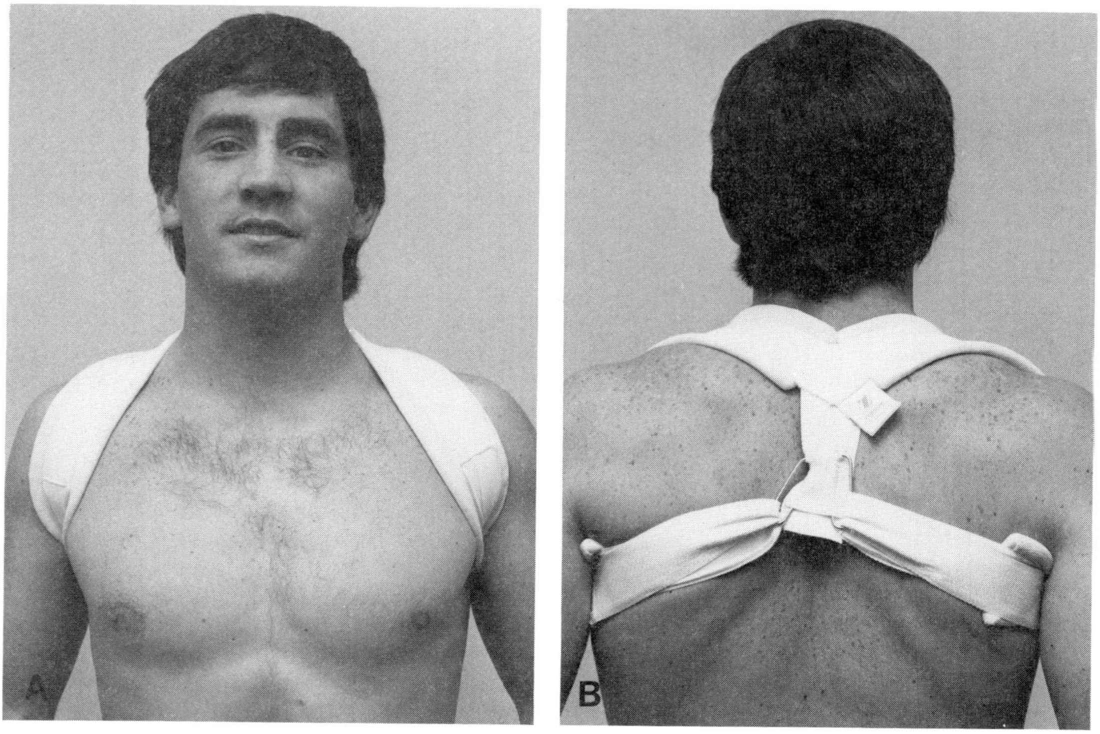

Figure 32-19. Figure-of-eight splint.

formed under general anesthesia using towel clips percutaneously.

Open reduction is rarely indicated because bony union generally occurs even with significant displacement. The patient who is dissatisfied with the cosmetic appearance caused by displacement should realize that open reduction is associated with a higher rate of nonunion and simply means trading a bump for a scar.

There are, however, certain indications for operative treatment of acute clavicle fractures. Open fractures should always be debrided surgically, but they do not necessarily require internal fixation. Type II fractures of the distal clavicle (Fig. 32-20) are associated with a high nonunion rate and are most appropriately treated with internal fixation. If the viability of the overlying skin is compromised by protruding fracture fragments that cannot be reduced, then open reduction may be indicated.

The vast majority of clavicle fractures, including nearly all fractures involving the middle and medial third of the bone, can be treated satisfactorily with a figure-of-eight splint. The splint should be worn for about 6 weeks in adult patients.

Type I and III distal clavicle fractures require only symptomatic treatment with a sling. Resection of the distal clavicle can be done acutely to prevent late-onset osteoarthritis of the acromioclavicular joint in the patient with Type III fracture.

ACROMIOCLAVICULAR JOINT INJURIES

Acromioclavicular joint injuries occur as a consequence of blunt trauma to the shoulder. The force is directed either straight into the shoulder or obliquely from above. Stability of the acromioclavicular joint is provided by two sets of ligaments. The superior and inferior acromioclavicular ligaments are reinforcements of the joint capsule and confer horizontal stability on the acromioclavicular joint. Restraint of vertical translation of the distal clavicle on the acromion is provided by the coracoclavicular ligaments, the conoid and trapezoid. The conoid ligament is a direct connection from the coracoid to the surface of the clavicle immediately superior to it. The

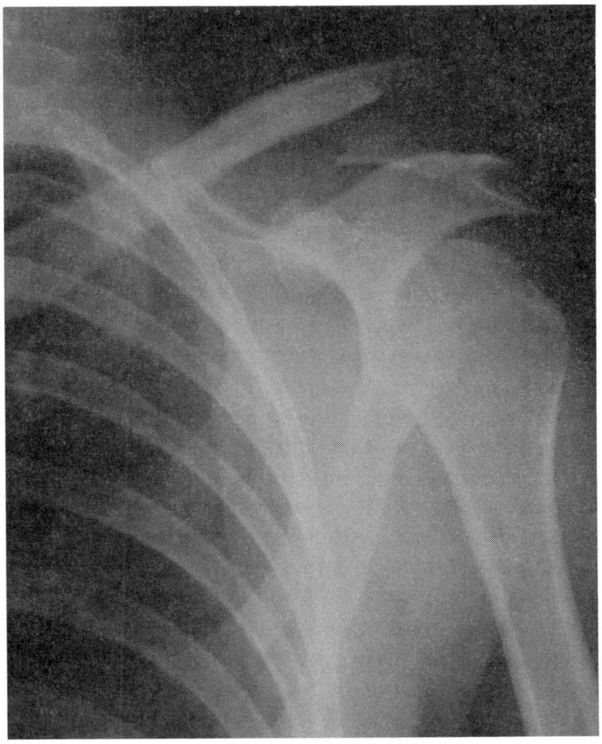

Figure 32-20. Type II fracture of the distal clavicle with third-degree acromioclavicular separation.

trapezoid ligament attaches to the clavicle more laterally near the acromioclavicular joint. Ligamentous injuries involving the acromioclavicular joint are called separations. They are graded according to the amount of trauma to the stabilizing ligaments, which is inferred from the amount of displacement. A Type I injury is a mild sprain of the AC joint capsule without complete disruption of the stabilizing ligaments. In Type II injuries there is significant disruption of the acromioclavicular ligaments evidenced by a subluxation of the joint surfaces. A Type III injury is a complete dislocation of the acromioclavicular joint that occurs as a result of complete rupture of the acromioclavicular ligaments from the coracoclavicular ligaments. As a result of ligamentous disruption the distal clavicle is typically translated superiorly in relation to the acromion. However, it is possible for the clavicle to translate directly posteriorly, which would not be as well visualized on plain x-rays. This would represent a variant of the Type II injury. In rare cases the distal end of the clavicle and the acromion may be widely displaced, such that the distal end of the clavicle is buried within the fibers of the trapezius muscle. This is a Type IV injury.

Diagnosis

Typically, the patient complains of pain localized in the region of the acromioclavicular joint and gives a history of blunt trauma to the shoulder. Acromioclavicular separations can also be caused by a sudden downward pulling force on the adducted upper extremity. The degree of pain and physical findings correlate with the severity of the injury. A patient who strikes his shoulder against a wall while playing racquetball may not even notice pain in the acromioclavicular joint region until several hours later. Patients with Type III and IV separations, however, have immediate severe pain and obvious deformity. Since any downward force on the upper extremity exacerbates the pain, the patient generally presents supporting the elbow of the injured extremity with the opposite hand. Any shoulder motion, especially abduction, causes pain. There may be some evidence of direct trauma to the shoulder, such as abrasions or contusions. Acromioclavicular joint injury should be suspected whenever the patient gives a history of blunt shoulder trauma.

The type of acromioclavicular separation is usually determined on radiographic examination. The acromioclavicular joint region is typically overpenetrated by a routine AP shoulder film. Superimposition of the acromioclavicular joint over the acromion obscures it even more on an AP film. Tilting the x-ray tube 15 degrees cephalad and decreasing the exposure allows adequate visualization of the joint. Comparison with the uninjured side can be done if a large cassette is used and both sides are visualized simultaneously. In large patients two cassettes can be used simultaneously. No radiographic abnormalities are observed in a Type I injury. Type II injuries are defined as a subluxation (incomplete dislocation) of the acromioclavicular joint. In Type III injuries a complete dislocation is present. Because of the configuration of the acromioclavicular joint it may be difficult to determine precisely the type of injury based on the amount of displacement of the joint surfaces alone. In such cases the distances between the coracoid and the clavicle can be measured and compared with the opposite side. A side-to-side difference of 5 mm or greater indicates a complete rupture of the coracoclavicular ligaments. The validity of this measurement may be affected somewhat by the size of the individual. But an increase in the coracoclavicular distance on the injured side of 40% to 50% over the uninjured side correlates with a Type III injury. In cases where the amount of radiographic displacement is not thought to correlate well with the other clinical findings, stress radiographs may be useful to find the true extent of the instability. A stress radiograph is performed with 10 pounds to 15 pounds of weight strapped around each of the patient's wrists. These weights are not held in the hand because contracting the forearm musculature may increase the tone of the shoulder muscles and negate to some extent the effect of the weight. In cases in which the initial films show a Type III injury, stress films are unnecessary because the amount of instability has already been clearly demonstrated on the routine films and physical exam. Similarly, with a mild Type I injury a stress film is usually not indicated. Stress films are uncomfortable for the patient and increase the amount of radiation exposure. They should be ordered for a specific reason. An axillary lateral radiograph should be a routine part of the evaluation of an AC separation, as it is with any other significant shoulder injury. On this view translation of the distal clavicle in the transverse plane can be detected.

Treatment

The treatment of acromioclavicular joint injuries is controversial. Paradoxically, there appears to be, if anything, an inverse relationship between the amount of displacement and the degree of chronic symptoms. Untreated Type III injuries have been shown not to cause significant long-term shoulder dysfunction. Their only effect is on the cosmetic appearance of the shoulder, which is left with a bump. Type I and II injuries treated only symptomatically are more likely to be associated with degenerative AC joint arthritis and chronic pain. The best explanation for this is that Type I or II injuries result in significant joint surface damage or incongruity and yet leave the two surfaces at least partially articulating. In contrast, in Type III (Fig. 32-21) injuries where the two surfaces no longer are opposed, incongruity of the surfaces is inconsequential. In light of the preceding it seems reasonable to treat nearly all AC joint injuries

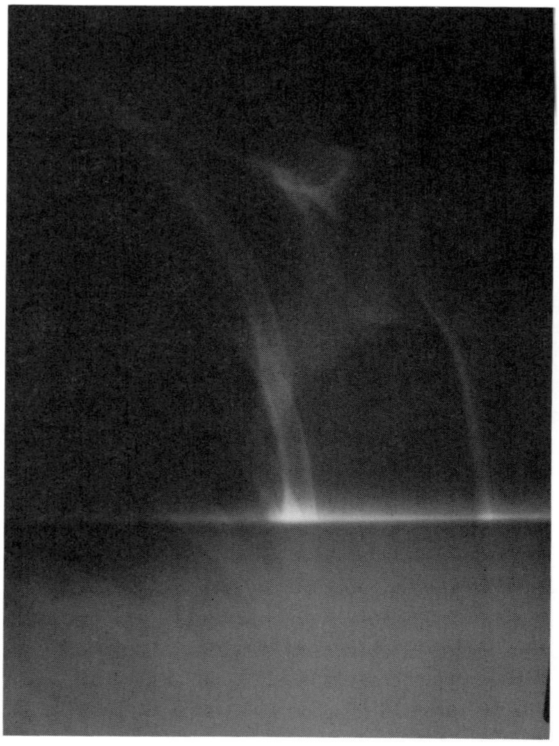

Figure 32-21.

symptomatically initially. If the patient develops degenerative arthritis at the acromioclavicular joint, with chronic pain, the distal 2 cm of the clavicle can be resected with the expectation of satisfactory pain relief and minimal effect on shoulder function. Placing the upper extremity in a sling or shoulder immobilizer and doing range-of-motion (ROM) exercises for about 3 weeks are recommended, as symptoms dictate. This is then followed by a course of physical therapy for regaining motion and strength.

There are several relative indications for surgical repair of acromioclavicular joint injuries. The female patient, for example, with a Type III injury may be displeased with cosmetic appearance. Such a patient should consider whether a scar is more appealing than a bump. Surgical repair may be indicated in athletes who must throw, where even a small disturbance in shoulder function could have a significant detrimental effect. Type IV injuries may interfere with shoulder function enough to justify surgical repair. The technique of repair of acromioclavicular joint separation usually involves securing the clavicle to the coracoid process by a variety of techniques or fixing the end of the clavicle to the acromion, usually with pins passed across the acromioclavicular joint. The latter technique has been complicated by pin breakage and migration.

SCAPULA FRACTURES

The scapula is a complex bone with multiple muscular attachments. The overlying muscles provide protection against injury and allow the scapula to recoil in response to a blow. Thus a relatively large amount of force is necessary to produce a scapula fracture. The vast majority of scapular fractures occur in motor vehicle accidents, but they can also occur as a result of indirect force, such as a fall on the elbow or the outstretched hand. The latter mechanism usually results in a fracture of the acromion or the glenoid. Approximately 75% to 80% of all patients with scapula fractures have other significant injuries. Therefore scapular fractures should be looked for in the multiple-trauma patient and other injuries should be suspected in the patient with a scapula fracture.

Fractures of the scapula are divided into two main groups: those that do not compromise shoulder motion and those that result in decreased shoulder motion. Those fractures involving the body, neck, and spine of the scapula nearly always heal uneventfully without much compromise of shoulder function. In contrast, fractures involving the acromion and glenoid fossa commonly lead to decreased shoulder motion. Intra-articular fractures of the scapula with the significant displacement can also cause premature degenerative arthritis of the glenohumeral joint. The common sites of scapula fractures are illustrated in Figure 32-22.

Diagnosis

Patients with scapula fractures complain of pain that is typically well localized to the area of the injury. There are usually other signs of trauma as well, such as overlying contusions and abrasions. Active shoulder abduction is extremely painful. Occasionally, the patient may display marked weakness of the rotator cuff muscles that is indistinguishable from a rotator cuff tear. In this setting the dysfunction is believed to be due to hematoma formation within the rotator cuff muscles causing spasm and the reflex inhibition.

Scapular fractures can usually be diagnosed radiographically on a routine AP chest radiograph. To define the fracture adequately, however, it may be necessary to obtain true AP and lateral views in the scapular plane. To obtain a true AP view of the scapula the x-ray tube should be angled approximately 30 degrees to 45 degrees lateral to the sagittal plane.

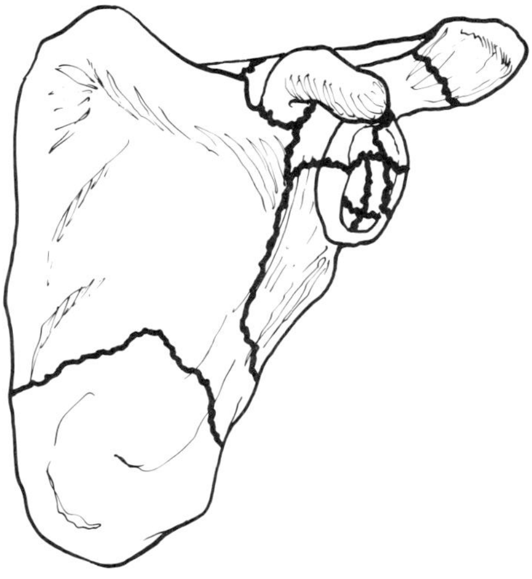

Figure 32-22. Common sites of fractures of the scapula.

The scapular lateral is obtained by positioning the tube at a 90-degree angle to the AP view. An axillary lateral view should also be obtained to visualize the lateral part of the scapula including the acromion, coracoid process, scapular neck, and glenoid.

Treatment

Nearly all scapular fractures are appropriately treated nonoperatively. The shoulder region has excellent vascularity and even significantly displaced fractures of the body and spine usually heal uneventfully. The patient should be placed initially in a shoulder immobilizer for comfort and then ROM exercises should be instituted as soon as the symptoms permit.

Fractures of the coracoid process are most often due to avulsion of the attached muscles and are most appropriately treated conservatively. Fractures of the acromion can be confused with an os acromiale, which represents a failure of fusion of a secondary ossification center in the scapula. Radiographically, this can be distinguished by the irregularity and radiodense cortical margin adjacent to the lucent line, in contrast to a fracture, which is usually a sharp line with no adjacent change in density. Acromion fractures can generally also be treated symptomatically. If, however, the lateral fracture fragment is displaced inferiorly and unites in that position, it may interfere with normal glenohumeral motion. Closed reduction can be attempted by flexing the elbow and pushing superiorly in line with the humerus. If this is unsuccessful, open reduction is indicated. Fractures of the acromion with superior displacement are associated with rotator cuff tears. A patient with this type of acromion fracture should have an arthrogram to rule out a cuff tear. Scapular neck fractures may appear ominous on x-ray films, but like most other scapula fractures, they can be treated very effectively nonoperatively. Again, the preferred treatment is shoulder immobilization until symptoms subside, followed by early ROM. Uneventful healing and return of function usually occur even with significant displacement.

PROXIMAL HUMERUS FRACTURES

Etiology

Proximal humerus fractures in adults occur most commonly in the sixth and seventh decades of life. Osteoporosis is considered one of the prime etiologic factors. In a younger individual the bone is stronger, and if failure occurs it is usually in the soft-tissue restraints, which results in a dislocation. A proximal humeral fracture can lead to debilitating loss of shoulder motion in a previously productive individual.

The common sites of fractures and avulsions of the proximal humerus are shown in Figure 32-23. The anatomic neck of the proximal humerus is located just proximal to the tuberosities, whereas the surgical neck is just distal to the tuberosities. The blood supply to the humeral head comes mainly from the ascending branch of the anterior humeral circumflex artery, which enters the head proximal to the surgical neck. Fractures to the anatomic neck can interrupt this important blood supply. The usual mechanism of proximal humerus fractures in adults is a fall on the outstretched upper extremity. Occasionally, tuberosity fractures occur as a result of forceful contracture of the attached muscles, resulting in avulsion. Fracture dislocations of the proximal humerus occur by the same mechanism as shoulder dislocations in younger individuals, and they occur most commonly in a slightly younger age group than fractures without dislocation.

Proximal humerus fractures are classified according to the anatomic site and displacement of the involved fragments. Displacement is defined as translation of the involved fragment more than 1 cm or angulation of more than 45 degrees. The standard classification places proximal humerus fractures into six groups. Group I is composed of "one-part fractures," which are defined as those with no significant displacement of any of the fracture fragments. All other fractures contain at least two parts, which means at least one of the fracture fragments is displaced. Group II fractures are through the anatomic neck without any displacement of the tuberosities. Fortunately, this is a rare injury, but it can be complicated by aseptic necrosis. Fractures of the surgical neck with displacement are placed in Group III. The prognosis for vascularity of the proximal fragment is much better for these fractures than for those in Group II. Group IV fractures are characterized by displacement of the greater tuberosity. If the tuberosity is displaced more than 1 cm, there is presumed to be a tear in the rotator cuff. In this group there

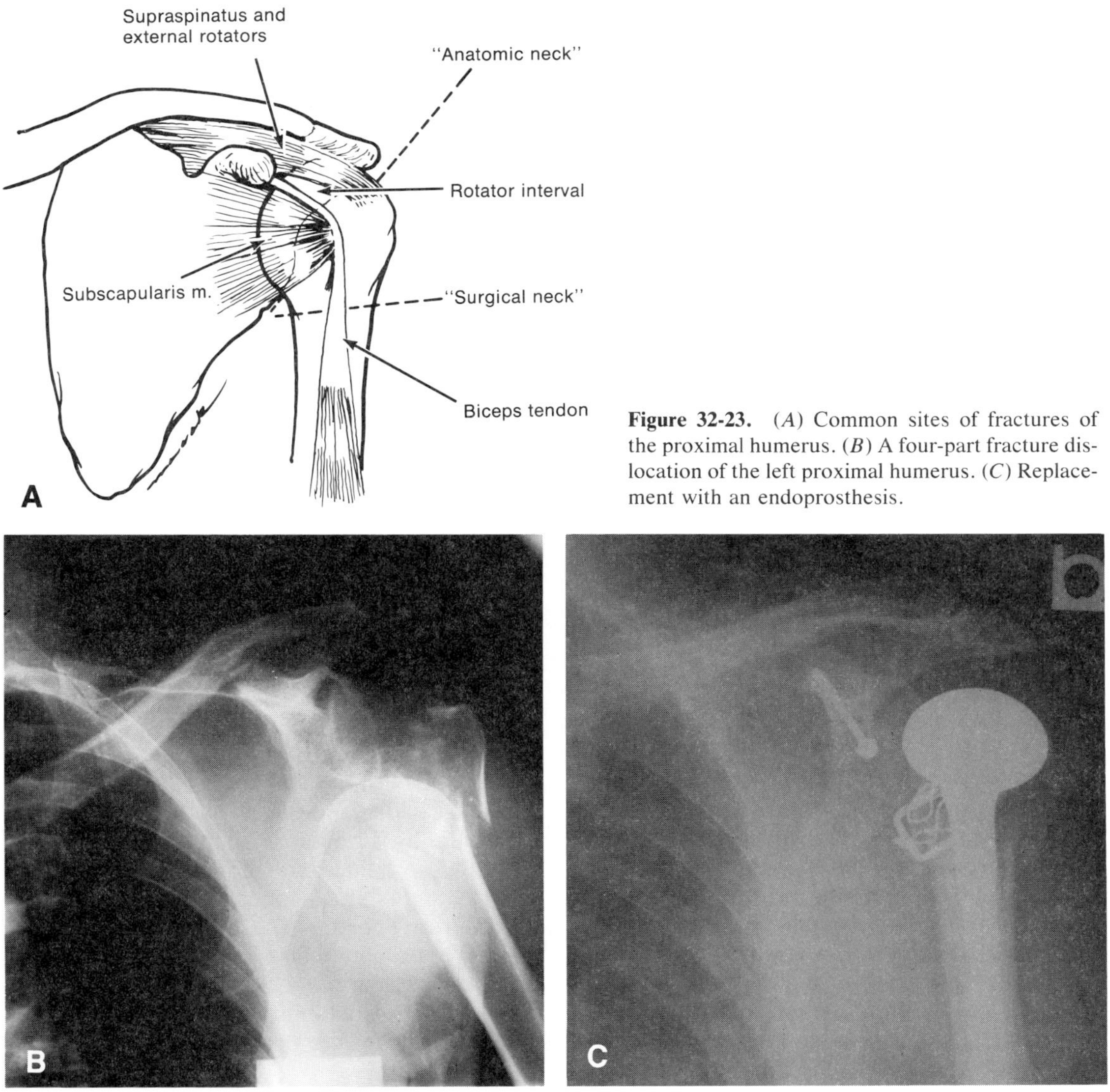

Figure 32-23. (*A*) Common sites of fractures of the proximal humerus. (*B*) A four-part fracture dislocation of the left proximal humerus. (*C*) Replacement with an endoprosthesis.

can also be associated displaced fractures of the lesser tuberosity and/or surgical neck, which are called three- and four-part fractures. Four-part fractures interrupt all the blood supply to the humeral head and have a poor prognosis. Group V fractures are defined as those with displacement of the lesser tuberosity. A three-part fracture in this group has an associated displaced surgical neck. A four-part fracture in this group is the same as a four-part fracture in Group IV. Group VI fractures include anterior and posterior fracture dislocations. Two-part fracture dislocations involve the lesser or greater tuberosity, depending on the direction of the dislocation. Anterior dislocations are associated with greater tuberosity fractures, and in posterior dislocations the lesser tuberosity is usually displaced. A three-part fracture dislocation consists of a displaced fracture of the surgical neck in addition to the tuberosity fracture with dislocation of the humeral head. In a four-part fracture dislocation the humeral head is dislocated and is separated from its vascular supply by the fractures (Fig. 32-23A).

Diagnosis

The patient with a fracture of the proximal humerus complains of severe pain on motion and has severe swelling and tenderness about the shoulder. A history of direct or indirect trauma in the appropriate age group is a strong indication of this type of injury. As with any other significant upper-extremity injury, the neurovascular status should be assessed initially. A thorough radiographic examination should be performed, including AP and lateral views in the scapular plane. An axillary lateral view is also mandatory to rule out dislocation of the humeral head, which may not be evident on the other projections.

Treatment

The previously described classification is useful because it provides a rational approach to treatment. Group I fractures are treated symptomatically with initial immobilization until symptoms subside followed by early ROM. Two-part fractures can be treated closed unless the displaced fragment is the greater tuberosity, in which case open reduction, internal fixation, and rotator cuff repair are indicated. In three-part fractures the muscle pull on one of the tuberosities is no longer counterbalanced by the pull on the other tuberosity. The result is rotational displacement of the humeral head fragment caused by the unopposed muscle pull. Most authorities agree that three-part fractures are associated with unacceptable deformity and are best treated surgically. Open reduction with internal fixation (ORIF) is the treatment of choice, but prosthetic replacement of the humeral head is also acceptable in some cases. Four-part fractures have a uniformly poor prognosis; a prosthetic replacement is the treatment of choice. This approach, together with aggressive postoperative physical therapy, gives the patient the best chance for return of shoulder function (Fig. 32-23B).

Reduction of fracture dislocations of the proximal humerus is difficult to achieve by closed methods. Direct fingertip pressure on the displaced head fragment can sometimes be used to improve the ease of the reduction. This should be done in the controlled environment of the operating room under general anesthesia with muscle relaxation. If the closed reduction cannot be achieved, open reduction should be undertaken without delay.

GLENOHUMERAL DISLOCATIONS

Glenohumeral dislocations account for 30% of all shoulder injuries. The glenohumeral joint is the most commonly dislocated joint of the body, probably because of its lack of inherent bony stability. The main contribution to glenohumeral instability is made by the capsule and surrounding muscles. The strength of the capsule decreases with age and reaches its peak in about the third decade. Dislocations in older persons usually result in tears of the capsule, whereas those in patients younger than 30 usually cause avulsion of the glenoid labrum by pulling the capsule. This defect in the attachment of the labrum is called a Bankart lesion and is thought to be the most specific anatomic correlate to recurrent shoulder instability.

Several types of instability have been described and a fairly specific terminology has evolved. *Acute instability* is the term reserved for the initial instability episode, which is usually posttraumatic. The term *recurrent instability* is used to describe repeated episodes of instability that may not always have associated trauma. *Chronic instability* is a term reserved for a fixed or permanent dislocation. The patient with chronic instability has a dislocated shoulder that has not been reduced for some time, in contrast to the patient with recurrent instability, whose shoulder is generally in a reduced position.

Shoulder instability is also described by the direction in which the abnormal translation of the humeral head occurs. Translation can be anterior, posterior, superior, inferior, or multidirectional. Before undertaking any surgical reconstruction of the shoulder, the exact nature of the instability must be defined so that the appropriate procedure can be undertaken.

Shoulder instability is also classified according to the degree of the instability. The term *subluxation* refers to displacement of the articular surfaces from their normal position without complete loss of contact. A dislocation is a complete displacement of the two articulating surfaces. A subluxation is a transient event, and the diagnosis is frequently made from the patient's history.

More than 90% of all shoulder dislocations are anterior. Instability is recurrent in about one third of all cases. Posterior dislocations are rare but are notorious, because the diagnosis is frequently missed. This is most often attributed to the fact that the radiographic appearance on the AP view of the shoulder can appear near normal in the presence of a posterior dislocation. An even less common type is the inferior dislocation, which is also called luxatio erecta.

Diagnosis

The mechanism of an anterior dislocation most often involves forced external rotation of the abducted shoulder. The patient usually gives a history consistent with this mechanism and complains of acute severe pain. Usually the patient is aware that the shoulder is dislocated. A history of any previous dislocations or other shoulder problems should always be obtained.

Examiners should also be alert to the patient with psychiatric problems who is a recurrent voluntary dislocator. These patients are manipulative and dislocate their shoulders for secondary gain (e.g., to obtain narcotics).

On physical examination the patient with an acute anterior dislocation is obviously uncomfortable. The arm is usually held in slight to moderate abduction and the lateral border of the acromion is prominent on palpation. Any active or passive movement of the shoulder is painful, especially adduction and internal rotation.

The most common mechanism of a posterior dislocation is a combination of forceful internal rotation, adduction, and flexion. Occasionally, a direct blow to the anterior humeral head can produce a posterior dislocation. The most common cause of posterior dislocation is an accidental electrical shock or a convulsive seizure. In any patient with any dislocation induced in either of these settings a posterior dislocation should be strongly suspected.

The physical signs of posterior dislocation are classic and should not be missed. Diagnosis should not depend on radiographic evaluation alone. The patient with posterior dislocation holds the arm in fixed adduction and internal rotation. Active and passive external rotation are markedly limited because of mechanical block of the humeral head impinging on the posterior lip of the glenoid. The posterior aspect of the shoulder is more prominent when compared to the normal side, and the anterior aspect is less prominent. The coracoid process is also more prominent than on the normal side. Another typical finding is that when the elbow is extended, the forearm cannot be fully supinated, also because of the mechanical impingement of the humeral head on the glenoid.

Luxatio erecta, or inferior dislocation (Fig. 32-24), is caused by forced hyperabduction of the shoulder, which results in impingement of the neck of the humerus against the acromion. The head is levered inferiorly and can "button-hole" through the inferior capsule. The clinical findings are unmistakable. The arm is fixed in more than 90 degrees of abduction and the patient is in extreme pain. The humerus is sometimes palpable, overlying the lateral chest wall. Neurovascular complications, especially brachial plexus injuries, are commonly associated with this type of dislocation.

The radiographic evaluation is important for both the diagnosis and treatment of glenohumeral instability. It is absolutely essential that

(*Text continues on p 614.*)

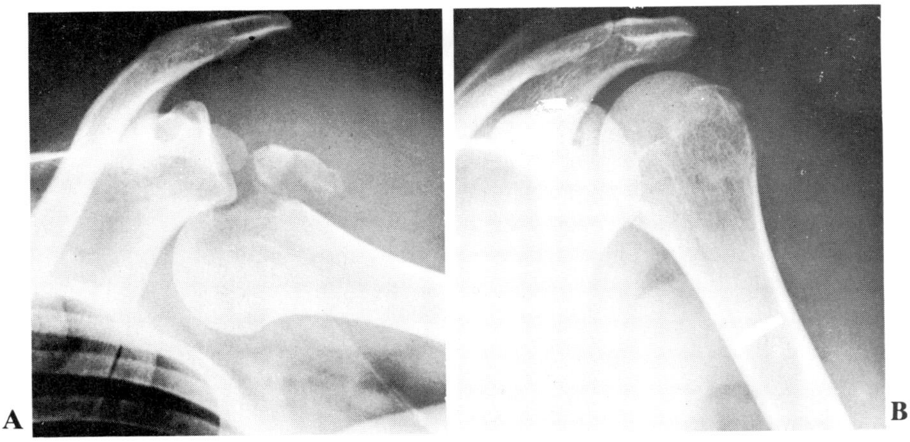

Figure 32-24. Luxatio erecta complicated by a fracture of the greater tuberosity.

the glenohumeral joint be imaged in two orthogonal planes. The patient with a shoulder dislocation always has discomfort on abduction of the shoulder. For this reason x-ray technicians are reluctant to perform an axillary lateral view of the shoulder, which requires abduction. Several alternative techniques have been developed to obtain a reliable lateral view of the shoulder in patients with suspected dislocations. In our experience, however, an adequate axillary lateral view can be obtained in any patient with any shoulder injury if positioning is done slowly and gently. The traditional technique of positioning for an axillary lateral view involves placing the cassette in the axilla and directing the x-ray beam toward it from above. However, if the positions of the x-ray tube and the cassette are reversed so that the beam is directed into the axilla from below, an adequate axillary lateral view can be obtained with the shoulder abducted as little as 30 degrees (Fig. 32-25A). Other methods of obtaining satisfactory lateral views of the shoulder have been developed but are technically more difficult and are reliable only in experienced hands. One such technique is the transscapular view. To obtain this view the x-ray cassette is placed to the side of the shoulder perpendicular to the plane of the scapula (Fig. 32-25C). The x-ray beam is then directed obliquely in line with the scapula. In this view the scapula is Y-shaped and the normal (reduced) humeral head should be centered where the arms of the Y meet (Fig. 32-25D,E,F).

Treatment

All shoulder dislocations should be reduced as soon as possible after a neurovascular examination and radiographs are obtained. This is generally undertaken in the emergency room. The patient is premedicated with narcotics and muscle relaxants, which can be given either by the intravenous or intramuscular route. In either case it is important to have an intravenous line in the uninvolved extremity. Regardless of the technique used to reduce the dislocation, the goal should always be to achieve the reduction as gently as possible.

A simple technique for reducing anterior dislocation involves using traction with countertraction. Countertraction is applied through a sheet looped through the patient's axilla. Traction is gently and gradually applied in line with the humerus. After the soft tissues are felt to be out to length, the arm can be gently internally and externally rotated. When the shoulder reduces there is usually a palpable "clunk." If the technique is done properly and gently, the patient may hardly be aware initially that the shoulder is reduced. Another commonly used technique of reduction involves placing the patient prone and hanging the involved extremity over the side of the table. A weight is then tied to the wrist and the shoulder reduces spontaneously after a variable period of time. The amount of weight can vary with the size and musculature of the individual, but 5 pounds is usually adequate.

Posterior dislocations can be reduced closed by applying traction in line with the deformity and gently lifting the head back into the glenoid fossa. Under no circumstances should the arm be forcefully externally rotated.

The reduction of an inferior dislocation is performed using the same traction–countertraction technique described earlier. The folded sheet should be placed across the top of the shoulder to apply countertraction in the proper direction. Again, when the soft tissues are out to length, reduction may be facilitated by gentle internal and external rotation.

Reduction of a dislocated shoulder should always be preceded by x-ray views as described earlier and a neurovascular examination of the upper extremity. Anterior dislocations are associated with injuries to the axillary nerve. It is important to document whether the injury or deficit was present before the reduction. Another purpose of the prereduction x-rays is to document the direction of the dislocation. Not only is this important for reduction, but it also documents the direction of the dislocation, which aids the orthopaedic surgeon in planning reconstruction should the instability become recurrent.

HUMERAL SHAFT FRACTURES

Etiology

The most common mechanism of fractures of the humeral shaft is direct violence, such as occurs with a fall or an automobile accident. As with other upper-extremity injuries, the mechanism can also be an indirect force, such as a fall on the outstretched hand. Rarely, a humeral shaft fracture can be caused by throwing a heavy object.

Diagnosis

The patient with a humeral shaft fracture has marked tenderness and swelling at the fracture site. The arm is shortened by the accompanying muscle spasm. In some cases an angular deformity may be visible. Manipulation is usually not necessary to make the diagnosis, but when performed it elicits instability and crepitation at the fracture site.

The fracture pattern is determined on radiographic examination and is described, as for any other long bone fracture. A spiral pattern implies a rotational mechanism, whereas a transverse fracture is usually caused by a direct blow. Simple transverse fractures are associated with less force and soft-tissue injury than comminuted fractures. The radial nerve courses near the humeral shaft and is at risk of injury, especially with spiral fractures of the distal third.

Treatment

Open humeral shaft fractures are surgical emergencies and are treated according to the same principles applied to other open fractures. The vast majority of humeral fractures can be treated effectively by closed means with a satisfactory union rate in excess of 90%. Up to 20 degrees of apex anterior and 30 degrees of apex lateral angulation with up to 3 cm of shortening can be accepted. One popular method of treating humeral shaft fractures is the hanging cast. The cast should be as lightweight as possible and extend above the elbow while immobilizing the wrist in neutral position (see Fig. 32-9). The elbow should be immobilized at a right angle, and the forearm should be suspended by a sling. Posterior angulation can be corrected by lengthening or shortening the sling. ROM exercises can be performed with the cast on. There are several disadvantages to the hanging cast. The weight of the cast plus the upper extremity can be great enough to actually cause distraction at the fracture site and lead to nonunion. The cast immobilizes the shoulder and the wrist, which can lead to stiffness after the cast is removed. If the cast extends only up to the level of the fracture, it can actually act as a long lever arm and increase motion at the fracture site.

Another popular method of managing humeral shaft fractures is to use a coaptation splint. As with hanging casts angulation at the fracture site can be corrected somewhat by shortening or lengthening the sling. This technique has the advantage of allowing some elbow and full wrist motion during the period of immobilization of the arm. A relatively new method of mobilization of humeral shaft fractures is the functional brace. The brace consists of two half-shells of polypropylene with Velcro straps. Functional braces can be either custom made or prefabricated. They are lightweight and easily adjustable. They are also designed to allow full elbow motion. The results of treatment using these devices are comparable to those using other closed methods.

ELBOW DISLOCATIONS

Dislocations of the elbow are fairly common injuries. They are commonly associated with neurologic and vascular injuries. As with other dislocations they should be reduced as soon as possible to avoid excessive swelling, circulatory compromise, and articular cartilage damage. Although they can occur in any direction, over 80% are posterior or posterolateral. The usual mechanism is a fall on the outstretched hand with hyperextension of the elbow. The distal end of the humerus pierces the anterior joint capsule and the brachialis muscle is torn.

DIAGNOSIS

If the injury is acute the diagnosis can be made by palpation. However, if swelling is severe it is difficult to distinguish an elbow dislocation from a fracture in the same area. The elbow is usually held in about 45 degrees of flexion and the forearm appears shortened. The distal humerus may be palpable in the antecubital fossa. The olecranon process tenses the skin posteriorly. The nature of the dislocation and associated fractures can be detected on routine AP and lateral radiographs of the elbow.

TREATMENT

The first step in management is careful neurovascular examination of the upper extremity. It is important to document any deficits before a reduction is attempted. The preferred form of anesthesia is intravenous or intramuscular narcotics and muscle relaxants. The only other effective form is an I.V. regional anesthetic. The latter technique has two important

(*Text continues on p 616.*)

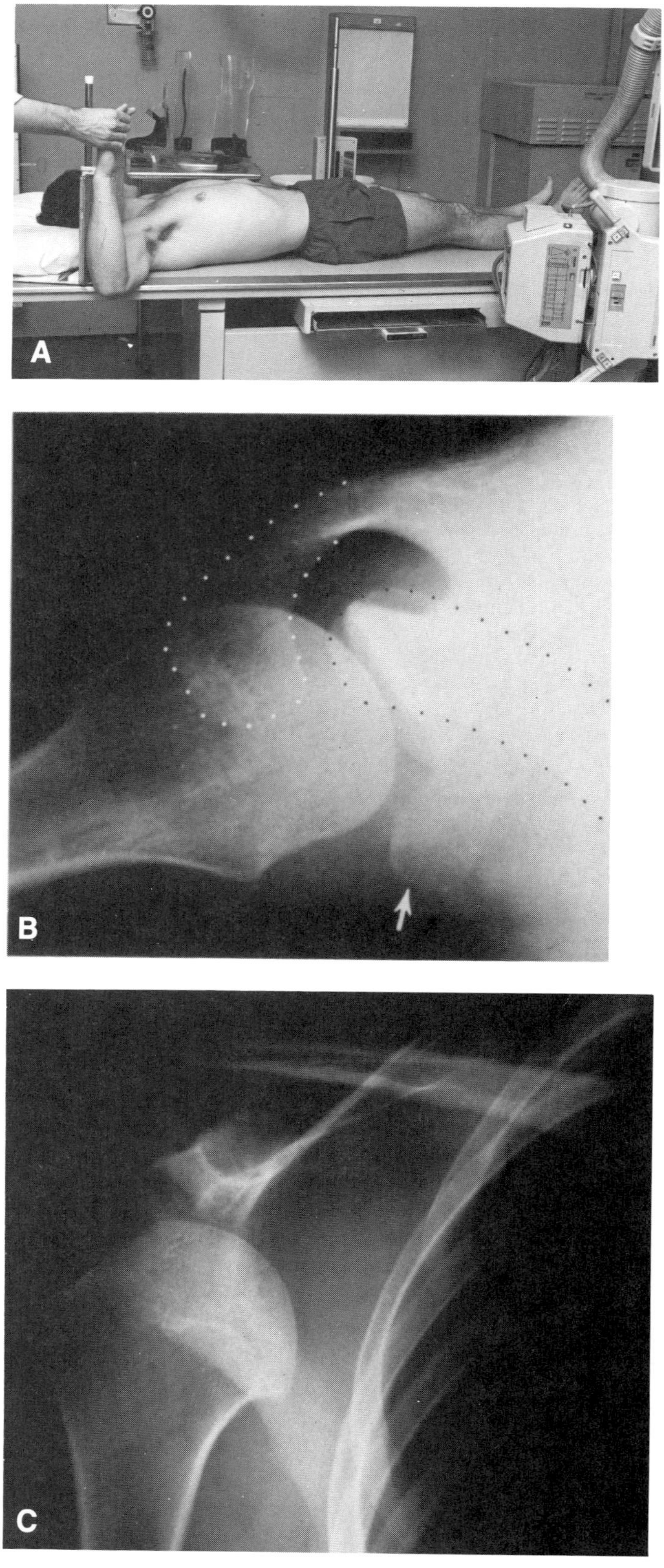

Figure 32-25. (*A*) Positioning for an axillary lateral radiograph. (*B*) Axillary lateral radiograph of the shoulder. The acromion is outlined in white dots and the clavicle in black dots. The arrow points to the tip of the coracoid. (*C, D*) AP and axillary views of an anterior shoulder dislocation. (*E, F*) The same views of a posterior dislocation. Note that the dislocation is not obvious on the AP view. (*B*, Rosse C: The shoulder region and the brachial plexus. In Rosse C, Clawson DK: The Musculoskeletal System in Health and Disease p 81. Hagerstown, Harper & Row, 1980)

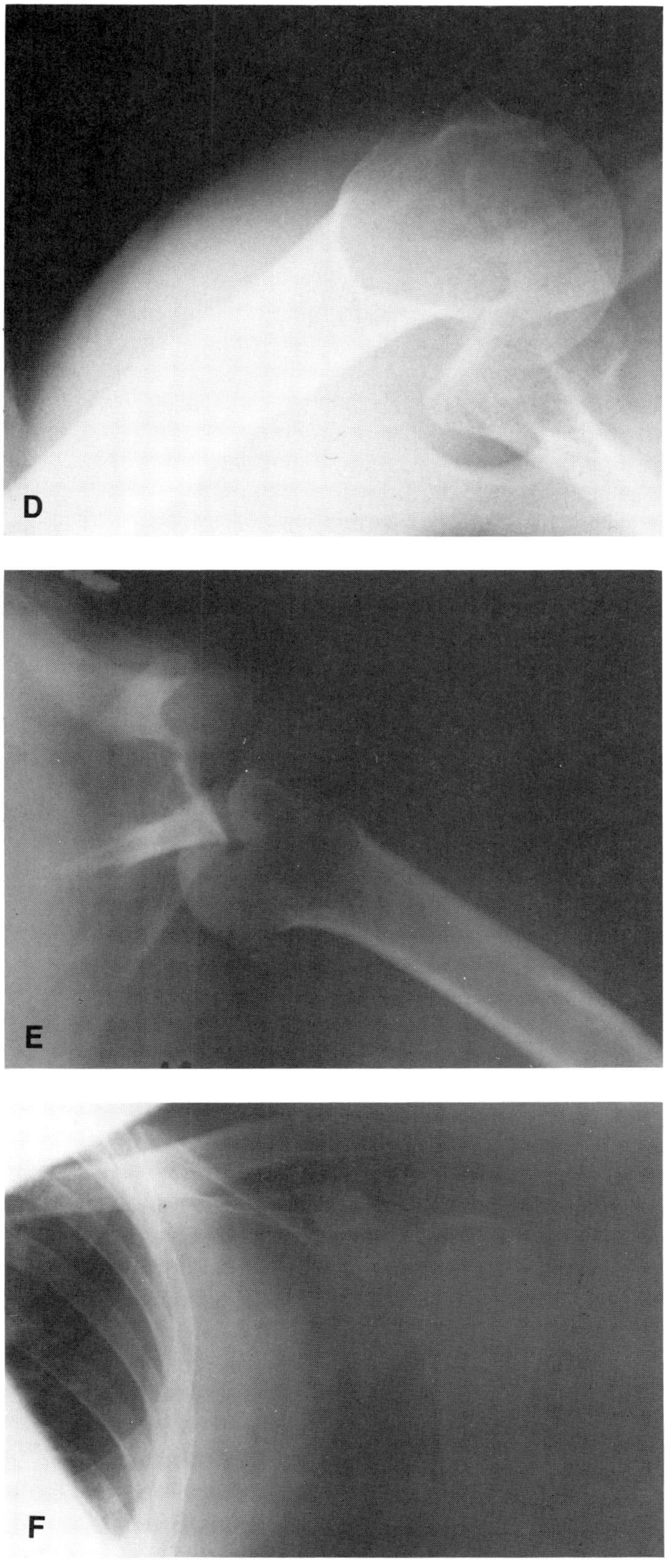
D
E
F

disadvantages: (1) The tourniquet around the arm may trap the arm muscles, making reduction difficult; (2) the regional anesthetic prevents an accurate neurologic examination following the reduction.

If reduction is performed soon after the injury, it can be done with a minimal amount of force. The simplest method is to apply traction to the forearm in line with the deformity while countertraction is applied to the distal humerus. Any medial or lateral displacement should be corrected before traction is applied. Hyperextension should always be avoided because it can compromise the anterior neurovascular structures. If no assistant is available the reduction can be performed by placing the patient prone on the examination table and applying downward traction. Either countertraction can be applied with one hand or the extremity can be positioned so that only the forearm is hanging down and the arm is stabilized by the examination table or the back of a chair (Fig. 32-26). The reduction usually occurs with a palpable and audible "clunk." After the reduction the examiner should gently move the elbow through a full range of motion to be sure that a satisfactory reduction has been achieved. Postreduction x-ray films are performed to confirm a satisfactory reduction and to detect intra-articular fracture fragments. A neurovascular examination should follow the reduction to be sure that no neurovascular structures have been caught in the elbow joint or otherwise damaged as a result of the manipulation.

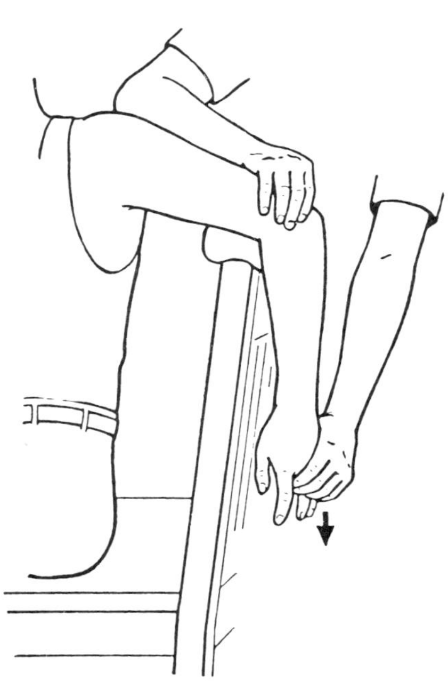

Figure 32-26. Reduction of a posterior elbow dislocation. (Lavine LS: J Bone Joint Surg 35A:786, 1953

After reduction the extremity is immobilized in an above elbow posterior molded plaster splint that includes the wrist. Immobilization is continued for 3 to 4 days until swelling subsides. After that the splint can be removed for gentle active ROM several times a day. After about 2 weeks the splint can be discontinued and substituted by a sling. Passive ROM is thought to be contraindicated for elbow dislocations because it is associated with a high incidence of elbow stiffness and heterotopic ossification.

RADIAL HEAD FRACTURES

Fractures of the radial head are common injuries in young adults and are frequently caused by a fall on the outstretched hand. A less common mechanism is a direct blow to the elbow.

DIAGNOSIS

Acute elbow pain exacerbated by motion is the main presenting symptom. Soft-tissue swelling is often minimal. Tenderness is localized over the radial head, which is easily palpable. The fracture is demonstrated radiographically on routine AP, lateral, and oblique views of the elbow.

Radial head fractures are radiographically classified into four types:

Type 1: Undisplaced fractures
Type 2: Marginal fractures with displacement or angulation
Type 3: Comminuted fractures involving the whole head (Fig. 32-27)
Type 4: Fractures associated with elbow dislocations

The radiographic findings in Type 1 fractures may be subtle. A positive fat pad sign indicates intra-articular hemorrhage, which is nearly always present.

TREATMENT

The main goal of treatment of radial head fractures is to avoid elbow stiffness, a frequent complication of prolonged immobiliza-

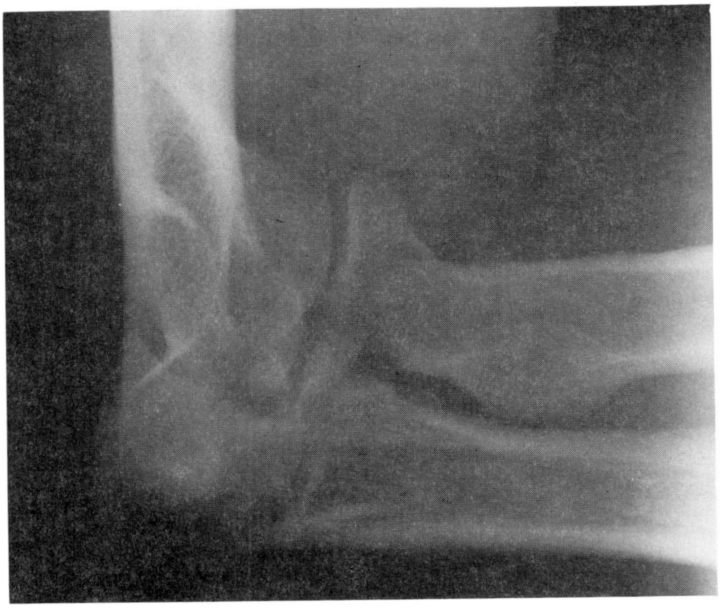

Figure 32-27. Type 3 radial head fracture. This patient was treated with a radial head excision.

tion. The treatment of Type 1 fractures is straightforward and consists of early protected motion that can be started as early as 24 to 48 hours after the injury. Aspirating the hematoma using sterile technique and injecting local anesthetic can dramatically relieve the initial pain and allow immediate motion for diagnostic purposes.

Treatment of Type 2 fractures is controversial. Closed treatment is indicated if displacement is minimal. Indications for early radial head excision include angulation of more than 30 degrees, depression of more than 3 mm, and involvement of more than one third of the head. If there is a mechanical block to passive motion or loose bodies within the joint on x-ray examination, surgery is also indicated. Type 3 fractures are usually best treated by early excision of the radial head. Type 4 fractures are placed in a separate category because of their association with complications such as myositis ossificans.

FRACTURES OF THE ULNAR SHAFT

ETIOLOGY

Fractures of the ulnar shaft, like other upper-extremity injuries, may be caused by either direct or indirect force. Those caused by a direct blow are called "nightstick" fractures. Because it is subcutaneous, the ulna is at relatively increased risk for open fractures. This situation represents a surgical emergency that should be treated according to the principles applied to all open fractures. The isolated minimally displaced ulnar shaft fracture results from a relatively mild force and is a straightforward injury to treat. However, if greater force is applied, a comminuted or displaced ulnar shaft fracture with an injury to the radius is usually found. The dissipation of force into the radius produces either a radial shaft fracture, which is evident on x-ray examination, or a more subtle dislocation of the radial head. The latter combination has been given the eponym Monteggia fracture, after the Italian surgeon who described it (Fig. 32-28). In Monteggia fractures the ulnar shaft fracture is typically in the proximal third of the diaphysis or proximal metaphysis. Although the radial head can dislocate in any direction, anterior dislocation occurs in the majority of cases. The apex of the accompanying angulation of the ulnar shaft is in the direction of the radial head dislocation.

DIAGNOSIS

The diagnosis of ulnar shaft fractures is easily made, both on physical examination and by radiographs. The patient usually is able to give a typical history such as a fall on the outstretched upper extremity or a direct blow to the forearm. The classic history is that the pa-

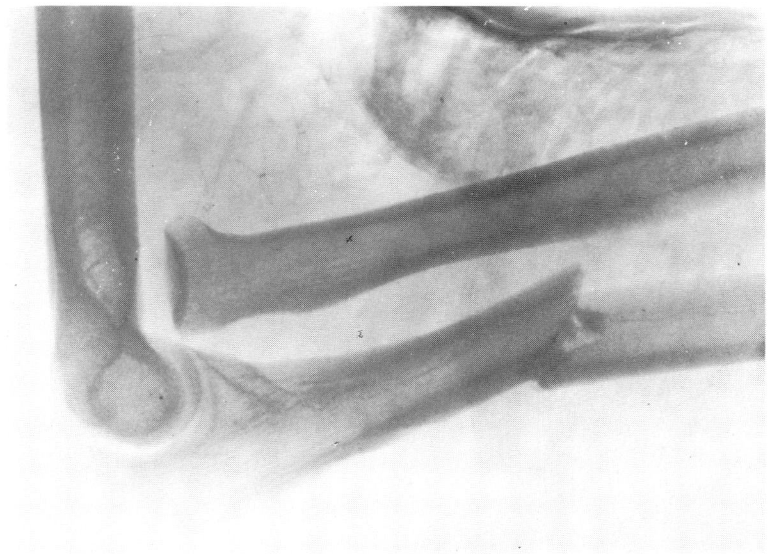

Figure 32-28. Monteggia fracture.

tient raises the forearm to protect against a blow with a club, hence the name *nightstick fracture*. Pain and swelling and tenderness are well localized to the fracture site. In the case of a Monteggia fracture the radial head may be palpable either in the antecubital fossa, if dislocated anteriorly, or subcutaneously, if dislocated laterally or posteriorly. Associated neurovascular injuries are uncommon with truly isolated ulnar shaft fractures, but injuries to the posterior interosseous (motor) branch of the radial nerve are common with Monteggia lesions. Injuries to this branch do not cause sensory deficits, but result in weakness of the thumb and finger extensors.

Ulnar shaft fractures are usually well visualized on both AP and lateral views of the forearm. Obviously, it is critical that the elbow be well visualized as well. In its normal position the radial head lies opposite the capitellum of the distal humerus. If the radial head is subluxated or dislocated, a Monteggia lesion is present.

TREATMENT

Several methods have been used to treat isolated minimally displaced ulnar shaft fractures, all of which result in satisfactory union in the vast majority of cases. Fractures immobilized in an above elbow cast, a fracture brace, or simple elastic bandage have been reported to heal uneventfully in the vast majority of cases. The length of mobilization required is usually 6 to 10 weeks. The best treatment for displaced ulnar shaft fractures and Monteggia fractures is ORIF, usually with compression plating. The radial head should always be reduced by whatever means is necessary.

FRACTURES OF THE DISTAL RADIUS

ETIOLOGY

Fractures of the distal radius nearly always occur as a result of a fall on the outstretched hand. Several eponyms have been ascribed to distal radius fractures, including Colles, Barton, and Smith. In communicating regarding these fractures confusion can be minimized by avoiding the use of eponyms and simply describing the radiographic appearance of the fracture. Distal radius fractures can be intra-articular or extra-articular involving either the radiocarpal or distal radioulnar articulation. An associated fracture of the distal ulna may be present and should be noted. Intra-articular fractures of the distal radius can also be associated with volar or dorsal dislocations of the carpus. Dorsal fracture dislocation (Barton's fracture) is one of the spectrum of injuries caused by a fall on the outstretched hand with the wrist dorsiflexed. The palmar fracture dislocation (Smith's fracture) is also associated with falls on the outstretched hand, but the exact mechanism is unclear.

DIAGNOSIS

Distal radius fractures in adults most commonly occur in the elderly. Osteoporosis is a predisposing factor. Typically, these fractures result in dorsal angulation of the distal radial articular surface and the classic ''silver fork'' deformity. There is always marked tenderness at the fracture site and the amount of swelling is variable, depending on the force of the injury. In elderly patients this injury typically occurs as a result of a minor fall. Swelling may be minimal and there is seldom any associated neurologic compromise. However, in younger adults a substantial amount of force is required to cause a distal radius fracture. Severe swelling is commonly present and an acute carpal tunnel syndrome may be precipitated. The elbow and shoulder should always be examined as part of the assessment of a distal radius fracture to rule out associated injuries.

Routine AP and lateral radiographic views of the wrist are usually sufficient to assess these injuries adequately. The distal radial articular surface is normally inclined volarward and from radial to ulnar about 10 degrees to 15 degrees. The radial styloid process normally projects distally about 1 cm past the end of the ulnar styloid. Distal radius fractures commonly are associated with dorsal angulation of the articular surface with proximal displacement of the radial styloid. Ulnar styloid fractures are commonly associated with all the different types of distal radius fractures.

TREATMENT

The goals of treatment of distal radius fractures are to restore the anatomic configuration of the distal radius as well as possible. With intra-articular fractures the highest priority is restoring the integrity of the articular surface. With extra-articular fractures treatment is aimed toward restoring the length of the radial styloid and the inclination of the articular surface. Usually a satisfactory reduction can be achieved by closed means. No reduction is necessary for minimally displaced fractures with no deformity. Extra-articular fractures can nearly always be reduced in the emergency room setting. Satisfactory anesthesia can be provided by hematoma block or IV regional block. Longitudinal traction is applied using Chinese finger traps with a countertraction weight hanging from the arm (Fig. 32-29). The distal fragment can be additionally manipulated by direct pressure, usually on the dorsal cortex (Fig. 32-30). Displaced intra-articular fractures may be reduced by simple closed manipulation, but maintenance of the reduction in a cast is very difficult. This type of distal radius fracture is usually best managed by external or internal fixation (Fig. 32-31A, B,C), both of which must be performed in the operating room under optimal anesthesia.

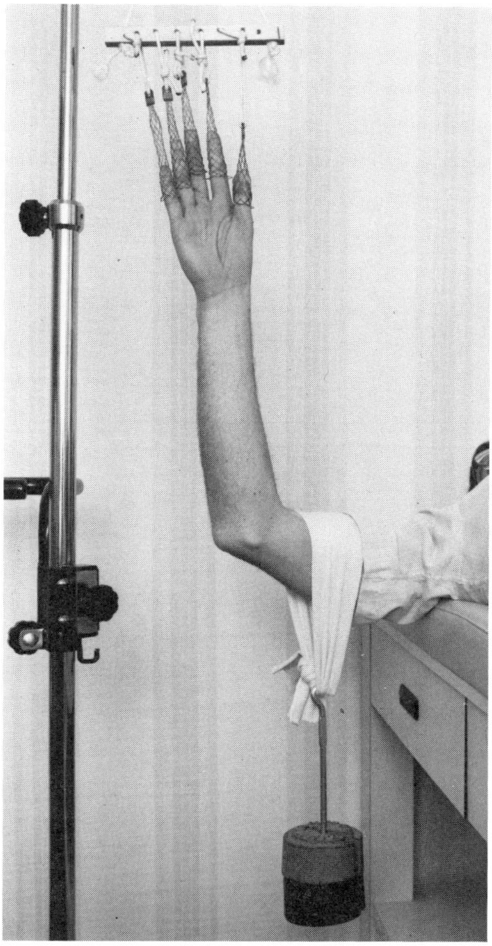

Figure 32-29. Chinese fingertraps with counterweight to apply traction to the forearm.

DEGENERATIVE AND OVERUSE SYNDROMES

IMPINGEMENT SYNDROMES OF THE SHOULDER

Etiology

Impingement is a common cause of shoulder pain in all age groups. It is associated with

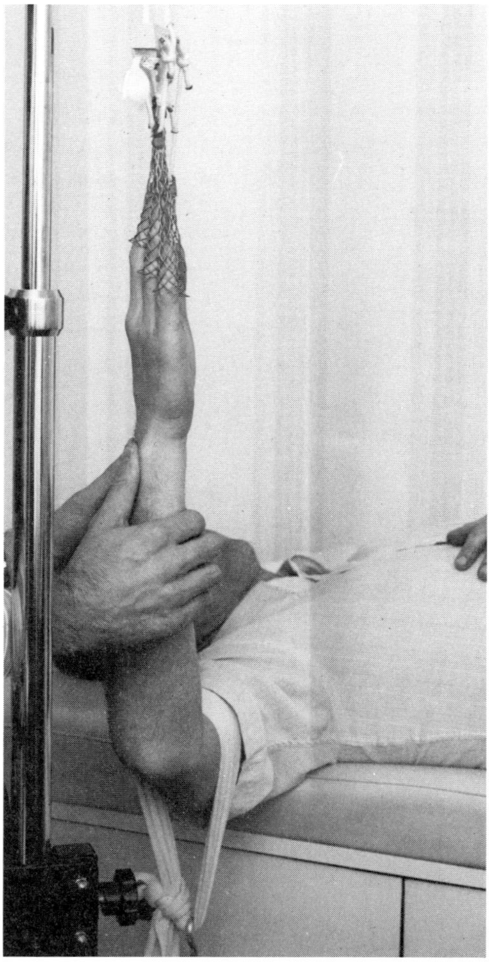

Figure 32-30. Fracture reduction with traction applied.

repetitive upper-extremity overhead activities. Young athletes involved in sports, such as swimming, tennis, and baseball, are at risk, along with those involved in occupations such as painting and carpentry. The specific lesion is inflammation of the rotator cuff tendons. The tendons are vulnerable to injury with overuse because of the narrow space available for gliding between the humeral head and the acromion and because of their relatively poor vascularity. The inflammatory process is probably initiated by repetitive impingement of the greater tuberosity against the anterior edge of the acromion. As the process continues and becomes chronic, the rotator cuff becomes thin and degenerated. Complete tears of the rotator cuff can then occur with relatively minor trauma. Shoulder impingement is pathologically classified in three stages: The first stage is edema and hemorrhage in the rotator cuff, which can occur at any age. Stage II is fibrosis and tendinitis, reflecting a more chronic process. Patients with Stage II impingement are usually over 25 years of age. In the third stage tendon degeneration, bony changes, and rotator cuff tears are found. Usually these patients are over 40 years of age.

Diagnosis

The clinical presentation of shoulder impingement is divided into three stages, which correspond with the pathologic classification. Stage I impingement may be found in competitive athletes, especially swimmers, as young as 12 years of age. A typical history is aching shoulder discomfort in the region of the anterior acromion that is precipitated by overhead activities. The supraspinatus tendon is a primary site of inflammation, as indicated by point tenderness over the greater tuberosity and the anterior acromion. Other typical physical findings include a painful arc of abduction and a positive impingement sign (Fig. 32-32), which is considered the most specific finding of shoulder impingement. This sign is elicited by passively flexing the shoulder fully until the greater tuberosity impinges against the anterior acromion. The result is pain and the typical facial grimmace. The diagnosis is confirmed by complete relief of pain, with the impingement test, after an injection of 10 ml of 1% lidocaine under the anterior acromion. The biceps tendon may also be involved in the Stage I impingement. Physical findings specific to biceps tendinitis are a tenderness over the biceps tendon, pain in the region of the biceps tendon on resisted forward flexion of the shoulder with the forearm supinated and elbow extended (Speed's test), and pain on resisted forearm supination (Yergason's sign). Stage I impingement is usually reversible with conservative measures such as shoulder flexibility and strengthening exercises, nonsteroidal anti-inflammatory medications, and avoidance of the inciting activity.

Stage II impingement is a more chronic process that generally occurs in an older age group. Symptoms are similar to Stage I, but the aching discomfort is more severe and persistent, leading to the inability to perform work and daily living activities. Crepitation on shoulder motion in the region of the subacro-

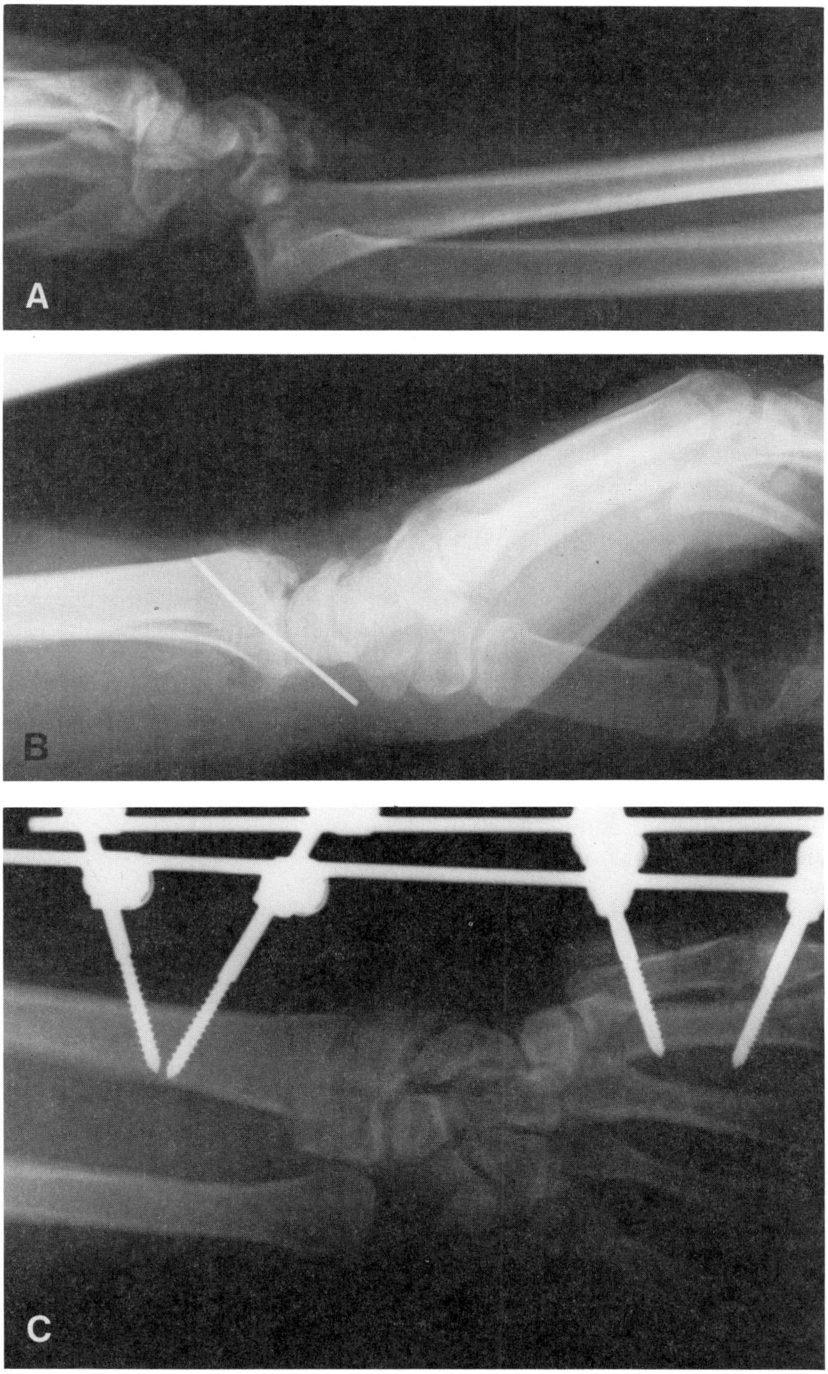

Figure 32-31. (*A*) Posterior fracture dislocation of the wrist (Barton's fracture). (*B*) Radiography following open reduction and pin fixation. (*C*) Comminuted intra-articular fracture of the distal radius treated with an external fixator.

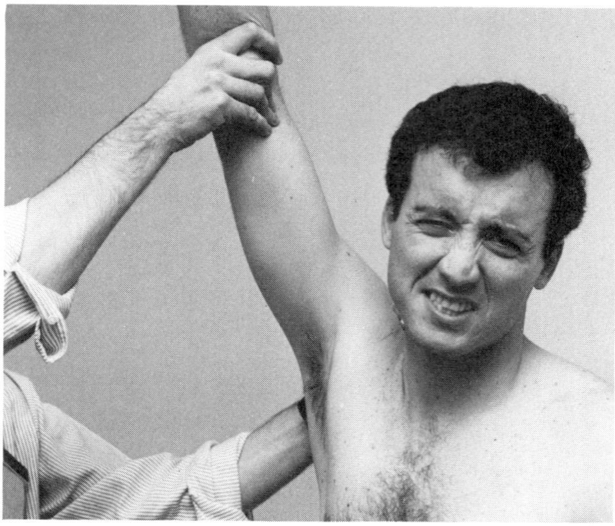

Figure 32-32. Positive impingement sign.

mial bursa is a common finding in this stage. Stage II impingement is frequently not a reversible lesion. Stage III impingement occurs in middle-aged or elderly persons, who frequently have a prolonged history of shoulder symptoms. Partial rotator cuff tears occur at an average of 50 years of age. The biceps tendon is frequently involved. A history of night pain is typical. At this stage minor shoulder insult can cause a severe tear of the rotator cuff. If the patient presents with a history of an acute insult superimposed on chronic complaints and is unable to move the shoulder fully because of pain, an injection test may be helpful to determine the integrity of the rotator cuff. If good pain relief is achieved by subacromial injection but the patient is still weak, particularly in shoulder rotation, a rotator cuff tear can be inferred. The diagnosis is confirmed by an arthrogram, which demonstrates contrast material outside the normal confines of the shoulder joint. The most important physical signs of Stage III impingement are atrophy of the infraspinatus and supraspinatus muscles, which is manifested as loss of normal soft-tissue bulk overlying the posterior scapula, marked weakness in abduction and rotation, limited active ROM with full or passive ROM, and rupture of the biceps tendon. At this stage, degenerative changes in the acromioclavicular joint are also common.

Significant radiographic abnormalities are usually not found until the disease has progressed to Stage III. At this stage sclerosis and osteophyte formation on the anteroinferior acromion and degenerative changes in the acromioclavicular joint are common findings. The distance between the acromion and the humeral head is also frequently diminished. If this distance is less than 5 mm, there is a high likelihood that a rotator cuff tear is present. The diagnosis of rotator cuff tear is confirmed with an arthrogram that shows radiographic contrast outside the shoulder joint (Fig. 32-33).

Treatment

In young athletes impingement syndrome can be prevented by careful warm-up exercises and avoiding use past the point of fatigue. Again, Stage I impingement is usually a reversible process and can be effectively managed by flexibility exercises and avoiding the inciting activity. For example, a young swimmer can use a different stroke for a short time, or a carpenter can avoid hammering above his head. Other effective nonoperative modalities include icing after overhead activities, ultrasound, and anti-inflammatory medications. The same methods are used for nonoperative treatment of Stage II and Stage III impingement. However, in these stages more emphasis is placed on shoulder flexibility, which is frequently compromised. Patients with impingement in either of these stages are sometimes forced to modify their activities permanently. Surgical treatment for impingement is reserved for patients with longstanding symptoms, usually greater than 1 year in duration. Patients with chronic impingement and no rotator cuff tear are candidates for surgical decompression, which involves resecting the

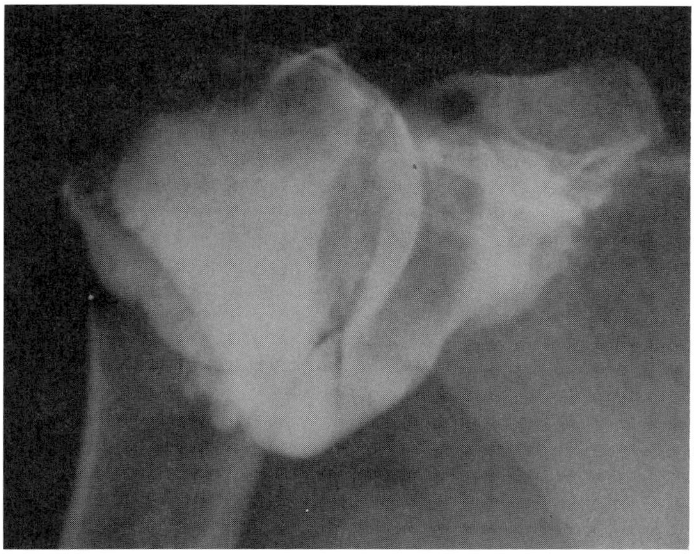

Figure 32-33. Shoulder arthrogram illustrating dye outside the shoulder joint, indicating a rotator cuff tear.

coracoacromial ligament and the undersurface of the anterior acromion. Repairing rotator cuff tears is effective for pain relief but frequently does not restore shoulder motion and strength. Therefore incapacitating pain is the main indication for surgical repair of the rotator cuff.

OVERUSE SYNDROMES OF THE ELBOW

Etiology

Elbow overuse syndromes fall into three broad catagories: lateral epicondylitis, osteochondritis dissecans, and medial epicondylitis. Lateral and medial epicondylitis result from overuse of the forearm extensors and flexors, respectively. The inflammatory changes involve the common extensor and flexor tendons, which attach to the lateral and medial epicondyles. Osteochondritis dissecans of the capitellum occurs most often in children but has also been reported in adults. In this disease an osteocartilaginous fragment of the articular surface of the capitellum becomes separated from the remainder of the bone and loses its blood supply. This disorder is sometimes called "Little League elbow" and is found in throwing athletes.

Diagnosis

Medial and lateral epicondylitis should be suspected in any patient with a history of overuse and pain in these regions. As the pain progresses it becomes more severe and persistent with continued activity. Patients sometimes complain of weakness, but especially with lateral epicondylitis the weakness is usually pain related. Patients with medial epicondylitis can develop symptoms of ulnar nerve entrapment, but these are usually mild. Other signs of lateral epicondylitis are pain with resisted dorsiflexion of the wrist and pain on full extension of the elbow, especially with the forearm pronated. Medial epicondylitis has corresponding findings of pain on resisted wrist flexion. Radiographs are usually normal. They may show calcifications within the common flexor or extensor tendons.

The main symptoms of osteochondritis dissecans of the elbow are activity-related elbow pain and decreased ROM. If there is a free fragment within the joint, the patient may complain of intermittent elbow popping or locking. The physical examination may reveal crepitation and decreased ROM in elbow flexion and in pronation and supination. There may be tenderness to palpation over the radial humeral joint. The diagnosis of osteochondritis dissecans is confirmed with radiographs that reveal a separate osteocartilaginous fragment in situ with sclerotic edges or an empty crater in the articular surface. Tomography is sometimes helpful to define the lesion more clearly.

Treatment

As for most overuse syndromes the initial treatment for all three of these disorders is nonsurgical and begins with avoiding the offending activity. In addition to rest, application of ice and use of nonsteroidal anti-inflammatory medications are recommended for initial treatment. In more refractory cases of epicondylitis the inflamed tendon can be injected with steroids. Steroid injections can be repeated several times at 2- to 3-week intervals if necessary. Usually a combination of conservative methods is used to achieve symptomatic relief. In osteochondritis dissecans of the capitellum similar conservative methods are recommended initially. If a loose body within the elbow joint is identified and is causing symptoms, then surgical removal is indicated. Other forms of surgical therapy, however, including drilling of the osteochondyle defect, do not seem to improve symptoms enough to be justified. Only approximately 5% of cases of epicondylitis are refractory to conservative treatment. In these cases lengthening or recession of the tendons at the epicondyle is the usual surgical treatment.

OLECRANON BURSITIS

Etiology

Olecranon bursitis can result from direct trauma or from repetitive pressure, such as leaning on the elbows. It is also associated with playing football, especially on artificial turf. Systemic inflammatory processes such as rheumatoid arthritis and gout may also cause olecranon bursitis. Septic olecranon bursitis is a relatively common problem that usually presents with more inflammatory signs and a more fulminant course than bursitis from other causes.

Diagnosis

In nonseptic olecranon bursitis the elbow may be surprisingly pain-free. The swollen bursa is subcutaneous and easily visible. Pain with motion usually occurs past 90 degrees of flexion. Aspiration of the swollen bursa reveals bland, clear synovial fluid.

Treatment

Initial therapy for acute nonseptic olecranon bursitis is immobilization in a compressive dressing, such as a posterior splint and elastic bandage. If the swollen bursa is large or painful, aspiration is indicated, followed by immobilization. Chronic bursitis is treated similarly with aspiration of the bursa carried out nearly always as part of the initial treatment. In recalcitrant cases operative therapy may be indicated, which consists of excision of the bursa.

33 Lower Extremity

AARON A. HOFMANN AND JAMES B. MANNING

In practice, most major lower-extremity injuries are appropriately managed by orthopaedic surgeons. Patients with these injuries, however, frequently present to emergency or other primary care physicians. In order to expedite care and communication it is important for the primary care physician to have an appreciation of the severity of a given lower-extremity injury and the ability to perform an initial assessment. If certain basic principles of lower-extremity injury care are understood, major errors in emergency management should be avoided.

Important principles of lower-extremity fracture and dislocation management are as follows:

Initial assessment of lower-extremity injuries begins with evaluation of the neurovascular status of the injured extremity. The principles of the screening neurovascular exam are discussed in the previous chapter. Figure 33-1 shows the sensory distribution of the lower extremities.

Open fractures are surgical emergencies and require irrigation and debridement in the operating room.

X-ray films of a lower-extremity fracture should be taken in two orthogonal (perpendicular) planes. The radiographic evaluation of shaft fractures should include the joint above and below the injury.

An AP pelvis radiograph should be obtained in any patient with a history of significant lower-extremity trauma, especially if there is an associated head injury and the patient is unable to identify the hip as a source of pain.

All lower-extremity fractures should be effectively immobilized, even if emergent surgical stabilization is planned. This should be done after the assessment of the neurovascular status of the involved extremity and can also frequently be postponed until adequate radiographs are taken.

Lower-extremity dislocations are surgical emergencies and reductions should be performed as soon as possible. Knee and ankle dislocations are obvious and should be reduced prior to obtaining radiographs if any significant delay is anticipated.

All intra-articular fractures in a lower extremity with significant displacement (step-off) of the joint surface require anatomic reduction and frequently rigid internal fixation if possible.

RADIOGRAPHIC DESCRIPTION

It is important for the primary care physician who sees the patient initially to be able to communicate accurately with an orthopaedic surgeon regarding the exact nature and extent of the lower-extremity injuries. The implications of a given lower-extremity fracture dislocation are frequently not evident until radiographs are taken. Therefore the primary care physician must be able to describe the radiographs in meaningful terms.

The term *dislocation* (Figure 33-2) implies that the two opposing articular surfaces of a given joint have lost contact completely. A subluxation is an incomplete dislocation in which the articular surfaces maintain some contact. Both dislocations and subluxations are described by the direction of the translation of the distal articular surface on the proximal surface. For example, an anterior knee dislocation is an anterior translation of the proximal tibia on the distal femur with no remaining joint surface contact.

Intra-articular fractures are described by indicating the articular surfaces involved and the amount of displacement or step-off. The tibial plateaus are unique in that depression of their articular surface is frequently not evident on plain x-ray films. If there is any doubt, tomograms should be obtained.

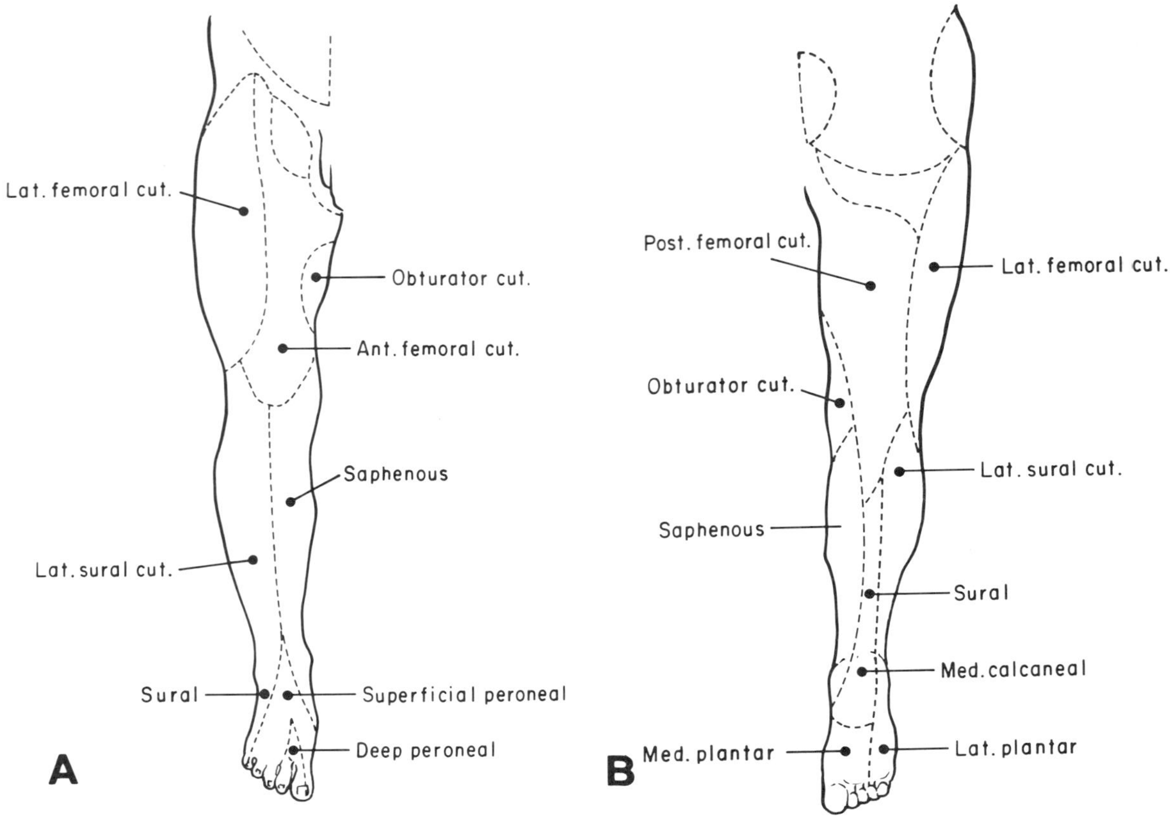

Figure 33-1. Sensory distribution of the lower extremity.

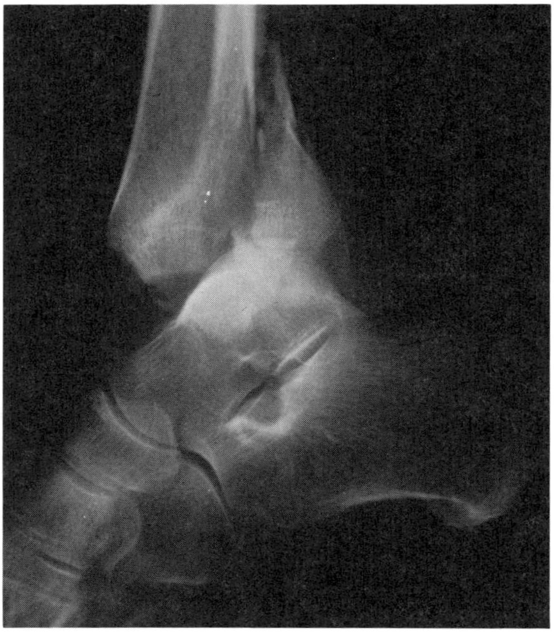

Figure 33-2. Posterior dislocation of the ankle with an attached articular fragment. This type of injury is properly termed a *fracture dislocation*.

In the case of extra-articular shaft fractures of the long bones, several radiographic features are important. The first is the fracture pattern, the simplest of which is the transverse fracture. Other common patterns are oblique and spiral, which can have two oblique components. If there are more than two major fracture fragments, the fracture is said to be comminuted. There is a direct relationship between the amount of comminution and the amount of soft-tissue damage. Two other important features are angulation and displacement. The only unequivocal way to describe angulation is to state the direction of apex at the fracture site. An example of apex medial angulation is shown in Figure 33-3A. Displacement is described by the amount of loss of apposition at the fracture site and is usually expressed in percentage. Accurate quantitation of displacement requires AP and lateral radiographic views (Fig. 33-3B).

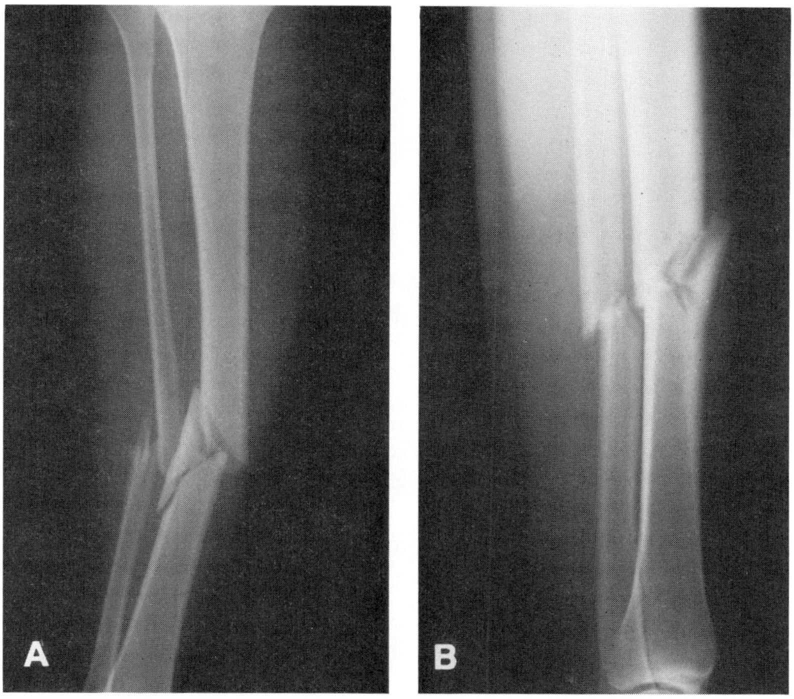

Figure 33-3. (*A*) Midshaft comminuted fractures of the right tibia and fibula with apex medial angulation of about 20 degrees and lateral displacement of about 50%. (*B*) On the lateral view the displacement and the angulation are not evident, illustrating the need for two views.

METHODS OF IMMOBILIZING THE LOWER EXTREMITY

As stated earlier, one of the important principles of emergency treatment of fractures is adequate immobilization. This prevents further hemorrhage and soft-tissue injury and helps control painful muscle spasms. Femoral shaft fractures cannot be adequately immobilized nonsurgically without traction. Traction can be effectively applied temporarily using a splint of the type shown in (Fig. 33-4). The semicircular proximal pad rests against the ischium and traction is applied through a stirrup placed around the foot using a crank at the end of the splint. The splint is stabilized around the extremity with Velcro fasteners. Use of this splint is recommended only for short periods because the pressure exerted by the proximal pad can cause sciatic nerve injury.

The traditional mainstay of immobilization of lower-extremity fractures is the bulky dressing. This can be used for injuries from the level of the distal femur to the foot. It is a simple dressing that can be properly applied by almost anyone. Our version of the bulky dressing is applied as follows (Fig. 33-5A): First, 5 to 10 layers of cast padding are evenly applied, beginning at the toes and extending proximally as far as appropriate (Fig. 33-5B). This is followed by a posterior slab of plaster also extending to the toes and immobilizing the ankle in neutral position (90 degrees) (Fig. 33-5C,D). A second thin layer of cast padding is then applied to increase the ease of removing the dressing. An elastic bandage or bias-cut stockinette is applied as the outside layer (Fig. 33-5E). The ankle is held in neutral position until the plaster hardens. Application of the bulky dressing usually requires at least two persons. The extremity should be carefully held by one or two persons while the other applies the dressing. Great care should be taken not to displace the fracture while the dressing is applied. The plaster should be thoroughly wet before application, with warm, not hot water to avoid giving off excessive heat during hardening. The posterior slab should be at least 15 thicknesses and should not be allowed to touch the skin at any point, since this can cause full-thickness burns during hardening. Support of the ankle can be augmented by

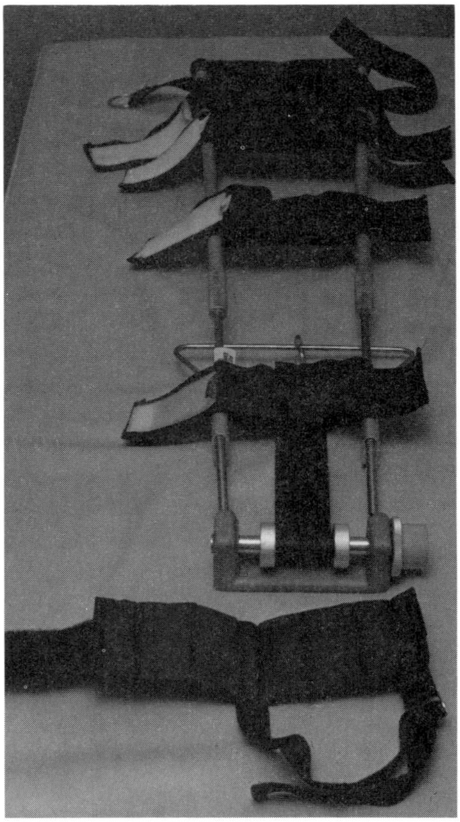

Figure 33-4. A splint can be used for temporary mobilization of femoral shaft fractures.

placing a second slab in the shape of a stirrup around the heel in contact with the posterior slab (Fig. 33-6). The elastic bandage can be applied snugly at first to mold the splint to the contours of the leg. It should then be loosened, however, since it can act as a venous tourniquet. As the plaster is hardening, the limb should not be placed directly on a rubber pillow because this can decrease the dissipation of heat and also cause burns.

OPEN FRACTURES

The presence of any opening in the skin no matter how small near a lower-extremity fracture is a sign that the fracture site may be contaminated from the external environment. In this setting the burden of proof that the fracture is not open is with the treating physician. If there is any doubt, the fracture should be treated as an open injury. Adult osteomyelitis can be a chronic and sometimes incurable disease. The main goal of emergency treatment of open injuries is the prevention of osteomyelitis.

Several factors conspire to increase the risk of infection in an open injury. The most obvious, of course, is bacterial contamination. Other factors include compromise of local defense mechanisms due to soft-tissue injury and a devitalization of bone and soft tissue. Although antibiotics are an important adjunct to treatment of open fractures, there is no substitute for surgical debridement and irrigation, which should always be done in the operating room.

INITIAL MANAGEMENT

Over half of open fractures are contaminated, as demonstrated by positive cultures taken on initial assessment. The value of these cultures is somewhat controversial and some experts feel that they are unnecessary and can even be misleading. However, because pretreatment cultures are the most likely to be positive, they may provide useful information, and there is no contraindication to obtaining them.

Initial management starts with a sterile dressing containing antiseptic solution (e.g., povidone-iodine) followed by appropriate immobilization. Intravenous antibiotics should be administered as soon as possible. The initial regimen should include a first-generation cephalosporin and an aminoglycocide (tobramycin or gentamicin). If soil or farm contamination has occurred, penicillin should be given to cover for clostridium contamination. All should be given in maximal safe dosages. Tetanus toxoid should be given as a booster, or Hypertet should be administered if there is no current tetanus immunization.

COMPARTMENT SYNDROMES

A compartment syndrome is defined as a condition in which high pressure within a closed fascial space causes reduced capillary blood flow below the level necessary for tissue viability. General causes of increased compartment pressure are bleeding into the compartment and increased capillary permeability. Clinical settings associated with the compartment syndromes include lower-extremity frac-

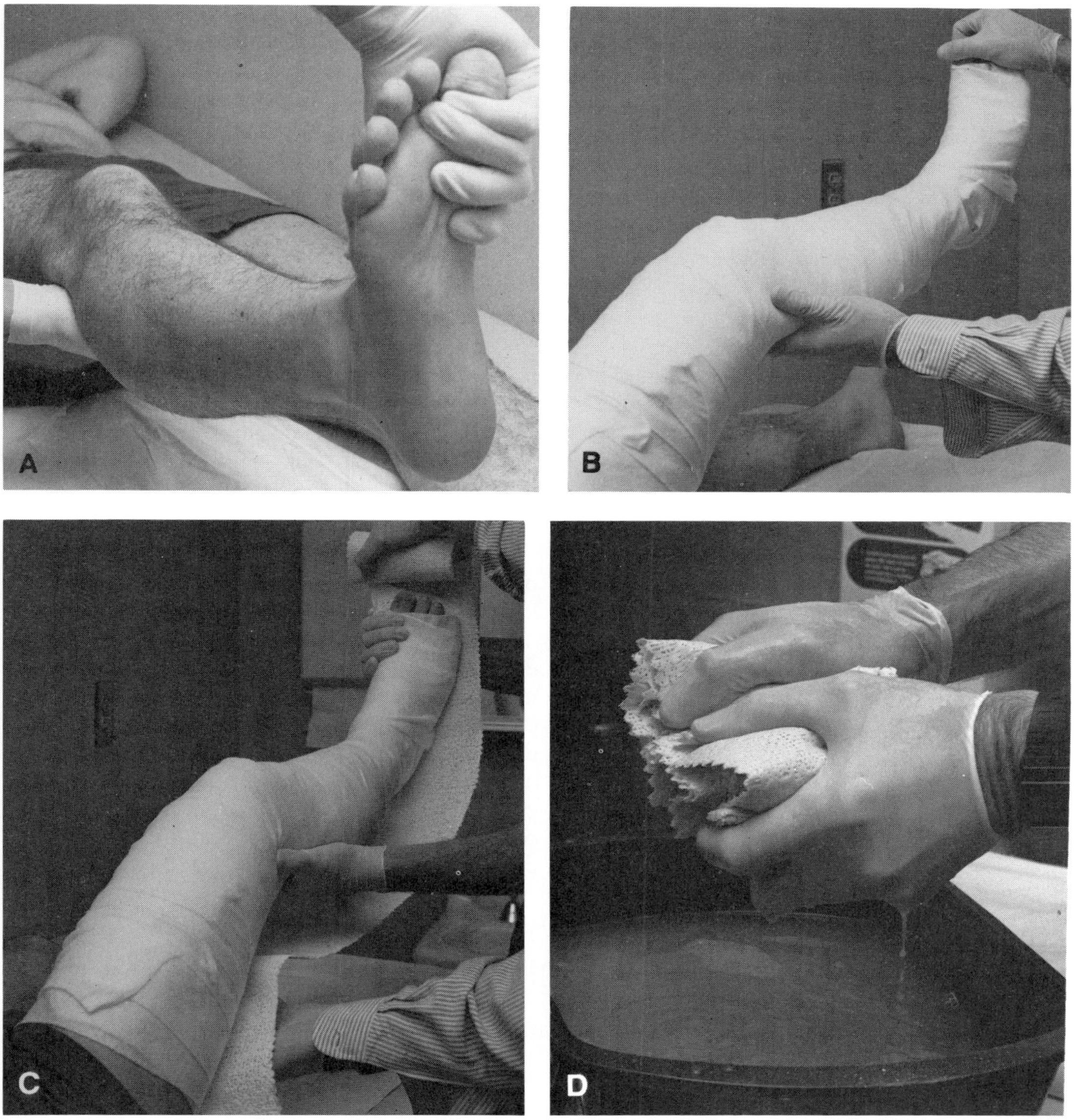

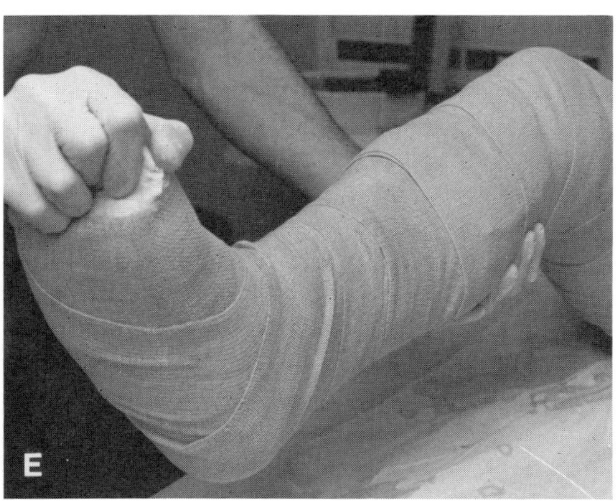

Figure 33-5. (*A*) Application of a bulky dressing for lower-extremity injuries. The injured part is carefully held by an assistant. (*B*) A thick layer of cast padding is applied. (*C*) The length of the splint is measured. (*D*) The splint is dipped and squeezed. (*E*) The splint is applied followed by a layer of cast padding and an elastic bandage.

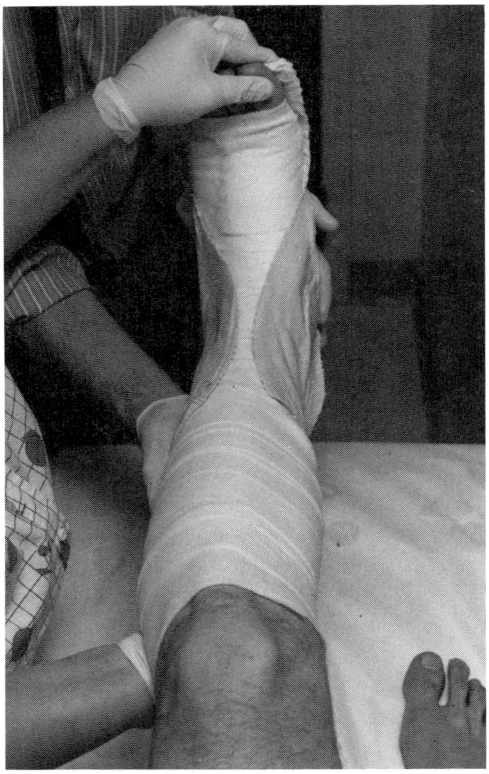

Figure 33-6. Plaster stirrup for augmentation of ankle support.

tures, osteotomies, crush injuries with or without associated fractures, prolonged limb compression as is seen in certain injuries and drug overdoses, and postischemic swelling from arterial occlusion. Compartment pressures can also be increased by applying tight compressive dressings. Any external pressure applied to the compartment is directly transmitted in equal magnitude to the tissues of the compartment.

Normal capillary pressure is approximately 25 mm Hg. The postcapillary venule pressure is about 16 mm Hg. Rather than causing collapse of the postcapillary venules, an increase in compartment pressure is simply transmitted to the postcapillary venules, increasing their intravascular pressure. The net result is a decrease in capillary blood flow and muscle ischemia.

Compartment syndromes have been reported in all the muscular compartments of the lower extremities, but they are most common in the leg. An anatomic cross section of the leg is shown in Figure 33-7. Of the compartments in the leg those most commonly involved with compartment syndromes are the anterior and deep posterior compartments. These compartments contain the toe and ankle flexors and extensors. Any one or all of the compartments of the leg can be involved simultaneously in a compartment syndrome.

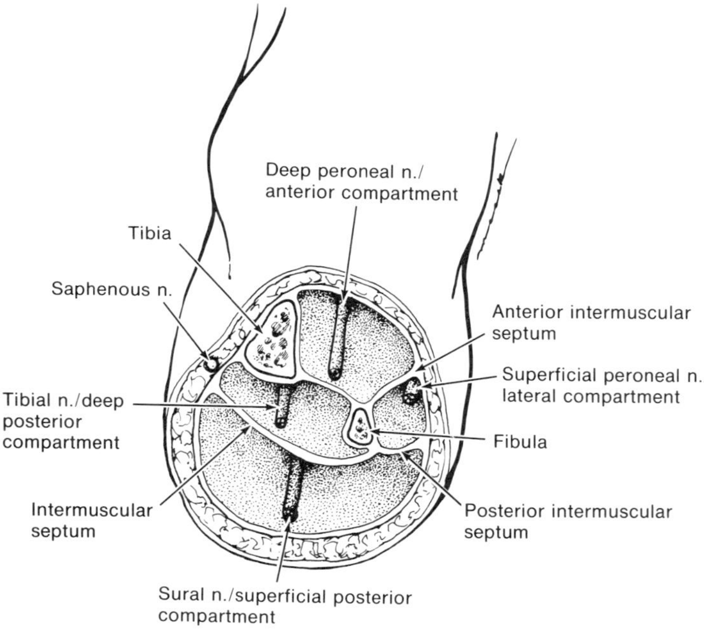

Figure 33-7. Compartmental anatomy of the leg.

SYMPTOMS

The first symptom of a compartment syndrome is pain that is increasing for no apparent reason or out of proportion to the magnitude of the injury. The pain is caused by muscle ischemia. Passive stretch of the muscles in the involved compartment causes a marked increase in the pain. For example, with an anterior compartment syndrome, flexing the toes stretches the anterior compartment muscles, producing excruciating pain. This procedure should be performed gently to avoid confusing pain on passive stretch with the pain from manipulating an injured leg. In addition to pain, the patient may complain of decreased sensation in the foot.

DIAGNOSIS

The first sign of compartment syndrome is a tense swelling of the leg. If all the compartments of the leg are soft to palpation, the patient is probably not in any immediate danger. Pain with passive stretch may or may not be a specific finding for the reasons previously described. In the patient without significant head injury or loss of consciousness the most reliable physical finding is a sensory deficit of the nerves in the involved compartments. Diminished sensation is the first sign of ischemia of a peripheral nerve. This may be detected by decreased sensation to light touch, pinprick, or two-point discrimination in the foot compared with the opposite side. A paradoxical finding of lower-extremity compartment syndromes is that, although there is ischemia on the capillary level, the arterial pressure exceeds the intracompartmental pressure, and distal pulses are routinely intact along with capillary filling in the foot. Compartment syndromes must be differentiated diagnostically from deep vein thrombosis, cellulitis, achilles tendon ruptures, and muscular tears in the legs, which can present with pain and swelling but rarely cause compartment syndromes. Nerve injuries may present with similar sensory deficits but do not cause the pain and swelling typical of compartment syndromes (Table 33-1.)

In certain situations the diagnosis of compartment syndrome cannot be made clinically. Those classically described include compartment syndrome in unresponsive or uncooperative patients and in patients with peripheral nerve deficits from other causes. For these situations quantitative pressure measurements can be obtained using several techniques all of which involve inserting a needle or catheter into the involved compartment. Values for elevated compartment pressures vary according to the technique used. These techniques are well described elsewhere and can have pitfalls. Performance of compartment pressure measurements should be left to those experienced with the techniques.

TREATMENT

The only effective treatment for an established compartment syndrome is surgical fasciotomy. However, if a compartment syndrome can be detected in the incipient stage, it is possible to obviate the need for fasciotomy in certain circumstances. An example would be a case of an incipient compartment syndrome caused by an excessively tight cast. Splitting the cast may decrease compartment pressure and relieve the tissue ischemia. The cast should always be split in two places (on either side). Splitting the cast anteriorly alone may not be adequate. The padding underlying a cast can also act as a compressive dressing and should always be cut as part of splitting

TABLE 33-1. Differential Diagnosis of Compartment Syndrome

DIAGNOSIS	PAIN WITH STRETCH	PARESIS OR PARALYSIS	PARESTHESIA OR ANESTHESIA	INCREASED COMPARTMENTAL PRESSURE	PULSES INTACT	TREATMENT
Compartment syndrome	Yes	Yes	Yes	Yes	Yes	Fasciotomy
Arterial injury	Yes	Yes	Yes	No	No	Repair or remove thrombosis
Nerve contusion (neurapraxia)	No	Yes	Yes	No	Yes	Observe

(Reproduced by permission from Mubarak, Scott J., and Hargens, Alan R.: Diagnosis and management of compartment syndromes. In American Academy of Orthopaedic Surgeons: Symposium on trauma to the leg and its sequelae, St. Louis, 1981, The C. V. Mosby Co)

the cast. Positioning of the limb is also important in treating an incipient compartment syndrome. There is experimental evidence that elevating an involved leg reduces arterial pressure and the blood flow to the affected compartment. For this reason it is recommended that the involved limb not be excessively elevated but be held at the level of the heart. There is no evidence to suggest that sympathetic blockade, either surgical or chemical, affects the pathophysiology of compartment syndrome. Again, it is emphasized that for an established compartment syndrome, the only effective treatment is emergent surgical fasciotomy.

HIP DISLOCATIONS

Hip dislocations are considered major injuries because of the extreme force required to cause them. The femoral head can dislocate in any direction in relation to the acetabulum, depending on the type of force applied. One of the most common long-term complications of hip dislocation is aseptic necrosis and collapse of the femoral head, which frequently results in early osteoarthritis. Prompt reduction of a dislocated hip gives the patient the best chance at retaining a viable femoral head, since there is a direct relationship between the incidence of avascular necrosis and period of time the hip has remained dislocated. Neurovascular injuries can occur acutely as a complication of hip dislocations. Direct pressure on the femoral neurovascular bundle can be exerted by a superior hip dislocation. Posterior dislocations can cause impingement on the sciatic nerve. Initial radiographic assessment includes both AP and lateral views of the involved hip to identify precisely the location of the femoral head. The position of the femoral head determines the maneuver used to reduce the hip. Dislocations are commonly associated with fractures of the acetabulum or femoral head. These should be identified if possible on the prereduction x-ray films. Patients with dislocated hips frequently have multiple system trauma and compromised mental states. In this setting an AP pelvis x-ray is considered an essential part of the initial radiographic evaluation to rule out hip trauma.

The diagnosis of a hip dislocation can usually be made clinically. In the patient with a posterior dislocation the hip is held in flexion, adduction, and internal rotation. If both hips are flexed about 45 degrees, the height of the knee on the dislocated side will be lower than that on the normal side (Galeazzi's sign). An anterior dislocation forces the hip into extension, abduction, and external rotation.

A special case of hip dislocation is dislocation of a total hip prosthesis. The usual imputed causes of a dislocated total hip are

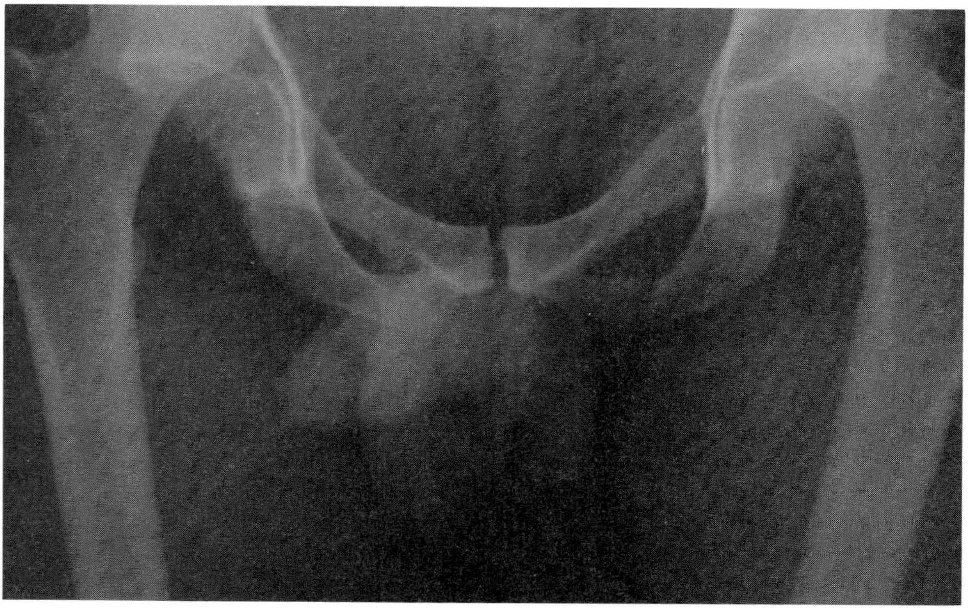

Figure 33-8. Bilateral posterior dislocations.

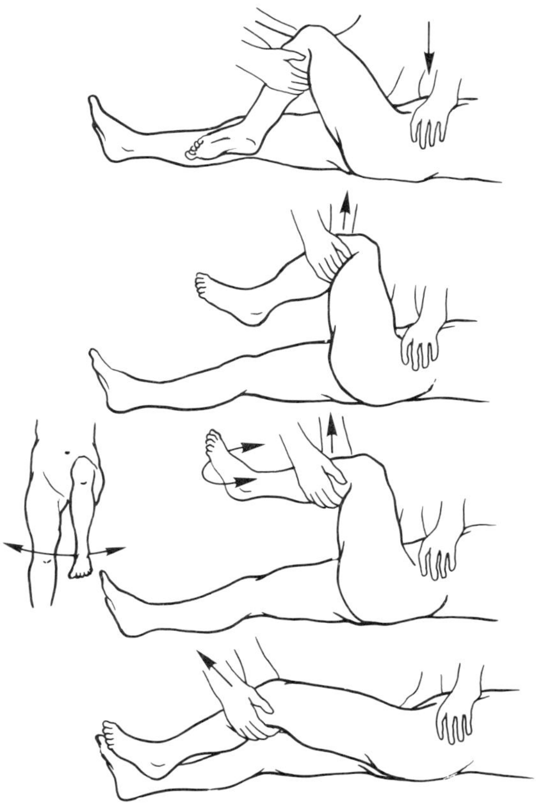

Figure 33-9. Allis maneuver for reduction of posterior hip dislocation.

improper placement of the prosthetic components or a lack of patient compliance. A total hip patient is most prone to a dislocation in the early postoperative period because performing the surgical approach for the procedure compromises the normal soft-tissue stability until healing is complete. Recurrent dislocations are common in patients with compromised mental status or improperly positioned components.

The history is important in evaluating a patient with a dislocated total hip. Frequently, the dislocation is caused by some innocuous activity such as sitting on a low chair. If there has been any significant trauma, one should suspect that the prosthesis could have been loosened as a result. A dislocated total hip is completely different from, and much less serious than, a dislocated, previously normal hip. Since no femoral head is present there is no risk of the long-term complications of avascularity. The hip generally dislocates in the direction of the surgical approach and there is seldom an associated neurovascular injury.

The treatment of a posteriorly dislocated hip (Fig. 33-8) is reduction, which can usually be accomplished in the emergency room under sedation. Our preferred technique of reduction is the Allis maneuver (Fig. 33-9), which is performed with the patient in the supine position. The knee is flexed to relax the hamstrings and the pelvis is stabilized by an assistant. The

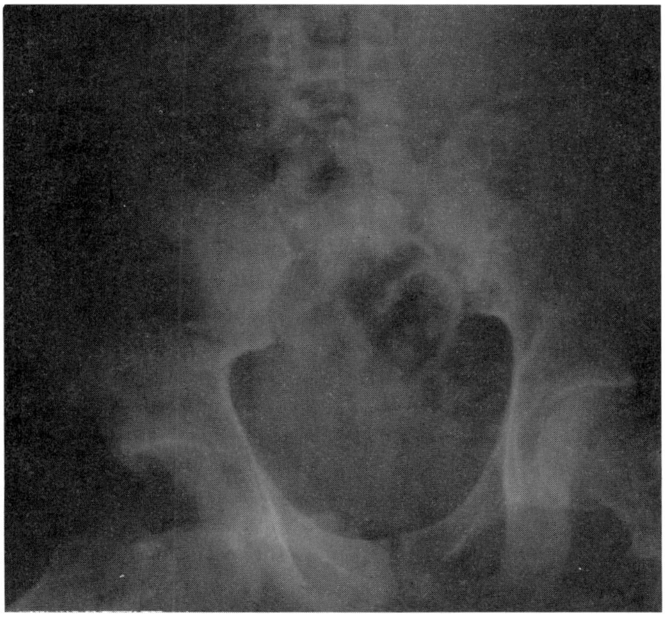

Figure 33-10. Anterior dislocation of the right hip.

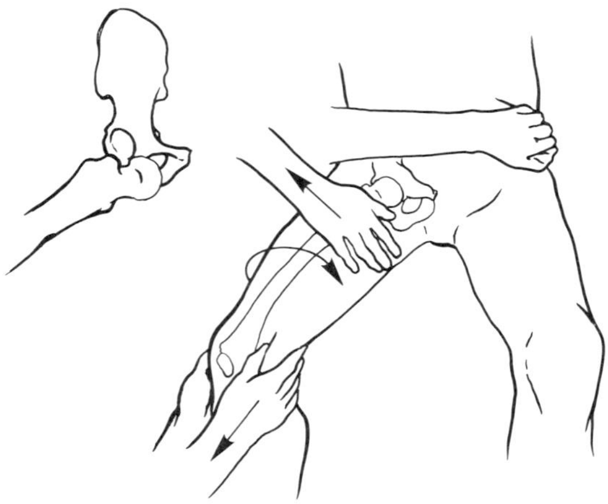

Figure 33-11. Allis maneuver for reduction of anterior hip dislocation.

hip is then flexed to 90 degrees with continued traction and gently externally rotated until reduction occurs. When the hip is reduced, a "clunk" will be felt. Further evidence of reduction is equal height of the knee on the involved side with contralateral knee when both hips are flexed to about 45 degrees (negative Galeazzi's sign). Anterior dislocations (Fig. 33-10) can be reduced using a similar maneuver also described by Allis. Longitudinal traction is applied in line with the femur while an assistant stabilizes the pelvis. The hip is then rotated gently back and forth until reduction is achieved. Reduction can be facilitated by pulling laterally on the proximal end of the femur (Fig. 33-11).

KNEE DISLOCATIONS

Dislocation of the knee is among the most devastating of all lower-extremity injuries. It occurs most commonly as a result of motor vehicle trauma and occasionally athletic injuries. The treating physician should be aware that the amount of translation at the time of injury was probably much greater than indicated by the initial radiograph. Because the popliteal artery is tethered by soft tissues above and below the knee joint, it is at high risk for injury with knee dislocation (Fig. 33-12). The treating physician's initial chief concern should be the vascular status of the leg and foot. Intact distal pulses initially are no assurance that the artery is undamaged, since an intimal injury can occur without initially compromising blood flow and eventually cause thrombosis.

A dislocation renders the knee completely unstable so that reduction is easily performed. Reduction should be done at the scene of the injury by the person administering first aid. Obviously, it is critical that the emergency room physician be made aware that the knee was dislocated when the patient was found and in which direction the dislocation occurred. Anterior dislocations are by far the most common and are usually produced by hyperextension of the knee. Posterior dislocations are much less common and are caused by extreme force applied to the anterior proxi-

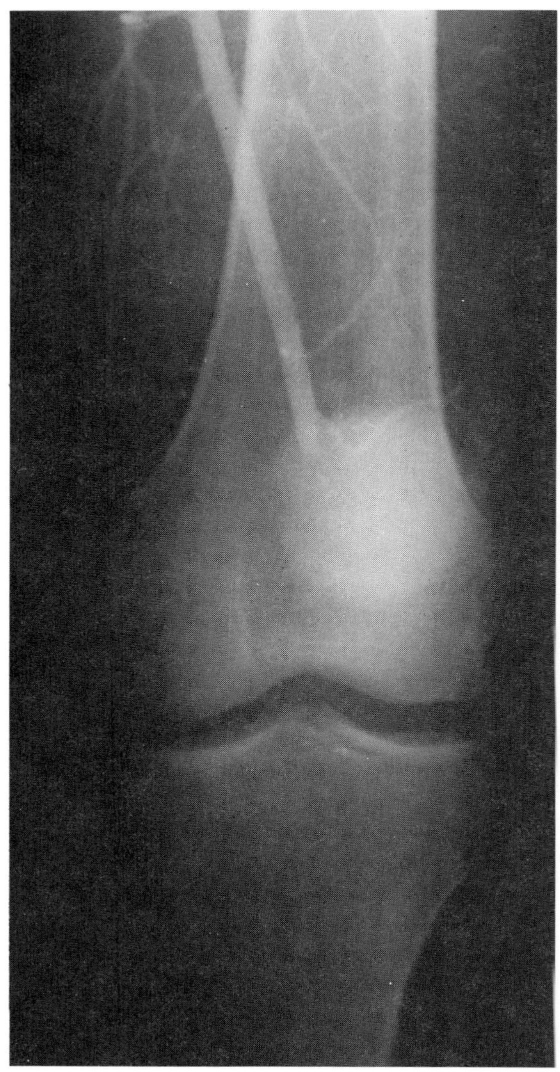

Figure 33-12. Arteriogram showing arterial injury following knee dislocation.

mal tibia. Medial and lateral dislocation are caused by extreme rotatory forces.

Neurologic injuries do occur as a result of knee dislocations, although they are less common than vascular complications because the nerves are not as tethered by the soft tissues as is the popliteal artery. The peroneal or tibial nerves may be involved. Differentiating nerve compromise due to direct injury or ischemia can be difficult in the patient with vascular injury.

Postreduction radiographs should always be taken to demonstrate the adequacy of reduction and the presence of associated fractures. Arteriography is usually indicated. If there is obvious vascular compromise, immediate surgical repair of the vessel is indicated. In this setting the arteriogram is done in the operating room just prior to the surgical procedure. It should be emphasized that if any doubt exists as to the patency of the popliteal artery, surgical exploration should not be delayed.

TREATMENT

As stated earlier, all knee dislocations should be reduced as quickly as possible. Anterior dislocations are reduced by applying longitudinal traction and lifting the distal femur until it is reduced. Hyperextension of the knee should be avoided to prevent further neurovascular injury. Posterior dislocations are reduced by applying longitudinal traction and lifting the proximal tibia upward. Medial and lateral dislocations are similarly reduced. Posterolateral dislocations may be difficult to reduce because of button-holing of the medial femoral condyle through a rent in the medial knee joint capsule. Adequate closed reduction in the other positions may also be prevented by soft-tissue interposition. Indications for emergency operative treatment include open dislocations, irreducible dislocations, and popliteal artery injury. After the knee is reduced it should be immobilized in slight flexion with a full-length bulky dressing.

TIBIAL SHAFT FRACTURES

ETIOLOGY

Fractures of the tibial shaft can be caused by direct or indirect violence, such as vehicular trauma or skiing injuries. With direct trauma the fracture pattern is most likely to be transverse or comminuted. Torsional forces produce an oblique or spiral pattern. Open fractures of the tibia are common because the entire anterior border is subcutaneous. Any skin disruption, no matter now insignificant, in the region of a tibial fracture should alert the physician to the possibility of the fracture being open and contaminated. When the tibia alone is fractured the fibula may act as a splint and prevent displacement and shortening. An intact fibula is also associated with varus angulation of the tibia, which is difficult to control by closed manipulation and may require operative treatment.

DIAGNOSIS

Tibial fractures present with pain and swelling in the region of the fracture with occasional visible angular deformity. For examination the legs should be placed parallel to each other on the table or bed and longitudinal or rotational malalignment noted. Tenderness due to tibia fracture is acute and well localized except in spiral fractures, where it extends over the length of the fracture site. Detailed definition of the fracture type usually depends on radiographic examination. The radiographic features of the fracture should be defined by the treating physician.

TREATMENT

Treatment of tibial shaft fractures is usually under the purview of the orthopaedic surgeon. Reduction and casting technique in closed fractures is demanding and requires considerable experience (Fig. 33-13). Even with meticulous technique some degree of deformity is frequently accepted. Unstable tibial fractures require operative stabilization, usually with an intramedullary nail or plate and screws. With these techniques significant deformity can usually be avoided. The attendant risks of infection should not be taken lightly.

FRACTURES OF THE SHAFT OF THE FIBULA

Fibular shaft fractures most frequently occur in combination with ankle or tibial shaft fractures. Isolated fractures of the fibular shaft generally result from a direct blow to the fib-

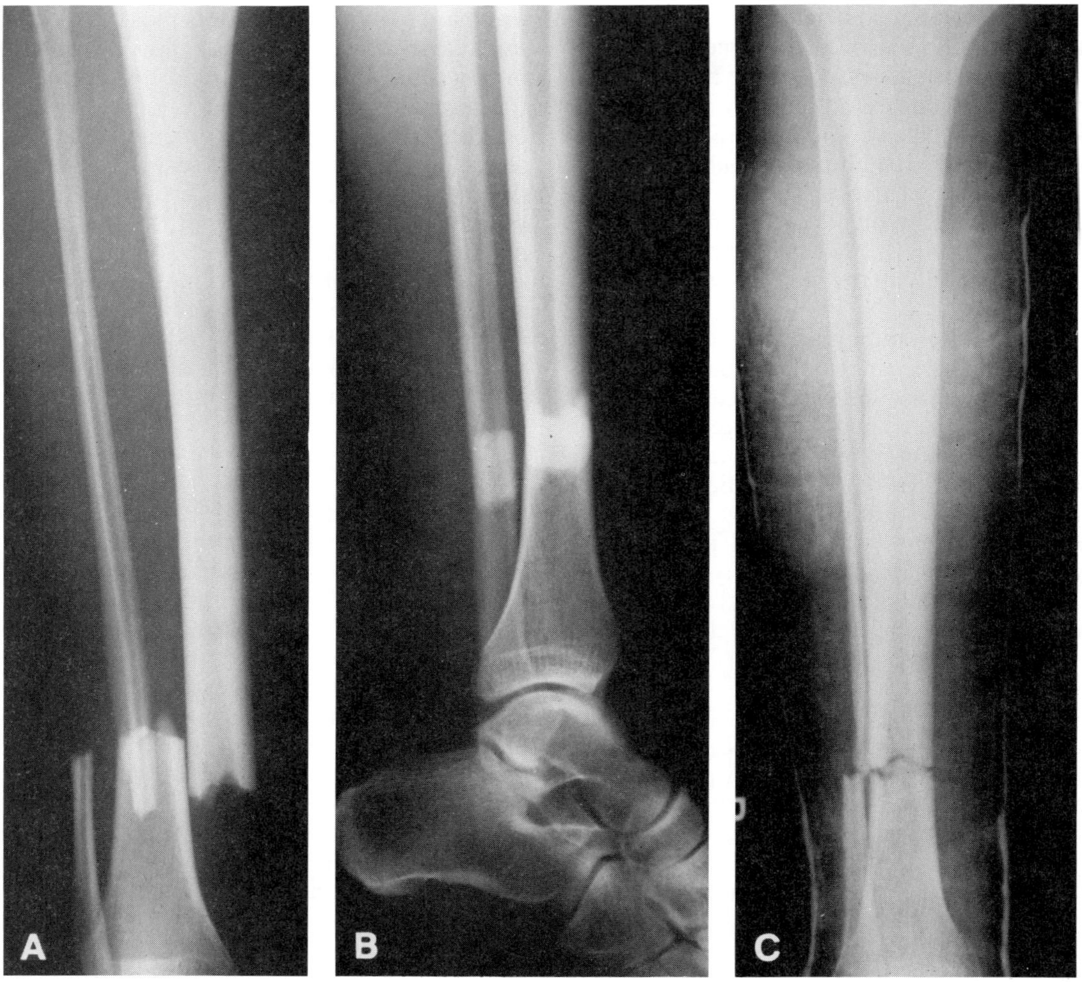

Figure 33-13. (*A,B*) Completely displaced and shortened fracture of the distal tibial shaft. (*C*) Satisfactory closed reduction.

ula. Clinical findings include local tenderness, swelling, and difficulty in ambulation. Neurovascular injuries are uncommon except with fractures next to the proximal fibular neck, which is in close proximity to the peroneal nerve. For fibular shaft fractures with minimal displacement the treatment is symptomatic. A below-knee cast or brace is adequate protection and the patient can be allowed immediate weight-bearing as tolerated. For certain patients with minimal tenderness and swelling even a cast or brace may be unnecessary. Healing is usually uneventful and complete by 6 weeks after the injury. A special type of fibula fracture (Maisonneuve fracture) involves the proximal tibial shaft in combination with an injury at the ankle (Fig. 33-14). The mechanism is rotation, which tears the ankle syndesmosis and interosseous membrane between the ankle and the fibular fracture. Occasionally, this fracture occurs with only a soft-tissue injury to the medial side of the ankle, making the diagnosis subtle. The treatment is surgical stabilization of the ankle.

EVALUATION OF KNEE INJURIES

HISTORY

A detailed history is absolutely essential and sometimes nearly diagnostic in the evaluation of knee injuries. Since knee injuries fall into two broad categories, chronic and acute,

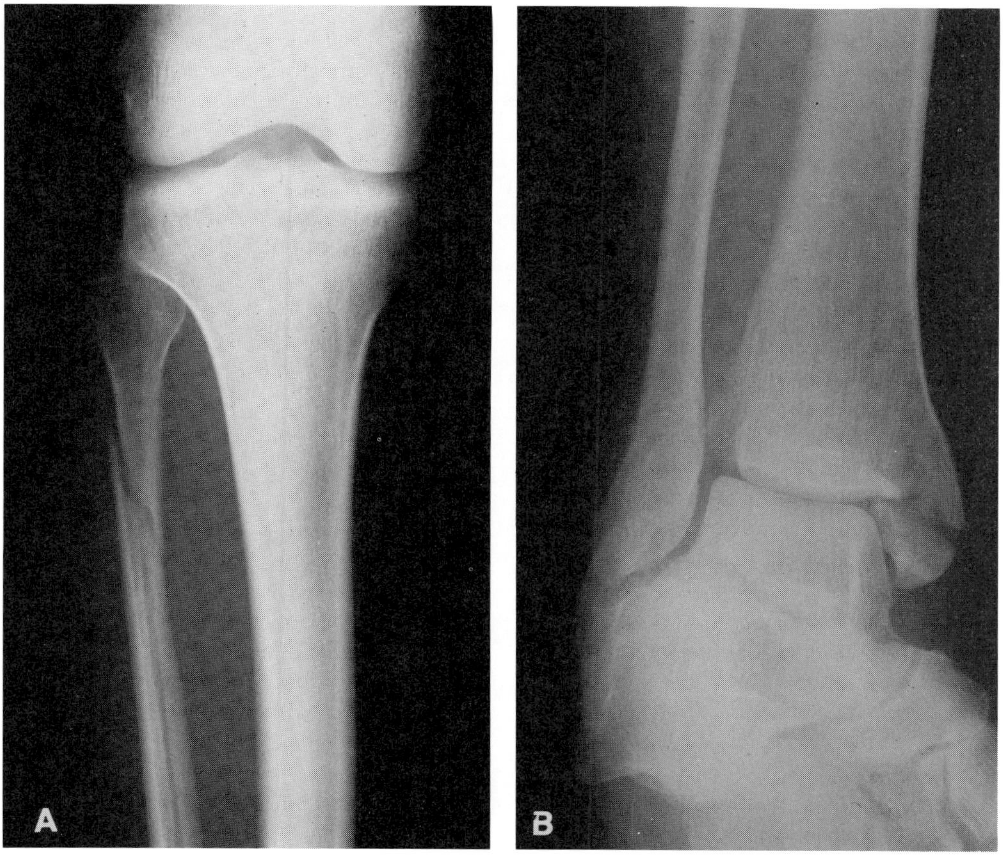

Figure 33-14. Maisonneuve fracture. (*A*) Spiral fracture of the proximal tibia. (*B*) Fracture of the medial malleolus with widening of the syndesmosis.

the examiner should initially determine the clinical course of the symptoms. If the symptoms are chronic and progressive associated with continued activity, the patient most likely has an overuse syndrome. Since most overuse syndromes are associated errors in training, the physician should inquire about the training habits of the patient. For example, in the case of running injuries, questions regarding mileage, terrain, type of shoes worn, stretching program, and any recent change in running habits frequently provide useful information.

In acute injuries the first question to be asked is whether the patient has had a previous injury to the involved knee. It is well known, for example, that patients with anterior cruciate deficient knees are at risk for recurrent instability and meniscus tears. In these patients the initial injury may have occurred almost incidentally and been untreated.

The mechanism and circumstances of the injury also provide important information. Specifically, the examiner should note whether the injury resulted from a direct externally applied force or an indirect force. If the patient has a history of a previous injury, the original mechanism should also be noted.

Classic symptoms of knee injuries include giving way, locking, localized pain, effusion, and an audible or palpable "pop" associated with the injury. Giving way or "going out" of the knee is usually a symptom of either ligamentous instability or patellar dislocation. Locking of the knee is associated with acute or chronic meniscal tears in which the torn portion is displaced and caught between the articulating surfaces of the femur and tibia. Localized pain is a typical feature of several knee injuries that will be discussed in detail in the following sections. If an effusion is present, the time period over which it accumulated is extremely important. Intra-articular fractures usually cause tense acute effusion, whereas the effusion associated with a torn anterior cruciate ligament is more delayed but usually occurs by the first 4 hours after injury. A tear of the medial collateral ligament and capsule associated with an anterior cruciate ligament may not result in a tense effusion because the capsular rent allows the fluid to escape the knee joint. An effusion that is substantially more delayed is indicative of a less severe injury, such as a meniscal tear.

PHYSICAL EXAMINATION

Examination of the knee involves using the same techniques used elsewhere in the body. A great deal of information can be obtained from simply observing and palpating the knee. Percussion and auscultation are also sometimes employed. Specific techniques involve evaluating range of motion and stability of the joint.

There are two prerequisites for performing an adequate examination of an injured knee. First, the patient must be relaxed and in the supine position. If possible, the room should be quiet and the patient's head should be resting on a pillow. Second, if the contralateral knee is normal, it must be examined first to act as a reference for examination of the injured knee. The entire sequence of the examination should be performed on the normal side. Examination of the injured knee begins with observation. First, the alignment of the extremity is observed and compared with the opposite side. There should be no significant difference in varus–valgus alignment between the two. Visible evidence of effusion consists of loss of the normal hollows around the patella. Collateral ligament injuries are usually associated with corresponding soft-tissue swelling and tenderness. Abnormal superior or inferior translation of the patella may be indicative of acute injury to the quadriceps mechanism. Lateral translation is seen with patellar dislocation. Palpation of the knee should be gentle and systemic. The adductor tubercle is an important anatomic landmark used for distinguishing between medial collateral ligament sprain and patellar dislocations. Tenderness proximal to the adductor tubercle indicates a tear of the oblique portion of the vastus medialis that occurs with patellar dislocation. The tenderness associated with medial collateral ligament sprain can be found anywhere along the course of the ligament, but it is always distal to the adductor tubercle. Palpation on the lateral side of the knee should be along the lateral collateral ligament from its femoral attachment on the condyle to the fibular head. The joint lines are then palpated around the entire circumference of the knee (Fig. 33-15). In a swollen knee the joint line may be difficult to locate precisely by palpation. A helpful anatomic landmark is the inferior pole of the patella, which is normally near the level of the joint line. Joint line tenderness is a characteristic finding of meniscal tears. It should also be remembered that the collateral ligaments can be torn at the level of the joint line, and differentiating between the two injuries by palpation is difficult. The patello-

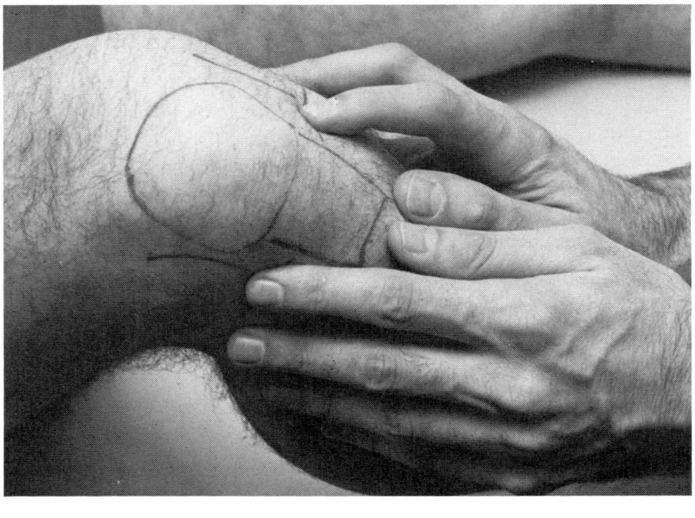

Figure 33-15. Joint line palpation.

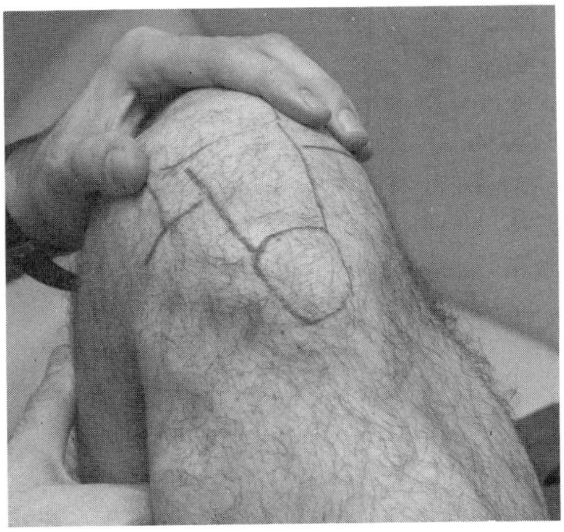

Figure 33-16. Palpation for patellofemoral crepitation on active motion.

femoral articulation and the surrounding soft tissues are then palpated. Tenderness just proximal or distal to the patella indicates inflammation or injury to the quadriceps mechanism, whereas tenderness along the medial retinaculum is found in patellar dislocation. The medial and lateral femoral condylar ridges along with the margins of the patella should be carefully palpated for bony defects found with osteochondral fractures. Knee range of motion is then tested. This should be done both actively and passively. Normal knee motion is from 5 degrees of hyperextension to approximately 135 degrees of flexon. The most comfortable position for the patient with an acute tense effusion is approximately 30 degrees of flexion. Knee range of motion will always be diminished with a tense effusion due to pain. Active range of motion is tested by flexing the hip approximately 45 degrees and having the patient actively flex and extend his knee fully. As this is performed the examiner should palpate the patellofemoral joint for any crepitation (Fig. 33-16). The patient with an acute knee injury may not tolerate this maneuver. Several diagnostic tests are employee to evaluate the patellofemoral joint and quadriceps mechanism. First, the alignment of the quadriceps mechanism is observed by measuring the quadriceps angle (Q-angle) (Fig. 33-17). The Q-angle is formed by one line drawn along the femoral shaft to the center of the patella and a second line drawn from the center of the patella to the tibial tuberosity. The normal Q-angle is 8 degrees to 12 degrees. Since with the knee fully extended the patella can subluxate laterally, the best position for measuring the Q-angle is with the knee in 20 degrees of flexion, which places the patella in the femoral groove. The patellar apprehension test (Fig. 33-18) is very helpful for distinguishing patellar dislocations from other knee injuries. This test is performed with the knee fully extended. The patella is then gently pulled laterally by the examiner. If a patellar dislocation has occurred, this maneuver will elicit extreme discomfort because it reproduces the sensation of dislocation.

Many knee injuries can be diagnosed without performing a ligament exam. For example,

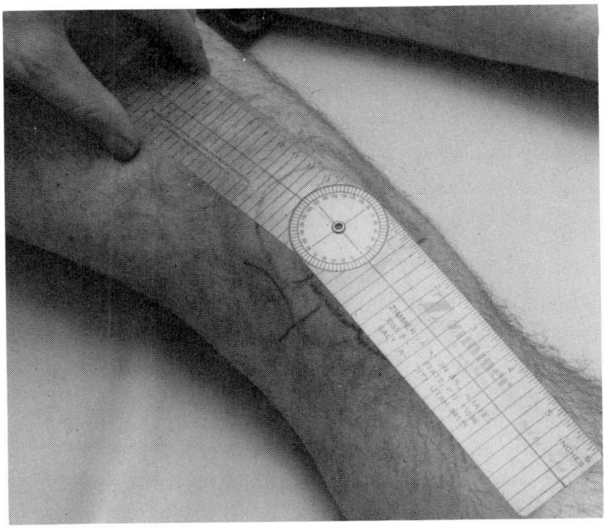

Figure 33-17. The Q-angle.

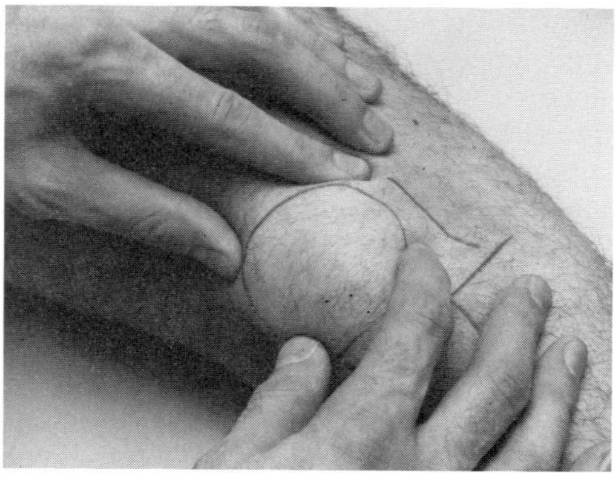

Figure 33-18. Patellar apprehension test.

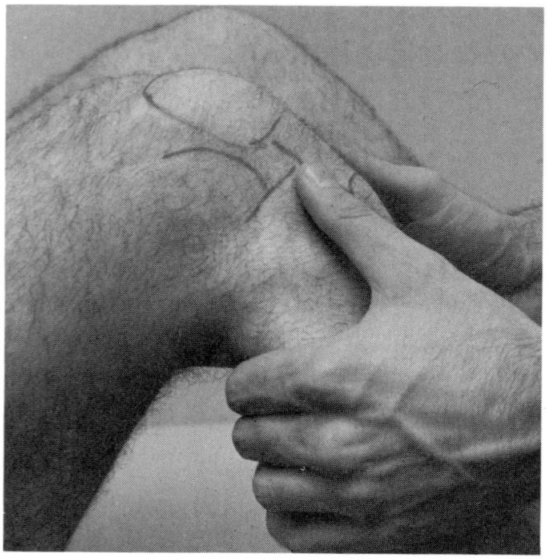

Figure 33-19. Anterior drawer test.

tenderness and soft-tissue swelling overlying the medial collateral ligament are good presumptive evidence of an MCL sprain. The treatment of ligament injuries, however, depends on the amount of laxity, which can be determined only by manipulation of the knee. If the primary care physician has determined that the knee is sufficiently lax to require immediate orthopaedic consultation, the ligament exam should be stopped at that point. Repeated manipulations, especially by inexperienced examiners, can cause increased pain and muscle spasm, which can compromise the examination of the orthopaedic surgeon.

The goal of the ligament examination is to evaluate the integrity of the primary and secondary restraints of the knee. Functional knee stability is presumed to correlate with the amount of translation or joint opening demonstrated on exam. The traditional mainstay for testing anterior cruciate function is the anterior drawer test (Fig. 33-19). With the knee flexed 90 degrees and the foot fixed the examiner places an anterior displacement force on the proximal tibia. More recent biomechanical data indicate that the best position for evaluating the integrity of the collateral and cruciate ligaments is 30 degrees of flexion. Posterior cruciate ligament function can be evaluated by reversing the maneuvers used for the anterior cruciate. The Lachman test is an anterior drawer performed at 30 degrees flexion (Fig. 33-20). The findings may be misleading, however, if the tibia is initially subluxated anteriorly. The 90–90, or Godfrey's, test (Fig. 33-21) is more specific for the posterior cruciate. With the hip and knee flexed 90 degrees the examiner can observe a slight indentation distal to the patella indicating posterior sag of the tibia and posterior cruciate ligament incompetence. Medial and lateral ligament laxity are examined by stressing the knee in valgus and varus. The best position for isolating the collateral ligament is in 30 degrees flexion (Fig. 33-22). As the stress is applied the joint line is palpated to detect the amount of opening, which is measured in millimeters.

Although ligament tests are fairly simple conceptually, in practice a fair amount of experience is necessary to achieve accurate results. Again it is emphasized that if the other knee is normal it should be examined first and

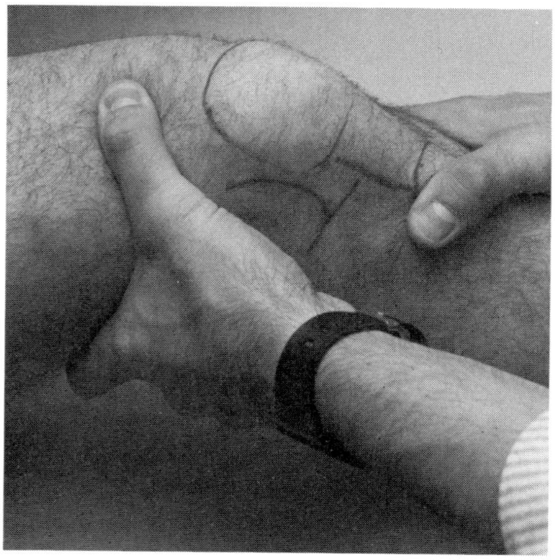

Figure 33-20. Hand position for performing the Lachman test. The upper end stabilizes the distal femur while anterior translation force is applied with the distal hand on the proximal tibia.

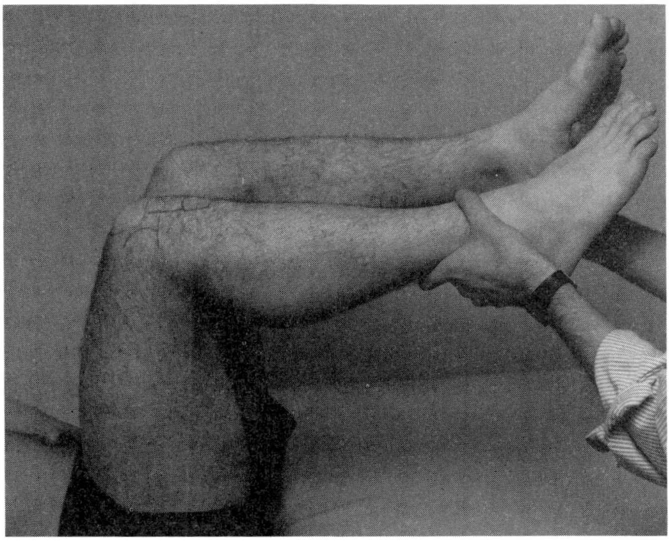

Figure 33-21. Godfrey's test in the PCL-deficient knee. A visible posterior sag in the proximal tibia would be evident just below the level of the patella.

used for comparison. Other more complex tests have been described for evaluating the rotatory stability of the knee. These are described elsewhere and are beyond the scope of this text.

Knee ligament laxity is graded according to the amount of opening or translation demonstrated as follows:

Grade 1: 0 mm to 5 mm
Grade 2: 6 mm to 10 mm
Grade 3: 11 mm to 15 mm
Grade 4: more than 15 mm

A 5-mm increase in laxity compared with the opposite side indicates complete loss of function of the primary restraining ligament. Any laxity beyond 5 mm implies that other restraining structures are damaged as well. The grade of laxity is used to determine the degree of ligament rupture, as discussed in the following sections.

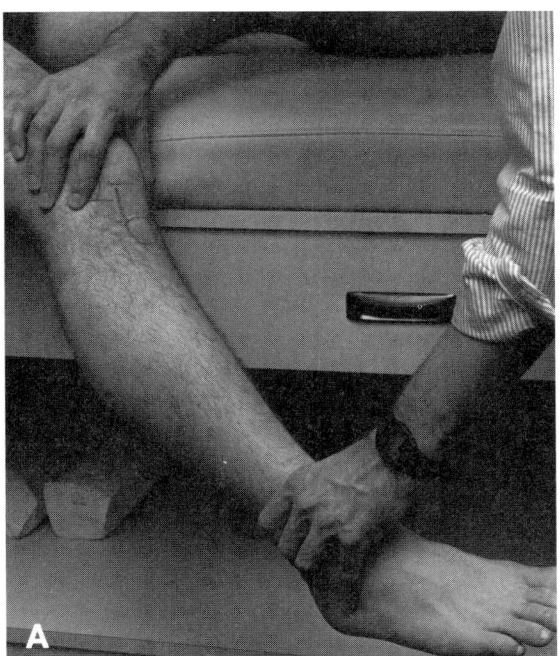

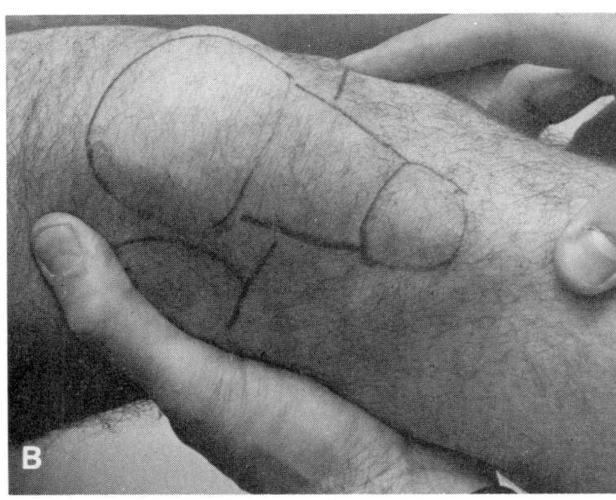

Figure 33-22. *(A)* Varus–valgus testing. The examiner's finger is on the joint line to allow quantitation of the amount of opening. *(B)* Hand position for an alternative method of valgus laxity testing. The fingertip is again on the medial joint line. The distal leg is held in the examiner's axilla while a valgus stress is applied.

MENISCUS TEARS

ETIOLOGY

Meniscus tears occur in a variety of circumstances and age groups. They frequently result from what is thought by the patient to be very minor stress on the knee. The mechanism is almost always rotation between the femur and tibia. The opposing articular surfaces move in opposite directions and the meniscus is caught in between. Meniscus injuries are commonly associated with ligament injuries, especially anterior cruciate ligament tears, which also frequently have a rotational mechanism.

DIAGNOSIS

Meniscal tears can be acute or chronic. The history of an acute rotational injury with a "locked knee" is classic for an acute meniscal tear. Chronic tears are associated with intermittent effusion, chronic popping or clicking in the knee joint, and intermittent locking. The most important physical finding both in acute and chronic meniscal tears is joint line tenderness. The joint line should be thoroughly palpated around the entire circumference of the knee. Because joint line tenderness is a nonspecific finding, other tests have been developed to diagnose meniscal tears. Of these tests McMurry's maneuver is the most popular. To perform this test the examiner stabilizes the thigh with one hand and holds the foot with the other. The knee is then flexed and extended with application of external rotation and varus. The maneuver is then repeated while applying internal rotation. Any palpable or audible popping or clicking is noted. Although this is a popular test it is poorly tolerated by patients and false positives are common. A more useful test in our hands is a modification of Apley's grinding test. In this test the knee is fully flexed and then extended while applying a valgus stress. This results in compression of the medial meniscus during knee motion. Patients with medial meniscal tears have pain during this maneuver. A similar technique is used to test the lateral meniscus.

Plain radiographs of the knee show no specific findings with an acute meniscal tear. The traditional method of radiographic diagnosis is by arthrography. With the advent of arthroscopy of the knee arthrography is now used less frequently.

TREATMENT

For many years it was thought that the menisci served no important function. Therefore the preferred treatment of a meniscus tear was complete excision. Now the important role of the menisci is appreciated and a more conservative approach is preferred.

The initial treatment of meniscus tear depends on whether the knee is locked. A locked knee must be unlocked within 48 to 72 hours to prevent pressure necrosis of the articular cartilage. Closed manipulation to unlock the knee is not necessary and can actually extend the tear. In any case, a history of an acutely locked knee is an indication for either arthroscopic repair or partial excision. If the patient has findings consistent with an acute meniscal tear but full range of motion, the appropriate initial treatment is nonoperative. It consists of ice, compressive dressing, and non-weight-bearing crutch ambulation. If the symptoms subside within 4 to 7 days, graduated weight-bearing can begin. Rehabilitation should then include quadriceps and hamstring strengthening exercises and a gradual increase in activity. If the patient is then free of symptoms, no further intervention is necessary. If, however, typical symptoms recur the patient should undergo arthroscopy on a semielective basis (within 3 months) to avoid further damage to the articular cartilage.

MEDIAL LIGAMENT INJURIES

Medial ligament injuries are caused by either a pure valgus force on the knee or a combination of valgus and rotation. The pure valgus force usually results from a blow to the lateral side of the knee and frequently occurs in football. Medial sprains by this mechanism are the most common knee ligament injuries.

As a valgus force is applied, a sequential rupture of restraints occurs in order from superficial to deep. The superficial medial collateral ligament, which is the primary restraint to valgus force, is the first structure to fail. With continued force, the deep medial ligament, and remainder of the medial capsule, and the cruciates (secondary restraints) will fail because this injury is caused by pure valgus stress. Intrasubstance meniscal tears are uncommon.

The other major mechanism of medial ligament sprain involves a rotational mechanism and is associated with tears of anterior cruciate ligament along with meniscal tears. This is a common skiing and football injury. The combination of anterior cruciate ligament, medial ligament, and meniscal tears has been termed "the unhappy triad." Both medial and lateral meniscal tears are commonly associated with this combination of injuries.

DIAGNOSIS

The history is a very important part of evaluating medial ligament sprains. The mechanism of injury should be elicited in detail. If an effusion is present, the time course should be documented. Medial soft-tissue swelling and tenderness are present and located distal to the adductor tubercle. The joint line should be carefully palpated for meniscal tears. The most important part of the physical evaluation is the ligamentous exam. Laxity on valgus stress should be assessed both in 30 degrees of flexion and in full extension. The amount of laxity is compared with the opposite side if it is normal. A side-to-side difference of 5 mm indicates a complete failure of the superficial medial collateral ligament. If there is Grade III laxity on valgus stress, especially in full extension, there is a high likelihood of rupture of one or both of the cruciate ligaments in addition to the medial collateral ligament. After valgus laxity is tested, the other ligamentous structures of the knee should also be evaluated, especially the cruciate ligaments (see the following discussion).

Medial ligament injuries are categorized according to the amount of joint opening or valgus stress as follows:

First degree: Grade I laxity
Second degree: Grade II laxity
Third degree: Grade III laxity
Fourth degree: Grade IV laxity

Plain radiographs of the knee should always be obtained with a history of a valgus mechanism of injury and should precede the ligament exam. In older persons a valgus force may result in a lateral tibial plateau fracture. Associated cruciate injuries have characteristic radiographic signs (see the next section).

TREATMENT

In recent years clinical and experimental evidence has accumulated to support nonoperative treatment of isolated medial ligament tears. If the two ends of the ligament return to satisfactory apposition after the injury, then little benefit is obtained from surgery. In the presence of Grade I or II medial laxity and no evidence of cruciate injury, satisfactory results have been obtained with nonoperative therapy. This approach also has the advantage of avoiding the risks of surgery.

Any form of nonoperative therapy for isolated medial injuries should allow some degree of continued knee motion. Motion of the knee is essential for diffusion of synovial fluid and nourishment of articular cartilage. It also minimizes muscle atrophy, which always results from immobility.

First-degree medial injuries are treated symptomatically. Full motion is allowed and the ligament is protected with a hinged brace (Fig. 33-23A). Crutches are used initially but full weight-bearing is usually restored by 7 to 10 days. Isometric and progressive resistive muscle exercises are started immediately to prevent atrophy. The patient is then allowed a gradual increase in his activities beginning at about 2 weeks after the injury. The brace should be worn for 2 or 3 months for any significant physical activity. In second-degree injuries with 1 mm to 5 mm of medial laxity the same treatment program is followed, except the patient is kept non-weight-bearing for up to 3 weeks and returned to activity over a longer period of time, based on the persistence of tenderness and swelling. In a second-degree major injury (6 mm to 10 mm of increased laxity) there has been significant damage of the secondary restraints. For this reason a considerably longer period of bracing is necessary. The cast brace is worn for 4 weeks with the hinges set to allow motion from 30 degrees to 50 degrees (Fig. 33-23B), a range that will not stretch the medial collateral ligament. Extension is increased by 5 degrees and flexion by 10 degrees each week. The patient is kept non-weight-bearing, but isometric and progressive resistive exercises are performed. After the range of motion is from about 10 degrees to 90 degrees, the treatment continues as for a first-degree injury. A short knee brace is worn for an additional 4 weeks after the cast brace is discontinued. The short brace is then worn for all physical activity for at least 4 months. As indicated previously, the degree of laxity associated with a third-degree medial sprain indicates severe damage to the secondary restraints. The status of the cruciate ligaments should be thoroughly evaluated. If the integ-

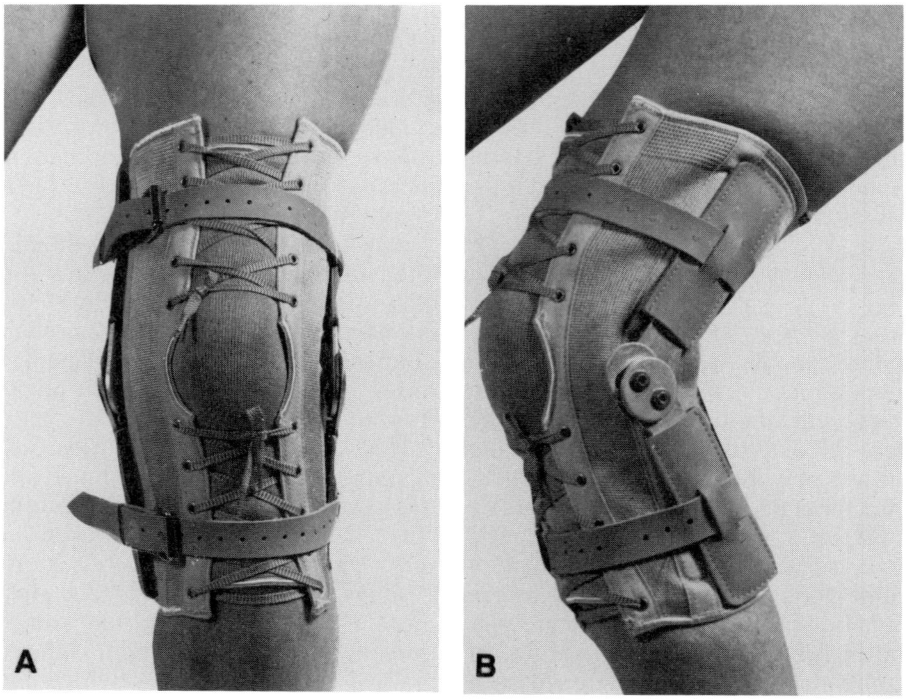

Figure 33-23. A hinged knee brace used for the treatment of medial ligament injuries.

rity of the cruciate is intact, third-degree medial sprains can be treated nonoperatively. The patient is initially placed in an above-knee cast with the knee at 40 degrees of flexion and the tibia in slight internal rotation. At the end of this period of cast immobilization the treatment is continued as for a second-degree major sprain. The total time to full weight-bearing after a third-degree sprain is about 3 months.

Combined injuries of the medial collateral ligament and anterior cruciate ligament are usually treated by surgical repair and reconstruction. This should be undertaken in the acute postinjury period (7 to 10 days) to allow better identification and repair of the injured structures. During the surgery the menisci are thoroughly examined and tears are appropriately treated, either by partial excision or repair.

LATERAL LIGAMENT INJURIES

ETIOLOGY

Lateral injuries are relatively rare. They usually result from an indirect varus force on the knee. They can also be caused by a rotatory mechanism in which the cruciates are at risk as well. The most severe associated injury with the lateral sprain is a traction injury of the peroneal nerve. Variable degrees of injury to the nerve can result and complete return is uncommon.

DIAGNOSIS

Physical examination reveals tenderness and swelling over the lateral collateral ligament. The capsule frequently remains intact, and if there is an associated intra-articular injury, an effusion may be present. Again, the most important part of the physical examination is assessment of ligamentous laxity compared with the contralateral knee. As with medial injuries laxity is checked in both full extension and 30 degrees of flexion applying a varus stress. Since the cruciate ligaments are at risk, their status should be carefully assessed. Significant findings on plain radiographs are not uncommon with lateral injuries. The lateral capsule may avulse a small fragment of the tibial plateau, which is an important indicator of ligamentous disruption. Avulsions of the fibular head can also be seen along with occasional medial tibial plateau fractures.

TREATMENT

Because of the rarity of lateral injuries, little is known about their natural history. It is generally believed that injuries associated with Grade I or II laxity and no evidence of cruciate injury can be treated nonoperatively, as previously described for medial injuries. Third-degree lateral injuries have a high association with intra-articular pathology, especially cruciate and meniscal tears. The potential for spontaneous healing of a lateral ligament is also probably not as great as that for the medial ligament. For this reason third-degree lateral injuries are usually treated surgically.

ANTERIOR CRUCIATE LIGAMENT INJURIES

ETIOLOGY

Anterior cruciate ligament tears can occur by a rotational mechanism, which usually involves one of the collateral ligaments as well, or by straight anterior translation of the tibia on the femur. A rupture of the anterior cruciate with minimal associated injuries can result from hyperextension of the knee or sudden deacceleration, which is a common mechanism in athletic injuries. The ligament can be torn at any point along its course, or its bony attachments can be avulsed. Meniscus tears occur with anterior cruciate tears in 65% of cases, with lateral meniscus most commonly involved.

DIAGNOSIS

Again, the history can be very important in diagnosing anterior cruciate ligament tears. The mechanism should be elicited in as much detail as possible. The patient commonly reports a palpable or audible pop in the knee at the time of the injury. Occasionally, the pain is minimal and the athlete may continue playing after the injury. The presence and timing of a tense effusion are indicative of the type of injury. Seventy-five percent of acute hemarthrosis is associated with anterior cruciate ligament tears. Although some feel that aspiration of a bloody effusion is beneficial, it cannot be justified on therapeutic grounds because the effusion will recur. The additional information gained from examining following aspiration is probably not worth the risk of infection. The collateral ligaments should be thoroughly evaluated because they are at risk, especially with rotational injuries. Range of motion is important. With a hyperextension mechanism the injured knee will extend farther than the normal contralateral knee. Also, if the injured knee cannot extend fully it may be "locked," indicating a meniscus tear. The most important maneuver in physical exam is the Lachman's test. A side-to-side difference of 3 mm indicates probable complete anterior cruciate disruption. Less than 5% of the normal population have a 3-mm side-to-side difference. Associated meniscus tears can be difficult to diagnose. McMurry's test is usually not well tolerated by patients with acute anterior cruciate ligament injuries. Radiographs play an important role in the initial evaluation of anterior cruciate ligament injuries. They may show avulsion of a small piece of the lateral tibial condyle attached to the lateral capsule, the so-called lateral capsular sign. This is a highly specific radiographic sign of anterior cruciate ligament injury. Plain radiographs may also show an avulsion of the tibial spine, which can be repaired surgically and has an excellent prognosis compared with a midsubstance tear.

TREATMENT

The treatment of combined anterior cruciate ligament and collateral ligament injuries is nearly always surgical. High-performance athletes usually undergo repair or reconstruction of isolated anterior cruciate ligament tears as well. For the remainder of patients with anterior cruciate ligament tears, nonoperative treatment is acceptable. It is estimated that the majority of these patients will not require further treatment if they limit their activities. A substantial percentage, however, will develop significant laxity and other complications, such as meniscal tears. If major giving-way episodes occur more than three times per year, an acceleration of joint degeneration can be expected. Symptomatic instability usually correlates with clinical instability on ligamentous examination. Other important prognostic factors are the age and activity level of the patient. The older and less active the patient is, the less likely he or she is to develop symptomatic instability and early joint degeneration. Adequate conservative therapy for anterior cruciate ligament injuries involves aggressive muscle rehabilitation and bracing of the knee. Another major component is modification of the patient's activity level. If symptomatic instability results despite conservative therapy, ligament reconstruction can be performed.

POSTERIOR CRUCIATE LIGAMENT INJURIES

ETIOLOGY

The posterior cruciate ligament is the strongest ligament in the knee. Compared with the other knee ligaments, a greater amount of force is usually required to rupture it. Posterior cruciate ligament injuries are more typically associated with motor vehicle and industrial accidents than with athletics. The most common mechanism of injury is blunt trauma directed toward the anterior proximal tibia, causing posterior displacement. This is one type of motor vehicle "dashboard injury." Since the posterior cruciate ligament acts as a secondary restraint to varus and valgus stress, it may be torn in combination with one of the collateral ligaments. Another common mechanism of a combined injury is rotation. Hyperextension can also cause posterior cruciate ligament injury, but this is thought to occur after rupture of the anterior cruciate and posterior capsule.

DIAGNOSIS

The history may be strongly suggestive. Any patient with a history of a strong blow to the proximal tibia should be thoroughly evaluated for a posterior cruciate ligament tear. In an acute situation the diagnosis may be subtle and a high index of suspicion is necessary. The mechanism of the injury should be elicited in detail. On physical exam signs of a blow to the proximal tibia, including contusions and abrasions, may be found. Although an effusion may be present it is typically not as tense as that associated with an anterior cruciate tear. Tenderness is not a specific finding of posterior cruciate ligament injuries but may indicate associated injuries. The most sensitive position for testing the functional stability of the posterior cruciate ligament is with the knee in 90 degrees of flexion. The Lachman test is helpful but can be misleading, especially if the tibia is subluxated posteriorly before the test is performed. The unaware examiner may interpret anterior translation of the tibia in this setting as indicative of an anterior cruciate tear. The most specific test for posterior cruciate ligament incompetence is Godfrey's test. It should be performed on anyone who demonstrates increased laxity with the Lachman's test. Even in cases where both cruciates are ruptured, Godfrey's test will indicate a posterior cruciate ligament injury.

TREATMENT

The natural history of posterior cruciate ligament deficient knees is unclear, probably because of the rarity of the injury and because of the difficulty of diagnosis. Symptomatic instability is less pronounced than with anterior cruciate ligament–deficient knees and usually occurs with the knee in the flexed position, such as walking down an incline. The most significant long-term complication of a posterior cruciate ligament tear is degenerative arthritis, which has been reported in up to 50% of cases. As with anterior cruciate ligament injuries the tendency to develop instability and other complications depends on the age and activity level of the patient.

In contrast to anterior cruciate ligament injuries, acute repair of the posterior cruciate ligament seems to produce good results. If augmentation of the repair is necessary, the semitendinosis tendon is frequently used. In the chronic posterior cruciate–deficient knee or the acute injury treated nonoperatively, quadriceps strengthening is a most important component of rehabilitation. By dynamically preventing posterior translation of the tibia the quadriceps can act as a substitute for the posterior cruciate ligament. Custom knee bracing and reasonable limitation of activities are also important in nonoperative therapy. If this regimen fails, surgical reconstruction may be performed.

FRACTURES OF THE PATELLA

ETIOLOGY

Patella fractures are common injuries and nearly always result from a direct blow. This is another type of "dashboard injury." Fractures of the patella can result in disruption and incompetence of the extensor mechanism, loose osteochondral fragments in the knee joint, and incongruity of the patellofemoral articulation. These fractures have implications similar to other intra-articular fractures, and anatomic restoration of the articular surface is a fundamental goal of treatment. The distal 25% of the patella is extra-articular. Fractures in this portion do not necessarily require anatomic reduction. The fracture pattern varies, but is usually transverse through the midportion of the patella. Comminution at the fracture site is not uncommon.

DIAGNOSIS

Patellar fractures are usually easily diagnosed. The patient complains of extreme pain and swelling, localized at the patella. Again, history of blunt trauma is most common. However, occasionally an indirect mechanism is implicated. On physical examination, trauma to the overlying soft tissues is frequently found because of the subcutaneous position of the patella. Open patella fractures are not uncommon. If the knee capsule remains intact, a tense hemarthrosis can develop. Palpation reveals soft-tissue swelling and extreme localized tenderness.

The most important determination to be made in the physical examination is the functional integrity of the extensor mechanism. Patients with significant disruption may be able to extend the knee partially but may be unable to extend it actively and fully (''extensor lag''). If it is unclear whether the patient is unable to extend fully because of quadriceps incompetence or pain, the knee can be fully extended passively by the examiner and the patient can then be asked to maintain this position. If the patient is able to do this for even a few seconds, the quadriceps mechanism is probably intact. Complete inability to maintain full extension indicates a significant disruption. This latter maneuver is performed with the patient's limb elevated off the examining table. Routine radiographic evaluation of patella fractures include AP, lateral, and sunrise views. Distraction at the fracture site and articular stepoff are noted (Fig. 33-24). Acute patella fractures must not be confused with a bipartite patella, which is a congenital anomaly. A bipartite patella appears as a separate patellar fragment that is nearly always located in the upper lateral portion of the patella. Radiographically, the edges of the fragment are smooth, with a radiodense rim as opposed to the sharp edges of a fracture. This condition is frequently bilateral, so views of the contralateral knee may be helpful.

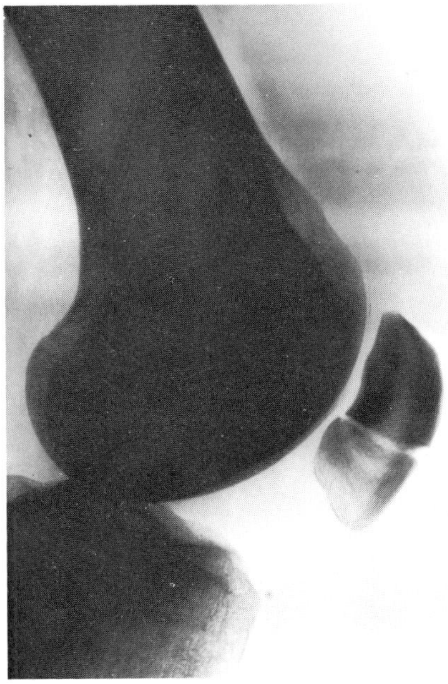

Figure 33-24. Transverse patella fracture.

TREATMENT

If the integrity of the extensor mechanism is intact and there is no significant stepoff of the articular surface, nonoperative treatment is appropriate. If either of these two conditions exists, surgery is indicated. Nonoperative therapy consists of application of a cylinder cast with the knee in slight flexion. Since the weight-bearing surfaces are not involved, progressive ambulation can be allowed. After about 4 weeks the amount of allowed flexion is increased by 10 degrees to 15 degrees per week. The surgical treatment of patella fractures includes examination of the patellofemoral joint for articular cartilage injury, irrigation of the knee to remove these osteocartil-aginous fragments, anatomic reduction, and internal fixation. In severely comminuted fractures partial or complete excision of the patella may be necessary. The important biomechanical role of the patella mandates salvage if possible.

EXTENSOR MECHANISM RUPTURES

ETIOLOGY

The less common sites for rupture of the extensor mechanism of the knee are the quadriceps and patellar tendons. There is usually some predisposing cause, such as systemic disease. Patients with acute rupture usually describe a variable degree of previous symptoms relating to the quadriceps mechanism. Degenerative changes and evidence of tendon repair are found in biopsy specimens of torn quadriceps tendons.

DIAGNOSIS

Quadriceps tendon ruptures are frequently undiagnosed initially. The absence of fractures can give the examiner a false sense of security. The usual mechanism of extensor mechanism rupture involves forceful quadriceps contraction. A typical history is of an elderly individual who stumbles and forcibly contracts the quadriceps in an effort to regain balance. Occasionally, bilateral acute ruptures may occur. Blunt trauma is an unusual mechanism, but it can occur, especially with patellar tendon ruptures.

The history usually reveals the mechanism of injury, either direct or indirect. On further questioning the patient may relate antecedent symptoms. A history of systemic disease, such as connective-tissue disease, atherosclerosis, or hyperparathyroidism or other diseases associated with steroid ingestion, is pertinent. Evidence of blunt trauma may be found on physical examination. The patella may be in abnormal position, especially with patellar tendon ruptures that result in patella alta. Patella baja can occur with quadriceps tendon ruptures, although this is usually a less impressive finding. Palpation reveals soft-tissue swelling and tenderness in the area of the injury. A defect in the quadriceps mechanism may also be palpable. Patellar mobility to manipulation is usually increased. The most important physical sign of extensor mechanism rupture is inability to extend the knee fully against gravity (extensor lag). If the medial and lateral retinacula are intact, the patient will be able to extend the knee partially but not fully. The deficit is confirmed by demonstrating the ability to passively extend the knee fully. Plain radiographs of the knee should always be obtained to rule out patella fracture, which is another form of quadriceps mechanism rupture.

TREATMENT

If extensor mechanism disruption is demonstrated, surgical repair is indicated. Even in patients who are debilitated or have some severe systemic disease, surgery is a treatment of choice because this group is most likely to be severely debilitated by an incompetent extensor mechanism. The site of the rupture is usually near a bony attachment to either the proximal or distal pole of the patella or the tibial tuberosity. The repair is performed by reattaching the tendon using sutures passed through bone. Most authorities have recommended 6 to 10 weeks of immobilization.

TRAUMATIC DISLOCATIONS OF THE PATELLA

ETIOLOGY

Traumatic dislocations of the patella can result from either a direct blow or indirect trauma. Indirect mechanism usually involves an external rotation force combined with strong quadriceps contracture. In patients with normal patellofemoral anatomy, a large amount of force is usually required to produce a patellar dislocation. These patients also have a higher likelihood of osteochondral fractures of the patella associated with their dislocation. Other patients, especially young women, may have predisposing abnormalities that place them in greater risk for patellar dislocation, such as an abnormally high patella (patella alta), a shallow femoral groove, or genuvalgum with an excessive Q-angle. The vast majority of patellar dislocations are lateral.

DIAGNOSIS

If the patient presents with the patella dislocated, the diagnosis is obvious. A more common situation, however, is that the dislocation reduces spontaneously, sometimes without the patient being aware of what actually happened. Typically, the patient will report that the knee "went out of joint." On physical examination there is typically a tense hemarthrosis with marked tenderness over the medial patellar retinaculum. There may also be marked tenderness over the lateral femoral condyle. The most classic physical finding of acute patellar dislocation is the positive Fairbank's test, or apprehension sign. Classically, when this test is done, the patient anxiously grabs the knee, because the test duplicates the original sensation of the dislocation. The differential diagnosis of acute patellar dislocation includes medial meniscus injuries and medial collateral ligament injuries. The tenderness in patellar dislocation, however, is usually proximal to the adductor tubercle and closer to the patellar margin than the tenderness of the medial ligament injuries and meniscus tears, which is distal to the adductor tubercle. A history of an acute tense effusion would also be more consistent with a patellar dislocation. Routine radiographic views should be obtained and include a standing anterior/posterior and lateral view of both knees and a sunrise, or Merchant's, view. Positive findings with acute patellar dislocations include osteochondral fractures of the patella or femoral condyles, abnormal patellar tilt, and a patellar subluxation.

TREATMENT

Some first-time dislocators may be treated initially with immobilization. A cylinder cast is applied and worn for 6 weeks. While in the cast the patient should perform quadriceps strengthening exercises as soon as symptoms permit. Surgical repair of the torn retinaculum or removal of loose osteochondral fragments may be indicated. Patients with recurrent dislocations may be candidates for surgical correction of their patellar malalignment.

OVERUSE SYNDROMES

TROCHANTERIC BURSITIS

Etiology

The trochanteric bursa lies between the fascia lata and the greater trochanter of the femur. Inflammation of this bursa is associated with running or prolonged sitting. The mechanism of the inflammation is mechanical irritation of the bursa as the fascia lata repetitively passes over it or places prolonged pressure against it. There may be an associated snapping sensation as fascial bands pass over the bursa. The pain is exacerbated by the inciting activity. In severe cases the hip can be extremely painful, even mimicking septic arthritis.

Diagnosis

The diagnosis of greater trochanteric bursitis is most often made on physical examination. Although the tenderness may involve a large area, the main focus is directly over the greater trochanter. Pain on gentle range of motion in trochanteric bursitis is much less than that associated with septic arthritis. The patient is usually still able to ambulate, although with some discomfort. The typical laboratory tests for infection, including sedimentation rate, are normal in greater trochanteric bursitis. X-rays usually show no specific findings, but they should not show evidence of an acute intra-articular process. The differential diagnosis includes hip pain of radicular origin and, in runners, for example, stress fractures about the hip, including those of the pubic rami, femoral neck, and a subtrochanteric region of the femur. X-rays are typically negative during the first 2 or 3 weeks following a stress fracture. Bone scans are more sensitive during this early period.

Treatment

The first step in treatment of an overuse syndrome such as trochanteric bursitis is to avoid the precipitating activity. Nonsteroidal anti-inflammatory agents may also be effective. In severe cases a bursal injection of local anesthetic and steroid can provide a lasting relief. Crutch ambulation with limitation of weight-bearing is indicated for severe cases.

Presence of trochanteric bursitis can indicate an abnormality in gait that may be corrected. The patient should be examined for limb length inequality, which can cause a pelvic obliquity and prominence of the greater trochanter during gait. In runners, contracture of the tensor fascia lata muscle can result in snapping of the iliotibial band over the greater trochanter. Physical therapy can be effective in stretching out these contractures. Minor limb length inequality can be corrected with a shoe lift. On rare occasions if symptomatic treatment fails, a surgical release of the fascia lata over the greater trochanter can be performed.

BURSITIS OF THE KNEE

Etiology

There are several bursa in the region of the knee. These are synovial compartments that are separate from the knee joint itself. They are located over bony prominences such as the patella and at other areas of friction between tendons. The most common bursae involved are the prepatellar and infrapatellar bursae. Prepatellar bursitis is caused by repetitive trauma or prolonged kneeling. Hence the traditional name *housemaid's knee*. Infrapatellar bursitis is caused by a similar mechanism with the symptoms located slightly inferior to the prepatellar bursa.

Diagnosis

When a bursa becomes inflamed, the lining cells secrete synovial fluid. This results in a localized swelling that is very characteristic and easily distinguished from an effusion of the knee joint. This physical finding together with a typical history usually confirms the diagnosis. If the overlying skin is inflamed and the presentation is acute, a gram stain and culture of an aspirate from the bursa should be obtained to rule out infection. The diagnostic work-up is completed by an examination of the bursal fluid under polarized light to detect the presence of crystals.

Treatment

Bursitis about the knee is treated similarly to bursitis elsewhere in the body and consists initially of avoiding the aggravating activity and the use of nonsteroidal anti-inflammatory medications. Symptomatic treatment usually results in significant improvement within 2 to 3 days. Injection of steroid preparations is generally not advised.

If the activity causing the bursitis is continued or repeated, a syndrome of chronic bursitis can result. Adhesions and calcium deposits may develop secondarily within the bursa. Repeated episodes of swelling may occur. If this condition becomes chronically symptomatic, the bursa can be excised surgically.

PATELLAR TENDINITIS (JUMPER'S KNEE)

Etiology

Patellar tendinitis is an overuse syndrome typical of athletes involved in running, jumping, or kicking activities. It is characterized by pain felt just distal to the inferior pole of the patella. The pain is insidious and presents initially as aching that occurs after running or jumping. With continued activity the pain may persist during periods of inactivity. In severe cases stair climbing may be associated with extreme pain. Athletes who have been immobilized for an injury and who suddenly return to vigorous activity are especially susceptible to this condition. With continued activity in the face of patellar tendinitis the athlete will develop feelings of weakness or giving way of the knee.

Diagnosis

Physical examination reveals swelling below the inferior pole of the patella. Knee range of motion is usually full but may be slightly limited because of pain. There is focal tenderness at the inferior pole of the patellar, which is best elicited by palpating the distal patella and applying pressure with the thumb and index finger on either side of the proximal end of the tendon (Fig. 33-25).

Abnormalities in patellar alignment may also be present, such as patella alta, patella baja, or an abnormal Q-angle. Functional shortening of the patellar tendon from previous Osgood–Schlatter's disease may also be found. Radiographic examination of the knee may reveal traction spurs or stress fractures of the patella and calcifications within the patellar tendon. The characteristic findings of Osgood–Schlatter's disease may also be present.

Treatment

Treatment of patellar tendinitis depends on the clinical phase of the condition. In the early phase the patient has pain during activity and may also have mild pain during periods of inactivity, neither of which interferes significantly with athletic participation. These patients are treated symptomatically with anti-inflammatory medication, stretching, activity modification, and ice after participation. The patient's activity level must be limited to the point where clinical improvement continues. A patellar restraining brace may be a successful adjunct to treatment. Steroid injection is strictly contraindicated because it has been shown to weaken the tendon and predispose it to complete rupture.

The next phase of patellar tendinitis is characterized by pain that is severe enough to interfere with participation. These patients also

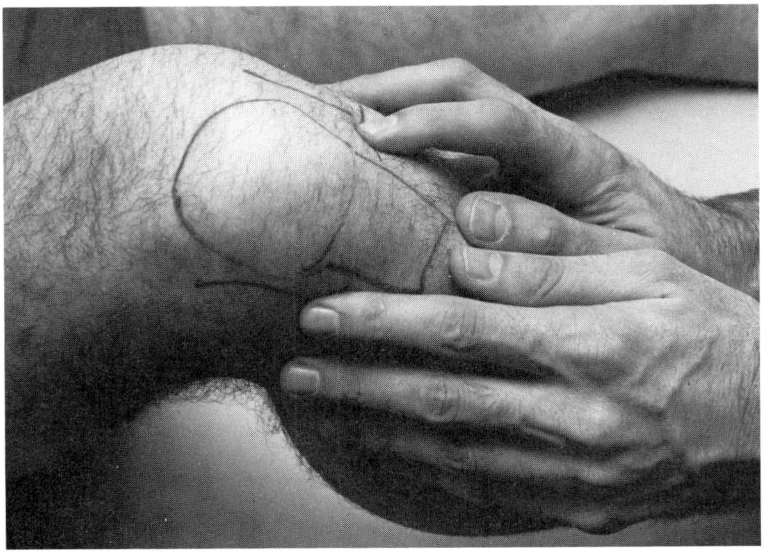

Figure 33-25. Method of palpating the patella to detect patellar tendinitis.

typically have significant discomfort with daily activities such as stair climbing. Effective treatment usually requires a prolonged period of inactivity in addition to the conservative measures described previously. Disabled chronic patients may be candidates for surgery, which may include resection of the distal pole of the patella, excision of the degenerated portion of the tendon, or drilling of the inferior patellar pole. The fact that several procedures are advocated implies that none is extremely successful. At this phase tendinitis can be a chronic disabling problem. The last phase of patellar tendinitis is complete disruption of the tendon. This is most common in athletes in the fourth and fifth decades. Patient's with patellar tendon rupture may present with only a minimal extensor lag on straight leg raising, if the capsule is intact on either side of the tendon. A high degree of suspicion is helpful in making the diagnosis.

OSGOOD–SCHLATTER'S DISEASE

Osgood–Schlatter's disease is a syndrome of pain, tenderness, and prominence in the region of the tibial tuberosity in adolescence. The etiology is uncertain, but it may be due to an avulsion fracture of the tibial tuberosity. The disease is associated with repetitive activities that involve contraction of the quadriceps muscles, including running, jumping, and climbing stairs. As the disease progresses, the tibial tuberosity becomes more prominent (Fig. 33-26). This phenomenon has been explained as a consequence of callous formation.

Treatment

The treatment of Osgood–Schlatter's fracture disease is similar to that for adult patellar tendinitis and includes the typical conservative measures, including stretching exercises for tight muscles, nonsteroidal anti-inflammatory medication, and limitation of activity.

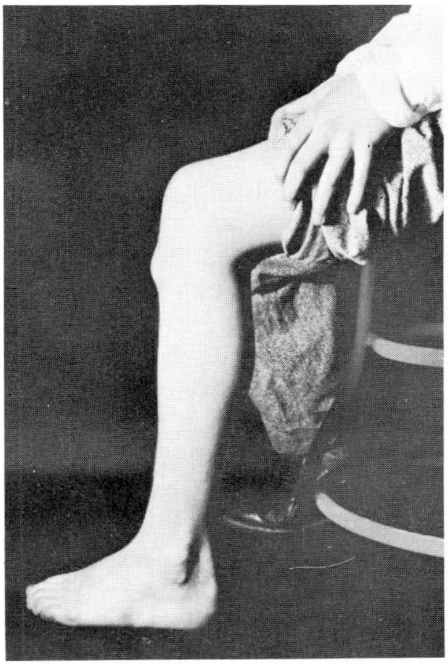

Figure 33-26. Osgood–Schlatter's disease.

Immobilization is not necessary unless the patient has pain with ambulation. Gaining adequate flexibility is considered a prerequisite to resuming athletic participation. Surgery is rarely necessary.

STRESS FRACTURES

Stress fractures of the tibia and fibula are not uncommon and occur in very characteristic clinical settings. Historically, they were most often reported in military recruits after prolonged marching. Today they are perhaps more typically associated with athletes, especially ballet dancers and runners. In military recruits stress fractures of the tibia are more common than those of the fibula and typically occur in the upper third. The location of the fractures in runners is reported to be most often in the distal third of the tibia, whereas in ballet dancers it is most common in the middle third.

Diagnosis

The most common symptom is pain of insidious onset. At first the pain is associated only with activity and later occurs with rest as well. There is usually focal tenderness at the site of the fracture.

The differential diagnosis of stress fracture includes chronic compartment syndrome (see the following discussion) and in the young athlete, osteoid osteoma, a benign bone tumor. The diagnostic difficulty can be compounded by the fact that x-rays of a stress fracture taken within the first 2 to 4 weeks after the onset of the pain may show nothing abnormal. Stress fractures can usually be differentiated from a compartment syndrome by the region of tibial shaft tenderness. In a chronic compartment syndrome tenderness is usually located only over the posteromedial border of the tibia where the muscles attach. The rest of the bone is nontender. Differentiation can be achieved by plain x-rays if abnormal findings are present and by a bone scan, which will show increased uptake in the region of the stress fracture and no abnormalities in the chronic compartment syndrome. Plain x-ray findings of a stress fracture can be difficult to differentiate from those associated with an osteoid osteoma. Bone scan findings are similar for the two entities. Osteoid osteomas can sometimes be differentiated from stress fractures on the basis of age, since they are very rare over the age of 30, and by the symptomatic response to taking aspirin, which dramatically relieves the pain caused by an osteoid osteoma.

CHRONIC COMPARTMENT SYNDROME

Etiology

The etiology of chronic compartment syndrome is thought to be the same as that of acute compartment syndrome, although the clinical presentation is much different. This syndrome is nearly always associated with repetitive activities such as running or volleyball.

Diagnosis

Patients usually report pain in the region of the involved compartment. The pain is described as a deep cramp or ache. Typically, it abates completely between periods of activity. Bilateral involvement is not uncommon. Symptoms may be present for months prior to presentation. The diagnosis is confirmed with compartmental pressure measurements. Measurements are made as the patient performs active plantar flexion and dorsiflexion. Patients with chronic compartment syndrome have been shown to have high resting pressures and much higher peak pressures during exercise than normal controls.

Treatment

The treatment for chronic compartment syndrome is fasciotomy. This procedure can be performed by subcutaneous dissection without making long incisions. Conservative treatment of chronic compartment syndrome is ineffective.

SHIN SPLINTS

Etiology

Musculotendinous inflammation in the leg is a common complication of repetitive exercise such as running. The term *shin splints* is specific to this disorder. It should not be used for other syndromes. The cause of the inflammation is thought to be rupture of individual collagen and elastin fibers within the musculotendinous unit. This is commonly associated with an abrupt increase in training activity. Patients who have been immobilized for a previous injury are at increased risk of developing shin splints on returning to full activity. The main symptom is pain, the location of which corresponds to the involved muscles. Any of the muscles of the legs can be involved. A history of inadequate shoewear or a change in running surface is also typical.

Diagnosis

Tenderness is found in the involved muscles. Pain can also be elicited on flexion and extension of the ankle.

Treatment

Treatment of shin splints begins with discontinuing the inciting activity. Ice application with massage two or three times a day can also be helpful. In severe cases anti-inflammatory medication can be effective. Alternate aerobic exercises such as swimming should be allowed to maintain a sense of physical and psychological well-being. After the period of acute symptoms has passed, a stretching program especially involving the antagonistic muscles is recommended. When the symptoms have completely resolved, the patient should be allowed to return gradually to full activity. Running should initially be allowed only with proper shoes on a rubberized level surface. If this is well tolerated, the patient may return to full activity.

RUPTURE OF THE MEDIAL HEAD OF THE GASTROCNEMIUS

Etiology

Rupture of the medial head of the gastrocnemius is commonly called tennis leg. It may occur in any sport involving lateral motion. Although this problem has been attributed to rupture of the plantarus tendon, in fact this structure is probably not involved in the majority of cases.

Diagnosis

The history is similar to that of an Achilles rupture. The patient describes acute calf pain that feels like a firm, painful blow. The injury usually occurs during sudden deceleration while running. On physical examination, swelling, ecchymosis, and tenderness are localized to the region of the tear and a palpable defect may be present (Fig. 33-27). The patient may be more comfortable standing on his toes on the affected side allowing the contracted soleus muscle to relieve the stress on the gastrocnemius.

Treatment

Initial treatment is symptomatic and consists of ice, elevation, and immobilization in a compressive dressing for 24 to 48 hours. After the acute symptoms have subsided a stretching program should be instituted to prevent contracture of the musculotendinous unit by the scar. No athletic activity should be allowed until normal motion and strength have returned. Recovery is usually complete in 8 to 12 weeks.

ACHILLES TENDINITIS

Etiology

The Achilles tendon is the most common site of tendinitis. Predisposing factors include tight calf muscles, excessive femoral anteversion, and hindfoot valgus. As with other overuse syndromes Achilles tendinitis is frequently associated with a sudden increase in training activity.

Diagnosis

The pain usually occurs 3 to 4 hours after exercise. It is exacerbated by climbing stairs but usually not by normal ambulation. On physical examination, tenderness is found usually a few centimeters above the insertion of the tendon. Occasionally, crepitation can be found on motion.

Treatment

The initial treatment of Achilles tendinitis is discontinuation of the causative activity and anti-inflammatory medications. After the acute symptoms have subsided an aggressive muscle-stretching program should be followed. The patient can then be allowed to return gradually to full activity. A syndrome of chronic Achilles tendinitis can develop with persistence of symptoms despite adequate conservative therapy. A period of at least 3 to 6 months should pass before surgery is recommended. A short (4- to 6-week) period of cast immobilization may be effective. Surgery for this condition consists of exposing the tendon then excising any defective portions. If possible the tendon is not completely transected.

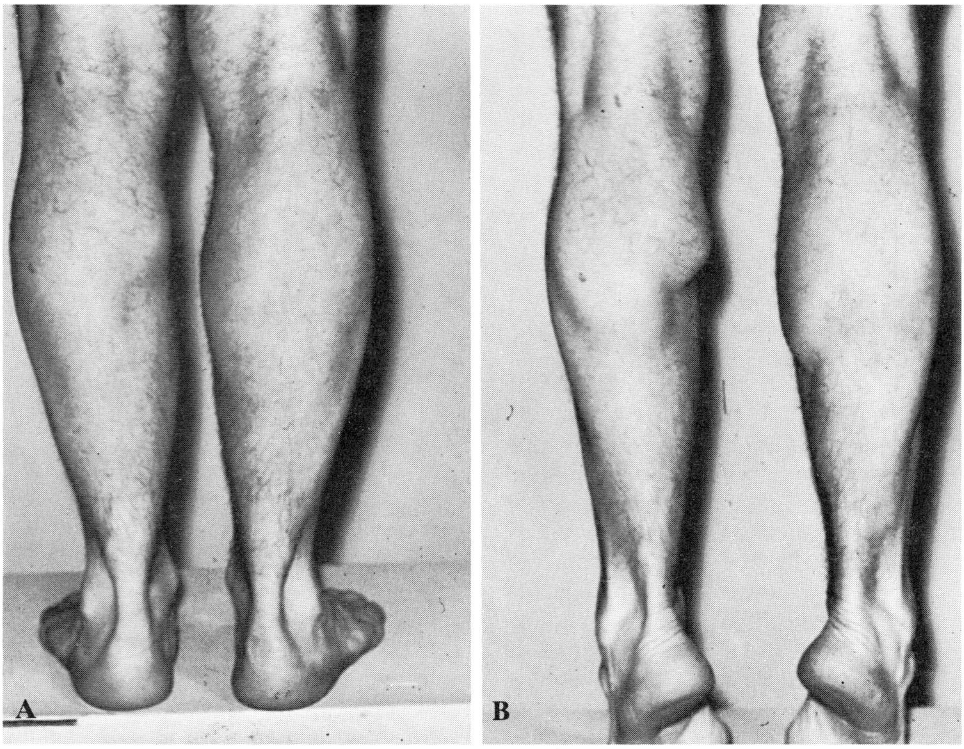

Figure 33-27. Tennis leg.

ACHILLES TENDON RUPTURES

Etiology

An Achilles tendon rupture occurs as an acute event but is thought to result from a preexisting degenerative process. The rupture can occur at any level from the musculotendinous junction to the insertion on the calcaneus. The typical patient with an Achilles rupture is a weekend athlete in the third or fourth decade of life. Sports associated with Achilles ruptures are those requiring rapid accelera-

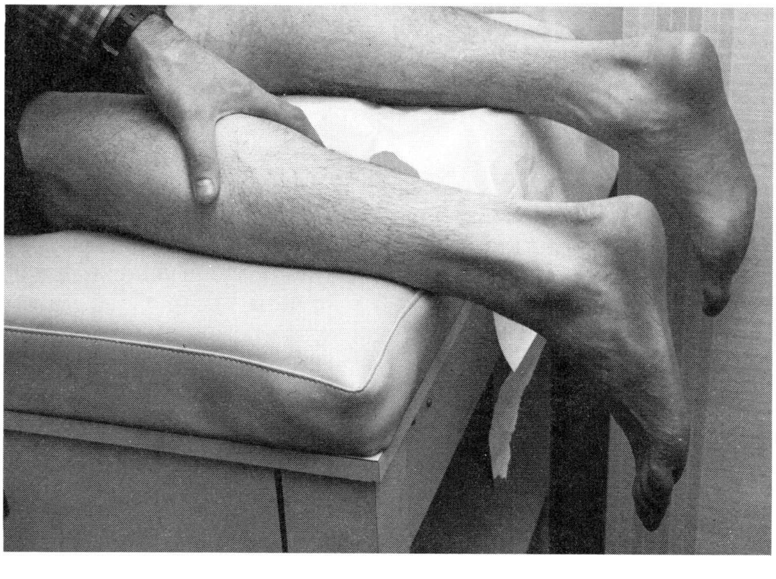

Figure 33-28. Thomas test.

tion, especially court sports such as racquetball, tennis, and basketball.

Diagnosis

The patient with an Achilles rupture usually has a vivid memory of the mechanism of the injury. Typically, the tendon tears during pushoff associated with rapid acceleration while running. The patient relates the sensation of a firm, painful blow to the heel. After the injury the patient may be able to walk but is unable to run because of pain and weakness. If the patient presents acutely, the diagnosis is usually easily made. With a delayed presentation the presence of the leg may be consistent with other diagnoses, such as deep venous thrombosis and cellulitis.

A patient with a suspected Achilles tendon rupture is examined in the prone position with the legs hanging over the end of the table. Ecchymosis, swelling, and tenderness will be localized to the level of the tear. If the rupture has occurred in the midportion of the tendon, a palpable defect may be present. The resting tone of the calf muscles will hold the uninvolved ankle in slight plantarflexion at rest. If the injured side is held more dorsiflexed, an Achilles rupture is implied. By far the most specific test for an Achilles rupture is the Thomas test. Performing this test simply involves squeezing the calf while observing the ankle. If the Achilles tendon is intact, squeezing the calf always illicits passive ankle plantarflexion (Fig. 33-28). With a ruptured Achilles, no ankle motion is observed.

Treatment

Satisfactory results have been achieved treating Achilles ruptures by both operative and nonoperative means. The main complication of nonoperative therapy is rerupture, which has been reported to occur in 20% to 30% of the cases. The rerupture rate with surgical repair is only about 2%, but other complications, such as deep infections and skin necrosis, can occur. The athletic individual presented with the options frequently chooses operative therapy. Nonoperative therapy is probably satisfactory for the majority of patients.

34 Arthroscopic Surgery

ALAN P. NEWMAN

Over the last 15 years the arthroscope has evolved from an awkward, seldom-utilized instrument to an indispensable tool in the surgical treatment of many large- and small-joint problems.[31,35,58] Although this technique was originally applied to the knee joint, instruments and methods have been developed for use in many other joints. Originally confined to a diagnostic role, the variety of procedures that can be performed arthroscopically has increased tremendously. In the knee, for example, virtually every intra-articular procedure, excluding total joint replacement, is amenable to the arthroscopic approach.

However, it should be stressed that arthroscopy is a *technique,* not a *procedure,* such as a meniscectomy or synovectomy. An intra-articular procedure can be performed either open (via an arthrotomy) or closed (arthroscopically), but regardless of the technique employed, the same indications and contraindications for the particular procedure exist. Although it is often possible to perform a more precise and thorough operation with the arthroscopic technique, its primary advantage over open surgery is the significant decrease in postoperative morbidity. Arthroscopy is associated with decreased hospitalization and recovery times, less pain, lower infection rates, and less derangement of normal anatomy. In effect, it has shifted the risk–benefit ratio by usually decreasing the risk, and often increasing the benefit, thereby allowing some conditions to be treated surgically earlier in their course than previously.

Although there were scattered early attempts at applying endoscopic principles to the examination of joints, the first suitable arthroscopic system was devised by Takagi of Tokyo in 1931.[58] The same year, Burman[58] of New York described a cadaver study on arthroscopic joint visualization, and in 1934 he published a clinical study of the use of the arthroscope in the diagnosis of knee disorders. The modern era of arthroscopy began in 1958, when Watanabe developed his No. 21 arthroscope, technically superior to its predecessors.[58] He performed his first arthroscopic partial meniscectomy in 1962. Jackson[31] of Toronto went to Japan in 1964 and studied with Watanabe and is credited with introducing the modern arthroscopic era to North America in 1965. In the 1970s a number of Americans, including O'Connor, Cascells, Metcalf, McGinty, and Johnson, pioneered many new techniques. Johnson helped develop the first motorized instrumentation in 1976, and from that point on, arthroscopic surgery became a dynamic, rapidly expanding field highlighted by dramatic improvements in patient care.

ARTHROSCOPIC ENVIRONMENT

The technical skills required to perform arthroscopic surgery are not extremely difficult; many other fields of surgery call for more manual dexterity and/or operative finesse. Nonetheless, arthroscopy is most often a very difficult technique to master. The key to understanding this seeming paradox lies with the realization that arthroscopy relies on a set of technical abilities very different from those used in most other surgical techniques. Traditional open surgery is performed in a familiar three-dimensional world, viewed directly through our eyes. Arthroscopic visualization is accomplished through the interface of a lens system, transmitting two-dimensional information. Furthermore, most arthroscopists utilize a technique called *triangulation.*[11,42] In this approach the arthroscope is inserted through one portal; an operating instrument, through a second portal; and frequently a second instrument, through a third portal. Bringing together the arthroscope and either one or two additional instruments into the same field of view may prove challenging. These facts and the physical removal of the surgeon from the operative field often produce a difficult psychomotor impasse for the novice arthroscopist. Thus the learning curve for mastery of the arthroscope is very gradual. Over 200 to 300 cases must be dealt with before competence is achieved, and more may be required to achieve excellence.

These problems demand that arthroscopic procedures be carried out in a well-planned, comfortable, familiar environment.[63] Furthermore, there are so many "moving parts" (fluid inflow–outflow, light source, arthroscopes, manual and motorized instrumentation, video transmission systems, etc.) that a small problem with one of them can completely halt the procedure. The only way to avoid being mired in innumerable technical hitches is to set up and initiate each procedure *identically*. Only by thoroughly and repetitively standardizing the technique can one hope to master it. There are many successful approaches to setting up a system; the important thing for an individual is to pick one routine and use it until it is habitual.

Most arthroscopic procedures can be done on an outpatient basis.[51] Exceptions are for more complex procedures (e.g., arthroscopic-aided cruciate ligament reconstruction) and for patients representing greater surgical and/or anesthetic risks. Currently, many hospitals have separate outpatient surgery units, although outpatients may share a common operating room with inpatients. Free-standing ambulatory surgery centers offer an alternative to hospital-based units and are becoming increasingly popular. They generally provide lower-cost care in a pleasant environment, since they are geared to caring for a healthy population undergoing elective procedures. This pleasant and relaxed environment usually is enjoyed by the surgeon also, as he is free from the scheduling pressures of lengthy procedures and trauma cases.

Just as a surgeon must strive to make every step of the arthroscopic procedure routine, so too must the other members of the operating team. It is imperative to have circulating and scrub personnel who are well acquainted with the equipment and techniques. Furthermore, particularly in knee arthroscopy, the use of an experienced surgical assistant is mandatory. The assistant, by positioning the knee and applying various stresses, can facilitate passage of instruments and visualization of the various compartments. His contribution can largely determine the relative ease or difficulty of a case.

Local anesthesia has been used with some success; it is perhaps the ideal anesthetic for outpatient procedures.[16] However, it has important limitations, and its use is therefore restricted. Tourniquets are commonly employed during arthroscopy, and tourniquet pain becomes a limiting factor with local anesthesia. Furthermore, since arthroscopic procedures have become more complex, and some require combined open and arthroscopic exposure (e.g., cruciate ligament reconstruction and meniscal repair), the anesthetic requirements often demand more than the cutaneous portal and limited synovial anesthesia that local anesthesia provides.

Therefore regional and general anesthesia are preferred over local anesthesia in most instances. For young, healthy, low-risk patients, general anesthesia is usually selected.[51] It provides a more predictable, rapid recovery in ambulatory patients. Spinal (subarachnoid) and epidural techniques are appropriate (especially in the presence of any contraindications to general anesthesia) but have some drawbacks. Spinal headaches are occasionally a problem, as are urinary retention—incontinence and prolonged recovery. Sometimes tourniquet pain during a longer procedure may require an intraoperative switch from regional to general.

Arthroscopy is carried out in either a gas (CO_2) or fluid medium. There are some technical points in favor of CO_2, the most important being that articular cartilage surface irregularities are more easily seen than with fluid.[18,54] A fluid tends to disperse light more evenly, making contours and shadows less prominent. However, there are other technical problems with gas, and numerous advantages with a fluid medium, and the latter is much more commonly used, with either normal saline or Ringer's lactate.

A fluid medium requires an inflow–outflow system, which can be accomplished by two different methods. Inflow can occur through the arthroscopic cannula itself and outflow can be through another cannula in a separate portal, or the direction of flow can be reversed.

Outflow is usually accomplished via gravity drainage. Inflow can be delivered by a gravity system (where the height of the fluid bottle relative to the joint determines the pressure head) or by an infusion pump[7] (where pressure

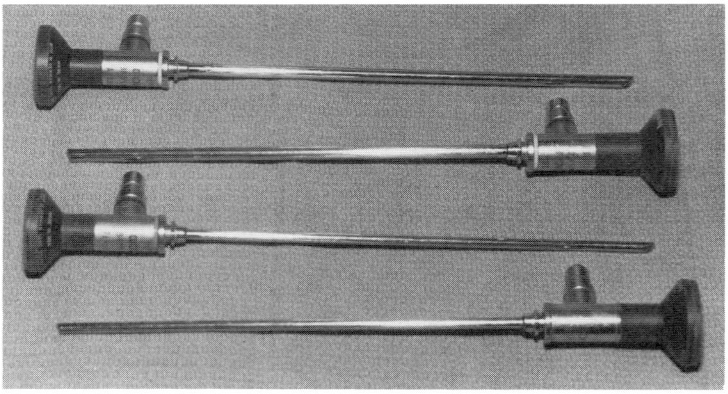

Figure 34-1. The most commonly utilized arthroscopes employ angles of inclination of 30° and 70°, in both 4-mm and 5-mm sizes.

and flow rate can be independently set). The important parameters to control with either approach to inflow–outflow are flow rate (important in clearing debris, blood, etc.) and pressure (important for capsular distention). The methods used to achieve optimum pressure and flow are a matter of individual preference.

For limb arthroscopy (other than shoulder and hip) tourniquets are routinely employed. Except in the simplest of diagnostic procedures, visualization is usually enhanced in the absence of blood. One situation in which this may be counterproductive is in the visualization of an inflammatory process, where the extent of synovial hyperemia is important to document and may be underestimated with the use of a tourniquet.

The heart of the equipment utilized in arthroscopy is the arthroscope itself.[35,54] The scope is a rigid tube enclosing a series of lenses that transmit an image from the joint to the eye (or camera). Surrounding the lens systems are glass fibers that transfer light from the light source to the joint. Arthroscopes range in size from 1.7 mm to 7.5 mm, with 4 mm and 5 mm being the most commonly used sizes (Fig. 34-1).

The objective lens can be angled away from the long axis of the scope. Thus rotation can increase the conical field of vision, the magnitude of increase depending on the angle of inclination (Fig. 34-2). The most common angles of inclination are 30 degrees and 70 degrees, although 0-degree, 90-degree, and 120-degree arthroscopes are occasionally used.

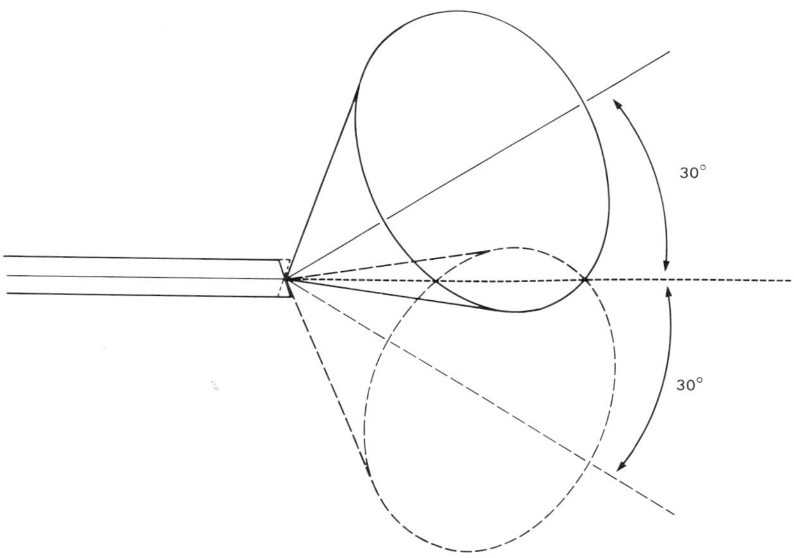

Figure 34-2. When the objective lens is placed at an angle to the long axis of the arthroscope, rotation of the scope can greatly increase the conical field of vision.

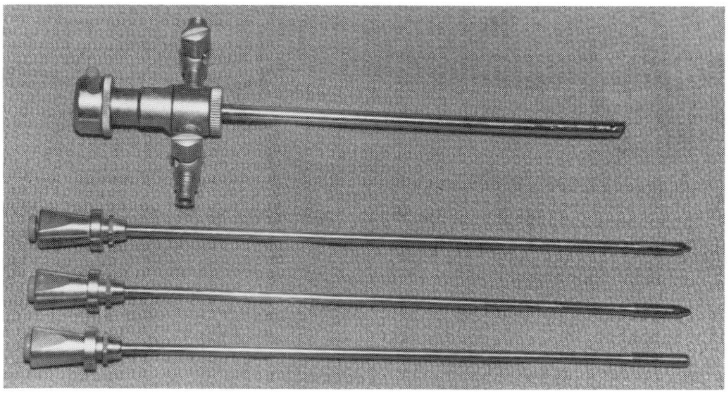

Figure 34-3. An arthroscopic cannula, with sharp, conical, and blunt obturators.

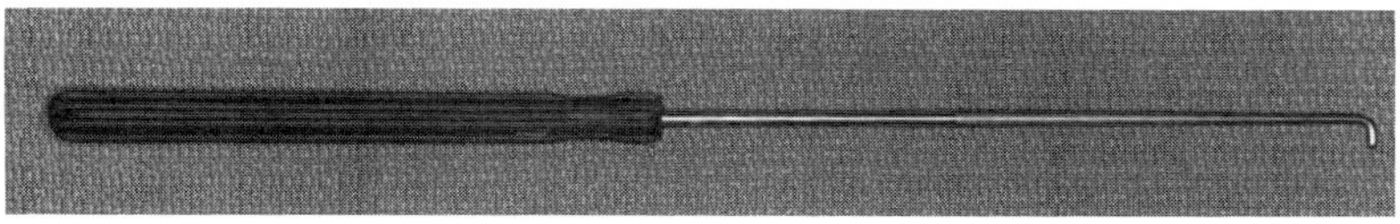

Figure 34-4. An arthroscopic probe.

Illumination is provided to the arthroscope by a light source and light cable. A number of different light sources exist, with higher-intensity (such as tungsten or metallic halogen or xenon arc) sources required for adequate illumination during most procedures.[35] The most popular light cables are flexible bundles of fiberglass strands. These cables are relatively fragile, with strand breakage or thermal injury diminishing the effective light delivered to the arthroscope.

For use in the joint, the arthroscope is placed in a sheath or cannula, with an outer diameter slightly larger than the scope itself (Fig. 34-3). This allows fluid to flow through the cannula and around the scope. Side-arms with spigots are placed proximally on the cannula for fluid inflow–outflow. To insert the cannula into the joint, a number of obturators are used, with either blunt, conical, or sharp tips. After joint entry, the obturator is removed and replaced by the arthroscope.

There has been a virtual explosion of instrumentation developed for arthroscopy, and this has been primarily responsible for the tremendous increase in the variety of procedures that can be accomplished arthroscopically. Instruments generally fall into two categories, either manual or motorized.[35,54]

The simplest and most frequently used manual instrument is the probe (Fig. 34-4). This is a modified nerve hook and adds important tactile feedback and reinforcement to the sensation of sight. Palpation aids greatly in diagnosis by helping to assess tissue consistency and mobility.

Basket (or punch) forceps have been borrowed and modified from other endoscopic disciplines. The metal bridge at the base of the basket has been removed, allowing the cut tissue to fall through the open hole and float free in the joint (Fig. 34-5). At the conclusion of the procedure the joint is then irrigated and/or suctioned free of these fragments. These instruments come in a variety of sizes and either are straight or have angled shafts and cutting tips (Fig. 34-6).

Various knife configurations and styles have been designed. The blades are either straight, angled, curved, or hooked (for retrograde cutting). Retractable blade-sheath systems allow for ease and safety of use. If the retractable blades are not used, the knives should be inserted through cannulas, to avoid joint damage. Scissors have also been designed specifically for arthroscopy, available in a variety of sizes, shapes, and angles.

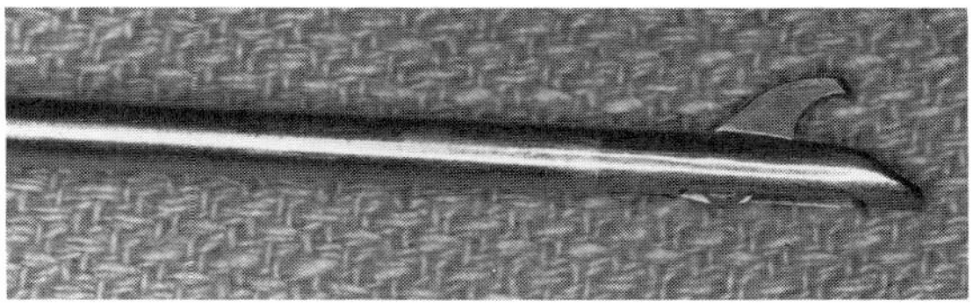

Figure 34-5. A punch forceps used for piecemeal resection of tissue.

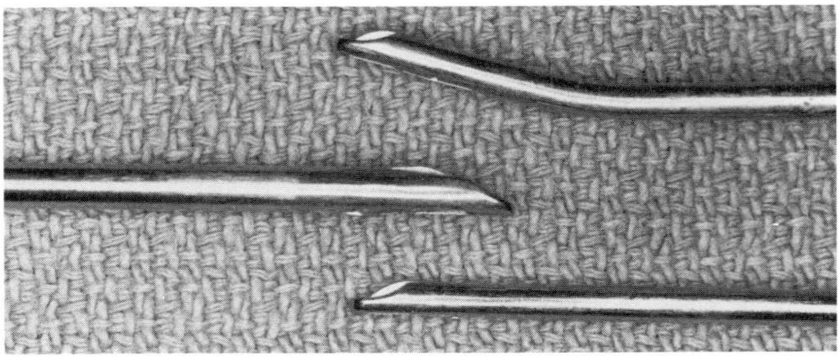

Figure 34-6. An upcurving 2.75-mm punch forceps, with 3.4-mm and 2.75-mm straight forceps below it.

Grasping instruments complete the spectrum of manual instrumentation for arthroscopy. Although hemostats and small Kocher clamps can be used, their radius of opening is so large that they are not generally useful inside a joint. Special grasping instruments have been designed with their axes of opening very close to their tips, allowing the jaws to open widely, even in tight corners. Other manual instruments, such as small curettes, rasps, and osteotomes, are occasionally used in arthroscopy but have not required any special modifications.

The application of arthroscopy to more and different procedures has been possible because of the development of effective motorized instrumentation.[35] These systems are composed of a motor, a hand-held unit, and a variety of interchangeable cutting heads. The motors are usually powered by electricity, but some run on compressed air.

The cutting heads all share a common design. They consist of an outer hollow sleeve with a window near the tip and an inner rotating cutting head driven by the motor. Usually these are attached to in-line suction. The suction pulls the tissue to be cut into the window, and the inner cutting head then resects the tissue, which is cleared by suction. The designs of the cutting heads vary, depending on their intended use. Specific instruments exist for the removal of synovium, fibrous tissue, meniscal and articular cartilage, and bone (Fig. 34-7).

Finally, drill and suture guides have been devised that allow precise intra-articular placement of guide pins, drill bits, and suture under arthroscopic visualization.

One recent change in the arthroscopic environment is the advent of video equipment to view the operative procedure on a television monitor, with the ability to record the surgery simultaneously on videotape.[35,57] Although not mandatory, this does provide significant advantages over direct viewing through the ocular lens. When one looks directly through the arthroscope, the eyepiece is always considered nonsterile. This is a distinct problem when changing from one arthroscope to another and particularly in more complex, combined open–arthroscopic cases, where there is a greater risk of infection. The ability to maintain sterility by attaching a sterile video camera directly to the eyepiece is a major improvement. Furthermore, using a camera improves surgeon comfort and maneuverability, as opposed to having to lean constantly and twist one's head in proximity to the eyepiece.

Video equipment is expensive, but the investment must be balanced against the ability to perform better procedures and provide improved patient care. Required components are special camera systems, an adequate light source, and a video monitor. Videotape recording equipment is optional but is valuable in documentation for records, patient education, and teaching.

Figure 34-7. A motorized instrument specifically designed to cut meniscal tissue. The smaller-diameter cutting head fits inside the larger hollow sleeve and rotates, allowing the blades to resect tissue that has been pulled into the window by inline suction.

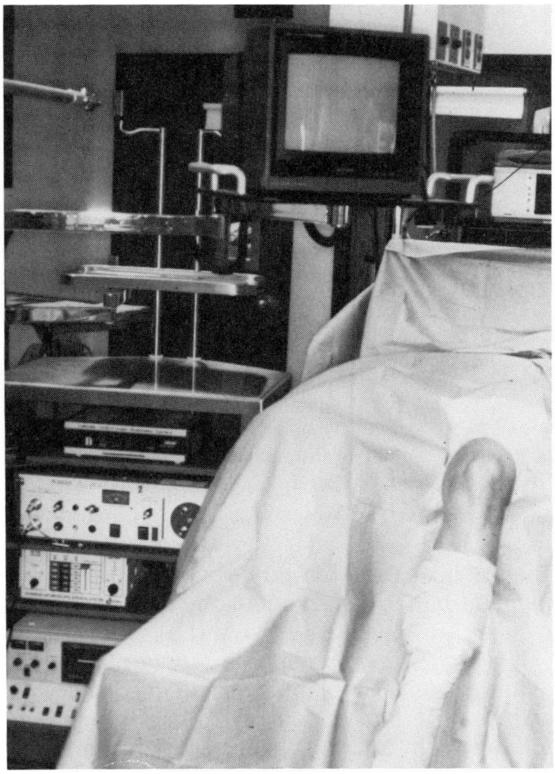

Figure 34-8. A knee sterilely prepared and draped for arthroscopy.

KNEE ARTHROSCOPY

Knee surgery has truly been revolutionized by the arthroscopic approach. Formerly requiring painful and morbid arthrotomies, most intra-articular processes can now be handled efficiently and with less discomfort and quicker recoveries. This represents better patient care, with significant economic benefits. The decreased cost of treating the problem arthroscopically is augmented by decreased time lost from the workplace.

BASIC SETUP

The patient is brought to the operating room, placed supine on the table, and given appropriate anesthesia (Fig. 34-8). Generally a tourniquet is placed about the proximal thigh, which is then placed into a leg holder (Fig. 34-9).[35] A number of commercially available devices serve the purpose of stabilizing the thigh during the procedure while the surgical assistant places varus and valgus forces on the knee to open up the lateral and medial tibiofemoral compartments, respectively. Routine sterile preparation and draping are then carried out.

Portal selection is perhaps the most critical technical aspect of arthroscopy. Improperly positioned portals make maneuvering within the joint difficult, if not impossible. There are six primary portals in knee arthroscopy. The two most commonly used sites are anterolateral and anteromedial (Fig. 34-10). They are located just lateral and medial (respectively) to the patellar tendon, within 5 mm to 10 mm of its border. The skin incision is made approximately 1.5 cm to 2 cm proximal to the edge of the tibial plateau, at or slightly distal to the inferior pole of the patella. The lateral and medial suprapatellar portals are made 1 cm to 2 cm proximal to the superior patellar pole,

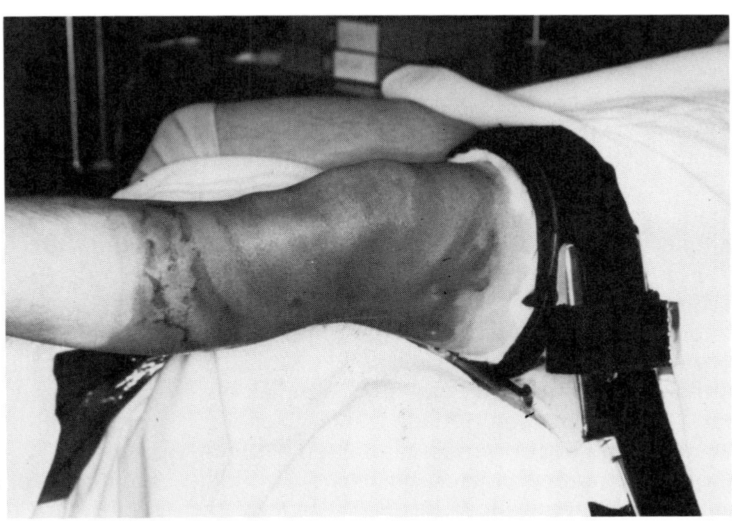

Figure 34-9. An arthroscopic leg holder.

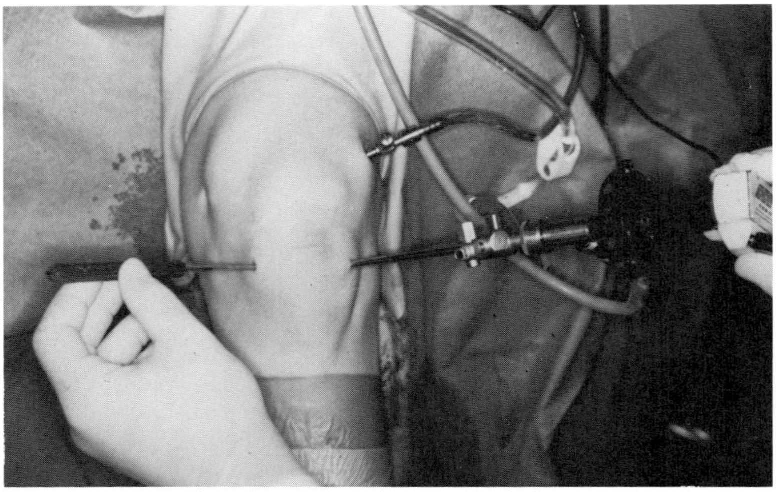

Figure 34-10. In this knee arthroscopy, the arthroscope is placed in the anterolateral portal and a probe is utilized through the anteromedial portal.

and just off the patellar border. The other two common portals are posterior. The posteromedial site is proximal to the joint line, posterior to the femoral condyle and medial collateral ligament, and anterior and proximal to the semimembranosus tendon. Posterolaterally the portal is located proximal to the joint line, posterior to the lateral collateral ligament and popliteus tendon, and anterior to the biceps femoris tendon. The posterior portals are occasionally difficult to place and can be facilitated by visualizing the proper location from inside the joint, with the 70-degree arthroscope inserted through the intercondylar notch looking around the back of the condyle. The portal is then made by sequentially visualizing placement of an 18-gauge spinal needle, a No. 11 blade, and finally the instrument or cannula.

Any number of secondary portals may be needed. The midpatellar portal is usually located lateral, at the level of the middle of the patella.[47] The transpatellar tendon portal directly penetrates the patellar tendon in the midline, 1 cm distal to the patella.[24,46] Occasionally, other portals are originated, for example, opposite a trapped loose body.

For routine diagnostic arthroscopy, the arthroscope is usually inserted in the anterolateral portal, the probe in the anteromedial portal, and the inflow (or outflow) cannula, in either the lateral or medial suprapatellar portal. The skin incision is made just large enough to insert the arthroscopic cannula. Two techniques for cannula insertion exist. The incision can be made only through skin and the sharp trocar used for cannula insertion, or the incision can be continued down through the capsule, followed by the blunt obturator.

The first step in any procedure is a thorough examination of the intra-articular space. The arthroscope is first positioned in the suprapatellar pouch, and the anterior compartment is observed for loose bodies and synovial changes. The articular surface of the patella is carefully examined for acute or chronic changes. The anteromedial joint wall is then visualized to characterize the constant medial synovial plica.

Next, the arthroscope is moved to the lateral gutter and the popliteus tendon hiatus is identified. This is an excellent location to find loose or foreign bodies.

The next step involves moving the scope back into the anterior compartment, sweeping it down into the medial gutter and into the medial compartment. This is a coordinated action, done in concert with the assistant placing the tibia in valgus, external rotation, and approximately 40 degrees of flexion to facilitate viewing the medial compartment. The articular surfaces and meniscus are visualized, taking care to probe the meniscus thoroughly in order to avoid missing small or occult tears.

The intercondylar notch is best seen with the knee in about 45 degrees flexion. The anterior cruciate ligament is usually well visualized, from its tibial attachment to its femoral insertion. Usually there is a good deal of synovium overlying the posterior cruciate ligament, with the anterior cruciate ligament obscuring much of the posterior cruciate ligament from the front.

The lateral compartment is entered with the tibia in varus, internal rotation, and approximately 20 degrees to 30 degrees flexion. The joint surface, meniscus, and popliteus tendon should be well seen.

Routine visualization of the posterior compartments should be carried out.[24] The posterolateral compartment is entered by passing the arthroscope from the anteromedial portal and through the intercondylar notch (between the anterior cruciate ligament and the lateral femoral condyl). In a similar fashion the posteromedial compartment is entered with the arthroscope in the anterolateral portal and passed between the posterior cruciate ligament and medial femoral condyle.

Only after a *thorough* diagnostic tour of the joint interior is any procedure undertaken. Otherwise, important pathology may be missed if the procedure is interrupted to address therapeutically the first lesion encountered. The only exception would be to remove a loose body, which might float away and be difficult to find later. Therefore such bodies are removed when first visualized.

MENISCUS TEARS

Meniscal tears are common, usually occurring after a twisting injury, with or without an associated ligament injury. In the older population, acute tears can occur, but are usually superimposed on preexisting attritional changes within the meniscal substance. There is a horizontally oriented, midline plane of increased shear stress in the posterior aspect of the meniscus, secondary to the frictional forces applied by the articular surfaces during flexion–extension and axial rotation. With time this excess strain can cause a horizontal cleavage within the meniscal substance (Fig. 34-11). Subsequent to a twisting injury, the cleavage may propagate to the inner free edge, resulting in the classic horizontal tear of a degenerative meniscus.[19,56]

Although originally viewed as superfluous structures, recent work has shown that the menisci serve important functions in the proper transmission of load in the knee and act to prevent the development of osteoarthritis. Therefore the attitude toward the treatment of meniscal lesions has shifted from one favoring complete meniscectomy for any lesion to a more conservative approach. Partial meniscectomy is attempted whenever feasible. In this procedure, only torn, unstable, or abnormal meniscal tissue is removed, leaving behind as much normal peripheral meniscus as possible. Some normal tissue is generally removed in order to leave behind a tapered and smoothly contoured C-shaped structure, but every attempt is made to preserve the peripheral meniscus. Studies have shown that the residual peripheral rim functions better mechanically than a complete meniscectomy.

There has been a great deal of interest lately in the subject of meniscal repair. The peripheral 10% to 30% of the meniscus has a vascular supply adequate to support healing[5] (Fig. 34-12). Longitudinal tears in this vascular region can heal, as shown by both animal models[6] and clinical studies.[13] Although only 10% to 15% of tears occur in this region, appropriate tears should definitely be repaired.

An acute meniscus tear can frequently be managed conservatively at first, unless the patient presents with a locked knee (which should be treated arthroscopically within 48 to

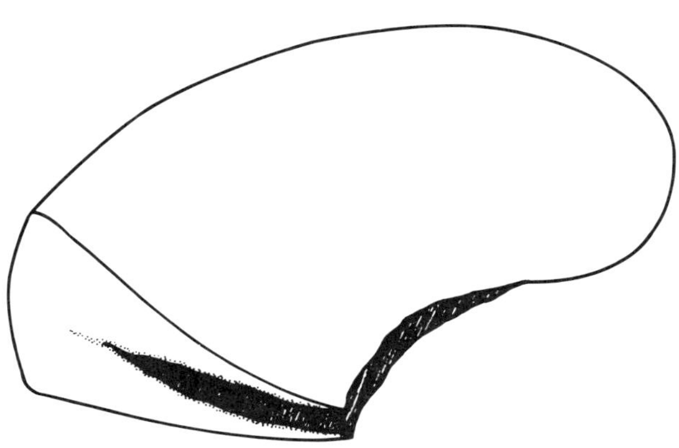

Figure 34-11. A cut-away drawing of the medial meniscus illustrating a degenerative, horizontal cleavage within the plane of increased shear stress.

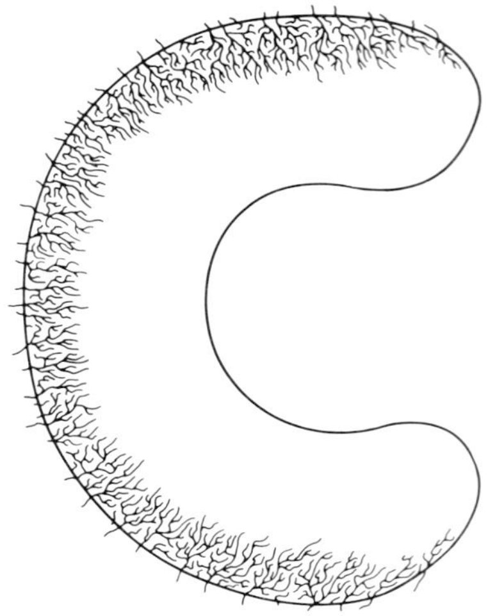

Figure 34-12. A drawing of the medial meniscus from above, illustrating the arborization of the perimeniscal capillary plexus.

72 hours). Rest, ice, and anti-inflammatory medications sometimes result in the return to a symptom-free state. If symptoms persist (such as pain, swelling, catching, or locking), then arthroscopy is indicated. Arthrograms are not obtained as often today as previously, since the findings will not strongly influence the treatment plan. A positive arthrogram in an asymptomatic meniscus tear will be managed conservatively, and a negative arthrogram in a patient with symptoms suggestive of a meniscus tear will still undergo arthroscopy, to rule out an occult tear or other pathology.

There are many different tear patterns[56,64] (radial, longitudinal, flap, horizontal, complex), but the treatment principle is the same for all of them.[59] All torn or unstable meniscus must be removed back to a stable border. The easiest patterns to treat are bucket-handle tears (longitudinal tears with anterior and posterior attachments) and flap tears (flaps of meniscus attached to the periphery by one pedicle). In each case, the attachment (or attachments) to the periphery is amputated by a scissors, knife, or basket forceps. The free fragment is then removed with a grasper. It is important to probe the peripheral rim carefully to check for tears not evident previously and to make sure that there is no pedicle left at the site where the attachment was cut. Further resection is accomplished with basket forceps and motorized cutters.

Other tear patterns usually require a combination of basket forceps and motorized instruments. Patience is required to ensure that the goals of resection are achieved: a stable rim with resection of as little normal meniscus as possible.[59] This often requires switching the arthroscope and cutting instrument between the two anterior portals, and occasionally utilizing some of the other portals.

Postoperative care following an arthroscopic meniscectomy consists of ice, elevation, and compression wrapping. Crutches are used, and progressive weight bearing is instituted the first postoperative day. Usually crutches are needed for 3 to 5 days. They are discarded when the patient is pain-free and can ambulate without a limp. A return to full activity is possible in 2 to 3 weeks.

If a longitudinal meniscal tear is in the peripheral vascular zone, repair should be carried out. Meniscal repair requires adherence to two principles: preparation of the peripheral rim to stimulate healing[29] and stabilization of the central fragment by secure sutures. It is thought that roughening and excoriation of the perimeniscal synovium stimulates a vascular response that increases the likelihood of healing. This is accomplished either manually with rasps or with motorized synovial resectors.

A number of different arthroscopic techniques have been devised for meniscal repair.[30,35,50] These usually involve the percutaneous passage of needles through cannulae, under arthroscopic visualization. These are generally safe and efficient methods, except when the tears extend to the extreme posterior attachments. The blind passage of needles in these regions can jeopardize the posterior neurovascular bundle, the saphenous nerve medially, and the peroneal nerve laterally. Some techniques have been developed specifically to minimize these risks,[43] or the repair can be done open.[12]

Some questions exist in the treatment of small (less than 1 cm) tears, or partial (not extending through the full meniscal thickness) tears. If they are stable and cannot be translated with the nerve hook into the region of the joint not normally occupied by meniscus, they should be left alone. If they are unstable, they probably will tear further and should be treated by excision, or repair if they are in the peripheral vascular zone.

CHONDROMALACIA

Softening and basal degeneration of the patellar articular surface, commonly referred to as chondromalacia, is an attritional condition due to chronic overload and malalignment.[21] Patellar malalignment can have many underlying structural (lateral retinacular tightness, patella alta, lateral femoral condyle hypoplasia, etc.) and dynamic (vastus medialis hypoplasia, quadriceps atrophy, etc.) causes, but the end result of malalignment is the tendency for the patella to track laterally. This culminates in hyperpressure under the lateral patellar facet and hypopressure under the medial facet. Articular cartilage is a unique tissue in that it requires intermittent pressure within a safe range. Pressures above or below that range are not tolerated well. This induces poor cartilage nutrition, chondrocyte damage, and matrix dissolution, starting in the deeper layers and moving superficially. Eventually the cartilage ulcerates, fibrillates, and is shed into the joint. The cartilage fragments are entrapped by the synovium, inducing a synovitis, effusion, and increasing levels of pain. This pain causes disuse quadriceps atrophy, exacerbating the malalignment. A vicious cycle ensues.

All patients with patellofemoral pain syndromes warrant a thorough trial of nonoperative treatment to include anti-inflammatory medications, physical therapy, and avoidance of bent-knee activities. If, after 3 to 6 months, this fails, surgery should be considered.

Part of the pain, effusion, and pseudolocking seen in this condition is due to the fibrillated cartilage in the patellofemoral joint (Fig. 34-13). Arthroscopic debridement is efficiently carried out by motorized chondral planers.[20] This can markedly reduce symptoms; however, it usually is of only temporary benefit. Unless the underlying cause of the malalignment is addressed, the fibrillation (and the symptoms) will recur.

One component of malalignment that is amenable to arthroscopic treatment is lateral retinacular tightness. Pathologic tightness of the lateral patellar retinaculum can pull the patella laterally. Open lateral retinacular release has been successful in altering the natural history of this condition. The lateral retinaculum can be incised percutaneously under arthroscopic visualization, using either scissors or knives.[35] Cutting the superior lateral geniculate vessels occasionally produces a large hemarthrosis. Because of this, work has been done in the use of electrocautery in arthroscopy.[22,23] Hemostasis can be achieved in this fashion but requires use of a nonconductive fluid medium, such as glycine or glycerol.

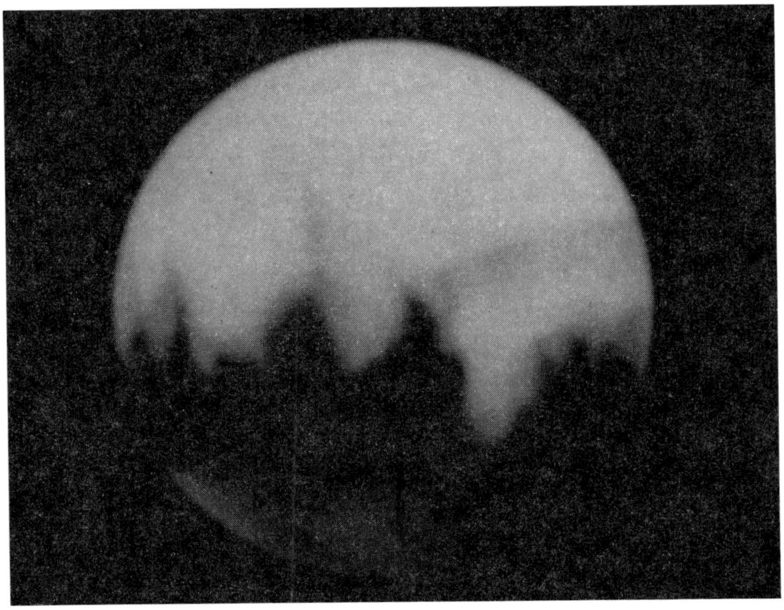

Figure 34-13. An arthroscopic view of the patellar undersurface, demonstrating the fibrillated articular cartilage seen in advanced chondromalacia.

If more than lateral retinacular tightness exists as part of a malalignment picture, then a lateral release alone usually is not enough. In this situation open surgery may be needed to correct the other components of the malalignment.

SYNOVIAL DISEASE

Diseases of the synovium can be either primary (as in rheumatoid arthritis) or secondary (as in hemophilia). Although not curative of the disease process itself, surgery has often been beneficial in the management of these conditions. Gross visualization of the involved tissue and biopsy have been helpful in diagnosis,[1,15] and lavage and synovectomy have proved to be therapeutically beneficial in slowing down the disease processes, although not in eradicating them. Arthroscopy offers several advantages over open surgery for each of these procedures.

Visualization of the joint interior can be more thoroughly completed with the use of the arthroscope, particularly in the posterior compartments, and in the medial and lateral gutters. Inspection of the synovium and articular cartilage changes may help distinguish between primary inflammatory versus degenerative involvement of the knee (Fig. 34-14).

The synovium in rheumatoid arthritis is boggy and hyperemic, with edematous, hypertrophic villi. This is to be contrasted with osteoarthritic synovium, which, although it may be mildly hyperemic, is usually less markedly involved, with slender villi. Frequently in osteoarthritis, entrapped cartilage debris is present. Other synovial disorders, such as pigmented villonodular synovitis, synovial osteochondromatosis, and hemophilic arthropathy, present with a typical arthroscopic appearance, although in these conditions the diagnosis is usually made preoperatively.

The gross articular cartilage changes are also important to characterize. Hyaline cartilage in rheumatoid joints is frequently soft and friable, but devoid of the focal ulcerations seen in osteoarthritis, until very late in the disease process. Rheumatoid pannus formation, growing in from the chondrosynovial junction to engulf the articular cartilage, is a classic finding. In osteoarthritis, hyaline cartilage may be soft, but this is usually at the border of a fibrillated, ulcerated region. It is thinned and shallow, with advanced cases exposing eburnated, subchondral bone (Fig. 34-15). Osteophytes, rather than pannus, are present at the chondrosynovial junction. Frequently, cartilaginous debris shed from the fibrillated regions is seen floating in the joint.

The other important diagnostic use of the arthroscope is in synovial biopsy. Although

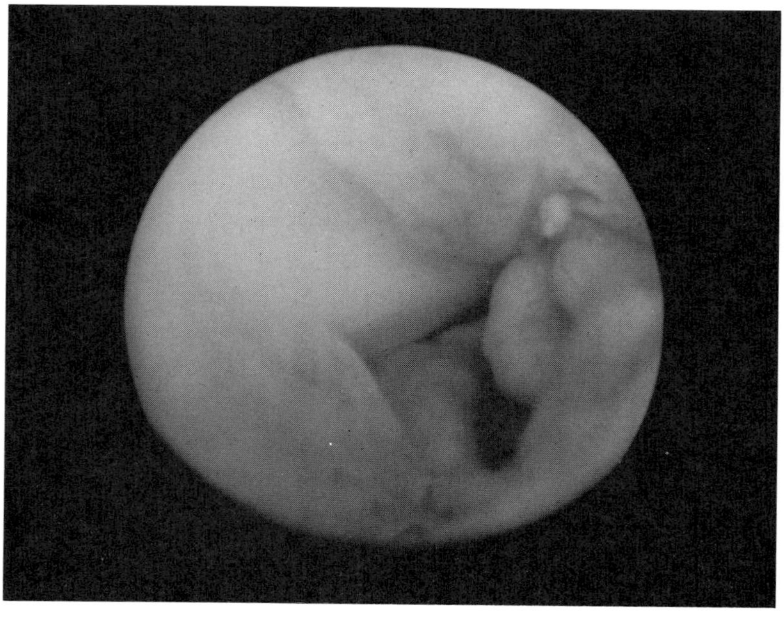

Figure 34-14. The plump, hyperemic villous hypertrophy typical of rheumatoid arthritis.

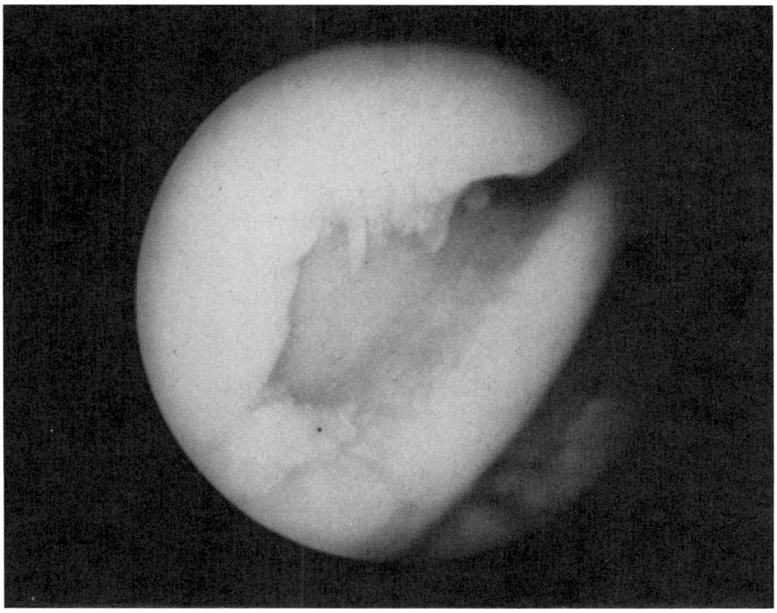

Figure 34-15. A severe case of osteoarthritis, with complete loss of the articular cartilage on the tibial plateau, exposing the underlying bone.

gross examination of the synovium is helpful, many conditions require a tissue diagnosis, and biopsy is a time-honored diagnostic procedure, either via open or percutaneous needle biopsy. However, arthroscopy avoids the higher morbidity of an open arthrotomy and the "blind" aspect of the needle biopsy. Under direct vision the biopsy instrument (such as a pituitary rongeur) can be directed to the precise location of the most florid pathologic changes. Frequently this occurs on the floor of the suprapatellar pouch, over the distal femur.

The simplest therapeutic procedure to be performed arthroscopically is lavage of the joint space. This is most effective in cases of crystal-induced synovitis and osteoarthritis.[45] Pain, swelling, and stiffness may be much less following simple lavage, although the relief is usually temporary. The effect is probably mediated by clearing the joint of floating crystals or debris, thereby diminishing the volume delivered to the synovium.

When medical management of a primary inflammatory synovitis fails, synovectomy can be a very important therapeutic modality. Open synovectomy has been performed for many years, and it can be effective in diminishing pain and swelling and retarding disease progression. However, it has substantial morbidity, primarily that of pain, decreased motion, and prolonged hospitalization and physical therapy. These problems are due to the postoperative hemarthrosis and pain that combine to limit early postoperative motion and favor the formation of fibrous adhesions. Arthroscopic synovectomy, although usually requiring six portals, is still a closed technique, without any large incisions or disruption of the extensor mechanism. Postoperative pain is markedly diminished, and immediate postoperative active and passive motion can be instituted, with maintenance of, and sometimes improvement in, the preoperative range of motion.

Arthroscopic synovectomy also provides for a more complete synovial excision. With an open technique, the posterior compartments of the knee could not be addressed, unless additional posteromedial and posterolateral incisions were made. Furthermore, the parameniscal synovium could not be removed without a meniscectomy,[40] which is contraindicated if the meniscus is structurally normal. Arthroscopy provides ease of access to the posterior compartments, the parameniscal synovium, and every corner and recess of the knee. A more complete excision is possible, and this advantage of the arthroscopic technique also holds for the ankle and shoulder.

The technique of arthroscopic synovectomy is tedious and demanding. It requires nothing more than basic triangulation skills, but due to the sheer volume of diseased synovium, it necessitates extreme patience and persistence. Arthroscopic synovectomy is made possible by very efficient motorized synovial resectors.

Hemophilic arthropathy represents a special situation where the advantages of the arthroscopic technique are most apparent.[37,62] Unlike rheumatoid arthritis, the synovium of a hemophiliac is intrinsically normal, until it is involved secondarily by recurrent hemarthroses. It becomes engorged with hemosiderin, hypertrophic, and friable, decreasing the threshold for future bleeds. The presence of the hemosiderin and the synovial hypertrophy frequently lead to severe, disabling degenerative changes. Following synovectomy, a normal synovium regrows, and if the patient is able to avoid significant trauma to the joint, he may be able to avoid the vicious cycle of recurrent bleeds and the disastrous sequelae. Since the morbidity of the arthroscopic technique is so much lower than that for an open synovectomy, hemophiliacs currently are being surgically treated earlier, prior to the initiation of the chronic, progressive degenerative changes.

Any condition that has been treated by open synovectomy in the past is amenable to the arthroscopic approach. This includes rheumatoid disease, pigmented villonodular synovitis, synovial osteochondromatosis, Reiter's syndrome, and chronic nonspecific monarticular synovitis.

Synovial Plica

There are many folds of synovium within the knee, and occasionally they become inflamed and symptomatic.[33,36,53] The medial synovial shelf is the most common of these, although still a rare cause of knee pain. It runs obliquely between the infrapatellar fat pad and medial synovial wall, attaching opposite the midportion of the patella (Fig. 34-16). It is occasionally subject to blunt trauma and can become pathologically thickened and fibrotic, initiating a region of wear-induced medial femoral chondromalacia. In the presence of a classic history and physical examination, and with arthroscopic confirmation of chondral changes, excision of the plica by a localized synovectomy can be very successful in relieving symptoms.

INTRA-ARTICULAR LOOSE BODIES

Intra-articular loose bodies are generated in a variety of conditions and can be osseous, chondral, fibrous, or any combination of these tissues. They can cause pain, swelling, and a variety of mechanical symptoms (locking, catching, etc.). Their removal is quite gratifying, but attempting that removal by an arthrotomy can be one of the more frustrating surgical experiences. They tend to hide in remote recesses and folds. In the knee they frequently are found in the medial and lateral re-

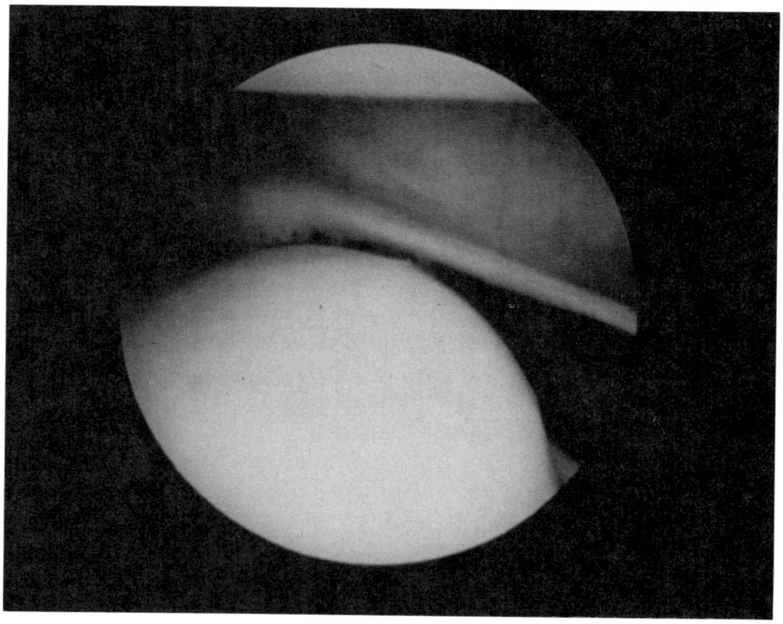

Figure 34-16. A large medial synovial plica, which extends as a shelf obliquely across the top of the medial femoral condyle.

cesses, the posterior compartments, and even within the sheath of the popliteus tendon. Since the arthroscope can probe all these areas with relative ease, loose body removal is reduced to a matter of systematic analysis of the joint space, as opposed to an often exasperating and unsuccessful open search of a limited portion of the joint.[41,54]

OSTEOCHONDRITIS DISSECANS

Osteochondritis dissecans is a spontaneous condition in which a segment of articular cartilage and subchondral bone becomes separated (fractured) from the adjacent, surrounding bone. Controversy exists as to its exact etiology; speculation has centered around hereditary causes, ischemia, or trauma. It typically occurs in adolescent males and can be a cause of significant pain and swelling. The most common location is on the lateral aspect of the medial femoral condyle, adjacent to the attachment of the posterior cruciate ligament.

Classification is based on the amount of mobility and separation of the fragment.[28] Intact fragments have no break in the overlying articular cartilage. Early separation refers to those fragments that have a break in the articular cartilage that allows slight mobility but cannot be displaced. Partially detached lesions can be displaced from the crater, but are not free, held in place by a hinge of articular cartilage. A loose body is a fragment floating free in the joint, and these lesions can be further subclassified as salvageable or unsalvageable. A salvageable lesion has relatively preserved articular cartilage and can be reduced into a congruous crater, or bed. An unsalvageable lesion lacks these qualities.

The treatment of osteochondritis dissecans is based on the classification of the lesion and age of the patient.[28] In a child under the age of 12, the intact lesion can be treated with immobilization and non-weight-bearing. In an older patient with an intact lesion, or any patient with a break in the articular cartilage, operative intervention is indicated.

Arthroscopic visualization greatly aids in the staging and treatment of osteochondritis dissecans. In an intact or early separated lesion, simply drilling with Kirschner wires or fixing with a specially designed cannulated cancellous screw set is feasible under arthroscopic control. The same treatment is recommended for partially detached and loose fragments where, after the bony surface of the fragment and the crater have been debrided of fibrous tissue, the fragment is reduced and fixed with wires or screws (Fig. 34-17). However, some authors advocate bone grafting of detached and loose fragments, especially in older, skeletally mature patients.[28] Unsalvageable loose bodies are removed, with debridement of the crater.

LIGAMENT INJURIES

Ligament injuries (sprains) are common injuries in the young, active population and require aggressive, although not always operative, treatment. It must be emphasized that a ligament is evaluated functionally, by manual stress testing during the physical examination. One of the important functions of a ligament is to restrain abnormal joint motion, and testing its mechanical function is more important than its visual appearance during open or arthroscopic surgery. Furthermore, ligaments frequently undergo in-substance failure, appearing grossly intact but no longer capable of restraining abnormal motion because its collagen fibers have undergone microscopic failure. In this instance the *appearance* of a ligament can actually be misleading. Although there are infrequent instances of arthroscopy aiding in the diagnosis of a ligament injury (e.g., arthroscopy demonstrating a torn anterior cruciate ligament following an acute hemarthrosis where the physical examination failed to demonstrate any instability), the diagnosis should usually be made *prior* to arthroscopy.

Collateral ligament injuries are, in general, not amenable to arthroscopic treatment. They are extracapsular structures, so their repair usually requires an open dissection. Furthermore, capsular tears occur in association with collateral ligament injuries and represent a relative contraindication to arthroscopy in the acute phase. The capsular rent allows soft-tissue extravasation of the arthroscopic fluid, which can cause compartment syndromes, large-vessel compression, and so forth. Additionally, leaking of the fluid impairs visualization.

Cruciate ligament injuries can be evaluated arthroscopically. The type of injury (bony avulsion vs. midsubstance tear) can be identified, and associated meniscal pathology can be diagnosed and treated. Recently, techniques

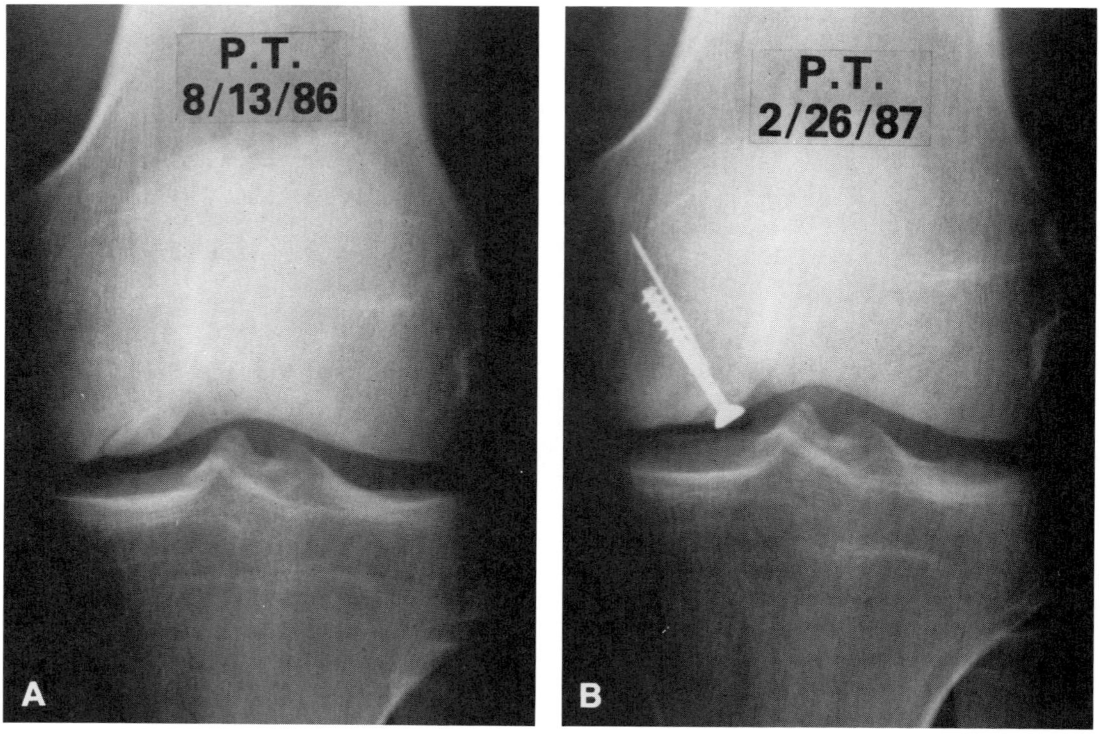

Figure 34-17. (*A*) A symptomatic osteochronditis dissecans lesion in the medial femoral condyle of a 24-year-old male. (*B*) The lesion went on to heal uneventfully after arthroscopic placement of a screw and wire.

and equipment have been developed that allow cruciate ligament injuries to be repaired and/or reconstructed with arthroscopic visualization. A staple system can be used to attach the anterior cruciate ligament stump back to the lateral femoral condyle.[35] However, significant questions exist as to the efficacy of acute repair of a torn anterior cruciate ligament, whether by open or arthroscopic technique. A true bony avulsion off the lateral femoral condyle may be an appropriate lesion for this approach, but these are extremely rare. Most anterior cruciate ligament injuries have substantial intrasubstance damage, which apparently does not heal, and residual instability follows in a high percentage of acute anterior cruciate ligament repairs without some type of augmentation.

Most cruciate ligament surgery involves either augmentation of an acute repair or replacement.[61] The substances utilized are autogenous tissues, allografts, and prosthetic materials. Arthroscopic techniques have been developed to aid in placement of all these materials. These usually represent combined open and arthroscopic techniques, as proximal and distal incisions are made for the passage and anchorage of the graft material. The procedures usually involve widening of the intercondylar notch with a motorized burr, identification of the correct tibial and femoral attachment sites, and placement (with the aid of special drill guides) of guide pins exiting at the attachment sites. Cannulated reamers then create bony tunnels of preselected size to allow passage of the ligament grafts.

The postoperative recovery is very much the same following arthroscopic-aided cruciate ligament reconstruction as it is following open surgery, since the biologic healing parameters are the same. However, the morbidity and risk of joint infection is much less with the arthroscopic technique.

OSTEOARTHRITIS

Arthroscopic debridement of osteoarthritic joints has met with mixed reviews.[49] Synovectomy is not generally successful in decreasing symptoms in these patients, and certainly does not alter the natural history. Osteophyte removal, unless palpably tender or implicated as a cause of limitation of motion, is similarly unrewarding. Lavage does decrease the cartilaginous load to the synovium, as does motorized shaving of loose, fibrillated articular cartilage, decreasing synovitis and providing some symptomatic, but usually temporary, relief.

The treatment of meniscal lesions in the older population has been somewhat controversial.[10] It is recognized that routine excision of meniscal tears in patients with established degenerative articular changes frequently leads to little or no resolution of symptoms, probably because the preoperative symptoms were more related to the arthritis than the meniscal tear. However, degenerative meniscal tears (horizontal cleavage tears) in the absence of associated osteoarthritis do occur in the older population and can be a source of considerable symptoms. If a patient presents with a relatively short history of joint line pain following a traumatic episode, has a physical examination suggestive of a meniscal tear, and radiographs indicating minimal degenerative disease, then a partial meniscectomy correlates well with relief of symptoms. Lacking these critical indicators of success, indiscriminate arthroscopy of patients with degenerative joint disease will reveal many meniscal lesions, few of which are directly related to the level of symptoms.

One area of recent interest concerns attempts to stimulate regrowth of cartilage in areas of eburnated bone.[34] Drilling or complete removal of exposed cortical bone has been advocated in an attempt to stimulate the underlying vascular cancellous bone to provide both a matrix and new cells, which might undergo metaplasia to form fibrocartilage. This has been performed by open technique for many years, and recently arthroscopic instrumentation has been developed for this purpose. A high-speed burr is applied to the sclerotic cortical surface, and approximately 2 mm of bone is removed evenly, until fresh bleeding is encountered. Some early series of abrasion arthroplasties have been reported, with mixed results. Repeat arthroscopies have demonstrated coverage of the surface with a fibrocartilaginous material, with some improvement in symptoms. However, the percentage of patients improved with this procedure is unclear, as is the fate and longevity of the fibrocartilaginous material.

SEPTIC ARTHRITIS

The treatment of septic arthritis is predicated on appropriate antibiotic management and adequate joint drainage. Although there is controversy over whether closed or open drainage is superior, the principle of *adequate* drainage is universally accepted. Advocates of repeated needle aspiration point to the significant morbidity associated with a large arthrotomy and open treatment, as well as the many successful results with closed treatment, especially in certain joints and with particular organisms. Advocates of open drainage argue that after 48 to 72 hours, the fibrinous exudate and loculations that form make adequate drainage by closed means impossible.

Some recent studies[32,55] have suggested that arthroscopic treatment of septic joints can be successful and have specifically addressed the issues raised by both open and closed drainage advocates. Arthroscopic drainage certainly minimizes the operative morbidity, with the risk of anesthesia the only significant consideration. On the other hand, the arthroscopic instrumentation developed to remove synovium and other tissue is very capable of removing all loculations and infected synovium. That capability and better visualization than that afforded by arthrotomy offer some practical reasons for arthroscopy providing more effective drainage and lavage than arthrotomy. Although larger and longer clinical series need to be performed to document the efficacy of this approach, it has exciting potential.

SHOULDER ARTHROSCOPY

The arthroscope is beginning to change shoulder surgery in much the same way that it has knee surgery. Arthroscopy in the shoulder may be a few years behind the knee in terms of development of techniques and procedures, but there is no question that the applications are expanding rapidly. Both the glenohumeral joint and the subacromial bursa have been successfully approached with the arthroscope.

BASIC SETUP

The patient is placed in the lateral decubitus position, with the operative side up.[9,27] A suction-molded bean bag is helpful in maintaining patient position. The forearm and hand are placed in skin traction, and the shoulder is placed in 70 degrees abduction to view the glenohumeral joint, and 30 degrees abduction for the subacromial bursa. Care is taken to minimize the length and amount of traction, because brachial plexus traction injuries have been described following shoulder arthroscopy.[38]

Following sterile preparation and draping, it is helpful to trace out the bony landmarks. The initial portal is posterior, 2 cm distal and 1 cm medial to the junction of the posterior acromion and scapular spine. An 18-gauge spinal needle penetrates the skin at this point, aiming for the coracoid process anteriorly. After entering the joint, the capsule is distended with 50 ml of Ringer's lactate. A skin incision is made, and the cannula with sharp trocar are advanced through the tissue, following the previous course of the spinal needle toward the coracoid process. After penetrating the capsule but not the synovium, the sharp trocar is changed for the conical obturator, which is then advanced into the joint.

After the arthroscope is placed inside the cannula and the joint interior is visualized, a number of secondary portals can be made. A superior portal, utilized for inflow or outflow, is located posterior to the acromioclavicular joint and just medial to the inner curve of the acromion. It is easy to penetrate the supraspinatus tendon at this point with a cannula.

Anterior portals are difficult to establish from the outside-in direction. Instead the arthroscope is advanced anteriorly over the glenoid, and between the biceps and subscapularis tendons. It is pressed against the anterior capsule at this point, the scope is removed from the cannula and replaced by a Wissinger rod.[35] This is a long, thin rod with a dull point on the end. It is pushed bluntly through the capsule and anterior soft tissues until it tents the skin. A skin incision is made over the point, and it is advanced through the skin. Next, a cannula is placed anteriorly over the Wissinger rod and advanced into the joint. This establishes a permanent anterior portal for fluid, manual or motorized instruments, and the arthroscope. Other anterior portals can be fashioned similarly, taking care that the Wissinger rod always exits the skin lateral to the coracoid process, to ensure the safety of the neurovascular structures.

To view the subacromial space, the same posterior portal can be utilized, simply redirecting the cannula more superiorly, to a position just under the acromion. Accessory subacromial portals are lateral and anterior, and they can be made by direct penetration with cannulae.

As with knee arthroscopy, it is important to inspect the joint in an orderly fashion.[2,14] The biceps tendon is a good orienting structure, and it should be viewed in its entirety, from the supraglenoid tubercle to its disappearance out the bicipital groove. Next, the anterior capsule, with the subscapularis tendon and middle and inferior glenohumeral ligaments are visualized. The glenoid fossa is observed next, followed by the anterior and posterior glenoid labra. The anterior and posterior recesses and the axillary pouch are inspected; occasionally, they house loose bodies. The condition of the humeral head is noted, especially for the existence of a Hill–Sachs lesion, the posterolateral humeral head impaction fracture seen after anterior glenohumeral dislocations. Finally, the rotator cuff insertion into the humeral head can be studied.

There are not as many anatomic features to be seen in the subacromial bursa, and generally motorized debridement of fine, adventitial strands of fibrous tissue must be carried out before inspection of the bursa is possible. The under surface of the entire acromion can be seen, as well as the coracoacromial ligament and acromiaclavicular joint. Most important, the bursal side of the rotator cuff should be inspected for small or partial tears.

As was mentioned in regard to the knee, arthroscopic visualization of the shoulder is quite helpful diagnostically. Generalized synovial and/or degenerative disease can be quantitated. Observation of Hill–Sachs and Bankart lesions, evidence of glenohumeral instability, can help confirm a tentative diagnosis. Loose bodies, glenoid labral tears, and rotator cuff pathology are all well seen through the arthroscope.

The remainder of this section will deal with entities and procedures unique to the shoulder. The use of the arthroscope in a number of other shoulder procedures, such as lavage, loose body removal, synovectomy, and so forth, is conceptually very similar to the description of these procedures in the preceding section on the knee.

GLENOHUMERAL INSTABILITY

The glenohumeral joint is a remarkable articulation. It has an extremely large range of motion, enabling the hand to be positioned virtually anywhere in space. However, it pays a high price for this motion, that of significant instability. It is the most frequently dislocated joint in the body and accounts for 31% of all shoulder girdle injuries.[52] Both the motion and instability are due to the same facts of functional anatomy. The glenohumeral articulation is a ball-and-socket joint, but unfortunately, the socket (glenoid fossa) is extremely small and shallow. Shoulder stability is therefore dependent on ligamentous and neuromuscular contributions, and these soft-tissue restraints are frequently overcome by trauma. Recurrent shoulder instability (subluxation and dislocation) is a common functional problem, and occasionally this represents a dilemma in diagnosis, both in differentiating from other conditions and in determining the direction of instability (anterior vs. posterior). Arthroscopy is helpful in both the diagnosis and treatment of this entity.

As with ligamentous injuries of the knee, the examination under anesthesia is critical in the evaluation of the unstable shoulder. However, there are still occasions when there is some question as to the extent and/or direction of instability. Visualization of a posterolateral humeral head compression fracture (the Hill–Sachs lesion) is pathognomonic of an anterior shoulder dislocation. A Bankart lesion represents an avulsion of the anterior capsular–periosteal sleeve from the scapular neck (with or without an associated labral tear) and is also indicative of anterior instability.

If a Bankart lesion exists, its repair will restore glenohumeral stability. An arthroscopic stapling technique has been developed for repair of these lesions.[35] Viewing from the posterior portal, a motorized burr directed from the anterior portal can debride and roughen the exposed anterior scapular neck. A staple can then pick up the capsule and inferior glenohumeral ligament, advance it superiorly, and reattach it to the prepared anterior glenoid lip.

Another technique that has been described attempts to reconstruct the inferior glenohumeral ligament, thought to be critical in the prevention of anterior instability.[8] Under arthroscopic control a guide pin is placed from anterior to posterior through the scapular neck, with the anterior entry point at the attachment site of the inferior glenohumeral ligament. A cannulated reamer is then passed over the guide pin, creating a tunnel through which a graft (autograft or allograft) can be passed. It is secured at the posterior exit point, then passed anteriorly and inferiorly, re-creating the path of the inferior glenohumeral ligament, and secured to the proximal humerus through a small open incision.

Both these procedures are innovative and share the arthroscopic advantage of smaller incisions (or, as in the case of stapling, only portals are used). Nonetheless, they do not represent substantial improvements in the risk–benefit ratio over traditional open surgery. The healing times, and therefore the recovery times, are analogous for both open and arthroscopic techniques. Neither arthroscopic technique has been used widely enough to know what the success rates are. However, since traditional open shoulder repairs are about 95% successful in controlling recurrent dislocation, it is unclear whether the arthroscopic techniques will match, let alone, exceed, this success rate.

GLENOID LABRAL TEARS

Both the anterior and posterior glenoid labra can tear and may cause mechanical symptoms of catching and clicking (much like torn knee menisci) in addition to chronic pain.[4,65] These symptoms may be relieved by excision of the torn fragment, but it is important to determine if the labral tear exists in conjunction with glenohumeral instability. If it does, labral excision may worsen the instability, and repair rather than excision is indicated.

Although the history and examination under anesthesia will help uncover the association of instability with a labral lesion, there are certain features of the tear that indicate whether it is an isolated lesion in a stable shoulder. In general, a torn labrum in association with a Bankart-type lesion is evidence for instability and warrants repair of the capsular lesion, with or without salvage of the labrum. If the anterior capsular mechanism is attached flush with the anterior glenoid lip, the examination under anesthesia demonstrates a stable shoulder, and the labral tear resembles a bucket-handle meniscus tear (with superior and inferior attachments), then its excision will relieve the patient's symptoms and will not result in increased instability.

Excision of a torn anterior labrum is easily carried out with the arthroscope in the posterior portal and the cutting instrument in the anterior portal. Basket forceps can cut the two attachments of a bucket-handle tear (or the single attachment of a flap tear) and the free fragment removed by a grasper. Alternatively, one attachment can be cut, converting the bucket-handle to a flap, and the flap can be removed with a motorized meniscal cutter or synovial resector.

The technique for cutting a posterior labral tear is quite similar. Often the arthroscope can be left in the posterior portal, but occasionally the instruments need to be reversed, with the scope anterior and the cutting instrument posterior.

Postoperatively, the patient is placed in a sling, which can be discarded in 2 or 3 days, as comfort permits. Active and passive exercises are instituted immediately, and full activity is allowed by 3 weeks.

IMPINGEMENT SYNDROME

Impingement syndrome is a spectrum of disorders showing a common pathophysiology. Included in this spectrum are subacromial bursitis, biceps tendinitis, and rotator cuff tendinitis and ruptures, in addition to a variety of clinical syndromes, such as painful arc and some cases of frozen shoulder. Central to the pathophysiology are the mechanics of shoulder elevation[44] and the vascularity of the rotator cuff and biceps tendons.[48]

When the shoulder is raised in the functional arc of elevation, the biceps tendon and insertion of the supraspinatus tendon pass directly under the coracoacromial arch (the coracoid process, coracoacromial ligament, and anterior acromion). With repetitive overhead activities, pressure and friction cause wear and attritional changes within this critical zone of the tendons. Healing and recovery could occur, except that this region has a very marginal vascular supply, located in a watershed region between contributions from the greater tuberosity and the more medial extent of the tendons. Thus the potential for healing is limited, and patients who repetitively perform overhead tasks (baseball pitchers, swimmers, carpenters, etc.) are at risk for this problem.

Initially, the pathologic changes are reversible, with inflammation in the subacromial bursa. If the overuse is continued, irreversible changes may occur, leading to fibrosis, tendon degeneration, and ultimately tendon rupture. It may take years to progress through the entire spectrum, and treatment is certainly more successful if rendered early in the process.

The diagnosis is made by the history, a physical examination demonstrating pain with forward elevation and internal rotation, and a positive therapeutic response to an injection of 10 ml of lidocaine in the subacromial space. Many patients respond to initial management with anti-inflammatory medications, rest, and physical therapy, but if this fails, surgical decompression of the subacromial space is indicated.

Removal of the anterior–inferior acromion and attached coracoacromial ligament gives the critical zone of the biceps and supraspinatus tendons more room without experiencing compression.[44] This has been performed by open techniques for many years with gratifying results. However, the approach requires taking down some of the attachment of the anterior deltoid, and that requires a recovery of 3 to 4 months.

Recently, arthroscopic acromioplasty has been advocated as an alternative to open surgery, and the early results appear promising. The arthroscope is placed in the subacromial bursa from the posterior portal, and the motorized synovial resector in the lateral subacromial portal. Initially, the resector must remove the fibrous strands present in the bursa, and after adequate visualization is obtained, a motorized burr replaces the resector in the lateral portal. Starting at the anterior tip of the acromion, bone is removed from the acromial undersurface to achieve an adequate decompression. This requires a smoothly tapering resection, taking less bone as the decompression proceeds posteriorly. The coracoacromial ligament can be cut under direct vision, with either basket forceps or motorized instrumentation. A large branch of the thoracoacromial artery may be encountered, so this step is usually reserved for last.

Hemostasis can be achieved by electrocautery (see section on *lateral release*) or by the use of dilute solutions of epinephrine. A 1 : 100,000 epinephrine solution can be injected into the subacromial space prior to the procedure, or some of the inflow fluid can contain a 1 : 300,000 concentration of epinephrine. Either approach can minimize bleeding, but care must be taken to keep the total epinephrine dosage within safe ranges.

Treatment of a rotator cuff tear must be individualized according to the patient's functional demands, but frequently the level of symptoms (pain, weakness) warrant surgical intervention. Although there are some investigations into arthroscopic repair of cuff tears, the traditional open repair of a complete cuff tear is still the treatment of choice.

There are some things that arthroscopy does offer in the treatment of rotator cuff tears. Visualization of both the bursal and articular surface of the cuff will reveal partial tears that can be missed on arthrograms. Arthroscopic debridement of these partial tears in conjunction with an acromioplasty may prevent these lesions from progressing to full-thickness lesions.

Some older patients have symptomatic full-thickness tears but may not be good candidates for repair. In these instances arthroscopic acromioplasty and debridement of the edges of the tear may provide pain relief.

ARTHROSCOPY IN OTHER JOINTS

Although shoulder and knee cases comprise the vast majority of arthroscopic procedures, many other joints are suitable for this approach. The development of improved techniques and equipment has greatly extended the possible applications to smaller joints and those that are not as superficial as the knee.

ANKLE

The ankle is perhaps the third most commonly arthroscoped joint, and a number of operative procedures on the ankle can now be carried out, in addition to simple diagnostic arthroscopy.

Ankle arthroscopy is done with the patient supine, and usually under tourniquet control. A number of different positions can be used. One of the best is with the foot of the table flexed approximately 45 degrees and the knee flexed about 15 degrees to 20 degrees. The calf is placed in the arthroscopic leg-holder. This allows the surgical assistant to apply longitudinal traction and inversion and eversion forces; it also makes posterior portals feasible.

There are five portals described in ankle arthroscopy: anterolateral, anterocentral, anteromedial, posterolateral, and posteromedial.[26] The posteromedial portal is mentioned only to be condemned; the neurovascular bundle is at too great a risk to justify its use. Although occasionally helpful, the anterocentral portal is also risky, being very close to the dorsalis pedis artery, and should be avoided. Most, if not all, ankle cases can be done using the other three portals.

The joint is first insufflated with fluid by use of an 18-gauge spinal needle in the anterolateral portal. This is located at the joint line, lateral to the peroneus tertius tendon. The 4-mm cannula is inserted next, with the sharp trocar penetrating the capsule and the blunt obturator entering the joint. An inflow–outflow cannula can be inserted through the anteromedial portal. This portal is at the level of the joint line, medial to the tibialis anterior tendon and lateral to the saphenous nerve and vein (usually palpable percutaneously).

Visualization of the anterior compartment is increased by alternate dorsi- and plantar flexion and by the use of traction. About two thirds of the talar dome can be seen, extending anteriorly to the chrondrosynovial junction on the talar neck. From the anterolateral portal the interval between the talus and medial malleous can be inspected, particularly with use of the 70-degree scope. The talofibular joint is best inspected from the anteromedial portal. From either portal the distal tibia can be seen (about 5 mm is intra-articular), a common location of osteophytes.

With longitudinal traction the scope can be advanced over the talar dome, through the tibiotalar space, and into the posterior compartment. Depending on the patient and portal placement, passage from either the anterolateral or anteromedial portal may be easiest. Usually the majority of the posterior compartment can be visualized, by a combination of scope rotation and alternating between the 30-degree and 70-degree inclined lenses. While viewing posteriorly, an 18-gauge spinal needle can be used to establish the posterolateral portal. It pierces the skin just lateral to the Achilles tendon and is advanced obliquely in an anteromedial direction.

With a systematic approach to ankle arthroscopy, more of the interior can be seen than with multiple arthrotomies, and some procedures are greatly facilitated. Loose body removal is feasible, and synovectomy is more easily and thoroughly accomplished than with an open technique.

Treatment of osteochondritis dissecans is substantially improved over open techniques. Lateral lesions usually occur anteriorly and are accessible arthroscopically. These lesions actually require only a small arthrotomy if addressed by an open technique, so the real benefit of arthroscopy is evident with medial lesions. These are generally posterior and require medial malleolar osteotomies to treat by open methods. The morbidity of an arthroscopic approach is substantially less.

Intact osteochondritis dissecans lesions can be treated with multiple drill holes, placed percutaneously under arthroscopic visualization. This is followed by immobilization and partial weight-bearing for 6 to 12 weeks. Many lesions treated in this fashion will go on to heal. Detached and loose fragments are best removed, with debridement of the donor site.

ELBOW

There are relatively few reported series on elbow arthroscopy, and most of these are limited in number of patients.[3] Once again, this reflects the risk–benefit ratio of this procedure, because the potential complications from elbow arthroscopy are great. Of the four major corners of the joint (anterolateral, anteromedial, posterolateral, posteromedial), only one allows a "safe" portal, the other three being perilously close to major neurovascular elements.[39] The posteromedial portal is *never* used, owing to the position of the ulnar nerve. The anteromedial portal lies 2 cm distal and 2 cm anterior to the medial epicondyle, and the cannula passes within 4 mm of the median nerve and 9 mm of the brachial artery. The anterolateral portal is made 3 cm distal and 1 cm anterior to the lateral epicondyle. On its path to the joint a cannula placed in this location comes within 4 mm of the radial nerve. The posterolateral is the safest and is placed 3 cm proximal to the olecranon tip, just lateral to the triceps tendon. Portal safety can be increased by entering the posterior portal in extension and the anterior portals in flexion and by distending the joint prior to cannula insertion. Joint distention elevates the neurovascular elements away from the borders of the joint.

The patient is usually positioned supine, with the shoulder abducted, the elbow flexed to 90 degrees, and skin traction applied to the forearm from above. A tourniquet and limb holder are placed about the midarm.

The primary indication for arthroscopy in the elbow is in the removal of loose bodies. Additionally, chondral debridement can be accomplished and subtotal synovectomies performed. Osteochondritis dissecans lesions can be visualized, helping in the decision on either arthroscopic removal of the fragment or reduction and fixation by an open procedure.

OTHER JOINTS

Virtually any joint can be arthroscoped, with the indications for this technique based on an examination of the relative advantages and disadvantages compared with open surgery. Simply possessing the ability to perform a procedure does not justify its use. Investigators have compiled small clinical series on arthroscopy of the temporomandibular,[35] hip,[17,25] wrist,[60] and finger[35] joints. Further work in these areas and development of joint-specific equipment may document advantages of this technique, but until then, arthroscopy in these joints must be considered investigational.

CONCLUSIONS

The arthroscope has revolutionized the treatment of joint problems. The technique is demanding and requires the investment of significant time and effort to master the requisite skills, but the dividends in terms of improved patient care are marked. Caution must be exercised against indiscriminate and overly liberal use of the technique. The fact that arthroscopy is a relatively low-risk operation is only half of the equation; one has to consider whether the potential benefit of the procedure justifies abandoning nonoperative treatment or justifies choosing arthroscopy over an open procedure of higher risk but correspondingly higher benefit. However, with the proper indications, arthroscopy is a safe, effective method of treating a wide variety of intra-articular processes.

REFERENCES

1. Altman RD, Gray R: Diagnostic and therapeutic uses of the arthroscope in rheumatoid arthritis and osteoarthritis. Am J Med 75:50–55, 1983
2. Andrews JR, Carson WG: Arthroscopic anatomy of the shoulder. In Jackson DW (ed): Shoulder Surgery in the Athlete, pp 25–30. Rockville, MD, Aspen Systems, 1985
3. Andrews JR, Carson WG: Arthroscopy of the elbow. In McGinty JB (ed): Arthroscopic Surgery Update, pp 183–190. Rockville, MD, Aspen Systems, 1985
4. Andrews JR, Carson WG: The arthroscopic treatment of glenoid labrum tears in the throwing athlete. Orthop Trans 8:44, 1984
5. Arnoczky SP, Warren RF: Microvasculature of the human meniscus. Am J Sports Med 10:90–95, 1982
6. Arnoczky SP, Warren RF: The microvasculature of the meniscus and its response to injury. Am J Sports Med 11:131–141, 1983
7. Bergstrom R, Gillquist J: The use of an infusion pump in arthroscopy. Arthroscopy 2:41–45, 1986
8. Caspari RB: Shoulder instability. Presented at Arthroscopic Surgery—1985. Salt Lake City, Utah, March 2, 1985
9. Caspari RB: Instrumentation and operating room organization for arthroscopy of the shoulder. In McGinty JB (ed): Arthroscopic Surgery Update, pp 155–160. Rockville, MD, Aspen Systems, 1985
10. Casscells SW: Gross pathologic changes in the knee joint of the aged individual. Clin Orthop 132:225–232, 1978
11. DeHaven KE: Principles of triangulation for arthroscopic surgery. Orthop Clin North Am 13:329–336, 1982
12. DeHaven KE: Meniscus repair—Open versus arthroscopic. Arthroscopy 1:173–174, 1985
13. DeHaven KE: Peripheral meniscus repair—An alternative to meniscectomy. J Bone Joint Surg 63B:463, 1981
14. Detrisac DA, Johnson LL: Arthroscopic Shoulder Anatomy. Thorofare, NJ, Slack, 1986
15. Dorfmann H: Arthroscopic recognition of synovial disorders. Contemp Orthop 10:19–29, 1985
16. Eriksson E, Haggmark T, Saartok T et al: Knee arthroscopy with local anesthesia in ambulatory patients. Orthopedics 9:186–188, 1986
17. Eriksson E, Arvidsson I, Arvidsson H: Diagnostic and operative arthroscopy of the hip. Orthopedics 9:169–176, 1986
18. Eriksson E, Sebik A: Arthroscopic surgery in a gas versus a fluid medium. Orthop Clin North Am 13:293–298, 1982
19. Ewing JW: Arthroscopic surgery: The pathogenesis, evaluation, and treatment of horizontal cleavage tears of the meniscus. Contemp Orthop 9:23–27, 1984
20. Ewing JW: Arthroscopic treatment of chondramalacia patellae. In McGinty JB (ed): Arthroscopic Surgery Update, pp 21–30. Rockville, MD, Aspen Systems, 1985
21. Ficat RP, Hungerford DS: Disorders of the Patellofemoral Joint. Baltimore, Williams & Wilkins, 1977
22. Fox JM, Ferkel RD, Del Pizzo W et al: Electrosurgery in orthopedics: Part I—Principles. Contemp Orthop 8:21–32, 1984
23. Fox JM, Ferkel RD, Del Pizzo W et al: Electrosurgery in orthopedics: Part II—Applications to arthroscopy. Contemp Orthop 8:37–44, 1984
24. Gillquist J: Arthroscopy of the posterior compartments of the knee. Contemp Orthop 10:39–45, 1985
25. Glick JM, Sampson TG, Gordon RB et al: Hip arthroscopy by the lateral approach. Arthroscopy 3:4–12, 1987
26. Gollehon DL, Drez D: Arthroscopy of the ankle. In McGinty JB (ed): Arthroscopic Surgery Update, pp 161–173. Rockville, MD, Aspen Systems, 1985
27. Gross RM, Fitzgibbons TC: Shoulder arthroscopy: A modified approach. Arthroscopy 1:156–159, 1985
28. Guhl JF; Arthroscopic management of osteochondritis dissecans. In McGinty JB (ed): Arthroscopic Surgery Update, pp 63–84. Rockville, MD, Aspen Systems, 1985
29. Henning CE, Lynch MA, Clark JR: Vascularity for healing of meniscus repair. Arthroscopy 3:13–18, 1987
30. Henning CE, Lynch MA, Jolly BL et al: Arthroscopic meniscus repair. In McGinty JB (ed): Arthroscopic Surgery Update, pp 97–108. Rockville, MD, Aspen Systems, 1985
31. Jackson RW: Memories of the early days of arthroscopy: 1965–1975. The formative years. Arthroscopy 3:1–3, 1987
32. Jackson RW: The septic knee—Arthroscopic treatment. Arthroscopy 1:194–197, 1985
33. Jackson RW, Marshall DJ, Fujisawa Y: The pathologic medical shelf. Orthop Clin North Am 13:307–312, 1982
34. Johnson LL: Arthroscopic abrasion arthroplasty historical and pathologic perspective: Present status. Arthroscopy 2:54–69, 1986
35. Johnson LL: Arthroscopic Surgery: Principles and Practice. St. Louis, CV Mosby, 1986
36. Joyce JJ, Harty M, Tetzlaff JE: Surgery of the synovial folds. In Casscells SW (ed): Arthroscopy: Diagnostic and Surgical Practice, pp 94–99. Philadelphia, Lea & Febiger, 1984

37. Kim HC, Klein K, Hirsch S et al: Arthroscopic Synovectomy in the Treatment of Hemophilic Synovitis. Scand J Haematol 33 (Suppl 40):271–279, 1984
38. Klein AH, France JC, Mutschler TA et al: Measurement of brachial plexus strain in arthroscopy of the shoulder. Arthroscopy 3:45–52, 1987
39. Lynch GJ, Meyers JF, Whipple TL et al: Neurovascular anatomy and elbow arthroscopy: Inherent risks. Arthroscopy 2:19–197, 1986
40. Marmor L: Synovectomy of the knee joint. Orthop Clin North Am 10:211–222, 1979
41. McGinty JB: Arthroscopic removal of loose bodies. Orthop Clin North Am 13:313–328, 1982
42. Metcalf RW: Meniscectomy by triangulation through medial and lateral portals. In Casscells SW (ed): Arthroscopy: Diagnostic and Surgical Practice, pp 131–146. Philadelphia, Lea & Febiger, 1984
43. Morgan CD, Casscells SW: Arthroscopic meniscus repair, a safe approach to the posterior horns. Arthroscopy 2:3–12, 1986
44. Neer CS: Anterior acromioplasty for the chronic impingement syndrome in the shoulder. J Bone Joint Surg 54A:41–50, 1972
45. O'Connor RL: The arthroscope in the management of crystal-induced synovitis of the knee. J Bone Joint Surg 55A:1443–1449, 1973
46. Oretorp N: Anterior midline or central approach for arthroscopic meniscectomy. In Casscells SW (ed): Arthroscopy: Diagnostic and Surgical Practice, pp 147–152. Philadelphia, Lea & Febiger, 1984
47. Patel D: Proximal approach to arthroscopic meniscectomy. In Casscells SW (ed): Arthroscopy: Diagnostic and Surgical Practice, pp 153–159. Philadelphia, Lea & Febiger, 1984
48. Rathbun JB, McNab I: The microvascular pattern of the rotator cuff. J Bone Joint Surg 52B:540–553, 1970
49. Richards RN, Lonergan RP: Arthroscopic surgery for relief of pain in the osteoarthritic knee. Orthopedics 7:1705–1707, 1984
50. Rosenberg TD, Scott SM, Coward DB et al: Arthroscopic meniscal repair evaluated with repeat arthroscopy. Arthroscopy 2:14–20, 1986
51. Rosenberg TD, Wong HC: Arthroscopic knee surgery in a free-standing outpatient surgery center. Orthop Clin North Am 13:277–282, 1982
52. Rowe CR: An atlas of anatomy and treatment of midclavicular fractures. Clin Orthop 58:29–42, 1968
53. Schonholtz GJ, Magee CM; The synovial plicae of the knee joint. Contemp Ortop 12:31–37, 1986
54. Shahriaree H (ed): O'Connor's Textbook of Arthroscopic Surgery. Philadelphia, JB Lippincott, 1984
55. Smith MJ: Arthroscopic treatment of the septic knee. Arthroscopy 2:30–34, 1986
56. Sprague NF: Arthroscopic surgery: Degenerative and traumatic flap tears of the meniscus. Contemp Orthop 9:23–46, 1984
57. Thayer AL, Jackson DW: Videoarthroscopy: What an orthopedist should know about video equipment. Contemp Orthop 6:51–58, 1983
58. Watanabe M: Memories of the early days of arthroscopy. Arthroscopy 2:209–214, 1986
59. Whipple TL: Arthroscopic surgery: The meniscus rim after operative arthroscopy. Contemp Orthop 9:25–32, 1984
60. Whipple TL, Marotta JJ, Powell JH: Techniques of wrist arthroscopy. Arthroscopy 2:244–252, 1986
61. Whipple TL: The role of exogenous materials in arthroscopic management of cruciate-deficit knees. In McGinty JB (ed): Arthroscopic Surgery Update, pp 139–154. Rockville, MD, Aspen Systems, 1985
62. Wiedel JD: Arthroscopic Synovectomy in Hemophilic Arthropathy of the Knee. Scand J Haematol 33 (Suppl 40):263–270, 1984
63. Zarins B: Arthroscopic surgery—Basic techniques and instruments. Contemp Orthop 6:25–31, 1983
64. Zarins B, McInerney VK: Lesions of the meniscus. In Casscells SW (ed): Arthroscopy: Diagnostic and Surgical Practice, pp 37–51. Philadelphia, Lea & Febiger, 1984
65. Zarins B, Matthews LS: Evaluation and treatment of glenoid labrum tears. In Jackson DW (ed): Shoulder Surgery in the Athlete, pp 31–44. Rockville, MD, Aspen Systems, 1985

35 Foot and Ankle

ANDREW C. RUOFF III

SOFT TISSUES

INFECTIONS

Infections of the foot correspond roughly to those of the hand, except that tenosynovitis is not a frequent lesion in the lower limb.

CELLULITIS AND LYMPHANGITIS

Etiology and Symptoms

A common infection in the foot is cellulitis with associated lymphangitis, which arises from an infection of the toes or from dermatophytosis between them. This is either primarily or secondarily streptococcal in origin, and the usual history is of some small, often insignificant, abrasion or crack in the skin followed by development of edema and cellulitis of the dorsum of the foot and of the typical red streaks due to lymphangitis up the leg. The subinguinal nodes overlying the saphenous opening are the ones involved most frequently, and these become enlarged and painful, often without apparent intervening lymphangitis. The same type of infection may arise from an infected blister over the heel or over the metatarsophalangeal joint of the great toe.

Treatment

The treatment of streptococcal infection of the foot consists of elevation, hot wet dressings over the foot, the leg, and the involved lymph nodes, and administration of antibiotics, usually penicillin. This therapy necessitates rest in bed, but usually it can be carried out safely at home and results in a rapid subsidence of the infection in 2 or 3 days. However, the possibility of later development of suppurative adenitis in the lymph nodes involved should be remembered, and the patient should be seen frequently, since this may demand incision.

INFECTED CALLUS

A second type of infection that is seen occasionally in the foot is a local one about a callus on the plantar surface. This lesion is similar to the collar-button abscess seen in the hand, and it is treated in the same manner.

Treatment

The overlying thickened skin is incised, and the subcutaneous abscess is drained by spreading the small opening through the true skin with a hemostat. Treatment with a small drain and hot wet dressings usually results in rapid subsidence of the infection. Antibiotics are useful adjuncts. During the course of this treatment the patient should be off his feet with the part elevated.

CHRONIC ULCERS OF THE PLANTAR SURFACE OF THE FOOT

Diagnosis

Chronic ulcers in the center of callosities on the plantar surface of the foot occur especially in older individuals, and most often in diabetics. They may develop in any foot in which there is a neurologic deficit, whether this is due to diabetic neuropathy or to other causes. These ulcers are characterized by a heaping up of thickened epithelium, in the center of which is a punched-out ulceration (Fig. 35-1). When they occur over the ball of the foot they extend sometimes to the heads of the metatarsal bones. In addition, there are often roentgen changes in the bone, and these are frequently misdiagnosed as osteomyelitis. In reality they are the changes of osteoporosis, although a secondary infection may lead to true inflammation of the bony tissue.

Treatment

These ulcers are very resistant to all forms of treatment, and they often become infected

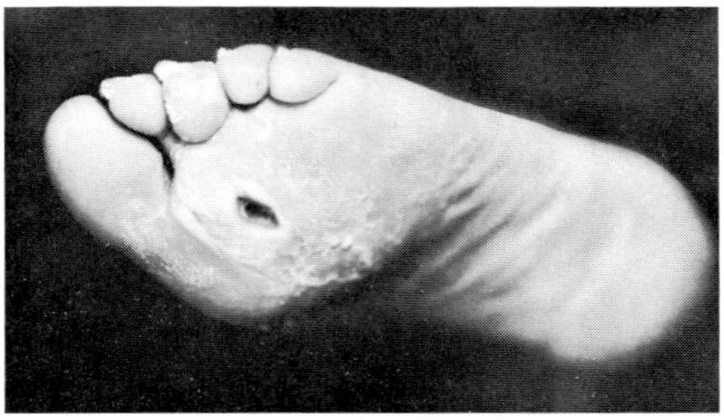

Figure 35-1. Chronic ulcer and callus of the plantar surface of the foot in a diabetic. Note the punched-out appearance of the ulcer, which extends deeply, even into the bone of the foot. This patient was treated with gelatin boots, and for more than a year and a half was able to get about on the foot. Eventually infection necessitated amputation.

secondarily. In diabetic patients they may have serious consequences leading to amputation.

The ulcer is probably the result of a reduced blood supply in the area, with a consequent decrease in healing power, even though pulsations may be palpable in the arteries in many cases.

Treatment by rest in bed is advised by some. The ulcer may heal but tends to recur with weight bearing. We have suggested the use of felt or sponge-rubber arch supports, with a high pad under the scaphoid bone to shift the excessive pressure from the prominent metatarsal head to the soft tissues of the instep. Operation has been found useful by Classen: excision of the metatarsal head and the base of the phalanx through a dorsal incision, packing, and drainage through the plantar ulcer. "A distressing aspect of the problem is the rapidity with which calluses develop under other metatarsal heads. Some go on to frank ulcerations." After-care and the need for foot supports to redistribute weight bearing are emphasized. Custom-fitted orthoses utilizing the new CAD-CAM (computer-assisted design, computer-assisted manufacture) may be a real advance in the near future.

TRAUMATIC LESIONS

INCISED WOUNDS

Incised wounds of the feet occur most commonly from stepping with the bare foot on some sharp object, such as glass or a razor blade.

Treatment

The care of such injuries does not differ from that for incised wounds elsewhere in the body. As a rule the preparation of the surrounding area, followed by cleaning of the wound itself, permits primary suture. A pressure bandage is applied, and the patient usually is provided with crutches for a time to limit weight bearing.

PUNCTURE WOUNDS

Etiology

Puncture wounds are probably more common in the foot than elsewhere in the body. Pointed objects may enter the foot through the shoe, as when one steps on a nail in a board, or needles or other sharp-pointed objects left lying on the floor may enter the foot directly when one walks barefoot about a room. Often the patient does not seek treatment for several hours or even days.

Treatment

Follow the recommendations of the American College of Surgeons Committee on Trauma (see Chapter 6). The treatment of the wound itself depends somewhat on its condition. At the time of the primary dressing it is usually unwise to probe the wound, and in a large majority of cases in which a simple protective dressing is applied, healing occurs without infection. If there is reason to believe that considerable contamination has been introduced with the puncturing object, it is wise to incise the wound under local anesthesia and to perform radical wound cleansing. Prophylactic use of antibiotics is the rule in such cases.

Many puncture wounds are complicated by the presence of foreign bodies (see Chapter 5). Needles and splinters are the most common offenders.

CONTUSIONS

Contusions of the foot and the toes are common industrial accidents, the foot being caught under heavy machines, rolling barrels, or trucks. Often there is fracture of the distal phalanx of the great toe and of other bones of the toes. Therefore such injuries should always be examined by roentgenography. The swelling is usually quite marked on the dorsum of the toes and on the dorsum of the foot. Frequently there is a subungual hematoma, or the base of the nail may be torn free and lie on top of the eponychium.

Treatment

Following roentgenography the lesion is cleaned if there are open wounds, and any part of the nail base that lies on the eponychium is excised. The wounds are then protected with petrolatum gauze, and the whole foot and ankle are enclosed in a compression dressing.

The advantage of this dressing is that it supplies comparative immobilization, as well as pressure, and with this therapy the swelling and the pain subside rapidly, and the patient, even in the case of severe contusion and fracture, may be able to walk without too much discomfort in 2 or 3 days to a week. The dressing is allowed to remain in place as long as it is in good condition. During this time the patient can be ambulant without much disability with a shoe cut out at the toe, or a commercially available walking boot may be applied.

CORNS

Description

Corns are a variety of callosity in which there is a central piling up of epithelial cells forming what is frequently called a corn. They are the result of pressure and friction, and they are seen most commonly over the lateral and the dorsal surfaces of the fifth toe, though they may occur also over any bony prominence. Corns are described as being either hard or soft. This differentiation is due only to the amount of moisture in the area. Those occurring between the toes become macerated and are called soft corns, whereas those on the dorsum of the foot and the toes have a hard, horny epithelial covering. Soft corns are often associated with dermatophytosis.

Treatment

In the treatment of corns the most important factor is the removal of the cause. Frequently, the correction of ill-fitting shoes or improper weight bearing of the feet permits the corn to disappear. However, if corns are to be removed a scalpel or electrocoagulation may be used. A conservative method, shaving away the hardened epithelium followed by application of trichloroacetic acid, is sometimes effective. Any local therapy without removal of the cause of the pressure is almost sure to be followed by reappearance of the corn.

SPRAINS AND RUPTURES OF LIGAMENTS ABOUT THE ANKLE JOINT

Etiology and Symptoms

Sprains at the ankle occur most commonly laterally (Fig. 35-2). Sudden inversion of the foot causes an injury to the lateral ligament, manifested by limping and pain and by swelling, ecchymosis, and tenderness at the side of the ankle. Ecchymosis may not appear for a day or two after injury. A similar condition may occur at the medial side of the ankle. Sprains can usually be differentiated from fractures by the location of the most acute ten-

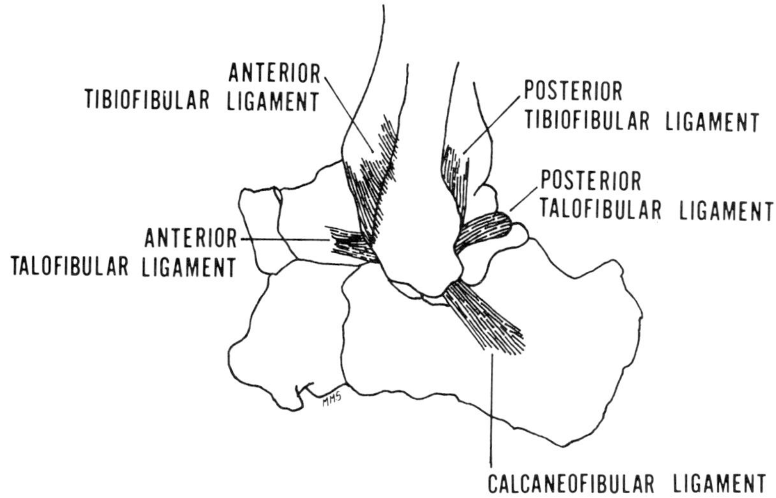

Figure 35-2. Ligaments of the ankle.

derness. In sprains this is the area in front of and below the lateral malleolus. In fractures it is definitely over the bone.

Very often the anterior tibiofibular ligament is found to be tender, and there may be tenderness over the dorsum of the foot in front of the ankle. Tenderness at these sites indicates sprains of the tibiofibular ligament and the ligaments of the dorsum of the foot. Occasionally, the lateral ligament tears away from the malleolus and takes with it a small portion of the tip of the bone. This condition is called a sprain fracture.

When the signs of sprain at the lateral or the medial side of the joint are severe, very extensive laceration of the involved ligament may be present. Similarly, great tenderness at the tibiofibular ligament indicates possible rupture. These lacerations are suspected more strongly when the foot can be inverted or everted forcibly beyond its normal limit and when the astragalus is felt to rotate excessively between the malleoli, indicating that the injury is a reduced dislocation. Normally, the astragalus does not move mediolaterally.

The test is performed best after the tender areas have been infiltrated with 10 ml of 1% lidocaine solution. When excessive mediolateral mobility is found or is suspected, it should be verified by making an anteroposterior roentgenogram of the ankle with the foot inverted or everted forcibly, as the case may require, so as to put the ligament affected on tension. Comparison should always be made with similar views of the normal ankle.

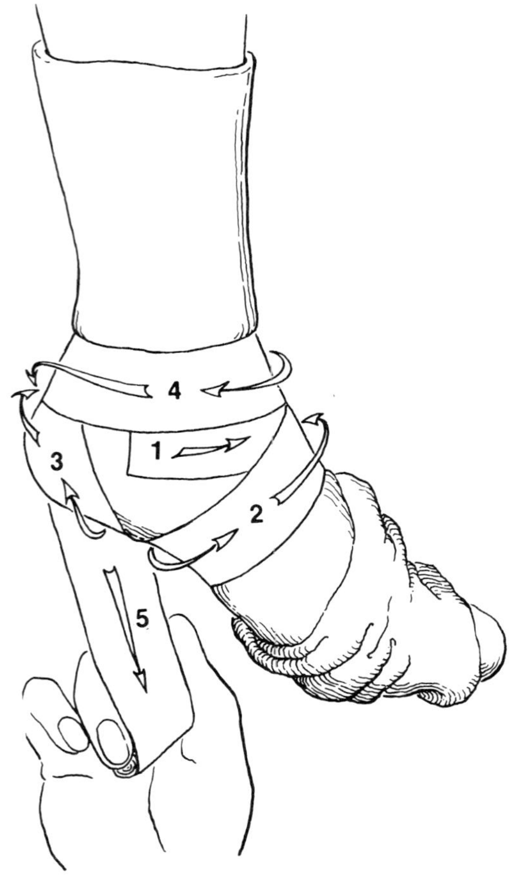

Figure 35-3. Technique of the ankle wrap.

Prevention of Ankle Injuries in Sports

Many players believe that "ankle wraps" afford some protection against injury. A nonelastic bandage is applied by the player or the trainer over the inner of two pairs of socks, with a turn around the heel (Fig. 35-3). Its purpose is to limit mediolateral mobility without restricting flexion-extension. Quigley pointed out that the incidence of ankle injuries can be reduced by 50% by the use of such a bandage.

Treatment

Sprains and sprain fractures without abnormal mobility of the astragalus require support of the ankle joint and measures to control swelling. A strapping provides a firm supportive dressing (Figs. 35-4 and 35-5). This is renewed when it becomes loose. Elevation and application of ice bags for 24 to 48 hours will control swelling. The patient continues his usual activities so far as possible. Recovery takes place in 3 to 14 days as a rule. Another method of treatment is to have the patient begin vigorous active use after the strapping has been applied. Often there is striking subsidence of symptoms after a few hours. Local anesthetic injections may be used in treating these injuries but are generally discouraged because of the possibility of introducing infection and allowing patients too much activity; if necessary, 6 ml to 10 ml of 1% local anesthetic solution is injected at the site of the most acute tenderness. The joint is then moved to find any other painful areas and is palpated for additional tender spots. Any such areas should be injected also with 5 ml to 10 ml of the local anesthetic solution. Immediate relief of pain and the ability to walk freely result. The pain may return after some hours. It may or may not be severe. Additional injections may be

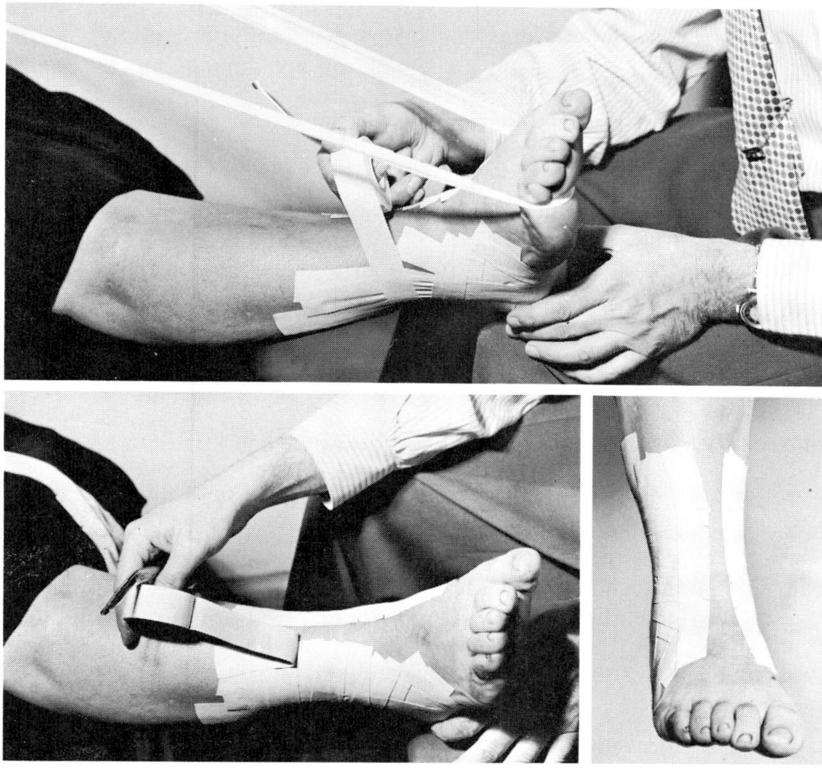

A B C

Figure 35-4. Ankle strapping (Gibney boot). (*A*) The heel is supported on the surgeon's knee, and the foot is held in a bandage loop at right angles to the leg by the patient. Alternate longitudinal and transverse strips of 1-in.-wide adhesive are applied from a roll. Each strip should lie flat on the part. Except for the dorsum of the foot, the entire area is covered by varying the direction of the adhesive strips. (*B*) Rolling of the adhesive edges is prevented by longitudinal binding strips; these are nicked with scissors to permit them to conform to the part. (*C*) Completed strapping.

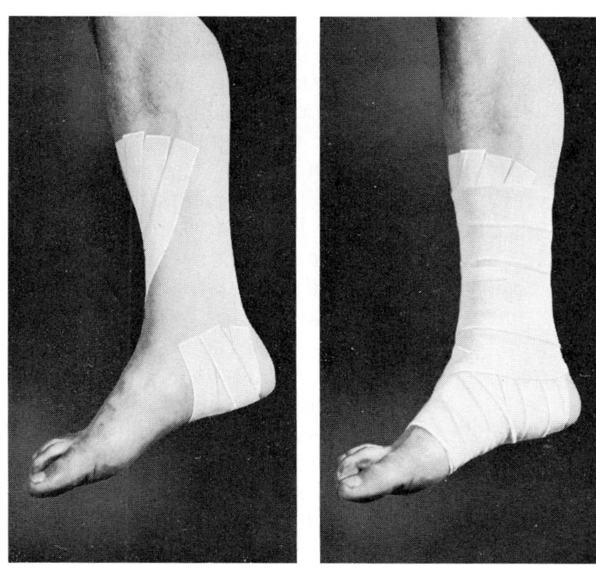

Figure 35-5. Simple strapping and elastic adhesive bandage dressing for sprains of the lateral ligament or sprain fractures of the tip of the lateral malleolus. Both injuries are caused by inversion, which the strapping prevents.

given at intervals of 24 hours or more. Recovery is expedited by strapping the ankle as described.

There is some question whether injection of procaine should be used in the treatment of ankle sprains in sports. Quigley, after a large experience with such injuries at the Harvard Athletic Association, felt that anesthetization with procaine produces a loss of a sense of timing and coordination that predisposes to other injuries if the player goes back into the game immediately.

Some advise plaster-cast immobilization for ankle sprains. However, Nevin, in a large experience with paratroopers, had much better results with immediate ambulation than with casting.

Caro and associates made a study of 172 patients with inversion injuries of the ankle; 14 of these were severe tears of the lateral ligament diagnosed roentgenologically after injection of the area with local anesthetic and 1500 IU hyaluronidase. There were 28 fractures. In these cases three types of treatment were used:

Hydrocortisone, 50 mg, injected into the site of maximum tenderness and spread into the injured ligament. An elastic bandage was applied and weight bearing and gentle exercise advised.

Strapping and elastic adhesive bandage to produce strong eversion of the ankle. Weight bearing and gentle exercise were encouraged.

Plaster of paris cast with walking rocker. Full weight bearing was permitted after 48 hours. The cast was worn for 2 weeks.

They found that the treatment by hydrocortisone injection gave the best results.

When signs of sprain are associated with abnormal mobility of the astragalus, rupture of the lateral ligament, the deltoid (medial) ligament, or the tibiofibular ligaments must be suspected and verified by means of roentgenograms. Prolonged immobilization is necessary to secure firm healing of the rupture. When the swelling subsides an unpadded case is applied from the toes to the knee, the malleoli being compressed firmly together with the flats of the hands and the plaster being molded well. A total of 6 weeks of immobilization is required. The patient begins to bear weight immediately after the cast is hard and the walking heel has been applied. The after-care is similar to that for ankle fractures without displacement. If prolonged immobilization and the prescribed walking are carried out the prognosis is usually good.

OVERUSE SYNDROMES

The development of sophisticated diagnostic tests and specialized clinical techniques to determine subtle injuries have made possible early identification and treatment of these often-missed problems. Bone scans, CT scans, and laminography may often identify problems that would otherwise be missed for some time.

The overuse syndrome may be manifested by the presence of a stress fracture, periostitis, myostitis, tendinitis, or even a compartment syndrome.

Improved techniques for the training of athletes, including the development of flexibility programs and equipment modifications, have helped in the prevention of many of these problems.

Treatment of overuse syndrome problems has changed drastically, and the approach for many of them includes short-time immobilization, prompt surgery if indicated, and very rapid rehabilitation. One successful technique for lower back and stress fracture problems is hydrotherapy, running in a swimming pool supported by a water ski jacket to assist flotation.

Stress fractures of the fifth metatarsal may heal slowly or go on to nonunion, whereas stress fractures of the middle metatarsals generally heal rapidly.

SPRAINS OF THE METATARSOPHALANGEAL JOINT

Treatment

Stubbing the toes, especially when walking barefoot or in soft slippers, often results in a sprain of a metatarsophalangeal joint, especially that of the great toe. This causes swelling and pain on motion. The pain may often be relieved by injection of a local anesthetic, usually procaine, 1% or 2%. Strapping applied along the dorsum of the foot and the toe provides relative immobilization, gives comfort, and results in rapid subsidence of the painful symptoms. It is essential that the patient bear his weight on the foot while the strapping is being applied; otherwise the toe often is strapped in the hyperextended position, which

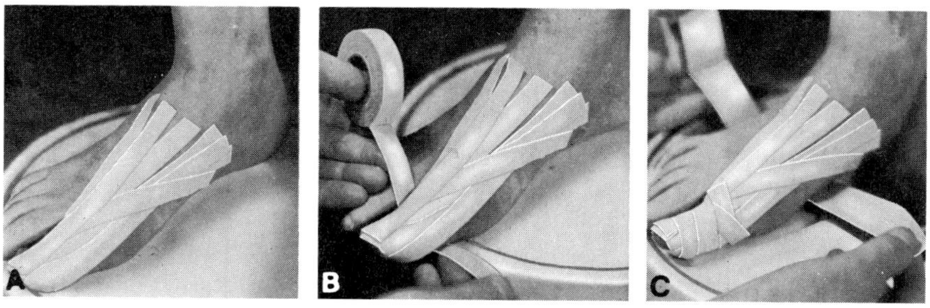

Figure 35-6. Adhesive strapping for sprains of the metatarsophalangeal joint and of the joints of the toes. This strapping also is used frequently for fractures of the phalanges of the toes. It is a most effective dressing and much better than any form of splint. It should be applied with the patient standing on a stool and bearing his weight on the affected foot. (*A*) Cross-strappings, extending from the dorsum of the foot to the end of the toe, are applied. (*B*) The longitudinal strips are anchored with circular turns of adhesive, applied with the patient extending his toes beyond the stool on which he is standing. A loop of adhesive is placed under the toe. The patient again places the entire foot on the stool and bears his weight on the foot, and the circular turn is completed. If these circular turns are put on while the patient's weight is borne on the foot, the strapping will be comfortable; otherwise the tendency is for the toe to be held in extension, making the patient uncomfortable. (*C*) The circular turns of the upper portion of the strapping are placed round the foot while it is lifted off the stool. With the patient's weight on his foot, the turns are completed.

gives more discomfort than the original lesion (Fig. 35-6). Local infiltration of 1% lidocaine may be all that is necessary. This may be repeated on several occasions.

LESIONS OF THE TOENAIL

SUBUNGUAL WARTS

Warts under the toenails are troublesome lesions (Fig. 35-7). By pressing on the undersurface of the nail they frequently cause pain and disability. Patients usually attempt to relieve their discomfort by cutting away the nail around the wart, but as the nail grows out it tends to cut into the wart, causing pain and sometimes infection.

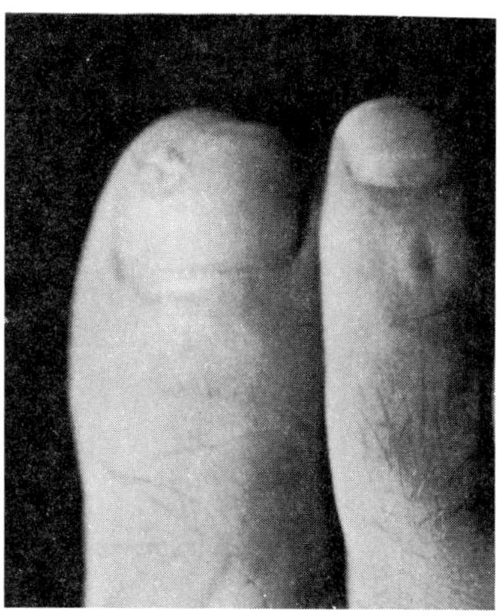

Figure 35-7. Subungual wart of the great toe. This wart was cured by electrocoagulation under local anesthesia.

Treatment

The warts may be removed either by cauterization with an electrocoagulating needle under local anesthesia or by injection into the base of the wart of a drop or two of a sclerosing solution, such as sodium morrhuate. The nail should be cut back from the area until the wart separates and comes away.

SUBUNGUAL EXOSTOSIS

In some patients a small bony spur projects off the dorsum of the distal phalanx, projecting up into the nail. Because of the pressures of the growth of the bone mass beneath the nail, this becomes a very painful affliction. This is often misdiagnosed as an ingrown toenail when in reality a simple lateral roentgenogram of the nail will show the bony projection beneath the nail.

Treatment

Conservative care with pads and spacers in the shoes is seldom of lasting benefit. Surgical

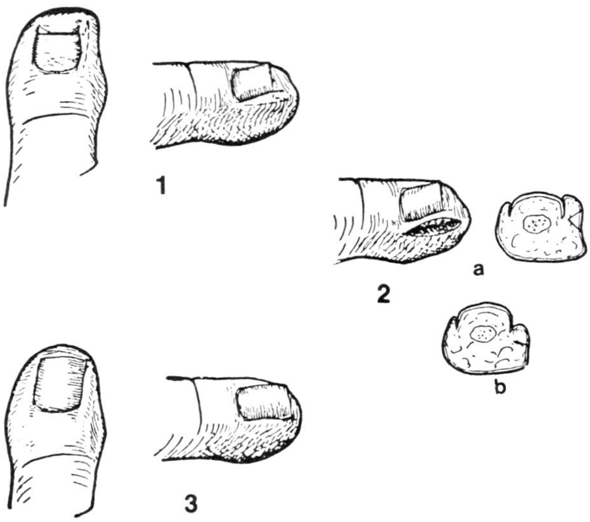

Figure 35-8. (*1*) Ingrown toenail, showing how cutting the nail too short permits a burned corner to remain and to grow upward as a point under the soft tissues. (*2*) Bartlett operation for ingrown toenail; this is especially valuable when there is no infection. A wedge of soft tissue is excised along the side of the toe (*a*), and the wound is sutured primarily (*b*). This pulls the soft tissues away from the edge of the nail. (*3*) Proper cutting of the nail; the entire nail edge is beyond the soft tissues.

removal of the bony mass is required, and this may be accomplished by simply making a transverse incision at the tip of the toe, gently elevating the tissues at a periosteal level away from the bony mass, which can then be filed off or removed with a rongeur. The wound is simply closed with interrupted sutures, and since the blood supply is usually extremely good, these wounds heal rapidly, requiring only soft-tissue dressings and protection.

INGROWN TOENAIL

Etiology

Ingrown toenail is a painful lesion caused by the pressure of tight shoes on the soft tissues at the edge of the nail of the great toe. The secondary, or exciting, cause of the difficulty is the frequent mistake of cutting the nail too short so that its corner may be overlain easily by the soft tissues at the edge of the nail. In teenaged boys, when wear and tear on the feet is high and foot care is poor, and when canvas shoes are frequently worn, ingrown toenails are especially common. As the nail grows out the uncut corner is pushed into the soft tissues (Fig. 35-8), and the pressure of the shoe on the tissues produces marked pain. Frequently, the sharp projecting tip of the nail produces an ulceration in the skin overlying the nail edge, and this causes a chronic infection (Fig. 35-9A). Granulations form over the nail edge, and there is constant discharge of a small amount of purulent secretion (Fig. 35-9B). In this type of lesion the discomfort is more or less con-

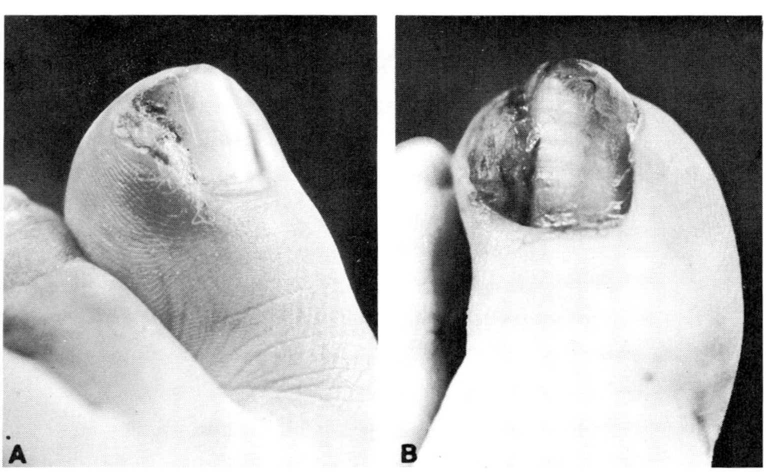

Figure 35-9. (*A*) Infection along the edge of the nail in a typical ingrown toenail. (*B*) Neglected ingrown toenail, with growth of hypertrophic infected granulation tissue along the edge of the nail.

stant, but it is made much worse by the pressure of shoes.

Treatment

The treatment of ingrown toenail may be conservative or operative.

In most minor cases of ingrown toenail the soft tissues may be pushed away from the projecting tip of the nail with the tip of a scalpel. When the offending corner of the nail has been demonstrated, a wisp of cotton may be introduced between the soft tissues and the nail to hold the soft tissues away from the nail. It should be packed under the projecting corner of the nail. We have used a small piece of cotton pulled from an alcohol sponge for this purpose. This elevation of the nail permits it to grow out beyond the soft tissues, and if the nail is permitted to grow so that its entire end appears, and if this is then cut at right angles to the axis of the toe, the symptoms are relieved and there is no recurrence. In some people the discomfort may be relieved without anesthesia by excising the side of the nail with the tip of a scalpel, thus removing the factor that causes the pain. It is important to remove the corner of the nail that projects into the soft tissues, which is often found as a sharp point. The overhanging granulations may be cauterized with a silver nitrate stick, and if precautions are taken to prevent pressure by wearing shoes that fit properly, the patient's symptoms may be relieved completely and often permanently.

In many cases some form of operative treatment may be wiser than conservative therapy. Two methods of operation have been employed, and we have found specific indications for each type. The operation described by Bartlett has been found to be of particular value in patients in whom the pain from the ingrown toenail is not associated with an in-

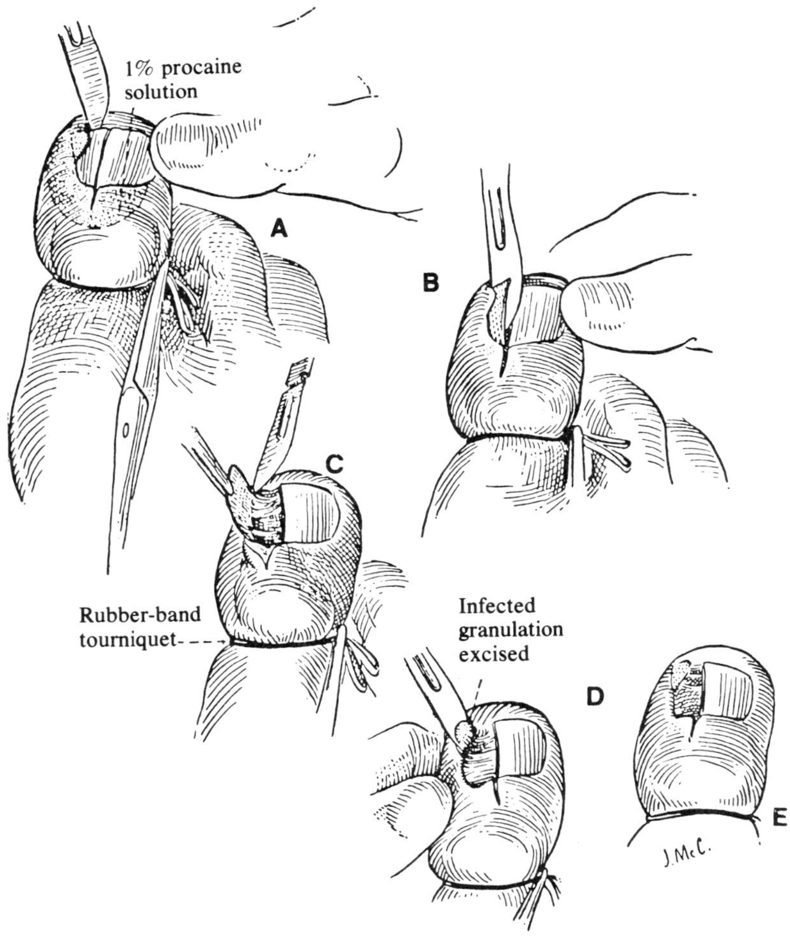

Figure 35-10. Operation for ingrown toenail. (*A*) The eponychium at the base and the sides of the nail is infiltrated with 1% procaine solution. The anesthesia should extend upward to the soft tissues at the tip of the toe. An incision is made through the nail and the eponychium with a knife or scissors. (*B*) The nail is reflected from the phalanx throughout its entire length, including the matrix. (*C*) The nail is dissected away, tension being kept upon it with forceps or a hemostat. (*D*) After the entire nail and its matrix have been removed the infected granulation tissue is excised. (*E*) Petrolatum gauze or a small piece of Gelfoam is applied.

fection along the edge of the nail (Fig. 35-8, 2 and 3). In this operation, using local anesthesia, an ellipse of skin and subcutaneous tissue is excised along the side of the toe. The wound is sutured primarily, and a simple pressure dressing is applied with adhesive. The sutures are permitted to remain in place for at least 7 days, and often the dressing is not changed until this time. The advantages of this operation are the rapid, usually primary, healing and the relatively short period of disability, not more than a day or two. Excellent permanent results are obtained by means of this treatment, which is designed to pull the soft tissues away from the edge of the nail.

For ingrown toenails in which there is a definite infection along the edge of the nail, with a heaping up of chronic granulation tissue, a much better operation is excision of the side of the toenail and of the overhanging soft tissues (Figs. 35-10 and 35-11). The operation is performed under a block anesthesia at the base of the nail and round the edges of the toe. A tourniquet at the base of the toe provides hemostasis. With a knife or scissors the toenail is divided down to and through the matrix. This includes also an incision through the eponychium, which is turned back with an Allis forceps. The scalpel is then inserted under the uplifted cut edge of the nail, and the offending portion of the nail is removed together with its matrix. The hypertrophic granulation tissue and the soft tissues that overhang the nail are excised, and a small piece of Gelfoam is laid over the resulting wound. A pressure dressing is applied. The gauze is changed in about 3

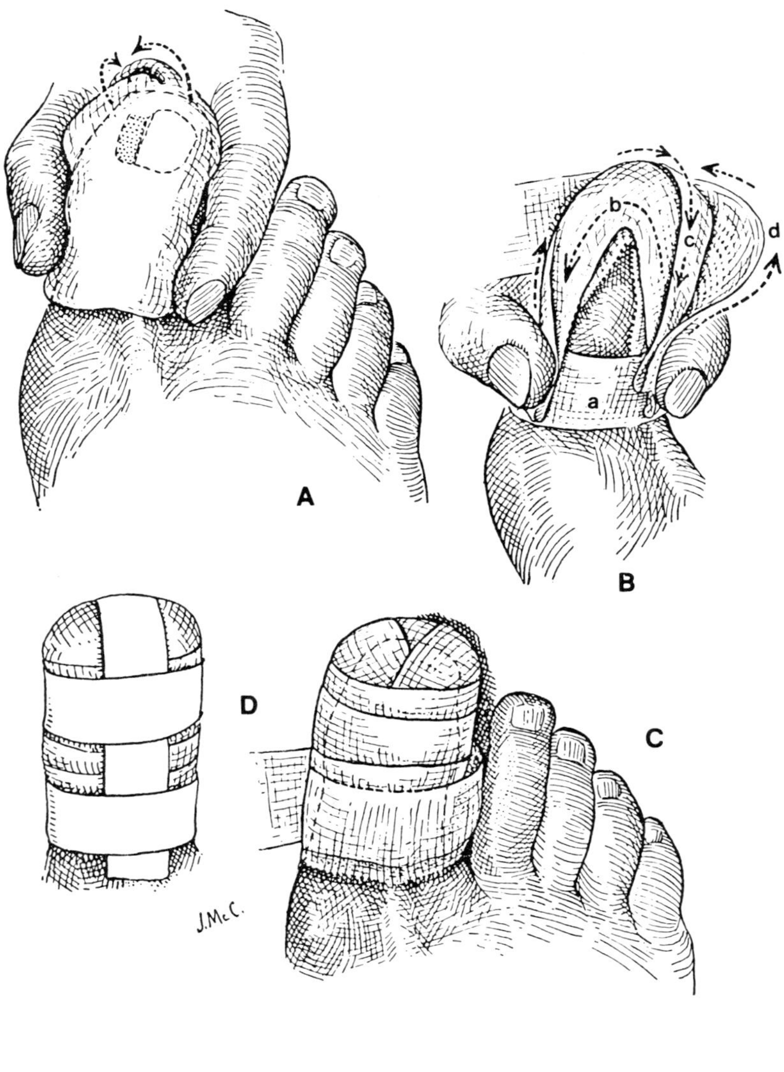

Figure 35-11. Dressing for use following excision of an ingrown toenail. (*A*) A gauze dressing 2 × 3 in. is cut at the top and folded over the end of the toe. (*B*) A circular anchor-turn of bandage is applied, followed by a reverse turn of the bandage over the toe. (*C*) The bandage is finished by making circular turns. (*D*) Adhesive strips are applied: one longitudinal strip, which extends beyond the bandage front and back; and two circular strips, which anchor the bandage and the longitudinal adhesive strip in place.

days. After that, small protective dressings are continued until the wound has healed. This occurs in about 2 to 3 weeks.

After operation the patient should be warned that the wearing of shoes that cause pressure on the edge of the nail may result in recurrence of the ingrown nail. Instructions should also be given about permitting the nail to grow so that the edge extends beyond the soft tissues.

HYPERTROPHIED TOENAIL (ONYCHOGRYPHOSIS)

Etiology and Symptoms

Hypertrophy of the toenail occurs most frequently in the great toe. As a rule the cause of the overgrowth is a subungual fungal infection, although trauma to the nail has been implicated; both result in very marked thickening of the nail. Often an almost hornlike nail develops, especially in older people who have a tendency to neglect themselves. The hypertrophy may result in pain by causing pressure on the toe by the shoe, and for this reason many patients seek treatment.

Treatment

If it is recognized that the symptoms may be relieved by relief of pressure, then conservative therapy, consisting of simple cutting away of the hypertrophied nail, may be tried. Bone-cutting forceps are used to cut off the excessive nail, and the patient is taught to file away the overgrowth as necessary. This will not produce a cure, but it will relieve the symptoms. Treatment with griseofulvin over an extended period is reputed to have alleviated many symptoms, but few patients will continue day-to-day medication for a period of 6 months or more.

Removal of the nail often is a disappointing procedure because the deformity sometimes recurs. For this reason careful excision of the nail matrix must be performed in addition to removing the nail as a further precaution against regrowth. Some authors advise cauterization of the nail base. This operation can be done under local anesthesia.

SUPERNUMERARY TOES

Supernumerary toes are not at all uncommon, and because of the difficulty they may cause in wearing shoes, it is frequently necessary to remove the extra digit. This is best done in childhood because the growing child is able to adjust to the joint deformity that may follow removal of the extra toe and its articulation.

Treatment

The operation is performed easily under local anesthesia. A roentgenogram is an aid in deciding which portion of the several toes should be removed. The toe is given a block anesthesia at its base for excision. It is wise to carry the skin incision fairly high along the toe to be removed. This flap of skin is reflected back sufficiently from the toe articulation to ensure that there will be sufficient skin and subcutaneous tissue to close over the defect resulting from the removal of the extra toe. Skin sutures that pass through the entire thickness of the underlying soft tissues and to the bone are necessary. Fine steel wire is an excellent suture material. A pressure dressing is applied without a splint. The patient may be ambulatory throughout the period of treatment.

PLANTAR WARTS

Etiology and Diagnosis

Warts occurring on the plantar surface of the foot are among the frequent and painful lesions of this area (Fig. 35-12). Dermatologists believe that they are due to a type of virus. However, their appearance at sites of irritation is not infrequent. Often they are associated with fallen arches. When they are associated with problems of faulty weight bearing, measures that improve the weight bearing

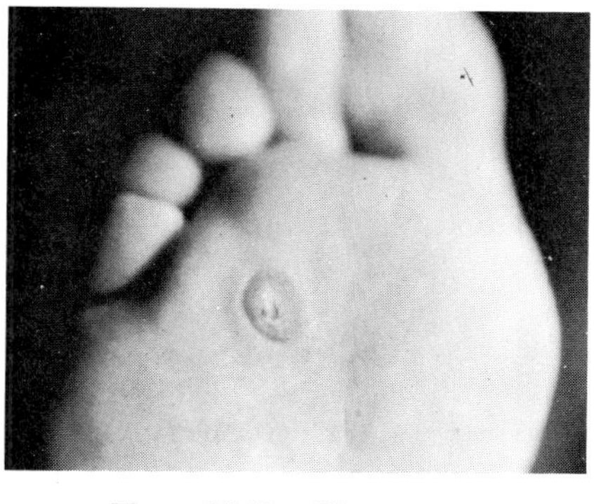

Figure 35-12. Plantar wart.

often relieve the discomfort, and the wart disappears; exercise may prevent recurrence. A very useful device is an L-shaped orthosis that extends under the first metatarsal head and then across the plantar surface proximal to the remaining metatarsal heads.

They occur more often in younger people, and they are important because of the pain produced by pressure upon them. Plantar warts may be small, or they may reach considerable size. Usually they are surrounded by an area of thickened epithelium, and in their center is a papillary growth that bleeds easily when it is pared with the scalpel. Pressure over this central core causes definite pain.

Treatment

There are several methods of treatment. The discomfort of a plantar wart is due to pressure on its central core. This can often be relieved by shaving the wart. We have used a double-edged safety razor blade for this purpose, bending it in the fingers so that the shaving may be done with the curved blade. After very thin slices of the epidermis have been shaved from the wart and the surrounding skin, the core of the wart can be plainly seen. There may often be a very slight capillary ooze from the core. After the surrounding skin has been protected with petrolatum, the core of the wart is treated with bichloracetic acid. This is applied with a toothpick that is dipped in the solution and is worked into the soft tissues of the core carefully and deeply. This may cause slight discomfort. After the bichloracetic acid has had a chance to be absorbed into the tissues the area is covered with a bandage. There may be slight soreness in the area for a day, but when the patient returns in 6 or 7 days the core of the wart is black and can be removed with the tip of a knife or a small curette. This treatment may have to be repeated if the entire wart cannot be removed after one treatment.

An ointment of 20% linseed oil and 20% podophyllin in lanolin has been used with success by British authors. They claim that the linseed oil disrupts the keratin layer of the skin and allows podophyllin to destroy the wart. The ointment is applied to a piece of gauze a little larger than the wart, placed on the wart, and retained in place by waterproof adhesive. This dressing is not changed for a week. Thereafter the foot is washed daily with soap and water.

Branson and Rhea inject 2 ml to 3 ml of 1% procaine, under pressure, with a 26-gauge needle at the base of the wart. If the needle tip is properly placed at the stratum germinativum there is marked blanching of the skin and elevation of the wart. The curative effect probably results from interruption of the blood supply of the wart.

The slight soreness produced by the injection disappears in 24 hours, and if the injection has been properly placed the wart may be lifted out of its site in about a week. We have used this method of treatment with success in several cases.

Other methods of therapy are removal of the wart by electrodesiccation after anesthetization with procaine solution and application of carbon dioxide snow. In many cases the wart disappears with a minimum of discomfort by injection into its base of a drop or two of quinine and urethane solution. The wart becomes dark or black in a few days and peels out of its crater without difficulty. Suitable arch supports should be prescribed when necessary. Often this alone will effect a cure.

INTERDIGITAL NEUROMA

Interdigital neuroma or so-called Morton's neuroma is caused by entrapment of an interdigital nerve. It commonly occurs in the third interspace, that is, between the third and fourth toes. The pain of a neuroma is most often confused with a metatarsal callosity or metatarsal strain, but this painful syndrome is characterized by the patient's desire to kick his shoes off and massage the painful foot. A better diagnostic test is to squeeze the foot from the side, thus compressing the neuroma between the third and fourth metatarsal heads. In some circumstances an actual click will be felt, and if the neuroma is large, sometimes it can be palpated between the metatarsal heads.

Treatment

Conservative treatment by injecting the interdigital neuroma with lidocaine (Xylocaine) and dexamethasone (Decardron) often will alleviate some of the symptoms, and a metatarsal pad to support the metatarsal heads often is of some comfort. However, surgical excision of the neuroma is often necessary. This is done by making a linear incision between the metatarsal heads and then delivering the neuroma to the dorsum of the foot by simple pressure on the plantar aspect. The nerve is transected both proximally and distally and then the neuroma is removed. The relief of pain is often dramatic and the postoperative convalescence can be extremely gratifying.

CALLOSITIES (CALLUSES)

Callosities are masses of hypertrophied epithelial tissue, hard and yellowish, that occur over areas subjected to long-continued pressure or friction. They are seen most commonly over the ball of the foot, and they arise in this area because of imperfect weight bearing. Frequently they become tender and painful as a result of continued trauma.

Treatment

The treatment of callosities is removal of the cause. Since there usually is defective weight bearing, suitable arch supports or pads must be prescribed. Painful areas subjected to pressure may be shaved with a razor blade or reduced by filing with an emery board.

BUNIONS

Etiology

Bunion is the name given to hypertrophy of the metatarsophalangeal joint of the great toe. This joint becomes deformed as a result of the wearing of shoes that do not fit properly and that cause lateral deviation of the great toe. As the joint becomes more and more prominent, pressure over the hypertrophied bone produces either a callus or a subcutaneous bursa. As the condition continues the joint becomes painful, and frequently the bursa becomes the site of an infection (Fig. 35-13).

Treatment

In conservative treatment of bunion, attempts are made to reduce the deformity by placing a pad of lamb's wool between the great and the second toes and by preventing pressure over the metatarsophalangeal joint with felt pads. The wearing of shoes with toes that are wide enough may relieve the symptoms, but it rarely relieves the entire pathologic process.

Surgery is usually necessary to produce a cure, and this may necessitate hospitalization.

PAINFUL HEEL

A heel that is painful in walking is a troublesome clinical entity for both patient and surgeon. This condition occurs in children and adults.

PAINFUL HEEL IN CHILDREN

Symptoms and Diagnosis

In the first group are the young children between 8 and 12 years of age, most of them boys. In this group there rarely is a history of injury, but the patient usually is active and vigorous. The pain is at the back of the heel.

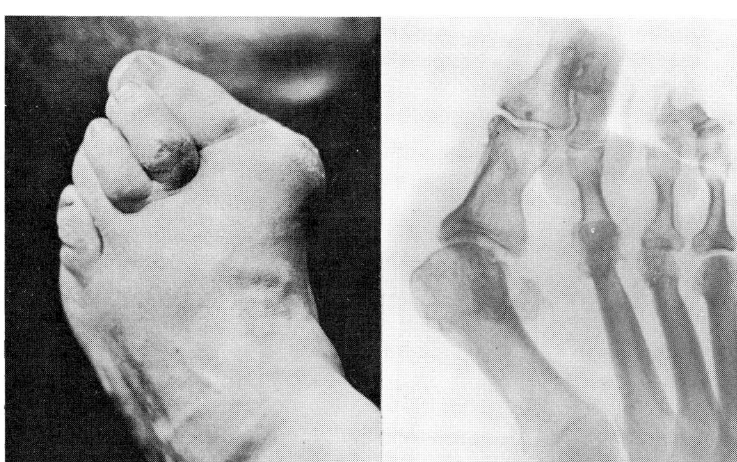

Figure 35-13. Typical deformity of a bunion. The photograph shows the infected callus over the prominence of the metatarsal head. The roentgenogram shows the marked bony deformity.

The patient walks with a slight limp and often notes that he is more comfortable when walking on his toes. On examination the heel is found to be tender posteriorly, and there is a slight thickening at the insertion of the Achilles tendon.

This symptom complex in children has been found to be due to an apophysitis of the heel. A lateral roentengogram may or may not show density of the apophysis with some irregularity of the posterior surface.

Treatment

In milder cases, elevation of the heel with pads relieves the pressure of the Achilles tendon, and if strenous exercise is avoided, usually the symptoms disappear rapidly. Local heat in the form of foot baths may be of value. As a rule the pain disappears spontaneously, but the patient should be warned that shoes with heels should be worn to avoid recurrence.

PAINFUL HEEL IN ADULTS

Etiology and Pathology

Painful heel in adults has been regarded as resulting from the development of a calcaneal spur. However, this finding in the roentgen film probably is of no great clinical significance, and its presence appears to be incidental. Current belief is that the pain is due either to the development of bursitis in the region of the spur or to painful inflammation of the plantar fascia and of the flexor digitorum brevis, which have their points of attachment near the site of the calcaneal spur. The pathologic process in this type of change may be similar to that occurring at the lateral epicondyle in tennis elbow. It is often seen following prolonged and unusual periods of time on the feet. It is worse on first arising in the morning and then improves as the day progresses, only to worsen later in the day as fatigue sets in. It should be noted that this syndrome is much more prevalent in the obese or heavily built patient.

Treatment

Various types of pads, springs, and other devices to relieve pressure have been used, but usually without much success. Two methods of therapy are of value—injection and needling or actual division of the fascia and the muscles attached to the os calcis.

In injection and needling the painful area is infiltrated with 5 to 10 ml of 1% lidocaine (Xylocaine) and 1 ml of dexamethasone (Decadron), the entry site being medial to the os calcis and paralleling the line of insertion of the plantar fascia. The needle is passed deeply across the origin of the plantar fascia from the os calcis, and the site is then covered with a simple bandage. In a fair percentage of cases this results in a cure of the painful heel.

Commercially available heel cups that are simply inserted in the shoes also result in relief of a high percentage of pain. Certainly if the patient is extremely heavy, a weight reduction regimen should be instituted.

Lapidus and guidotti recommend phenylbutazone, 0.1 g three times daily by mouth for a maximum of 20 doses.

Conservative treatment, including rest and avoidance of excessive standing, especially on hard surfaces, plus foot exercises, is usually successful.

FRACTURES

FRACTURES ABOUT THE ANKLE JOINT

ANATOMY

The tibia and the fibula are bound together just above the ankle joint by the tibiofibular ligaments (Fig. 35-2). These ligaments are often stronger than the fibula and resist widening of the space between the malleoli, which astragalus fits snugly. The astragalus tapers slightly from before backward. This tight mortise and tenon joint, between the tibiofibular unit above and the astragalus below, permits free flexion and extension but practically no mediolateral or rotary movement of the astragalus. Strong medial and lateral ligaments reinforce the sides of the capsule of the ankle joint. A strong posterior portion of the lateral ligament inserts on the posterior aspect of this bone to the fibula much stronger than those to the tibia. When the lateral malleolus is displaced the astragalus tends to move with it. The articular surface of the astragalus fits exactly into the articular surface of the distal end of the tibia. When the astragalus becomes displaced, the weight-bearing axis shifts, and if this is not corrected serious impairment of ankle function follows. When the space between the malleoli increases as the result of displacement, the astragalus wobbles with each step and, again, serious impairment of function results.

ETIOLOGY

Most fractures about the ankle joint are caused by indirect violence, the force usually being applied to the foot and transmitted to the astragalus. They are classified according to the violence causing them: fractures due to eversion and external rotation, fractures due to inversion and internal rotation, fractures due to forward or backward thrust against the articular surface of the tibia, and fractures due to upward thrust against the articular surface of the tibia.

FRACTURES DUE TO EVERSION (ABDUCTION) AND EXTERNAL ROTATION

Forcible eversion of the foot, that is, elevation of the lateral border, rotates the astragalus about its long axis so as to wedge the malleoli apart. The strain is applied to the tibiofibular ligament, which becomes a fulcrum at which the lever action works. The lateral malleolous is pressed outward. When it breaks there is tension on the deltoid (medial collateral) ligament (Fig. 35-14A). The ligament may tear, or the medial malleolus may be fractured. External rotation of the foot, that is, forefoot outward, forces the astragalus to rotate about a vertical axis, and it also acts to wedge the malleoli apart.

Eversion and external rotation are usually combined to cause typical fractures. When the force is not great there is fracture of the fibula at or above the tibifibular ligaments, the fracture line being irregularly transverse or from in front upward and backward, oblique. When the force is greater there is a fracture of the fibula complicated by disruption of the mortise because of fracture of the medial malleolus below the level of the ankle joint or rupture of the deltoid ligament.

FRACTURES DUE TO INVERSION AND INTERNAL ROTATION

Forcible inversion of the foot, that is, elevation of the medial border, acts to press the malleoli apart (Fig. 35-14B). The strain falls on the tibiofibular ligaments and the lateral ligament. Internal rotation may occur at the same time and add to the wedging action. When the force is not great the medial malleolus alone may be fractured, the fracture line running almost vertically upward. When the force is greater the fracture of the medial malleolus is complicated by fracture of the fibula below the tibiofibular ligament, rupture of the tibiofibular ligaments.

FRACTURES DUE TO FORWARD OR BACKWARD THRUST AGAINST THE ARTICULAR SURFACE OF THE TIBIA

When the foot is plantar flexed and is thrust backward (Fig. 35-14) the posterior margin of the articular surface of the tibia may be broken off, and the foot may be dislocated posteriorly. When the foot is dorsiflexed and thrust forward, the anterior margin of the articular surface of the tibia may be broken off, and the foot may be dislocated anteriorly. Fractures of an articular margin occur less frequently alone than in combination with fractures of the malleoli.

FRACTURES DUE TO UPWARD THRUST AGAINST THE ARTICULAR SURFACE OF THE TIBIA (EXPLOSION FRACTURE)

Fractures that result from upward thrust against the articular surface of the tibia are very rare, and they follow falls on the feet. The inferior tibiofibular ligaments may be ruptured and the astragalus driven up between the two bones. The articular surface of the tibia may be crushed or split and the astragalus displaced upward between the fragments that lie in front of it and behind it.

DIAGNOSIS

The history of an injury causing violent torsion of the foot, followed by severe pain and swelling of the ankle and inability to walk, suggests a fracture. The ankle must be examined with definite points in mind. Characteristic deformity indicating displacement of the foot may be visible before swelling becomes great. Lateral, medial, anterior, or posterior displacement indicates disruption of the mortise. The condition of the soft tissues, that is, swelling, ecchymosis, and bleb formation, should be noted.

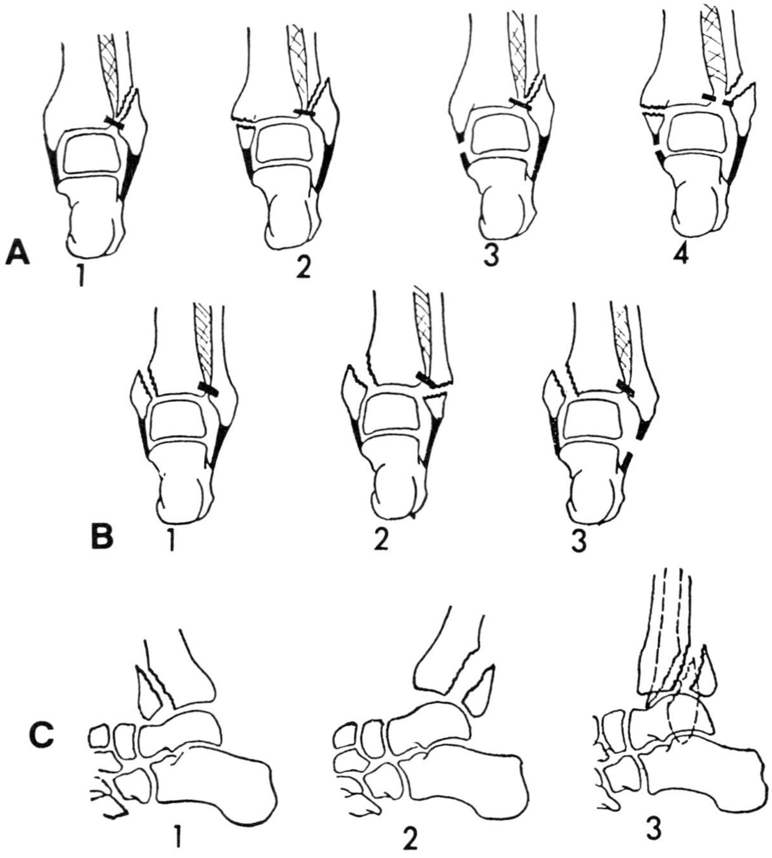

Figure 35-14. Types of ankle fractures.

(*A*) Fractures due to eversion-external rotation: (*1*) simple fracture of the fibula above the ankle joint; (*2*) fracture of the fibula with fracture of the medial malleolus at or below the level of the ankle joint; (*3*) fracture similar to *2*—the medial malleolus has not been fractured, but the deltoid ligament has been torn; (*4*) the most severe type of injury, fractures of both malleoli with rupture of the tibiofibular ligament and sometimes rupture of the deltoid ligament (*2, 3,* and *4*). These often are complicated by a posterior marginal fracture of the tibia as shown in *C, 2* and *3*.

(*B*) Fracture due to inversion-internal rotation: (*1*) simple fracture of the medial malleolus running upward from the joint; (*2*) similar fracture of the medial malleolus with fracture of the lateral malleolus below the level of the ankle joint; (*3*) fracture similar to (*2*)—the lateral malleolus has not been fractured, but the lateral ligament has been torn.

(*C*)(*1*) Fracture of the anterior margin of the tibial articular surface—this is caused by a forward thrust on the foot, excessive dorsiflexion, or a fall on the foot. (*2* and *3*) Fracture of the posterior margin of the tibial articular surface with posterior dislocation of the foot—this is caused by a backward thrust on the foot or excessive external rotation of the foot, and very often it is associated with *A, 1* through *4*.

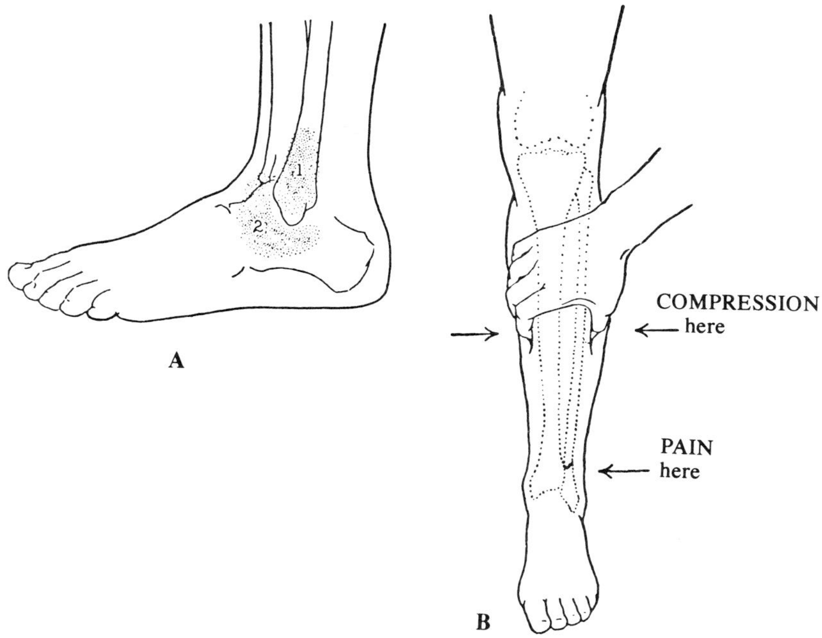

Figure 35-15. (*A*) The tender areas in ankle sprains and fractures. (*1*) The site of tenderness in fractures of the lateral malleolus; (*2*) the site of tenderness in sprains of the lateral ligament. (*B*) Compression of the bones at the middle of the leg causes pain at the ankle when the lower end of the fibula is fractured.

Points of acute tenderness indicate points of injury. Acute tenderness over the deltoid, lateral, or tibiofibular ligaments indicates sprain or rupture of these ligaments (Fig. 35-15); over the malleoli, below or above the level of the joint, it indicates fracture. The entire fibula should be examined, because it may be fractured high in its shaft. Acute tenderness in the space anterior to the insertion of the Achilles tendon suggests posterior marginal fracture of the tibia or fracture of the posterior lip of the astragalus. Similarly, the anterior margin of the tibia is tender when fractured.

Increased mediolateral mobility should be sought by grasping the heel, not the foot, and pressing it firmly to the lateral side, to the medial side, toward eversion, and toward inversion. Increased mobility points to disruption of the mortise. This may be checked in roentgenograms by having additional anteroposterior views made with the foot in forced eversion and forced inversion after the tender points have been anesthetized with local anesthetic solution.

The bowlike relation of the fibula to the tibia may be used to demonstrate the pain produced by movement at the fracture site. The test is performed by pressing the bones together in the middle of the leg. This causes no particular discomfort in the ankle in cases of sprain, but when the fibula is fractured there is definite pain at the fracture site (Fig. 35-15).

The roentgen examination is extremely important. Exact anterioposterior and lateral views from the lower third of the leg to the os calcis are the minimum requirement. These may be supplemented by views made with the foot in forced eversion and inversion. The films should be examined for fracture of the malleoli and of the articular margins of the tibia, for separation of the tibia from the fibula, and for mediolateral and anteroposterior displacement of the astragalus. Normally the articular surface of the astragalus lies exactly beneath the articular surface of the tibia, and it is fitted accurately between the malleoli. Widening of the space between a malleolus and the astragalus indicates disruption of the mortise. When there is any doubt, the uninjured side should be examined for comparison.

TREATMENT

Preliminary

When the examination has been completed, the ankle must be adequately splinted for transportation (Fig. 35-16). The foot, the ankle, and the lower third of the leg should be wrapped firmly in an elastic compression dressing to control swelling. Two well-padded or cardboard splints, long enough to reach from the heel to the knee, are secured to the medial and lateral aspects of the leg with wide adhesive straps. The foot should be secured to the splints with a figure-of-eight strap, and as a general rule, it is best to splint the injured ankle with the shoe in place. During the wait for further treatment, the leg should be elevated and ice bags applied. An inflatable plastic splint may be used if available. Air splints should never be inflated by mechanical means, but always by lung pressure.

For further treatment the fractures about the ankle are classified according to the severity of the injury as follows:

Fractures without displacement of the malleoli and without displacement of the astragalus. These include fractures of the lateral malleolus, the fibula above the tibiofibular ligaments, the medial malleolus, and both malleoli and the anterior or the posterior margin of the tibia.

Fractures with displacement of the malleoli and the astragalus. These include fractures due to eversion–external rotation, the astragalus being displaced laterally; fractures due to inversion, the astragalus being displaced medially; marginal fractures of the tibia, with anterior or posterior displacement of the astragalus; and fractures of the tibial articular surface, or tibiofibular separation, with upward displacement of the astragalus.

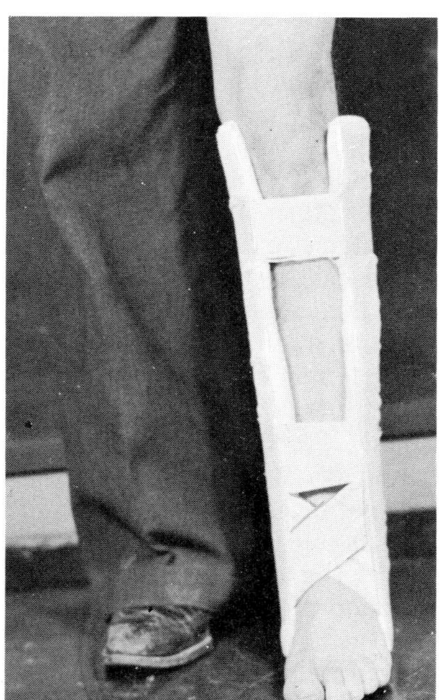

Figure 35-16. Application of splints for preliminary treatment of ankle fracture. The pressure dressing has been omitted for clarity.

Fractures of the Medial or Lateral Malleolus Alone

When they are in a good position and without torn ligaments, fractures of the medial or lateral malleolus alone (Fig. 35-17) require only support and a pressure dressing to maintain a useful extremity and to enable the patient to walk without crutches during treatment. When the fracture is slight, such as a fissure in the bone, a local anesthetic may be injected into the site of most acute tenderness. A firm adhesive strapping may be applied. An elastic adhesive bandage or gelatin boot may be all that is required to make the patient comfortable. Additional local anesthetic injections may be necessary at invervals of 1 or 2 days. After a few days the patient should be able to walk with little discomfort. The dressing is reapplied when it becomes loose, and after 3 or 4 weeks it may be replaced by an elastic ankle support.

If the fracture is comminuted or if displacement seems likely with active function, the strapping and the pressure dressing are replaced with a boot cast as soon as the swelling subsides.

Application of a Boot Cast. As a general rule the patient is allowed to sit with the injured leg flexed over the side of the table, and the surgeon sits on a low stool facing the patient. He may support the toes of the affected foot with his knee. Stockinet is placed over the leg from above the knee to beyond the toes. A strip of felt is placed about the proximal tibia and fibula to protect the fibular head. A thin layer of sheet wadding is wrapped about the malleoli and around the forefoot. With the knee flexed at 90 degrees and the ankle maintained at ap-

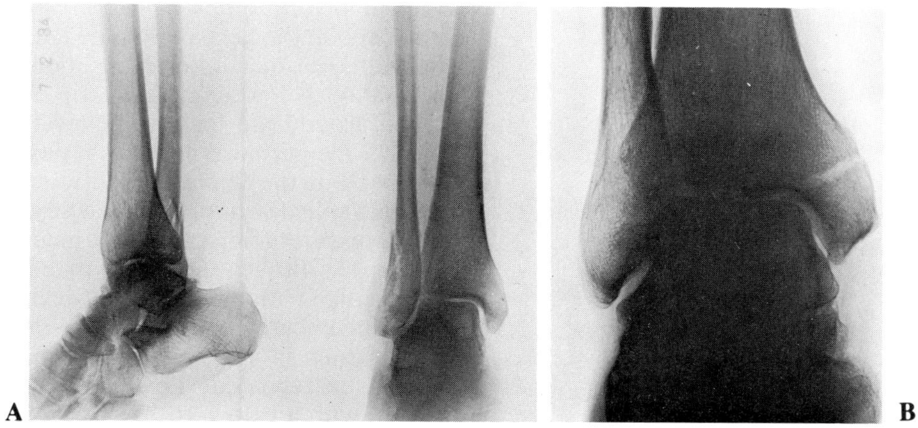

Figure 35-17. (*A*) Comminuted fracture of lateral malleolus caused by eversion-external rotation. (*B*) Fracture of medial malleolus in good position.

proximately neutral position between flexion and extension, a circular plaster cast is applied and is molded well behind and below the malleoli. The cast is allowed to extend beyond the toes and while still wet is cut back on the dorsum to allow toe extension. The stockinet is folded back over the cast proximally and distally and is held firmly with a small additional circular plastic bandage. The cast should be molded well to maintain a satisfactory plantar arch and for additional comfort and should also be molded slightly behind the second, third, and fourth metatarsal heads. A walking heel may be attached to the cast, and the patient may be allowed to begin to walk after the plaster is thoroughly set.

After 4 to 6 weeks the cast may be removed. Following removal of the cast, elastic support should be used from the toes to the knees until the circulation readjusts to its unprotected condition. These injuries rarely require any physiotherapy, but when they do, the patient is instructed to immerse the foot in hot water for 15 minutes and to massage it for 5 minutes twice daily at home.

Fractures of Both Malleoli in Good Position and of the Anterior or the Posterior Articular Margin of the Tibia in Good Position

Fractures in the next classification (Fig. 35-18) may also be treated with a boot cast applied with the foot and ankle in neutral position. The cast should be left in place for 6 to 8 weeks and follow-up care is similar to that described previously.

Fractures With Displacement of the Malleoli or the Astragalus or Both

Fractures with malleolar or astragalar displacement are serious injuries, since the mortise of the ankle is disrupted or the astragalus is moved from the weight-bearing axis; sometimes both occur. The soft tissues usually exhibit evidence of severe injury. Without extremely accurate reduction and careful aftertreatment there may be great disability. When there is any doubt concerning the ability to manage these patients on an ambulatory basis, they should be given hospital care. Closed reduction methods can fail, because of infolding of soft tissue between the fragments or bony irregularities. If necessary to obtain a good ankle mortise, open reduction is indicated.

The basic requirements for a good result are adequate roentgen study, accurate reduction, adequate measures for reducing the swelling, prolonged uninterrupted immobilization of the fragments until union occurs, and active use of the limb during the period of immobilization whenever possible.

Eversion–External Rotation Fractures With Displacement (Pott's Fracture)

The most common eversion–external rotation fracture (Fig. 35-19) is the so-called Pott's fracture. The fibula is broken at or above the tibiofibular ligament, the medial malleolus is fractured below the level of the joint, and the astragalus is shifted laterally. Reduction is performed without delay, each fracture site being infiltrated with local anesthetic solution,

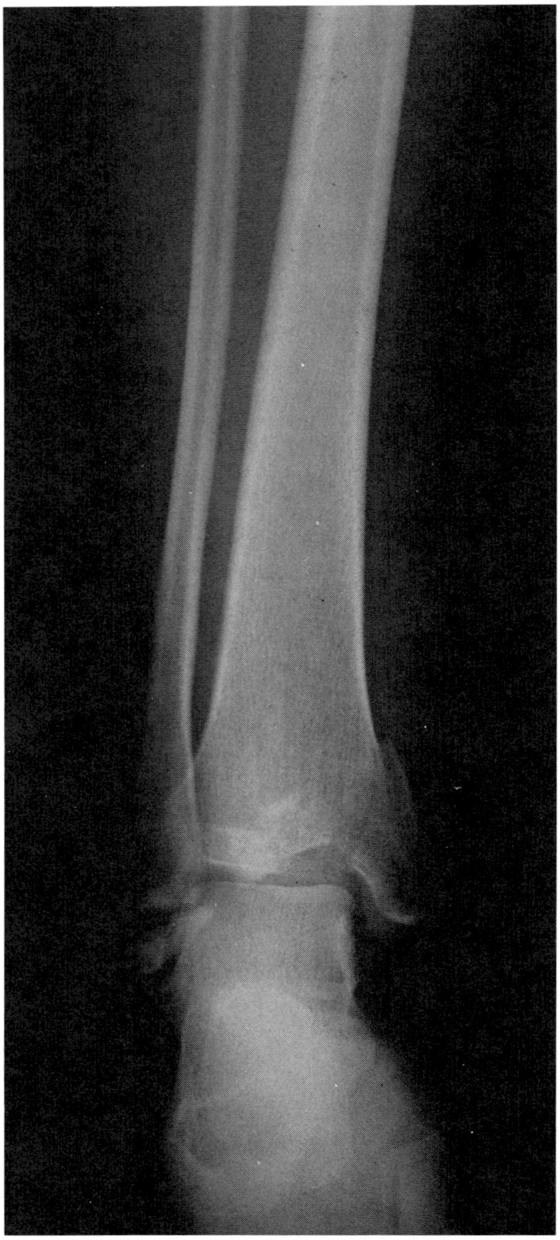

Figure 35-18. Bimalleolar fracture with fracture of the lateral half of the tibial plafond displaced proximally. (This fracture requires open reduction.)

and 10 to 15 minutes being allowed to elapse before proceeding; general anesthesia may be used if preferred.

The patient sits with the knee flexed and the leg hanging over the edge of the table; the surgeon grasps the medial side of the leg above the ankle with one hand and presses strongly medially on the heel and on the lateral malleolus with the other. Internal rotation of the foot is usually also necessary. A strip of felt is fastened around the leg just below the knee to protect the peroneal nerve as it passes around the neck of the fibula. A lightly padded boot cast is applied with the ankle at 90 degrees and firm pressure holding the foot medially. After the cast is firm it should be extended to the upper thigh with the knee in 30 degrees of flexion. Roentgen evaluation is then made, and if the position is not satisfactory, manipulation should be repeated. This cast should be replaced with a below-knee walking-cast in 4 to 6 weeks. At any sign of circulatory difficulty the cast should be bivalved to the skin, and it should be replaced with a snug above-knee cast when the initial swelling has subsided. Care must be taken to instruct the patient in proper elevation of the foot and in avoiding pressure on the heel.

The leg is kept elevated and ice bags are applied for from 24 to 48 hours after injury. Early weight bearing is not permitted.

When the cast is removed an elastic support should be used until the circulation adapts to the changed situation; alternate elevation and dependency should be allowed.

Inversion–Internal Rotation Fractures With Displacement

The medial malleolus is fractured along a line running upward from the articular surface, and the fibula is broken below the level of the ankle joint. The malleoli and the astragalus are displaced toward the medial side. When the lateral malleolus shows no fracture and the intermalleolar space is widened, rupture of the lateral and the tibiofibular ligaments must be suspected. This may be confirmed by taking an anteroposterior roentgenogram with the foot forcibly inverted, again using a local anesthetic.

The treatment of these fractures is similar in all respects to that for eversion–external rotation fractures, except that the reduction maneuvers are reversed. The surgeon strongly forces the heel and the medial malleolus laterally and repeats this pressure when the plaster is applied. Persistent displacement of the medial malleolus may be due to soft-part interposition and requires open reduction and internal fixation.

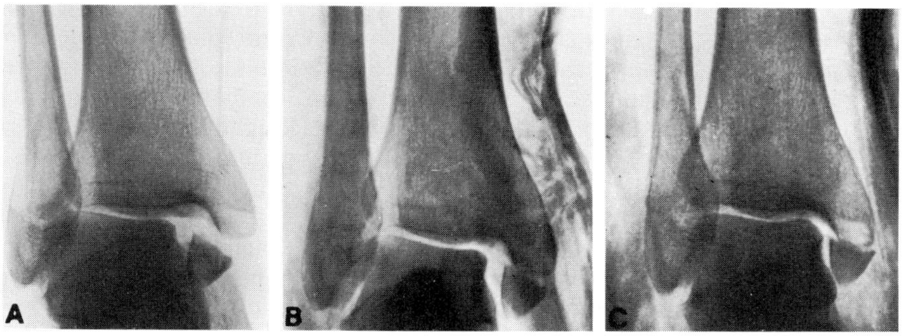

Figure 35-19. Fractures following eversion-external rotation. (*A*) An oblique fracture of the fibula and a fracture of the medial malleolus are seen. The astragalus has moved laterally, and the intermalleolar space has widened greatly. (*B*) The position of the fragments has been improved, but residual displacement still can be seen in the wide space between the medial margin of the astragalus and the unbroken portion of the medial malleolus. (*C*) Almost full correction by pressure 1 week after injury, when the swelling had subsided. An unpadded cast was applied. If the medial malleolus shows considerable residual displacement, it may be advisable to operate for reduction and fixation.

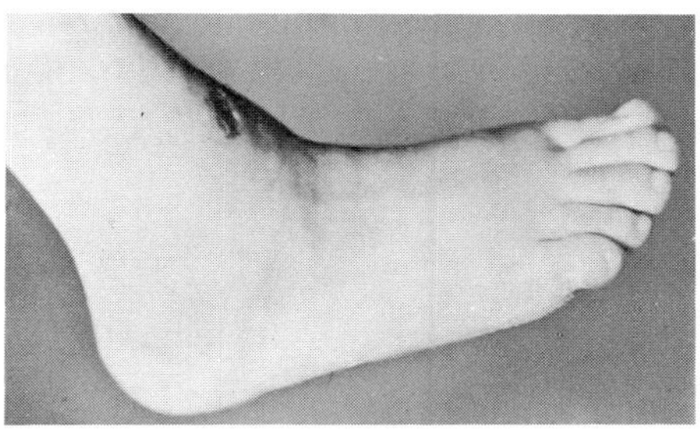

Figure 35-20. Typical deformity after a posterior marginal fracture of the tibia with posterior dislocation of the foot. An ulceration is present over the prominent lower end of the tibia; this was due to excessive pressure from a dressing that had been applied incorrectly.

Marginal Fractures With Anteroposterior Displacement of the Foot

Although fractures of the posterior margin of the articular surface of the tibia with posterior displacement of the foot (Figs. 35-20 and 35-21) are usually associated with fractures of the malleoli, they may occur without them. If the posterior fragment of the tibia includes less than 20% of the joint surface, the fracture may be treated by closed reduction, but if more of the articular surface is involved, accurate reduction is required and open reduction is usually necessary.

Reduction is obtained with the knee flexed, by making backward pressure on the leg above

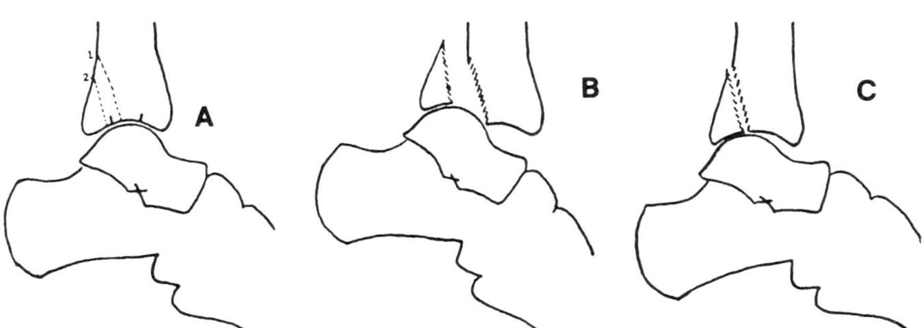

Figure 35-21. (*A*)(*1*) The "classical" type of posterior marginal fracture (after Nelson and Jensen); (*2*) the "minimal" type of fracture. (*B*) typical displacement. (*C*) Incomplete reduction. The articular surface of the astragalus is not concentric with the main articular surface. Unless the foot is brought forward to its correct position the result will be very unsatisfactory.

the ankle and a strong forward pull on the foot, accompanied by dorsiflexion. The displacement will tend to recur very easily. Immediate roentgenograms must show complete reduction of the posterior dislocation and complete or almost complete replacement of the posterior fragment. In rare instances there may be a fixed displacement of the fibula behind the tibia that blocks reduction and may require open reduction. Failure to maintain reduction indicates the need for hospitalization. Roentgenograms should be repeated in 7 to 10 days so that recurrent displacement may be identified and corrected. The after-care is similar to that for displaced malleolar fractures except that the cast remains in place for 8 weeks.

Fracture of the posterior margin of the articular surface of the tibia occurs frequently in parachute jumpers. It may occur alone or associated with malleolar fractures, as described above. When it occurs alone, displacement is apt to be slight and immobilization in a walking cast for 4 to 6 weeks seems to be sufficient.

Fractures of the anterior margin of the articular surface of the tibia with anterior displacement of the foot require that the foot be pushed posteriorly and plantar flexed while the leg above the ankle is pulled forward. Displacement recurs readily, and this makes it necessary to use the same precautions and roentgen criteria as are used in the treatment of posterior marginal fractures. When displacement of the astragalus tends to recur a Kirschner wire may be inserted through the heel, and traction distally and posteriorly may maintain reduction. The wire may be incorporated in a cast and traction posteriorly and distally maintained for 10 to 14 days. The after-treatment is similar to that described previously.

FRACTURES OF THE OS CALCIS

ETIOLOGY

The os calcis is fractured by falls on the feet from a height, rarely by other means. Bilateral fracture occurs frequently, and both heels must be examined when one is injured. Fractures of the lumbar spine are frequently caused by the same violence, and patients with fracture of the os calcis should always be examined for possible fracture of the spine and vice versa.

A properly functioning os calcis is ordinarily essential for painless weight bearing and walking. Violence may so compress (Fig. 35-22), widen, or shatter the bone that its articulations no longer fit, or they become roughened. Its weight-bearing axis is also distorted. Many fracture patterns occur. The constant pull of the gastrocnemius muscle often maintains the displacement. To reduce these displacements and to maintain good position, skeletal traction and pin transfixion may be required.

DIAGNOSIS

Pain in the heel after a fall or a jump from a height suggests fracture of the os calcis. Swelling occurs after a few hours, and ecchymosis appears later. Weight bearing on the heel causes severe pain. The bone is tender on mediolateral compression. Comparison with the uninjured side may disclose widening of the heel. Anteroposterior and lateral roentgenograms must be made.

TREATMENT

Only those cases of single- or multiple-fissure fractures without displacement (Fig. 35-23) and those of isolated fractures of a small portion of the bone are suitable for ambulatory treatment. Narrowing of the tuber-joint angle (Fig. 35-22), displacement, or depression of the joint surfaces and widening of the tuberosity require hospitalization and expert care.

Ambulatory patients receive a firm compression dressing immediately to control swelling. A thick flannel or elastic bandage is applied from the toes to the middle of the leg,

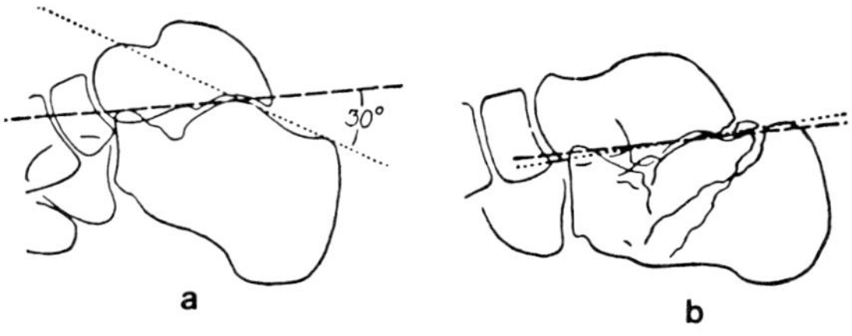

Figure 35-22. The tuberosity-joint angle. (*a*) The dotted line from the tuberosity to the posterior margin of the articular surface intersects the broken line from the anterior margin of the articular surface to the posterior margin. These lines make an angle of about 30 degrees. When the os calcis is crushed the angle is decreased or reversed, as shown in (*b*).

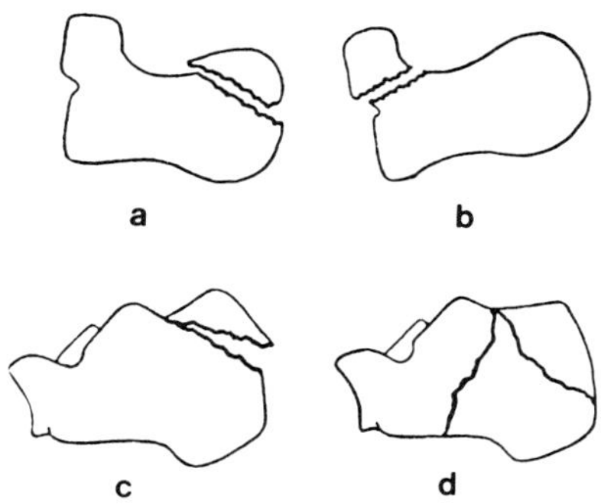

Figure 35-23. Some varieties of fracture of the os calcis that can be treated by ambulatory methods: (*a*) simple fracture of the posterior portion of the base; (*b*) fracture of the sustentaculum tali without displacement; (*c*) "beak" fracture of the tuberosity; (*d*) fissure fractures without displacement. (After Watson-Jones.)

or the part may be wrapped in a heavy layer of cotton and bandaged tightly with gauze or muslin. The leg is kept elevated and ice bags are applied for 24 to 48 hours after injury. After 5 to 7 days, when the swelling has subsided, a lightly padded cast from the toes to the knee and a walking heel are applied. No manipulation is required in the case of fissure fractures without displacement.

A "beak" fracture of the tuberosity (Fig. 35-24) is reduced by moderate plantar flexion of the foot and direct pressure of both thumbs above the fragment at the sides of the Achilles tendon. If the displacement cannot be corrected, operation may be required.

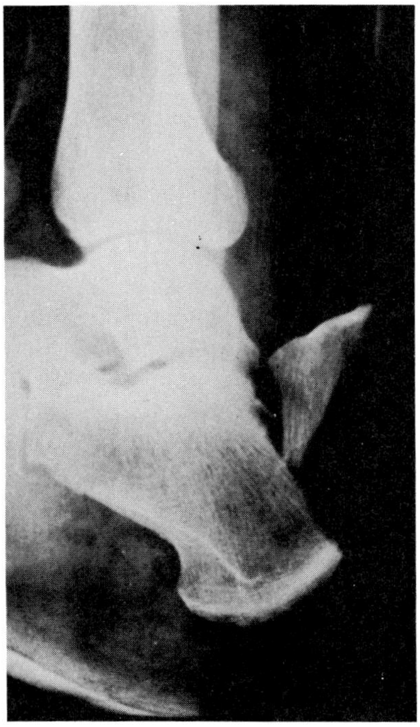

Figure 35-24. "Beak" fracture of the os calcis.

Medial displacement of a fragment of the sustentaculum tali or a fragment of the tuberosity may be reduced by strong pressure with the thumbs. The cast must be well molded about the heel and the ankle. The foot should be kept at a right angle to the leg, except after reduction of a beak fracture, in which case some plantar flexion is preferable. The cast should be maintained for 6 to 8 weeks. The after-care is similar to that for fractures about the ankle. If the plantar surface remains tender a pad of felt or sponge rubber may be worn in the heel of the shoe.

The prognosis in the simple types of fracture is usually good. Full return of function is usually anticipated.

SUBASTRAGALAR DISLOCATIONS

ETIOLOGY

Inversion and eversion of the foot take place at the subastragalar joint (Fig. 35-25). When the normal range of motion is exceeded suddenly there may be dislocation of the foot at this joint. The astragalus remains between the malleoli, while the os calcis and the scaphoid dislocate with the foot. The dislocation is usually to the medial or the lateral side, rarely forward. Fracture of the astragalus or of the surrounding bones may also be present.

DIAGNOSIS

There is severe pain at the ankle following a violent injury. The dislocation, lateral or forward, presents a striking deformity quite unlike that of ankle fractures. The malleoli are usually intact and painless. Roentgen study is required to exclude fractures.

TREATMENT

The dislocation must be reduced promptly. Under general or local anesthesia, the knee is flexed, the foot is plantar flexed, and strong traction is made on the foot, which is then pulled quickly and gently toward its normal position. A well-padded boot cast is applied and immediately bivalved. The leg is elevated and the ankle is surrounded with ice bags for

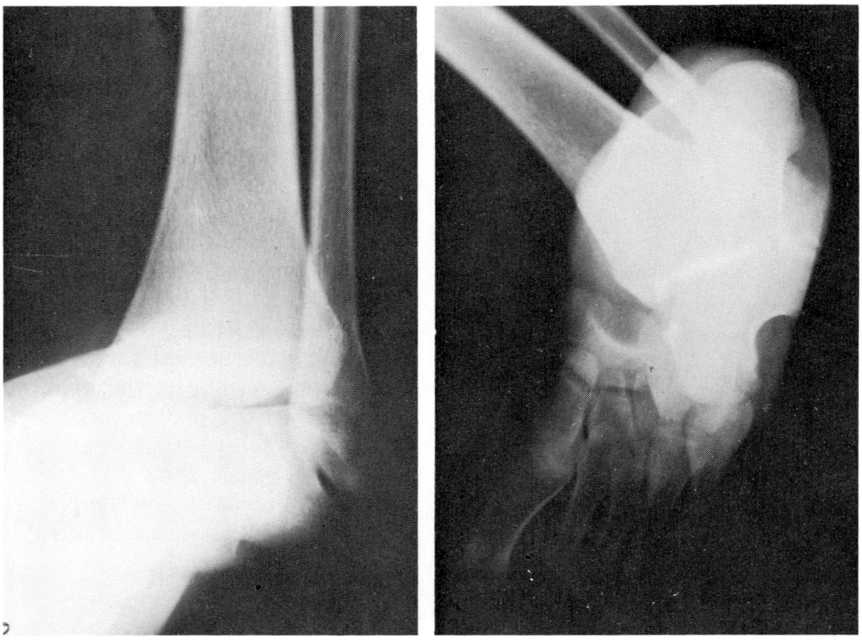

Figure 35-25. Subastragaloid dislocation. (*A*) Anteroposterior view of the ankle. The astragalus lies in its normal position between the malleoli, and the foot is dislocated to the medial side. (*B*) View with the foot placed flat on the film. The head of the astragalus lies over the tarsal bones on the lateral side of the foot and not in the concave facet of the scaphoid on the medial side.

24 to 48 hours. When the swelling subsides a lightly padded plaster cast and a walking heel are applied. The patient begins to walk as soon as the cast is hard and dry. The cast is removed after 6 weeks. After-care is similar to that for ankle fractures.

The prognosis is good if there are no complicating fractures of the astragalus. Failure to reduce the dislocation, associated fractures, or open wounds are indications for hospital care.

FRACTURES OF THE METATARSALS

ETIOLOGY

Fractures of the metatarsals (Fig. 35-26) often follow direct violence, such as the impact of a heavy object or being run over by a wheel. They may also be caused by indirect violence. Fracture of the base of the fifth metatarsal often follows sudden inversion of the foot. Most metatarsal fractures exhibit little or no displacement unless the violence has been very great.

DIAGNOSIS

A history of violence followed by pain, swelling, ecchymosis, and inability to bear weight is suggestive of fracture. There is acute localized tenderness over the fracture line and increased pain when the toe is pressed proximally in the long axis of the metatarsal. Fractures with great displacement swell very rapidly. The deformity is readily palpable. The site of the fracture becomes acutely tender. In children 11 to 16 years of age it is important to differentiate in the roentgenogram between a fracture and a normal epiphysis of the tuberosity at the base of the fifth metatarsal.

TREATMENT

When there is a fracture in good position, a felt pad is applied to the plantar surface to conform to the arch, and a firm flannel or elastic bandage or a gelatin boot is applied from the toes to the knee. Ice bags are then applied for 24 to 48 hours, and the leg is elevated until the swelling subsides. When there are multiple fractures, a snug boot cast and a walking heel

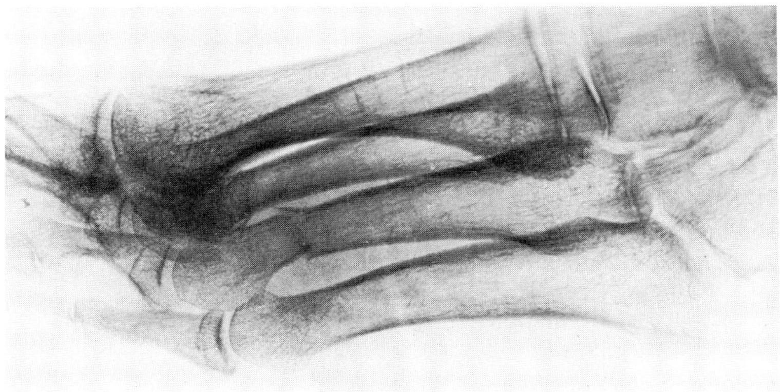

Figure 35-26. Fracture of the neck of the fourth metatarsal without displacement.

may be applied from the toes to below the knee. This should remain in place for 4 to 8 weeks. The longitudinal arch must be molded well, and the foot must be at right angles to the leg. Walking begins when the cast is hard. An arch support is used in the after care, in addition to the other measures for fractures of the ankle.

Many of these patients with metatarsal fractures may be treated well with nothing more than gelatin boot or an elastic adhesive bandage. The gelatin is applied in a heavy layer from above the ankle to include the toes. Felt pads are cut to conform to the plantar arch, and they are applied over the first layer of gauze-bandage. Usually two layers of gelatin are sufficient. The patient may wear a cutout shoe, which will allow him to walk comfortably after 7 to 10 days.

Fractures of the base of the fifth metatarsal (Fig. 35-27) may require only firm strapping with adhesive or with an elastic bandage, the foot being held in eversion while the bandage is applied. A procaine injection at the fracture site usually relieves pain and discomfort. Most of these patients walk without disability in 6 to 8 days.

When there is considerable displacement complicating fracture of a metatarsal, it must be reduced as accurately as possible. With the patient under local or general anesthesia, assistants make traction on the toe and countertraction on the foot and leg above the ankle. The toe or the toes may be wrapped in adhesive to obtain a better grip. The surgeon presses on the fragments to restore normal position. In the presence of great swelling, reduction may be deferred for a few days while the part is elevated. Oblique and unstable fractures require continuous skeletal traction, as is required for similar fractures of the metacarpals.

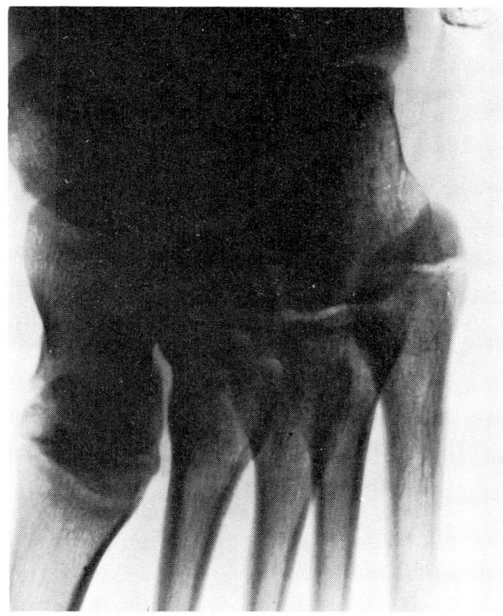

Figure 35-27. Fracture of the tuberosity of the fifth metatarsal.

Since the first metatarsal bears a large share of the weight of the body, it is particularly important to correct any angulation of its fragments. Some slight displacement of the other metatarsals is not of such importance.

PROGNOSIS

When there is no displacement the prognosis is excellent. When there is great displacement the prognosis depends on accurate reduction and adequate after-care. There may be prolonged discomfort in the foot when angulation remains, particularly when the angle is open toward the dorsum of the foot.

FRACTURES OF THE SESAMOID BONES

There usually are two sesamoid bones in the flexor tendons beneath the head of the first metatarsal. In rare instances a congentially divided, bipartite, sesamoid bone may be found. This should not be mistaken for a fracture. Occurring after a fall on the feet, the fracture of a sesamoid bone may be identified by acute tenderness on the plantar surface just to the medial side or to the lateral margin of the head of the first metatarsal. Treatment is identical with that for fracture of a metatarsal.

FRACTURES OF THE TOES

Fractures of the toes result from the impact of a falling object or from stubbing the toe. The great toe is involved most often by crush injuries. Displacement is seldom great. When present, it is seen in fractures of the proximal phalanges and is similar to the displacement seen in the phalanges of the fingers. There is a history of a characteristic injury followed by pain, swelling, and tenderness of the toe involved. The toe may be abnormally mobile, and crepitus may be felt.

TREATMENT

Unless there is considerable displacement that is likely to lead to deformity, reduction is not required. When the phalanges of the great toe are involved, a medial plaster splint may be molded about the toe, a small soft pad applied between the great toe and the second toe, and the forefoot bandaged with elastic adhesive. When the second to the fifth toes are involved these may be best treated by placing a small soft padding between the injured toe and the adjacent toe and bandaging the two toes together, using small strips of elastic adhesive bandage. Care must be taken when using regular adhesive to avoid abnormal pressure, and the rest of the foot may be protected with an elastic bandage. The uninjured toe can be used very successfully as a mold or a splint. Local anesthetic injections sometimes relieve pain and disability.

A shoe may be worn. A larger shoe, or a slit in the shoe, may be necessary to avoid pain due to pressure. Wearing the type of sandal that has a strap between the great toe and the other toes is excellent for these fractures.

Displacements of the distal or middle phalanges are reduced easily by traction and pressure or molding, and the position is maintained by a dressing similar to that mentioned above. Fractures of the proximal phalanges sometimes prove to be troublesome, but they rarely need dressings other than the simple ones described above.

Support should be continued until there is no tenderness or pain. A firm-soled shoe should always be prescribed, and if one is not available, an additional sole can easily be applied to a shoe that fits over the dressing. In simple fracture, only the adhesive dressing may be needed for 2 weeks, and the patient may wear his regular shoe if there is sufficient room for this foot.

BIBLIOGRAPHY

General

Edmondson EL, Crenshaw JB: Campbell's Operative Orthopedics, 6th ed. St Louis, CV Mosby, 1980

Rockwood CA Jr, Green DP: Fractures, 2nd ed, Vol 2, pp 1665–1820. Philadelphia, JB Lippincott, 1984

Plantar Ulcers

Classen JN: Neurotrophic arthropathy with ulceration. Ann Surg 159:891, 1964

Ankle Sprains and Injuries

Nevin JE: Immediate ambulation of ankle sprains. Surg Gynecol Obstet 117:368, 1963

Quigley RB: Management of athletic ankle injuries. JAMA 169:1431, 1959

Staples OS: Result study of ruptures of lateral ligaments of the ankle. Clin Orthop 85:50, 1972

Plantar Warts

Branson EC, Rhea RL Jr: Plantar warts: Cure by injection. N Eng J Med 248:631, 1953

Carslaw RW, Neill J, Thom JA: Linseed oil treatment of plantar warts. Br J Dermatol 75:380, 1963

Kerr PR: Care of the feet. Practitioner 206:626, 1971

Ingrown Toenail

Bartlett RW: A conservative operation for the cure of so-called ingrown toenail. JAMA 108:1257, 1937

Lloyd-Davies RW, Brill GC: Management of ingrown toenail. Br J Surg 50:592, 1963

Painful Heel

Lapidus PW, Guidotti FP: Painful heel: Report of 323 patients with 364 painful heels. Clin Orthop 39:178, 1965

Fractures of the Ankle

Ahstrom JP Jr: Epiphyseal injuries of the lower extremity. Surg Clin North Am 45:119, 1965

Bosworth DM: Fracture dislocation of the ankle with fixed displacement of the fibula behind the tibia. J Bone Joint Surg 29:130, 1947

Cave EF: Treatment of ankle injuries. General Practitioner 15:85, 1957

Lauge-Hansen M: Fractures of the ankle. Arch Surg 67:813, 1953

McDade WC: Treatment of ankle fractures. Instr Course Lect 24:251, 1975

Nelson MC, Jensen NK: The treatment of trimalleolar fractures of the ankle. Surg Gynecol Obstet 71:509, 1940

Overuse Syndromes

Sammarco LD et al: Symposium: Overuse syndromes of the leg, foot and ankle in athletes. Contemp Orthop 12:67, 1986

Torg JS: Fractures of the base of the fifth metatarsal distal to tuberosity—classification and guidance for nonsurgical management. J Bone Joint Surg 66A:209, 1984

Fractures of the Foot

Carey EJ, Lance EM, Wade PA: Extra-articular fractures of the os calcis. J Trauma 5:362, 1965

Fahey JJ, Murphy JL: Dislocations and fractures of the talus. Surg Clin North Am 45:79, 1965

Hawkins LG: Fracture of the lateral process of the talus. J Bone Joint Surg 47A:1170, 1965

Lindsay WRN, Dewar FP: Fractures of the os calcis. Am J Surg 95:555, 1958

36 Back and Neck

ANDREW C. RUOFF III

Back pain is one of the most common afflictions known to man. It is probably one of the leading causes of lost time from work. Its causes are protean, and its evaluation must include the knowledge of many conditions that can be the cause as well as the history, physical examination, and tests that can lead to an appropriate diagnosis.

Back pain may result from trauma in the form of a contusion, sprain, strain, fracture, or intervertebral disk derangement. It may also be caused by infection (acute or chronic), rheumatoid disease, or tumor. It may be secondary to abdominal or pelvic disease, or psychological problems. In some cases it is outright malingering.

Knowledge of the many factors that can precipitate an episode of low back pain, supplemented by a good history, well-performed physical examination, and careful observation of the individual patient, should lead the treating physician in the proper direction.

PHYSICAL EXAMINATION

Initial evaluation of a patient complaining of low back pain must be performed with the patient sufficiently disrobed to allow observation of the spine and back muscles. The patient should stand with his back toward the seated examiner, who should then note the posture, compare the height of the iliac crests bilaterally to determine whether or not there is a discrepancy of limb length, and note any deviations of the thoracic and lumbar spine either in the lateral or anteroposterior direction. Of particular interest would be the relation of the lumbar spine to the pelvis with the presence or absence of a list to either side and the presence or absence of normal lumbar lordosis. In the presence of acute back pain, the lumbar lordosis is quite often flattened. The patient is next asked to walk away from the examining physician and then walk back and the presence or absence of a limp or muscle guarding is noted.

With his back to the examiner the patient is then asked to forward flex, and the examiner should note whether there is normal reversal of the lumbar lordosis on forward flexion or any limitation of forward flexion. Even in the presence of marked restriction of lumbar motion most patients can still flex comfortably at the hips, and, if the patient is not trying to exaggerate his complaints, the buttocks will move toward the examining physician on forward flexion even in the presence of marked restriction of low back motion. In a patient who is exaggerating his complaints, this normal balancing mechanism is short-circuited, and the patient will tend to sway away from the examiner even to the extent of occasionally falling down. The presence of a *positive withdrawal sign* is a strong indication of a volitional element in the restriction of motion.

The range of motion in forward flexion, extension, lateral bending, and rotation should be noted.

The back should be palpated for specific localized points of tenderness, and these points, if identified, should be reexamined in the course of the remainder of the physical examination to ascertain whether or not they are consistently present.

The patient should be asked to walk on his toes and his heels to evaluate the comparative strength of the plantar flexors and dorsiflexors of the ankle. The patient should next be examined in the supine position on a firm examining table, and the range of motion of both hips ascertained to rule out hip disease. With the hip and knee flexed at 90 degrees, the knees should be gradually extended, and if necessary, the flexion of the hip gradually decreased to ascertain the amount of straight-leg raising that is possible, and the amount of straight-leg raising allowed on either side should be noted. If there is complaint of pain over the sciatic distribution at the limit of straight-leg raising

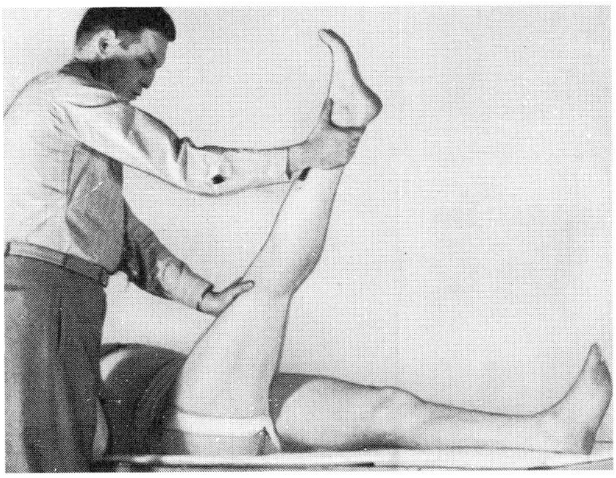

Figure 36-1. The straight-leg-raising test. This maneuver stretches the sciatic nerve and yields pain if one of its lower roots is compressed. Pain may be experienced in the back, leg, or both.

(Fig. 36-1), the knees should be slightly flexed and pressure applied to the popeiteal space to stretch the sciatic nerve; this "sciatic tension test" will give valuable information as to the presence or absence of compression of a nerve root as it emerges from the spinal foramen. Pain referred to the opposite sciatic distribution on straight-leg raising (contralateral sciatic pain) is often an indication of a massive intervertebral disk herniation.

The patient is next examined in the sitting position. While he is sitting, with the hips at 90 degrees of flexion, the knee is extended to check the point at which straight-leg raising produces low back or sciatic pain. Deep tendon reflexes of both the knee and ankle should be tested and compared at this time, after which the strength of dorsiflexion of the great toe extensors should be checked, the calves measured at their point of greatest circumference, and the thighs measured at a fixed distance above the superior pole of the patella. Areas of abnormal sensation should then be checked by a variety of methods, including blunt and sharp touch to see whether or not the abnormalities conform to specific dermatomes. A glove type of distribution of anesthesia is a good clue to the presence of hysterical or psychogenic basis for some of the complaints. It should always be kept in mind that even in the presence of overacting or clearly hysterical manifestations, real disease can exist, but it should also be appreciated that overtreatment or surgical intervention in the presence of clear evidence of psychological abnormalities frequently leads to an unsatisfactory result.

ROENTGEN EXAMINATION

In evaluating low back pain, roentgenograms of the low back should be obtained, and it is recommended that the views include anteroposterior (Fig. 36-2) and a 45-degree cephalic oblique. Figure 36-3 shows how to take a cephalic oblique view. The purpose of these roentgenograms is to identify developmental and congenital anomalies, traumatic manifestations, and the possible presence of infectious or neoplastic conditions. The cephalic oblique view (Fig. 36-4) gives a much clearer picture of the lumbosacral articulation and its transverse processes and the intervertebral space with its adjacent end-plates than is possible in another view and is strongly recommended as routine.

CONSERVATIVE CARE

Initially all patients with incapacitating low back pain, except for an occasional patient with neurologic abnormalities including some bowel and bladder problems, should be treated conservatively. The conservative regimen, regardless of cause (excluding infection and tumor), should consist of a period of complete bed rest on a firm surface, usually with the knees somewhat flexed. Analgesics should be used sparingly; use of a narcotic that dulls the pain too often allows the patient to become much more active than his condition would normally allow can prolong the period of irritation. Muscle relaxants may be prescribed, but their real usefulness is not clear. Heat to the low back may be of some use if given intermittently. Quite often real relief can be obtained by the use of ice packs for relatively short periods.

The patient should avoid the sitting position and from the first day should do abdominal sitting-up exercises and straight-leg raising alternately to a point just short of causing pain. As his condition improves the exercise should be increased but never to the point that causes back discomfort. As the acute situation subsides, ambulation should be allowed, but sitting should be precluded as much as possible during the early stages of recovery.

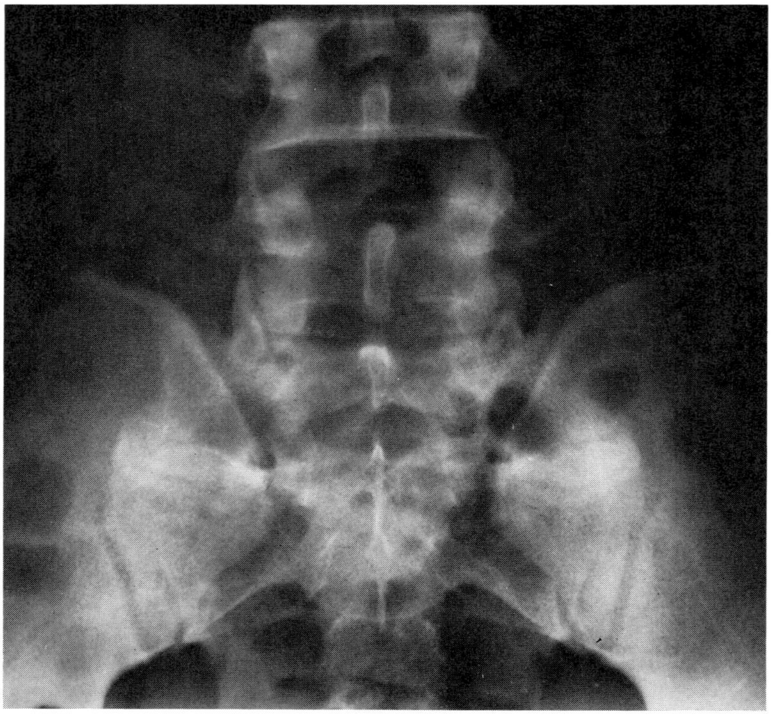

Figure 36-2. AP view. Note how clearly the L3–4 interspace can be seen and the progressively increasing overlap of L4–5 and S1 since the x-ray beam is coming at an increasingly oblique angle to the interspace.

Early use of a low back support may be necessary to allow more rapid return to productive activity, but it should never be used for a prolonged time since this type of protection tends to allow muscle atrophy, which is counterproductive. Recovery should always be accompanied by a gradually increased regimen of low back exercise.

ACUTE BACK STRAIN

Muscle and ligamentous strains do occur in the low back following sudden jerking movements, sudden lifting, straining in an awkward position, and with falls. Patients will show lumbar muscle spasm, often restriction of the normal reversal of the lumbar curve on forward flexion, and often point tenderness in the area of involvement whether along the iliac crest, over the muscle mass itself, or over an interspinous ligament. Radiation of pain into the legs is often absent in the presence of acute low back strain.

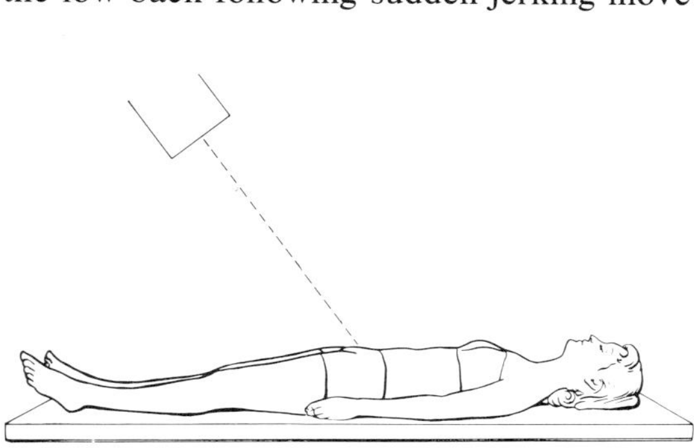

Figure 36-3. The x-ray beam should be aimed at the lumbosacral joint at about a 40- to 45-degree angle to obtain clear definition of the lumbosacral interspace.

TREATMENT

The conservative treatment outlined previously usually suffices in these cases. It can be augmented by injection of trigger points with a local anesthetic solution and possibly supplemented with some corticosteroid, although these should be avoided for the most part.

RHEUMATOID STATES

Patients with active rheumatoid disease commonly have back pain, but usually other joints are involved in addition. Sedimentation rates are usually elevated, and serologic tests for rheumatoid disease are positive. Roentgeno-

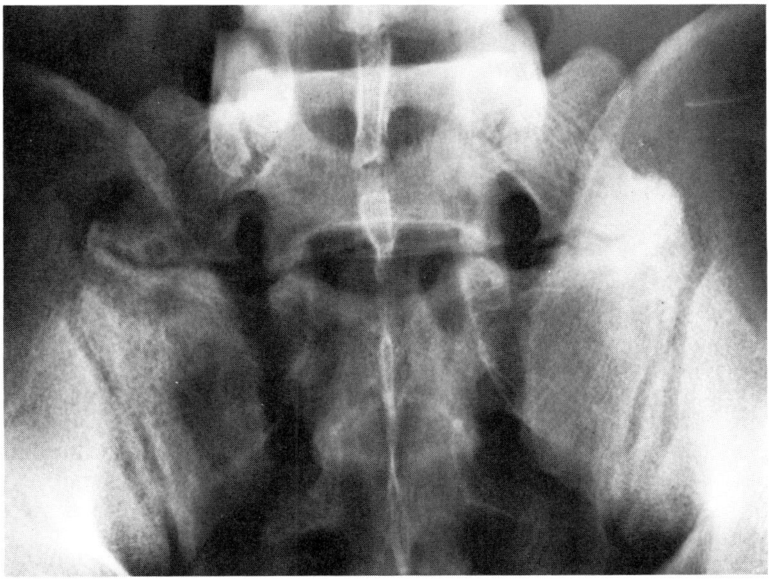

Figure 36-4. This cephalic-oblique view clearly delineates the transverse processes, their relationship to the alae of the sacrum, and the L5–S1 interspace.

grams of the back may reveal straightening of the lumbar curve due to muscle spasm.

Characteristically, patients complain of stiffness after being in one position for a long time and are usually stiff in the morning when they first get out of bed. They often complain primarily of back pain and stiffness of the back, and on examination there is usually some degree of limitation of back motion. There are usually no neurologic deficits. In more chronic cases the patient's complaints of disability are often more striking than any abnormalities on physical examination. Antiinflammatory drugs, exercise routine, and protection of the low back with a lumbosacral corset are all useful in the treatment of back pain secondary to rheumatoid arthritis.

Ankylosing spondylitis is not uncommon in young adults. It is often manifested at first by back pain in the thoracic, lumbar or sacroiliac area. Roentgenograms initially are completely within normal limits, but there is definite restriction of back motion. Marked decrease in chest expansion is often the first indication of this condition, and roentgenographic changes are often first seen in the sacroiliac area. When this diagnosis is considered in a patient with low back pain and limited chest expansion (less than 2 in.), tissue typing showing HLA-B27 is quite specific for ankyolosing spondylytis (about 90% to 95% positive).

OSTEOARTHRITIS

Degenerative arthritic changes are often associated with pain, limitation of motion, and paravertebral muscle spasm. The pain tends to be worse when the patient gets up in the morning and improves after the patient has limbered up. Severe degenerative changes in the low back are often asymptomatic, and when symptoms arise in patients with this condition, conservative treatment is appropriate unless there are prolonged radicular signs caused by stenosis of the spinal canal by osteophytes or encroachment on the intervertebral foramina.

CONGENITAL ABNORMALITIES OF THE LUMBAR SPINE

Congenital abnormalities of the lumbar spine may result in mechanical dysfunctions in the low back. Severe congenital anomalies can occur, however, without any symptoms.

SPONDYLOLYSIS AND SPONDYLOLISTHESIS

Spondylolysis is a relatively common defect that is first noted during the early years. It is most readily demonstrated on oblique views of the lumbar spine, which show a defect in the pars interarticularis, usually at the L4 or L5 level.

Spondylolisthesis is a complication following the presence of spondylolysis in which the vertebra slides forward on the vertebra immediately below because of the defect in the pars interarticularis. This can be present without any symptoms, but it can be the cause of back pain. The diagnosis can best be made with a lateral roentgenogram showing the anterior displacement of the body of the affected vertebra (Fig. 36-5).

Acute episodes should be treated conservatively, and increasing exercises are prescribed as acute symptoms subside. A low back support is frequently useful until the muscle power improves to the point where the weakness is compensated for. Surgery is indicated only in cases with prolonged symptoms or in adults with neurologic abnormalities and persistent postural deformity. This condition is often noted in the course of routine roentgenographic examination in a back that is completely symptom-free.

EXAGGERATED LUMBOSACRAL ANGLE

Many patients with chronic low back pain have a marked increase in the lumbar lordotic curve due to increased lumbosacral angle.

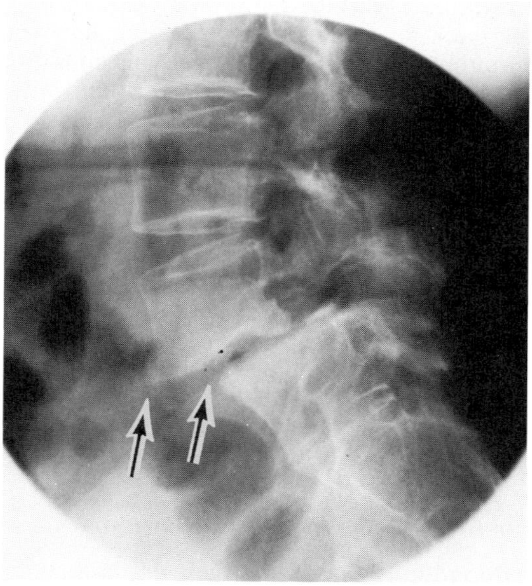

Figure 36-5. Spondylolisthesis. Laterial view of the lumbosacral spine of a 45-year-old female with complaint of low back pain. There is marked forard displacement of the L5 vertebra over the S1 vertebra (*arrows*). (R and G Orthopedic Supplies, Washington, D.C.)

This results in mechanical instability and chronic low back pain that is aggravated by activity, prolonged walking, and standing. The results of examination are usually normal except for the exaggerated lumbar lordosis. A back exercise routine is usually the treatment of choice.

CHRONIC BACKACHE OF UTERINE, PROSTATIC, RECTAL, OR PELVIC MUSCLE ORIGIN

Lesions of the uterus and adenexa, such as malposition, inflammation, and tumors, may cause dull aching discomfort in the low back. Examination of the back shows little to account for the pain, but a check on the history may reveal exacerbations associated with menstruation or leukorrhea, and vaginal examination may disclose significant lesions.

Prostatic inflammation or congestion sometimes causes pain in the region of the lumbosacral joint or the sacrum. The pain is apt to be dull, aching, a nonradiating. Examination of the back shows little, but rectal examination may show a distended and tender prostate. Satisfactory relief of the back pain often follows suitable treatment of the prostate condition.

Rectal lesions such as cryptitis and fissure in ano that cause sphincter spasm may also produce pain over the sacrum. The patient is often aware of the association. Digital and proctoscopic examination of the rectum is in order, and treatment of the anal or rectal lesions should precede measures for relief of the back pain.

Spasm of the perineal muscles may cause pain over the coccyx and upper buttocks with radiation down the thigh.

FRACTURES OF THE TRANSVERSE PROCESSES OF LUMBAR VERTEBRAE

The transverse processes in the lumbar region may be fractured by indirect violence due to muscular action, such as a sudden jerking movement of the back or a fall that causes extreme twisting or lateral bending of the back. Direct violence such as a kick or a blow may also be a cause. The quadratus lumborum muscle is attached to the transverse processes and is often torn when the fracture occurs.

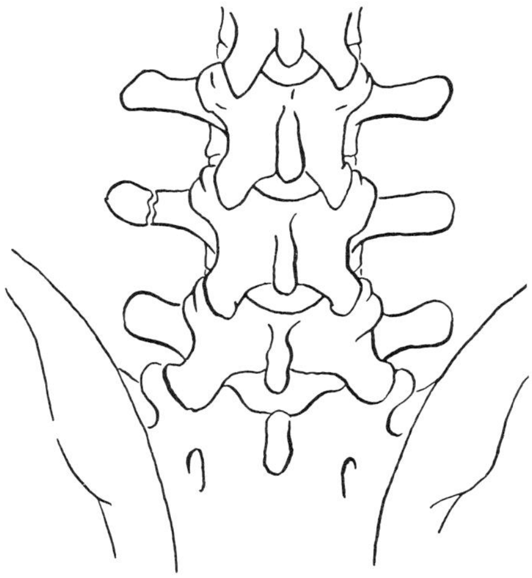

Figure 36-6. Fracture of left transverse process, fourth lumbar vertebra. (Ferguson LK, Erb WH: Ann Surg 114:304, 1941)

DIAGNOSIS

The history of acute violence followed by severe pain on one side of the lower back, intense muscular spasm, tenderness on one side of the lumbar region, and severe pain on lateral bending to the opposite side will indicate the diagnosis. There is often pain on flexion of the thigh of the affected side, especially when resistance is offered. The diagnosis is made by roentgen examination (Figs. 36-6 and 36-7).

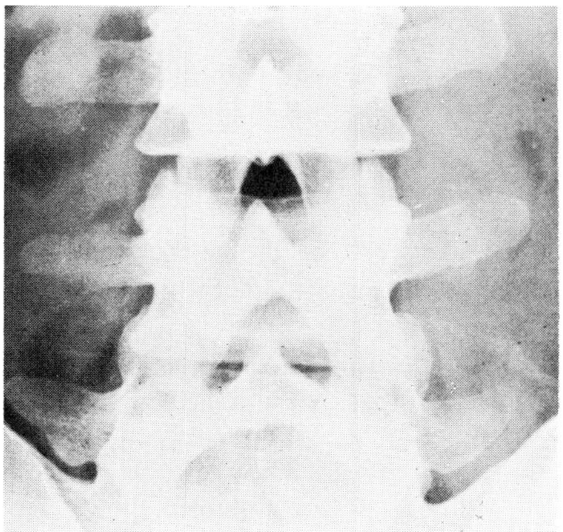

Figure 36-7. Fracture in Fig. 36-6 18 days after fracture, showing early callus formation. (Ferguson LK, Erb WH: Ann Surg 114:304, 1941)

TREATMENT

When pain is very acute, bed rest is indicated for a short period, but ambulatory treatment is usually quite satisfactory. Injection of a local anesthetic into the area around the fracture can give marked relief of symptoms, and a low back support can be of use for the first week or 10 days. When several transverse processes are involved, soft-tissue damage may be more extensive, and it is occasionally necessary to apply a light body cast for a short period after a period of bed rest.

LESIONS OF THE COCCYX

ETIOLOGY

Pain in the region of the coccyx most often arises as a result of trauma. Because the ischial tuberosities are separated somewhat more in females than in males, the coccyx is less protected and more often traumatized in females. Trauma producing this local injury may be a fall on the back. More often, some projecting object is struck in the fall, that is, a stair or a child's block, or it may be the result of a kick. In such instances the coccyx is driven forward, and if the force is sufficient, dislocation or fracture may occur.

DISLOCATIONS AND FRACTURES

Diagnosis

Injuries of the coccyx, either dislocations or fractures, cause acute pain that is noted especially on sitting, on rising from the sitting position, and on walking. It is less notable when the patient is lying down.

On examination there is tenderness over the area of the coccyx, especially on pressure. If the finger is inserted into the anal canal and the coccyx grasped between the thumb and forefinger, there is marked tenderness when the coccyx is manipulated.

Treatment

In cases of dislocation the displacement may be palpated in the preceding manner, and reduction may be effected by gentle manipulation, often with relief of pain. In case of fracture, however, little can be done in the way of reduction and there is no known method of fixation.

Coccygeal injuries should be treated by avoidance of pressure, bed rest when very acute, and the use of a lightly inflated rubber ring when sitting cannot be avoided. Injection of a local anesthetic after careful preparation of the skin with an antiseptic can give marked relief.

COCCYGODYNIA

Coccygodynia is a throbbing, aching, or stabbing pain occurring in the region of the coccyx. It may occur spontaneously but is aggravated by any movement that brings into action muscles attached to the coccyx.

Etiology

Although the initiating cause of coccygodynia may be trauma, the duration of the pain suggests that its persistence must be due to some other factor, perhaps secondary trauma such as that due to involvement of some of the muscles or nerve fibers in scar tissue formation, causing persistent neuralgia in the region of the coccyx.

Diagnosis

The patient gives a history of definite pain in the coccygeal region made worse by sitting. Such discomfort is experienced that the patient is unable to sit very long; he twists and squirms, sitting first on one ischial tuberosity and then on the other. For pain relief, the patient frequently places his feet underneath his chair and sits forward, holding himself on the ischial tuberosity and thighs.

On examination there is usually tenderness and pain over the coccyx, especially along its edges. On rectal examination no particular pain is caused by movement of the coccyx, but pain is caused by pressure of the index finger along the muscles attached to it.

Treatment

It is often difficult to relieve this condition. In many cases the marked pain caused by pressure along the edge of the coccyx with the finger in the rectum suggests spasm of the muscles attached to the coccyx, and relief has been obtained by daily massage of these muscles with a long, sweeping stroke of the finger per rectum and local applications of heat in the form of sitz baths or hot compresses.

Injections of local anesthetic into the tender area and occasionally a corticosteroid may be of some use.

Surgical removal of the coccyx may be indicated in cases in which prolonged conservative care gives no relief whatsoever.

RUPTURED INTERVERTEBRAL DISK

Acute back pain associated with radiating pain over the sciatic distribution may accompany many pathologic conditions, but the most frequent cause is pressure on a nerve root at the level of the intervertebral foramen from a bulging or herniated nucleus pulposus (Fig. 36-8). Although lumbar intervertebral disk lesions often produce a characteristic clinical syndrome, there does tend to be significant variation from patient to patient. The patient often gives a history of recurrent low back pain related to minor degrees of trauma, but following a specific incident; this low back pain may be accompanied by pain radiating down the posterior aspect of the thigh and into the foot.

The severity varies from patient to patient, and the attack may be extremely acute and sudden in onset. When this is the case the patient usually has marked spasm of the paravertebral muscles. He may also have a list of the lumbar spine to one side, usually opposite the side of the sciatic pain. Characteristically, coughing, sneezing, and movement intensify the pain. There may be associated areas of numbness and paresthesias over the distribution of the nerve root involved (Fig. 36-9). There may be more severe neurologic problems, including bowel and bladder dysfunction. Occasionally, pain radiating over the sciatic distribution is not accompanied by low back pain.

EXAMINATION

During an acute attack the patient with a ruptured intervertebral disk will show spasm of the paravertebral muscles and decrease in normal lumbar lordosis and often a tilt of the lumbar spine away from the affected leg. Movements of the lumbar spine are often limited. Straight-leg raising usually demonstrates pain over the sciatic distribution (Fig. 36-1). Pain referred to the contralateral sciatic nerve distribution on straight-leg raising often indi-

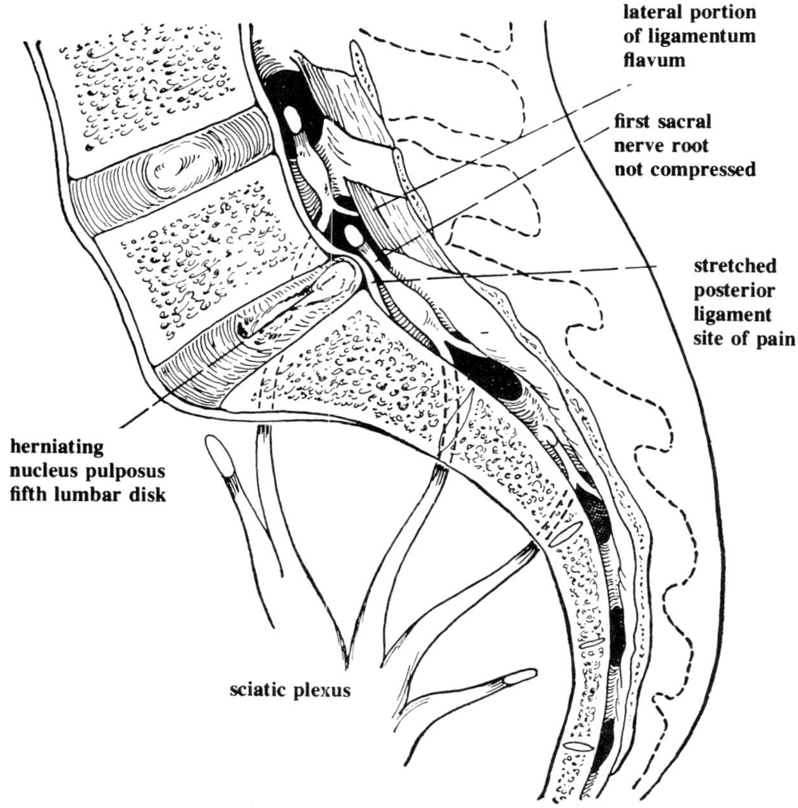

Figure 36-8. Posterior herniation of the nucleus pulposus of the fifth lumbar disk giving rise to low back pain without nerve root irritation. (Keegan JJ: JAMA 126:868, 1944)

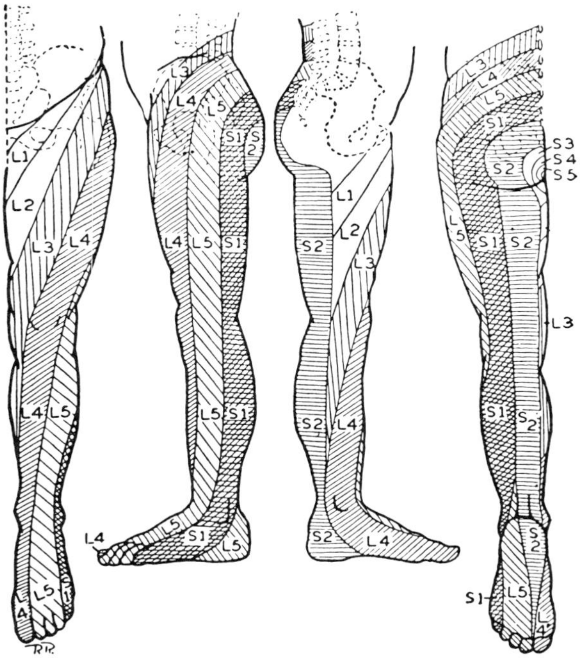

Figure 36-9. Composite dermatome chart of the lower extremity. (Keegan JJ: Arch Neurol Psychiatr 50:81, 1943)

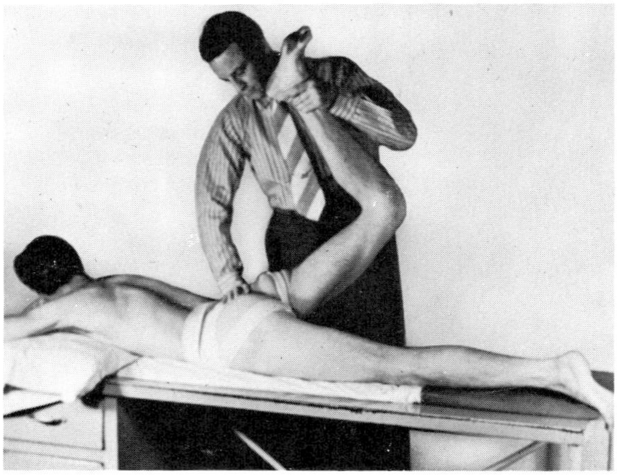

Figure 36-10. Femoral stretch test. This maneuver yields pain in the anterior aspect of the ipsilateral thigh when the L3 or L4 nerve root is compressed.

cates a large herniation. When the lesion is at the L3–4 level straight-leg raising may cause no discomfort and there may be discomfort on stretching the femoral nerve as illustrated in Figure 36-10.

Neurologic examination may be normal, or it may show varying degrees of neurologic deficiency, depending on the degree of nerve root compression. Most lumbar disk protrusions occur at the L5–S1 or L4–5 level. With lesions at the L5–S1 level, the S1 nerve root is usually compressed. If sensory loss is present it occurs in the S1 root distribution, namely, the lateral aspect of the leg and foot, including the lateral three toes. If weakness is present it involves plantar flexion and eversion of the foot and toes. The Achilles reflex may be depressed or absent. In lesions of the L4–5 interspace the L5 root is compressed, and the sensory loss involves the lateral aspect of the calf and the dorsum of the foot, including the great toe. Weakness, when present, is noted on dorsiflexion of the great toe and occasionally of the foot. Usually there is no reflex abnormality. In protrusion at the L3–4 level, the L4 nerve root is compressed, and the leg pain is usually on the anterior aspect of the thigh. When present, sensory loss is over the anteromedial aspect of the lower thigh and the proximal portion of the lower leg. Weakness and atrophy of the quadriceps muscle may be present. The patellar reflex may be diminished.

Roentgen examination should be done to rule out other pathologic processes. Narrowing of intervertebral spaces in the regular roentgenograms is of no real significance since it could have been present previously.

TREATMENT

Except in the presence of severe neurologic abnormalities, particularly bowel or bladder dysfunction, all acute intervertebral disk problems should be treated conservatively. Rest in bed for 1 to 4 weeks with the knees flexed in a semi-Fowler position should be utilized. If relief is not obtained with bed rest at home, treatment in the hospital is sometimes necessary. If symptoms subside after a reasonable period of bed rest, exercises should be started while the patient is in bed and then continued indefinitely.

Exercises should be, when possible, instituted under the direction of a physiotherapist. The basic early exercise should consist of abdominal setting to flatten the lumbar spine against a firm support, and while the abdominal muscles are held firm, straight-leg raising should be instituted alternately with the leg elevated to the point of beginning discomfort. Well-functioning abdominal muscles are the key to adequate functioning of the reciprocal back muscles.

A low back support may be useful in the early stages of ambulation following a period of bed rest but should not be continued for prolonged periods. The key to successful conservative treatment is prolonged use of exercise to increase the protective function of the back musculature.

If prolonged conservative treatment does not give relief, or in the presence of significant and increasing neurologic dysfunction, electromyography, CT scan, or myelography may be indicated, and surgical intervention must be considered.

LUMBAR STENOSIS

Progressive or congenital narrowing of the lumbar spinal canal and/or the lateral nerve root canals may result in a rather specific clinical syndrome manifested by pain in the back with either claudication or sciatic distribution of pain in the legs; pain on standing, relieved by sitting; cramping and pain in the calves on walking for short distances with decreased ability to walk; walking that leads to paresthesias or numbness in one or both legs, which may become unbearable; increased pain when walking uphill; relief of pain when walking downhill; no difficulty with bicycle riding; hyperextension of the low back, causing severe pain; and normal circulation to the legs.

With progressive symptoms surgery to relieve the stenosis may be the only alternative, but early ambulatory care should consist of training in routine care of the low back, including instructions on how to stoop and lift and the appropriate sleeping posture. Isometric abdominal strengthening exercises often help. An elastic back support may be useful to give some protection but allow motion. Occasionally, epidural injection of steroids has been useful and anti-inflammatory, nonsteroidal drug therapy may be of value. Conservative treatment should be carried out indefinitely as long as pain is tolerable.

The CT scan and MRI have been a tremendous aid in the definition of stenotic areas if clinical findings and routine roentgenograms are suggestive of the diagnosis.

CERVICAL SPINAL INJURIES

Any sudden, unguarded, flexion, extension, or torsion involving the head and neck may result in minor or more severe soft-tissue injury. The most frequent injury of this nature results from a rear-end collision when a car that is stationary is struck from the rear by another vehicle. Since these incidents usually occur without warning the victim is not prepared, and without the protection of a head rest, the head is forcibly hyperextended, then snaps back into hyperflexion, and returns toward the upright position. This is the mechanism leading to a "whiplash injury."

The symptoms of whiplash injury vary greatly. Often the patient has very little immediate pain in the neck but sometime during the next 12 to 24 hours experiences increasing neck pain frequently associated with occipital headaches. Discomfort in the neck and limitation of motion of the head and shoulders are characteristic. The pain is usually poorly localized but is often mostly occipital and in the posterior cervical thoracic area. The symptoms may persist for a period of weeks or months or may disappear, only to recur.

In addition to these local symptoms it is not uncommon for patients to develop profound emotional reactions such as nervousness, anxiety, nervous tension, insomnia, and sweating of the hands. It is believed by some that many of these symptoms are psychosomatic and exaggerated by the litigation incidental to the accident and that they are resolved to a great extent by settlement.

In most cases there is little or minor evidence of trauma. On examination there is tenderness on pressure on the back of the neck, at times with spasm of the cervical spinal muscles. Often the muscle spasm is more pronounced on one side than on the other, which accounts for tilting of the head forward or to one side.

Roentgenographic findings are usually normal, but flattening of the normal cervical lordosis may be noted. One often overlooked more serious finding is divergence between two of the spinous processes posteriorly (Fig. 36-11). This divergence is secondary to a tear of the interspinous ligament and at least a portion of the capsules of the facets and possibly the posterior longitudinal ligament. If this divergence is noted on a lateral film it is an indication for active treatment since, untreated, these injuries tend to heal with scar tissue that is not stable. This finding requires immediate consultation, and segmental spinal fusion may be necessary.

Previously present asymptomatic changes in the vertebral bodies, such as lipping or spurring, may be noted. These may become symptomatic in a patient in the older age group following a cervical spine injury and may be persistent.

TREATMENT

In severe cases of cervical spinal injury, hospital admission is advised, but for others, treatment may be given on an ambulatory basis. Halter traction given in a horizontal position can be arranged at home (Fig. 36-12). De-

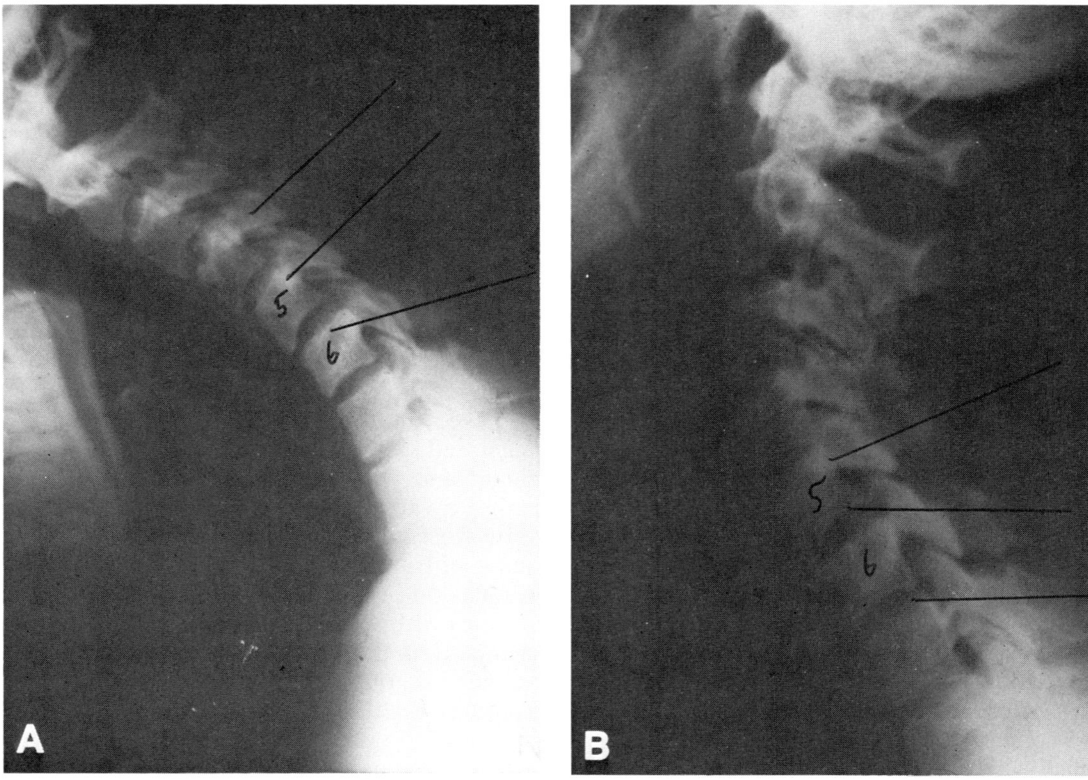

Figure 36-11. Divergence between spinous processes. (*A*) This lateral view in flexion shows marked divergence of the spinous processes of C5 and C6 as compared with the normal roughly parallel arrangement between all the other cervical vertebrae. This finding indicates tearing of the interspinous ligament, capsules about the facets, and injury to the posterior longitudinal ligament. (*B*) This view shows progression in a similar case, untreated, with gross instability, marked divergence of the spinous processes, and subluxation of the facets and bodies of C5 and C6.

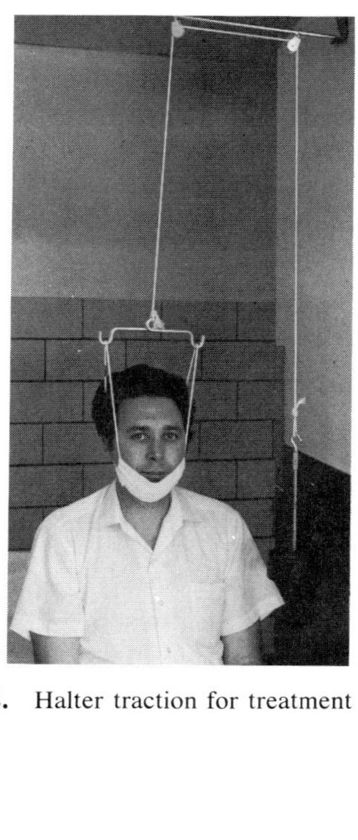

Figure 36-12. Halter traction for treatment of whiplash injury.

pending on the patient, 5 to 15 pounds of traction is applied for 30 minutes at a time two or three times a day until acute symptoms subside. When the patient is upright, the neck may be protected by a folded turkish towel wrapped around the neck and pinned in place. More formal cervical collars are commercially available but tend to be worn for too long; use of the less aesthetic and more cumbersome towel collar is more likely to be discontinued fairly promptly. Use of a towel collar is less likely to impress the patient with the fact that he is going to require prolonged care. Hot moist packs may be helpful in relieving muscle spasm and soreness.

Most of these patients have relatively minor injuries that with conservative treatment disappear within a few days or weeks.

TRACTION INJURY TO THE BRACHIAL PLEXUS

ETIOLOGY

In severe injuries to the neck and shoulder area, particularly when the shoulder is forced down away from the neck or severe traction is placed on a shoulder against resistance, the brachial plexus may be stretched and injured to a greater or lesser degree.

SYMPTOMS

The symptoms of brachial plexus stretch are usually extreme tenderness and pain over the entire shoulder and often down the arm. Muscles of the shoulder region, especially the trapezius, are frequently in painful spasm with the most marked tenderness along the sides of the neck. The pain becomes worse on bending the head toward the opposite side and may be relieved somewhat by bending toward the side of injury. The cervical spine and shoulder area should be examined roentgenographically, and in the presence of marked paresis, a myelogram is often indicated early to rule out avulsion of the cervical spinal roots.

TREATMENT

It is important to relieve the shoulder of the weight of the arm. This may be done by placing the arm in a triangular sling supported by the uninjured shoulder or using an abduction cast or splint. The abduction splint in particular is useful in the presence of muscular paralysis. In most cases with brachial plexus injury, unless complete, the prognosis for eventual recovery is good if adequate early treatment is given.

BIBLIOGRAPHY

Harris JH Jr et al: A practical classification of acute cervical spine injuries. Orthop Clin North Am 17:15–30, 1986

Kornberg M: Upper cervical spine injuries: A review. Contemp Orthop 121:61–68, 1986

Wiltsie LL et al: The treatment of spinal stenosis. Clin Orthop 115:83–91, 1976

Index

Page numbers followed by f indicate figures; followed by t, tables.